THEORETICAL NURSING 6TH EDITION

DEVELOPMENT AND PROGRESS

THEORETICAL NURSING 6TH EDITION

DEVELOPMENT AND PROGRESS

AFAF IBRAHIM MELEIS, PhD, FAAN, LL

Dean Emeritus
Professor of Nursing and Sociology
School of Nursing
University of Pennsylvania
Philadelphia, Pennsylvania

and

Professor Emeritus
School of Nursing
University of California, San Francisco
San Francisco, California

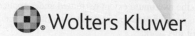
Wolters Kluwer

Philadelphia • Baltimore • New York • London
Buenos Aires • Hong Kong • Sydney • Tokyo

Acquisitions Editor: Christina C. Burns
Development Editor: Helen Kogut
Editorial Assistant: Hilari Bowman
Production Project Manager: Cynthia Rudy
Design Coordinator: Teresa Mallon
Illustration Coordinator: Jennifer Clements
Manufacturing Coordinator: Karin Duffield
Marketing Manager: Todd McKenzie
Prepress Vendor: S4Carlisle Publishing Services

Sixth edition

9 8 7 6 5 4 3 2 1

Printed in China

Library of Congress Cataloging-in-Publication Data
Names: Meleis, Afaf Ibrahim, author.
Title: Theoretical nursing: development and progress/Afaf Ibrahim Meleis.
Description: Sixth edition. |Philadelphia: Wolters Kluwer Heath, [2018] |
Includes bibliographical references and indexes.
Identifiers: LCCN 2016031581|ISBN 9780060000424
Subjects: |MESH: Nursing Theory
Classification: LCC RT84.5|NLM WY 86|DDC 610.7301–dc23 LC record available at https://lccn.loc.gov/2016031581

CCS1116

Dedicated to an inspiring past
Soad Hussein Hassan, RN, PhD

A maverick—
for exemplifying humanism and commitment,
for encouraging feminism and autonomy,
for accepting challenge and diversity,
for tolerating rebellion,
for sponsoring inquisitiveness,
for teaching me about the courage
to face a life of challenges
and an end of life with Alzheimer's
and
for being my mother.

And dedicated to an exciting future

Exemplified by my grandchildren—
Karim, Amani, Alia, Samir, Alex, and Nile.

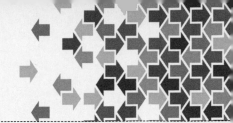

Contributor

Eun-Ok Im, PhD, MPH, RN, CNS, FAAN
Professor and Mary T. Champagne Professor
Duke University School of Nursing
Durham, North Carolina
Chapter 17, Developing Situation-Specific Theories

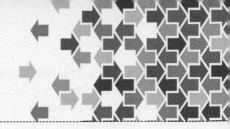

Reviewers

Claudia Beckmann, PhD, RN, WHNP, BC, CNM
Associate Dean
Graduate and Professional Programs
Associate Professor
Rutgers University School of Nursing-Camden
Camden, New Jersey

Miriam Bender, PhD, RN, CNL
Assistant Professor
Nursing Science
University of California, Irvine
Irvine, California

Franco Carnevale, PhD, RN
Assistant Director
Ingram School of Nursing (Master's Program
   Director)
McGill University
Montreal, Quebec, Canada

**Linda Carmen Copel, PhD, RN, CNS, BC, CNE,
NCC, FAPA**
Professor of Nursing
Villanova University
Villanova, Pennsylvania

Leslie L. Davis, PhD, RN, ANP-BC, FAHA
Assistant Professor
University of North Carolina Greensboro
Greensboro, North Carolina

Ellen D'Errico, PhD, RN
Associate Professor of Nursing
Loma Linda University
Loma Linda, California

Joseph DeSantis, PhD, ARNP, ACRN, FAAN
Associate Professor
University of Miami School of Nursing and
   Health Studies
Coral Gables, Florida

Nancy Dluhy, PhD, RN
Adjunct Faculty PhD Nursing Online
University of Massachusetts
Dartmouth, Massachusetts

Bobbe Ann Gray, PhD, RNC-OB, CNS-BC
Associate Professor
Wright State University
Dayton, Ohio

Susan Sweat Gunby, PhD, RN
Professor of Nursing
Mercer University
Atlanta, Georgia

Debra R. Hanna, PhD, RN
Professor of Nursing
Molloy College
Rockville Centre, New York

Brenda Hosley, PhD, RN
Clinical Associate Professor
Arizona State University
Phoenix, Arizona

Cynthia Jacelon, PhD, RN-BC, CRRN, FAAN
Rehabilitation Clinical Nurse Specialist
University of Massachusetts
Amherst, Massachusetts

Norma Kiser-Larson, PhD, CNE
Associate Professor
North Dakota State University
Fargo, North Dakota

Deborah Lindell, DNP, RN, CNE, ANEF
Associate Professor
Case Western Reserve University
Frances Payne Bolton School of Nursing
Cleveland, Ohio

Rozzano Locsin, PhD, RN, FAAN
Professor Emerita
Florida Atlantic University
Boca Raton, Florida

Star Mahara, MSN, RN
Associate Professor
Thompson Rivers University
Kamloops, British Columbia, Canada

Ruth McCaffrey, DNP, ARNP, FNP-BC, GNP-BC
Professor and Coordinator—Doctor of Nursing
   Practice Degree Program
Mercer University
Atlanta, Georgia

Karen H. Morin, PhD, RN, ANEF, FAAN
Professor Emerita
PhD Program Director
University of Wisconsin-Milwaukee
Milwaukee, Wisconsin

Jennifer Robinson, PhD, RN, CNE, FAHA
Professor of Nursing
University of Mississippi Medical Center
Jackson, Mississippi

Beth Rogers, PhD, RN, FAAN
University of New Mexico (Retired)
VCU School of Nursing
Professor and Chair of the Department of Adult
   Health and Nursing Systems
Albuquerque, New Mexico

Jacqueline R. Saleeby, PhD, RN
Associate Professor
Maryville University
St. Louis, Missouri

Anne Thomas, PhD, MSN, BSN
Dean, Associate Professor
University of Indianapolis School of Nursing
Indianapolis, Indiana

Joan Tilghman, PhD, RN, CRNP
Associate Dean of Masters Education in Nursing
   Education
Coppin State University
Baltimore, Maryland

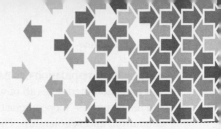

Preface

Why produce a sixth edition of the book? And why at this particular time? The answers to these two questions are both simple and complex. The simple answers are because faculty who teach theory are continuing to use it, graduate students are both inspired and challenged by its content, and it has become a valuable resource for clinicians and researchers. Their unsolicited comments and evaluations provided the impetus for me to revise, update, and expand the content of this revised volume. The rest of the simple answer is also because based on reviews, evaluations, and demands, my publisher requested a new revised edition. I am grateful for all these reasons that prompted embarking on this sixth edition journey.

But there are even more compelling rationales warranting the time and energy to produce a much updated and revised version of the fifth edition. This could be summarized in two equally compelling rationales. The first is my own passion and deep conviction that theories are powerful tools that empower members of our discipline in making an even more positive impact on the health of populations globally. The second compelling rationale is that this is the most significant turning point in the history of our discipline, where the stars are all aligned for what our predecessors set the stage to achieve, which is the best access to quality health care for all, including the most vulnerable of populations.

Let me explain more about my two-prong rationale for why I again bring this book to you, the readers, whether students, faculty, clinicians, research, policy makers, or all the above. My passion for theoretical nursing was ignited from the day I started reading and learning about our first-generation theorists: Virginia Henderson, Dorothy Johnson, Myra Levine, Florence Nightingale, Dorothea Orem, Ida Orlando, Hildegard Peplau, Martha Rogers, and Ernestine Wiedenbach. What added fuel to the flame of theorizing was when I taught that first theory course, designed by Dorothy Johnson, and I added to it an analysis of

the paradigms that influenced these early pioneering theories—Systems, Symbolic Interaction, and Adaptation, among others. The students' reactions were phenomenal and ranged from total excitement to bewilderment. Excitement that nurses can theorize and that they can use these coherent frameworks to actually name what they have done so well for so long, but could not find the right words to describe. They also expressed bewilderment about grappling with philosophic and theoretic ideas they felt were reserved for others who were more "intellectually inclined" because "nurses are hands-on" and are not theorists or philosophers. The outcomes of that era piqued my interest even more and nurtured the theory flame. Some of the outcomes, as you will see throughout the pages of this book, were theory-based curricula (too soon, too much, with too little initially), theory-based research, and the stimulation of even more theoretically sophisticated second-generation theorists—Imogene King, Betty Neuman, Margaret Newman, Rosemarie Parse, Josephine Paterson and Loretta Zderad, Callista Roy, and Jean Watson. Then a very complicated dialogue ensued about theory development and its strategies that stimulated a third generation of theorists who focused on strategies to develop and evaluate theories. From all that, the fourth generation of theorists who developed middle-range theories evolved and enriched our literature with more research and practice-friendly theories.

This brings me to my second rationale for why this volume and why at this time. As I mentioned above, the stars are aligned for making in the immediate future an incredible impact on population health, driven by nurses' voices and nurtured by the discipline's mission and values. It goes without having to belabor it that we as nurses are far better prepared educationally and have demonstrated our expertise. But there are other stars that are aligned: there is global health care reform that brings the attention to access to health care, to disparities, to community-based practices, to home care, to marginalized populations, to patient-centered care and precision medicine, all of which are congruent and reflect nurses' scope of practice, goals, expertise, education, and scholarship. There is an alignment between nursing history, mission, and goals (including the 2015–2030 Sustainable Development Goals). There is also heightened realization, of legislators and health care policy developers, of the centrality of nurses in enhancing access to health care, coupled with the global shortage of nurses as a workforce. All of the above provides a rich platform for nursing organizations to garner the public's support and the financial resources for developing and implementing creative care models that insure equitable access to quality care throughout the life cycle of populations.

You, the reader, may wonder at this point and question the role of theory and why that theoretical thinking may be contributing to the star alignment. Theory brings order to the galaxy of stars. It is the orbit that defines their movements and interactions. It provides the language, the principles, the evidence, and the goals for policy recommendations. Several major events support nurses' roles in policy change: focused strategic goals developed by the National Institute of Nursing Research in the United States; the appointment of a commission for nursing by the United Nations to make recommendations about the nursing workforce; the bold move made by the Robert Wood Johnson Foundation's President, Risa Lavizzo-Mourey, to invest in and promote a culture of health; and a voiced movement toward more gender, cultural, and sexual orientation equity. All of these, along with the development of health care commissions in many countries to implement health reforms, provide golden opportunities for nurses to make the health care impact that they always wanted to make. There is a momentum, and nurses equipped with theories and research can, and must, support this momentum.

This brings me back to this sixth edition of the book before you. This book comes to you as many assumptions about theory development have been debunked, such as that theory development is an elitist endeavor and that it is an academic exercise; that nurses cannot engage in developing theories; that nursing as a discipline is practical and is not amenable to theorizing; and that theory, research, practice, and education must exist in siloes. While these are old assumptions, I am deeply concerned about a few of the new assumptions that substitute for these old ones, such as we need not include theory in our curricula, there is no room in our

nursing educational systems to include theoretical dialogues, that we should not be teaching these old theories that are too abstract, and that advancing the discipline of nursing requires investments *only* in growing research programs that produce the evidence for practice.

The intent of this book, then, is to demystify theory, to chart the different strategies to use in developing and advancing theory, and to provide tools and best practices in evaluating progress in the discipline. It provides both an open invitation to embark on a journey without the many preconceived assumptions that may have been a barrier to pursuing knowledge development. Demystifying theory and dispelling assumptions are essential but not sufficient conditions for empowerment. The metaphors that describe the current stage in theory development are *epistemic diversity* and *integrative process*, both of which are an acknowledgment and valuation of nursing history, heritage, and practice. Both of these metaphors reflect and accept the central role of practice in advancing nursing knowledge and nurses' ways of knowing as vital in uncovering and developing knowledge. Empowerment is also about believing in one's own abilities and capacities to advance knowledge and about using these capacities to become an agent for continuous learning and creating. It is about being a critical thinker, a theoretical thinker, an innovative advocate, and an agent for change. Our discipline is ready to invest in and nurture *fifth-generation theorists*.

In this book, I provide support for our domain as we see it today. The future progress of the discipline depends on the extent to which members of the discipline will embrace our disciplinary identity, our theoretical progress, and our epistemic diversity, and utilize integrative approaches to theory development. The scholars of the future, along with fifth-generation theorists, are those who are as comfortable with theorizing as with researching, practicing, and teaching. They will be able to understand and speak the languages of different disciplines, translate their findings to the different practice fields, and engage in changing policies.

In short, the major goals of this book are to make a contribution to raising the consciousness of the reader and to acknowledge our theoretical history and pave the way for our future. It is to place the present in the context of our history and to develop an awareness of the potential for theory advancement by members of the discipline, both men and women, old and young, clinicians and academicians, researchers and theorists, students and faculty. It is about the pride we must have in the contributions our discipline makes to the health and well-being of people.

I offer the ideas in this book as tentative thoughts to provide an even platform to enforce self-agency in students, faculty, clinicians, researchers, and theoreticians to drive the development of new coherent frameworks to advance nursing science. By knowing equally, they may be empowered to leverage their competency and use their expertise. A democratization of the processes in developing theory is an empowering process to you, the reader, to believe in your own voice, to respect and value the voices that came before you, but to challenge and build on them.

Every time I work on a new edition, I feel renewed, inspired, and regenerated. It has been a privilege for me to be a nurse, and it is an incredible privilege to write this book honoring the past and envisioning the future. I continue to be inspired by the many questions and comments I hear from you in global meetings and through the new, more convenient digital media. Thank you for the work you do, the thoughtful questions you raise, and the comments you have made. I have tried to reflect all of them in this new edition. To readers far and near, thank you for continuing to dialogue with the ideas in this text. And keep dialoguing with me!

Afaf Ibrahim Meleis, PhD, FAAN, LL

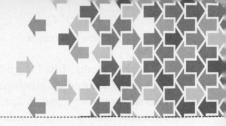

Acknowledgments

Writing and/or revising a book is an experience that is only understood through the author's relationships and repertoire of interactions. It is based on much thinking, plenty of reading, many opportunities for creativity, a pinch of stamina, and a large dose of persistence, all wrapped together in layers of engagement and support from others. To start with, if it were not for my husband's (Mahmoud) patience and lifelong support, I would not have written the first edition of *Theoretical Nursing*, followed by five more editions. He provided support at all levels, from the tangible to the emotional. He empowered me through consistent dialogues and controversial debates, as well as many political disagreements. While affirmations of ideas are always helpful, debates are even more powerful, as through them I learned how to separate or connect the personal and the political and to sharpen negotiation through controversial and competing ideas, which this book is about. Our sons Waleed and Sherief continue to provide incredible joy and support as they create and define their new roles as fathers and successful professionals.

To revise a major textbook such as this one, I needed thinking time, literature updates, expert typing, sharp editing, project coordination, art work, and copy editing. I received a Rockefeller Foundation /Bellagio fellowship that gave me a month of thinking and writing time. Though the goals of this fellowship were about global women's health in the changing urban landscape rather than for developing the plans for this sixth edition, the scope of thinking cannot be contained to the specific identified goals. Invariably I found myself thinking and planning for this edition. I am grateful to The Rockefeller Foundation for providing me with the environment to decompress from 12½ years Deanship, for giving me the gift of an environment where I had uninterrupted thinking and writing time, and for helping me to jump-start this sixth edition. My Bellagio cohorts were an incredible sounding board as well as a source of inspiration about economics, art, music, law, civic responsibilities, and philosophic discourse.

The management of my schedule for this project and the monumental task of reviewing and selecting the right literature to use in revising this sixth edition were left to the executive coordinator of my office, Kim Freeman. I am most grateful for her tireless, expert, and thoughtful efforts. It was she who provided the organizational and coordinating structure for this extensive project. In addition, I give her complete credit for ensuring that Chapter 21 updates reflect the most recent literature and that they match the new citations in all of the 20 other chapters.

Maria Marconi typed both my fifth and sixth editions. She provided continuity and a filter that eliminated redundancies and insured consistency. Her availability, timeliness, and attention to detail are a dream for authors who are always facing many deadlines. I truly appreciated her partnership and passion on this project.

Wolters Kluwer also provided me with continuity. Helen Kogut and I successfully completed the fifth edition, and similarly the sixth edition, on schedule. Her organization and coordination ensured timely reviews, critiques, and revisions. I give her much credit for the edited quality of the manuscript. Her support and affirmation throughout the project are appreciated not only by me, but equally by Kim and Maria.

Though I have never met Dan Alt, his sharp critical eyes, the seriousness by which he handled the editorial critique, and the thoughtful questions he posed always gave me pause and the rationale to revise.

Christina Burns also coordinated and facilitated legal and marketing processes while expecting her first child.

Inspiration for the continuity of discourse that started in previous editions as well as for tackling new themes in this edition came from many sources. Over the years and across many continents, in person or through media, I had the privilege globally to engage in short and long dialogues with colleagues who read, reviewed, and critiqued or affirmed ideas presented in my writing. Whether they realized it or not, they have influenced my thinking. Their enthusiasm, creativity, and dedication to the discipline of nursing have made a lasting impact on my decision to review, revise, and update my thinking about the theoretical bases of our discipline.

In short, this sixth edition is a product of the thought and loyal team mentioned above as well as the many volunteer comments I have received over the years. Without all of the above, I would not have been able to produce this edition. I am absolutely grateful for the contributions of all.

Afaf Ibrahim Meleis

Contents

Part Six

OUR THEORETICAL FUTURE

Part Seven

OUR HISTORICAL AND CURRENT LITERATURE

Part One

OUR THEORETICAL JOURNEY

I invite you, in this first part of the book, to embark on a journey that will introduce you to the rich theoretical underpinnings of our discipline. Uncovering the role that theory plays in our daily experiences as nurses is the first step in the theoretical journey proposed in this book. In the three chapters in Part One, the theoretical journey, along with its symbols and scholarly destinations, is described. In Chapter 1, you will find assumptions on which the journey is planned, the organizational plan for the journey, and some of the supporting material. Chapter 2 includes scholarly goals and the different possible destinations for the journey. The context for the journey is then set in Chapter 3, where the key definitions of theoretical symbols and terms are provided.

As with any long journey, planning is essential, but it is equally important to allow flexibility for personal goals to emerge from the experience, side trips that may distract or enrich you, and serendipitous opportunities that may attract you. It is the totality of these experiences that will lead to immersion, understanding, and innovation.

1

Positioning for the Journey

Disciplines should be dynamic to respond to emerging and changing needs of societies and to the new demands imposed by population movements, health care reforms, and transformation of global order. However dynamic disciplines are, each has a core set of values, assumptions, a perspective, a domain that includes its major concepts, and a mission, all of which maintain its stability and effectiveness. This core is what provides continuity and drives progress in disciplines.

Quality care pertaining to health and illness for all people continues to be nursing's top priority. In the 21st century, attending and realizing this goal is even more urgent than it has been in the past because of increasing population diversity and better awareness of inequities in meeting the needs of the different groups in societies, the majorities and the many minorities, the conflicting priorities in health care systems, and the emergent costs and reimbursement issues that patients, insurance companies, the health care industry, and health care professionals are confronting. Theory and theoretical thinking may have been promoted in the past as answers to the undefined roles of nursing or the diffused nature of the profession of nursing. However, in this era in which unequal access to health care continues to persist, where disparities in provision of health care services are becoming more recognized, where there are emerging challenges in treating chronic illnesses and infections, where there is a proliferation of health care professionals and nonprofessionals, and where there are many global dialogues about health care reforms, the role of theory and the utilization of a coherent framework in providing care have become even more urgent and more compelling.

By examining history we shape the present and future dialogues related to our world. When we visit Independence Hall, where statesmen wrote the U.S. Constitution, when we listen to Martin Luther King's "I Have a Dream" speech, or when we are in the presence of the pyramids built by Egypt's pharaohs, we are provided with interpretive reminders about how historical individuals and events continue to shape discourse, legislation, equity, life and afterlife, and other aspects of our society. In the same way, to fully appreciate the role of nursing theory in shaping the future of equitable and accessible quality health care, we must review and analyze our theoretical past and its influence on the present and future of health care.

By uncovering and understanding a discipline's theoretical journey, members of the discipline learn to build on it. By unfolding the processes used in developing our theoretical past, we gain insights that improve our understanding of our current progress, and we are empowered to achieve our disciplinary goals. When we take a critical and reflective stance on the current theoretical discourse, or lack thereof, as the case may be, we see shadows of past issues and accomplishments, as well as visions of the future of our discipline and profession. Therefore, reconstructing our theoretical heritage is a process that involves interpreting our present reality and shaping our future. The intent of the historical-to-future journey proposed in this book is to demonstrate the progress of nursing through analyses of the philosophical assumptions, theoretical processes, and patterns that have influenced the development of the discipline. We will perform these analyses in ways that value our experiences as nurses, in ways that support and enhance our progress, and in ways that allow us to proactively develop abstractions, exemplars, conceptualizations, and theories that reflect and guide our nursing assessments and actions. Synthesizing insights from and about the past, considering the current reality of the health care systems, analyzing the societal context, and considering the potential future visions of quality care can enhance creativity in the discipline of nursing, which could further its development and progress.

Despite many crises along the path toward providing quality care, the development of the discipline of nursing has progressed by leaps and bounds during the last 50 years. The first two decades of the 21st century brought with them many challenges, some new and some merely shadows of the past. Few would dispute the notion that theory in general has been responsible for this development; yet, some continue to question the specific role of theory in the development of the discipline and its effects on the discipline's scientific bases and clinical practice. The thesis of this book is that the evolution of the discipline of nursing and its scholarliness is greatly intertwined with its focus on theory. The movement in our discipline to incorporate vigorous philosophical and theoretical discourses is a credit to those who theorized about nursing practice: thinkers who dared to conceptualize in a practice discipline and educators who pioneered theory development, all of whom were instrumental in defining and advancing the discipline of nursing. These thinkers framed the discussions and the discourse about the mission and the boundaries of the discipline of nursing. The discussions in this book go beyond this thesis to delineate the core of the domain of knowing as well as the permeable boundaries of nursing knowledge, the sources used to advance that knowledge, the different approaches to knowing, the theories that guided the development of nursing's scientific base, and the criteria of truth that the discipline may or may not use. Although the dialogues in this book intend to provide the reader with a sense of history, the process itself helps to unfold a futuristic course that may inspire the readers to develop their own agendas for advancing nursing knowledge. The readers of this text are the active agents who will shape the future of the discipline.

Theory is not a luxury in the discipline of nursing. Using theory as a way to develop conceptual frameworks to be used to guide curriculum development is part of our past. Theory has become an integral part of the nursing lexicon in education, administration, and practice. Members of the nursing discipline should understand its role in the development of nursing and in the delivery of quality evidence-based nursing care. Theory is vital for guiding coherent and influential programs of research. Theory drives policies that are congruent with the assumptions, values, and evidence of a discipline. Theory guides the impact that members of the discipline plan to make.

BEGINNING THE JOURNEY

Like all journeys, the journey proposed for you, the reader, could be short or long, detached or involved, superficial or profound, simple or complex, preplanned or spontaneous, or structured or discovered. Like all journeys, this one has maps, destinations, lamp posts, detours, setbacks, surprises, disappointments, and insights. Like all journeys, you will get out of it what you put into it. It has been my experience in sharing this journey with many fellow travelers through teaching, research, and practice, that the insights gained and progress achieved coincide with the extent to which there is complete openness and flexibility in the discoveries experienced and developed during the journey, to the extent to which there is true engagement in all aspects of the journey, and to the extent that there are opportunities to integrate this journey with personal and professional experiences.

Journeys are meaningful when they become personal. Therefore, you are invited to embark on a long personal journey that spans the theoretical past, present, and future of our discipline. And, you are also encouraged to reflect on your own theoretical journey and to compare and contrast your experience and responses with that of other members of the discipline, as well as with the journey of the discipline itself. All journeys will take on different meanings—the insights from one journey will enhance the insights from another. For your journey, take some time to question your values about theory, your own assumptions about theoretical thinking, your biases against theory, your goals for reviewing theoretical writings, and your goals for the discipline of nursing. For the discipline's journey, ask questions about the discipline's focus and ultimate goals, who establishes and drives these goals, which discipline's perspective is shaping these goals, in what ways these goals may be congruent with overall health care goals and issues, and whether these goals are the same for all health care professionals. Questions that include "if then," and "so what," could help in promoting critical thinking about the discipline and its role in the overall health care of populations.

ASSUMPTION, GOALS, AND ORGANIZATIONS

This book is designed to provide tools and strategies to unfold the thought processes inherent in nursing, analyze the origins of nursing concepts, and contribute to the ongoing dialogue about the role of theoretical thinking in the development of the discipline of nursing. Its intent is to provide the reader with the knowledge base necessary to fully engage in and understand the current situation in health care, and to begin to formulate ideas about how to shape a future for nursing that is more theoretically coherent and effective. This book is about theory, theorizing, and theoretical thinking. Critical thinking is essential for theoretical thinking. Clinicians, theoreticians, and researchers use different forms of theoretical activities in their work. When theory is discussed, the discussion should include how nurses have been theorizing and using theory in the different components of the discipline of nursing, perhaps without attaching the label of "theory" to these activities. It is also about how we can continue to advance the discipline of nursing through knowledge development, enhance professional nursing through the processes that nurses use in conceptualizing their actions, and facilitate better care for clients through theory-based policies and theory-driven practices. This book does not provide recipes for achieving these goals; instead, it provides ideas, questions, processes, and some strategies to enable you to pursue your own goals, develop your own action plans, and share your own insights and wisdom with your colleagues.

The ideas contained in this book are articulated to compete vehemently with any work that denigrates the theoretical history of nursing—past, present, or future. At the same time, the ideas complement and are intended to collaborate with all other writings of colleagues on theory and metatheory. When I provide critique, I attempt to voice it from a nursing perspective, place the critique within a historical context, and analyze the contributions, allowing for the contextual forces and constraints.

This book is not intended to promote a certain epistemological perspective, a certain theory, or a certain set of ontological propositions over any others. Instead, this book explores, discusses, analyzes, critiques, compares, and contrasts different epistemologies, theories of truth, and nursing theories. It delineates components of theory and criteria for theory critique. It describes different strategies used in the development of nursing theories and the consequences of each strategy. This book is intended to be used by those who want to understand significant aspects of the discipline of nursing that may have been dichotomized with practice and shadowed by an emphasis on education of nurses. The ideas presented in this book attempt to promote understanding, not to dissect the discipline of nursing into separate compartments, but

rather to emphasize nursing as a discipline that is based on the integration of philosophical dialogues, theoretical frameworks, practice knowledge, and research findings. Although the focus is on nursing theories, the relationships and interdependence among research, art, philosophy, and practice are highlighted and explicated. The ultimate goals of the different chapters are to stimulate critical thinking, inspire robust dialogue, and challenge the status quo.

The development of the ideas for this book is based on several assumptions:

- Understanding theory and its role is enhanced by exploring the origin of ideas and the processes by which ideas develop into theories.
- Pluralism in nursing theories is desirable and inevitable; therefore, an exploration of existing theories is essential for improving the utility of theory and for continuing the development and progress of the discipline.
- A critical assessment of the history of theoretical thought will pave the way for the development of theories that further describe and prescribe nursing practice. This understanding will help delineate issues that could be resolved in the future.
- No evidence can exist without a coherent theoretical framework that drives the questions and answers for practice.

ORGANIZATION OF THE BOOK

To improve the potential of achieving the goals of understanding the role of theory in the development and progress of the discipline, and of understanding the role of members of the discipline in developing and constructing theory, this book is organized into parts and chapters according to potential illuminations throughout the journey. It is divided into six major parts.

Part One describes terms of the theoretical journey, assumptions to guide the journey, the lamp posts that define key elements of the journey, and the destinations of the journey, as well as scholarship and what it means within the context of the 21st century.

The second chapter in Part One focuses on the agents and producers of knowledge—the scholars in the discipline. Different frameworks for scholarship are analyzed, and scholarship is defined within the context of the practice properties of the discipline. Scholarship includes giving careful attention to the development of nursing theories and to ways in which nursing theories are viewed and analyzed. Chapter 3 provides definitions of major components of the journey and the journey outcomes.

Part Two presents a historical analysis of the discipline's progress toward its present theoretical perspective. Chapter 4 provides a discussion of the forces and barriers that may have influenced theory development, and therefore indirectly affected the scholarly evolution of the discipline of nursing. Chapter 5 presents the evolution of the discipline of nursing and the various stages that have been marked by significant turning points or milestones. It provides trends and patterns of progress intended to stimulate dialogue and reflection among the readers.

In Part Three, I provide an epistemological discussion of our discipline as it is perceived and articulated by theorists and thought leaders in our discipline. The dialogue and analysis provided reflect the thinking about our discipline at the end of the second decade of the 21st century. This part contains three chapters focused on defining the discipline of nursing, the sources of its theoretical bases, and the major philosophical paradigms that has influenced its knowledge base. More specifically, in Chapter 6, the structure of the discipline of nursing is analyzed and discussed. The reader will find definitions of the domain of nursing that provides the impetus for programs of research, and the perspective of clinical practice that provides us with assumptions and values. It is proposed that both the domain and the perspective differentiate the discipline of nursing from other disciplines. The discussion provides an analysis of the permeable boundaries of the discipline. Readers are encouraged to reflect on whether those boundaries are expandable or retractable in light of the many changes that are happening in patterns of population's health as well as in the delivery of health care. Chapter 7 provides an analysis of the sources and resources used to develop theory, and it dispels the myth that only research can be a source of theory. Chapter 8 provides a proposed approach to analyzing the structural components of the discipline and the different ways by which we claim knowledge. The different paradigms that influenced theoretical development of the discipline are explored. In addition, I provide a discussion of several theories that guide how truth and evidence are considered.

Part Four focuses on the analyses of those theory pioneers who provided the tipping point for initiating a robust theoretical and philosophical dialogue. In Chapter 9, I provide an overall perspective on the theories by putting them through magnifiers, telescopes, and microscopes. The result is an integrative synthesis providing support for emerging categories. In Chapter 10, I provide a discussion of the different analysis and critique models for evaluating the quality and effectiveness of theories. The model provided differentiates between strategies and processes for describing, analyzing, critiquing, and testing theories. The remainder of Part Four is devoted to the use of the model for theory description, analysis, critique, and testing for analyzing the selected nursing theories. The selections, based on the theories' central questions, are matched with domain concepts. Therefore, the five chapters in Part Four are organized around an integrative analysis of the theories, focusing the analysis on three categories of theories: needs and self-care, interactions, and outcomes theories.

Part Five is devoted to the future, without losing track of our past or the context of our discipline. Frameworks and strategies for developing concepts and theories are provided as processes and guideposts for a future of influencing health care policies. This part focuses on processes of developing theories, beginning in Chapter 14 with strategies for developing concepts, followed by identifying sources for developing theories in Chapter 15. Subsequently, Chapters 16 and 17 provide more specific strategies for developing middle-range and situation-specific theories.

Part Six continues with a focus on the future. The question that I propose to answer in Chapter 18 is "How do we measure progress in our discipline?" Three theories of progress are discussed and analyzed for their utility in a human science discipline that is dynamic and that continues to respond to societal changes. Chapter 19 provides the challenges we must consider and the paradoxes we must face to continue in our theoretical journey, to insure that nursing science is growing and nursing practice models are making a difference.

Part Seven contains two chapters. Chapter 20 presents an abstracted analysis of selected central writings on metatheory and nursing theory. It is not intended as a comprehensive compilation of abstracts of everything that has been written about metatheory and theory; rather, it is intended as a beginning—but central—collection that you are encouraged to use as a model for your own collection of analytical abstracts. The analyses are intended to provide a starting point for discussion and debate.

The last chapter of the book, Chapter 21, contains an extensive bibliography on metatheory, on paradigms that have been used in nursing, and on nursing theory. Sections 1 through 12 of this chapter contain the metatheory literature and are organized around common themes in nursing and theory, such as philosophy and methods, theory development in nursing, forces and constraints in theory development, theory and science, theory and research, theory and practice, theory and education, and theory analysis and critique. Sections 13 through 37 contain writings about nursing theories by theorists or others who have used the theories for research practice, education, or administration. You can find all the writings related to a theory—to the best of my knowledge—by looking under the theorist's last name in this section. In addition, there are two new sections on middle-range and situation-specific theories, with many references reflecting both.

Asterisked citations in this chapter indicate citations that have been abstracted and analyzed in the previous chapter under metatheory or theory. Sections 38 through 48 contain writings on several central paradigms that have influenced the discipline of nursing, including psychoanalytical theory, symbolic interaction, developmental systems, adaptation, and role theories. Sections 49 through 53 provide a descriptive list of audiotapes and videotapes that have been created to explain the theorists' ideas.

This book is designed to be used sequentially or nonsequentially. This free use of each chapter and each part necessitates a slight repetition of ideas. The repetitions emphasize and expand on significant themes and present the same or similar ideas with a different analytical posture. This book ideally should be used in five teaching/learning units: the first focusing on Part One and Part Two, the second on Part Three, the third on Part Four, and the fourth on Part Five which is devoted to strategies for developing theories. The fifth unit of study should be devoted to dialogue about the future, and Part Six provides the bases for such dialogue and reflections. Part Seven provides the necessary supportive material for each of the parts and should be introduced at the outset of utilizing the book.

ON A PERSONAL NOTE

Writing and reading books are both existential experiences and ongoing, evolving processes. Neither the reader nor the writer is the same person after reading or writing a book, nor are their ideas and viewpoints the same. A book is never complete because ideas are never complete. Yet, at some point, a project needs to be abandoned so that others can explore its ideas to modify, extend, affirm, refine, or refute their own—all of which, if shared with the author, will allow her to do the same. Sometime ago, I decided to abandon the notion that this book is an individual endeavor. It is *our* book, a dynamic project; it belongs to the readers as much as it belongs to me, and as much as it reflects my thinking, engagement of the readers' ideas and their constant discourse is the ultimate goal. These assumptions continued to guide the current edition.

I urge you to consider this book complete as well as incomplete, a temporarily abandoned project that represents my own thinking and analysis at a particular juncture. It incorporates my past, present, and future, intermingled with the past, present, and future of nursing, of nurse theorists, and of the historical and most recent literature. It is from all of this that my present interpretation of theoretical nursing has evolved, but this continuous, dynamic, and evolving process is presented here with temporal boundaries. Therefore, if I misinterpreted any theorists' or metatheorists' admonitions, it was unintentional, and my critique should be viewed as an honest epistemological interpretation bounded by cognitive, historical, and sociocultural meanings of the time.

I firmly believe that without the theorists and metatheorists and their writings, this book would not have been written, and it would not have been necessary. Interpretations and selections of theorists and metatheorists and their ideas were not guided by a desire for omission, but rather by limitations imposed by time and space. The conceptualizations of all theorists and all the analyses of the metatheorists, whether included in this text or not, provide the tapestry that depicts the future of theoretical nursing.

Finally, I have tried to avoid language that suggests stereotypical views of the nurse, patient, and physician, but at times comprehension, clarity, and simplicity have taken precedence. Because the majority of nurses are women, I have used "she" to encompass both "she" and "he."

REFLECTIVE QUESTIONS

The following are some questions to guide a reflective approach to your journey:

1. Comment on this statement that is often heard: "I have practiced (or taught) nursing for many years without the need to use theory, so why do I need theory in a practice discipline?"

2. How did you come to define theory, nursing, human beings, and health? What values and assumptions do these definitions hold, and what courses of action are dictated by those values?

3. What theories guided you in your assessment of your patients, in your research projects, and in your teaching methods? Why did you select these theories? How congruent are the ontological beliefs of these theories with your own and with those of the discipline of nursing?

4. What criteria do you use in selecting or rejecting theories developed in other disciplines to guide your actions? Compare and contrast these criteria with those used in selecting or rejecting nursing theories.

5. How do you measure progress in theoretical and scientific nursing? Are these measures illuminated by an understanding of the daily experiences of nurses caring for people? Are they guided by a nursing perspective? Define that perspective. (Then respond to this question again after reading Chapter 18.)

6. In what ways does your conception of the nursing perspective match or not with your practice environment? With a curricular framework? With a research framework?

2

On Being and Becoming a Scholar

Theory and theoretical thinking are intrinsically intertwined with advancing scholarship in any discipline. Established disciplines provide an intellectual environment that nurtures and promotes scholarly inquiry, and theory and theoretical propositions drive that inquiry. Theory development encompasses these goals and outcomes of inquiry in the discipline that claims scholarship.

The goal for scholarly work is to make a difference in the lives of the people we are entrusted to care for. These may be individuals, families, communities, populations, or whole societies. Scholarship is about making that difference, either directly or indirectly, through developing evidence and advancing knowledge.

There are several questions to consider when we think of the role of scholarship in nursing. Some of these are:

- Is nursing a scholarly discipline?
- Do nurse scholars have the same attributes as other scholars?
- If there are differences, what might these differences be?
- Have there been changes in how the scholarly community views scholarly work?
- In what ways did these changes shape scholarliness for the 21st century?
- Are there historical lessons that may shed better light on contemporary views of scholarship?

These are a few questions to keep in mind as you, the readers, are critically dialoguing with the ideas in this chapter.

SCHOLARLINESS IN NURSING

A scholarly discipline has a focus that is evident and significant as well as a sustainable core of values and principles that guide its members' goals and actions. *Scholarship* in a discipline refers to the degree to which its mission is defined and based on rigorous and credible research and on well-developed, supported, and significant theories. Scholarship is evident in disciplines in which knowledge and its progress are easily articulated, and in which research and philosophical inquiries explore, examine, and answer significant domain questions. *Scholarliness* in a discipline is defined by the extent to which phenomena are articulated, and by the presence of a dynamic discourse and debate about the scope and the boundaries of the discipline's theoretical assumptions and frameworks. *Theory* is an essential component of scholarly disciplines; it provides members of the discipline with the means to articulate their focuses. Theories in nursing and about nursing helped in defining the focus of nursing. They gave nurses the concepts and the language to describe its activities and roles.

Nursing theories to describe, explain, and predict the quality and outcomes of nursing practice and nursing interventions were developed during the decades of the 1960s to the 1980s to answer broad questions that were central to the field of nursing. Although these questions at the time may have been driven by an interest in curricula, they nevertheless addressed practice indirectly. These questions concerned what knowledge is essential for students, how to organize curricula, and what to include and what not to include in a nursing curriculum. Answers were developed in the form of theories that addressed the relationships among the nursing client, environment, transitions, nursing process, nursing therapeutics, strategies for nursing care, and health care goals and outcomes. The theories attempted to describe the phenomenon of nursing and chart a theoretical course for nursing actions. Thus, the beginnings of a scholarly discipline were created.

Rogers, in the late 1960s and early 1970s, used electromagnetic concepts to explain human reactions to health and illness and to give philosophical guidelines to nurses' interventions. She talked about holism before holism became part of our health care language (Rogers, 1970). Orem (1971) spoke of self-care before the initiation of the self-care movement. Travelbee (1966) pioneered the role of a nurse as the explorer of perceived meanings of suffering, and she discussed the significance of spirituality in nursing care. The humanists in the discipline articulated the meaning of the experience of loss and death before it became part of our media lexicon, and clinicians used creative therapeutics such as touch, imagery, and acupressure as alternative health care interventions before the National Institute of Complementary and Alternative Health Practices was instituted to legitimize these practices.

When compared to the study of purely physical phenomena, disciplines oriented to human responses may require a different set of criteria to judge their scholarly progress and development. These criteria evolve from the people-oriented nature of the clinical and human sciences, as well as from the struggles that women have endured to achieve equity and to receive acknowledgment for their work and respect for their credibility. Scholarliness in such disciplines may, by necessity, take different routes and reach different destinations.

Nursing falls into this latter category of disciplines. Besides being defined by its perspective and domain, the nursing discipline is defined by its historical association with women and the propensities of most societies to assign the work and labor of caring to women. These definitional characteristics may be reflected in the philosophical perspectives adopted by its members, both women and men, who often represent a scholarliness that is more congruent with the nature of nursing and less with the nature of other disciplines. The characteristics drive the way in which members of the discipline approach the frameworks they develop or use to define the curricular content and the educational strategies used, and they may also define the ethical decision-making frameworks that govern knowledge development and utilization. Analysis of any of these frameworks, their organization, their level of development, and their impact must consider the history of nursing as a discipline and as a profession that relied heavily on the work of women. When considered within these lenses, nursing is a scholarly discipline.

Indications of Scholarliness in Nursing

Scholarliness is a hallmark of nursing in the 21st century because research and theory help explicate major agreed-on nursing phenomena; because nursing is able to articulate its mission in theoretical terms and with scientific data (Fagin, 1981; Grady and Gough, 2015); because nursing has well-established organizations, scientific journals, and scientific arenas in which to express its views, using both scientific and philosophical methods; because it has authoritative reference groups, all of which helped in establishing agreed-on, well-defined intellectual goals; because it believes in the autonomy of its clients; because it has a pluralistic view of truth that encompasses internal coherence of premises and propositions, external correspondence of truth through sense, and pragmatic truth through metaphysical processes; because it deals with significant problems; because it deals with humanity; because its constituents have both a passion for advancing knowledge and a flair for practice; and, finally, because it offers cumulative wisdom. Nursing goals are generally congruent with those of the recipients of its care; nursing operates from a health and holistic approach and purports to enhance coping and harmony with one's environment.

Seven specific indicators serve as examples of the scholarly maturity of nursing: continuity, concatenation, the National Institute of Nursing Research (NINR), cumulative work, centers of research and centers of excellence, clinical scholars, and the research of unique nursing phenomena.

The first indicator of scholarly maturity, *continuity*, is manifested by those important and fundamental questions in the field that are addressed within a conceptual or theoretical scheme to refine and modify ideas over generations of scholars (Gortner, 1980). Answers are not the isolated incidents with which nursing is confronted (NINR, 2006). The relationship of mechanostimulation on primary or secondary pain; therapeutic touch as a modality for communication, assessment, and intervention; or the consequences of reality testing on the elderly are linked to other answers to form a whole that belongs to a theory of stimulation or person–environment interaction.

Scholarliness is the ability to delineate the premises on which one's decisions and questions are based; the ability to engage in, complete, and communicate the results of research projects that are supported and documented; the ability to critically assess the objective and subjective components in their inquiry; and the ability to relate the results to existing theory and to participate in the development of theories. Our scholarly efforts are concentrated on sharpening and refining our knowledge of the theory-making process identified as central to the discipline and on using the frameworks that define a nursing perspective.

Scholars in nursing use quantitative and qualitative analyses to define, refine, and sharpen concepts, and to test basic propositions for the purpose of adding to substantive knowledge. We must not forget, however, that a significant mission of the discipline is not only the better care of patients, but the emergence of our clients from transition situations equipped with the tools to cope with similar or different transitions in life, with the ways to promote their health, with the means to prevent further illness episodes, and with the techniques to deal with stress in life. In doing so, we help to merge research, theory, and practice—the concatenation realized as we handle clinical problems more and more with the same ease as we handle theoretical and research problems (Barnard, 1980).

The second indicator, *concatenation*, therefore, is demonstrated through nursing theories that evolve from practice and are used in education. As practice joins with education (Schlotfeldt, 1981), the distance between creation of knowledge, corroboration, and translation of knowledge in practice is diminishing. I call this process concatenation, which is the condition under which that shortening of distances is occurring. Joint appointments for nursing faculty that bridge practice and academic systems, as well as regular clinical rounds conducted by faculty and clinicians, are examples of achieving a collaboration that drives the translation of knowledge in practice areas. Concatenation also involves joining with the public media to inform the public of nursing's mission and to modify its goals based on public needs. As we near the end of the second decade of the 21st century, the local and national media are cooperating in modifying the negative image the public had of nursing experts, and, more importantly, nurses are speaking up, their messages are loud and clear, and they are being heard within organizations (Garon, 2012), and locally, nationally, and globally (Cipriano, 2015). Articles and broadcasts have highlighted themes such as the role of nurse-to-patient ratio requirements in helping lower death rates and the Institute of Medicine's recommendation that nurses take on more advanced responsibilities that reflect their education, training, and capacities (Brown, 2010; Kingsbury, 2015; Moore, 2015; Tavernise, 2015). In addition, the story lines of several prime-time television programs in the United States have focused on nurses as the central figures, depicting them in leadership and decision-making positions. Furthermore, scholarship

related to speaking up is driving research and theory development (Rainer, 2015).

The third indicator of scholarliness is the *development of the NINR*, which was authorized under the Health Research Act of 1985 and was established in 1986. This represented a significant milestone in nursing scholarliness, and it affirmed two significant aspects of the discipline of nursing. First, quality nursing care depended on a careful and systematic program of investigation; and second, nursing defined its domain and its thematic characteristics. The Act made us hopeful of increased support and commitment to knowledge development. However, successful funding through the National Institutes of Health (NIH), which has become the gold standard for scholarship, in and of itself is an inadequate indicator. It is merely a means to an end, and better indicators are the quality and significance of the area of scholarship, the quality of publications, the venue for dissemination of knowledge, and the manner by which knowledge is translated (El-Masri and Fox-Wasylyshyn, 2006; Meleis, 2001).

The fourth indicator of nursing's growing scholarly maturity is the *cumulative work* through research and theory that is being done on the central concepts in nursing. For example, when considering the environment's impact on health, **environment** is considered to be the patients' environment, the sociopolitical environment, the administrative environment, and the environment for students. The growing interest in considering the roots of violence and the connection between violence and the environment—at home, at school, in public places, and at work—and how violence, injury, and human safety are related and are the business of nursing, further demonstrates a disciplinary maturity leading to more effective programs of research (Chinn, 2008). Studies also were developed to explain different components of environment that add to our understanding of a safe environment. The concept may be the same, but the different settings help in the development of all components and all properties of the concepts of environment, violence, and safety. One example is Dr. Jianghong Liu's research, which examines how environmental interactions with risk factors, such as nutritional deficiencies and prenatal toxin exposure in early life stages, impact developmental and behavioral problems in children and adults, as well as what environmental interventions can improve development (Liu, Zhao, and Reyes, 2015). In another example, an innovative study related to environment conducted by Holzemer and Chambers (1986) found a significant relationship between faculty perceptions of the environment's scholarly excellence, available resources, student commitment, and motivation and faculty productivity. They helped us conceptualize properties of healthy environments for students in the same way that we conceptualize healthy environments for patients. Similarly, a whole issue of *Advances in Nursing Science* was devoted to violence, injury, and human safety in schools, homes, workplace, global war, and military areas, as well as in different age groups (Chinn, 2008).

The fifth indicator is the development of *centers of research and centers of excellence* that house scholars with expertise, interest, and research methodologies focused on a particular area for knowledge development. These research centers have been the force for advancing knowledge related to central problems in the field of nursing, such as women's health, vulnerable populations, disparities in health care, care for elder adults, symptom management, and transitions and health. Prominent research centers include the Women's Health Research Center at the University of Washington, as well as the Center for Health Outcomes and Policy Research, the NewCourtland Center for Transitions and Health, and the Center for Global Women's Health at the University of Pennsylvania. Each is an example of a critical mass of scholars united to collaborate on developing knowledge that is connected by theoretical assumptions, values, and goals. Research centers also train and mentor future scholars, as well as provide continuity in training postdoctoral scholars. Similar to research centers are centers of excellence, which not only conduct research but integrate it with education and practice. Centers of excellence are used globally as instruments to strengthen nursing scholarship, as well as to improve health care. Two examples are the Nursing Center of Excellence (CoE), the first of its kind in Italy that was established as a strategy to advance the role of professional nursing as a model for other countries (Rocco, Affonso, Mayberry, et al., 2015), and the Perinatal Nursing Care Research Center, which is one section of the Research Institute of Nursing Care for the Community at the University of Hyogo in Japan (Yamamoto, 2015). Both of these centers are potential vehicles for enhancing scholarship globally.

The sixth indicator of scholarship in the 21st century is the movement toward the valuation and respect accorded to *clinical scholars*, who integrate clinical and academic goals and who are offered joint clinical and faculty appointments (Bauer-Wu, Epshtein, and Ponte, 2006).

The seventh indicator of maturity of the discipline of nursing is the acceptability of exploring and *researching unique nursing phenomena*. Phenomena that are unique to nursing, which in previous times were not deemed as worthy of scientific investigation, are now taken seriously. A new generation of scholars are studying, for example, spirituality and well-being (Campesino and Schwartz, 2006; Lewis, 2008); comfort (Arruda-Neves, Larson, and Meleis, 1992; Morse, 1983); and self-management to improve quality of life (Grady and Gough, 2014). Such studies are indications of changes in the outlooks of nursing pacesetters and confidence in the significance of our nursing phenomena and goals.

NURSES AS SCHOLARS

The word *scholar* has been used since around the 12th century (Conrad and Pape, 2014). It was traditionally reserved for individuals who had a depth of knowledge in a particular area of study. In more contemporary times, it is reserved for individuals with advanced degrees (Meleis, 1992).

The common themes in defining scholars are that a scholar is a person who has a high intellectual ability, is an independent thinker and an independent actor, has ideas that stand apart from others, is persistent in her quest for developing knowledge, is systematic, has unconditional integrity, has intellectual honesty, has some convictions, and stands alone to support these convictions. A scholar is a person who is flexible and who respects all divergent opinions (Armiger, 1974; Diers, 1995; Meleis, Wilson, and Chater, 1980; Parse, 1994; Roe, 1951). In addition, of course, a scholar is a person who is deeply engaged in the development of knowledge in the field (Johnson, Moorhead, and Daly, 1992). Not all scientists are scholars, and not all scholars are scientists. Scholarliness concerns having a sense of history about a discipline and knowing how one's work fits within the larger framework and goals of the discipline. Scholarship is enhanced by obtaining advanced degrees; while such degrees are essential, they are not sufficient for scholarship.

Nursing is a human science focused on the health of human beings, and the trajectory of its development as a discipline is unique to its nature and goals. The context for nursing as a discipline and as a profession influences how scholarliness may have evolved and been defined. Because of the discipline's focus on human beings and their health, defining its scholarliness may be dynamic and changeable. There are also some indications that the nature of those disciplines that are oriented to human responses and the nature of those disciplines that focus on clinical matters may differ considerably from other disciplines that focus on physical phenomena or that are purely theoretical in nature (Holmes, 1990; Sarvimki, 1988; Watson, 1990). There are also historical indications that women's history and their lived experiences may provide them with different voices, different cognitive styles, and different ways of knowing (Belenky, Clinchy, Goldberger, et al., 1986; Gilligan, 1984; Anderson, Reimer–Kirkham, Browne, et al., 2007).

Although nursing is a field of study open to men and women, the predominance of women in nursing must not be ignored when considering nurses as scholars. Scholarship is based on knowledge, and women are agents of knowledge whose characteristic activities provide a grounding that is different from and in some respects (in some disciplines based on human science) preferable to men's grounding (Harding, 1988). Harding makes this argument:

> *What it means to be scientific is to be dispassionate, disinterested, impartial, concerned without abstract principles and rules, but what it means to be a woman is to be emotional (passionate), interested in and partial to the welfare of family and friends, concerned with concrete practices and contextual relations. (Harding, 1988, p. 83)*

The question that forms the basis for this section is: Are nursing's approaches to scholarship, knowing, understanding, and formulating conceptualizations unique? There are indications in the literature from the 1980s through the present comparing men and women and supporting the uniqueness of women's developmental processes and women's ways of describing their experiences, and the unique ways by which women experts tend to make decisions. But let us look at history first.

When I think of scholarship in nursing, I think of two renowned individuals from ancient times who made an impact on the meaning of scholarship— *Hypatia and Hatshepsut*. I choose these two historical women because they reflect women who were innovators and risk takers, and because they are part of my own heritage—Egypt in general and Alexandria in particular (where Hypatia flourished and died). Though they were very different types of scholars, they continue to inform modern thought.

Hypatia was a renowned Greek philosopher and scholar of the fifth century (Osen, 1974) who lived in Upper Egypt, in Alexandria. *Hatshepsut* was the only ruling queen among pharaohs in Egypt. She was born in 1508 BC and reigned for more than 20 years, from approximately 1478 BC until her death in 1458 BC (Holmes, 1959; Wells, 1969). Hypatia and Hatshepsut demonstrated commitment, persistence, innovation, leadership, and intelligence. Both developed new theories in mathematics and architecture with implementable, coherent frameworks that reflected values, assumptions, and goals for action, and both made a lasting impact. Both followed similar paths in their lives, different from the universal and mainstream paths that existed during their respective times. Both were resisted by different constituents of oppressors, mostly religious men, and both met with deaths that were said to be untimely and violent, and that may have been preceded by torture, simply because they charted different paths for their people, were forceful in expressing their views, and were successful in making impactful changes.

Hypatia left her mark on the world in the form of innovative devices to study astronomy and to determine the specific gravity of liquids—devices that were praised highly by Socrates. Hatshepsut left her mark in the form of architecturally beautiful temples for her people. She ensured peace both within her country and, by promoting exchanges and partnerships, between Egypt and neighboring countries (Holmes, 1959). She empowered her own people and people from other lands.

Both women demonstrated a unique brand of scholarship; however, scientists had to dig deep to learn about their work and their stories. The question is, was that because of their gender (Rahayu, 2011)? Were they judged by the same criteria used to evaluate and judge male mathematicians and pharaohs? These are questions to consider in more contemporary times as we review how scholarship of nurses, theorists, researchers, and clinicians are judged.

Contemporary literature demonstrates and supports ways to consider scholarship through uniqueness in uncovering knowledge and in decision-making that are different from discovery and research findings. In using Dreyfus and Dreyfus' (1985) framework for analysis and decision-making by pilots, Benner and Tanner (1987) demonstrated how nurses use intuition in expert clinical judgment. Six key aspects of intuitive judgment were identified and discussed in a study that included 21 nurses who were defined by their colleagues as experts. Nurses demonstrated their ability to make judgments by using their intuitive expertise to recognize patterns of relationships in situations that are not readily recognizable to others, by detecting similarities between situations through common-sense understanding, by "knowing how" in a way that is not definable in common scientific terms, by having a "sense of salience" (i.e., recognizing priorities), and by using "deliberative rationality" (shifting perspectives for better understanding) (Benner and Tanner, 1987). These processes involved a level of intuition that has been, in the past, devalued by nurses for its lack of scientific bases. Are any of these characteristics for caring congruent with those needed for knowing and understanding? The uniqueness of nurses' capacity to know and the unique ways by which they demonstrate that knowing and understanding are proposals that should be seriously considered.

That there are different processes of knowing is a proposal that has been supported by a number of key publications from the 1980s. For example, Belenky et al. (1986) identified five different types of knowers. Schultz and Meleis (1988) theorized that these types could be found in nursing. Types of theories and levels of theory development may be influenced by the ability of nursing theorists to uncover knowledge of the different types, to be able to hear and reflect the voices of the different knowers in theoretical development.

If the five types of knowers identified by Belenky et al. (1986) are defined from a nursing perspective, the following is what we might find:

1. **Silent knowers** are nurses who tend to accept the voices of authority and thus learn to be silent. These nurses know their practice, their teaching, or their administrative practice, but they may not be able to articulate what they know through abstract thought for theoretical development and may not have the language to express their analysis or interpretation of the phenomenon. Their work, insights, and wisdom are invisible because they are not represented or because theorists have not been able to retrieve them for further theoretical development. Could these silent knowers conceptualize their understanding of phenomena in ways that are more congruent with their propensity to develop theories?

2. **Received knowers** believe others are capable of producing knowledge that they can follow and reproduce. They believe in external authorities' abilities to generate knowledge, but not in their own or their peers' abilities

to do the same. These people depend on and value the expertise of others. Many nurses have contented themselves with using the works of others, believing those works to be far superior to anything they themselves could create. Examples are the different theories and paradigms that we have bought into and used for years without questioning.

3. **Subjective knowers** depend on their personal experiences. These knowers believe and depend on their own inner voices and inner feelings. Knowledge to them is "personal, private, and subjectively known and intuited," and truth "is an intuitive reaction— something experienced, not thought out, something felt rather than actively pursued or constructed" (Belenky et al., 1986, p. 69). Although these knowers find it difficult to articulate the processes used to arrive at knowledge, they have the wisdom to look holistically and explain complete situations. Knowledge from nursing practice as articulated by subjective knowers could inform the discipline of nursing in ways that no other knowledge could. This is the knowledge that Carper (1978) referred to as *personal knowledge* and Benner (1984) as *expert knowledge*.

4. **Procedural knowers** depend on careful observations and procedures. They are the rationalists among us. These are the people who communicate procedures, rules, and regulations, and thus may be best suited for developing empirical or procedural theories.

5. **Constructed knowers** view all "knowledge as contextual, they experience themselves as creators of knowledge and value both subjective and objective strategies of knowing" (Belenky et al., 1986, p. 15). These knowers integrate the different ways of knowing and the different voices (including the silent voice). To them, "all knowledge is constructed, and the knower is an intimate part of the known" (Belenky et al., 1986, p. 137). To subscribe to this view is to accept the never-ending process of knowledge development, to accept that theories are always in process, to accept that frames of reference are constructed and reconstructed, and to accept that situations, as well as knowledge, are contextual and subject to different interpretations (Schultz and Meleis, 1988).

Observing nurse scholars over many decades, let me risk proposing for dialogue and critique that those who theorize in nursing, those who go beyond a particular clinical situation, findings for a particular project, or beyond themes they uncover from teaching, fall into one of the following categories:

The conceptualizers are those who are discovering, identifying, and exploring the discipline's concepts. These concepts may be central or tangential.

The synthesizers are conceptualizers who are able to connect already developed ideas, analyze them, and arrive at new "wholes." These new wholes make for a more effective explanation and interpretation of already existing knowledge.

The leap theorizers are those who amass research or clinical data and reduce these data to abstract ideas. They are the conceptualizers who are able to make leaps to generalizations, to create challenging theoretical questions and answers.

The bush describers are those who know how to describe relationships that have been empirically identified and verified. They usually are reluctant to go beyond these specific findings.

The out-of-discipline theorizers are those who see the world of nursing through glasses tinted by other disciplines. Therefore, when engaging in conceptualizing and answering questions, they select those that are more accepted and more central to other disciplines. At the same time, however, their findings and conceptualizations shed some light on nursing problems, however minor those problems are to the core of nursing.

The integrated theorizers are those who are as comfortable with theorizing as with researching or practicing. More importantly, these are individuals who have synthesized the different aspects of their problem of interest and have been able to develop conceptualizations in which clinical, research, and theoretical insights are contained.

Tools of Scholarliness

Established disciplines provide intellectual environments that nurture and promote scholarly inquiry, and theory and theoretical propositions drive such inquiries. Over the decades, different approaches have been used to support the scholarly development of nurses. Among them are higher education and mentorship. These tools purport to foster innovation and creativity and develop nurses as agents for advancing knowledge.

Creativity in nursing is manifested in many ways. Creativity is the ability to link seemingly unrelated concepts and variables (Bronowski, 1956), just as Einstein linked time with space and Newton linked mass with energy. Creativity is the discovery of hidden likenesses. Bronowski (1956) said that the act of creation is original but does not stop with the originator. Kepler's laws, which describe the movements of the planets, were not arrived at by mounds of corresponding facts that he collected himself or by corresponding readings, although both are significant. He speculated, dreamed, used metaphors, and made analogies (e.g., with music), all of which helped to give conceptual order to the data. In the same fashion, Rogers (1970) used the analogy of symphonic harmony to describe a human being's relations with his environment. Creativity is a leap of imagination, and scholarliness is characterized by leaps that enhance the explanation and understanding of phenomena.

Communities also enhance scholarship. Cash and Tate (2008) used a community development approach to build scholarship capacity among faculty by creating a community of scholars. By using a nursing practice approach (community development) as a tool, they demonstrated the connection between strategies for nursing practice and their use for nursing scholarship. Scholarliness is a process and a state that encompasses the norms and tools of science and the norms and tools of theorizing and philosophizing. It includes not only creativity but also the communication of ideas through teaching to enhance the scholarly socialization of its members. Over the decades, nursing added the necessary pieces to the puzzle of scholarliness. Nursing continues to have a high commitment to improve its curricula, its teaching and learning strategies, its methods of evaluation, and its administrative styles. It is one of the few disciplines that isolates the components of research design and methodology and helps students to develop necessary skills to undertake a research career.

Scholarliness necessitates the use of *local models of excellence* and the promotion of sponsorship of novices by experts or mentors and mentees as essential. To preach scholarship without demonstrating it in a close working relationship between mentor and mentee leaves a lot to the imagination of the mentee that may not be tangible and attainable (Meleis, Hall, and Stevens, 1994). Participation in a mentoring relationship with a person who is pursuing scholarship in practice, theory, or research tends to promote the potential development of the same characteristics in the mentees. Scholarliness in a discipline not only depends on the definition of the discipline by those who are inside it; it also depends on how the discipline is viewed by those outside it. We need to make our discipline more *public*—demonstrate its significance to the health and care of the public. We also need to become involved in the political and policy-making processes and to make a point of speaking to the public directly.

Scholarliness in nursing includes the *collaborative efforts* of all the resources within nursing, working together to develop critical and reflective thinking in students, academicians, and clinicians. According to Dewey (1922), *critical thinking* is defined as the ability to suspend judgment on matters of interest. Critical thinking should be fostered by cognitive and affective approaches in the educational and clinical arenas. The cognitive approach is enhanced by the provision of frameworks for teaching, discussion, and clinical practice. The affective approach is enhanced by providing frameworks that allow for dialogue, analysis, and reflection on experience.

Examples of critical thinking in nursing include the awareness and inclusion of a focus on systems of patriarchy and domination and their influence on knowledge development (Thompson, 1987). Scholarship in nursing must reflect the type of critical thinking that generates awareness of unequal resources, of relationships that are distorted because of domination, and of the influence of marginalization on members of the discipline and on those who are the recipients of care (Hall, Stevens, and Meleis, 1994; Thompson, 1987). A scholar in nursing demonstrates a *passion for making a difference*, for dismantling old patterns that are based on unequal power and reconstructing patterns that are based on equity, resources, shared power, and on collaboration in decision-making.

A balance should be struck between *providing a framework* that enhances critical thinking and one that may lead to other created frameworks. If only one framework is provided, it could be a stifling act that prevents a person from seeing other potential avenues to understanding the situation. Critical thinking lies in the balance between framework thinking and the flexible viewing of a situation. Critical thinking can also be enhanced by using effective approaches—for example, through the creation of dialogues about patient care situations that are open to debates and critiques. Critiquing

existing theories or research is also appropriate for developing critical thinking. Scholarship includes the creativity needed to consider ways to develop knowledge in a human science, ways that do not stifle the richness of its phenomena.

Scholarship Redefined

The definition of scholarship has changed. Rules once were clear. Scholarship meant research, and research meant one type of research. Scholars were defined as academics who conduct research, publish, and then perhaps convey their knowledge to others, and/or apply what they have uncovered to practice (Boyer, 1990).

Scholarship was confined only to those involved in the discovery of knowledge and was limited to innovative discoveries that made contributions to knowledge development and progress. Scholarship in nursing, within this prevailing framework, was defined as having an academic rank and as being engaged in basic research and in publication (Hofmeyer, Newton, and Scott, 2007). Furthermore, the sentiment prevailed that those who applied knowledge were not scholars; rather, they were practice-oriented folks who must leave scholarship aside and focus on their own practice.

Nurses who value practice as the essence of the discipline have always known something is missing in this definition. It robbed nurses of their rich clinical heritage, and it stifled the processes needed to integrate knowledge and relate it to practice. And practice, we suspected, was the heart and the soul of the discipline. As nurses, we were, however, afraid to rock the "ivory towers" in an attempt to change these definitions. After all, we were just the new kids on the block, with no clout and with a lot of vulnerability. Beginning rumblings were manifested in the writings of many nurses who questioned this status quo. But these rumblings became louder when Ernest Boyer, in his Carnegie Foundation report, "Scholarship Reconsidered: Priorities of the Professoriate" (Boyer, 1990), urged that scholarship be redefined.

Boyer inspired disciplines to engage in robust dialogues about the meaning of scholarship in modern times, and his publication continues to resonate in academic institutions. Boyer discussed the origin of the most prevalent definition of scholarship, as research and discovery corresponding with an emphasis on higher education and on increasing grant support that nurtures the research enterprise. Increasingly, in Boyer's opinion, scholarship was becoming synonymous with academic work, and professors were expected to compete for grant funding and focus on research, thereby creating a dichotomy between teaching and research. Many groups in the U.S. society had begun to question this de-emphasis on teaching in universities, and analyses such as those done by Boyer (1990) and Glassick, Huber, and Maeroff (1997) fueled the call for a redefinition of scholarship.

Boyer proposed that there are four different categories of scholarship. The first and most familiar is the *scholarship of discovery* that is tied to original research. This type of scholarship calls for activities that enhance a deeper understanding of research processes in a quest to answer a discipline's pressing questions. The emphasis in this type of scholarship is on research, and research attracts funding from such institutions as the NIH through the R01 program, among other sources of similar funding. In the U.S. scientific community, the R01 designation is considered the gold standard for research funding, denoting the significance of the research, the credibility of the investigation, and the standing of the investigator in the academic community. However, disciplines, and students within the various disciplines, needed other kinds of scholarship to advance and flourish (Meleis, 2001). Therefore, a second area of scholarship, the *scholarship of integration*, was proposed. This is the quest to find connections between different discoveries, leading to new wisdom and insights about an area of investigation or a discipline. Scholarship of integration is achieved when innovative insights are realized that are larger than the smaller disconnected facts produced by research. The exceptional discoveries in sciences in the late 20th century and the complexity and interrelationship between the different disciplines makes the scholarship of integration more timely (Strober, 2006).

Scholars who excel more at the *integration of knowledge* rather than at the discovery of knowledge tend to focus on conceptualizing and theorizing; they not only describe findings, but also interpret and ascribe meanings to these findings within the context of the discipline. Their scholarship is thus manifested in presenting thoughtful analyses of profound, philosophical, and theoretical changes in the discipline. This form of scholarship is manifested but continues to be overshadowed by the scholarship of discovery. The language of integration increasingly penetrated academia and practice, and there are indications that it is being accepted and valued as an acceptable form of scholarship (Hofmeyer et al., 2007).

The third type of scholarship as defined by Boyer is the *scholarship of application*. This type of scholarship builds bridges between theory, research, practice, and recognizes and rewards nurses' contributions to knowledge development. Scholarship of application encompasses the translation of knowledge to solve problems for individuals, families, or societies. This type of scholarship requires the integration of knowledge of best practices in achieving best outcomes (Shapiro and Coleman, 2000). With the increasing acknowledgment of this interdependence between academic institutions and society, there comes an expectation that relevant knowledge must be translated to benefit societies, and, conversely, the knowledge that is developed must emanate from the needs of society (Limoges, Acorn, and Osborne, 2015). Scholarship of application has gained more support in nursing and beyond. It is honored in institutions of higher education through professional appointments in the clinical and practice ladders (Barnsteiner, Lipman, Spatz, et al., 2014).

Other authors have provided their own definitions of scholarship of application. Palmer (1986) defined it as:

a complex activity and synthesis of observations of clients and patients . . . a complex activity that has as its purpose, the discovery, organization, analysis, synthesis, and transmission of knowledge resulting from client-centered nursing practice. (p. 318)

Diers (1995) defined *clinical scholarship* (which is the equivalent of Boyer's scholarship of application) as:

. . .certain habits of mind. Clinical scholarship modifies the noun only by focusing on observations in and of the work, including the perception of one's own participation in it. To these observations are applied disciplined habits of analysis (including careful attention to sources) and analogy, that are carefully described and even more carefully edited so that, when written, the activity produces new understanding, new knowledge. (p. 25)

Clinical scholarship is reflected in the careful analyses of situations and critical assessment of responses; it requires a certain intellectual maturity that comes from expertise and repeated experiences. The explanations and reflections offered by the clinical scholar are contexted in her personal history and are enhanced by her well-supported interpretations.

The fourth type of scholarship is that of *teaching*. Boyer's conceptualization of teaching as scholarship resonated with what nurse educators emphasized for many years. Teaching was traditionally set aside as an application of knowledge, and accepted as secondary to knowledge discovery. We all spent hours developing innovative curricula, creative teaching strategies, and learning modules, and we discovered new ways to help students understand their practice roles, defined ways by which we could create synthesis and integration in student's knowledge, and watched with admiration how seasoned clinicians assisted the inexperienced to become transformed.

Shulman and colleagues provided more conditions to clarify what is meant by teaching scholarship. They suggested that good teaching should be differentiated from scholarly teaching and from scholarship of teaching (Glassick, 2000; Hutchings and Shulman, 1999; Shulman, 1999). Shulman states that for teaching to be scholarship, the work must be communicated and public, should be peer reviewed critically, should be compared to some accepted standards for quality control, must be reproduced, and must be cumulative, building on other scholars' work.

I believe that what began in nursing decades ago—that is productive researchers inspiring, guiding, and mentoring novice researchers—and that nurses have long attempted to demonstrate as scholarship, is now acknowledged as such. There has been a growing realization for the need for scholarly educators who ask questions and research best practices for educating, evaluating, and testing innovations in all teaching, learning, and curricular matter (Oermann, 2014). This need may have been driven by shortages in faculty members, as well as the growing concern for systematic approaches to advancing knowledge in nursing education (Fiedler, Degenhardt, and Engstrom, 2015). An indicator of the acknowledgment of teaching scholarship is the Josiah Macy Jr. Foundation's support for grant sponsorship of nurse and physician scholars who focus on innovative curriculum and technology projects (Macy, 2015). However, it is important to note that turning teaching into scholarship of teaching requires an infrastructure that facilities experiences of faculty and supportive systems to change or supplement university policies, criteria, and benchmarks for scholarship (Heinrich, 2010).

The question before us to discuss: In what ways will these redefinitions of scholarship reshape scholarship in nursing? These redefinitions of scholarship, which are more friendly to the nature of the discipline of nursing, the practice of nursing, and the mission of nursing, have affirmed what nurses believed was essential to a human science but reluctantly ignored for many decades. These new acknowledged approaches to nursing as a discipline value the need for nurses to have a "group of fields" that are related to nursing but are outside nursing (Diers, 1995). There remains the need for dialogue on how these different scholarships are considered equal, nurtured, and rewarded (McBride and Kanekar, 2015; Probert, 2014). Similarly, much dialogue is needed to determine how social media and online publishing influence scholarship. As Greenhow and Gleason (2014) indicated, social media can facilitate the connection between scholars and the public, but it also raises many questions about how to shift entrenched practices in how scholarship is considered through academic and public lenses.

Our discipline is scholarly if members of the discipline engage in the development of knowledge that has some significance to humanity and to human beings, if they open doors for those who have the most difficulty in accessing the health care system, and if they encompass and include the underserved population. Nursing scholars deal with human beings, and they not only pursue explanation and prediction, they also address an understanding of clinical phenomena that may result from clinical as well as theoretical knowledge. Therefore, perhaps our discipline of nursing may be at the scholarship of integration stage.

Scholarship of Integration

A hallmark of nursing in the 21st century is in its focus on the scholarship of integration. An analytical view of the normative structure of the discipline of nursing that focuses on education and practice came together during the 1970s and 1980s. Some institutions tried and succeeded in having their faculty maintain joint appointments. Theory infiltrated practice, and, from practice, theories evolved. Instead of occurring only within the curriculum, tests of theories were done in practice. Research findings demonstrated significant outcomes of nursing care through changes in morbidities, mortalities, and quality of life (Fagin, 1981), and there were indications as well of more tolerance for the use of multiple theories (Newman, 1983).

The use of many theories and the acceptance of pluralism were accompanied by an attempt to derive meaning from their relationship to nursing practice. Representative examples of excellent theoretical frameworks of nursing phenomena appeared increasingly in the nursing literature (Mercer, 1981; Millor, 1981; Mischel, 1990; Norbeck, 1981; Tilden, 1980; Weiss, 1979; Younger, 1991). These conceptualizations represented openness to multiple approaches (Armiger, 1974; Schlotfeldt, 1981); they comprised a pluralism that was neither addressed nor advocated during the previous stages.

Authors of these new conceptualizations combined the traditional view that concepts were not accessible to empirical testing with the view that concepts did, however, generate variables that *were* testable. Other nursing concepts, such as maternal role attainment, touch, and temperament in battered children, were based on research and premises from interactionist and developmental models, and were drawn from natural and physical science. These new propositions allowed for the divergence of thought and approach that was essential for the development of further testable propositions and, eventually, the development of theories.

This process was analogous to other processes in the history of science. Johannes Kepler, for example, developed the four laws of planetary motion by using careful observations painstakingly collected by Tycho Brahe (Bernstein, 1978). By doing so, Kepler opened up new avenues and brought up new questions. Therefore, he used a convergence of Brahe's data and his own ideas to evolve his laws and to allow for more questions and propositions to develop. Extensions and refinements of early data produced refined and usable laws.

There are more indications that nursing scholarliness became even more integrated in the 1980s and 1990s (Table 2-1). A review of nursing practice literature demonstrated a growing awareness of a stronger relationship between theory and practice. In clinically oriented national meetings, there was an outgrowth of presentations that were theory based, and there were discussions of questions that lent themselves to theory and theory development. We moved away from "how to" to "why," "what if," and "when" in an attempt to generalize, document, and verify phenomena in nursing practice.

Nursing theories tended to address imaginative and ideal nursing practice. These theories were visions of what nursing ought to be and what care should be; they were necessary visions of how nursing should move forward to establish its identity and its boundaries. Once the ideal goals were established, these theories were modified as nurses described and documented real-world scholarliness, combining theory, research, philosophy, and, in disciplines such as nursing, practice. Scholarliness is also reflected in the synthesis and integration between a discipline's different components. Characteristics of the integrative approach to knowledge in a discipline are that the relationships among theory, research, philosophy, and practice become more apparent; that clinical scholarship is expected and practiced; and that clinical research, as well as fundamental research, is required (Diers, 1995). Integrative knowledge is also indicated by engaging in societal issues and achieving partnerships to deal with pressing civic, moral, and social issues (Boyer, 1990). When questions arise about how nurses are or are not engaged in making a difference in communities, they indicate that our discipline has achieved a new milestone toward becoming a scholarly discipline based on integrative knowledge (Duke and Moss, 2009). We would not have been able to reach this current stage without having gone through previous stages in which the focus was on practice only or teaching only, theory only, or research only.

History provides a comparative context to more contemporary analysis of knowledge development, providing support for progress toward integration. In the early 1960s, nursing theorists developed theories in isolation, researchers pursued questions of interest only to educators or administrators, investigators asked isolated questions, and practitioners pursued their practices while remaining somewhat oblivious to what the other groups were doing. Today, significant changes have occurred in the relationships among educators, researchers, theoreticians, and practitioners from the different disciplines making the scholarship of integration more of a reality (McGaghie, 2015). These groups are now partnering with each other, writing for each other, and working with each other. Note the increasing involvement of clinicians in educational

TABLE 2-1	Characteristics of the Stage of Scholarship of Integration

- Relationships among theory, research, practice, and philosophy become more apparent.
- Pluralism in paradigms is encouraged.
- Boundaries of domain become more identified.
- Domain guides nursing practice, research, and theory.
- Knowledge is developed that makes a difference in health care.

programs, the increasing commitment of academics to practice, and the emerging research collaboration between both groups. Clinicians and academics are crossing the boundaries to work together and, more importantly, most of them believe that practice is the *raison d'être* of nursing. As a result, middle-range and situation-specific theories are being developed to answer clinical questions that evolve from the partnerships forged between academic institutions and academic health centers. These may encompass more inclusive questions such as: Who are our nursing clients? When does a client need nursing care in addition to or instead of medical care? And, when do we discharge a client from our care? Or, they may include more specific questions pertaining to ways in which we make our patients comfortable, strategies for pain relief, symptom management, care of wounds, culturally competent nursing therapeutics, and transitions and health promotion.

These questions should be compared with those related to teaching strategies (such as those related to modular or individualized instruction) or with questions about leadership styles (such as those related to developmental or transformational styles of leadership). Both of these sets of questions were the forms of inquiry pursued in the past; the answers they provided led to knowledge that was not as central to clinicians' concerns about providing quality nursing care but were more congruent with nursing management and teaching missions. However, these types of questions also can be related to the scholarship of practice if they include outcomes, such as the discovery of the effects of teaching strategies and leadership styles on patients, families, or communities. The current generation of scholars in nursing ask questions central to practice and explore phenomena emanating from and influencing practice outcomes. New generations of scholars are being educated to provide answers that drive and shape the future of nursing practice (Lusk, 2014). Nurses became more comfortable with looking at their own practice, describing it, and allowing theoretical formulations to emanate from it (Benner, 1984), without abandoning their commitment to teaching or to management. Acknowledging and valuing practice as a source of theory, and nurses as agents for developing integrated and coherent theoretical descriptions of nursing practice, resonates in some ways with Boyer's definition of scholarship of practice.

There are also many indications that professional organizations speak a language congruent with that spoken by theorists and clinicians; an example is the social policy statement issued by the American Nurses Association (ANA) in the 1980s and updated most recently in 2010. The statement provided the profession of nursing with a national definition of nursing and a direction for practice, and was another indication of agreement on nursing concepts and issues. Nursing was defined as "the diagnosis and treatment of human responses to actual or potential health problems," which is congruent with the focus that emerged on human responses (versus nurses' functions, interactions, or relationships, and versus symptoms, signs, and behavior) (ANA, 1980, p. 9). This definition was reviewed, affirmed, and supplemented by an ANA task force (ANA, 1995). The policy statement affirmed that, "The nursing profession remains committed to the care and nurturing of both healthy and ill people, individually or in groups and communities" (ANA, 2010, p. 6). This definition that was expanded in 2003, has maintained the essence of the earlier definitions but was made more specific:

Nursing is the protection, promotion, and optimization of health and abilities; prevention of illness and injury; alleviation of suffering through the diagnosis and treatment of human response; and advocacy in the care of individuals, families, communities, and populations (ANA, 2010, p. 6).

The definition of nursing provided in the ANA policy statement acknowledges several essential features of nursing practice. These are that nursing: focuses on the full range of human responses; places less emphasis on problem-focused evaluation; emphasizes the integration of knowledge based on objective data, as well as on knowledge that reflects subjective experiences; stresses the application of knowledge related to diagnostic and interventional processes, caring relations, and the goal of facilitating and promoting health and healing. This document also defines the nurse's function as incorporating a responsibility to develop theories from evidence provided through research. These theories are expected to guide nursing practice (Hobbs, 2009).

The definition of human responses to health and illness includes need, condition, concern, event, dilemma, difficulty, occurrence, and fact—as well as lived human experiences that can be described within the target area of nursing. It considers the diversity of human responses in the health/illness situation. In the social policy statement (ANA, 1995), one can see the influence of a number of theories from the 1960s and 1970s on the concepts selected for inclusion, such as interaction, self-care, and affiliation, as well as on the inclusion of the goals for advancing nursing theories. Human responses to health and illness provide us with phenomena on which to base further research and theory development.

A positive relationship between theory and research is not as foreign and unattainable as it was in previous stages of nursing scholarship. More specifically, up until the late 1970s, only a limited relationship existed between research and theory. Later, more links were established (Batey, 1977), with links between theory and research preceding links between theory and practice. The literature is replete with suggestions of how nurses can use theory to guide research and how they can use research to build theories (Fawcett and Downs, 1986). These links between theory, practice, and research continued to build on early indications, culminating in the full realization of the scholarship of integration in the 21st century.

CONCLUSION

Scholarship matters in advancing knowledge, in developing educational programs, and in providing care. One does not develop knowledge to gain scholarliness in a discipline. Being a scholar is a means toward an end and not an end in itself; it is a means toward the empowerment of nursing as a profession, and of nurses as scientists, clinicians, educators, and policy-makers. The end goal is patient care based on socially relevant knowledge that is developed with social consciousness. It is to provide, enable, and empower nurses to make the changes they want to make in the quality of patient care. It is to participate in the development of policies that affect the care that is given. That influence is possible only if it comes from a socially relevant knowledge base. Such a knowledge base can be developed if reflective attention is given to patterns of knowing that are most congruent with the discipline of nursing as a human science, to the phenomena relevant to nursing, and within a value system that accepts and respects a nursing perspective. Scholarship of integration evolving over many years of silos in scholarship has become the prevailing and more accepted and utilized framework in the disciple of nursing.

REFLECTIVE QUESTIONS

1. After you review the chapter, reflect on this statement: "A scholarly discipline must engage in societal concerns, in dialogues about pressing issues, and in shaping health care reform." Considering the above as conditions for scholarship, what would be your assessment of the level of scholarship in nursing?

2. Scholarship is defined in terms of science, discovery of knowledge, verification of knowledge, empirically and by the extent to which these processes render the research competitive for funding. Discuss the aforementioned within the context of nursing as a human science.

3. If you think the definition of scholarship in question 1 is the best in reflecting the discipline of nursing, discuss the outcomes on nursing science of using such a definition.

4. What are the advantages and disadvantages of utilizing norms of scholarship that reflect scholarship of integration in advancing the discipline of nursing?

5. Give examples of the different types of scholarship within your field of interest.

6. Identify key scholars in your field of interest who represent each type of scholarship as discussed in this chapter.

7. In what ways is theoretical thinking related to scholarship?

8. What criteria, milestones, and outcomes should be used in nursing to evaluate progress for scholars who are engaged in the scholarship of application and the scholarship of integration? What strategies would you use to influence the gold standard criteria for scholarship that are embodied in academic institutions?

9. In this chapter, the scholarship of integration is presented as the type of scholarship that has evolved as the choice scholarship. Some may argue that in fact there are more recent indications about the primacy of the scholarship of application. What is your opinion? Defend with indictors and evidence.

ACKNOWLEDGMENTS

This section, dealing with scholarliness, norms of scholarliness, and tools of scholarliness, was adapted, with extensive revisions, from the Helen Nahm Lecture that I delivered at the University of California, San Francisco, in 1981; and from (by permission) Meleis, A.I. (1983). The evolving nursing scholarliness. In P.L. Chinn (Ed.), *Advances in Nursing*. Rockville, MD: Aspen Systems.

REFERENCES

American Nurses Association. (1980). *Nursing: A social policy statement* (Publication No. NP-63). Kansas City, MO: Author.

American Nurses Association. (1995). *Nursing's social policy statement* (Publication No. NP-107). Washington, DC: Author.

American Nurses Association. (2010). *Nursing's social policy statement* (p. 6). Washington, DC: Author.

Anderson, J.M., Reimer–Kirkham, S., Browne, A.J., and Lynam, M.J. (2007). Continuing the dialogue: Postcolonial feminist scholarship and Bourdieu–discourses of culture and points of connection. *Nursing Inquiry*, 14(3), 178–188.

Armiger, B. (1974). Scholarship in nursing. *Nursing Outlook*, 22(3), 162–163.

Arruda-Neves, E., Larson, P., and Meleis, A.I. (1992). Comfort: Immigrant Hispanic patients' views. *Cancer Nursing*, 15(6), 387–394.

Barnard, K. (1980). Knowledge for practice: Directions for the future. *Nursing Research*, 29(4), 208–212.

Barnsteiner, J., Lipman, T., Spatz, D., Stringer, M., and Walsh-Brennen, A.M. (2014). 25 Year Retrospective of the Clinician Educator Role at the University of Pennsylvania School of Nursing. University of Pennsylvania School of Nursing Report.

Batey, M.V. (1977). Conceptualization: Knowledge and logic guiding empirical research. *Nursing Research*, 26(5), 324–329.

Bauer-Wu, S., Epshtein, A., and Ponte, P.R. (2006). Promoting excellence in nursing research and scholarship in the clinical setting. *Journal of Nursing Administration*, 36(5), 224–227.

Belenky, M.F., Clinchy, B.M., Goldberger, N.R., and Tarule, J.M. (1986). *Women's ways of knowing: The development of self, voice, and mind*. New York: Basic Books.

Benner, P. (1984). *From novice to expert: An excellence and power in clinical nursing practice*. Menlo Park, CA: Addison-Wesley.

Benner, P. and Tanner, C. (1987). Clinical judgment: How expert nurses use intuition. *American Journal of Nursing*, 87(1) 23–31.

Bernstein, J. (1978). *Experiencing science*. New York: Basic Books.

Boyer, E. (1990). *Scholarship reconsidered: Priorities of the professoriate* [special report]. Princeton, NJ: The Carnegie Foundation for the Advancement of Teaching.

Bronowski, J. (1956). *Science and human values*. New York: Harper Colophon Books.

Brown, T. (2010). Is there a nurse in the house? *The New York Times*, June 18, 2010, p. A21.

Campesino, M. and Schwartz, G.E. (2006). Spirituality among Latinas/os implications of culture in conceptualization and measurement. *Advances in Nursing Science,* 29(1), 69–81.

Carper, B. (1978). Fundamental pattern of knowing in nursing. *Advances in Nursing Science/Practical Oriented Theory*, 1(1) 13–23.

Cash, P.A. and Tate, B. (2008). Creating a community of scholars: Using a community development approach to foster scholarship with nursing faculty. *International Journal of Nursing Education Scholarship*, 5(1).

Chinn, P.L. (Ed.). (2008). Violence, injury, and human safety. *Advances in Nursing Science*, 31(2), 93.

Cipriano, P.F. (2015). Nurses at the table: In the United States and around the world. *American Nurse*, 47(5), 3.

Conrad, P.L. and Pape, T.T. (2014). Roles and responsibilities of the nursing scholar. *Pediatric Nursing*, 40(2), 87–90.

Dewey, J. (1922). *Human nature and human conduct*. New York: Henry Holt.

Diers, D. (1995). Clinical scholarship. *Journal of Professional Nursing*, 11(1), 24–30.

Dreyfus, H. and Dreyfus, S. (1985). *Mind over machine: The power of human intuition and expertise in the era of the computer*. New York: Free Press.

Duke, J. and Moss. C. (2009). Re-visiting scholarly community engagement in the contemporary research assessment environments of Australasian universities. *Contemporary Nurse*, 32(1–2), 30–41.

El-Masri, M.M. and Fox-Wasylyshyn S.M. (2006). Scholarship in nursing: What really counts? *Nurse Researcher*, 13(4), 79–80.

Fagin, C. (1981, September). *Nursing's pivotal role in achieving competition in health care*. Paper presented at American Academy of Nursing meeting, Washington, DC.

Fawcett, J. and Downs, F.S. (1986). *The relationship of theory and research*. East Norwalk, CT: Appleton-Century-Crofts.

Fiedler, R., Degenhardt, M., and Engstrom, J.L. (2015). Systematic preparation for teaching in a Nursing Doctor of Philosophy Program. *Journal of Professional Nursing*, 31(4), 305–310.

Garon, M. (2012). Speaking up, being heard: Registered registered nurses' perceptions of workplace communication. *Journal of Nursing Management*, 20(3), 361–71.

Gilligan, C. (1984). *In a different voice: Psychological theory and women's development*. Cambridge, MA: Harvard University Press.

Glassick, C.E. (2000). Boyer's expanded definitions of scholarship, the standards for assessing scholarship, and the elusiveness of the scholarship of teaching. *Academic Medicine*, 75(9), 877–880.

Glassick, C.E., Huber, M.T., and Maeroff, G.I. (1997). *Scholarship assessed. The Carnegie Foundation for the Advancement of Teaching*. San Francisco, CA: Jossey-Bass Publishers.

Gortner, S.R. (1980). Nursing science in transition. *Nursing Research*, 29(3), 180–183.

Grady, P.A. and Gough, L.L. (2014). Self-management: A comprehensive approach to management of chronic conditions. *American Journal of Public Health*, 104(8), e25–e31.

Grady, P.A. and Gough, L.L. (2015). Nursing science: Claiming the future. *Journal of Nursing Scholarship*, 47(6), 512–521.

Greenhow, C. and Gleason, B. (2014). Social scholarship: Reconsidering scholarly practices in the age of social media. *British Journal of Educational Technology*, 45(3), 392–402.

Hall, J.M., Stevens, P.E., and Meleis, A.I. (1994). Marginalization: A guiding concept for valuing diversity in nursing knowledge development. *Advances in Nursing Science*, 16(4), 23–41.

Harding, S. (1988). Feminism confronts the sciences: Reform and transformation. In V.C. Bridges and N. Wells (Eds.), *Proceedings of the fifth nursing science colloquium: Strategies for theory development in nursing: V.* Boston, MA: Boston University.

Heinrich, K.T. (2010). Passionate scholarship 2001-2010: A vision for making academe safer for joyous risk-takers. *Advances in Nursing Science,* 33(1), E50–E64.

Hobbs, J.L. (2009). Defining nursing practice: The ANA Social Policy Statement, 1980–1983. *Advances in Nursing Science,* 32(1), 3–18.

Hofmeyer, A., Newton, M., and Scott, C. (2007). Valuing the scholarship of integration and the scholarship of application in the academy for health sciences scholars: Recommended methods. *Health Research Policy and Systems,* 5(5), 1–8.

Holmes, C.A. (1990). Alternatives to natural science foundations for nursing. *International Journal of Nursing Studies,* 27(3), 187–198.

Holmes, W. (1959). *She was Queen of Egypt.* London, UK: G. Bell & Sons.

Holzemer, W. and Chambers, D. (1986). Healthy nursing doctoral programs: Relationship between perceptions of the academic environment and productivity of faculty and alumni (research). *Research in Nursing and Health,* 9(4), 299–307.

Hutchings, P. and Shulman, L. (1999). The scholarship of teaching: New elaborations, new developments. *Change,* 31(5), 10–15.

Johnson, R.A., Moorhead, S.A., and Daly, J.M. (1992). Scholarship and socialization: Reflections on the first year of doctoral study. *Journal of Nursing Education,* 31(6), 280–282.

Kingsbury, K. (2015). Call (back) the Midwife! *The Boston Globe,* September 2, 2015.

Lewis, L.M. (2008). Spiritual assessment in African-Americans: A review of measures of spirituality used in health research. *Journal of Religion and Health,* 47(4) 458–475.

Limoges, J., Acorn, S., and Osborne, M. (2015). The scholarship of application: Recognizing and promoting nurses' contribution to knowledge development. *The Journal of Continuing Education in Nursing,* 46(2), 77.

Liu, J., Zhao, S.R., and Reyes, T. (2015). Neurological and epigenetic implications of nutritional deficiencies on psychopathology: Conceptualization and review of evidence. *International Journal of Molecular Sciences,* 16(8), 18129–18148.

Lusk, P. (2014). Clinical scholarship: Let's share what we are doing in practice to improve outcomes. *Journal of Child and Adolescent Psychiatric Nursing,* 27(1), 1–2.

Macy Jr., J. (2015). *The Josiah Macy Macy Jr. Foundation.* Retrieved from macyfoundation.org

McBride, L.G. and Kanekar, A.S. (2015). The scholarship of teaching and learning origin, development, and implications for pedagogy in health promotion. *Pedagogy in Health Promotion,* 1(1), 8–14.

McGaghie, W.C. (2015). Varieties of integrative scholarship: Why rules of evidence, criteria, and standards matter. *Academic Medicine,* 90(3), 294–302.

Meleis, A.I. (1992). On the way to scholarship: From master's to doctorate. *Journal of Professional Nursing,* 8(6), 328–334.

Meleis, A.I. (2001). Scholarship and the R01. *Journal of Nursing Scholarship,* 33(2), 104–105.

Meleis, A.I., Hall, J.M., and Stevens, P.E. (1994). Scholarly caring in doctoral nursing education: Promoting diversity and collaborative mentorship. *Image: Journal of Nursing Scholarship,* 26(3), 177–180.

Meleis, A.I., Wilson, H.S., and Chater, S. (1980). Toward scholarliness in doctoral dissertations: An analytical model. *Research in Nursing and Health,* 3, 115–124.

Mercer, R. (1981). A theoretical framework for studying factors that impact on the maternal role. *Nursing Research,* 30(2), 73–77.

Millor, G.K. (1981). A theoretical framework for nursing research in child abuse and neglect. *Nursing Research,* 30(2), 78–83.

Mischel, M.H. (1990). Reconceptualization of the uncertainty in illness theory. *Journal of Nursing Scholarship,* 22, 256–262.

Moore, M. (2015). The nursing shortage and the doctor shortage are two very different things. *The Washington Post,* June 5, 2015.

Morse, J.M. (1983). An ethnoscientific analysis of comfort: A preliminary investigation. *Nursing Papers,* 15(3), 6–19.

National Institute of Nursing Research (NINR). (2006). *Changing practice, changing lives: 10 landmark nursing research studies.* Bethesda, MA: National Institutes of Health.

Newman, M. (1983). The continuing revolution: A history of nursing science. In N. Chaska (Ed.), *The Nursing Profession: A Time to Speak.* New York: McGraw-Hill.

Norbeck, J. (1981). Social support: A model for clinical research and application. *Advances in Nursing Science,* 3, 43–59.

Oermann, M.H. (2014). Defining and assessing the scholarship of teaching in nursing. *Journal of Professional Nursing,* 30(5), 370–375.

Orem, D. (1971). *Nursing concepts of practice.* New York: McGraw-Hill.

Osen, L.M. (1974). *Women in mathematics.* Cambridge, MA: MIT Press.

Palmer, I.S. (1986). The emergence of clinical scholarship as a professional imperative. *Journal of Professional Nursing,* 2, 318–325.

Parse, R.R. (1994). Scholarship: Three essential processes [editorial]. *Nursing Science Quarterly,* 7(4), 14.

Probert, B. (2014). *Why scholarship matters in higher education* (Discussion paper 2). Sydney, Australia: Australian Government Office for Learning and Teaching.

Rahayu, M. (2011). The representation of women scientist in Agora. *LiNGUA,* 6(2).

Rainer, J. (2015). Speaking up: Factors and issues in nurses advocating for patients when patients are in jeopardy. *Journal of Nursing Care Quality,* 30(1), 53–62.

Rocco, G., Affonso, D., Mayberry, L., Sasso, L., Stievano, A., and Alvaro, R. (2015). Center of Excellence to Build Nursing Scholarship and Improve Health Care in Italy. *Journal of Nursing Scholarship,* 47(2), 170–177.

Roe, L. (1951). A psychological study of eminent biologists. *Psychological Monographs,* 65, 1–67.

Rogers, M.E. (1970). *An introduction to the theoretical basis of nursing.* Philadelphia, PA: F.A. Davis.

Sarvimki, A. (1988). Nursing as a moral, practical, communicative, and creative activity. *Journal of Advanced Nursing,* 13, 462–467.

Schlotfeldt, R.M. (1981). Nursing in the future. *Nursing Outlook,* 29, 295–301.

Schultz, P.R. and Meleis, A.I. (1988). Nursing epistemology: Traditions, insights, questions. *Image—Journal of Nursing Scholarship,* 20(4), 217–221.

Shapiro, E.D. and Coleman, D.L. (2000). *Redefining scholarship in contemporary academic medicine* (pp. 25–28). Washington, DC: Association of American Academic Medicine Council of Academic Societies (CAS).

Shulman, L. (1999). The scholarship of teaching. *Change,* 31(5), 11.

Strober, M.H. (2006). Habits of the mind: Challenges for multidisciplinary engagement. *Social Epistemology*, 20(3–4), 315–331.

Tavernise, S. (2015). Doctoring, without the doctor. *New York Times*, May 25, 2015.

Thompson, J.L. (1987). Critical scholarship: The critique of domination in nursing. *Advances in Nursing Science*, 10(1), 27–38.

Tilden, V. (1980). A developmental conceptual framework for the maturational crises of pregnancy. *Western Journal of Nursing Research*, 2, 667–677.

Travelbee, J. (1966). *Interpersonal aspects of nursing*. Philadelphia, PA: F.A. Davis.

Watson, J. (1990). Caring knowledge and informed moral passion. *Advances in Nursing Science*, 13(1), 15–24.

Weiss, S. (1979). The language of touch. *Nursing Research*, 28(2), 76–80.

Wells, E. (1969). *Hatshepsut*. Garden City, NY: Doubleday.

Yamamoto. (2015). Personal Communication.

Younger, J.B. (1991). A theory of mastery. *Advances in Nursing Science*, 14(1), 76–89.

3

Theory: Metaphors, Symbols, and Definitions

THE DESTINATION: THEORY AND THEORETICAL THINKING

Every journey has its own symbols and metaphors that shape the experience and the destinations. Students of theory, as well as of the discipline's history, should clarify the metaphors, symbols, and definitions along the way, being sure to take into account dynamic changes in meaning. Metaphors reflect estimation of value of events and concepts. A number of metaphors have been attributed to theory in nursing, and these metaphors have shaped the development, progress, and the use of theory in the discipline. Some of these metaphors have contributed to either the promotion or the decline in the theoretical progress of the discipline. Among the metaphors that have constrained progress are theory attributed to ivory towers; theory as an academic exercise; theory for curriculum; conceptual frameworks that are not considered theories; theories that are too esoteric; theories borrowed from non-nursing disciplines; and theories as a framework for research questions. When metaphors reflect curricula or ivory towers, they tend to derail progress in theoretical discourse among clinicians and for clinical practice. When metaphors reflect practice and research, they move the discipline forward, refining and building on its theoretical progress. Metaphors that help to advance theoretical discourse are theories and interpretations of responses or results; shared theories; integrated theoretical frameworks; theories in nursing and for nursing; practice theories; and theories from practice.

New antitheory metaphors within the discipline are related to nurses progressing from being novices to becoming experts, a progress that is erroneously perceived by some to denote that becoming an expert is based solely on a nurse's own personal and clinical experiences and insights. The wisdom gained in the process of moving to expert status is reflected in

articulating clinical exemplars, and these exemplars are then used to guide the work of future novices. Other metaphors that tend to substitute for theories are evidence-based practices (with evidence being equated with research), best practices (defined as based on experience), and inductive reasoning as far more effective than deductive reasoning. However, theory may be either the driving force or the outcome of all these metaphors. One metaphor that could shape the discipline of nursing during the 21st century is the *cyclical integration of theory, research, and practice*. Evidence for practice then becomes viewed as being based on a set of principles and assumptions, as well as on research processes and outcomes. Interpretations of the findings are driven by the theory that framed the research questions as well as by the meanings imputed on the data by the researcher's own wisdom, views, and experiences. Therefore, whether the agent of knowledge or the agent of practice is aware of theory, some level of theory shapes the questions and the interpretations that the agent uses in research or practice. In short, theory metaphors that dominate a discipline shape how students, faculty, and clinicians tend to accept, reject, use, or refute the use of theory in their work.

A metaphor that may be useful in understanding the role of theory in knowledge development is that of a painting that requires a coherent vision of a completed tapestry. It includes the right canvas to translate a vision, the painter to execute his or her vision, the tools to make the painting happen, the viewer who perceives the painting based on his or her context, the public who may or may not value the painting, and the media that may make or break the artist or the painting. Theory is the coherent vision of the context, process, and outcome. Theory is the goal of all scientific work; theorizing is a central process in all scientific endeavors, and theoretical thinking is essential to all professional undertakings. However, the painter (the nurse/theoretician), the viewer (the student of theory and the translating clinician), and the public (including the patient, other professions, the public at large, and the researchers) have their own perspectives and interpretations of the theory. The media (all constituencies) may promote, refute, or obstruct the use of theory.

Think of all components that make up a painting or a school of thought in art as you read about theory and theoretical thinking in the next few pages. Despite the tremendous progress made in the theoretical development of the discipline of nursing, as demonstrated in the explosion of theoretical writing, some confusion remains regarding the role of theory in the development of knowledge and the role of researchers and clinicians as theorists (creator of a painting school of thought, interpretation, and translation of art). More recently, the explosion in programs that prepare nurses as nurse practitioners is matched by a decline in theoretical and philosophical dialogues as reflected in decreasing theory courses in Masters programs. It is natural and expected for some nurses to declare themselves only clinicians, only theoreticians, or only researchers. However, it should be of great concern to nurses when theorization, theory development, and theory utilization are seen as "ivory tower" activities, removed from other scientific and professional processes, or when theoretical nursing or nursing theories are totally substituted with medical sciences (Fawcett, 2006). It is of concern and should be alarming because, without a coherent view of what nursing is, what goals are to be accomplished, and how to evaluate consequences, how do we expect to provide lifestyle changes that promote health, maintenance of healthy behaviors, and healing and recovery? Activities that clinicians and researchers perform and should perform in some form or other, with varying degrees of intensity throughout their careers, are dependent on coherent views of outcomes. Without a vigorous theoretical discourse about our practice, research, profession, and outcomes, we would not be able to build a cumulative knowledge base, which is the basis for established disciplines and expert knowledge. Claiming expert and advanced clinical practice is predicated on a coherent body of knowledge and evidence of outcomes of quality care—the markers for established disciplines and expert knowledge. None of it would be possible without theoretical dialogues and coherent theories that reflect existing evidence and lead to the development of more evidence for practice.

On one level, nurses have demonstrated more commitment to the activities associated with theory, as manifested in the language nurses use to describe the activities that occupy them. Healthy skepticism, evaluation and revisions of theories are equally as important and essential in advancing theoretical knowledge. However, skepticism and non–criteria-based critiques founded on limited knowledge and paucity of criteria are not helpful in making changes or in developing knowledge. Therefore, examples of criteria-based evaluations demonstrate more maturity in any field. One example in nursing is the use of well-defined adjectives to describe theory utilization (Cormack and Reynolds, 1992; Fawcett and Madeya, 2013) such as scope, usefulness, or goodness of fit of theory with one's values or with clients' clinical problems. Im (2015) found out that there are still relatively limited robust theory-based evaluations. Another is the increasing literature about theories in books, in clinical journals, and in research publications (Im, 2013; Im and Chang, 2012; Meleis, 2015).

Theory and theoretical thinking are not limited to theoreticians in the discipline. Theoretical thinking is integral to all the roles played by nurses, including those of researcher, clinician, consultant, and administrator. In research, for example, theoretical thinking could be demonstrated in all aspects of the research process, from conceptualizing the research questions to interpreting the meaning of data (Wolf, 2015). *First*, it is demonstrated in identifying the phenomenon within the domain of nursing, in differentiating between relevant and irrelevant phenomenon, and in deciding how the research questions are related to the theoretical domain of nursing and to the focus of nursing practice. In human science, theoretical thinking is also demonstrated when and if the researcher attempts to determine the importance of the research questions to the discipline of nursing, as well as to society at large (Clarke and Fawcett, 2014). Theoretical thinking helps to raise questions about the investigator as an agent of the research and to determine the meaning of the investigation to the researcher personally. Theory provides a framework from which to consider those personal meanings that drive the research, as well as from the researcher's personal commitment to the research process. When these questions are asked, discussed, and answered, a process of theoretical thinking has already occurred.

Second, theoretical analyses guide the process of phenomenon definition, as well as the research process (Quinn, 1986). The researcher seeks theories that can help in describing the phenomenon or its relationships to other phenomena, or that can prescribe a nursing action for it. If theories are available, then the researcher evaluates them to determine the most useful theory for the research process—one that will expand knowledge. Theory evaluation is as much the business of the theoretician as it is the business of the researcher and clinician. The researcher evaluates whether a theory should be tested as well as whether, and in which ways, the findings of the research can help refine and extend the theory. The clinician evaluates theories for use in practice. Therefore, even the process of theory evaluation for use in research or practice demonstrates another component of theoretical thinking. Unfortunately, Im (2015) has documented a decline in systematic theory evaluation, which may impact the continuous development of theoretical knowledge.

Third, after a theory is evaluated, a hunch may evolve and propositions may be developed to guide the research process or to test the theory. *Fourth*, after testing a theory or the propositions of a theory, the researcher may complete the task by simply describing the findings or by interpreting those findings in relationship to the original theory, perhaps choosing to refine, extend, or modify the original theory. Each of these activities is theoretical in nature and represents a vital component of theoretical thinking and theory building; each of these activities should be acknowledged as an aspect of engaging in the work needed to develop theoretical nursing.

The professional clinician goes through a similar process in deciding what to assess in clients, the timing of assessment, how to define the needed actions, and what interventions are best for the situation. He or she develops hunches, pursues some, accepts others, and refutes others. The clinician develops priorities, modifies them, and reorders them in the process, making some "automatic" decisions and others that require careful consideration and deliberation. Some of these decisions are based on theory; others could be the impetus for theoretical development. These processes reflect those activities of theoretical analysis and development that are described in this book. In engaging in any or all of these processes, a clinician is experiencing theoretical thinking, but may not be aware of the process, may not label it as such, or may not allow the theoretical process to progress enough to culminate in knowledge development. To understand these processes of evaluation of use of theory for research and practice, which are essential for continuous progress and to use the criteria presented

in Chapter 10, definitions of some key concepts are first proposed as a baseline.

DEFINITIONS

Concepts used in developing, evaluating, and operationalizing theories can be defined in a number of different ways. Definitions are influenced by one's world view, as well as by the particular theoretical heritage of the concept. Language tends to shape the discourse about a particular problem or a specific care situation. Kramer (2002) demonstrated how informal caregiving for patients with dementia was described in terms of burden, and thus questions raised about such care tended to be built on assumptions of passivity in patients with dementia and oppression by caregivers. It is significant for theory students to be critical of any definitions provided and to recognize that they are based on a variety of frameworks and a number of different truths.

With that caveat, I encourage you to familiarize yourselves with the definitions provided in the subsequent text. Recognize that a variety of options exist, and perhaps one of them will be most congruent with your own philosophical values. The following definitions (Meleis, 1997a) are influenced by a feminist perspective, which shapes the fabric of tentative realities (Bleier, 1990). Another major influence on my thinking and writing about theory is the tradition of symbolic interactionism (Mead, 1934). The definitions that I provide here are given as guidelines and are, therefore, limited in depth and scope. I encourage the reader to engage in dialogue about these definitions, as well as their origins, their meanings, and the biases they impose, all of which frame the outcomes of their use. It is essential, however, to decide on a set of definitions that guide your subsequent practice, research, teachings, or theory advancement.

Assumptions

Assumptions are statements that form the bases for defining concepts and framing propositions. Assumptions provide the context for a theory. They are accepted as truths, and they represent values and beliefs. These statements represent the thread that holds different aspects of knowledge together. Assumptions are the taken-for-granted statements of the theory, the concept, or the research that preceded the subsequent investigation. When assumptions are challenged, they become propositions. Assumptions emanate from philosophy; they may or may not represent the shared beliefs of the discipline. The values in a theory and/or about the profession and discipline of nursing are reflected in the theory's explicit or implicit assumptions.

Concept

Concept is a term used to describe a phenomenon or a group of phenomena. A concept denotes some degree of classification or categorization. A concept provides us with concisely summarizing and communicating thoughts related to a phenomenon or a group of phenomena; without such concise labeling, we would have to go into great detail to describe them. Notice the difference between describing the phenomena of what happens to individuals who travel from one time zone to another through detailing their sleep disturbances, and the changes in their moods, eating habits, bowel movements, and routines, and summarizing all those details through the concept of "jet lag." The latter is a more concise and a more efficient way of communicating the ideas contained in, and related to, jet lag. Labeling a concept may make it more feasible to analyze and to develop it further. A labeled phenomenon or a set of phenomena is a concept, and a concept could be operationalized further and is more amenable to be translated into a research tool. Concepts are the building blocks in a discipline.

Domain

Domain is the territory of the discipline. It contains the subject matter of a discipline, the main agreed-on values and beliefs, the central concepts, the phenomenon of interest, the central problems of the discipline, and the methods used to provide some answers in the discipline. A domain includes the players and actors who help to ask and answer the questions. The actors in the domain of nursing are clinicians, researchers, theorists, metatheorists, philosophers, teachers, consultants, and ethicists. Domains are discussed further in Chapter 6.

Epistemology

Epistemology is a branch of philosophy that focuses on the reflection on and investigations about the nature and foundation of knowledge. Questions about how knowledge is defined, developed, verified, believed, or became certain are epistemological questions

(Przylebski, 1997). Epistemology also addresses notions about the extent to which knowledge is limited or expansive. Epistemology is the theory of and about knowledge, and it is also about the methods by which knowledge is developed (White, 1999).

Evidence-Based Practice

Evidence-based practice is a concept that was initially developed in Canada, in the 1980s, for medical education with the intent of using and valuing research findings over data-generated dichotomy and opinion. The Cochrane Collaboration, an organization with global influence, helped sustain the momentum by developing and propagating meta-analyses. Evidence-based practice is based on the comprehensive review of research findings, with emphases on intervention, randomized clinical trials as a gold standard, the integration of statistical findings, and making critical decisions about the findings based on evidence hierarchies, tools used in studies and in meta-analysis, and cost (Jennings, 2000; Jennings and Loan, 2001).

Evidence-based practice is based on research data that suggests a basis for the choice of a particular practice and the consequences and outcomes that are likely to occur. It is the implementation of findings from the most recent investigations for the purpose of providing quality care (Banner, Janke, and King-Shier, 2015). Decisions that a nurse makes in caring for her patients may depend on the best solutions derived from her experiences or from the best research findings that are substantiated through publication in public or academically peer-reviewed forums. The latter choice reflects evidence-based practice (Ervin, 2002).

What guides the nature of the questions and the evidence must not be forgotten (Melnyk, Fineout-Overholt, Gallagher-Ford, et al., 2012). Similar meta-analysis of theories that drive the questions, analysis, and interpretation should become part of the meta-analysis (Fawcett, Watson, Neuman, et al., 2001). Therefore, although evidence-based practice rarely refers to theoretical underpinnings, evidence based on research that is not theoretically driven limits the utility of that evidence to limited sets of variables that may lack a coherent framework.

Ontology

Ontology is the fundamental assumptions about the nature of beings, the relationships between the parts as they exist. It is a theory of "what there is"

(Lejewski, 1984). Ontology provides the basis for analyzing and understanding nature and the relationship between human beings and nature (Rawnsley, 1998), as well as the laws that are behind these categories (Burkhardt and Smith, 1991). It is the discipline that provides the logical tools to analyze the nature of basic and fundamental categories (Grossman, 1983). An ontological analysis of a conceptualization is an analysis of the nature of its existence, the categories it encompasses, and the relationship between those categories and what they mean. Ontology has been referred to as a science, a theory, and/or a specific conceptualization (Gracia, 1999; Jacquette, 2002). It is a concept used in the philosophical tradition, as *formalized ontology*. It is a branch of metaphysics, and it has a variety of meanings (Hartmann, 1953). Among them are describing the nature of theoretical formulations as they exist, an analysis of the qualities of beings, and postulations about relationships (Burkhardt and Smith, 1991). *General ontology* focuses on the study of such concepts as space, time, and event, and *special ontology* studies social systems and structures (Dictionary of Philosophy, 1999, pp. 200–201).

However, in nursing we use ontology to mean a study and critical analysis of the very nature—the core—of beings, relations, and concepts. It is an internal analysis of the core of an entity. The analyses utilize logic as a tool. Ontology as a concept has been used to describe the nature of development and analysis of theories (Rawnsley, 1998), and it has been used to dialogue about the nature of nursing (Reed, 1997) and the differences between viewing nursing as an innate human process of well-being and its service orientation (Bryant, 1998).

Paradigm

The definition of paradigm is closely associated with Kuhn (1970), who introduced the concept to those members of the scientific community who were interested in philosophical analyses of disciplines and their development. Critics and supporters of Kuhn's work have created a multitude of meanings for paradigm, which were further confused by the many uses of the term that Kuhn demonstrated in his own writings. Kuhn reported a critic's finding of "22 different" uses of *paradigm* in his writings (Kuhn, 1977, p. 294). *Paradigm* is defined as those aspects of a discipline that are shared by its scientific community. To dispose of the confusion created by his multiple use of *paradigm,* Kuhn (1977, p. 297)

proposed to replace it with *disciplinary matrix*. A disciplinary matrix includes the shared commitments of the community of scholars, its shared symbolic generalizations, and its exemplars, which are the shared problems and solutions in the discipline. The varied, and at times conflicting, definitions of paradigm within and among disciplines make its use in nursing problematic. (See Chapter 18 for further discussion of paradigms.)

Parsimony

Parsimony is the presenting of ideas succinctly, under the premise that explanations should be clearest when made using the fewest statements. Parsimony requires the elimination of redundancies. Parsimony is also known as the "principle of economy of thought" (Marenbon, 1999, p. 411).

Phenomenon

A phenomenon is an aspect of reality that can be consciously sensed or experienced. Phenomena within a discipline are those aspects that reflect the domain or the territory of the discipline. A phenomenon is the term, description, or label given to describe an idea about an event, a situation, a process, a group of events, or a group of situations. A phenomenon may be temporally and geographically bound. Phenomena can be described from sense-based evidence (e.g., something seen, heard, smelled, or felt) or from evidence that is grouped together through thought connections (e.g., the observation that more children die in pediatric intensive care units during the 3 PM to 11 PM shift than on other shifts). In this example, simply observing the deaths does not make the phenomenon; it is grouping them and considering a connection between them—considering a connection between the deaths and the specific staff shift—that makes it a phenomenon. As another example, taking a certain amount of time to adjust to new time zones, having trouble remembering, experiencing foggy thinking, and being indecisive may all be part of the phenomenon related to flying or flying across time zones. Another discussion of phenomena appears in Chapter 14.

Philosophy

Philosophy is a distinct discipline in its own right, and all disciplines can claim their own philosophical bases that form guidelines for their goals. Philosophy is concerned with the values and beliefs of a discipline and with the values and beliefs held by members of that discipline. An individual's values and beliefs may or may not be congruent with those of the discipline. Philosophy focuses on providing a framework and worldview for asking both ontological and epistemological questions about central values, assumptions, concepts, propositions, and actions of the discipline. Philosophy also provides the assumptions inherent in the discipline's theoretical structure.

The philosophy of a science deals with those values that govern the scientific development and justification of a discipline. It helps in defining or questioning priorities and goals. Philosophical inquiries help members of the discipline to uncover issues surrounding priorities and to evaluate these priorities against societal and humanistic priorities.

Praxis

Action theory or action research was introduced with more frequency to the nursing lexicon in the 1980s, as critical inquiry based on social criticism and nursing practice. Actions are predicated on interactions between the theorist and the researcher, and knowledge and action are intricately connected. Feminist praxis is based on the premises of mutual interaction: nurses working on changing situations while developing knowledge, and incorporating emotions and reciprocity in the knowledge that is being developed. Theories based on praxis allow for action, activity, development, and constant dynamic changes, but, most importantly, on the dialectic relationship between theory, action, and critical reflection (Powers and Knapp, 2006, p. 135). Perhaps a purist view of praxis may negate the development of theoretical thoughts (O'Toole, 2003, p. 1421), which is more ordered and could be viewed as more structured and static. Purist praxis followers, the creators of emancipatory knowledge through a dynamic process of critical reflection and practice changes, would argue vehemently against what they view as the more static nature of theory and theory development.

Science

Science is a unified body of knowledge about phenomena that is supported by agreed-on evidence. Science includes disciplinary questions and answers to the questions that are central to the discipline. These answers represent collective wisdom based on patterns in the results of the data that have been obtained through different designs and methodological approaches. These answers are also the impetus from which science evolves and develops. There are different approaches to evaluating and judging scientific findings: support of truth through repeated findings, tentative consensus among a community of scholars supporting aspects of evidence, tentative consensus among other subcommunities attesting to descriptions of reality, and the use of objective criteria by members of the community (Brown, 1977; Kuhn, 1962; Popper, 1962).

Tautology

Redundancies, repetitions, and circular statements are described as tautological (Mautner, 1999).

Teleology

This is the branch of philosophy that deals with ends or consequences. It postulates that the purpose of any action must be understood in terms of final causes. It is an inquiry into the consequences of the phenomenon being studied. Phenomenon could only be studied in terms of purpose. There is an element of predetermination and determinism. Teleology allows for looking at the effect of a phenomenon as the cause (Collins English Dictionary, 2000).

Theoretical Frameworks

A theoretical framework is a basic structure developed to organize a number of concepts that are focused on a particular set of questions (O'Toole, 2003).

The terms *theoretical frameworks, conceptual frameworks, conceptual models*, and *theories* have been used interchangeably in the literature. The distinction between them occupied much of the discourse and debates of the mid-1980s. Theories are developed to answer specific questions. Frameworks and models are developed to provide direction for research projects. Models are developed to represent theories and to provide direction for research projects. Theoretical and conceptual frameworks evolve from theory, theories, or research. Theories differ from frameworks in coherence, a connection between concepts, and the nature of propositions.

Theory

A theory is an organized, coherent, and systematic articulation of a set of statements related to significant questions in a discipline and communicated as a meaningful whole. It is a symbolic depiction of those aspects of reality that are discovered or invented for describing, explaining, predicting, or prescribing responses, events, situations, conditions, or relationships. Theories have concepts that are related to the discipline's phenomena. These concepts relate to each other to form theoretical statements.

Nursing Theory

Nursing theory is defined as a conceptualization of some aspect of reality (invented or discovered) that pertains to nursing. The conceptualization is articulated and communicated for the purpose of describing, explaining, predicting, or prescribing nursing care, as well as for defining the outcomes of nursing care.

Nursing theories are reservoirs in which are stored those findings that are related to nursing concepts, such as comfort, healing, recovering, mobility, rest, caring, enabling, fatigue, transitions, and family care. They are also reservoirs for answers related to significant nursing phenomena, such as levels of cognition after a stroke, process of recovery, refusing a rehabilitation regimen for myocardial infarction patients, and revolving admissions.

The definition of nursing theory has been most problematic, as demonstrated by many exchanges in the nursing literature. Many concepts have been used interchangeably with the term theory, such as *conceptual framework*, *conceptual model*, *paradigm*, *metaparadigm*, *theorem*, and *perspective*. The use of multiple concepts to describe the same set of relationships has resulted in more confusion and perhaps in less use and development of nursing theory.

Several types of theory definitions (Table 3-1) are identified by Chinn and Jacobs (1987), Chinn and

Kramer (2011), and Fawcett and Madeya (2013). Each of these definitions drive different criteria for utilization and evaluation of theories:

1. The first type of definition focuses on the structure of theory, as exemplified by McKay (1969), who defined theory as "logically interrelated sets of confirmed hypotheses" (p. 394). This definition incorporates research as a significant step in theory development and discounts conceptualizations that are based only on mental processes. Therefore, using this definition would not allow the consideration of any of the current nursing theories as theories and as it dictates the requirement of research confirmation.

2. The second type of definition focuses on the goals on which the theory is based. Different theorists, such as Dickoff and James (1968), define nursing theory as "a conceptual system or framework invented for some purpose" (p. 198). Not only do they focus on outcomes and consequences because of their premise that prescriptive theory should be the ultimate goal for all theory activities in nursing, but they also do not distinguish between conceptual framework and theory. Indeed, theory is defined in terms of a conceptual framework. This definition also brings to our attention the potential for inventing nursing reality (Chinn and Jacobs, 1987); mental images are therefore not restricted to the discovery of reality but to the construction of reality.

3. The third type of definition alludes to the tentative nature of theory, as exemplified by Barnum (1998). Barnum defines theory as "a construct that accounts for or organizes some phenomena" (p. 1). Barnum emphasizes that the source of nursing theory is not "what is" but "what ought to be," and that existing conceptualizations are indeed nursing theories because, she asserts, quibbling over labels of theory, concept, framework, and so forth are "mere splitting of hairs" (p. 1). Barnum's definition is significant in a number of ways: It acknowledges that theories are always in the process of development (Chinn and Jacobs, 1987), that existing conceptualizations are theories, and that invention is as much an arena for theory development in nursing as is discovery.

4. The fourth type of definition focuses on research and is exemplified by Ellis (1968).

TABLE 3-1	Types of Theory Definitions

Chinn and Jacobs (1987) identify four types:
1. Definitions focusing on structure
2. Definitions focusing on practice goals
3. Definitions focusing on tentativeness
4. Definitions focusing on research

From these, Chinn and Kramer (2011) present a fifth type:
5. Definitions focusing on creativity in developing and connecting concepts and the use of theory in practice as well as research

Fawcett and Madeya (2013) provide a sixth type:
6. Definitions focusing on progression from conceptual framework to theory

Ellis defines theory as "a coherent set of hypothetical, conceptual, and pragmatic principles forming a general frame of reference for a field of inquiry" (p. 217). Ellis' definition reminds us that theory is developed for the purpose of guiding research. This definition assumes that practice guides theory development, theory guides research, and research guides theory.

5. A fifth definition emerged from the previous four and was articulated by Chinn and Kramer (2011). They define theory as "a creative and rigorous structuring of ideas that projects a tentative, purposeful, and a systematic view of phenomena" (p. 257). According to this definition, imagination and a coherent vision are important, but a rigorous process of ordering of these imaginative ideas is essential. Tentativeness in putting these ideas together is essential. Also, according to this definition, when concepts are defined and interrelated in some coherent whole for some purpose, we have a theory. The definition leaves the door wide open for using theory in practice and research, and it does not restrict theory to research-verified propositions. This definition exemplifies the multiple usages of theory.

6. A sixth definition of theory is exemplified by Fawcett and Madeya (2013), who differentiate between conceptual models and theories, indicating that few nurses present their ideas as theories. For example, Newman (1994) and Parse (1996) did present their ideas in the form of a theory, whereas others such as Orlando (1987), Peplau (1992), and Watson (1989) are a few, according to Fawcett and Mandeya, who spoke about their ideas as theories, whether grand or middle-range. She defines theory as "one or more relatively concrete and specific concepts that are derived from a conceptual model, the propositions that narrowly describe these concepts, and the propositions that state relatively concrete and specific relations between two or more of the concepts" (Fawcett and Madeya, 2013, p. 15). This definition and differentiation adds another dimension to how theories are viewed in nursing.

The definition of nursing theory adopted in this text is based on the work and definitions of previous theorists. I have considered the common themes that evolved from these definitions and incorporated them into the definition offered here. Theorists and utilizers of theory used labels interchangeably to describe their conceptualizations, and sometimes different labels were used to describe the same structures. The criteria for the selection of the different labels (model, paradigm, science, theory, and framework) are not always entirely clear. For example, the utilizers of theory have used *models* and *theories* interchangeably; and, although some usage differentiated between models and theories, such differentiation was not completely clear. For some, models are considered structures of concepts that precede the development of theory. They are also used as structures of concepts evolving from theories. (Refer to Chapter 21, wherein a cursory review of the section titles will document this multiple usage.)

A deliberate decision was made to avoid fine-line debates about how to label existing conceptualizations about nursing. These differences are tentative at best, and hair-splitting, unclear, and confusing at worst. Some theorists who differentiate between theory, metaparadigm, conceptual framework, and model have provided analyses that tend to overlap the properties of each of these concepts. If, indeed, conceptual models are more abstract, less specific, and contain fewer defined concepts and testable propositions, then their linkages with research and practice should not be expected. Because the utility of these models in practice and research has in fact been evaluated, and the linkages between theory and practice, research, education, and administration have been addressed by the utilizers, the properties of the existing conceptualizations do not lend themselves to the label "conceptual models." (See Chapter 7 for further discussion.) Therefore, the differences between the different labels (theory, metaparadigm, conceptual frameworks, and so forth) are differences in emphasis rather than substance and may not be worth continued debate or the creation of new esoteric entities to describe the mental images of nurse theorists. There is limited support that the use of one label over another has helped in the differentiation of the type of knowledge developed, and it may have managed to create more ambiguity for the novice and the experienced alike. Perhaps we need to debate *more substance and less form!*

When comparing nursing theories with theories in other fields, such as role theory in sociology or psychoanalytical theory in psychology, we often find that some of our nursing theories may be as specific or as nonspecific as those theories, or as abstract or as concrete. However, the tendency is to be more critical of nursing theories and to prefer the use of other discipline theories which at times may be informative for nursing phenomena. That being said, perhaps this may have been some of the reasons that we continue to unwittingly downgrade nursing theory by relegating it to a conceptual framework status when other conceptualizations have been called theory. The early reluctance of nurses to designate their work or the work of others as theories changed in the mid-1990s (Lenz, Suppe, Gift, et al., 1995). Indicators of this progress are manifested in the proliferation of the many books written about nursing theories.

Theories are always in the process of development. Therefore, a theory in process should not be considered a conceptual framework just because it is in progress or in process. It is simply in an expected stage in the process of development, and, in a human science, it will always be in process and in progress.

Some theorists and theory utilizers may prefer the use of one particular label, such as conceptual framework, middle-range theory, or grounded theory. However, they may find that the use of the labels may actually not be consistent nor does it reflect the level of abstraction or specificity of the conceptualization. Theories could be used as conceptual frameworks when concepts from different theories are linked together to form a new whole. They could be used as theoretical frameworks when concepts from one theory are given new meanings or when they are linked with another theory to form a new structure that will be tested. They could be labeled a conceptual model when a theory is used as a prototype and is modeled in form or structure.

Nurse theorists (such as Martha Rogers, Dorothy Johnson, and Virginia Henderson) developed coherent, systematic, and organized visions of what nursing is and what the nursing mission ought to be. To consider these conceptualizations as models and frameworks for nursing as a whole is to convey the idea that nursing is conceptualized in one way and according to one model. Therefore, other conceptualizations may be excluded prematurely by the one-particular-model advocate. Proponents may ask: How can we see the world through different pairs of glasses simultaneously?

The position taken in this book is that existing nursing conceptualizations are theories that could be used to describe and explain different aspects of nursing care. They are not competing models; they are complementary theories that may provide a conceptualization of different aspects, components, or concepts of the domain. They reflect and represent different realities. They also address different aspects of nursing; thus, nursing theory is defined as a *conceptualization of some aspect of reality (invented or discovered) that pertains to nursing. The conceptualization is articulated and communicated for the purpose of describing, explaining, predicting, or prescribing nursing care, as well as for defining the outcomes of nursing care.*

Nursing theories evolve from extant nursing reality, as seen through the mind of a theorist who is influenced by certain historical and philosophical processes or events. These theories also may evolve from a perception of ideal nursing practice, tinted by one's history (personal, professional, and disciplinary) and philosophy. Furthermore, they may reflect a coherent representation of nurses' daily work. Theory is a tool for the development of research propositions (see the left side of Fig. 3-1). Theory is also a goal, a reservoir in which findings (both quantitative and qualitative) become more coherent and meaningful. The cyclical nature of theory, practice, philosophy, history, research, and science is depicted in Figure 3-1. Taken together, and in relationship to each other, theories constitute the knowledge base for the discipline of nursing.

Examples of the phenomena and relationships depicted in nursing theories are:

- A nursing client is conceptualized as a self-care agent.
- A nursing client is a biopsychosocial and cultural being.
- A nursing client is a system with a number of behavioral subsystems.
- A nursing client is conceptualized as a conglomerate of needs.
- A nursing client is a system of such modes as interdependence, self-concept, roles, and psyche, among others.
- Person–environment interactions are the focus of nursing care.
- Health and illness behavior is a product of person–environment interactions.
- Communication is a tool for diagnosis and intervention in nursing.
- An efficient, functional, productive interaction has several components: sensing, perceiving, and conceiving.
- A goal of interaction is to develop rapport, which in turn enhances patient care.
- The focus of intervention is the client's environment.

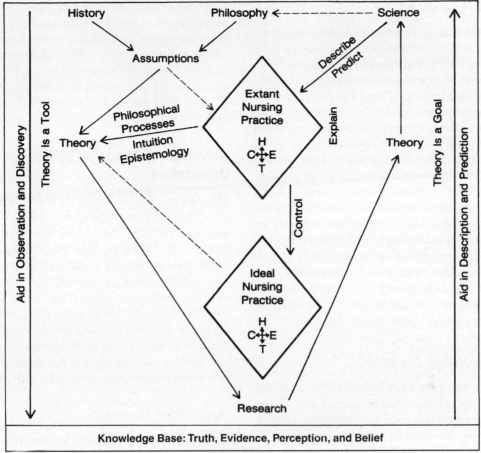

Figure 3-1 Knowledge Base: Truth, Evidence, Perception, and Belief.
(H, health; C, client; T, transitions; E, environment; 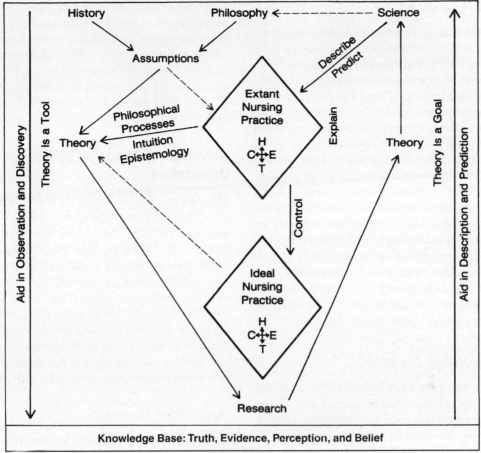, interactions and process).

- Environment is a composite of energy fields.
- Nursing care deals with manipulation of environment.
- Nursing provides self-care needs only until the client or a significant other is capable of providing self-care.
- A nurse is conceptualized as performing a number of functions designed to meet the patient's needs.
- Nurses deliver care that focuses on patients' outcomes; these outcomes reflect medical and/or nursing perspectives.
- Nurse–patient interactions are a framework for assessment or intervention.

TYPES OF THEORIES

Theories are reservoirs in which related knowledge is articulated and organized into meaningful wholes. Theories answer significant questions and help investigators and clinicians to focus on raising questions in a systematic and a coherent way. Tentative theories reflect growth in disciplines. They reflect the wisdom of articulating disparate facts in a meaningful whole and the challenge of answering new questions as they arise. To accomplish its goals of optimum health for its clients, the discipline of nursing must have theories to describe its phenomena, to explain relations, to provide a framework for interventions, and to predict outcomes. Theories may be described in terms of their levels of abstraction or in terms of their goals.

Definition of Theories by Level of Abstraction

When considered in terms of their levels of abstraction, three types of theories emerge in nursing: grand theories, middle-range theories, and situation-specific theories. Each is described in the subsequent text.

Grand Theories

Grand theories are systematic constructions of the nature of nursing, the mission of nursing, and the goals of nursing care. Grand theories are constructed from a synthesis of experiences, observations, insights, and research findings. Grand theories reflect the broadest scope and provide relationships between a large number of abstract concepts. Because grand theories are the highest in abstraction, they do not lend themselves to empirical testing; even so, some argue that grand theories can be relevant to policy making under certain conditions, such as when there is consensus among policy makers on values (Eriksson, 2014). Early theorizations in nursing are considered grand theories. Examples are Roger's theory of energy fields and King's theory of goal attainment. These theories are considered by some international colleagues to have implications for quality patient care and to enhance the image of nursing (Shah, Abdullah, and Khan, 2013).

Middle-Range Theories

Theories that have more limited scope, have less abstraction, address specific phenomena or concepts, and reflect practice (administrative, clinical, or teaching) are considered middle-range theories. The phenomena or concepts tend to cross different nursing fields and reflect a wide variety of nursing care situations. Middle-range theories lend themselves to empirical testing because the concepts are more specific and can be readily operationalized. Examples of middle-range theories are uncertainty, incontinence, social support, quality of life, community empowerment, comfort, social support, and unpleasant symptoms. Many middle-range theories were developed during the first two decades in the 21st century (Smith and Liehr, 2014). (See Chapter 16 for more discussion about middle-range theorizing.)

Situation-Specific Theories

Situation-specific theories focus on specific nursing phenomena that reflect clinical practice and that are limited to specific populations or to a particular field of practice. These theories are socially and historically contexted; they are developed to incorporate—not transcend—time, social, or political structures (Meleis, 1997b). Therefore, their scope and the questions driven by them are limited and encompassing of the context. Examples are menopausal experiences of Korean immigrants, lived experiences of Asian American women caring for their elderly relatives, and preventive models for HIV among adolescents. Situation-specific theories may be developed from middle-range theories (Im, 2014) or from research findings (Riegel and Dickson, 2008), and they could also inform the development of middle-range theory (Riegel, Dickson, and Faulkner, 2016; Riegel, Jaarsma, and Stromberg, 2012). (See Chapter 17.)

Definition of Theories by Goal Orientation

Theories can also be classified in terms of their goals. As such, there are *descriptive* and *prescriptive* theories. Descriptive theories describe relationships between phenomena, describe nurses' and patients' relationships, and describe guidelines for interventions. Processes of assessing, diagnosing, and intervening must be considered in the development of nursing theories (Kritek, 1978). To accomplish their goals of supporting and promoting optimum health and well-being, nurses also need theories to capture efficient and effective clinical therapeutics to use in achieving health care outcomes for their patients.

Descriptive Theories

Descriptive theories are those that describe a phenomenon, an event, a situation, or a relationship; they identify its properties and its components; and they identify some of the circumstances under which it occurs. Although descriptive theories have an element of prediction (e.g., predicting when a phenomenon may occur and when it may not occur), their contribution to knowledge is mainly to help sort out observations and meanings regarding the phenomenon. Descriptive theories describe a phenomenon, speculate on why a phenomenon occurs, and describe the consequences of that phenomenon; therefore, they have explanatory, relating, and predicting utility. Descriptive theories are complete theories and have the potential to guide research.

There are two types of descriptive theories. The first type is the *factor-isolating, category-formulating*, or *labeling theory*. This theory describes the properties and dimensions of phenomena. The second type is the *explanatory theory*, which describes and explains the nature of relationships of certain phenomena to other phenomena. Examples of descriptive theories are the descriptions of the life processes of a nursing client, person–environment interactions in health and illness, health status, ways of assessment, types of diagnosing, disruptions of life processes, and outcomes and interventions. Descriptive nursing theories are those that help describe, explain, and predict nursing phenomena and relationships between nursing phenomena. Descriptive theories are not action oriented and do not attempt to produce or change a situation.

Prescriptive Theories

Prescriptive theories are those that address nursing therapeutics and the outcomes of interventions. A prescriptive theory includes propositions that call for change and predict the consequences of a certain strategy for a nursing intervention. A prescriptive theory should designate the prescription and its components, the type of client to receive the prescription, the conditions under which the prescription should occur, and the consequences. It articulates the conditions in the life process, person–environment interactions, and health status that need the prescription and the effect on the client's life process, health status, and interaction with the environment. Prescriptions may also be focused on the environment.

In summary, all theories used in nursing to understand, explain, predict, or change nursing phenomena are nursing theories, whether they evolved out of other theories, other paradigms, other disciplines, nursing experiences, diagnoses, nursing processes, or nursing practices, and whether they were developed by nurses. If we must differentiate between different types of theory, then such differentiation is meaningful only in terms of levels and goals, not in terms of the source of the theory. Theories that are developed to understand and explain human processes in health and illness are pure or basic theories. In other words, they are theories with a descriptive focus. Theories that are developed to control, promote, and change are nursing practice theories or prescriptive theories (Crowley, 1968).

THEORY COMPONENTS

Theories are structures that include assumptions, concepts, narrative descriptions, propositions, and exemplars. The structural components of descriptive and prescriptive theories are somewhat different.

Structural components of *descriptive* theories include:
Client's state or condition
Patterns of responses to conditions, situations, or events

Analyses of contexts of conditions, situations, or events and patterns of responses
Analyses of conditions that promote and inhibit contexts
Structural components of *prescriptive* theories include:
Definition of client's situation
Nursing therapeutics
Process by which therapeutics are implemented
Patterns of responses for desired status or outcomes
Context for desired/undesired responses and outcomes

USES OF THEORY

Theory and Research

The objective of theory is to formulate a minimum set of generalizations that allow one to explain a maximum number of observable relationships among the variables in a given field of inquiry. Theories set limits on what questions to ask and what methods to use to pursue answers to the questions. Relationships between theories and research are cyclical in nature; the results of the research can then be used to verify, modify, disprove, or support a theoretical proposition. Nursing theories have provided nurse researchers with new propositions for nursing research that could not have been as well articulated if theories from other disciplines were used. Nursing research has been driven in the past by educational, sociological, and psychological theories and less by nursing thought. Nursing theories stimulate nurse scientists to explore significant responses in the field of nursing such as eating, feeding, pain monitoring, sleeping, and resting. In doing so, the potential for the development of knowledge that informs daily activities of patients and nurses increases.

Theory and Practice

The primary uses of theory are to provide insights about nursing practice situations and to guide research. Through interaction with practice, theory is shaped and guidelines for practice evolve. Research validates, refutes, and/or modifies theory as well as generates new theory. Theory then guides practice. Until empirical validation, modification, and support are completed, theory can be given support through clinical utilization and validation and can therefore be allowed to give tentative direction to practice. Nurses gain wisdom from their practice experiences and formulate theories that were generated from their experiences. However, until such theories are articulated and communicated, they cannot be subjected to systematic tests and, therefore, do not inform the practice of other nurses.

Theory provides nurses with the framework and the goals for assessment, diagnosis, and intervention. Nurses working as part of health care teams focus on those aspects of care that are described theoretically for a more effective judgment of patients' situations and conditions. If the goals of the care provided are health maintenance, promotion of self-care, and enhancement of stability and integrity during the illness, then a nurse has an intellectual checklist by which the levels of health and well-being, self-care needs and abilities, and integrity and stability are assessed. Diagnosis is related to those areas in which health and wellness are compromised, self-care is problematic, or integrity of the human being is undermined. Evaluation of care and its consequences focus on patient care outcomes.

Theory is a tool that renders practice more efficient and more effective and helps in identifying outcomes. Simply by being goal-directed through a theoretical perspective, a nurse's energy and time spent in assessing extraneous areas are minimized. If nursing goals are not articulated from a nursing perspective, a nurse's time is used inefficiently, and the nature and quality of care are compromised. By considering areas of assessment or intervention that may be handled more efficiently and expertly by other members of the health care team, the nurse conserves her own energy, time, and talent for those areas and phenomena for which she is well prepared, such as processes of adherence to a regimen, mobilizing support, or monitoring pain. Patients and their families are more likely to seek and respond more effectively to nursing care when nursing goals driven by nursing knowledge are clearly articulated.

Theory has other uses. The language of theory provides us with common ground for communicating effectively and efficiently. More effective and efficient communication can eventually lead to further theory development as concepts are refined, sharpened, extended, and validated. Well-defined concepts with conceptual and construct validity enhance cyclical communication among practitioners, theorists, clinicians, and educators. The world of nursing can become more coherent, more goal-oriented, and more effective. Building evidence depends on a common language and symbols, and using evidence is predicated on a common language. Articulating outcomes and linking these outcomes with nursing actions and interventions are enhanced by naming concepts.

Professional autonomy and accountability are supported by the use of theory in practice. Being able to practice through the use of scientific principles allows nurses the opportunity to accurately predict those patterns of responses that are consequences of care. Articulation of actions, goals, and consequences of actions empowers nurses and enhances their accountability. If we can talk clearly about our purpose and what we hope to accomplish, perhaps other professionals and patients will also be able to describe or articulate nursing actions and goals more accurately and comprehensively, and even seek and demand the type of care nurses are capable of providing. Defining the focus and the means to achieving that focus, and being able to predict consequences increase a nurse's control of nursing practice and therefore increase a nurse's autonomy. As stated by Fuller many decades ago (1978),

The autonomy of a profession rests more firmly on the uniqueness of its knowledge, knowledge gathered ever so slowly through the questioning of scientific inquiry. Nursing defined by power does not necessarily beget knowledge. But knowledge most often results in the ascription of power and is accompanied by autonomy. (p. 701)

In summary, theory helps to identify the focus, means, and goals of practice. Using common theories enhances communication, thereby increasing autonomy and accountability to care. Theory helps the user gain control over subject matter (Barnum, 1998). All these in turn help bring about further refinements of theory and better relationships among theory, research, and practice. Figure 3-1 identifies the relationships among theory, research, practice, and philosophy.

REFLECTIVE QUESTIONS

1. Why does practice-based discipline need theories?

2. For some clinicians, theories seem to be such esoteric notions for a profession that has functioned well for decades. Could our practice history guide our practice future without theories? Why? Why not?

3. For each definition of theory components, there are different views on how the component is defined and used. Find two opposing definitions for each and argue for what difference this particular definition makes in our practice profession. Ultimately, how could developed knowledge be different, and in what ways is the practice of nursing differently informed?

4. What difference do the different levels and types of theory make in advancing nursing knowledge?

5. Give an example of theory-based intervention and another example of an intervention that you believe is atheoretical. Compare, contrast, and dialogue about the relationship between practice and theory.

REFERENCES

Banner, D., Janke, F., and King-Shier, K. (2015). *Making evidence-based practice happen in 'real world' contexts.* In M. Lipscomb (Ed.), *Exploring evidence-based practice: Debates and challenges in nursing* (pp. 11–28). New York: Routledge.

Barnum, B.J.S. (1998). *Nursing theory: Analysis, application, and evaluation* (5th ed.). Philadelphia, PA: Lippincott Williams & Wilkins.

Bleier, R. (1990). *Feminist approaches to science.* New York: Pergamon Press.

Brown, N.H. (1977). *Perception, theory and commitment: The new philosophy of science.* Chicago, IL: University of Chicago Press.

Bryant, L. (1998). Commentary: A challenge to Reed's perspective. *Nursing Science Quarterly,* 11(4), 145–148.

Burkhardt, H. and Smith, B. (Eds.). (1991). *Handbook of metaphysics and ontology* (pp. 640–641). Munich, Germany: Philosophia Verlag.

Chinn, P.L. and Jacobs, M.K. (1987). *Theory and nursing: A systematic approach* (2nd ed.). St. Louis, MO: C.V. Mosby.

Chinn, P.L. and Kramer, M.K. (2011). *Integrated knowledge development in nursing* (8th ed.). St. Louis, MO: C.V. Mosby.

Clarke, P.N. and Fawcett, J. (2014). Life as a nurse researcher. *Nursing Science Quarterly,* 27(1), 37–41.

Collins English dictionary. (2000). HarperCollins Publishers.

Cormack, D.F.S. and Reynolds, W. (1992). Criteria for evaluating the clinical and practical utility of models used by nurses. *Journal of Advanced Nursing,* 17, 1472–1478.

Crowley, D.M. (1968). Perspectives of pure science. *Nursing Research,* 17(6), 497–501.

Dickoff, J. and James, P. (1968). A theory of theories: A position paper. *Nursing Research,* 17(3), 197–203.

Dictionary of philosophy. (1999). (pp. 200–201). Amherst, NY: Prometheus Books.

Ellis, R. (1968). Characteristics of significant theories. *Nursing Research,* 17(3), 217–222.

Eriksson, J. (2014). On the policy relevance of grand theory. *International Studies Perspectives,* 15, 94–108.

Ervin, N.E. (2002). Evidence-based nursing practice: Are we there yet? *Journal of the New York State Nurses Association,* 33(2), 11–16.

Fawcett, J. (2006). The state of nursing science: Where is the nursing in the science? *Theoria, Journal of Nursing Theory,* 15(4), 3–10.

Fawcett, J. and Madeya, S.D. (2013). *Contemporary nursing knowledge: Analysis and evaluation of nursing models and theories* (3rd ed.). Philadelphia, PA: F.A. Davis.

Fawcett, J., Watson, J., Neuman, B., Walker, P., and Fitzpatrick, J. (2001). On nursing theories and evidence. *Journal of Nursing Scholarship,* 33(2), 115–119.

Fuller, S. (1978). Holistic man and the science and practice of nursing. *Nursing Outlook,* 26, 700–704.

Gracia, J. (1999). *Metaphysics and its task. The search for the categorical foundation of knowledge* (pp. 147–148). Albany, NY: State University of New York Press.

Grossman, R. (1983). *The categorical structure of the world* (pp. 3–5). Bloomington, IL: Indiana University Press.

Hartmann, N. (1953). *New ways of ontology.* Chicago, IL: Henry Regnery Company. Translated by Henry Regnery Company.

Im, E-O. (2013). *Theory in transitions.* In M.J. Smith and P. Liehr (Eds.), *Middle range theory for nursing* (3rd ed., pp. 253–277). New York: Springer.

Im, E-O. (2014). Situation-specific theories from the middle-range transitions theory. *Advances in Nursing Science,* 37(1), 19–31.

Im, E-O. (2015). The current status of theory evaluation in nursing. *Journal of Advanced Nursing,* 71(10), 2268–2278.

Im, E-O. and Chang, S.J. (2012). Current trends in nursing theories. *Journal of Nursing Scholarship,* 44(2), 156–164.

Jacquette, D. (2002). *Ontology* (pp. 2–3). Montreal & Kingston, Ithaca: McGill-Queens University Press.

Jennings, B.W. (2000). Evidence-based practice: The road best traveled? *Research in Nursing and Health,* 23(5), 343–345.

Jennings, B.W. and Loan, L.A. (2001). Misconceptions among nurses about evidence-based practice. *Journal of Nursing Scholarship,* 33(2), 121–127.

Kramer, M. (2002). Academic talk about dementia caregiving: A critical comment on language. *Research and Theory for Nursing Practice: A International Journal,* 16(4), 263–280.

Kritek, P. (1978). The generation and classification of nursing diagnosis: Toward a theory of nursing. *Image,* 10(2), 33–40.

Kuhn, T.S. (1962). *The structure of scientific revolutions,* Chicago, IL: University of Chicago Press.

Kuhn, T.S. (1970). *The structure of scientific revolutions* (2nd ed.). Chicago, IL: University of Chicago Press.

Kuhn, T.S. (1977). *The essential tension.* Chicago, IL: University of Chicago Press.

Lenz, E.R., Suppe, F., Gift, A.G., Pugh, L.C., and Milligan, R.A. (1995). Collaborative development of middle-range nursing theories: Toward a theory of unpleasant symptoms. *Advances in Nursing Science*, 17(3), 1–13.

Lejewski, C. (1984). On Lesniewski's ontology. In T.J. Srzednicki, V.F. Rickey (Eds.), *Leśniewski's systems. Ontology and mereology* (pp. 123–148). The Hague: Martinus Nijhoff.

Marenbon, J. (1999). Parsimony. In *Dictionary of philosophy* (p. 411). London, UK: Penguin Books.

Mautner, T. (Ed.). (1999). *Dictionary of philosophy* (p. 556). London, UK: Penguin Books.

McKay, R. (1969). Theories, models and systems for nursing. *Nursing Research*, 18(5), 393–399.

Mead, G.H. (1934). *Mind, self, and society.* Chicago, IL: University of Chicago Press.

Meleis, A.I. (1997a). Theoretical nursing: Definitions and interpretations. In J. Fawcett and I.M. King (Eds.), *The language of nursing theory and metatheory*. Indianapolis, IN: Sigma Theta Tau.

Meleis, A.I. (1997b). *Theoretical nursing: Development and progress* (3rd ed.). Philadelphia, PA: Lippincott Co.

Meleis, A.I. (2015). Transitions theory. In M. Smith (Ed.), *Nursing theories and nursing practice* (4th ed.). Philadelphia, PA: FA Davis Co.

Melnyk, B.M., Fineout-Overholt, E., Gallagher-Ford, L., and Kaplan, L. (2012). The state of evidence-based practice in US nurses. *Journal of Nursing Administration*, 42(9), 410–417.

Newman, M.A. (1994). *Health as expanding consciousness* (2nd ed.). New York: National League for Nursing Press.

Orlando, I.J. (1987). Nursing in the 21st century: Alternate paths. *Journal of Advanced Nursing*, 12(4), 405–412.

O'Toole, M.T. (Ed.). (2003). *Miller-Keane encyclopedia & dictionary of medicine, nursing, & allied health* (7th ed., pp. 1421, 705). Philadelphia, PA: Saunders.

Parse, R.R. (1996). The human becoming theory: Challenges in practice and research. *Nursing Science Quarterly*, 9(2), 55–60.

Peplau, H.E. (1992). Interpersonal relations: A theoretical framework for application in nursing practice. *Nursing Science Quarterly*, 5, 13–18.

Popper, K. (1962). *Conjecture and refutations.* New York: Basic Books.

Powers, B.A. and Knapp, T.R. (2006). *Dictionary of nursing theory and research* (3rd ed.). New York: Springer.

Przylebski, A. (1997). Roman Ingarden. In L. Embree et al. (Eds.), *Encyclopedia of phenomenology* (pp. 348–349). Dordrecht, Netherlands: Kluwer.

Quinn, J.F. (1986). Quantitative methods: Descriptive and experimental. In P. Moccia (Ed.), *New approaches to theory development*. New York: National League for Nursing.

Rawnsley, M.M. (1998). Ontology, epistemology, and methodology: A clarification. *Nursing Science Quarterly*, 11(1), 2–4.

Reed, P.G. (1997). Nursing: The ontology of the discipline. *Nursing Science Quarterly*, 10(2), 76–79.

Riegel, B. and Dickson, V.V. (2008). A situation-specific theory of heart failure self-care. *Journal of Cardiovascular Nursing*, 23(3), 190–196.

Riegel, B., Dickson, V.V., and Faulkner, K.M. (2016). The situation-specific theory of heart failure self-care (revised and updated). *Journal of Cardiovascular Nursing*, 31(3), 226–235.

Riegel, B., Jaarsma, T., and Stromberg, A. (2012). A middle-range theory of self-care of chronic illness. *Advances in Nursing Science*, 35(3), 194–204.

Shah, M., Abdullah, A., and Khan, H. (2013). Compare and contrast of grand theories: Orem's self-care deficit theory and Roy's adaptation model. *International Journal of Science and Research*, 4(1), 1834–1837.

Smith, J.J. and Liehr, P.R. (2014). *Middle range theory for nursing* (3rd ed.). New York: Springer Publishing Company.

Watson, J. (1989). Watson's philosophy and theory of human caring. In J. Riehl-Sisla (Ed.). *Conceptual models of nursing practice* (3rd ed.). Norwalk, CT: Appleton & Lange.

White, A. (1999). Epistemology. In *Dictionary of philosophy* (pp. 174–176). England: Penguin Books.

Wolf, L.A. (2015). Research as problem solving: Theoretical frameworks as tools. *Journal of Emergency Nursing*, 41(1), 83–85.

Part Two

OUR THEORETICAL HERITAGE

The discipline of nursing has established itself as a field with both a practice and a theoretical base and with programs of research that are making an impact in health care. This part of the book is focused on the discipline's theoretical heritage. The process of the evolution of the discipline and its theoretical base follows a unique path, a path that may not be clearly understood by those who attempt to measure the progress and development of the discipline by the same criteria used to measure the progress of the physical and natural sciences (see Chapter 18 on evaluating progress in the discipline). The origins of the developmental path for nursing can be traced through an analysis of both its research tradition as well as its theory traditions. This part, which includes Chapters 4 and 5, traces, in particular, the **historical development** of nursing theory and theoretical nursing, and the course of the evolution of nursing as a theoretical discipline is mapped and discussed.

Changes trigger transition processes, and along the way there are forces and barriers that promote or hinder outcomes. Therefore, forces and barriers in the development of theory in nursing are identified and discussed. The **roles of nurses**—as nurses, as predominantly women, and as nurse theorists who developed nursing theories against many odds—are explored and discussed. The development of the discipline of nursing is conceptualized as evolving in stages. The premise on which the discussion proceeds is that all stages preceding the most current stage made major contributions to the maturity of the discipline. Milestones in every stage are delineated, and the influence of each milestone on nursing theory is explored. The relationships among theory, science, practice, and philosophy are also explored.

4

From Can't to Kant: Barriers and Forces Toward Theoretical Thinking

The journey from the days of Florence Nightingale to scholarly nursing has been long, hard, and bumpy. Nightingale's attempts to establish professional nursing based on nursing's unique concern with the environment for the promotion of health were preempted by an illness-oriented training that depended on other professions for existence and on hospitals for training and sustenance. Nursing has traveled from apprenticeship to education, from hospital service and training to the university, from mere implementation of doctors' orders to accountability and autonomy, from practical to theory- and research-based applications.

The journey has included a major detour through the land of "Can't": a land of perceived inability to conceptualize or generalize; a land that espoused practice, concreteness, and practical relevance as antithetical to some generalizations, common propositions, and theoretical statements. The decades of the 1970s, 1980s, and 1990s marked our emergence from this land and, as the first two decades in the 21st century demonstrate, we are back on course to where Nightingale began. On our return journey, however, we are more experienced, more assured, and more trusting in our perceptions. We are more accepting of the significance of patients' and nurses' experiences and of the varied meanings of experience in the development of nursing knowledge. Many global reports support the centrality of nurses in providing quality care and the significance of nursing knowledge in health care (Institute of Medicine, 2011; Prime Minister's Commission, 2010).

We are reminded in this journey of Immanuel Kant, a dominant 19th-century philosopher, who maintained that reality is not only a thing in and of itself but is also constructed by those who experience it. Reality in nursing history has been a synthesis of conditions that predisposed nurses to a nontheoretical existence and an a priori perception that helped to promote a lack of acceptance of theoretical themes.

Kant aptly distinguished between perception of experience and sensation of experience. *Perception of experience*, the basis of knowledge, has, in nursing, depended on this or that procedure as performed at a certain moment, or on the knowledge of this or that patient occupying a certain space and existing at a certain moment. Therefore, the s*ensation of experience* is confounded by temporal and spatial limitations. Although knowledge begins with experience, Kant maintained that this does not mean that all knowledge evolves from experience. To him, our experiences have two components: an a priori impression of what may be experienced, and impressions as they are actually received. Understanding is a synthesis of both. Therefore, a human being—a knowing, active, and experiencing subject, not a passive recipient—interprets and analyzes impression data in a certain way. That certain way—the a priori form by which experiences are shaped—is a synthesis of something that is out there and something that is constructed by the person experiencing it (Copleston, 1964).

During the journey of nurses from early to modern times, experience assumed different meanings with more profound explanations. Experience provided the impetus for describing and explaining phenomena central to nursing and perhaps was responsible for the development of new therapeutics to promote health, change environments, or control unwanted events related to health care. During this journey, some nurses were more accepting of the role of clinical experience in the development of clinical knowledge, others were reluctant to acknowledge that experience had any role in theoretical nursing, and still others preferred to rely on the experiences of scientists in other fields to shape their clinical knowledge. Some pioneering thinkers in nursing assumed that nurses can conceptualize, and they allowed themselves the luxury to consider that patients' responses and experiences could help them, and others, better understand clients and their health care experiences. These thinkers helped the theoretical journey move forward. The journey is still in progress, and will continue to advance in a human and dynamic discipline such as nursing. Within the discipline of nursing, evidence suggests that this long journey will lead to more effective and useful theorizing. To continue to support the journey toward a more systematic development of nursing knowledge, it is necessary to value our history, to recognize the present context, and to envision our future.

Therefore, to enhance the development of theoretical knowledge, we must pause and ask why the journey was long and complex. Why did nursing go through such detours of seemingly nontheoretical periods and, more importantly, why did nurses appear to reject theory and theorizing during the journey, practically forcing the detour into a nontheoretical existence? Even when a small handful of nurses attempted to return, to put nursing on course by providing a theoretical view of what nursing is, it was almost two decades after the development of these conceptions that their notions and their stance became part of a more serious discourse. Why is it that some skeptics in nursing were still saying, at the beginning of the 21st century, that theory or theorizing in nursing is antithetical to the nature of nursing, and that nursing practice is practical and not amenable to theorizing nor to be driven by theory, and therefore choosing one standpoint leaves no room and no need for the other? Why have others held that only research evidence must be the framework for practice? The tension among theory, practice, and research continues to be an important impetus for disciplinary dialogues.

This chapter considers, historically, those forces that have hindered and fostered the development of nursing scholarship and more specifically nursing theory. Kant's writing on the synthesis between reality as a separate entity and reality as constructed by the subject who is experiencing it helps us understand the dialectical meanings of these forces. Human and knowledge barriers and human and knowledge forces are two sides of the same coin. We can analyze these as both negative and positive forces in the development of nursing theory. The content may be the same (the sensation in Kant's analysis), but the form distinguishes between forces as barriers and forces as resources. Together, content and form (provided by sensation and mind) enhance the knowledge and understanding of the dynamics of the journey from no theory to theory.

As we begin to perceive constraints in a new light and through a new lens, we can shift the negative power of constraint to a positive force, and we can reconstruct new realities and develop new blueprints that are more congruent with the mission of nursing and health care needs nationally and internationally. Knowing our history empowers us for a future in which we can better deal with barriers and change them into assets.

BARRIERS TO THEORY DEVELOPMENT

Human Barriers: Nurses as Nurses

The type of student who selects a nursing career, the kind of education nursing students receive, and the nature of nursing are all related to the paucity of developments in nursing theory or to the rejection of the theoretical nature of nursing, particularly when nursing education was confined to hospitals, before baccalaureate programs became the norm and before second-degree students began to enter the field of nursing. Evidence of these relationships varies from speculative to more empirical and verified. Historically, nursing and teaching were the default choices for women. Before the 1970s, women who entered nursing may have done so because of its gender and service orientations, rather than its professional potential. Nursing may have attracted non–career-oriented individuals who were looking for an occupation that allowed them to get in and out conveniently, as their families demanded. A decision to become a nurse may have depended on an image of nursing that was glamorized in the media but that was also paradoxically servile.

Whether nursing still attracts a unique group of individuals who are substantially different from students entering other fields is becoming increasingly debatable. Students are becoming attracted to nursing for its financial potential, its career possibilities, and its potential to make a difference in the lives of people and to societies in general. It is apparent to educators that there is an increasing applicant pool of qualified students, and that the attitudes of nursing students are changing drastically as changes occur in other spheres of life, in other professions, and in economic status. As we enter the third decade of the 21st century, many more nursing programs have been specifically developed to attract graduates from other disciplines. Similarly, more nurses are seeking university-based degrees, and fewer students are enrolling in diploma programs, although this still differs by state and country. At least three countries—Australia, Spain, and Norway—educate nurses only at the baccalaureate level. It is anticipated others will continue to move toward making the Bachelor of Science in Nursing (BSN) degree the entry level in practice for nurses.

One example of this shift in attitude toward nursing as a career option is the influx of graduate students (from other fields) into community college nursing or baccalaureate nursing programs in the United States. These students are often women (and increasingly men) who are older and therefore more developmentally mature and more intellectually sophisticated. They have already experienced academic life, they have experienced different occupations based on their first degrees, and they knowingly and deliberately selected a different educational path, one that has the potential to lead to financial independence and a new career. What they expect of their education, however, may not be completely congruent with the ideas of faculty who are used to teaching younger and less experienced students (D'Antonio, Beal, Underwood, et al., 2010). More men are also changing careers and choosing nursing. These differences between nursing students of the past and present may suggest a difference in attitudes toward nursing and its professional status, as well as its theoretical underpinnings, and are likely to create a different future for the discipline of nursing.

Although differences between students who select nursing and those who select other professions are inconclusive because of the sparseness of research, indications are that nursing education itself has created differences between nursing students and other students. Education plays a major role in training the mind to think beyond immediate action, to question situations, to link events, to generalize and, in short, to conceptualize.

Analyzing and understanding the history of nursing educational levels and the status of nursing is important in dialogues about knowledge development (D'Antonio, 2004). Nursing education has a long history of squelching curiosity, replacing it with conformity and a nonquestioning attitude. Nursing education in the past prepared nurses to think of themselves as the handmaidens of physicians, the executors of doctors' orders, and the implementers of hospital policy. It socialized students to roles that are not congruent with scholarship and discovery. Any independent thinking or critical attitude was the antithesis of what was expected of a nurse. Because nursing education was based

more on apprenticeship, training, and experience than on ideas, knowledge, and learning, the nurse graduated only to find herself far more dependent on medical and hospital systems than on her own problem-solving and clinical judgment abilities. The educational system in nursing did not help nurses see themselves as sources of knowledge. The discourse that nurses engaged in was one of techniques and skills (Canam, 2008).

Theory development is an active process, and early research characterized nurses as passive (Cleland, 1971; Edwards, 1969). In addition, the social climate in which nurses practiced did not encourage debate or freedom to experiment. In fact,

> [T]he subculture of nursing has encouraged the perpetuation of a feminine world that has been perceived to emphasize routine and repetition, intuition and magical thinking, respectful obedience for authority, and covert rather than overt methods of control. Such a subculture does not provide a fertile field for the growth and development of curiosity and challenge of the status quo, both so necessary to scientific inquiry and scholarship. As a result, a number of nurses . . . have chosen to move to other disciplines for the substantive background and the mental stimulation so necessary to scholarly development. (Benoliel, 1975, p. 25)

In addition, the *functional orientation* of nursing—the act of performing procedures rather than thinking, reflecting, and solving problems—is a theme apparent in the history of our discipline (Loomis, 1974). This orientation originated in the early inclusion of nursing training programs in hospital settings, in which nurses were socialized to become intellectually subordinate.

The hospital's role was to provide service within its means; apprenticeship and service were two sides of the same coin, and while clinical practice was emphasized, theoretical and philosophical discourses were not the norm. Therefore, when hospitals agreed to take on the education of nurses, they did so to provide patient care and save money. It was acceptable to have nurses work long hours and to allow them to attend lectures only when education did not interfere with the service they were providing. Nursing students were the lowest on the totem pole; they were taught how to respect physicians, how to believe in physicians, and how to totally submit to hospital routine. Essentially, nurses were taught "intellectual subordination" (Bullough, 1975, p. 229) even though they were also technically skilled.

Nursing students worked 12-hour shifts and were even further exhausted by being sent on home visits to bring in more revenue, which was sorely needed by the hospital. Decisions about home care were not predicated on the goals of nursing or on the outcome of nursing care but rather on the need for an economic boost through the use of students as cheap labor. As a result, nurses developed a task-oriented attitude and, for the most part, could not take time to think or reflect or, better put, were not given the necessary time to think or reflect, which maintained nursing at the practical and immediate level of functioning. Doing and thinking are not mutually exclusive, but they were promoted as such. And, unfortunately, the education that nurses received fostered an unquestioning acceptance of authority and a subservient attitude.

The weight of past tradition, the subordination of nurses, the sex segregation, and the apprenticeship model in nursing education may have left a mark on the attitudes of nurses historically (Bullough, 1975, pp. 229–230). This is reflected in many parts of the world where nurses are still trained in hospital settings.

The qualities necessary for theory development are thinking, reflecting, questioning, and perceiving the self as being capable of developing knowledge, through a discourse focused on relationships, caring, and the psychosocial determinants of the nursing act. The education that nurses received may not have honored the clinical aspects of nursing and therefore did not nurture the development of the educational qualities. It also did not reinforce critical thinking in those who came to nursing with critical-thinking abilities.

Nursing has also suffered from the paternalism of hospital administration and medical staff (Ashley, 1977), and remnants of that mind-set persist in different forms in the 21st century in many parts of the world, under the guise of economic constraints in the health care system. This paternalism has been internalized as the rules and regulations created by others have been replaced in recent years with rules and regulations created by nurses for nurses. Nurses may be following the rules unquestioningly, or they may only be controlling their questioning because, as Street (1992) discovered in a critical ethnography of nursing practice, nurses are aware of the negative and punitive consequences of thinking or speaking critically. Therefore, questioning may still be discouraged, rebelliousness is unthinkable,

and disobedience is punished, but leaving the discipline—attrition—is a personal option and many, indeed, resort to it. Shifting to other careers that feature less subordination has also been used as a coping strategy. The choice of attrition from the profession may be exacerbated by nurses' increasing awareness of their rights as nurses and as workers and their unwillingness to put up with oppression.

Early on, this patriarchal framework formed the context for the nurse's role, equated with a woman's or mother's subordinate role in the family, whereas the physician's role was equated with that of the father, the head of the family (D'Antonio, 2010). Therefore, just as wives and mothers were relegated to certain prescribed roles, the nurse was also plagued by the image of the sacrificing, altruistic, submissive placater, the fixer of all—a role detrimental to the creativity essential for theoretical thinking. Thinking, creating, and questioning were reserved for the head of the family. It is perhaps that same image that has helped perpetuate the duality of science and practice. Compassion (a characteristic of nurses in practice) cannot be replaced by the rigor, calculation, objectivity, and coolness of the scientist or the theoretician, although perhaps it could be complemented by such characteristics. Unfortunately, all these personal attributes of compassion, altruism, submissiveness, and sacrificing, cultivated by educational and practice environments, were often antithetical to theorizing and scientific endeavors.

Academic nurses suffered from this concept of nursing just as greatly but in a different way. Because they were far removed from patient care, they were more interested in theorizing about student learning or curricula than about patient environments. Being new themselves to the halls of academia, they dissipated their energies in the struggle to prove they belonged there. They competed with others in more established disciplines and shied away from those in practice who pointed fingers at these "ivory tower" colleagues and said, "Your theories are too theoretical and your research is too esoteric; what do you know about practice anyhow?" or "Stick to teaching and leave practice to us."

The reward structure of the nursing profession also helped shape nurses' attitudes about theory development. Recognition for nurses was based on immediate actions, and rewards were based on expedient doing. Rewards were more easily bestowed on nurses in clinical roles or on nurses in teaching roles than on those engaged in research or theory development. Rewards for scholarliness were not as tangible as rewards for these other roles; they were slow to come, and the rationale for the rewards was not as well defined, especially as the discipline was still developing and had no agreed-on standards for reward (Gaston, 1975). In addition, the subculture of nursing had not promoted constructive debates and competition, which could have been helpful in discussing and developing theoretical ideals. What Benoliel said in 1973 about competition in research applies to theory development in the 21st century:

If scientific inquiry and production of knowledge are dependent on individuals who thrive on open competition, then perhaps the slow development of research in nursing is tied to a lack of competitive spirit among nurses in idea development. Reflecting on nursing's origins as a form of women's work, I find this slow development not too surprising. Compliance with the rules rather than challenge of authority has been an organizing theme in much of nursing's history, and a subculture that places high value on conforming behavior is not fertile soil for the development of practitioners who are comfortable with the aggressive rivalry of scientific endeavors. The subservient and self-effacing posture that nurses have traditionally held in their working relationships with physicians is not an effective stance for nurses engaged in scientific study. Rather, those who seek to be purveyors of new nursing knowledge can only do so when they carry a sense of self-confidence that permits them to see and experience the positive values of open competition in the world of ideas. (Benoliel, 1973, p. 8)

Practitioner's orientation—the educational movement toward becoming nurse practitioners and nurse anesthetists—also contributed to the construction of barriers in the development of theory. "Why should there be other frameworks to assessing, diagnosing, treating, and evaluating disease, symptoms, and responses to illness when medical science and models of care are used?" asked my theory students who are nurse practitioners and nurse anesthetists. "If anything," they continued to argue, "we should be contributing to the development of medical science," not the use and development of theoretical nursing and the use of nursing knowledge. Although some are concerned about the dominant discourse of evidence-based practice, labeling it as the "colonial patronage" of the biomedical ideology (Holmes, Roy, and Perron, 2008), a kinder view may be that a need exists for nursing knowledge to drive the development of theories dealing with the daily responses, activities, and lived experiences of patients—such as eating, sleeping, mobility, relating, and interacting—responses and activities

that are central to nursing practice but less central to the practice of other disciplines. The best answers, however, emerge from those who are able to integrate nursing and medical sciences, as well as synthesize their practitioner's role with their nursing role (Fairman, 2008).

The development of the Doctor of Nursing Practice (DNP) degree in the United States, which is a practice doctorate as opposed to the research-oriented PhD, may be contributing to a more friendly relationship between nurses whose role is primarily clinical and the theoretical bases of nursing. Some advanced practice nurses and clinical nurse specialists who are pursuing the DNP consider theory as the bases for their practice (Gatti-Petito, Lakatos, Bradley, et al., 2013), use nursing theory (Eldridge, 2013), and develop theory that is driven both by their clinical expertise and by existing theoretical frameworks (Davidson, 2010).

Human Barriers: Nurses as Women

The slow development or acceptance of theory development and utilization in and for practice can also be attributed to sex-role stereotyping. Theory development is a laborious process that requires flexibility in time, access to leisure time, access to resources, and freedom from oppressions, none of which women possessed or obtained as readily as men did in the past (Keller, 1979). Many around the world still view a woman as a hard-working, home-bound, emotional person whose energies should primarily be directed to rearing children and caring for a family. Many women have internalized this role ascribed to them by society, and college-age students in the 21st century may be concerned about balancing roles in their lives and therefore prefer a return to that view. Even when women tried to break away from societal stereotypes, they were beset by the need to both fulfill new employment roles while maintaining their function in old roles. The result has been overload—hardly conducive to reflecting, questioning, and cumulatively developing theory. As Cole (1981) noted, "It is in the domain of informal activities in science that the biggest gaps between men and women remain" (p. 388).

As we move into the third decade of the 21st century, the number of male registered nurses has grown from 57,000 in 1983 to 330,000 in 2011, representing an increase from 4% of all registered nurses to 9.6%, with a similar increase in the number of men admitted to schools of nursing in the United States (Landivar, 2013). (At the University of Pennsylvania, 8.6% of the freshman class in 2015 consisted of men.) Although this increase is significant, approximately 91% of nurses are still women (Landivar, 2013). The sex-role identity of nurses cannot be ignored when we discuss theory development and the potential for theoretical thinking. In addition, two other barriers maintain this status quo. Although men have historically participated in nursing during times of war and acute shortages in some countries (e.g., Yemen and Jordan), there is still a failure to fully recognize that nursing should be gender neutral (Evans, 2004). This failure to acknowledge the historical trends and geographical patterns of men in nursing is a barrier to more effective gender-balanced recruitment in nursing. The net result of this failure is that nursing has always been an occupation with predominantly feminine characteristics, and it is still stereotyped by the nurturing and caring roles attributed to wives and mothers. Whether the image of nursing as a feminine role evolved from the recruitment of women into nursing or whether women were recruited into nursing because of its feminine image is a moot question. Ever since Nightingale recruited only women to accompany her to the Crimean War area to care for the wounded, the image of the nurse was fused with the ministering, sacrificing, and altruistic image of women. The same pattern also was demonstrated in the Eastern image of a nurse. Rufaida al-Aslamiya, considered the mother of nursing in the Middle East, recruited other women to tend to war victims in early Islamic history (Jan, 1996). There is little doubt that many of the issues facing nursing emanated from the feminine image of nursing and the idea of nursing as a profession for women, particularly in societies in which women are relegated to secondary status (Dachelet, 1978; Heide, 1973; Sandelowski, 2000; Wren, 1971).

Many of the characteristics of women have been considered antithetical to creativity and scientific productivity. Ample evidence indicates that women are reared and socialized differently than men from the minute they utter their first cry of life, which may lead to some differences in their cognitive structures. Women are perceived by many members of different societies (including the United States), rightly or wrongly, to be more affective, more subordinate, more emotional, less aggressive, and less achievement oriented, and they are generally expected to apply rather than to create. Because ours, like many others, is a patriarchal society, these differences, which could have been considered simply as differences without any value judgments, have been judged as negative when applied toward women. In addition to this attitude, which has been more than devastating and an impediment to women's progress, many women find themselves juggling multiple roles, and many struggle to survive in career-oriented jobs with limited resources to support them, issues that continue to be true and even more documented in the second decade of the 21st century (May, Meleis, and Winstead-Fry, 1982; Meleis, 1975; Nowak and Bonner, 2013; Valian, 2000). Women tend to be engaged or relegated to many time-consuming tasks (e.g., housekeeping and/or office calls and meetings) and busyness that deprives them from the time and energy required for building a thinking-driven career (Shambaugh, 2016). Generally, women also are conditioned and expected to consider a professional career as secondary to family and home. This has not allowed them to direct their energies toward more creative endeavors, such as theory development and theory testing, which are considered antithetical to practice (Hodges and Park, 2013; Sonnert and Holton, 1995).

Creativity and scholarly productivity embody curiosity, intellectual objectivity, the ability to be engaged in decision-making, and independent judgment. These are socially desirable attributes—so long as they are not adopted by women. Because nursing did not insist on independence or an active striving for success, it has generally been perceived as a profession congruent with what is "expected of women." Furthermore, nursing embodies subjectivity in caregiving, dependence on others for decision-making, and expressiveness in relationships—all considered female traits. Street (1992), in a critical ethnography of nursing practice, describes how nurses are aware of the potential negative consequences of thinking and speaking critically. Therefore, nurses may have been socialized against thinking critically, questioning, and changing the status quo (Group and Roberts, 2001).

Even when women broke from the mold, they suffered ambivalences. Horner (1972) demonstrated that anxiety in many women is created by achievement-related conflicts. Those qualities that are essential for "intellectual mastery," such as independence and active striving, are not female qualities. Therefore, women who defy the conventions of sex-appropriate behavior usually pay the price in anxiety.

Until recently, the message was that, because women are biologically different, they are inferior to men. Nursing is a profession for women, and the attributes that women should strive for and maintain are epitomized in nursing. Therefore, women believed the congruence between societal expectations of women and nurses. A self-fulfilling prophecy, of what education women should have and how they should act as women and nurses, lingered. As a result, women who entered nursing in the near past identified strongly with the roles of wife and mother and either believed that nursing would prepare them for the natural roles of women or that the nursing role was a way to earn a living until a knight came along and rescued them from the drudgery of full-time work. For most women, a career was not supposed to coexist with marriage and motherhood, so a woman had to choose between the two. Men, however, could easily combine career, fatherhood, and marriage. Career advancement for women continues to be less than for men as women fail to enter senior management positions because of second-generation gender bias and its impact on pipeline issues, because leadership qualities tend to be associated with men, and because female nursing students, like other young college-age women, may be unaware of gender discrimination (Ibarra, Ely, and Kolb, 2013). In addition to having less opportunity for advancement, women in nursing typically earn less money than men in the field (Muench, Sindelar, Busch, et al., 2015). Nurses who work part-time, and thus they stay in lower nursing positions, are typically women (Tracey and Nicholl, 2007).

The self-identity of nursing students lay in their womanhood rather than in their profession or in their discipline. Women in nursing were different from women studying other professions in other ways as well. The self-concept of women who selected nursing, teaching, and dental hygiene included a perception of low autonomy, less chance for advancement, and less need for intellectual stimulus. They also asserted, by selecting nursing, that they had more favorable attitudes toward marriage and family. Students in nursing in the late 1960s and early 1970s ranked home and family roles as number one and career roles as number two, with their own identity being attached more to the former and less to the latter roles (Cleland, 1971; Olesen and Davis, 1966). The increasing demands on families of the 21st century, the continuing limited resources for employed women, and the gender issues women encounter are not making it easier for this pattern to change (Hochschild and Machung, 1997).

On the job, nurses' productivity was measured by their constant doing, by their sense of urgency, and by their appearing busy. However, their identity remained first and foremost ascribed to simply being women. Their type of productivity was devalued because women were socialized to believe that what they do is of less worth than what men do (Reverby, 1990). Their identity also suffered because they were allowed to receive validation mainly through the capacity to attract a marital partner and to bear and rear children, rather than through intellectual achievement, career advancement, or financial gain. Male productivity was valued, and a man's identity was measured by his job, career, achievements, and financial gains. The male identity, therefore, was measured by what men did in society and female identity by what women did for the family (Langer, Meleis, Knaul, et al., 2015). Women learned to play the game of being less smart, less effective, and less expert to maintain an identity congruent with society (Gordon, 2005).

Other perceived differences between men and women might have constrained the development of nursing theory. For one thing, women in science were, in general, engaged in less scholarly production than men (Cole, 1981). Also, because nursing was fairly new to the scholarly arena, it was apparent that

> *New scholars in the field have more obstacles and ambivalence to overcome in their attempt to integrate the scholarly role with the repertoire of other roles that constitute the self-concept. (May et al., 1982, p. 23)*

Sex-role stereotyping has also impeded the theoretical development of nursing in one more way. Many women came to believe the stereotypes that they were unintellectual, subjective, and emotional (Keller, 1979, 1985) and thus were less vocal in confronting those claims, preferring invisibility and the careers that allowed them to do so (Ehrenreich and Hochschild, 2002). Women became prejudiced against each other, reinforced the myths against each other, and perpetuated the myth about their inability to think theoretically and to develop theories (Goldberg, 1968).

Collaboration, a hallmark of success in nursing practice and an activity about which nurses are most familiar, has not been attached to the scholarly development of disciplines. So, even this, which nurses can do well, was not acknowledged as a significant characteristic of development and progress in scientific disciplines until the late 1980s, when Gilligan (1984) and others described and explained the differences in development between men and women. Women's development was described in terms of connection and collaboration.

Several patterns of responses reflect barriers toward theory development:

- Slow acceptance of the acts of theorizing in nursing
- Devaluation of the work of nurse theorists
- Uncritical acceptance of theories developed by non-nurses
- Valuation of evidence-based practice (defined in terms of empirical research)
- Use of biomedical outcomes

Is it possible that the slow adaptation and utilization of nursing theories may have occurred because these were theories developed by women and nurses, as compared with other theories that were developed by men who were not nurses? This and other questions are worthy of further exploration by those interested in sex-role identity and perceptions and knowledge development in nursing. These issues may present different dialogues and answers depending on the context of the particular decade.

The influence of gender in nursing may be emerging in the populations used for research studies in nursing. Polit and Beck (2008) reviewed research publications during 2005–2006 and reported that about 75% of the study participants were female. Although the review is limited in scope, they provide a different view of gender bias in nursing, one that may be attributed to the nature of the questions that researchers ask or to the gender imbalance that has been the hallmark of the discipline of nursing.

Human Barriers: Nurses as Theorists

Nurse theorists have sometimes acted unwittingly as barriers to the further development of theory. In the minds of practitioners, theorists who were associated with educational institutions were castigated for being far removed from practice. The language that theorists used separated them from their colleagues in practice and other nursing arenas. The language of theories appeared esoteric to the rest of the nursing world, to say nothing of the outside world. A nursing client as an energy field, a system of behavior, or a self-care agent were all new and poorly defined concepts. To complicate matters, educators translated nursing theory to curricula rather than to propositions for testing. This intensified the schism between theory and practice and supported the perceived lack of relationship between theory and practice.

Nurse theorists, easily accessible to their immediate colleagues, appeared to practitioners to be remote and inaccessible. Academics in general are perceived to represent the "ivory tower" of academia and are perceived far less to represent the real world. The lack of intertheory discussions and debates added a new dimension to the many intradisciplinary schisms. Schisms also appeared between disciples of various theorists.

Most theorists believe that members of the discipline of nursing need to agree on the phenomena, perspectives, and problems that are central to the field and to the mission of nursing. But to select only caring, or adaptation, or homeostasis, or self-care, or need fulfillment, or effective nurse–patient interactions as the mission of nursing may mean concentrating exclusively on one mission to the exclusion of others. Defining a nursing mission, advocated by the early nurse theorists, may have been interpreted to mean an exclusive mission. Therefore, the perception was that those who theorize tend to preach for one binding philosophy, one theory, or one conceptual model to guide nursing's research and practice. To accept one theory (argued the practitioners, educators, and researchers) that has not evolved from practice, or has not been subjected to practice application, research validation or the test of time (to the exclusion of others) was unacceptable. Misconceptions, such as believing it was necessary to have only one theory, drew the few believers further away from theoretical nursing.

Although there is no published documentation for this analytical posture, the lack of debate about and among nurse theorists, and the limited discourse involving multiplicity of theories, in the 1960s and 1970s may be indications of such misconceptions. There were numerous debates, though, among and between faculty members and clinicians regarding which theory to use and the inadvisability of such a choice. These debates were more ideological than substantive. Therefore, we can propose that nurses have been harsh in critiquing nursing theories, perhaps because (1) the theories did not appear to evolve from an empirical base; (2) the theories were developed by women; (3) each theory in itself was not able to describe, explain, and predict all nursing phenomena; and (4) the theories were not perceived to reflect the complexities of nursing practice. Harshness was also apparent in criticism of the nurse theorists for taking risks, which is another manifestation of what Ryan (1971) called "blaming the victim."

Nurses have been admonished for contributing to their own oppression and inhibiting nursing from achieving the status of a profession (Stein, 1972).

Much energy and time has been wasted, through intradisciplinary battles between nursing service and nursing education and over types of educational programs and levels of entry into practice. Nurses invalidate other nurses by bringing in "experts" from other disciplines to dictate to nurses rather than to dialogue and exchange ideas about actions, outcomes, and theories with nursing "experts." This blaming, self-flagellation, and infighting must be recognized by nurses as deriving from the more general gender inequities that women encounter globally. And, like women generally, nurses must understand that they alone are not to blame for these problems (Yeaworth, 1978, p. 75) and that the biases they encounter are experienced by other women. (Ely and Rhode, 2010)

Knowledge Barriers

Knowledge barriers also inhibit development in theoretical nursing. Knowledge barriers are manifested in the uncritical use of knowledge developed by other disciplines, the reluctance to use nursing theory developed within the discipline by members of the discipline, and the further development of knowledge that is more pertinent to the fields of preparation of nurses (i.e., disciplines from which nurses may have received their doctoral education or from where their primary mentorship was provided).

An interesting phenomenon persisted for decades in nursing—the *what is imported is superior* phenomenon—in which imported knowledge is far more meaningful than that which is domestic and developed by nurses. By "imported" we mean theories developed by individuals other than nurses and those developed in a field other than nursing. Sometimes this importing of theories was done for legitimate reasons, but many times it was done with no rationale other than the obvious: someone who was not a nurse—and therefore was unfamiliar with the theoretical bases of our discipline—developed it, or it emerged from a non-nursing paradigm; therefore, it must be accepted, and its effectiveness must not be questioned. Other forms of "conceptual imperialism" have been described that perpetuate the institutional worldview (Smith, 1990). This is apparent in the unquestioning use of theories from other disciplines, the lack of reluctance to attribute the label of theory to conceptualizations that evolve from a non-nursing discipline (e.g., role theory, when sociologists are still debating whether role is a concept, a construct, or a theory), and the concomitant reluctance to attribute the label of *theory* to nursing conceptual schemes.

Nursing has been shadowed first by the biomedical model and then by numerous other models, theories, and paradigms; therefore, theory development was left to those in different fields that are related to nursing. Few in those related fields saw fit to support nurses' efforts to look for their own individualized "umbrella," their own perspective, their own paradigm. As expected, disciplines that opened their academic doors to nurses perpetrated the notion that these disciplines are best suited to provide the intellectual framework for nursing theoretical development. In addition, what Yeaworth declared in the late 1970s shaped the historical theoretical dialogues.

Sociologists, psychologists, and physiologists are much more comfortable with the idea of providing members of their discipline to do the research for nursing than with the idea of providing doctoral preparation for nurses who then return to nursing to apply their knowledge. (Yeaworth, 1978, p. 75)

Because nurses had few role models who combined nursing and another field in their graduate programs, and because nurses were away from nursing practice while studying theory and research, those with doctoral education from non-nursing fields tended to explore phenomena using their new field's binoculars and neglected to synthesize their findings into theoretical nursing. The result has been to explore propositions from sociology, psychology, education, or physiology. These explorations often have implications for nursing practice but not for nursing theory. Many of these nurses educated in other disciplines may have believed that nursing had nothing unique to offer and, therefore, maintained that the quest for a unique domain is a quest for separation and noncollaboration. To some, to condone nursing theories and nursing's need to develop theories was to support a separationist notion. This view continues to persist among some members of the discipline in the 21st century, thus creating an ideal discourse less useful in furthering the advancement of nursing's theoretical underpinnings (Hofrochs, 2000; Thompson, 1999). As more nurse scholars are educated in nursing PhD programs, this discourse has moved toward embracing and integrating theories from different disciplines including more friendly dialogues with nursing theories.

Theory itself was a barrier. First, nurses said they needed theories to prove that nursing is a profession, not simply an occupation. They argued that what nursing lacked in its quest for professionalism was a systematic, coherent body of knowledge with set boundaries. Theories fulfilled this requirement. As a result, theorists were suspected of developing theories for professionally selfish reasons. This turned off practitioners, and theorists found themselves spending a great deal of energy trying to justify their theories rather than revising, further developing, or making them more clinically useful.

Another misguided goal evolved. Educators began to believe that theory—which was then called "conceptual framework"—was needed to develop conceptually based curricula. In fact, the National League for Nursing required that a curriculum should have a well-articulated conceptual framework as a requirement for accreditation. The rationale was that if students were prepared in these programs, they would emerge as agents of change in practice. Therefore, from 1965 to 1975, faculty members of nursing schools tried to fit square pegs into round holes. The result was curricula that overwhelmed students with esoteric content that was rarely used in practice after graduation. The schism that existed between the languages of clinicians and educators convinced students of the uselessness of the esoteric content, even before they graduated and assumed clinical positions in the workforce.

Many graduate students have tried to revive the knowledge of nursing theory they gained in their baccalaureate years, knowledge that, to them, had not been useful in practice. Many of them believe that a theoretically based curriculum both confined and liberated their thinking. It confined it to one approach, but it liberated them to experiment with theory utilization. The decrease in the number of nursing theory–based programs, which may have started as an exercise in intellectual rebellion, may actually be a sign of progress. Curricula have become more coherent, systematic, and theoretical, and therefore do not need to be limited to any one framework. The academic need for theory may have been already established. However, when theory-based curricula were first introduced, faculty focus on curricula may have caused them to lose sight of the reason for theory, which is quality nursing practice and patient care. Theory-based research continued to suffer, as manifested by the limited number of nursing theory–based dissertations (Spear, 2007).

Another goal was that nursing have a disciplinary status based on scientific foundations. This required the utilization of theories. Theories, then, appeared to be a means to establish nursing as an academic discipline, one distinct from medicine

and deserving of professional status. All these are worthy goals for nursing. They will not be achieved, however, by developing theories to only guide curricula; theories are developed through asking and answering significant questions in the profession and in the discipline. The ultimate goals of nursing in any society are to provide quality and effective nursing care for clients and populations, to prevent illness, to promote well-being, and to enhance the ability of people to function up to their full capacity through self-care. Significant research questions arise in the quest to realizing these goals, and theories help us understand, explain, predict, and prescribe nursing care that helps in meeting these goals. Since the 1980s, nurses realized and used these goals to guide research programs and theory development. Secondary gains from a focus on the primacy of these goals are the gains in the status of the profession and the discipline.

Conceptual and Perceptual Barriers

All the previously discussed barriers—considered within a context of history, culture, and environment—contribute to the lack of conscious use of nursing theories, inhibit the potential for developing theories, and may have created conceptual barriers for nurses. Conceptual blocks are those closed gates that prevent nurses from perceiving or developing nursing phenomena beyond the immediate problem-solving need. According to Adams (1974), conceptual blocks are caused by perceptual, cultural, and environmental obstacles. Cultural and environmental blocks were discussed previously; the following section discusses perceptual blocks.

Perceptual blocks are obstacles that prevent the problem solver from clearly perceiving either the problem itself or the information that is necessary to solve the problem. (Adams, 1974, p. 13)

When used as a framework to describe the nursing situation, perceptual blocks may appear in the following six forms, as described by Adams (1974). First, a nurse may have difficulty delineating a phenomenon that is worthy of pursuance theoretically. She may be unable to perceive meaningful clues; she may focus on tangential issues, use a priori paradigms that do not permit a nursing perspective, or fail to see a phenomenon because of the lack of a defining framework.

Second, some nurses may put closer boundaries on a phenomenon—more acceptable boundaries in terms of societal expectations—to the detriment of understanding the phenomenon. For example, suppose an immigrant was admitted to the emergency room three times in the 6 weeks after his successful triple bypass surgery. Each time, there was a question of another myocardial infarction, and each time the infarction was unsubstantiated. The causes of the unwarranted emergency room appearances were recorded as noncompliance, diagnostic problems in the emergency room, or inability to communicate signs and symptoms. In this case, a premature closure on the phenomenon of repeated appearance prevented a careful exploration of the phenomenon within the context of the immigrant's experience and the cultural meanings attached to heart problems. Another example is the discovery of the first Ebola case in Texas in 2014 where the diagnostics decisions did not consider the patient's recent arrival from Ebola territory. The protocol for handling the patient resulted in delayed isolation and treatment.

Similarly, a third perceptual block is the lack of experience in considering a phenomenon from different perspectives. The ability to take the role of others, walk in their shoes, see the world through their eyes, and thus consider responses and experiences from different perspectives is a skill that needs to be developed. Without this skill, the nurse may experience and manifest a perceptual block.

Nurses also fall prey to a fourth type of perceptual block, one related to paradigms that have guided us for many generations and make us see what we expect to see. If we see the world through the biomedical model, we tend to see signs, symptoms, and biomedical antecedents. Our stereotypes of cultures and social classes, and our likes and dislikes in values, limit our perceptions and create blocks.

Immersion and experience are two-edged swords in theoretical development. Although both are essential in describing theoretically clinical practice, they also tend to prevent us from seeing a phenomenon from a fresh perspective. Anthropologists and sociologists have discussed this fifth perceptual block, and they advise distancing to allow a return to a fresh start. Another strategy is to consciously keep a journal of events related to the phenomenon. Putting the journal aside and picking it up again later permits distancing and diffuses what Adams calls the problems of "saturation" (1974, p. 25).

The final perceptual block to be aware of is the nurse's potential inability to permit and accept all senses and intuitive inputs in delineating and developing a phenomenon theoretically.

Research Enterprise as a Barrier

As the nursing discipline became defined as a research-based discipline, the movement toward evidence-based practice came to be regarded as the ideal goal for nursing practice (Goode, 2000). Evidence was equated with research, and research was equated with empirical investigations (Farquhar, Stryer, and Slutsky, 2002). Speaking the language of evidence, best models of care, and practice based on best research findings has become a substitute for the language of theory, theoretical thinking, and practice based on the expertise of clinicians, as if these two sets of discourse are antithetical or a substitute for each other, rather than being intricately connected in the production of quality practice (Doane and Varcoe, 2008). They are not. The framework for evidence-based practice did not include questions about the origin of the questions asked or the theoretical assumptions and rationale for interpretations. It further disconnected nursing research from nursing theory and oversimplified the dialogue and the meaning of evidence (Thorne and Sawatzky, 2014). Outcomes research became the panacea; it did not matter whether a disconnection existed between nursing care interventions driven by nursing thought and nursing care outcomes mostly driven by biomedical, social, and behavioral sciences, rather than by a new perspective within a nursing domain. Big data sources have become more utilized for answering nursing research questions about outcomes of care; however, the questions and the data require agreement on standardized language. The lack of this agreed-upon language in health records may continue to be a barrier for advancing nursing knowledge.

RESOURCES TO THEORY DEVELOPMENT

Human Resources: Nurses as Nurses

Theory is a mental image and conception of reality. Tools for theory development are similar to those tools that nurses use in their clinical practice and with which they are most experienced. Some of the most significant tools for theorizing are the abilities to observe, to discern patterns, and to make connections. Nurses have ample opportunity to learn how to observe, to sharpen their observations, and to use all their senses in collecting data. They further have the opportunity to hone the other tools in categorizing and interpreting that data. Observation is central to nursing practice; observation comes easily to the experienced clinician, and the abilities to discern patterns and make connections based on observations are acquired with education and practice.

Another significant tool for theorizing is the ability to record what actually is happening in a nursing care situation. Nursing records offer a wealth of information. They are patient specific, temporally limited, and have space boundaries that do not allow for generalization. With other tools—thinking and reflecting—providing legitimization for developing theories, the observation and recording of data could become the impetus for more general descriptions. Each one of these nursing care situations could become an exemplar for further generalization.

Examples from our theoretical history substantiate these abilities and their relationship to theory development. Nightingale reflected on the many functions and activities that nurses performed during the Crimean War. While in bed (Nightingale spent the last 30 years of her life in bed), she had uninterrupted time and resources to collate observations, critique actions, analyze perceptions of nursing, and arrive at the first systematic, comprehensive concept of nursing (Nightingale, 1992).

The field of nursing itself, as a source for theory development, is a gold mine for those who wish to articulate its many components and connect them theoretically. On a daily basis, nurses are dealing with many phenomena that need describing and explaining, and they are responsible for helping clients achieve their health goals through a wide range of activities, ranging from assessing to evaluating, from the technical to the highly abstract. A world of information exists in nursing, which needs to be described and put into order. Clinical stories from nurses' daily practice provide rich accounts of what nursing is about. These stories could provide the necessary data for developing exemplars and models for practice.

Unlike other disciplines that have doubtful social significance, nursing is needed as a human service and is sanctioned for its significance to health care. Nurses in practice settings spend a good deal of time with patients, and because practice is one of the most significant sources of theory, the central ingredient for theory development is therefore available.

In the 1960s, in the wake of changes in nursing education and its attempt at integration, the Yale school of thought evolved to represent developing theories by observing patients, cajoling nurses into articulating what they had accomplished in patient care, and composing a view of nursing—its mission, its goals, and its prescription. These nurse educators used observation and recording skills they had mastered as nurses, and they used nursing clinicians' abilities to do the same. The result was an early conceptualization of nursing as an interpersonal process, a conceptualization that remains useful to this day. One must consider, however, that federal funding at the time allowed those nurses the free time and flexible schedules to think, reflect, and develop theories.

Whereas earlier nursing education had been a deterrent to theory development, nursing education since the beginning of the 1980s has been a force toward its enhancement. When faculty of doctoral nursing programs in the United States were asked what they considered the core content in their respective programs, highest in rank order were nursing theory, theory development, and conceptual formulation (Beare, Gray, and Ptak, 1981). Students and recent graduates from doctoral programs in nursing, beginning in the 1980s, were practically the first purebreds in the science of nursing. The generation immediately preceding them had experienced a truly hybrid education, one comprising a multitude of programs. Therefore, it is natural that these purebred individuals address the central questions in the field by engaging in the much needed processes of theory development and organization of nursing knowledge. Many master's programs in the United States also offer nursing theory, and a few undergraduate programs are beginning to orient their students to the need for theorizing and for using nursing theory in practice. These patterns of education about theoretical nursing are found as well in many parts of the world. How the development of the clinical nurse leader and the doctorate of nursing practice programs will influence theory development and nursing knowledge remains to be seen (DeMaio and Jones, 2006).

Other quests make the nature of nursing a moving force in theory development. Theoretical knowledge is viewed as a "basis for power" (Chinn and Jacobs, 1987). Therefore, as nurses attempt to achieve their professional autonomy and gain recognition for their role as an equal member of the care team, theory becomes a most significant tool. When novices recognize that they can defend ideas better when they approach the argument or debate from a coherent theoretical basis, they may tend to utilize theory more. As the experienced push to have their organizations acknowledge nursing care outcomes as distinguishable from outcomes of other kinds of care, they will use theory to articulate their mission, their goals, and their focus. A move toward autonomy is indeed a moving force toward theory development and utilization (Fairman, 2008).

Autonomy is linked to communication about patient care among nurses and between nursing and other health care professions. Communication is enhanced when it is in an understandable language that is common, if not to all health care professionals, then at least among nurses themselves. Communication is enhanced when it evolves from some guiding framework. As nurses value and respect each other's observations and diagnoses, and as they search for a common language with which to communicate, a language that represents nursing's overall goals and missions more so than the immediate patient care issue, then theory becomes a means to achieve better communication. Therefore, improving communication about patient care goals and about patient care outcomes is a quest for theory development. Nursing practice and nursing education are present-day forces toward theorizing in nursing.

Finally, experiences of nurses as experts in nursing practice were formally acknowledged in the 1980s as a most significant source for nursing knowledge (Benner, 1984; Benner and Wrubel, 1989). Describing expert nursing practice, as seen and practiced by nurses, was considered a valued source if not the most significant source for articulating in a meaningful and coherent whole the fundamental and practice aspects of nursing.

Human Resources: Nurses as Women

Theorists and researchers are beginning to produce evidence to refute some of the myths surrounding female identity and the capacity of women to produce science. Recent empirical investigations and theories do not show sex-role differentiation in sensitivity to social cues, affiliative behavior, or nurturing behavior. Women are neither more empathic nor more altruistic than men. Although the myth surrounding these differences still lingers, data are increasingly refuting them (Meeker and Weitzel-O'Neill, 1977). Therefore, some of the attributes of women that have been linked to lower productivity and paucity in theoretical thinking are questioned by more contemporary researchers (Bleier, 1990). Although new findings have demonstrated that there are sex differences in brains (McCarthy, Arnold, Ball, et al., 2012), the findings

are still limited in distribution and in their power to support, refute, or reinterpret earlier findings about how men and women tend to conceptualize, manage special functions, or advance knowledge. In the future, more research in gender and sex differences in the brain and its functions, and greater awareness of the conclusion of that research, may contribute valuable knowledge to better understand productivity-oriented female attributes (McCarthy and Arnold, 2011). This knowledge could then drastically alter educational and socialization practices.

In the meantime, the feminist movement has done a great deal of consciousness raising among women in general and among nurses in particular. It has attempted to dissipate some of the long-held myths that have formed true barriers to career advancement of women. As early as the 1970s, nurses began to identify more with feminist ideals and with a view of nursing as a career rather than merely as a stepping stone toward motherhood (Moore, Decker, and Dowd, 1978; Stein, 1972). Research supports the presence of that shift. Graduate, baccalaureate, and associate-degree students had self-images more in harmony with the image of professional nursing (Stromborg, 1976). The shift is toward an image of independence, competence, and intellectual achievement, characteristics more congruent with a person who engages in idea development.

Research findings demonstrated that nursing students are not qualitatively different from other female college students in their sex-role identity and personality constructs (Meleis and Dagenais, 1981). These studies either dispelled earlier myths that nursing students manifest more feminine characteristics than other women in college or demonstrated that drastic changes have occurred for women, and particularly for nurses.

When the feminine characteristics of nursing students in programs at three educational levels (diploma, associate, and baccalaureate) were compared with normative data of women in general, results demonstrated that nurses are generally similar to female college and university students in a number of personality constructs. When there were differences, they were congruent with what is expected in practice professions; that is, they did not differ in autonomy but rather in practical aspects (Meleis and Dagenais, 1981). Education plays a more significant role in perception of self than in sex-role identity. Changing sex-role identities through dispelling some of the myths surrounding women's abilities makes the environment more receptive to women's creativity in knowledge development.

Changing society's expectations of women and science are other forces working in nursing theory development. Women possess some attributes that may have been perceived in the past as inappropriate and incongruent with creativity but that are becoming more accepted in today's society (Weedon, 1991). Women have been described as intuitive. Increasingly, as Eastern and Western modes of knowledge development merge, intuition is seen in a more positive light and, indeed, as essential in idea development, as a component in different patterns of understanding reality, and as an accepted method for scientific inquiry (Carper, 1978; Silva, 1977). Intuition is part of the philosophical process, the mental labor central to the process of developing theories. Intuition played a significant role in Einstein's discoveries and in Darwin's articulation of the evolutionary theory. Intuition, the "curse" of women's abilities, was recognized in the 1990s as a force for women's potential. Intuitive awareness of personal and social phenomena is a resource for women in nursing (Adams, 1972). Intuition has also been considered from the perspective of practice that is both information-based and deliberate, as well as on nursing science (Effken, 2001; Hams, 2000). And as Kahneman (2011) asserts in his groundbreaking book, *Thinking Fast and Slow*, ". . .accurate intuitions of experts are better explained by the effects of prolonged practice than by heuristics" (p. 11). While he maintains that skill and heuristics are both sources of intuitive "judgment and choices," he does not address them in terms of gender.

Although women may have been caught in a "compassion trap" of always being available as helpers in the past, Adams (1972) suggests that, as a result, women possess an attribute that is significant in today's world: flexibility. Women, as an oppressed minority, learned to deal with difficult situations when others controlled access to resources. In the process, they learned how to be flexible and innovative in finding alternative resources essential for their development and for accomplishing their goals. Persons with these sensitive capacities undoubtedly perceive reality differently from those who occupy positions of social power and dominance, yet their perceptions have much to contribute to knowledge about nurturing and the caretaking process (Benoliel, 1975, p. 26).

Changes in sex-role identity, changes in the image of women, and a growing respect for intuition as a pattern of knowing, flexibility, and resourcefulness are all significant forces in theory development, and they all influence women's contextual cognitive styles. Juggling roles is congruent with more contemporary consideration of contextual analyses.

Women in nursing have an added advantage over women in other disciplines. Women scientists—in physics, chemistry, and social and behavioral sciences, among others—are a minority in their own fields. They have experienced prejudices, less support, and outright discrimination in resource allocation, among other social ills that result from the competition with a dominant group. In such unfair competition, men tend to win, to the detriment of women's progress in these disciplines (Cole, 1981; Keller, 1985; National Science Foundation, 1996; Sonnert and Holton, 1995; Valian, 2000).

Most nurses are women; therefore, conflicts resulting from intradisciplinary sex-role competition are nonexistent. Female nurses have full citizenship within their own discipline. Moreover, we hope that the lessons we have learned from other disciplines will not permit prejudices against male nurses. Creative energy can be freed from the sex-role struggle for the benefit of theory development.

Women and nurses have exhibited a sense of humility as a corollary to humanity, which may have previously prevented them from generalizing beyond the immediate situation (Dickoff, James, and Wiedenbach, 1968). This sense of humility is now being replaced by self-assurance, as nurses articulate their own conceptualizations of the different clinical realities they encounter (Parker and MacFarlane, 1991).

Knowledge as a Force and a Resource

Having a knowledge-based discourse helps in further advancing knowledge; the more knowledge there is to advance, the more we are stimulated and challenged to further develop an understanding of phenomena. Theory development in nursing is enhanced by the wealth of theoretical knowledge and solid research findings we already have. The theories developed by nurse scholars provide an impetus for further refinement and development, and the evidence that evolved from research programs drives the development of theories. The theories and the evidence lead to an agreed-on set of concepts that are central to nursing and point to phenomena that need further development. They have set the stage for the next steps.

Debates surrounding which theories to develop, how to develop them, and whether or not to develop them have helped to clarify the mission of nursing. With a preliminary identification of content and a beginning articulation of methodology, the course is now clear for smoother sailing. All this has set the stage for shaping skills in analytical and critical thinking and has stimulated more nurse scholars to pursue development in theoretical nursing. Nursing has the potential for developing a feminist approach to science, or even a nonsexist science, by converting "value-free technology" to a "humane technology" that incorporates self-care (Ardetti, 1980).

Old paradigms of knowledge are being challenged by new paradigms, prompted by two significant social movements: the feminist movement and the women's health movement (McPherson, 1983). Essential components of the new paradigm represent a shift to include humanitarianism, holism, the incorporation of sociocultural content, perceptions of subjects of research, subjects and researchers collaborating in the research process, and a qualitative approach. The "new paradigm" is not new to nursing. Its newness stems more from social acceptance, as the public becomes more aware of ways to develop knowledge and demands participation in the process. The newness is in the congruence, rather than in a shift in thinking. There is wider acceptance of components of the "new paradigm" by consumers who care. That is a force that will help nurses further develop knowledge. The energy once expended by those defending components of a paradigm that was incongruent with a prevailing scientific perspective can now be channeled from the creativity of reaction to the creativity of action.

A new worldview emerged, a view that had even changed physics from the mechanistic conceptions advanced by Descartes and Newton to a more holistic and ecological view (Capra, 1983). The new worldview is congruent with women's views of science and nurses' views of health. It is a view that has shifted focus from the causative to the more interpretive. It is heightened by phenomenology and qualitative research.

Conceptual Resources

To use all senses, experiences, and intuition requires involvement and immersion in situations as a whole, and to describe patterns of responses theoretically requires longer periods of engagement in those situations where nursing phenomena occur. The nature of nursing, the process of nursing care, the history of the profession, and the predominant gender orientation of the profession enhance the conceptual

resources for nurses. Nurses are trained to observe, record, analyze, and solve problems. Whether we admit it or not, we tend to use our own and others' experiences in providing care, and in doing so, we rely on all our senses and intuitions, just as we rely on scientific principles to guide our action.

Nurses spend long hours with patients, families, and communities; this time allows an understanding of patterns of behaviors rather than isolated incidents. Diversity in caregivers, in some instances considered problematic, could become a useful resource for theoretical development. Diversity in nurses and in their cultural, educational, and socioeconomic backgrounds can be a resource to allow for diverse views and a safeguard against premature closure on a phenomenon and against narrow perspectives. This resource could help remove perceptual blocks which are discussed above under conceptual barriers.

Nurses have effective interviewing skills for which they have been meticulously educated and trained. They have mastered questioning and assessing, they know how to prioritize, and they know how to participate in dialogue. They have opportunities to confirm observations and hunches during clinical rounds at the end or beginning of shift reports, during impromptu meetings at the nurses' stations, in meetings with other members of the family, and during their many regular daily roles and activities that involve talking, listening, questioning, answering, and writing. Each one of these tasks enhances perception, and each is a resource and an asset for conceptualization.

Other Forces for Theory Use and Development

The journey to theoretical thinking has been a progression through self-effacing stops, self-doubt detours, humility delays, collisions with opposing and dominating paradigms, and near misses due to embarking into unfamiliar territory or unpaved terrain. Nursing and nurses are emerging theoretically stronger and far better prepared to embark on a task of theoretical clarification. The quality of the journey could be enhanced by coaching, mentorship, and sponsorship toward the development of the theoretical insights attached to the scholarly role.

Nurses who learn about theoretical nursing, who are groomed to think conceptually, are not resistant to the use of nursing theory in their practice or to their potential involvement in theory development. Rather, they are asking how they can use theory, and they are looking for those they can emulate in the process. One example of nurses' interest in theory was several national conferences held in the 1980s and 1990s by clinical specialists, in which the topic of theory development and utilization dominated a full half-day of the 2-day conference (e.g., a Clinical Nurse Specialists Annual Conference, 1983). Another institutional example is the credentialing review criteria, used for granting a hospital the designation and recognition as a Magnet Hospital, which requires coherent theoretical approaches driven by the discipline of nursing, to improve the environment for nurses and patients and which influences patient health care outcomes (Kutney-Lee, Stimpfel, Sloane, et al., 2015). Many more examples are demonstrated in the increasing numbers of nurses who are members of organizations established to honor such nurse theorists as Dorothea Orem, Callista Roy, Imogene King, and Martha Rogers (see Chapters 11–13).

Planners of one of these conferences were concerned about the responses of attendants to what might appear as highly abstract ideas not directly related to everyday care issues. The results were astonishing, the evaluations were heartening, and the request came for another session the following year, focusing on how to bring acceptance to theory utilization and development in clinical areas (Clinical Nurse Specialists Annual Conference, 1984). In short, nurses were asking for role modeling, role clarification, and role rehearsal—all properties of mentorship.

Mentorship is an intense relationship calling for a high degree of involvement between a novice in a discipline and a person who is knowledgeable and wise in that area. . . . In the process of helping the beginning scholar to fit resources to her needs and capabilities, the mentor provides options, opens up new opportunities, and helps to make corrections. This means that, on cognitive and affective levels, the mentor is involved with the novice as a whole person and feels a sense of responsibility for her. (May et al., 1982, p. 23)

Role modeling, which is teaching by example and emulation, then fosters the learning of these behaviors (Bandura, 1962; Meleis, 1975). Role clarification provides an opportunity to understand the subtle intricacies of the role to be emulated. What does it mean to have a role in the theoretical development of nursing? What cues are needed to perform that role? Role clarification in theory use and development may include spelling out the differences between the various theories, the different strategies in theory development, the different barriers to the use of theory, and some strategies for handling all of these. Mentorship also includes opportunities for role rehearsal. Use of theory in theoretical patient care studies and use of different strategies in theory development are examples of staged situations in which to practice behaviors central to the use and development of theory (May et al., 1982; Meleis and May, 1981).

Time and sociocultural conditions are right for the development of theoretical nursing, which in turn is significant for patient care, and nurses are "going for it." If, indeed, there is a woman's way to understand the world, and if there are areas of knowledge that are better understood when seen through the eyes of women and through the use of feminine logic, then nursing is ready on all of these accounts, and nurses are prepared to pursue that knowledge.

Nursing education can provide enabling environments through programs that focus on scholarly productivity (Meleis and May, 1981; Meleis, Wilson, and Chater, 1980). Theory and theory development should not be limited to graduate programs. Theoretical thinking should be the modus operandi for conscientious patient care from day one in nursing education. Nursing practice has an equal commitment to provide avenues by which nurses can communicate their findings in theoretical terms and can have the opportunity to translate their hunches into theoretical terms. Within the appropriate atmosphere, nurses should be able to try using different theories in practice for the purpose of refining and extending them.

Similar supportive and enabling environments could be provided by nurse administrators to help in the development of a theoretical culture that allows dialogues, debates, and discussions that go beyond immediate day-to-day problem solving and decision-making. Strategies to be used by nurse administrators and educators for the enhancement of theory development include creating a theoretical culture, supporting critical thinking, refocusing dialogues and discussions on concepts, defining nursing territory, exploring ambiguous ideas, allowing uncertainty about phenomena to linger, avoiding premature closure on ideas, facing views of phenomena from different perspectives, and providing such resources as library time, observation time, and writing time (Jennings and Meleis, 1988; Meleis and Jennings, 1989; Meleis and Price, 1988).

REFLECTIVE QUESTIONS

1. Explain the barriers and forces that led to utilizing theoretical thinking in your area of clinical practice (or education, administration, or consultation).

2. Discuss how the changes toward women's and men's roles may have influenced nursing knowledge development. What changes would you like to see in the future that you believe could make an impact on advancing theoretical thinking in nursing? Be specific in identifying changes and influences.

3. Identify and discuss one more constraint and one more force that may have influenced the theoretical journey in the discipline.

4. In what ways do the different waves of the nursing shortage and the reduction in the work-force that is local and global support or constrain theoretical work? Why? Why not?

5. Are there ways to influence the cycle of shortage through coherent theoretical approaches? Discuss.

6. As gender, ethnic, and sociocultural diversity increases in nursing, what might be some impli-cations for scholarship in nursing? Envision and discuss outcomes. Provide support for your arguments.

7. Discuss the current situation in the use of theoretical nursing. How are theories used? What are the outcomes of use or nonuse of nursing theoretical thinking?

8. In what ways did the discourse of evidence-based practice contribute to or hinder the devel-opment of nursing theories?

9. In your view, what are some of the current dominant discourses in nursing? What evidence do you have for this assertion? In what ways did this dominant discourse influence knowl-edge development?

10. If and when theory is used in practice such as in Magnet hospitals, to what extent or in what ways is it used?

11. Should theoretical frameworks be a requirement for achieving a Magnet designation? Why? Why not?

CONCLUSION

Nurses are now in the land of Kant rather than the land of "Can't." Kant maintained that knowledge depends on experience and experience depends on observation, but observations by themselves do not form experience or give meaning to experience. Observations have to be organized a priori by the mind to develop into knowledge. In so organizing our observations, we tend to reflect and reconstruct reality.

Nurses may have reconstructed the meaning of theoretical constraints into forces that foster the further development of theoretical nurses. They can use the tools of practice in theory development, relying on the same abilities they have used for practice, research, teaching, and administering, and translating these skills into theorizing and the use of theory, perhaps thereby becoming convinced that their experiences comprise the appropriate impetus for theory development.

REFERENCES

Adams, J. (1974). *Conceptual block busting: A guide to better ideas*. San Francisco, CA: W.H. Freeman.

Adams, M. (1972). The compassion trap. In V. Goernick and B.K. Moran (Eds.), *Women in sexist society*. New York: Signet Books.

Ardetti, R. (1980). Feminism and science. In R. Ardetti, P. Bren-nan, and S. Cavrak (Eds.), *Science and liberation*. Boston, MA: South End Press.

Ashley, J.A. (1977). *Hospitals, paternalism, and the role of the nurse*. New York: Teachers College, Columbia University.

Bandura, A. (1962). Social learning through imitation. In M.R. Jones (Ed.), *Nebraska symposium on motivation*. Lincoln, OR: University of Nebraska Press.

Beare, P.G., Gray, C.J., and Ptak, H.F. (1981). Doctoral curricula in nursing. *Nursing Outlook*, 29(5), 311–316.

Benner, P. (1984). *From novice to expert: Excellence and power in clinical nursing practice*. Menlo Park, CA: Addison-Wesley.

Benner, P. and Wrubel, J. (1989). *The primacy of caring, stress and coping in health and illness*. Menlo Park, CA: Addison-Wesley.

Benoliel, J.Q. (1973). Collaboration and competition in nursing research. In *Communicating nursing research: Collaboration and competition.* Boulder, CO: Western Interstate Commission for Higher Education.

Benoliel, J.Q. (1975). Scholarship: A woman's perspective. *Image,* 7(2), 22–27.

Bleier, R. (1990). Sex differences research: Science or belief. In R. Bleier (Ed.), *Feminist approaches to science* (pp. 147–164). New York: Pergamon Press.

Bullough, B. (1975). Barriers to the nurse practitioner movement: Problems of women in a woman's field. *International Journal of Health Services,* 5(2), 225–233.

Canam, C.J. (2008). The link between nursing discourses and nurses' silence: Implications for a knowledge-based discourse for nursing practice. *Advances in Nursing Science,* 31(4), 296–307.

Capra, F. (1983). *The turning point: Science, society, and the rising culture.* New York: Bantam.

Carper, B.A. (1978). Practice oriented theory: Part 1. Fundamental patterns of knowing in nursing. *Advances in Nursing Science,* 1(1), 13–23.

Chinn, P.L. and Jacobs, M.K. (1987). *Theory and nursing: A systematic approach* (2nd ed.). St. Louis, MO: C.V. Mosby.

Cleland, V. (1971). Sex discrimination: Nursing's most pervasive problem. *American Journal of Nursing,* 71(8), 1542–1547.

Clinical Nurse Specialists Annual Conference. (1983, February 17–18). San Francisco, CA.

Clinical Nurse Specialists Annual Conference. (1984, February 16–17). San Francisco, CA.

Cole, J.R. (1981, July/August). Women in science. *American Scientist,* 69, 385–391.

Copleston, F. (1964). *A history of philosophy. Modern philosophy: Kant* (Vol. 6, Part II). Garden City, NJ: Image Books.

Dachelet, C.Z. (1978). Nursing's bid for increased status. *Nursing Forum,* 17(1), 18–45.

DeMaio, D.J. and Jones, D.A. (2006). Letter to the editor. *International Journal of Nursing Terminologies and Classifications,* 17(3), 127–128.

D'Antonio, P. (2004). Women, nursing, and baccalaureate education in 20th century America. *Journal of Nursing Scholarship,* 36(4), 379–384.

D'Antonio, P. (2010). *American nursing: A history of knowledge, authority and the meaning of work.* Baltimore, MD: The Johns Hopkins University Press.

D'Antonio, P., Beal, M.W., Underwood, P.W., Ward, F.R., et al. (2010). Great expectations: Points of congruencies and discrepancies between incoming accelerated second-degree nursing students and faculty. *Journal of Nursing Education,* 49(12), 713–717.

Davidson, J.E. (2010). Facilitated sensemaking: A strategy and new middle-range theory to support families of intensive care unit patients. *Critical Care Nurse,* 30(6), 28–39.

Dickoff, J., James, P., and Wiedenbach, E. (1968). Theory in practice discipline: Part 1. Practice oriented theory. *Nursing Research,* 17(5), 415–435.

Doane, G.H. and Varcoe, C. (2008). Knowledge translation in everyday nursing: From evidence-based to inquiry-based practice. *Advances in Nursing Science,* 31(4), 283–295.

Edwards, C.N. (1969). The student nurse: A study in sex-role transition. *Psychology Report,* 25(3), 975–990.

Effken, J.A. (2001). Information basis for expert intuition. *Journal of Advanced Nursing,* 34(2), 246–255.

Ehrenreich, B. and Hochschild, A.R. (2002). *Global woman. Nannies, maids, and sex workers in the new economy.* New York: Metropolitan Books.

Eldridge, C.R. (2013). Nursing science and theory: Scientific underpinnings for practice. In M. Zaccagnini and K. White (Eds.), *The doctor of nursing practice: A new model for advanced practice nursing.* Burlington, MA: Jones and Bartlett.

Ely, R.J. and Rhode, D.L. (2010). Women and leadership: Defining the challenges. In N. Nohria and R. Khurana (Eds.), *Handbook of leadership and theory practice* (Ch. 14). Boston, MA: Harvard Business Publishing.

Evans, J. (2004). Men nurses: A historical and feminist perspective. *Journal of Advanced Nursing,* 47(3), 321–328.

Fairman, J. (2008). *Making room in the clinic: Nurse practitioners and the evolution of modern health care.* New Brunswick, NJ: Rutgers University Press.

Farquhar, C.M., Stryer, D, and Slutsky, J. (2002). Translating research into practice: The future ahead. *International Journal for Quality in Health Care,* 14(3), 233–249.

Gaston, J. (1975). Social organization, codification of knowledge, and the reward structure in science. *Journal of Social Psychology,* 18, 285–303.

Gatti-Petito, J., Lakatos, B.E., Bradley, H.B., Cook, L., Haight, I.E., and Karl, C.A. (2013). Clinical scholarship and adult learning theory: A role for the DNP in nursing education. *Nursing Education Perspectives,* 34(4), 273–276.

Gilligan, C. (1984). *In a different voice: Psychological theory and women's development.* Cambridge, MA: Harvard University Press.

Goldberg, P. (1968, April). Are women prejudiced against women? *Trans-Action,* 5, 28–30.

Goode, C.J. (2000). What constitutes the "evidence" in evidence-based practice? *Applied Nursing Research,* 13(4), 222–225.

Gordon, S. (2005). *Nursing against the odds.* Ithaca, NY: Cornell University Press.

Group, T. and Roberts, J. (2001). *Nursing, physician control, and the medical monopoly.* Indianapolis, IN: Indiana University Press.

Hams, S.P. (2000). A gut feeling? Intuition and critical care nursing. *Intensive and Critical Care Nursing,* 16(5), 310–318.

Heide, W.S. (1973). Nursing and women's liberation—A parallel. *American Journal of Nursing,* 73(5), 824–827.

Hochschild, A.R. and Machung, A. (1997). *The second shift: Working parents and the revolution at home.* New York: Avon.

Hodges, A.J. and Park, B. (2013). Oppositional identities: Dissimilarities in how women and men experience parent versus professional roles. *Journal of Personality and Social Psychology,* 105(2), 193–216.

Hofrocks, S. (2000). Hunting for Heidegger: Questioning the sources in the Benner/Cash debate. *International Journal of Nursing Studies,* 37(3), 237–243.

Holmes, D., Roy, B., and Perron, A. (2008). The use of postcolonialism in the nursing domain: Colonial patronage, conversion, and resistance. *Advances in Nursing Science,* 31(1), 42–51.

Horner, M. (1972). Toward an understanding of achievement-related conflicts in women. *Journal of Social Issues,* 28(2), 157–175.

Ibarra, H., Ely, R., and Kolb, D. (2013). Women rising: The unseen barriers. *Harvard Business Review,* 91(9), 60–66.

Institute of Medicine. (2011). *The future of nursing: Leading change, advancing health.* Washington, DC: The National Academies Press.

Jan, R. (1996). Rufaida al-Aslamiya, the 1st Muslim nurse. *Image: Journal of Nursing Scholarship,* 28(3), 267–268.

Jennings, B. and Meleis, A.I. (1988). Nursing theory and administrative practice: Agenda for the 1990s. *Advances in Nursing Science,* 10(3), 56 69.

Kahneman, D. (2011). *Thinking fast and slow.* New York: Farrar, Straus and Giroux.

Keller, E. (1979). The effect of sexual stereotyping on the development of nursing theory. *American Journal of Nursing*, 79(9), 1585–1586.

Keller, E. (1985). *Reflections on gender and science*. New Haven, CT: Yale University Press.

Kutney-Lee, A., Stimpfel, A.W., Sloane, D.M., Cimiotti, J.P., Quinn, L.W., and Aiken, L.H. (2015). Changes in patient and nurse outcomes associated with Magnet hospital recognition. *Medical Care*, 53(6), 550–557.

Landivar, L.C. (2013). *Men in nursing occupations: American community survey highlight report*. Washington, DC: U.S. Census Bureau, Industry and Occupation Statistics Branch. Retrieved from www.census.gov/people/io/files/Men_in_Nursing_Occupations.pdf

Langer, A., Meleis, A., Knaul, F.M., et al. (2015, June). Women and health: The key for sustainable development. *The Lancet*, 386(9999), 1165–1210.

Loomis, M.E. (1974, November). Collegiate nursing education: An ambivalent professionalism. *The Journal of Nursing Education*, 13(4), 39–48.

May, K.M., Meleis, A.I., and Winstead-Fry, P. (1982). Mentorship for scholarliness: Opportunities and dilemmas. *Nursing Outlook*, 30(11), 22–28.

McCarthy, M.M. and Arnold, A.P. (2011). Reframing sexual differentiation of the brain. *Nature Neuroscience*, 14(6), 677–683.

McCarthy, M.M., Arnold, A.P., Ball, G.F., Blaustein, J.D., and DeVries, G.J. (2012). Sex differences in the brain: The not so inconvenient truth. *Journal of Neuroscience,* 32(7), 2241–2247.

McPherson, K.I. (1983). Feminist methods: A new paradigm for nursing research. *Advances in Nursing Science*, 5(2), 17–36.

Meeker, B.F. and Weitzel-O'Neill. (1977, February). Sex roles and interpersonal behavior in task-oriented groups. *American Sociological Review*, 42, 91–95.

Meleis, A.I. (1975). Role insufficiency and role supplementation: A conceptual framework. *Nursing Research*, 24(4), 264–271.

Meleis, A.I. and Dagenais, F. (1981). Sex-role identity and perception of professional self in graduates of three nursing programs. *Nursing Research*, 30(3), 162–167.

Meleis, A.I. and Jennings, B. (1989). Theoretical nursing administration: Today's challenges, tomorrow's bridges. In B. Henry, C. Arndt, M. DiVincenti, and A. Marriner (Eds.), *Dimensions and issues in nursing administration*. Boston, MA: Blackwell Scientific Publications.

Meleis, A.I. and May, K.M. (1981). Nursing theory and scholarliness in the doctoral program. *Advances in Nursing Science*, 4(1), 31–41.

Meleis, A.I. and Price, M. (1988). Strategies and conditions for nursing: An international perspective. *Journal of Advanced Nursing*, 13, 592–604.

Meleis, A.I., Wilson, H.S., and Chater, S. (1980). Toward scholarliness in doctoral dissertations: An analytical model. *Journal of Research in Nursing and Health*, 3, 115–124.

Moore, D.S., Decker, S.D., and Dowd, M.W. (1978). Baccalaureate nursing students' identification with the women's movement. *Nursing Research*, 27(5), 291–295.

Muench, U., Sindelar, J., Busch, S, and Buerhaus, P. (2015). Salary differences between male and female registered nurses in the United States. *Journal of the American Medical Association*, 313(12), 1265–1267.

National Science Foundation. (1996). *Characteristics of doctoral scientists and engineers in the United States-1993*. Arlington, VA: National Science Foundation.

Nightingale, F. (1992). *Notes on nursing: What it is, and what it is not*. Philadelphia, PA: J.B. Lippincott Company.

Nowak, M.J. and Bonner, D. (2013). Juggling work and family demands: Lifestyle career anchors for female healthcare professionals. *International Journal of Healthcare Management*, 6(1), 3–11.

Olesen, V.L. and Davis, F. (1966). Baccalaureate students' images of nursing: A follow-up report. *Nursing Research*, 15(2), 151–158.

Parker, B. and MacFarlane, J. (1991). Feminist theory and nursing: An empowerment model for research. *Advances in Nursing Science*, 13(3), 59–67.

Polit, D.F. and Beck, C.T. (2008). Is there gender bias in nursing research? *Research in Nursing & Health*, 31(5), 417–427.

Prime Minister's Commission on the Future of Nursing and Midwifery in England. (2010). *Front Line Care: the future of nursing and midwifery in England*. Retrieved from http://cnm.independent.gov.uk/wp-content/uploads/2010/03/front_line_care.pdf

Reverby, S.M. (1990). *Ordered to care, the dilemma of American nursing, 1850–1945*. Cambridge, NY: Cambridge University Press.

Ryan, W. (1971). *Blaming the victim*. New York: Random House.

Sandelowski, M. (2000). *Devices and desires: Gender technology, and American nursing*. Chapel Hill, NC: The University of North Carolina Press.

Shambaugh, R. (2016, March 7). The time-consuming activities that stall women's careers. *Harvard Business Review*. Retrieved from https://hbr.org/2016/03/the-time-consuming-activities-that-stall-womens-careers

Silva, M.C. (1977). Philosophy, science, theory: Interrelationships and implications for nursing research. *Image*, 9(3), 59–63.

Smith, D. (1990). *The conceptual practices of power: A feminist sociology of knowledge*. Toronto: University of Toronto Press.

Sonnert, G. and Holton G. (1995). *Gender differences in science careers. The project access study*. New Brunswick, NJ: Rutgers University Press.

Spear, H.J. (2007). Nursing theory and knowledge development: A descriptive review of doctoral dissertations. *Advances in Nursing Science*, 30(1), E1–E14.

Stein, L.I. (1972). Liberation movement: Impact on nursing. *AORN Journal*, 15(4), 67–85.

Street, A.F. (1992). *Inside nursing: A critical ethnography of clinical nursing practice*. Albany, NY: State University of New York Press.

Stromborg, M.F. (1976). Relationship of sex-role identity to occupational image of female nursing students. *Nursing Research*, 25(5), 363–369.

Thompson, C. (1999). A conceptual treadmill. The need for "middle ground" in clinical decision making theory in nursing. *Journal of Advanced Nursing*, 30(5), 1222–1229.

Thorne, S. and Sawatzky, R. (2014). Particularizing the general: Sustaining theoretical integrity in the context of an evidence-based practice agenda. *Advances in Nursing Science,* 37(1), 5–18.

Tracey, C. and Nicholl, H. (2007). The multifaceted influence of gender in career progress in nursing. *Journal of Nursing Management*, 15(7), 677–682.

Valian, V. (2000). *Why so slow? The advancement of women*. Cambridge, MA: MIT Press.

Weedon, C. (1991). *Feminist practice and post-structuralist theory*. Cambridge, MA: Basil Blackwell.

Wren, G.R. (1971). Some characteristics of freshman students in baccalaureate, diploma, and associate degree nursing programs. *Nursing Research*, 20(2), 167–172.

Yeaworth, R. (1978). Feminism and the nursing profession. In N. Chaska (Ed.), *The nursing profession: Views through the mist*. New York: McGraw-Hill.

5

On the Way to Theoretical Nursing: Stages and Milestones

Despite the barriers against theoretical thinking and theorizing identified in the previous chapter, nurses, in caring for human beings in an orderly and organized way, have always been involved in some form of theorizing. Concepts of care, comfort, communication, protection, healing, and health, among others, were used to guide clinical practice before they were labeled as concepts and before they were linked together to form nursing theories. However, between 1950 and 1980, a process of serious labeling and a more systematic communication of concepts and theories occurred. This process continues to enrich the discipline of nursing.

First attempts in theoretical nursing were made by Florence Nightingale in the late 19th and early 20th centuries to describe nursing focus and action in the Crimean War. Nightingale was prompted to articulate her ideas in numerous publications, with different goals. Among these goals were gaining support for a national need for nurses, achieving acceptance for the development of educational programs for nurses, and exposing the unhealthy environmental conditions that were endured by English soldiers during wars.

Subsequent attempts in theorizing were published by American nurse educators in the mid-1950s, prompted by the need to justify different educational levels for nurses and the need to develop curricula for each of the educational levels in nursing. To differentiate curricula, and to enhance the quality of education in each curriculum, a few pioneer nurses combined their clinical expertise with their theoretical thinking and forward vision to answer such questions as "What are the goals for nursing care?" and "What ought to be the aims of nursing?" These early theorists were aware that by developing programs that represented a nursing perspective, they would help nursing students—that is, future

clinicians—to focus on nursing phenomena and problems rather than on medical phenomena and problems. Groups of nurse educators were formed in different parts of the United States (and subsequently or simultaneously in other parts of the world) and curricular committees reframed their dialogue to focus on the nature of nursing, the nature of nurses' work, and the unique aspects of nursing. The goals of these early efforts were also focused on differentiating nursing from other health science disciplines. In the process it became more apparent that there is a need to explore the nature of nursing knowledge.

Perhaps the best way to consider the history of nursing theory and to analyze nurses' current interest in theory is to consider dominant themes in the different stages of the development of nursing knowledge (see discussion on the evolved Nursing Perspective in Chapter 6). The implicit assumption here is that the themes discussed in the literature are indicative and representative of what members of the discipline were interested in at different times during the transition process of its development. In addition to delineating these themes, a historical analysis of the theory literature provides us with an understanding of the specific milestones that may have supported or hindered the development of theoretical nursing. Both approaches provide insights into how nursing evolved into its current status, as well as shedding light on why new challenges may be interpreted differently when considered within the prism of history.

In this chapter, the themes are articulated as stages that have influenced progress in knowledge development. Stages are complemented by milestones, which characterize the turning points in the progression from one stage to the next. Each of these stages and milestones inform the current level of progress in the discipline.

STAGES IN NURSING PROGRESS

Since the time of the Crimean War, nursing has gone through many stages in its search for a professional identity and in defining its domain. It is interesting to note that our analysis and evaluation of nursing's theoretical thought, within the context of patriarchal societies and the position, and the status accorded nurses and nursing should provide support that each stage was not a deviation from the goal of establishing the structure of the discipline of nursing. Each of these stages has indeed sharpened and clarified the dimensions needed for the establishment of the scientific aspects of the discipline, promoting or leading to the scholarly evolution of the nursing discipline. Each stage has helped nurses come closer to identifying the domain of nursing, defining its mission, and defining its theoretical base. Progress in the transition toward the development of theoretical nursing is definable in terms of eight stages: practice, education and administration, research, theory, philosophy, integration, interdisciplinarity and interprofessionalism, and technology and information systems.

Stage of Practice

During this stage, the beginning of nursing was defined by its practice and considered as women's work during times of unrest. The Western version of nursing as an occupation dates from the late 19th century and the early 20th century, a product of the Crimean War. Because of the need to care for wounded soldiers, Florence Nightingale organized a group of women to deliver care under her supervision and that of the war surgeons. Nightingale focused on hygiene as her goal and environmental changes as the means to achieve that goal.

The Eastern version of the beginning of nursing gives credit to Rufaida Bint Saad al-Aslamiya (also referred to as Koaiba Bint Saad), who accompanied Prophet Mohammed in his Islamic wars. She, too, organized a group of women and focused on hygiene and environment in caring for the wounded. She established special moving tents to attend to the sick, the wounded, and the disabled. She modeled first aid, emergency care, and long-term healing and caring. She cared for patients and trained women in the arts of first aid and nursing (Fangary, 1980; Hussein, 1990). Like Nightingale, al-Aslamiya established the first school of nursing in the Muslim world. In addition, she conceptualized a code of ethics for nurses and inspired young women to be educated (Jan, 1996). Like Nightingale, her role in nursing did not end with the war. Al-Asalmiya continued to advocate for health care, preventive care, and health education.

Hussein (1981) described al-Aslamiya's devotion to nursing and her success in establishing new rules and traditions for quality nursing care as precursors to modern nursing in the Middle East. In both Eastern and Western versions of the beginnings of nursing, a woman saw the need for organizing other women to care for the wounded in wars; in both, they provided emergency care as well as long-term care. They both focused on caring, healing, promoting healthy environments, and on training other nurses. They both were driven by moral commitments to alleviate suffering and enhance healing. They both may have, inadvertently, established nursing as women's work, and may have limited care-giving to feminine characteristics.

The mission of nursing was defined, during this stage, as providing care and comfort to enhance healing and a sense of well-being, and to create a healthy environment that helps decrease suffering and deterioration. Nurses defined their domain to include the patient and the environment in which the care is offered. Both Nightingale and al-Aslamiya created and monitored the environment in which the care was being given. The stage of practice gave nursing its *raison d'être*, its focus, and its mission. Theoretical writings by Nightingale (1946) describing the care goals and processes are testimony to the potential for nurses to articulate practice activities theoretically. These writings also demonstrated that the practice of nursing could be described and articulated in theoretical terms.

Stage of Education and Administration

From that early focus on practice and the concomitant traditions of apprenticeship and service, there was a shift to questions related to training programs and nursing curricula. The "how to" of practice eventually was translated into what curriculum to develop to support different levels of nursing education and how to teach it. Almost three decades were spent experimenting with different curricula, ways of preparing teachers, and modes of educating and preparing graduates to be administrators for schools of nursing and for service. During this stage, the focus was on the development of functional roles for nurses. The dominant themes of this stage evolved from the educational and administrative roles of nurses.

The significance of this stage in the theoretical development of the discipline lies in the impetus it provided nurses to ask questions related to the domain of nursing. In developing curricula geared toward preparing nurses for different educational levels, nurses asked: What is nursing? How different is nursing care as provided by a diploma graduate, an associate-degree graduate, a bachelor of science graduate, or a master's-degree graduate? These questions prompted nurses to articulate the core of nursing practice in more theoretical terms (Henderson, 1966). In a curious way, it is during this stage that the theoretical ideas of the pioneering American nurse theorists were born. A focus on teaching and education, therefore, may have paved the way for the further development of theoretical nursing and for questioning where the education for the advanced nursing practice role fits. Returning to questions about the focus on nursing practice may have been the impetus for the development of curricula to prepare clinical nurse specialists, followed shortly with the birth of the nurse practitioner's program.

Stage of Research

The stage of research evolved through a series of events overlapping with the stages of practice and education. As Gortner (2000) indicated, during the 1920s, case studies were formulated as teaching tools, but they also were used as an impetus for standardization. Systematic evaluation of these cases triggered the need for graduate education during the post-Depression years in the United States. The war years required data collection and analysis, necessitating the establishment of the Division of Nursing Resources as part of the U.S. Public Health Services in 1948. The beginnings of a research enterprise were born. In the 1970s, commissions and councils of nurse researchers were established. Nurses increasingly were receiving graduate degrees in other disciplines, funds for National Research Service awards were established, and nursing research journals were initiated.

The momentum in nursing education, curriculum development, teaching and learning strategies, and in administration also led educators to pursue research. Experts in nursing curricula recognized that without

research and a systematic inquiry into, for example, the different teaching/learning modalities and the teaching/learning milieu on outcomes, the education of nurses could not be improved. Therefore, the research interest emerged from and focused on questions related to educational and evaluative processes. The scholarship in teaching dominated the early research enterprise.

How to teach, how to administer, how to lead, and which strategies would be more effective in teaching and administering were questions that led to the development and expansion of nursing research (Gortner and Nahm, 1977). The first nursing research journal in the world—entitled *Nursing Research*—was established in 1952, in the United States, and the Southern Regional Educational Board (SREB) and the Western Council for Higher Education in Nursing (WCHEN) were founded in the mid-1950s and mid-1960s, respectively. Their objectives called for improving nursing education, enhancing nursing research productivity, and raising the quality of research. The journal and the meetings of the SREB and WCHEN helped nursing develop its scientific norms—that "set of cultural values and mores governing the activities termed scientific" (Merton, 1973, p. 270).

Criteria for reviewing scientific papers were established, on the basis of the assumption that scientific inquiry must be judged by peers. Therefore, nurse researchers began to abide by Merton's norm of universalism, the impersonal evaluation of a research product by some objective criteria (Merton, 1973, p. 270). Universities also held the same expectations for nursing faculty that they held for other faculty; specifically, members of faculty in schools of nursing were required to develop their ideas and communicate them in the scientific arena through publications in refereed journals and scholarly presentations in meetings. Therefore, when seen in the context of science, the "publish or perish" dogma was not unrealistic but was rather another norm governing nursing science. Nurses were now involved in that communality—the sharing of ideas—and their research was subjected to the scrutiny of their peers and anonymous critics (Gortner, 1980; Merton, 1973).

Nursing's initial attempts at introducing ideas and sharing research results were met with severe and, at times, devastating critiques from other nursing colleagues. (Those who participated in early research conferences may remember the lengthy and harsh research critiques that traumatized researchers and audience alike. Authors of these critiques may not have considered that nursing research was still in its formative years.) As a result, and in addition to universality and communality, two other norms evolved: objectivity and detached scrutiny. Objective criteria for research evaluation, which were identified and shared, provided a turning point—a scholarly medium for research refinement and further development (Leininger, 1968).

The stage of research development made major contributions to contemporary scholarly nursing. It was also the stage in which tools of science left a major mark on curricula through the new offerings of research classes and statistics courses and through several publications in which major research tools and instruments were compiled and combined.

These stages have a global parallel. Progress in knowledge development is also influenced by international levels of education. Some countries, such as Australia and Germany, moved nursing education from hospital training to university training in the 1980s and 1990s, respectively. Other countries continued to follow, though many maintained different educational level programs. In the process, there has been a steady increase in philosophical and theoretical dialogues, as well as a cumulative trajectory of research productivity.

These, then, were the beginnings of nursing inquiry and science. During this stage, as in other sciences, researchers emphasized scientific syntax—the process rather than the substance of research (Kuhn, 1970). The binding frameworks or depositories of collected facts were still lacking. Nevertheless, the syntax of the discipline had been formulated.

Stage of Theory

Eventually, the fundamental questions about the essence of nursing—its mission and its goals—began to surface in a more organized way. An incisive group of leaders, nurses who believed that theory should guide the practice of nursing, wrote about the need for theory, the nature of nursing theory, philosophers' views of theory, and how nursing theory ought to be shaped. Although the conceptual schemata of nurse theorists for the discipline of nursing appeared during the education and administration stages of the discipline, it was not until the emergence of the stage of theory that they were taken seriously (Nursing Theory Think Tank, 1979).

During this stage, arguments arose about whether nursing was merely a chapter of medicine or whether it was part of the biologic, natural, or physical sciences (analogous to the earlier Cartesian concept

that biology is simply a chapter of physics). The Cartesian concept was rejected (biology is indeed a distinct and autonomous science), and nursing continued to resist the implication that it was a part of medicine. It became clear to a new breed of nurse leaders—the philosophers and the theorists (or conceptualists, as some referred to them)—that nursing could not be reduced to a single science that drives inquiries into just one aspect of human beings, just as biology is not reducible to physics. Nursing is complex, necessitating its intrinsic autonomy in content and methods.

The search for conceptual coherence evolved from a preoccupation with syntax to the disciplined and imaginative study of the realities of nursing and the meaning and truths that guide its actions. Its development from preoccupation with scientific method to speculation and conceptualization is reminiscent of the development of philosophical thought in the 18th and 19th centuries. The 18th century was greatly influenced by Newton and by Bacon, who was in turn influenced by Descartes. The 19th century was dominated by Kant, whose hypothetical, deductive, and metaphysical approach encouraged the speculative nature of science. The speculators in nursing began to construct realities as they saw them, and their imaginative constructs evolved from their philosophical backgrounds and from their educational inclinations.

It was natural for theory development to be influenced by the paradigms of other disciplines, by the educational background of nurse theorists, and by the philosophical underpinnings of the time. Therefore, we find premises stemming from existentialism, analytical philosophy, and pragmatism guiding the development of those theories, sometimes explicitly and often implicitly. Nurses also adopted concepts and propositions from other paradigms, such as psychoanalysis, development, adaptation, and interaction, as well as from humanism, to guide its assessment and its action. Theories were developed in response to dissatisfaction with isolated findings in research. The emerging theories addressed the nature of the human being in interactions and transactions with the health care system, as well as the processes of problem solving and decision-making for assessment and intervention.

Although certain theoretical concepts were synthesized from diverse paradigms, most nursing theories, such as subsystems of behavior, role supplementation, therapeutic touch, and self-help, were definable and analyzable only from the nursing perspective. Theories offered a beginning agreement on the broad intellectual endeavors and the fundamental explanatory tasks of nursing. This stage offered knowledge of relevant phenomena, but uncertainty continued about the discipline of nursing and its intellectual goals. Just as in nuclear physics—when the first achievement was not one of observation or mathematical calculation but one of intellectual imagination—conceptual schemata evolved before there was any clear recognition of nursing's empirical scope. In nursing, theories helped the discipline to focus on its concepts and problems.

Rogers (1970) offered a conception of nursing that focused on the constant human interaction with the environment. Johnson (1980) developed the notion that a human being—a biologic system—is also an abstract system of behavior centered on innate needs. Levine (1967) and Orem (1971) proposed guidelines for nursing therapeutics that preserve the integrity of the human being, the psychology, the community affiliation—in short—the entire person. Orem (1985) reminded us that the human being is perfectly capable of self-care and should progress toward that goal.

Because of the earlier focus on education and professional identity, because the National League for Nursing (NLN) stipulated a conceptual framework for curricula, and because the truth of a theory had not yet been established using the empirical positivists' criteria of corroboration, emergent theories were not used to guide practice or research but were instead used to guide teaching. Consequently, scientific energies were dissipated in developing curricula that corresponded to these theories.

Although theories may have influenced practice through students, such influence was not documented in the literature, which focused more on theory in educational programs. As an educator who was a member of a school that used nursing theory (also called a model) as a framework for the curriculum, I experienced firsthand, in the mid-1960s, the conflicts that graduates of the program encountered when they wanted to use a nursing framework, one that they studied and experienced in their educational program, in practice, and were unable to do so because of its novelty and its esoteric concepts. Whether the use of nursing models in education rendered nursing care more effective and efficient is a matter left to speculation and was evidenced only in isolated incidents and through experiential narrative analyses that were discounted for their lack of universality and generalization. The graduates of programs based on nursing theories in the early

and mid-1960s should be encouraged to write the stories of their experiences with these theoretically based programs and the ways by which their practice was informed or not informed by these programs.

The nagging questions continued:

- What frameworks enhance safety in nursing practice?
- What are the goals of nursing care?
- What are the desired outcomes related to nursing care?
- How do nursing interventions relate to desired outcomes?
- What are the quality care criteria by which to judge nursing practice?

These questions continued to lead to one type of answer: Let us find a guiding paradigm or search for a universal theory with explanatory power for all dimensions of nursing, and, once we find this all-encompassing theory, we will be able to answer questions related to the discipline. This approach reminds us that Galileo and Descartes talked of the scientist's task as that of being able to decipher once and for all the secrets of nature and to arrive at the "one true structure" of the nature of the world. However, that was a Platonic ideal rather than a plain description of the task of scientific research. Later, scientists began to discard this line of pursuit. Physicists and physiologists "now believe that . . . we shall do better in these fields by working our way toward more general concepts progressively, as we go along, rather than insisting on complete generality from the outset" (Toulmin, 1977, p. 387). Toulmin proposed that "human behavior in general represents too broad a domain to be encompassed within a single body of theory" (p. 387). When scientists accept the need for multiple theories, and when they accept the process nature of science, it will be a "sign of maturity rather than defeatism" (p. 387) within the discipline.

Because nurse scientists searched for one theory for the entire discipline, the task was either overwhelming and too highly abstract (Rogers, 1970), or too simplistic and reductionist (Orem, 1971). The sentiment of practitioners was to question the possibility and usefulness of an all-encompassing theory, as evidenced by the meager literature throughout the 1960s and 1970s on nursing practice using nursing theory. The desire for a single conceptual framework to guide the nursing curriculum was carried to nursing practice. Nurse practitioners came to believe that they were being asked to make a choice between theories, and then adhere to that one particular theory to address all of their practice and research work. Because none of the theories addressed all aspects of nursing, practicing nurses avoided nursing theory, ignored it, or refused to use it. Many nurses abandoned the notion of a universal theory to describe and explain nursing phenomena and units of analysis and to guide nursing practice.

Three themes in nursing that evolved during this stage were acceptance of the complexity of nursing and the inevitability of multiple theories; acceptance of the need to test and corroborate major propositions of differing theories before dismissing any of them; and the idea that concepts or theories remaining in the field, through a cumulative effect, become the basis for the development of a specific perspective. *Dualism* and *pluralism* were the norms during the stage of theory. It was also during this stage that nursing developed the boundaries necessary to focus its inquiry and the flexibility necessary to allow expansion through creative endeavor.

Stage of Philosophy

As nurses began reflecting on the conceptual aspects of nursing practice, on defining the domain of nursing, and on the most appropriate methods for knowledge development, they turned to philosophical inquiries. The focus during this stage was on raising and answering questions about the nature of nursing knowledge (Carper, 1978; Silva, 1977), the nature of inquiry (Ellis, 1983), and the congruency between the essence of nursing knowledge and research methodologies (Allen, Benner, and Diekelmann, 1986). During this stage, philosophy was considered an attempt to understand the philosophical premises underlying nursing theory and research (Sarter, 1987) and an attempt to develop philosophical inquiry as a legitimate approach to knowledge development in nursing (Fry, 1989).

This stage influenced profoundly the intellectual discourse in nursing literature. During this stage, epistemological diversity was accepted and the need for ethical, logical, and epistemological inquiries was legitimized, as evidenced in the numerous philosophically based manuscripts accepted for publication (Ellis, 1983).

This stage was also marked by a scholarly maturity in the discipline, as its members acknowledged the limitation of appropriate tools to investigate fundamental and practical issues. Assumptions about wholeness of human beings, contextual variables, and holism of care called for congruent investigative tools, and nurse scholars acknowledged the complexity of capturing nursing phenomenon

using existing tools (Newman, 1995; Stevenson and Woods, 1986). Accepting limitations while maintaining the reality of the contextuality and complexity of the phenomenon represents a marked scholarly maturity and the potential to focus on the development of appropriate tools.

Earlier during this stage, discussions encompassed the different "ways of knowing" in nursing and espoused a call for going beyond the empirical (Carper, 1978). These epistemological discussions focusing on the structure of knowledge, nature of theory, criteria for analysis, and justification of particular methodologies for knowledge development significantly contributed to the discovery and construction of an identity for the discipline of nursing. As theorists and metatheorists discussed the philosophical bases that shaped nursing knowledge (Allen et al., 1986; Roy, 1995), a new set of questions emerged. These questions reflected more the values and meaning of the knowledge being developed and the consequences of this knowledge on nursing practice, and focused less on the structure and justification of knowledge (Bradshaw, 1995; Silva, Sorrell, and Sorrell, 1995).

The emphasis on knowing was complemented by another emphasis on "being." The being was not limited to the nurse, or to the patient, but to each separately and to both joined in caring interactions (Benner, 1994; Newman, 1995). This philosophical stage, encompassing both components of epistemology and ontology, provided nurses with the legitimacy to ask and answer questions related to values, meanings, and realities using multiple philosophical and theoretical bases.

This philosophical stage persists, overlapping with the following stage of integration. Dialogues about postcolonialism provide the philosophical canons for understanding how domination, power, and resistance influence health care encounters at all different levels, from the individual to society (Kirkham and Anderson, 2002). The postcolonial scholarship in nursing was informed by the discourse in the discipline on race, culture, ethnicity, diversity, and power differential. It refers to and frames the theoretical and empirical work of people's experiences living under the oppression of colonial control. Using this philosophical stand, we can better understand the effects of diversity in skin color, religion, sexual preference, ethnicity, heritage, and class in shaping responses to health and illness. It allows health care professionals to access the meaning of marginalization. (See Chapter 8 for discussions about paradigms that influence nursing thought.)

Postmodernism, a reaction by philosophers to positivism, translated in nursing into a prevailing sentiment described by Whall as "Let's get rid of all nursing theory" (Whall, 1993; Whall and Hicks, 2002). Although the context is vital to postmodernism philosophy, universal totality is not possible. Other concepts that characterize postmodernism are relativism, deconstruction, context, atheoretical narratives, and structural influences.

Stage of Integration

This stage has seven universal characteristics, each described in the subsequent text. They should be used to stimulate thinking and discussions about the state of development of our discipline, both nationally and internationally. This stage differs from the next stage in its internal versus external integration with other disciplines. A first characteristic of this stage is the use of substantive dialogues and discussions focused on identifying coherent structures of the discipline of nursing at large and of its specific areas of specialization (Schlotfeldt, 1988). The structures include scientific, theoretical, philosophical, and clinical knowledge that is focused on the nursing domain and its phenomena. These dialogues take place in conferences, think tanks, and themed journal editions devoted to the development of middle-range and situation-specific theories focused on an aspect of nursing.

A second characteristic of this stage is the development of educational programs that are organized around substantive areas through the integration of theory, research, and practice—such as environment and health, symptom management, or transitions and health. It is also manifested in the ease by which nursing administrators, clinicians, and educators use theoretical nursing, and in the increasing dialogue among members of the discipline regarding matters related to knowledge, discovery, and development that is focused on and emanates from the domain of nursing.

A third characteristic of this stage is the evaluation of different aspects of theoretical nursing by members of the discipline—nursing clinicians, teachers, administrators, researchers, and theoreticians. Evaluation is not limited to theory testing; it includes description, analysis, and critiques as well. Each of these processes is important in the development and progress of our discipline because of its diverse philosophical bases.

A fourth characteristic of this stage is the attention that members of the discipline give to the strategies of knowledge development that are congruent with the discipline's shared assumptions and that consider the conditions of holism, patterning, experience, and meaning (Newman, 1995).

A fifth characteristic is the involvement of members of specialty fields in developing theories that are pertinent to the phenomena of that particular field. This involvement does not preclude similar attention to theories related to phenomena of the domain of nursing at large; for example, theories to describe and intervene in symptoms.

A sixth characteristic is the critical reappraisal of philosophical and theoretical underpinnings that have guided the definitions and conceptualizations of the central concepts of the nursing domain, as well as the methodologies used to generate knowledge. An example of such discourse is the reappraisal of the definition of *client* in the nursing literature and the congruency of these definitions with domain assumptions (Allen, 1987). Another example is the dialogue about melding different methods to generate knowledge that is more congruent to the tenets of a human science, such as grounded theory, feminist theory, and critical theory (Kushner and Morrow, 2003).

A seventh characteristic of this stage is the creative ways by which academic institutions in nursing become involved with patient care, either through academically run clinics (nursing clinics), or by developing clinically based faculty positions.

Stage of Interdisciplinarity and Interprofessionalism

The stage of integration leads to and overlaps the stage of interdisciplinarity and interprofessionalism. The road map for the National Institutes of Health (NIH) at the beginning of the 21st century provided a strong impetus for a different type of integration, one that challenged members of different disciplines to build programs of research that incorporate the theories and evidence from different fields. Although nursing has consistently depended upon, borrowed from, and shared the research and theories of other disciplines, the drive for interdisciplinary education and teaching research was now being promoted at leading research institutions. A central tenet of this stage is the forging of relationships between researchers and clinicians who are members of different disciplines, to develop joint institutes, advance research programs, or to provide more comprehensive education. Centers for sleep research, pain management, palliative care, complementary and alternative practices, safe practice, and gunshot injuries are examples of areas that require the expertise of members of different disciplines. A similar move to reflect the nature and complexity of science was initiated at the NIH. The question that drove these institutes was whether they should reflect discipline or an area of science. Time will tell whether a move away from disciplinary institutes will continue to support the development of disciplines horizontally as well as vertically. More discussion of disciplines and interdisciplines is provided in Chapter 19.

This stage is also reflected in the recruitment and hiring of faculty to teach across disciplines, as well as in educational reports that promoted changing curricula to incorporate interprofessional education. Many professors hold appointments in different departments and schools (e.g., schools of medicine, engineering, nursing, etc.), and that in itself exposes students to multiple disciplinary perspectives. At the University of Pennsylvania, the "Penn Integrates Knowledge" (PIK) University Professors program was developed to encourage schools to consider recruiting faculty members whose research and teaching transcends schools and can attract students from different fields. Simultaneously, an international commission was formed, *The Commission on Education of Health Professionals for the 21st Century*, with support from the Bill and Melinda Gates Foundation, the Rockefeller Foundation, and the China Medical Board, to review education for professional students, particularly those in public health, medicine, and nursing. One of its major recommendations in its report that was published in *The Lancet* is the development and implementation of innovative teaching and learning approaches that integrate educational experiences interprofessionally (Frenk, Chen, Bhutta, et al., 2010). Furthermore, the recommendations include giving attention to utilizing the most advanced, up-to-date, cutting-edge technology and information systems to enhance interprofessional and global education.

Stage of Technology and Information Systems

Health care records, robotic medication dispensers, tele-home care, long-distance monitoring, virtual surgeries, and voice mail reminders of appointments and medications are characteristic of this stage in the history of the development of the nursing discipline. Theories that incorporate variables and conditions related to informatics and technologic breakthroughs are necessary drivers for this stage. Self-care practices take on different meanings for individuals and families when they incorporate the most advanced and up-to-date information disseminated by scientists and clinicians to the public via the internet. Self-care practices and goals also incorporate the use of such new monitoring devices as home blood pressure apparatus, glucose kits, self-diagnosis protocols, and self-monitoring gadgets. The ability to sort among accurate and inaccurate information, and the alternative "if-then" scenarios that result, will need to be guided by situation-specific theories that incorporate guidelines for clinicians and consumers (An, Hayman, Panniers, et al., 2007).

MILESTONES IN THEORY DEVELOPMENT

The transitions in the trajectory of the development of theoretical nursing is marked by several milestones, which are identified through an analysis of theoretical literature that appeared in selected nursing journals between 1950 and 2015. These milestones substantially changed the position of theory in nursing and profoundly influenced the further development of theoretical nursing. Each milestone is defined and briefly described here (Table 5-1). Identifying and defining these milestones challenges others to explore the impact

TABLE 5-1	Theory Development in Nursing: Milestones
Prior to 1955	From Florence Nightingale to nursing research
1955–1960	The birth of nursing theory
1961–1965	Theory: A national goal for nursing
1966–1970	Theory development: A tangible goal for academics
1971–1975	Theory syntax
1976–1980	A time to reflect
1981–1985	Nursing theories' revival: Emergence of the domain concepts
1986–1990	From metatheory to concept development
1991–1995	Middle-range theories
1996–2000	Situation-specific theories
2001–2005	Evidence means research, not theory
2006–2010	Diversity in thought: Linking theory and practice
2011–2015	Voiced nurses

each milestone may have had on the progress and development of nursing knowledge.

Prior to 1955—From Florence Nightingale to Nursing Research

The significant milestone of the period before 1955, which has influenced the subsequent development of all nursing science, was the establishment of the journal, *Nursing Research*, with the goal of reporting on scientific investigations for nursing by nurses and others (Fig. 5-1). The journal's most significant goal was to encourage scientific productivity. The establishment of the journal confirmed that nursing is indeed a scientific discipline and that its progress will depend on whether nurses pursue truth through an avenue that respectable disciplines take, namely, research. Although Nightingale may

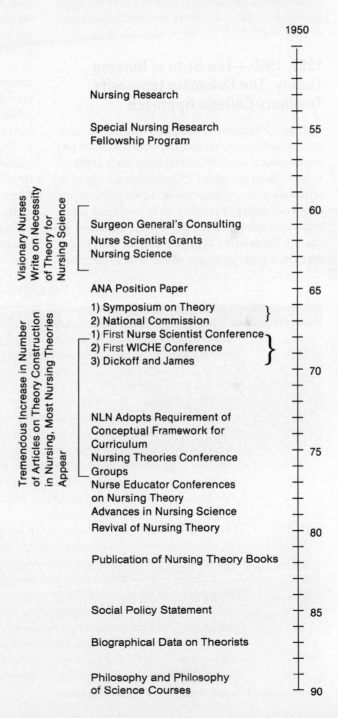

Figure 5-1 Chronology of the development of theoretical nursing.

have provided the beginning impetus for research and theory, initially, her impact was most keenly felt in nursing education. Education of nurses had predominantly occurred in diploma programs, but this period marked a beginning interest in providing different routes for nurses' education.

This period was otherwise uneventful for nursing theory, except that the establishment of nursing research publications provided the framework for a questioning attitude that may have set the stage for inquiries that led to more theoretical discourses in later years.

1955–1960—The Birth of Nursing Theory: The Columbia University Teachers College Approach

Although Florence Nightingale's ideas about nursing, focusing on the relationship between health and environment, were developed in the early 1900s, it was not until the mid-1950s that nurses began to articulate a theoretical view of nursing. Questions about the nature of nursing, its mission and goals, and about nurses' roles drove nurse educators to capture the answers to these questions and present them in a more coherent whole. These questions

grew out of an interest in changes in the educational preparation of nurses from diploma to baccalaureate programs, out of concerns about what to include or exclude in curricula, and about what nurses needed to learn to function as nurses.

Columbia University's Teachers College, where the first professor of nursing, M. Adelaide Nutting, was appointed, offered graduate programs that focused on education and administration, to prepare graduates as expert educators and administrators. Although the focus of that visionary program was not on nursing science or nursing theory, participants in this program must have felt that they were in an environment that promoted dialogue and debate of philosophical and theoretical questions. Of note, in 1999, the nursing education program celebrated 100 years of influence, a well-placed celebration given that most theorists who offered a conception of nursing during that decade were educated at Teachers College; these included Peplau, Henderson, Hall, Abdellah, King, Wiedenbach, and Rogers (Table 5-2).

Being prepared for functional roles and experiencing a sense of competency in preparing syllabi, setting staffing patterns, and so on may have freed the creative abilities of these scholars for other aspects

TABLE 5-2	Nursing Theorists: 1950–1980
1952	Hildegarde Peplau. *Interpersonal relations in nursing.* Also published 1962, 1963, 1969.
1955	Virginia Henderson. *Textbook of the principles and practice of nursing* (with B. Harmer). Also 1966, 1972, 1978.
1959	Dorothy Johnson. *A philosophy of nursing.* Also 1961, 1966, 1974.
1959	Lydia Hall. *A philosophy of nursing.* Also 1963 (and by others, 1975).
1960	Faye Abdellah. *Patient-centered approaches to nursing.* Also 1965, 1973.
1961	Ida Jean Orlando. *The dynamic nurse-patient relationship.*
1963	D. Howland and E. McDowell. *A hospital system model.*
1964	D. Howland and E. McDowell. *The measurement of patient care: A conceptual framework.*
1964	Joyce Travelbee. *Interpersonal aspects of nursing.* Also 1969, 1971, 1979.
1964	E. Wiedenbach. *Clinical nursing: A helping art.* Also 1967, 1969, 1970, 1977.
1966	Myra Levine. *Adaptation and assessment.*
1966	M. Harms and F. McDonald. *A new curriculum design.*
1967	Myra Levine. *An introduction to clinical nursing.* Also 1969, 1971, 1973.
1968	Imogene King. *A conceptual framework of reference for nursing.* Also 1971, 1975.
1969	Joyce Travelbee. *Interventions in psychiatric nursing.* Also 1971 (1979).
1970	Martha Rogers. *An introduction to the theoretical basis of nursing.* Also 1980.
1970	Sister Callista Roy. *Adaptation: A conceptual framework for nursing.* Also 1974, 1976, 1980, 1984.
1971	Imogene King. *Toward a theory for nursing: General concepts of human behavior.*
1971	Dorothea Orem. *Nursing: Concepts of practice.* Also 1981, 1982, 1985, 1991.
1972	Betty Neuman. *The Betty Neuman health-care systems model.* Also 1989.
1976	Josephine Patterson and L. Zderad. *Humanistic nursing.* Also 1988.

For complete citations, see Chapter 21 under appropriate authors.

of the scholarly process, such as theory or conceptual model development. And, although other experiences and programs may have directly influenced these scholars in their theoretical pursuits (e.g., Rogers' doctoral preparation at Johns Hopkins), it appears that the philosophy of Teachers College indirectly left an impact, not only on psychiatric theory and research, but also on theoretical thinking in all of nursing (Sills, 1977). Asking and answering questions about the influence of scholarly environments on preparing productive scholars may have stimulated the search for the nature of scholarship, which may have led to questions related to the nature of the nursing identity.

Peplau (1952), using Harry Stack Sullivan's theory title and concepts to develop her own, produced the first articulated concept of nursing as an interpersonal relationship, with components of interpersonal processes central to nursing needing to be elucidated and analyzed. The field of psychiatric nursing subsequently was substantially developed using Peplau's ideas. Other theories that evolved in the 1960s were based on those early conceptions of nursing. For example, Virginia Henderson, with Bershan Harmer, developed the early seeds of a nursing theory that was published in the mid-1950s in a textbook on the principles and practice of nursing.

The request from the International Council of Nursing (ICN) to define nursing and its mission led to the subsequent ICN statement in 1958 that appeared in a publication with wide distribution and that was adapted internationally (Henderson, 1966, p. 15). The message given by both Peplau and Henderson was that nursing has a specific and unique mission and that this mission has some order and organization that can be communicated. These articulated wholes represented the beginnings of theories in nursing.

Abdellah's nursing theory, evolving from her work at Columbia University, is another example of the influence of that school on theoretical nursing (Abdellah, Beland, Martin, et al., 1961). Abdellah's doctoral dissertation in 1953 at Teachers College, under the leadership of Hildegard Peplau, focused on determining covert aspects of nursing problems. The results of her research were subsequently published in *Nursing Research,* marking the beginning of her attempts at theorizing the nursing care process. Her conceptualization of nursing care evolved from her dissertation research and from another study completed in 1955, on the needs of patients for nursing care. The latter was based on data collected from patients, nurses, and doctors.

Abdellah developed her conception of what nursing is by focusing attention on patients rather than on techniques.

Ideas of other theorists were formulated around the need for a binding framework to guide curricula, but their writing and publications did not have the instant impact as that of Peplau, Henderson, and Abdellah on theoretical nursing. Their conceptions were slow to have an impact on nursing. Orem's ideas were first published in a guide for developing a curriculum for practical nursing in 1959. Patient needs were also the focus. Hall developed, in 1959, and implemented, in 1963, a concept of nursing based on needs and interpersonal relations at the Loeb Center for Nursing and Rehabilitation. One can see the influence of both Peplau and Henderson in her writing (Hall, 1963).

Independent of the Teachers College group of theorists, Johnson was beginning to play a central role in conceptualizing nursing. Johnson's (1959) analysis of the nature of science in nursing was undoubtedly a milestone in drawing attention to the potential of nursing as a scientific discipline and in advocating the development of its unique knowledge base. At that time, Johnson tentatively suggested that nursing knowledge is based on a theory of nursing diagnosis that is distinct and different from medical diagnosis. The substantive matter for such diagnosis, the beginning of Johnson's theory, was starting to be formulated at this time. (See Chapter 21 for appropriate citations for each theorist.)

1961–1965—Theory: A National Goal for Nursing

From a reduced conception of a human being as "an illness" or "a surgery," with signs and symptoms, nursing theory in the late 1950s refocused nursing attention on the individual as a set of needs and nursing as a set of unique functions. Still, a reductionist approach to nursing existed. The 1960s, with its turbulent social issues, the Camelot goals of harmony and coexistence, and the influence of Peplau may have prompted the refocusing of nursing from its stated mission of meeting patients' needs to the goal of establishing a relationship between the nurse and client. If relationships are effectively established through interpersonal interactions (as previously articulated by [Peplau, 1952], and as advocated by a new group of theorists), then nursing care can meet the needs of the patient—not as defined by nurses, but as perceived by the patient.

During this period, the Yale School of Nursing's position, influenced by the Columbia Teachers College graduates who became faculty members at Yale, was beginning to be formulated. To these scholars, nursing was considered a process rather than an end, an interaction rather than content, and a relationship between two human beings rather than an interaction between unrelated nurse and patient. Multiple social forces helped the Yale group to develop its ideas into concepts of nursing. Federal grant money was available for preparation ranging from psychiatric nursing to teaching positions, for identifying psychiatric concepts in nursing, and for developing an integrated curriculum. The availability of time and resources, therefore, was significant in providing the necessary push, as well as the appropriate environment in which to reflect on nursing's mission and goals.

Although the work of the faculty of the Yale School of Nursing may have profoundly influenced nursing research in the United States in the 1960s, its influence on theory was not as marked at the time. A revival of that impact came in the 1980s, as nurses acknowledged Yale's strategies for theory development; this is evidenced by the reconsideration of Orlando's work (Schmieding, 1983, 1987, 1988) and by the paradigmatic shift in nursing research to phenomenology (Oiler, 1982; Omery, 1983; Silva and Rothbart, 1984). These writers' conceptualization of nursing, therefore, was not the milestone that prompted the evolution of the next stage of theory. Rather, it was the position paper of the American Nurses Association (ANA)—in which nursing was defined as care, cure, and coordination, and in which theory development was identified as a most significant goal for the profession of nursing—that may have been influential in the further development of theoretical nursing (ANA, 1965).

Two other significant developments occurred during this period. First, federally supported fellowship programs were created to finance graduate studies for nurses interested in research careers, helping them pursue doctoral education in related fields such as biology, physiology, sociology, and anthropology. The graduates of these programs are those who, in the mid-1970s, further developed metatheoretical ideas. The second development was the inauguration of the journal, *Nursing Science*. Although short-lived, it was a medium for the exchange of ideas on theory and science in nursing and a confirmation that nursing is an evolving science with theoretical principles and underpinnings.

1966–1970—Theory Development: A Tangible Goal for Academics

With the ANA's recommendation that theory development was of highest priority in the profession, and with the availability of federal support, a symposium sponsored by Case Western Reserve University was held as part of the nursing science program. This symposium was divided into three parts. The part focusing on theory was held on October 7, 1967, and was considered a milestone during this period (Table 5-3). The papers were published in *Nursing Research* a year later. These publications supported what were previously considered simply perceptions and conceptions of theoretical nursing from an isolated number of theorists. Not only did a group of leaders in nursing get together to discuss theory in nursing, but the official scientific journal of the field recognized the significance of these proceedings by publishing them.

Nurses also received confirmation from two philosophers and a nurse theorist (who had been involved in teaching nurses at Yale for 5 years) that theories are significant for the practice of nursing, that the practice of nursing is amenable to theoretical development, and that nurses are capable of developing theories (Dickoff, James, and Wiedenbach, 1968a, 1968b). The presentations given at the October 1967 meeting and the subsequent series of publications by Dickoff and James (1968, 1971) and Dickoff et al. (1968a, 1968b) influenced the discipline of nursing profoundly, as evidenced by the classic nature of those publications and by the subsequent acceleration in publications related to theory. Nursing theory was defined, goals for theory development were set, and the confirmation of outsiders (people outside the field of nursing, non-nursing philosophers) was productive.

Although the insiders (the nurse theorists) may have charted the course of action for theory development, Dickoff and colleagues, by introducing their metatheory of nursing, helped ameliorate some of the skepticism regarding theory that still pervaded nursing at this time. Prior to the discourse initiated by the authors' work, critics had dominated the discussion of theory within nursing by maintaining that theories are scientific and as such should be developed through empirical and positivistic models. The evidence supporting that skepticism was derived from omission rather than commission. When theories were used during this period, they were used in conjunction with education and not in practice (except by faculty and students at New York

TABLE 5-3	Theory Development in Nursing: A Historical Perspective
1860	Florence Nightingale addresses the need for research and the educational preparation of nurses.
1900–1950	Diploma schools served as major source of nurses—the Flexner Report for Medicine.
1952	*Nursing Research* first published.
1955	Establishment of the Special Nurse Research Fellowship Program in the National Institutes of Health, Division of Nursing.
1959	D.E. Johnson. The nature of a science of nursing. *Nursing Outlook*, 7, 292–294.
1960	R.N. Schlotfeldt. Reflections on nursing research. *American Journal of Nursing*, 60(4), 492–494. (The primary task of nursing research is to develop theories that serve as a guide to practice.)
1961	Surgeon General's Consultant Group on Nursing appointed to advise the Surgeon General on nursing needs and to identify the appropriate role of the federal government in assuring adequate nursing services in the nation. This group strongly supported nursing research and recommended a substantial increase in funds.
1961	D.E. Johnson. Patterns in professional nursing education. *Nursing Outlook*, 9, 608. (Nursing science may evolve more easily through the identification of common but major problems of patients that are of direct concern to nursing.)
1962	Nurse Scientist Graduate Training Grants Program
1963	*Nursing Science* first published
1963	M.E. Rogers. Some comments on the theoretical basis of nursing practice. *Nursing Science*, 1, 11–13. (The theoretical base of nursing practice is nursing science . . . a body of scientific knowledge characterized by descriptive, explanatory, and predictive principles . . . developed through synthesis and resynthesis of selected knowledges from the humanities and the biological, physical, and social sciences. . . . It assumes its own "unique scientific" mix through selection and patterning of these knowledges.)
1963	M.E. Rogers. Building a strong educational foundation. *American Journal of Nursing*, 63(6), 941. (The explanatory and predictive principles of nursing make possible nursing diagnosis and knowledgeable intervention toward predictable goals . . . nursing science is not additive, but creative.)
1964	D.E. Johnson. Nursing and health education. *International Journal of Nursing Studies*, 1, 219. (Nurses must be socialized as scholars and must develop commitment to inquiry and skill in the use of scientific knowledge.)
	J.S. Berthold. Theoretical and empirical clarification of concepts. *Nursing Science*, 406–422.
	M.I. Brown. (Spring). Research in the development of nursing theory. *Nursing Research*, 13, 109–112. (Assess progress of theory development in nursing and emphasize need for explicit relationship of research to theory.)
	F.S. Wald and R. C. Leonard. (1964). Toward development of nursing practice theory. *Nursing Research*, 13(4), 309–313.
1965	American Nurses' Association. Educational preparation for nurse practitioners and assistants to nurses: A position paper.
	P. Putnam. A conceptual approach to nursing theory. *Nursing Science*, 430–442.
1967	V.S. Cleland. The use of existing theories. *Nursing Research*, 16(2), 118–121.
1967	L.H. Conant. (Spring). A search for resolution of existing problems in nursing. *Nursing Research*, 16, 115.
	Symposium on Theory Development in Nursing. (Reported in Nursing Research, 1968, 17[3].)
1967–1970	National Commission for the Study of Nursing and Nursing Education, Jerome F. Lysaught, director.
1968	First Nurse Scientist Conference on The Nature of Science in Nursing. Sponsored by University of Colorado School of Nursing, Dr. Madeleine Leininger, chair. (Reported in Nursing Research, 1969, 18[5].)
	First Annual WCHEN Communicating Research Conference

(continued)

TABLE 5-3	Theory Development in Nursing: A Historical Perspective (*continued*)
1968	J. Dickoff and P. James. A theory of theories: A position paper. *Nursing Research*, 17(3), 197–206. (Professional disciplines are obligated to go a step further than explanation and prediction in theory construction, to the development of prescriptive theory.)
	J. Dickoff, P. James, and E. Wiedenbach. Theory in a practice discipline: Part I. Practice oriented theory. *Nursing Research*, 17(5), 415–435.
	Idem. theory in a practice discipline: Part II. Practice oriented theory. *Nursing Research*, 17(6), 545–554.
	R. Ellis. (1968). Characteristics of significant theories. *Nursing Research*, 17(3), 217–222.
	D.E. Johnson. Theory in nursing: Borrowed and unique. *Nursing Research*, 17(3), 206–209.
	M. Moore. Nursing: A scientific discipline. *Forum*, 7(4), 340–347.
	J.L. Sasmor. Toward developing theory in nursing. *Nursing Forum*, 7(2), 191–200.
1969	G. Mathwig. Nursing science: The theoretical core of nursing knowledge. *Image*, 3, 9–14, 20–23.
	R. McKay. Theories, models, and systems for nursing. *Nursing Research*, 18(5), 393–399.
	C.M. Norris (Ed.). Proceedings: First, second, and third nursing theory conference. University of Kansas, 1969 and 1970.
1971	F. Cleary. A theoretical model: Its potential for adaptation to nursing. *Image*, 4(1), 14–20.
	I.M. Harris. Theory building in nursing: A review of the literature. *Image*, 4(1), 6–10.
	M. Jacobson. Qualitative data as a potential source of theory in nursing. *Image*, 4(1), 10–14.
	J.F. Murphy (Ed.). *Theoretical issues in professional nursing.* New York: Appleton-Century-Crofts.
	I. Walker. Toward a clearer understanding of the concept of nursing theory. *Nursing Research*, 20(5), 428–435.
1972	M. Newman. Nursing's theoretical evolution. *Nursing Outlook*, 20(7), 449–453.
	NLN Council of Baccalaureate and Higher Degree Programs approved its "Criteria for the Appraisal of Baccalaureate and Higher Degree Programs in Nursing," including criterion stating that curricula should be based on a conceptual framework.
1973	M.E. Hardy. The nature of theories. In M. Hardy (Ed.), *Theoretical foundations for nursing.* New York: MSS Information Corporation.
	The Nursing Development Conference Group. (1973). *Concept formulation in nursing: Process and product.* Boston: Little, Brown & Co.
1974	M.E. Hardy. Theories: Components, development, evaluation. *Nursing Research*, 18, 100–107.
	A. Jacox. Theory construction in nursing: An overview. *Nursing Research*, 23, 4–13.
	D.E. Johnson. Development of theory: Requisite for nursing as a primary health profession. *Nursing Research*, 18, 372–377.
1975	Nursing Theories Conference Group. (Formed out of a concern for the need for materials to help students of nursing understand and use nursing theories in nursing practice.)
1978	Advances in Nursing Science. S.K. Donaldson and D. Crowley. The Discipline of Nursing. *Nursing Outlook*, 26(2), 113–120.
1979	M.A. Newman. *Theory development in nursing.* Philadelphia: F. A. Davis.
1982	M.J. Kim and D.A. Moritz. *Classifications of nursing diagnosis.* New York: McGraw-Hill.
1983	L.O. Walker and K.C. Avant. *Strategies for theory construction in nursing.* New York: Appleton-Century-Crofts.
	J. Fitzpatrick and A. Whall. *Conceptual models of nursing: Analysis and application.* Bowie, MD: R.J. Brady Co.
	P.L. Chinn and M.K. Jacobs. *Theory and nursing: A systematic approach.* St. Louis: C.V. Mosby.
	H.S. Kim. *The nature of theoretical thinking in nursing.* New York: Appleton-Century-Crofts.
	I.W. Clements and F.B. Roberts. *Family health: A theoretical approach to nursing care.* New York: John Wiley & Sons.
	P.L. Chinn. *Advances in nursing theory development.* Rockville, MD: Aspen Systems.
1984	J. Fawcett. *Analysis and evaluation of conceptual models.* Philadelphia: F.A. Davis.

See Chapters 11–13 and 21 for evidence of increasing publications related to each of the theorists.

University and Yale University) or research. (Refer to the theory literature in Chapter 20 for documentation of the omission.)

The metatheorists in nursing did not acknowledge existing theories, instead focusing on questions about the types of new theories nurses should develop rather than to the nature of the substantive content of those theories. The metatheorists may have ignored existing nursing theories because of lack of awareness of their existence or they intentionally ignored them because they did not define them as theories. Some of these first metatheorists were Ellis (1968) and Wiedenbach (Dickoff et al., 1968a, 1968b). Dickoff and James (1968), who were philosophers by training, created debates about whether the theories should be basic or borrowed, pure or applied, descriptive or prescriptive. Existing conceptualizations were not used as examples.

Accomplishments at this stage can be summarized as:

- Nursing is a field amenable to theorizing.
- Nurses can develop theories.
- Practice is a rich area for theory.
- Practice theory should be the goal for theory development in nursing.
- Nurses' highest theory goal should be prescriptive theory, but it is acceptable to develop descriptive and explanatory theories.

1971–1975—Theory Syntax

There was a period, just before the research enterprise in nursing focused on answering significant questions in the field, when nurse researchers focused on discussing and writing about research methodology. A parallel exists in the area of theory. The period from 1966 to 1970 resulted in a beginning focus on theory development, which was followed by attempts at identifying the structural components of theory (see Table 5-3). Metatheorists dominated this period. The emphasis was on articulating, defining, and explicating theory components and on the processes inherent in theory analysis and critique. Nurse theorists were no longer questioning whether nursing needed a theory or whether or not theory could be developed in nursing; questions of this period focused on what is meant by theory (Ellis, 1968, 1971; Walker, 1971), on what are the major components of theory (Hardy, 1974; Jacox, 1974), and on ways to analyze and critique theories (Duffey and Muhlenkamp, 1974). Education of nurses in basic, natural, and social sciences through the federally supported nurse–scientist programs produced

a cadre of nurses who shared a common goal: the establishment of the unique knowledge base of nursing. Discussions of what constituted theory and the identification of theory syntax seemed to be the means to achieve that goal.

Just before the end of this period, a milestone was achieved. Just as the ANA acknowledged the significance of theory development during the previous period, the NLN not only acknowledged theory but also made theory-based curriculum a requirement for accreditation. Schools of nursing were expected to select, develop, and implement a conceptual framework for their curricula. This requirement for accreditation was both a moving force and a major barrier to theory development. To use theory for curriculum development further heightened awareness of academic nursing to the significance of theory and to the available nursing theories. However, this requirement diverted the goal of *developing theories for practice* (those theories that would answer significant questions related to practice) *to the goal of using theory for education.* Nevertheless, this milestone increased the use of theory and discussions about theory and prompted more writing about the syntax of theory to help academicians and students understand and use theories in curriculum and teaching. The limited number of journals that acknowledge and promote theoretical nursing, the focus on promoting the publication of empirical research findings, and the growing financial difficulties of some journals were barriers to written exchanges on theory and theorizing.

1976–1980—A Time to Reflect

Nurse theorists were invited to participate in presentations, discussions, and debates in conferences sponsored by nurse educators, marking a significant milestone in the progress of theoretical nursing. A national conference devoted to nursing theory and the formation of the Nursing Theory Think Tank in 1978 further supported the direction of the profession toward the utilization of existing theory and the development of further theory to describe and explain nursing phenomena, to predict relationships, and to guide nursing care (Preview, 1978). This was the time for nurse academicians, who had used nursing theories as guiding frameworks for curricula, to consider putting theory to other uses, particularly in practice.

The inauguration of the journal, *Advances in Nursing Science,* with its focus on "the full range of activities involved in the development of science," including "theory construction, concept, and analysis" and the application of theory, was another significant milestone during this period (Chinn, 1978) (see Table 5-3). The focus of the journal on theory and theory development added more support to the significance of theoretical nursing and simultaneously gave nurses who were interested in theory the necessary medium in which to present and discuss their ideas. It allowed for the questioning and debate that is necessary for the development of theoretical bases in any discipline.

This period was characterized by questioning whether nursing's progress would benefit from the adoption of a single paradigm and a single theory of truth (Carper, 1978; Silva, 1977). More sophisticated debates about what types of theory nursing needs (Beckstrand, 1978a, 1978b, 1980) and about issues in theory (Crawford, Dufault, and Rudy, 1979) appeared in nursing literature. A more solid commitment to the development of theory emerged, combined with a specific direction to nurses' efforts in theory development (Donaldson and Crowley, 1978; Hardy, 1978). The links between theory and research were considered and discussed (Batey, 1977; Fawcett and Downs, 1986), the path was charted for bridging the theory–research gaps between theory and practice (Barnum, 1990), theory and philosophy were examined (Silva, 1977), and the role of each in the development of nursing knowledge was clarified (see Fig. 5-1). Domain concepts were beginning to be identified, and their acceptance was demonstrated in the next period.

1981–1985—Nursing Theories' Revival: Emergence of the Domain Concepts

In this period, theory began to be questioned less and pluralism debated less. This period was characterized by an acceptance of the significance of theory for nursing and, furthermore, by the inevitability of the need for the development of nursing theory. Doctoral programs in nursing incorporated theory into their curricula and considered it a core content area, ranking it at the top of all other core content (Beare, Gray, and Ptak, 1981). This period was also characterized by enlightened international interest in theoretical nursing as manifested in conferences in Sweden and demand for consultations on theory teaching in Thailand, Korea, and Egypt, among other countries.

A review of theory literature during this period reveals the lack of debate on whether to use practice theory versus basic theory or borrowed versus nursing theory. Instead, there appeared to be more writing on the examination of nursing theories in relation to different research and practice problems and on comparisons between the different conceptualizations (Jacobson, 1984; Spangler and Spangler, 1983). Questions of this period included:

- What have we learned from theory?
- How can we use theory?

The second question was one that clinicians began to ask and for which there have been many useful dialogues.

The newly emerging syntax was used to analyze existing theories (Fawcett, 1984; Fitzpatrick and Whall, 1983). In addition, existing theories came to be thought of as the means to develop unique nursing knowledge. Concepts central to nursing were identified, and existing theory, the source of the identified concepts, was in turn reexamined in terms of further development and refinement (Crawford, 1982; Reeder, 1984).

This period was characterized by the nursing *theory advocates* who pleaded for the use of a nursing perspective in general or for the specific utilization of nursing theory (Adam, 1983; Dickson and Lee-Villasenor, 1982). (See *Advances in Nursing Science*, *Journal of Nursing Administration*, and *American Journal of Nursing* for examples of the American advocates and *Journal of Advanced Nursing* for examples of international advocates.) Another group also emerged during this period: the *theory synthesizers*. The difference between the advocates and the synthesizers was in the level of the scope of analysis. The advocates promoted nursing theory and demonstrated its use in research projects or in a limited practice arena. The synthesizers went beyond that limited use to describe and analyze how nursing theory had influenced nursing practice, education, research, and administration. The synthesizers are exemplified by, but not limited to, Fitzpatrick and Whall (1983, 1996) and Fawcett (1984, 1995). The Rogerian First National Conference (1983) and subsequent ones, in which theoreticians, practitioners, and researchers discussed the utility of Rogers' theory from different perspectives, is a different example of an effective synthesis of different uses of a theory. The planners of this conference belong to the group of theory synthesizers.

A few theory synthesizers graduated from New York University in the mid-1970s. One thing that cannot be ignored is the influence of New York

University's nursing program on advancing theoretical nursing. This is made evident by a review of the titles of doctoral dissertations in nursing from New York University from 1941 to 1983, which provide a clear example of how a school of nursing using a coherent theoretical framework can drive a coherent research agenda. Most of the titles of the dissertations indicate a nursing perspective, and there appears to have been an attempt at cumulative knowledge development. How and in what ways such a pattern may have influenced and may continue to influence theory development is an area worth further investigation and analysis; however, we do see a Rogerian conference every once in a while that brings many nurse scholars together to speak the same theory language and to show their research. The outcome of such gatherings on discovery, integration, and innovation of nursing knowledge is yet to be documented. (See the discussion of Rogers' theory in Chapter 13.)

This period was characterized by an acceptance of theory as a tool that emanates from significant practice problems and that can be used to guide practice and research. This period was also characterized by a greater clarity in the relationship between theory and research than between theory and practice.

One remaining confusion during this period was related to semantics. Conceptual models were referred to as conceptual frameworks, theories, metatheories, paradigms, and metaparadigms and, when differentiated, boundaries were not totally clear and properties not entirely distinct.

1986–1990—From Metatheory to Concept Development

Four characteristics of this milestone were epistemological debates, ontological analyses, an increase in concept development and analyses, and the acknowledgment of the gap between theory and practice. The epistemological debates included questions related to describing alternative approaches to knowledge development, such as the use of phenomenology, critical theory, and feminist or empiricist methodologies, and how to connect the dialectal approach to theory and practice (e.g., Allen, 1985; Allen et al., 1986; Hagell, 1989; Leonard, 1989). Although the debates were focused on knowledge development in general rather than on theoretical development of the discipline, these debates were related as well to the development of theoretical nursing. Concept development emerged as a potential link between the theoretical knowing and the practical doing.

Effective analyses were those that focused on ontological beliefs related to central nursing concepts, for example, environment (Chopoorian, 1986; Stevens, 1989) and health (Allen, 1985, 1986; Benner, 1984). These analyses added substantially to a more contextual approach to understanding each concept. These analyses also raised the awareness and the consciousness of nurses to the necessity of using frameworks that allow for an integrative, holistic, and contextual description of nursing phenomena, phenomena that go beyond the individual clients. Such frameworks, these authors demonstrated, maintained the integrity of the basic ontological beliefs that have historically guided nursing practice, for example, holism, integrated responses, and relationship with environment.

The third property of this milestone was an increase in writings related to concept development. These developments were different from earlier theory developments that included answers to such general questions as "What is nursing?" These analyses were more practice oriented, were integrative, and represented early attempts in the development of single domain theories. This was also the period in which a plea for substance was made (Chinn, 1987; Downs, 1988; Meleis, 1987; Woods, 1987). These authors echoed the sentiment of other discipline members by urging discourse that was more focused on substantive issues that were confronting health care recipients.

Process debates became more a potential force for theory development when and if they were grounded in substantive disciplinary content. Therefore, instead of debating whether critical theory or feminist theories were more appropriate as a philosophical base for the discipline, one may argue whether it was more effective to view environment or comfort from either or both perspectives. Such substantive debates then would add to or revise parameters and dimensions of that area of knowledge.

1991–1995—Middle-Range Theories

One significant milestone that marks the considerable progress in knowledge development in nursing is manifested in the numerous middle-range theories that evolved during this period. Some of these were labeled as theories (e.g., Younger's Theory of Mastery [1991] or Mishel's Theory of Uncertainty [1990]). Others were considered in the process of becoming theories. See Funk, Tornquist, Champage, et al. (1990) for discussions about key aspects of recovery and Hagerty, Lynch-Sauer, Patusky, et al. (1993) for their emerging theory of human relatedness. Middle-range theories focus on specific nursing phenomena that reflect and emerge from nursing practice and focus on clinical process (Meleis, 1987). They provide a conceptual focus and a mental image that reflect the discipline's values, but they do not provide prescriptions for practice or specific practice guidelines (Chinn, 1994).

1996–2000 Situation-Specific Theories

The emergence of situation-specific theories is a milestone for this period, although they were better defined in later years. They are theories that are more clinically specific and reflective of a particular context, and that may include blueprints for action. Although they were introduced first by Dickoff et al. (1968a, 1968b) as practice theories, they were further developed by Meleis in 1997. They are less abstract than middle-range theories but far more abstract than individual nurses' frameworks for practice designed for a specific situation (Meleis, 1997; Im, 2005; Im and Meleis, 1999). These situation-specific theories may emerge from synthesizing and integrating research findings and clinical exemplars about a specific situation or population with the intent of giving a framework or blueprint to understand the particular situation of a group of clients. They are theories that are developed to answer a set of coherent questions about situations that are limited in scope and limited in focus. For example, a conceptualization of patterns of responses to health–illness transitions of Middle Eastern immigrants could be developed from the results of research studies, the clinical exemplars, and the experience of nurses in their care of this population (Meleis, Isenberg, Koerner, et al., 1995). An example is work that has focused on Middle Eastern immigrants (Afghans, Iranians, Egyptians, and Arabs), supported by similar work on these populations in their native countries, which helps illuminate patterns of behavior and responses before immigration and helps in providing a historical and sociocultural context for the responses of immigrants in their new country. (See Chapter 17 for a full discussion about this type of theory.)

2001–2005—Evidence Means Research, Not Theory

Evidence-based practice evolved after much discourse in the literature from evidence-based practice to evidence-based nursing. During this milestone, the focus of the literature written about the discipline was on identifying the similarities and differences between utilizing models of care with best evidence, translating research into practice, and using applied research (French, 1999). To determine evidence, methodologies were discussed for defining the quality of individual studies, the methods for integrating study findings, and criteria for judging integrative findings and what constitutes evidence that could be used in the literature (Goode, 2000; McKee, Britton, Black, et al., 1999). Several properties distinguish this milestone. First, most of the dialogues were initially based on arguments from the medical field, which reduced "the evidence" to biomedical, empirical, and positivist variables and criteria (Lohr and Carey, 1999). A second property is a critical dialogue about eclectic views of evidence that may incorporate components that are more congruent with nursing science and emanate from how nursing knowledge and knowing have been defined. This critical dialogue includes discussions on widening the meaning of evidence to make it more pluralistic, to incorporate humanistic experiences as well as personal experiences as evidence of models of care to be used (Clarke, 1999). However, the criteria for judging evidence from within this framework have not been explored, and no definitive ideas been reached. A third property of this milestone is a focus on best strategies to implement the best evidence in health care institutions. Different models and approaches to utilizations are defined and explored utilizing teaching–learning theories as well as organizational change theories (Grol and Grimshaw, 1999).

The Cochrane Database of Systematic Review plays a major role in providing frameworks for rigorous reviews of data-based evidence, for integrating reviews for determining best-supported evidence, and for developing and implementing best organizational infrastructures to implement and promote best practices (Foxcroft, Cole, Fullbrook, et al., 2001).

The fourth property of this milestone is its global appeal and utilization of evidence-based concepts in different parts of the world. Nurses, researchers, and clinicians in different regions engaged in dialogues about integrative reviews and accessibility of research-based knowledge for clinicians (Thompson, McCaughan, Cullum, et al., 2001).

The last property of this milestone is the absence of a robust theoretical dialogue about the place of theory or philosophy in driving the nature of evidence, the premises supporting pluralism in methods, the framework for interpretation, and the principles behind the selection of outcomes. Shifting from an evidence-based discourse about practice to an inquiry-based dialogue could bring back a critical theoretical discourse to nursing practice (Doane and Varcoe, 2008; Holmes, Murray, Perron, et al., 2006; Holmes, Roy, and Perron, 2008).

2006–2010—Diversity in Thought: Linking Theory and Practice

A focus on diversity is a hallmark of this milestone in the ongoing journey toward the theoretical development of the discipline. As the agents of scholarship become diverse in identity, ethnicity, and heritage, and as they become more comfortable with their differences, their varices begin to appear in the literature, reflecting their different values, beliefs, and goals. Among the examples of the diversity in thought and in theories are those by nurses from different countries. Theorics were developed by nurses from Finland and Sweden and dialogues about more authentic theoretical formulations reflecting the realities of different countries gained more popularity (Salas, 2005).

Similarly, during this milestone, diversity of views on developing theories from a number of grounded theory research projects, as well as through integrating different theories, emerged with more robust dialogues than ever occurred before. Olshansky (2003), for example, conducted six grounded theory projects and developed a theory of "identity as infertile" and combined this theory with Miller's (1991) theory of "relational cultural" theory to explain potential vulnerability to depression of women whose identity is established as "infertile women." Both theories were integrated and provide a stronger explanation for identity shifts that occur post pregnancy for these women. The theory explains that although the women identified as "infertile women" were able to become pregnant, it is very difficult for them to perceive themselves as pregnant. This difficulty in identity is an obstacle to forming relationships with other pregnant women.

Diversity as a hallmark of this milestone was manifested in a variety of health–illness situations requiring a careful analysis of the factors that create diversity. Among these are age, race, ethnicity, country of heritage, gender, and sexual orientation. This awareness led theorists and researchers to critique prevailing approaches and assumptions and propose alternative and more contextually situated theoretical thoughts. Examples are Berman (2003) on the myths surrounding the power of children, Im and Meleis (2001) in their proposal for developing gender-sensitive theories that focus on health and illness, and Anderson, Perry, Blue, et al. (2003), who rewrote a conceptualization of cultural safety within postcolonial and postnationalist feminist theories.

Georges (2003) defined the prominent discourses that reflect this milestone. Her thesis is that there are two discourses in nursing that are shaping epistemic diversity in contemporary nursing. These are the discourses on science that are more broad and enlightened and a postmodernism discourse on marginalization. Both of these discourses provide a critique of dominant understanding and agreements on scholarship allowing freedom to represent the different perspectives on knowledge development. Epistemic diversity in an era that honors diversity in its broadest sense may free members of the discipline to be inclusive and may transform the discipline to make it truly reflective of the people nurses need to serve. Such diversity would also allow critique of power inequity as well as existing networks that support such inequities and transform social practices that tend to institutionalize dominant approaches to theory (Gustafson, 2005). Once again Hall (2003) reminds us in a powerful autobiographical note from her illness experience about how medicalization of illness experiences and the stronghold of the biomedical model are not in the best interest of patients and their families. Georges (2005) uses a critical feminist perspective to uncover her journey in rewriting her own identity as a clinician–theorist–academician–researcher. She provides a robust philosophical argument for the linking of theory and practice within the political and social context of the first decade of the 21st century. Such linking could occur through teaching theory using strategies that help students to develop their authentic voices about their practice. Properties of this milestone are critique of status quo, reconceptualization that is situated and contexted, and attention to analysis that honors diversity in cultures, ethnic backgrounds, heritage, language proficiency, gender, and sexual orientation.

With the diversity of thought came the decolonization of nursing from the biomedical model, from the patriarchal hierarchy, and from non-nursing institutional regulatory mechanisms (Holmes and Gastaldo, 2004; Holmes et al., 2008). Separating nursing from these paradigms is in itself liberating; however, a more compelling indicator of this liberation is the use of different paradigms to guide theory development and research, as is evident in the nursing literature produced at the end of the first decade of the 20th century (see examples in *Advances in Nursing Science*, *Nursing Inquiry*, and *Nursing Scholarship*).

2011–2015—Voiced Nurses

Theoretical discourses and the evidence generated by research gave nurses the language (concepts, theories) by which they can voice and support arguments for quality health care. Nurses are also more engaged in innovating health care through entrepreneurship. Theories and evidence are translated and disseminated in influencing health care delivery.

Two milestones are evident in this period. The first is the increasing visibility of nurses—both in the media and in the legislative halls—that accompanied the acknowledgment of their centrality to health care. The second is the engagement of nurses in entrepreneurship.

The first milestone—the increasing visibility of nurses—reflects nurses' confidence in sharing their stories publicly through letters to the editors, op-eds, columns, blogs, and social media. Researchers in nursing became more deliberate in translating their findings to the public through venues that are more readily accessible. As nurses continued to exercise their vices, the public's interest in nurses grew. Recognizing opportunity in this interest, the media began casting nurses as central characters in primetime television programs, depicting them as forceful clinicians (Garon, 2012).

The discourse surrounding health care reform (Patient Protection and Affordable Care Act, 2010, or "Obamacare") and the moral obligation of the government to provide safe, quality, and equitable health care for the U.S. population includes an acknowledgment that the nurse's role is central to the health care reform. The inclusion in the discourse of the need for increasing the number of nurses in the workforce, as well as ensuring the utilization of their full capacity, is in itself empowering for nurses. Therefore, the increasing dialogue about primary health care, patient-centered care, and collaborative partnerships between physicians and nurses, whether in conferences or in Institute of Medicine publications, honors and acknowledges the value of nursing knowledge and nursing care (Frenk et al., 2010; Institute of Medicine [IOM], 2011).

The second major milestone—the engagement in entrepreneurship—is evidenced in innovations made by nurses that reflect the nursing perspective and that impact nursing practice and research. Examples of these innovations include the launching of business models to provide interdependent care (Bowles, Chittams, Heil, et al., 2015), the development of mobile apps that facilitate patients' access to care and compliance with care regimens (Dougherty, Lipman, Hyams, et al., 2014), and the incorporation of telehealth and computers in nursing care and research programs (Im and Chang, 2013).

The juxtaposition of caring for the individual and her family within the environment of innovation and complexity of information and technology requires the nurse to develop new frameworks and models of care. This stage of the discipline's development is enriched by forging different and new partnerships between such disciplines as engineering, pharmacy, and the information sciences. Nurses are taking full advantage of the evidence produced through nursing knowledge and the use of technology and information systems to translate and disseminate nursing knowledge.

CONCLUSION

This chapter presented significant historical themes that are related to an interest in theoretical nursing. Progress and development in theoretical nursing was defined in terms of stages and milestones. A view of historical development offers a significant perspective on which current and future theoretical thinking can be built. Analysis of present development is deficient without tracing these historical themes.

REFLECTIVE QUESTIONS

1. In what ways does a review of the history of theoretical nursing development limit or promote progress in developing the discipline of nursing?

2. Which stages and milestones were vital for advancing nursing theory? Why?

3. Why do you think the environment and the culture of the schools of nursing at Columbia and Yale in the 1950s and 1960s contributed to the development of theoreticians and theoretical thinking?

4. Would the same properties of theoretical cultures contribute to creating gaps between theory research and practice? If so, how could these gaps be avoided within the political and social systems of the 21st century?

5. Can you identify more contemporary theoretical schools of thought? What environments may have led to each of these theoretical discourses?

6. Knowing about previous stages and milestones in the development of theoretical nursing, what would you predict about future stages and milestones? Provide strategies for creating these future stages and milestones.

7. What stages and milestones do you consider instrumental in understanding the history of theoretical nursing? Identify critical stages and milestones from your own perspective.

8. What insights have you gained about theoretical nursing from reading this chapter?

9. How would you describe the environment in your school (department)? In what ways does the environment in your school contribute to your scholarly development?

10. In what ways do you think the Affordable Care Act developed during President Barack Obama's administration may have contributed to furthering or hindering progress in theoretical development of the nursing discipline?

11. Reflect on the absence of men's voices in the development of theoretical nursing. How would the progress in nursing theory have been different, supported or hindered by men's perspectives and contributions?

12. What will patterns and pathways in nursing knowledge be in 2050 based on the history depicted in this chapter?

ACKNOWLEDGMENTS

The first part of this chapter is based on A.I. Meleis (1983). The evolving nursing scholarliness. In P.L. Chinn (Ed.), Advances in nursing theory development (pp. 19–34). Reprinted with permission of Aspen Publishers, 1983.

REFERENCES

Abdellah, F.G., Beland, I.L., Martin, A., and Matheney, R.V. (1961). *Patient-centered approaches to nursing.* New York: Macmillan.

Adam, E. (1983). Frontiers of nursing in the 21st century: Development of models and theories on the concept of nursing. *Journal of Advanced Nursing,* 8, 41–45.

Allen, D. (1985). Nursing research and social control: Alternative models of science that emphasize understanding and emancipation. *Image: The Journal of Nursing Scholarship,* XVII(2), 58–64.

Allen, D.G. (1986). Using philosophical and historical methodologies to understand the concept of health. In P.L. Chinn (Ed.), *Nursing research methodology: Issues and implementation.* Rockville, MD: Aspen Systems.

Allen, D.G. (1987). The social policy statement: A reappraisal. *Advances in Nursing Science,* 10(1), 39–48.

Allen, D.G., Benner, P., and Diekelmann, N. (1986). Three paradigms for nursing research: Methodological implications. In P.C. Chinn (Ed.), *Nursing research methodology: Issues and implementations.* Rockville, MD: Aspen Systems.

American Nurses Association. (1965). Educational preparation for nurse practitioners and assistants of nurses. *American Journal of Nursing,* 65(12), 106–111.

An, J., Hayman, L.L., Panniers, T., and Carty, B. (2007). Theory development in nursing and healthcare informatics: A model explaining and predicting information and communication technology acceptance by healthcare consumers. *Advances in Nursing Science,* 30(3), E37–E49.

Anderson, J., Perry, J., Blue, C., Browne, A., Henderson, A., Koushambi, K.B., Kirkham, S., Lynam, J., Semeniuk, P., and Smye, V. (2003). Rewriting cultural safety within the postcolonial and postnational feminist project: Toward new epistemologies of healing. *Advances in Nursing Science,* 26(3), 196–214.

Barnum, B.S. (1990). *Nursing theory: Analysis, application and evaluation* (3rd ed.). Boston, MA: Little, Brown.

Batey, M.V. (1977). Conceptualization: Knowledge and logic guiding empirical research. *Nursing Research,* 26(5), 324–329.

Beare, P.G., Gray, C.J., and Ptak, H.F. (1981, May). Doctoral curricula in nursing. *Nursing Outlook,* 29(5), 311–316.

Beckstrand, J. (1978a). The notion of a practice theory and the relationship of scientific and ethical knowledge to practice. *Research in Nursing and Health,* 1(3), 131–136.

Beckstrand, J. (1978b). The need for a practice theory as indicated by the knowledge used in conduct of practice. *Research in Nursing and Health,* 1(4), 175–179.

Beckstrand, J. (1980). A critique of several conceptions of practice theory in nursing. *Research in Nursing and Health,* 3(2), 69–80.

Benner, P. (1984). *From novice to expert: Excellence and power in clinical nursing practice.* Menlo Park, CA: Addison-Wesley.

Benner, P. (Ed.). (1994). *Interpretive phenomenology: Embodiment, caring, and ethics in health and illness.* Thousand Oaks, CA: Sage.

Berman, H. (2003). Getting critical with children: Empowering approaches with a disempowered group. *Advances in Nursing Science,* 26(2), 102–113.

Bradshaw, A. (1995). What are nurses doing to patients? A review of theories or nursing past and present. *Journal of Clinical Nursing,* 4, 81–92.

Bowles, K. H., Chittams, J., Heil, E., Topaz, M., et al. (2015). Successful electronic implementation of discharge referral decision support has a positive impact on 30- and 60-day readmissions. *Research in Nursing and Health,* 38, 102–114.

Carper, B.A. (1978). Practice oriented theory: Part 1. Fundamental patterns of knowing in nursing. *Advances in Nursing Science,* 1(1), 13–23.

Chinn, P.L. (1978). A model for theory development in nursing. *Advances in Nursing Science,* 1(1), 1–11.

Chinn, P.L. (1987). Response: Revision and passion. *Scholarly Inquiry for Nursing Practice: An International Journal,* 1(1), 21–24.

Chinn, P.L. (1994). *Developing substance: Mid-range theory in nursing* [preface]. Gaithersburg, MD: Aspen Systems.

Choporian, T.J. (1986). Reconceptualizing the environment. In P. Moccia (Ed.), *New approaches to theory development.* New York: National League for Nursing.

Clarke, J.B. (1999). Evidence-based practice: A retrograde step? The importance of pluralism in evidence generation for the practice of health care. *Journal of Clinical Nursing,* 8(1), 89–94.

Crawford, G. (1982). The concept of pattern in nursing: Conceptual development and measurement. *Advances in Nursing Science,* 5(1), 1–6.

Crawford, G., Dufault, K., and Rudy, E. (1979). Evolving issues in theory development. *Nursing Outlook,* 27(5), 346–351.

Dickoff, J. and James, P. (1968). A theory of theories: A position paper. *Nursing Research,* 17(3), 197–203.

Dickoff, J. and James, P. (1971). Clarity to what end? *Nursing Research,* 20(6), 499–502.

Dickoff, J., James, P., and Wiedenbach, E. (1968a). Theory in practice discipline: Part 1. Practice oriented theory. *Nursing Research,* 17(5), 415–435.

Dickoff, J., James, P., and Wiedenbach, E. (1968b). Theory in practice discipline: Part II. Practice oriented theory. *Nursing Research,* 17(6), 545–554.

Dickson, G. and Lee-Villasenor H. (1982). Nursing theory and practice: A self-care approach. *Advances in Nursing Science,* 5(1), 29–40.

Doane, G.H. and Varcoe, C. (2008). Knowledge translation in everyday nursing: From evidence-based to inquiry-based practice. *Advances in Nursing Science,* 31(4), 283–295.

Donaldson, S.K., and Crowley, D. (1978). The discipline of nursing. *Nursing Outlook,* 26(2), 113–120.

Dougherty, J.P., Lipman, T.H., Hyams, S., and Montgomery, K.A. (2014). Telemedicine for adolescents with type 1 diabetes. *Western Journal of Nursing Research,* 36(9), 1199–1221.

Downs, F. (1988). Doctoral education: Our claim to the future. *Nursing Outlook,* 36(1), 18–20.

Duffey, M. and Muhlenkamp, A.F. (1974). A framework for theory analysis. *Nursing Outlook,* 22(9), 570–574.

Ellis, R. (1968). Characteristics of significant theories. *Nursing Research,* 17(3), 217–222.

Ellis, R. (1971). Commentary on Walker's "Toward a clearer understanding of the concept of nursing theory." *Nursing Research,* 20(6), 493–494.

Ellis, R. (1983). Philosophic inquiry. In H. Werley and J. Fitzpatrick (Eds.), *Annual review of nursing research.* New York: Springer.

Fangary, A.S. (1980). *Rofaida: First nurse in Islam.* Kuwait: Dar el Kalaam.

Fawcett, J. (1984). *Analysis and evaluation of conceptual models of nursing.* Philadelphia, PA: F.A. Davis.

Fawcett, J. (1995). *Analysis and evaluation of conceptual models of nursing* (3rd ed.). Philadelphia, PA: F.A. Davis.

Fawcett, J. and Downs, F.S. (1986). *The relationship of theory and research.* East Norwalk, CT: Appleton-Century-Crofts.

Fitzpatrick, J. and Whall, A. (1983). *Conceptual models of nursing: Analysis and application.* Bowie, MD: Robert J. Brady Company.

Fitzpatrick, J. and Whall, A. (Eds.). (1996). *Conceptual models of nursing: Analysis and application.* Stamford, CT: Appleton & Lange.

Foxcroft, D.R., Cole, N., Fullbrook, P., Johnston, L., and Stevens, K. (2001). Organizational infrastructure to promote evidence based nursing practice (Cochrane Review). In *The Cochrane Library* (Issue 3). Oxford, UK: Update Software.

French, P. (1999). The development of evidence-based nursing. *Journal of Advanced Nursing,* 29(1), 72–78.

Frenk, J., Chen, L., Bhutta, Z.A., Cohen, J., Crisp, N., Evans, T., et al. (2010). Health professionals for a new century: Transforming education to strengthen health systems in an interdependent world. *The Lancet,* 376 (9756), 1923–1958.

Fry, S.T. (1989). Toward a theory of nursing ethics. *Advances in Nursing Science,* 11, 9–22.

Funk, S.G., Tornquist, E.M., Champage, M.T., Copp, L.A., and Wiese, R.A. (Eds.). (1990). *Key aspects of recovery: Improving nutrition, rest, and mobility.* New York: Springer.

Garon, M. (2012). Speaking up, being heard: registered nurses' perceptions of workplace communication. *Journal of Nursing Management,* 20(3), 361–71.

Georges, J.M. (2003). An emerging discourse toward epistemic diversity in nursing. *Advances in Nursing Science,* 26(1), 44–52.

Georges, J.M. (2005). Linking nursing theory and practice. A critical-feminist approach. *Advances in Nursing Science,* 28(1), 50–57.

Goode, C.J. (2000). What constitutes the "evidence" in evidence-based practice? *Applied Nursing Research,* 13(4), 222–225.

Gortner, S.R. (1980). Nursing science in transition. *Nursing Research*, 29(3), 180–183.

Gortner, S.R. (2000). Knowledge development in nursing: Our historical roots and future opportunities. *Nursing Outlook*, 48(2), 60–67.

Gortner, S.R. and Nahm, H. (1977). An overview of nursing research in the United States. *Nursing Research*, 26(1), 10–33.

Grol, R. and Grimshaw, J. (1999). Evidence based implementation of evidence based medicine. *Journal of Quality Improvement*, 25(10), 503–513.

Gustafson, D.L. (2005). Transcultural nursing theory from a critical cultural perspective. *Advances in Nursing Science*, 28(1), 2–16.

Hagell, R.I. (1989). Nursing knowledge: Women's knowledge. A sociological perspective. *Journal of Advanced Nursing*, 14, 226–233.

Hagerty, B.M.K., Lynch-Sauer, J., Patusky, K.L., and Bouwsema, M. (1993). An emerging theory of human relatedness. *Image: The Journal of Nursing Scholarship*, 25(4), 291–296.

Hall, B. (2003). An essay on an authentic meaning of medicalization: The patient's perspective. *Advances in Nursing Science*, 26(1), 53–62.

Hall, L.E. (1963). Center for nursing. *Nursing Outlook*, 11, 805–806.

Hardy, M.E. (1974). The nature of theories. In M.E. Hardy (Ed.), *Theoretical foundations for nursing*. New York: MSS Information Corporation.

Hardy, M.E. (1978). Practice oriented theory: Part 1. Perspectives on nursing theory. *Advances in Nursing Science*, 1(1), 37–48.

Henderson, V. (1966). *Nature of nursing*. New York: Macmillan.

Holmes, D. and Gastaldo, D. (2004). Rhizomatic thought in nursing: An alternative path for the development of the discipline. *Nursing Philosophy*, 5(3), 258–267.

Holmes, D., Murray, S., Perron, A., and Rail, G. (2006). Deconstructing the evidence-based discourse in health sciences: Truth, power and fascism. *International Journal of Evidence-Based Healthcare*, 4, 180–186.

Holmes, D., Roy, B., and Perron, A. (2008). The use of postcolonialism in the nursing domain: Colonial patronage, conversion, and resistance. *Advances in Nursing Science*, 31(1), 42–51.

Hussein, S.H. (1981). Rufaida al-Asalmiya. *Islamic Medicine*, 1(2), 261–262.

Hussein, S.H. (1990). Personal Communication.

Im, E-O. (2005). Development of situation-specific theories. An integrative approach. *Advances in Nursing Science*, 28(2), 137–151.

Im, E-O. and Chang, S.J. (2013). Web-based interventions in nursing. *CIN: Computers, Informatics, Nursing*, 31(2), 94–102.

Im, E-O. and Meleis, A.I. (1999). Situation-specific theories: Philosophical roots, properties, and approach. *Advances in Nursing Science*, 22(2), 11–24.

Im, E-O. and Meleis, A.I. (2001). An international imperative for gender-sensitive theories in women's health. *Journal of Nursing Scholarship*, 33(4), 309–314.

Institute of Medicine (IOM). (2011). *The future of nursing: Leading change, advancing health*. Washington, DC: The National Academies Press.

Jacobson, S.F. (1984). A semantic differential for external comparison of conceptual nursing models. *Advances in Nursing Science*, 6(2), 58–70.

Jacox, A. (1974). Theory construction in nursing: An overview. *Nursing Research*, 23(1), 4–13.

Jan, R. (1996). Rufaida al-Asalmiya, the first Muslim nurse. *Image: The Journal of Nursing Scholarship*, 28(3), 267–268.

Johnson, D.E. (1959). A philosophy of nursing. *Nursing Outlook*, 7(4), 198–200.

Johnson, D.E. (1980). The behavioral system model for nursing. In J.P. Riehl and C. Roy (Eds.), *Conceptual models for nursing practice* (2nd ed.). New York: Appleton-Century-Crofts.

Kirkham, S.R. and Anderson, J.M. (2002). Postcolonial nursing scholarship: From epistemology to method. *Advances in Nursing Science*, 25(1), 1–17.

Kuhn, T.S. (1970). The structure of scientific revolutions. In O. Neurath (Ed.), *International encyclopedia of unified science* (2nd ed., Vol. 2). Chicago, IL: University of Chicago Press.

Kushner, K.E. and Morrow, R. (2003). Grounded theory, feminist theory, critical theory: Toward theoretical triangulation. *Advances in Nursing Science*, 26(1), 30–43.

Leininger, M. (1968). The research critique: Nature, function, and art. *Nursing Research*, 17, 444–449.

Leonard, V.W. (1989). A Heideggerian phenomenologic perspective on the concept of the person. *Advances in Nursing Science*, 11(4), 40–55.

Levine, M.E. (1967). The four conservation principles of nursing. *Nursing Forum*, 6(1), 45–59.

Lohr, K.N. and Carey, T.S. (1999). Assessing "beat evidence": Issues in grading the quality of studies for systemic reviews. *Journal of Quality Improvement*, 25(9), 470–479.

McKee, M., Britton, A., Black, N., McPherson, K., Sanderson, C., and Bain, C. (1999). Methods in health services research: Interpreting the evidence: Choosing between randomised and non-randomised studies. *British Medical Journal*, 31(319), 312–315.

Meleis, A.I. (1987). Revisions in knowledge development: Being vs. becoming or being and becoming. *Health Care for Women International*, 8, 199–217.

Meleis, A.I. (1997). *Theoretical nursing: Development and progress* (3rd ed.). Philadelphia, PA: Lippincott.

Meleis, A.I., Isenberg, M., Koerner, J.E., Lacey, B., and Stern, P. (1995). *Diversity, marginalization, and culturally competent health care issues in knowledge development*. Washington, DC: American Academy of Nursing.

Merton, R.K. (1973). *The sociology of science: Theoretical and empirical investigations*. Chicago, IL: University of Chicago Press.

Miller, J.B. (1991). The development of women's sense of self. In J.V. Jordan, A.G. Kaplan, J.B. Miller, I.P. Stiver, and J.L. Surrey (Eds.), *Women's growth in connection* (pp. 11–26). New York: The Guilford Press.

Mishel, M.H. (1990). Reconceptualizing of the uncertainty in illness theory. *Image: The Journal of Nursing Scholarship*, 22, 256–262.

Newman, M.A. (1995). Theory for nursing practice. *Nursing Science Quarterly*, 7(4), 79–85.

Nightingale, F. (1946). *Notes on nursing: What it is and what it is not*. Philadelphia, PA: J.B. Lippincott.

Nursing Theory Think Tank. (1979). *Advances in Nursing Science*, 1(3), 105.

Oiler, C. (1982). The phenomenological approach in nursing research. *Nursing Research*, 31(3), 178–181.

Olshansky, E. (2003). A theoretical explanation for previously infertile mothers' vulnerability to depression. *Journal of Nursing Scholarship*, 35(3), 263–268.

Omery, A. (1983). Phenomenology: A method for nursing research. *Advances in Nursing Science*, 5, 49–63.

Orem, D.E. (1971). *Nursing: Concepts of practice*. New York: McGraw-Hill.

Orem, D.E. (1985). *Nursing: Concepts of practice* (3rd ed.). New York: McGraw-Hill.

Patient Protection and Affordable Care Act. (2010). Public Law 111–148, by the 111th Congress of the United States, March 23, 2010. Retrieved from http://www.gpo.gov/fdsys/pkg/PLAW-111publ148/pdf/PLAW-111publ148.pdf

Peplau, H.E. (1952). *Interpersonal relations in nursing.* New York: G.P. Putnam's Sons.

Preview: The Second Annual Nurse Educator Conference. (1978). *Nurse Educator,* 3(6), 37–39.

Reeder, F. (1984). Philosophical issues in the Rogerian science of unitary human beings. *Advances in Nursing Science,* 6(2), 14–23.

Rogerian First National Conference. (1983, June). New York: New York University.

Rogers, M. (1970). *An introduction to the theoretical basis of nursing.* Philadelphia, PA: F.A. Davis.

Roy, C.L. (1995). Developing nursing knowledge: Practice issues raised from four philosophical perspectives. *Nursing Science Quarterly,* 8(2), 79–85.

Salas, A.S. (2005). Toward a north-south dialogue. Revisiting nursing theory (from the south). *Advances in Nursing Science,* 28(1), 17–24.

Sarter, B. (1987). Evolutionary idealism: A philosophical foundation for holistic nursing theory. *Advances in Nursing Science,* 9(2), 1–9.

Schlotfeldt, R.M. (1988). Structuring nursing knowledge: A priority for creating nursing's future. *Nursing Science Quarterly,* 1(1), 35–38.

Schmieding, N.J. (1983). An analysis of Orlando's nursing theory based on Kuhn's theory of science. In P.L. Chinn (Ed.), *Advances in nursing theory development.* Rockville, MD: Aspen Systems.

Schmieding, N.J. (1987). Problematic situations in nursing: Analysis of Orlando's theory based on Dewey's theory of inquiry. *Journal of Advanced Nursing,* 12, 431–440.

Schmieding, N.J. (1988). Action process of nurse administrators to problematic situations based on Orlando's theory. *Journal of Advanced Nursing,* 13, 99–107.

Sills, G.M. (1977). Research in the field of psychiatric nursing 1952–1977. *Nursing Research,* 26(3), 281–287.

Silva, M.C. (1977). Philosophy, science, theory: Interrelationships and implications for nursing research. *Image: The Journal of Nursing Scholarship,* 9(3), 59–63.

Silva, M.C. and Rothbart, D. (1984). An analysis of changing trends in philosophies of science on nursing theory development and testing. *Advances in Nursing Science,* 6(2), 1–13.

Silva, M.C., Sorrell, J.M., and Sorrell, D.S. (1995). From Carper's patterns of knowing to ways of being: An ontological philosophical shift in nursing. *Advances in Nursing Science,* 18(1), 1–13.

Spangler, Z.S. and Spangler, W.D. (1983). Self-care: A testable model. In P.L. Chinn (Ed.), *Advances in nursing theory development.* Rockville, MD: Aspen Systems.

Stevens, P. (1989). A critical social reconceptualization of environment in nursing: Implications for methodology. *Advances in Nursing Science,* 11(4), 56–68.

Stevenson, J.S. and Woods, N.F. (1986). Nursing science and contemporary science: Emerging paradigms. In G.E. Sorensen (Ed.), *Setting the agenda for the year 2000: Knowledge development in nursing* (Publication No. G-a170, 3M, 5/86). Kansas City, MO: American Nurses Association.

Thompson C., McCaughan, D., Cullum, N., Shelton, T.A., Mullhall, A., and Thompson, D.R. (2001). The accessibility of research-based knowledge for nurse in United Kingdom acute care settings. *Journal of Advanced Nursing,* 36(1), 11–22.

Toulmin, S. (1977). *Human understanding: The collective use and evolution of concepts.* Princeton, NJ: Princeton University Press.

Walker, L.O. (1971). Toward a clearer understanding of the concept of nursing theory. *Nursing Research,* 20(5), 428–435.

Whall, A. (1993). Let's get rid of all nursing theory. *Nursing Science Quarterly,* 3(6), 164–165.

Whall, A.L. and Hicks, F. (2002). The unrecognized paradigm shift in nursing: Implications, problems and possibilities. *Nursing Outlook,* 50(2), 72–76.

Woods, N.F. (1987). Response: Early morning musings on the passion for substance. *Scholarly Inquiry for Nursing Practice: An International Journal,* 1(1), 25–28.

Younger, J.B. (1991). A theory of mastery. *Advances in Nursing Science,* 14(1), 76–89.

Part Three

OUR DISCIPLINE AND ITS STRUCTURE

Scholarship may be defined as a scholar's ability to focus and connect her inquiries to the discipline's ultimate mission and focus. The question is: How could members of a discipline engage in cumulative knowledge development without giving attention to the focus and nature of inquiry in the discipline or to the primary mission of that discipline? Therefore, Part Three is offered as a pause to reflect critically on our discipline's progress, which is significant to its continuous growth. This part of the journey focuses on an analysis of nursing as a discipline and the components that make it a coherent body of knowledge.

In this part, a bridge exists between past and present in three distinct areas: the meaning and structure of the evolved discipline, and the evolving epistemic diversity in the discipline.

Several components define the discipline of nursing. These are described in Chapter 6—a perspective, a domain, the existing and accepted definitions of nursing, and patterns of knowing in the discipline. In Chapter 6, the nursing perspective, which evolved from the nature of its defining characteristics, is presented. Next, the domain of nursing knowledge, its definitions, its components, and the unique characteristics of nursing are discussed. Last, several key definitions of nursing are presented and defined. In Chapter 7, sources, resources, and paradoxes in theory development are discussed. In addition, a theorist needs to engage in intellectual dialogues using strategies and tools for theory development. In Chapter 8, the different patterns of knowing and the human processes involved are discussed. These human processes—of the theorist, the nurse, and the client—are an integral part of nursing and its theory. Aspects of empiricism are still significant and useful for nursing, when added to other processes and aspects of knowing.

Two themes are apparent: a historical and a more contemporary view through the history of science, and a historical and a more contemporary view in nursing theory. The tension between the opposite poles of these two themes is healthy and effective, so long as work is not stunted while the tension is resolved. Perhaps the tensions—the challenges that members of the discipline are facing—should be considered as integral to nursing's theoretical progress, and the discipline of nursing and its scientific base could be considered as a process rather than as an end result. If this is true, then we can view the effectiveness of an epistemology in its process and in the number of problems in nursing that it has been able to solve.

No attempt is made in this part to discredit one philosophy and promote another; an attempt is made, however, to display our options in the development and progress of theoretical nursing. An attempt is also made to highlight the tensions, to demonstrate those aspects of the different paradoxes that are congruent with nursing and its mission, and, finally, to emphasize human aspects of nursing in general and theoretical nursing in particular.

6

The Discipline of Nursing: Perspective and Domain

t is important to define what is meant by *discipline* and *nursing discipline* because the nature of a discipline becomes embodied in its members and drives their thinking and actions. However complicated and variable these definitions are, they facilitate a sense of identity related to a body of knowledge. Understanding the structure of the discipline and defining its boundaries, however flexible, open, and permeable those boundaries are, is vital for focusing the scholarly work and the acquisition of new knowledge in the discipline, as well as in facilitating its growth and advancement. A question to ponder at the outset is, how could members of a discipline engage in cumulative knowledge development without giving attention to the focus and nature of inquiry in the discipline or to the primary mission of the discipline? A discussion about this question could help further an analysis of the meaning, structure, and mission of the discipline and clarify how individuals may become interdisciplinary but also maintain an identity in their own disciplines (Swoboda, 1979).

So what is meant when we speak of a discipline, and what does it mean when we speak of a nursing discipline?

A *discipline* is defined by its goals, structure, and substance. It is "a branch of knowledge or teaching" with a regulatory "set of rules or methods" that govern practice (*American Heritage Dictionary*, 1992). The concept *discipline* refers to "the tools, methods, procedures, exemplars, concepts, and theories that account coherently for a set of objects and subjects" (Klein, 1990, p. 104), and to methods of training (Turner, 2006). A discipline has a fundamental logic and an embedded thought process that connect its parts. In a discipline, experiences are organized into a coherent and well-articulated view of the world. Themes of reality recur to form an understandable pattern that is attributed to those who are members of the discipline. Disciplines encompass rhythm

and regularity of ideas. Disciplines differ in levels of specificity, codification, paradigmatic fields, and establishment. Mathematics is considered highly specific and highly codified, whereas sociology, political science, humanities, and social sciences are considered low-paradigm, less-codified, and less-specific disciplines (Klein, 1990). Toulmin, adding a term to define emerging disciplines, called them "would-be disciplines," and described behavioral sciences as falling into this category (Toulmin, 1972a).

A discipline provides the worldview by which phenomena are uncovered, organized, understood, and interpreted. A discipline is also "a unique perspective, a distinct way of viewing all phenomena," marking the boundaries that define the nature of the questions investigated (Donaldson and Crowley, 1978, p. 113; Moore, 1990). A discipline embodies a central unifying focus for knowledge (Willis, Grace, and Roy, 2008). A discipline includes the theories developed to describe, explain, and prescribe, as well as the research findings—related to the discipline's central phenomena and to other related disciplines—that are essential for the functioning of members of a discipline or for the continuous growth of the discipline.

How similar are the individuals pursuing education for scholarly careers in nursing—whether they are in the Karolinska Institute in Stockholm, Sweden, Mahidol University in Bangkok, Thailand, or the University of Alexandria in Alexandria, Egypt—is a question of the definition of structure and goals in a discipline. How different are the research questions, the way the questions are framed, and the methods by which members of the nursing discipline pursue scholarship as compared with those who are in other disciplines, such as sociology, psychology, or physiology? Some may answer that there are vast differences, some may deny any differences, and yet others may simply shrug their shoulders and say, "What difference does it make? Why even pursue these questions?" These are important questions, worth a robust dialogue and a critical discourse in any discipline, but particularly in a discipline such as nursing, which is attached to professional practice and tends to be eclectic, diffuse, and involving a high degree of receptivity to other disciplines. These dialogues are particularly cogent in the 21st century, where a move toward interdisciplinarity has been reinforced by the establishment of interdisciplinary departments in many halls of academia and in governments across the world (Hayes, 2005). Such receptivity to more permeable boundaries with other disciplines encourages heavy borrowing of theories, concepts, and methods and may decrease significantly enforcing and supporting an epistemological identity (Swoboda, 1979). Some consequences may be that the fundamental scholarly questions most pertinent to nursing are not asked and answered.

Discipline-specific inquiry, explorations, and theory development are vital for the development of nursing knowledge and become the foundation that drives nurses' actions. The discipline of nursing is an intellectual field, with a growing, distinctive knowledge, but it also incorporates the experiences of its members and the values that they espouse, as well as their specific goals and purposes (Northrup, Tschanz, Olynyk, et al., 2004). The discipline of nursing includes the content and processes related to all the roles that nurses play, including administrator, teacher, politician, clinician, and consultant (Banks-Wallace, Despins, Adams-Leander, et al., 2008). It could be understood through ways by which the structure and substance are viewed, organized, examined, researched, and understood. Three broad categories are delineated to analyze the discipline and to reflect on its focus and goals. These are a perspective, a domain, and the goals of the discipline as reflected in how the discipline of nursing in particular is defined.

NURSING PERSPECTIVE

We see the world through different lenses that shape how we understand and interpret it. These lenses provide us with a perspective through which we perceive, comprehend, and interpret situations and events in our lives. Disciplines are characterized by perspectives shared by the discipline's members, and these perspectives shape the way that members of a discipline tend to view phenomena within, as well as outside, the discipline. As nurses, we have developed some shared views that define the ways by which we come to assess our clients and their situations. Our individual and shared perspectives

reflect our culture, education, work experiences, and values, and these perspectives, in turn, influence our views of events and situations. A *perspective* is defined as the way that members of a group view and characterize a situation. It is the sum total of the attitudes and the outlook that help members of a defined group to develop a position or a viewpoint. A perspective provides a panoramic view of situations; it provides the signposts that characterize an outlook on the world. A perspective is based on a set of values that help in characterizing the nature of the world for members of a group. It contains the preferences for certain views and for certain ways of observing and reacting to situations. A perspective, according to Rosemary Ellis, is the prevailing view held by members of a discipline or a profession (Algase and Whall, 1993). A nursing perspective is defined by its unique aspects, the history of the profession, the sociopolitical context in which nursing care is provided, and the nature of the orientation of members of the nursing profession, as well as the discipline.

Although different nurses may perceive nursing somewhat differently and at different times, Sarvimaki and Lutzen (2004) found that Swedish nurses over several generations consider the discipline of nursing to have a unique perspective, and they agree on having a similar set of value systems.

The perspective of clinicians and scholars in nursing reflects their academic and professional approaches to knowledge development, a history of second-class citizenship, a history of devaluation of nursing's mission of caring, and a history of oppression of its members that reflects worldwide oppression of women and subordination of nurses to bureaucratic and professional structures. Therefore, nurses may be more experientially prepared to examine and analyze similar processes that may be encountered by nursing clients. By necessity, too, these experiences drive the kinds of analyses and interpretations of progress that are performed, as well as the development of the discipline. They shape the perspective that evolves and characterizes a discipline. A nursing perspective is shaped by many defining characteristics. It is the integration of these characteristics that defines the nursing perspective. Four important defining characteristics that determine our perspective are the

- Nature of nursing science as a human science
- Practice aspects of nursing
- Caring relationships that nurses and patients develop
- Health and wellness perspective

Each aspect of the nursing perspective is presented and discussed in the following sections.

Nursing: A Human Science

The science underlying the discipline of nursing has shifted away from an emphasis on only natural sciences, and nursing now tends to be described as a human science. A human science has many unique properties that define the ontology and epistemology of the nursing discipline and that shape its perspective. Meleis (1992), McWhinney (1989), Holmes (1990), and Cowling and Chinn (2001) identified some of these properties of human science.

1. A human science focuses on human beings as wholes, and advocates understanding the particulars in terms of the whole (Mariano, 2001; Owen and Holmes, 1993).
2. A human science incorporates a mode of perception based on holism (Stiles, 2011).
3. A human science has at its core an understanding of experiences as lived by its members. Kim (2000) proposed that nursing deals with "human living."
4. A human science does not separate the art and the science of nursing, which are the cornerstones on which nursing knowledge is built (Mitchell and Cody, 2002).
5. A human science deals with meanings as seen and perceived by its members. Meanings include those attached to responses, symbols, events, and situations, and thus guide its practice. Meanings are achieved from reflecting and processing experiences (Willis et al., 2008).
6. To be able to understand meanings and experiences, a scientist needs to enter into a meaningful dialogue with participants. Interaction is the prime source of meanings and perceptions of experiences, and participants in the activities of knowledge development are those who are developing and structuring knowledge and those about whom knowledge is developed. All participants have to verify the meanings of these experiences (Rolfe, 2015).
7. "The scope for generalization for a human science is limited" (McWhinney, 1989, p. 298). A generalization has to be made within a context; therefore, generalization may be presented in terms of patterns.
8. Responses and experiences form patterns. Patterns provide meaningful information about participants (Newman, 2002).
9. Some conditions, situations, behaviors, and events are reducible for purposes of description.

Nursing as a human science is concerned with the life experiences of human beings and their meanings, with health and illness matters and their significance in their lives, as well as with the experience of dying. It requires qualitative and quantitative research methodologies (Friedman and Rhinehart, 2000; Glaser and Strauss, 1964, 1967; Malinski, 2002; Rawnsley, 2003). Because these experiences are shaped by history, significant others, politics, social structures, gender, and culture, nurses also are concerned with how these perspectives shape the actions and reactions of human beings (Willis et al., 2008). It is precisely that concern that makes nursing a practice discipline, which in turn helps to define its perspective. However, a question that must be addressed is the extent to which this aspect of the nursing perspective—that is, the human science discourse—is incorporated in nursing education and practice (Pilkington, 2002). When does it get introduced, and what strategies are used to facilitate its integration into the student's identity as a prospective nurse? These questions beg a robust discussion by the readers of this chapter as well as within our literature. Do the curricula in nursing and educational programs that prepare future nurses reflect a distinguishable nursing perspective?

Nursing: A Practice-Oriented Discipline

The practice aspects of nursing are a second defining characteristic that shape its perspective. Nursing exists to provide nursing care for clients who experience illness, as well as for those who may experience potential health care problems. The discipline's perspective is shaped by the pragmatics of a nurse's work (Allen, 2014; Litchfield and Jonsdottir, 2008). Nursing has been described as a clinical discipline, an applied field, or a practice-oriented discipline. What do we mean when we say that nursing is a practice-oriented discipline? It means that it has a primary mission related to practice. Therefore, its members seek knowledge of what nurses as professionals do, why they do it, and when they do it. According to Weinberg (2006), even what nurses may consider the "little things" they do are really "big things for their patients" (pp. 42–43). Nurses deal with people's human condition and their responses to health and illness. Nurses help in monitoring the living experience of people as they deal with health and illness while caring for them. Nurses help in assisting individuals and families to care for themselves, and in empowering them to develop and use resources (Bottorff, 1991). Nursing may use basic and applied knowledge to achieve its goals, but it is still a practice-oriented discipline.

Nurses need basic knowledge to understand the basic phenomena related to the goals and mission of nursing; for example, how certain groups of people tend to seek help, how certain connections tend to maintain their balance and health, and how different patterns of responses to such events as pain, intrusive interventions, hospitalization, and discharge exert their influence (Mapanga and Mapanga, 2003). Basic understanding of such phenomena as comfort, touch, confusion, ambiguity, sleeplessness, and restlessness is essential for the subsequent development of applied knowledge. Applied knowledge is that which provides guidelines to maintain, ameliorate, develop, inhibit, support, change, advocate, clarify, or suppress some of these basic phenomena. Both basic and applied knowledge are the cornerstones of nursing as a practice-oriented discipline. Nurses also seek knowledge related to the practical care they provide. Practical aspects of nursing have been dichotomized with its theoretical aspects rather than integrating, incorporating, and using them as a springboard for further development of the discipline. The shift by nurse scholars away from practical aspects, and in particular from clinical skills, has been manifested in the limited research interest related to clinical concerns, in uncovering the daily work of nurses, in the conflicts between educators and administrators in defining educational end products, and in the decreasing emphasis on clinical skills, among others (Bjørk, 1995; Clarke, 1986; Titler, Buckwalter, and Maas, 1993). Such trends have slowly been replaced with more emphasis on biobehavioral and biomedical aspects of nursing, with more nurses prepared as nurse practitioners in the United States. With increasing realization of how biomarkers have become essential in providing quality care, they have become significant tools for advancing nursing knowledge (Kang, 2012).

The goal of knowledge development, then, is to understand the nursing care needs of people and to learn how to better care for them; therefore, the caring activities that nurses are involved in on a daily basis may be the focus for knowledge development and may be congruent with activities involved in knowledge structuring, particularly because the participants in both activities are human beings. Two types of knowledge development goals drive the activities and the progress in knowledge. There is "knowledge for the sake of knowledge" and knowledge to provide better nursing care to people through solving central problems of concern to the discipline (Laudan, 1977, 1981). Nursing as a discipline, and nurses as clinicians and scientists whose mission it is to care for people and enhance their well-being, cannot afford to participate only in developing knowledge for the sake of knowledge development.

Thus, the purposes of knowledge development in nursing are shaped by its practice orientation, which in turn shapes the nursing perspective. The nursing perspective reflects nurses' interest in

- Empowering members of the discipline of nursing with knowledge that makes a difference in the care of patients
- Empowering nurses to influence and enhance the well-being of clients, thereby decreasing their vulnerability to risks to their health
- Empowering clients with knowledge and experience to care for themselves and to manage their symptoms and their life transitions by fully utilizing available resources and creating new resources
- Supporting and facilitating activities of informal structures, such as families and communities who are engaged in caregiving

If these are the main purposes of developing knowledge in nursing, then we have to consider those approaches to knowledge development that make these purposes possible. To empower the discipline and its members, nurses look for and identify the same skills that made them effective and caring clinicians, and build on these as well as other skills that could enhance knowledge development. Empowering partnerships reflect the goals of nursing as a practice discipline. Such a perspective calls for competencies that emanate from nurses' work and may shape the nature of the questions that nurses investigate.

A unique aspect of nursing as a practice discipline that further defines its perspective is the around-the-clock care provided by nurses working in institutions. When nurses see patients around the clock, they tend to know more about their daily life processes and patterns, and therefore they are more likely to better understand their lived experiences and their health care needs. They possess a high level of continuity in their knowledge of their patients, which provides a more textured context for the clients' needs and responses. Nurses who care for patients in primary health care settings, including home care, may have to structure their encounters in more creative ways to increase their understanding of the daily life processes and the integrated patterns of their clients' responses to health and illness within a context of limited time and varying space. Whether in a hospital, a clinic, or a home, nursing encounters are characterized by continuity, intensity, and involvement in ways that other health care professionals do not experience. To nurse is to build relationships. Developing caring relationships has been considered a defining aspect of the nursing perspective by many theorists over many decades (Newman, Smith, Pharris, et al., 2008). Nurses also monitor and coordinate the care of their patients; this includes their own caregiving as well as the care offered by others in the health care team.

Nurses spend a great deal of time with clients (Masson, 1985). They conduct comprehensive assessments, including assessing family and medical histories, to establish a better care context and gain a better understanding of the client's responses. They perform daily activities such as giving bed baths, providing for daily hygienic needs, administering medication, and carrying out treatments. Therefore, the experiences and responses of clients to health and illness tend to be viewed within the context of the client's life relationships, culture, goals, and daily experiences. The ongoing relationship with nurses prompts clients to share their experiences in more narrative dialogues, allowing more details, meanings, and history that make their health and illness experiences more understandable and allow for more congruent plans of action. If patients are given indications that these experiences are important for the caring processes, they tend to share more freely with nurses the effects of their complaint, medical diagnoses, or intervention on their daily lives and on those of significant others in their lives. In other words, patients naturally are more interested in ways by which illness, altering conditions, or treatments affect their daily lives and daily routines. Nurses are optimally placed to get the benefit of hearing narratively about the experiences of their patients. Nurses tend to get to know their patients differently and more profoundly than do other health care providers (Jenny and Logan, 1992).

Another unique aspect of nursing practice is the nature and the properties of the environment and organizational structure in which nurses work. In addition, nurses' relationship with their work environment, the extent to which it values nurses and their work, whether or not it provides them with opportunities to have a voice, and whether or not they perceive they are well compensated for their efforts, all influence their work. In other words, the relationship between nurses and their workplace shapes the care nurses provide, as well as nurses' lived experiences. Therefore, as proposed by Willetts and Clarke (2014), the contextual nature of nurses' work defines their professional identity. And as a result, it also defines their caring activities.

Nursing: A Caring Discipline

The caring aspects of nursing also help define its perspective (Cook and Cullen, 2004). Many questions have been raised about the concept of caring. Is caring the essence of nursing, is it the field's special knowledge area, is it equal to the discipline of nursing, is it a central concept in nursing, or is it the core of its domain? Is it the goal *or* the mission of nursing, or is it a goal *and* a mission of nursing? Caring has been considered and discussed through each of these prisms, and there are enough writings in nursing to support each of these positions (Cohen, 1991).

Caring, which has been an integral part of the private domain of women, has been discussed recently as a component of both the public and private domains. Condon (1992) goes further by suggesting that caring may be the glue that will connect nurses' public and private domains and will decrease "the discrepancies between the demands of the private and public domains" (p. 19). She also proposes that caring and nursing are compatible, and that caring and feminist ideals are compatible. Caring, for Condon, is the foundational moral value for nursing. It is detrimental to nursing if it continues to be viewed as a component of public domains and is relegated only to women in society. She further proposes that we explore how the philosophy of professionalism may conflict with the ethics of caring.

Condon (1992) calls for a new metaphor for nursing caring to substitute for the metaphors of duty and religious calling. There are numerous such metaphors in nursing. Watson (1988, 1990) describes caring more from the perspective of an existential philosophy and reviews the spiritual bases of caring. To her, caring is the moral ideal of nursing. Leininger (1981) discusses caring from a cultural perspective. For Brody (1988), caring is the central virtue of nursing. Gendron (1988, 1994) provides innovative arguments, likening caring to the creativity that is woven on as a structure for the substance in nursing. The structure is based on the contextual knowledge of scientific facts as well as conceptual frameworks. The structure also includes skills, nursing interventions, and policies, among other aspects of structure. All these are brought to the patient's bedside or home through creative patterns used in an artistic way. To match nursing actions to people, a nurse needs to know how to synchronize with a person, and she must know when she is synchronized. The challenge is then not only in the development of the knowledge base required to provide these caring actions, but also in how to prepare clinicians to be able to develop a synchronized self–client relationship. A synchronized relationship is based on "sensing subjective tacit meaning" of experiences and situations and on attuning "one's self and others" to these experiences and their meanings. To develop and carry out these aspects of the caring processes, Gendron (1994) proposes using "reflective journals" and an "emphasis on dialogue in the sharing of students' experiences through narrative" (p. 29), storytelling, and analysis.

The art of nursing has also been used as a synonym for caring. An epistemological analysis by Johnson (1994) about the meaning of art in nursing identified five separate senses of art in nursing. Nursing art is exemplified when nurses are able to

1. Grasp the meaning that is inherent in their encounter with patients
2. Establish connections
3. Skillfully perform nursing activities
4. Choose between alternatives
5. Morally conduct nursing practice

Grasping meaning is attributed to perceptions rather than intellect; it depends on observations, feelings, imagination, and understanding that go beyond description—it depends on inner experiences and is holistic in nature. **Connecting with patients** is more than establishing a relationship; rather, it consists of the experiences in everything the nurse does with patients, including nonverbal communication. There is an authenticity to this communication that occurs between human beings. **Skill in nursing activities** is a behavioral ability in which there is an understanding about the skills needed for providing care and in which there is embedded understanding of these skills. The skills in such nursing activities can be learned, and they are expressed through ease and fluidity of movements, among other characteristics yet to be defined. **Determining a course of action** is expressed by the group of authors who contend that the nursing art is practical, and it is through assumptions derived

from a disciplinary structure that nurses are making decisions, based on a thorough understanding of all options. The nursing process proponents build their case on the artistic aspects of nursing as described in this category of definitions. **To practice morally** is a definition of nursing art that includes the view that skills are important, but are not a substitute for other aspects of practice, nor are they enough for the care that patients need. If a nurse does not make moral choices or address the moral dilemmas in her practice, then she is not using the artistic aspects of the discipline.

Morse, Bottorff, Neander, et al. (1991), and Morse, Solberg, Neander, et al. (1990) describe caring as human trait, moral imperative, affect, interpersonal relationship, and therapeutic intervention. Caring is further described in nursing literature in the following ways:

1. As a human trait, it should be considered from a personal, psychological, or cultural perspective.
2. As a moral imperative, Gadow (1985) and Watson (1988, 1990) view the fundamental essence of nursing as preserving the dignity of others. This meaning of caring provides the basis for all nursing interventions, assessments, and activities.
3. As an affect, this is manifested through emotional feelings or empathy, feelings of dedication. Demands on time may change this.
4. The nurse–patient relationship is the essence of caring.
5. Caring is also seen as a therapeutic intervention.

Caring for clients is a component of what defines a nursing perspective (Clifford, 1995; Sanford, 2000; Newman et al., 2008). It is one of the traditions handed down over the decades (Olson, 1993). It is another lens by which nurses as clinicians view their clients. It is the core activity in nursing practice (Benner and Wrubel, 1989; Leininger, 1978; Watson, 1985). It may also be the same lens through which nurses as scholars need to see the subject matter for their research or theory development. If caring is an integral part of a nursing perspective, it could also be an integral component of the subject matter of the theories developed (Newman, Sime, and Corcoran-Perry, 1991) or the guiding force for the strategies by which theories are developed and research is formatted (Feldman, 1993). A caring perspective has shaped the processes used for knowledge development. It is encouraging to observe that there is increasingly more openness in Western societies to acknowledge the caring aspects of relationships and to bring caring more into the public domain, a practice that has always been more prevalent in developing countries. The art of nursing and its caring aspects require time, energy, and skills that are not well acknowledged or rewarded through appropriate policies. Therefore, the question is: Are nurses rewarded for their caring activities? MacPherson (1989) contends that nurses are not rewarded for trying to care and for the time they spend in caring for their patient communities. Educators, clinicians, and administrators may have to hold and drive the notion that caring is not a negotiated commodity. Defining caring as a component of the nursing perspective may provide them with the rationale to support their quest for supportive and rewarding caring activities.

Nursing: A Health-Oriented Discipline

Nursing has been defined as work that focuses on "the human health experience" (Newman et al., 1991). To say that a nursing perspective is shaped by its health orientation is not to deny the work and the caring that nurses provide for clients who are sick, who are experiencing traumas, or who are recovering from illness. Nurses' orientation to the health of individuals and populations is historical, beginning with Nightingale's writings (1859), in which nurses' work is defined in terms of maintaining health and bringing a state of health back to the individual. Health has been considered integral to nursing (Allen, 1986), a goal (Rogers, 1970), a construct (Tripp-Reimer, 1984), an idea in nursing (Smith, 1981), a metaparadigm concept (Fawcett, 1995), a theory (Newman, 1986), and a concept (Reynolds, 1988).

Health is also a perspective that defines what we consider in our assessments, in making plans for interventions, in evaluating our interventions, or in considering changes in our interventions (Meleis, 1990). It is the lens through which we view our clients during the course of their illness, as well as when we attempt to maintain or promote their health. Divergent views of health have held it as dichotomous to illness or dynamic life experiences, a way to achieve one's potential, a unity of body and mind, a view of wellness, and a rhythmic fluctuation of life process (Newman et al., 2008). Moch (1989) provided a compelling argument for the development of the concept of health within illness, and demonstrated how such a perspective is receiving more support in health-related theory development.

Examples are Moss (1985), who described the transformational aspects of illness. Such a view is supported by many personal accounts of patients, particularly as discussed in the literature on patients with HIV and AIDS. The notion of "healthy dying" (Fitzpatrick, 1983) might be another supportive argument for health as an important component of the discipline's perspective.

There is also support for a health perspective in the daily work of nurses. Patients are assessed in terms of their perception of their well-being throughout their experiences with health care professionals, and are instructed in how to maintain their health despite a grave diagnosis or intrusive procedure. Many theorists speak of this perspective; Travelbee (1966, 1971) was a pioneer in encouraging nurses to help their clients find meaning in their illness experience. Paterson and Zderad (1976) described their nursing perspective in terms of health and connected interactions with clients. Although for Newman (1986) health may be the goal for caring, or seen as a process of expanding consciousness, and for Jones and Meleis (1993) as a process of empowerment, these analyses provide greater support for a more prevailing view of nursing as understood from within a health perspective. Through the process of nursing care, nurses uncover health strengths, mobilize these strengths, and support the available resources, so that the patient may take charge and fight their illness or injury.

Community health nurses provide useful examples of a health perspective in their work. They speak of positive resources, available support, healthful habits, and how to empower clients in using their healthy resources. Although nurses in the intensive care unit (ICU) may consider their approach more illness oriented, on careful analysis, we find that ICU nurses are concerned with patients' safety, well-being, promoting increasing health, maintaining healthful habits, and supporting as much normality in daily life as possible. These activities and goals reflect a health perspective.

DOMAIN OF NURSING KNOWLEDGE

A second essential component that defines the discipline of nursing is the domain of nursing knowledge. All disciplines are formed around a domain of knowledge. The concept domain as well as the nursing domain are extensively described

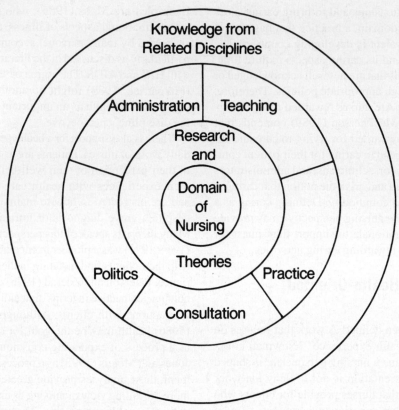

Figure 6-1   The discipline of nursing.

and discussed in the following text. A domain of knowledge is the crux of a discipline (Fig. 6-1). A *domain* is a territory that has both theoretical and practical boundaries. Domains of knowledge have a defined repertoire of principles, the rules used for applying and using these principles, and the constituencies to which these rules are applied (Gelman, 2000). The practical boundaries represent the current state of investigative interests that emerge from questions significant to members of the domain. The theoretical boundaries are formulated by the visionary questions proposed for exploration, as well as those that occupy the intellectual energies of members of disciplines. These visionary questions are not bound by, or limited to, current concerns of the members of the discipline. They are the main phenomenon of interest, and are of central concern to the members of the discipline. Core domains are those aspects of a discipline that represent universal knowledge structures (Gelman, 2000). Other aspects of the domain are more dynamic and changeable, such as the way phenomena are conceptualized; the nature of questions asked about the phenomena, as well as those phenomena that reflect societal or policy changes; and during

periods of transition, those phenomena that result from these changes. For example, some current questions that determine the territory of nursing include what is involved in caring for people who are not able to care for themselves because of illness or anticipated illness; how best to help individuals and populations to maintain their health and well-being; what is involved in self-care and how to support the promotion of self-care activities; and what are the best strategies that nurses could use to maintain or promote health, support recovery, and manage illness. In the future, theoretical boundaries may extend to include questions about caring for individuals who are in hemispheric transition or who may reside in a space shuttle for an extended period. Some elements of the domain may be maintained; for example, a focus on human beings and their environment. Others may require some modification; for example, the nature and the content of the surroundings may have to be changed considerably to reflect changing environments. The environment for clients living on Earth may be similar to as well as different from the environments of individuals living in space stations, or in the future, on other planets. The language used, the concepts defined, and the questions explored and examined are shaped by the structure of the discipline. The structure, in turn, shapes the nature of questions asked about the phenomena (Mitchell, 1994). Nurse scientists have made major contributions to the development of the domain of nursing using a focus on person and environment (Heitkemper and Bond, 2003), on patterns of behavior, and on health and lifestyles.

Domains: A Definition

Domains are defined differently by different philosophers of science. The following definitions of a domain synthesize some aspects of Kuhn (1970), Merton (1973), Parsons (1968), and Toulmin (1972b).

- It has some broad basic concepts.
- It contains the major problem areas of the field that make up the canons for significant statements.
- Some of its units of analysis that are used in research investigations are identified.
- It provides evidence of beginning agreement and a genealogy of ideas.
- Its members allow for the synthesis of a number of paradigms.
- Its members are knowledgeable about the different schools of thought, and they acknowledge and accept the use of different paradigms.
- It defines mechanisms to integrate and present the accumulated experiences of its members. These experiences are respected, critically assessed, and accepted. The grounds for analysis and critique are clear and subject to debate.
- The rules, norms, and tools for knowledge development are defined within the domain. These rules, norms, and tools emerge from the domain goals and are congruent with its shared assumptions.
- A domain informs and is informed by all outer circles of the discipline (see Fig. 6-1). That is, a domain is revised and developed through the wisdom and expertise of members of the discipline, through accumulated research and theory, and through knowledge developed in other disciplines. In sum, a domain has certain focal elements of stability, but the nature of its content is dynamic and responsive to changes occurring in other spheres.

A Nursing Domain

When we consider nursing analytically, we find numerous indications that nursing is indeed a discipline

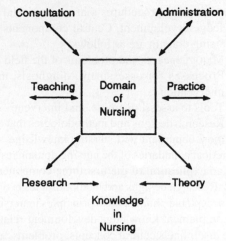

Figure 6-2   The domain of nursing.

with a particular perspective and a defined domain (Fig. 6-2). As you reflect on what constitutes our disciplinary domain, keep in mind that the central problems of the domain of nursing may be examined by other sciences; however, the centrality of these problems to the domain is what determines primary domain affiliation. Comforting patients during intrusive procedures may be of concern to a number of health science disciplines, but comfort of clients during all life processes related to health and illness situations, as well as the ways by which comfort is enhanced, are *central concerns of nurses and nursing*.

The interests of some disciplines overlap others. Engineering is an example of another discipline that may encounter such overlap. Premises on which the discipline of engineering is built may come from physics, chemistry, economics, and behavioral sciences, but the synthesis is uniquely engineering for the purpose of describing, explaining, and predicting phenomena central to engineering (e.g., the shielding of nuclear power plants). The problem of shielding is central to the field of nuclear engineering, but only peripheral to physics, chemistry, and other sciences.

The nursing domain does not simply encompass the results of research (i.e., nursing science), nursing theories, or nursing practice; rather it encompasses knowledge of nursing practice (Newman, 1983), which is based on philosophy, history, former practice, common sense, research findings, theory, and genealogy of ideas (see Fig. 6-2). The nursing domain encompasses units of analysis, congruent methodology, nursing processes, holistic approaches to assessment, and other practice and methodological procedures that are essential to knowledge development. Central components of the nursing domain are as follows:

- Major concepts and problems of the field
- Processes for assessment, diagnosis, and intervention
- Tools to assess, diagnose, and intervene
- Research designs and methodologies that are most congruent with nursing knowledge

Theoretical boundaries of the nursing domain result from an explication of the first three components listed. Research designs and methodologies evolve from acceptable philosophical principles in nursing and complement knowledge development related to the discipline's central concepts, problems, and goals. Research designs and methodologies also help identify and develop components of the domain of nursing. (Note the theory-specific research texts and methodologies that have evolved in nursing, including research texts by Rosemarie Parse and Patricia Benner, among others [references in Chapter 21].) Also note the revolutionary methodology of grounded theory that has been adopted in the discipline of nursing for its congruency with the domain of nursing (Glaser and Strauss, 1964, 1967). Nursing theories are a component of the domain of nursing, and they provide nurses with different perspectives on nursing and nursing phenomena.

In 1975, Yura and Torres delineated and described the major concepts used in baccalaureate programs that were central to the different conceptual models and frameworks used for nursing curricula. Four focal concepts emerged: person, society, health, and nursing (Yura and Torres, 1975). The centrality of these concepts in the discipline of nursing continued to be supported through the 1980s. For example, Newman (1983) asserted that the "domain of nursing has always included the nurse, the patient, the situation in which they find themselves, and the purpose of their being together, or the health of the patient" (p. 388). Therefore, she agreed that the major components of concern to nursing are "nursing (as an action), client (human being), environment (of the client and of the nurse-client), and health" (p. 389). Others modified the list to exclude environment (Barnum, 1994), or they expanded the meaning of "person" to encompass both human being and patient (Barnum, 1994), or they redefined "client" to mean "pluralities of persons and internal units, such as families, groups, and communities" (Schultz, 1987, p. 71).

Therefore, the structure of the discipline was further recognized in terms of these major concepts, most

of which evolved from nursing theories (Neuman and Fawcett, 2002). Many nurse scholars also agree about several points of convergence that define the structure of our discipline (Newman et al., 2008), and some argued that nursing theories could include one or more of the concepts that were identified by Yura and Torres (Fawcett, 1989). These are, for example, client, society, health, or nursing. Others, however, argued that nursing theories should include the concept of nursing as an activity, in addition to any of the other concepts (Flaskerud and Halloran, 1980) that are considered part of a set of "commonplaces" (nursing act, patient, health, nurse–patient relationships, nursing acts and health, and patient and health). These "commonplaces" differentiate nursing from other disciplines (Barnum, 1994, pp. 14–15). Still others emphasized that nursing theories should include health and the direction for nursing actions to facilitate the processes of health (Newman, 1983, p. 390). Although variations occurred in the recommendations of metatheorists in what, how many, and which central concepts should be included in nursing theories, none objected to the inclusion of all domain concepts—if indeed a theory is able to address them all. The position adopted in this text has its own unique features also, but it falls within general patterns of agreement within the discipline (Meleis, 1986). Concepts identified as central to the domain of nursing are included in Box 6-1.

It is proposed that the nurse interacts (interaction) *with a human being in a health/illness situation* (nursing client), *who is in an integral part of his sociocultural context* (environment), *and who is in some sort of transition or is anticipating a transition* (transition); *the nurse–patient interactions are organized around some purpose* (nursing process, problem solving, holistic assessment, or caring actions), *and the nurse uses some actions* (nursing therapeutics) *to enhance, bring about, or facilitate health and well-being* (health).

It is argued here that theories developed relative to any of the concepts listed in Box 6-1 are

BOX 6-1	CONCEPTS CENTRAL TO THE DOMAIN OF NURSING	
Nursing client	Nursing process	Nursing therapeutics
Transitions	Environment	Health
Interaction		

nursing theories when the ultimate goal is related to the maintenance, promotion, or facilitation of health and well-being, even though the theory may not specify nursing actions. It is also argued that nursing is an encompassing concept that includes all the concepts listed in Box 6-1 and is therefore defined by them. It would be an instance of tautological conceptualizing to define nursing by all its concepts and then include nursing as one of the concepts. Other disciplines may use nursing theories for different goals; as such, nursing theories lose their original goal, becoming adapted, "shared" theories (Barnum, 1994).

A conceptual definition is provided for each of the central concepts in nursing. These definitions, evolving from contemporary shared knowledge in nursing and from a current worldview, are provided as working definitions. The reader should use them as a springboard for further development and refinement.

The Nursing Client

The most central concept within the domain of nursing is the recipient of care or the potential recipient of care—the nursing client. Although a client is also central to a number of other disciplines, the perspective from which that client is considered is invariably different and evolves from the domain of the discipline. Please note that the nursing client has been used to define a patient and a consumer of care. Note also that, in the United States, a definition of professional nursing has in it a return to the concept of patient rather than client or consumer (American Nurses Association [ANA], 2010). Nurses have claimed that individuals are the focus of their actions ever since nurses began caring for patients and ever since they attempted to describe the care they provide. For example, Nightingale (1946) described nursing as having to "put the patient in the best condition for nature to act upon him" (p. 74). Others spoke of nursing in terms of helping individuals develop their self-care activities (Orem, 1988) and of doing what needs to be done to help individuals adapt to their illness or environment (Roy, 1984). Newman and her colleagues (2008) defined a client as a person who is primarily identified by a pattern of consciousness that also incorporates a sense of recognition of how they fit within a larger system.

To illustrate, when a physician thinks of a person, most often the image is one of a biologic system structure and function as well as genes and genetic biomarkers. Although that image may include a person's occupation, family, socioeconomic class, or other variables, the central image invariably is expected to be biophysiologic. When a sociologist thinks of a person, he or she thinks of the roles, status, interaction, and significant others of individuals as part of a society. When a psychologist thinks of a human being, he or she thinks in terms of intrapsychic processes. A human being to a cell biologist is made up of groups of cells.

Who the clients are and how they tend to define and interpret their patient status will drive theoretical nursing in the future. Clients have become more informed over the years, and they are vocal about what they need from their health care providers. Clients are embedded in multidimensional and dynamic contexts that are constantly changing (Reed, 1995). Theories that have defined clients as passive recipients of care or as human beings who are waiting for information, and those theorists who assumed that the nurse's role is to ensure compliance, are no longer congruent with how clients define themselves (Allen, 1987). Clients come to the health care system either with their consciousness raised about their rights to information, care, and participation in decision-making or with no such expectations; in the latter case, the caring encounter may then include opportunities for consciousness-raising. In either case, theories for the future must be developed to reflect changing assumptions about clients and their levels of awareness and consciousness, and they must also provide some strategies by which consciousness may be raised within the value and belief systems of these clients. These notions of a client are informed by their sociocultural and political contexts, and hence differ by levels of education, economics, age, and other variables.

Nurses deal with much more diversity in clients than they used to. Client diversity, with regard to gender, race, ethnicity, or religion, has always been, to a certain extent, a hallmark of health care practice; however, since the turn of the century, diversity has taken on another, more significant meaning because it comes with attached questions about the melting pot model of integration. Clients assert their identities, whether that identity is related to ethnic background or to sexual orientation. Clients are saying, "We like who we are, we do not want to assume or pretend otherwise, and we want to be respected and treated with sensitivity and with competence that includes our value systems and beliefs." This assertion requires different assumptions and different propositions that must be reflected in future nursing theories.

In addition, many world events are increasing transitions of people between countries and within countries through immigration and emigration. These transitions profoundly influence the health care and health outcomes of populations. The world's population is increasingly elderly, and this brings with it a corresponding increase in health care needs, because the elderly require different types of expertise from nurses. Nurses are also needed to help individuals live and cope with long-term illnesses. Who the clients are, how they respond to their situations, how society has defined them, and how they define and redefine themselves are questions that can be answered only within sociocultural, economic, and political contexts. Attention to these questions and their answers could increase the power of theories to explain responses to health care.

Nursing theories claim that nursing focuses on the person whose needs are not met because of illness or the person who needs help in maintaining or enhancing wellness. Nurse theorists provide us with several views of our clients. A nursing client probably is a composite of all of the conceptions provided by these nurse theorists, and perhaps the context determines which image is more central at any one time. Some of these conceptions are complementary, whereas others are based on conflicting value systems. The following are some examples of nurse theorists' conceptions of the nursing client:

- The nursing client has a set of basic human needs (Abdellah, 1969)—21 problems; (Henderson, 1966)—14 daily activities; (Orem, 1988)—the deficit between self-care capabilities and self-care demands. The focus of nursing is on assisting with activities to fulfill the client's needs.
- The nursing client is an open system, an adaptive being who changes to accommodate outside changes.
- The nursing client is conceptualized as a person in disequilibrium or at risk of disequilibrium due to insufficiency or incompatibility between one or more of his or her subsystems.
- The nursing client is a person who is unable or at risk of being unable, to be a self-care agent.
- The nursing client has a lifestyle that may render the person vulnerable or resistant to health risks.

These theories provided us with varied conceptions described in the social policy statement of the ANA (2010). These conceptions should be used as guidelines for analyses to determine their congruency with the values and mission of the discipline (Allen, 1987). A *nursing client* is defined in this book as a human being with needs, who is in constant interaction with the environment and has an ability to adapt to that environment but, because of illness, risk, or vulnerability to potential illness, is experiencing disequilibrium or is at risk of experiencing disequilibrium. *Disequilibrium* is manifested in unmet needs, inability to take care of oneself, and nonadaptive responses. More contemporary definitions are of "human living" (Willis et al., 2008) and "human dignity" (Jacobs, 2001).

Theoretical developments of phenomena related to nursing clients encompass, but are not limited to, six areas:

1. Research and theories to describe philosophical principles governing views of human beings in nursing, including analyses of values and norms related to human beings and their relationships
2. Research and theories that relate to the fundamental process of responses to human and environmental conditions that are considered within normal ranges
3. Research and theories to describe, explain, and predict responses of human beings' health and illness situations
4. Research and theories to describe human responses to nursing therapeutics
5. Research and theories to describe groups, communities, and organizational responses to health and illness and nursing therapeutics
6. Theoretical development of person models that are congruent with the disciplinary values

The nursing client is defined by his or her experiences (McIntyre, 1995). These experiences are expressed and related to others in continuous and discontinuous ways, in isolation or within a context, and are expressed through narration and various responses, whether verbal, written, nonverbal, or through silence. Experiences can be uncovered and understood through involvement and participation in dialogues and discourses.

One of the discipline's immediate goals is to discover and develop techniques and methodologies to capture the holistic nature of human beings and the nature of integrated responses to the environment that are considered central to the domain of nursing. To achieve this, nurses must develop ways by which the nature of the lived experiences of human beings can be accessed, captured, and used as the basis for caring for people (McIntyre, 1995). Until this goal is realized, nurses may have to continue to resort to a more reductionist approach to the study of clients. It is important to note that a focus on lived experiences must include the physical body in the analyses. For example, the experiences and responses to pain and illness are the embodied experiences of a person that include their physical being and an awareness of bodily sensations (McDonald and McIntyre, 2001). McDonald and McIntyre (2001) go even further with a warning that the body of patient and nurse included in the development of knowledge must *not* be objective and stripped from the synthesis of emotion and physicality. A focus on lived experiences must also incorporate the study of their genes. More recently, it became apparent that genomic concepts should be incorporated in defining clients and in advancing nursing knowledge (Conley and Tinkle, 2007; Williams, Prows, Conley, et al., 2011). Researching the biologic aspects of the client will inform nursing knowledge as well as reflect the discipline's ontological focus on holism (Stiles, 2011). Clients are also defined by the community of microorganisms that reside in different parts of a human body and influence their health and illness (Wright and Starkweather, 2015). How and in what way the interference of microbiomes' balance in the body is affected by interventions, and how clients' responses and needs inform the nature of nursing interventions are areas for further analysis and investigation.

Another goal for the discipline is to focus knowledge development on populations that have been marginalized in the health care systems in particular and in society in general. Minorities exist in every society because of differences in religion, ethnicity, culture, and sexual orientation, and additionally, wars have created other major groups of marginalized populations. These are the refugees, the displaced, the immigrants, and the trafficked populations, among others. The lived experiences of these populations and their responses to health and illness should be uncovered and utilized in advancing knowledge that informs culturally competent models of care.

Examples of the types of theories that need to be developed are as follows:

1. Descriptive theories (e.g., patterns of normal responses)
2. Explanatory theories (e.g., how and why different groups of clients respond in certain ways to noxious stimuli)
3. Prescriptive theories (e.g., how and in what ways nurses enhance a sense of comfort or well-being in clients)

Transitions

Nurses deal with people who are experiencing transition, anticipating transition, or completing the act of transition (Chick and Meleis, 1986; Meleis and Trangenstein, 1994). *Transition* denotes a change in health status, or in role relationships, expectations, or abilities. It denotes changes in the needs of all human systems. Transition requires the person to incorporate new knowledge, to alter behavior, and therefore to change the definition of self in the social context. Transitions are developmental, situational, or health/illness events (Meleis, 2010). Two significant developmental transitions may be associated with health problems (both psychosocial and biophysiologic): the transition from childhood to adolescence, which has the potential of being associated with ensuing problems such as substance abuse and teen pregnancies; and the transition from adulthood to mature adulthood, a period accompanied by gerontologic problems relating to identity, retirement, and chronic illness (Schumacher and Meleis, 1994). (See Chapter 16 for a comprehensive discussion of transition as a middle-range theory.)

Another transition falling within the domain of nursing is the situational transition, which includes the addition or loss of a member of the family through birth or death. Each situation requires a definition or redefinition of the roles that the client (a person or a family) is involved in. The transition from a nonparental role to a parental one, the change from double parenting to single parenting, and the attempts of women to move from the battered role to the nonbattered role are three examples of situational transitions that affect a human being in totality, although we are concerned with them in terms of health. Nurses are also concerned with the transition from institutional care to community care.

Nurses may also encounter the health/illness transition. This category includes such transitions as sudden role changes that result from moving from a well state to an acute illness, from wellness to chronic illness, or from chronicity to a new wellness that encompasses the chronicity (Tornberg, McGrath, and Benoliel, 1984). There is evidence that transitional care of patients who are discharged from hospitals and whose care requires advanced nursing practice enhances their healing and recovery (Naylor, 2002).

Finally, nurses may encounter the complex transition, in which multiple transitions occur simultaneously. An example is the transition from pediatric care to adult care of a patient suffering from a long-term illness such as sickle cell disease. Caring for patients and families during complex transitions presents challenges that must be carefully anticipated and dealt with (Crosby, Quinn, and Kalinyak, 2015).

The sociologist, psychologist, biologist, and physiologist are all interested in transitions at the micro- and macro levels, and the objective of their interest is to know. Because domains are identified not only by the types of objects that they deal with but also by the questions they ask, the different domain interests can be differentiated by considering the types of questions that nurses ask. Only the nurse is interested in articulating transitions that are biopsychosociocultural—not only to know, but ultimately to have knowledge of the utility of what we know and, in particular, to have ways to effectively use that knowledge in enhancing individuals' healthy transitions. Unlike other academic disciplines, nursing is accountable to the public; it is expected to meet the public's needs.

An example of a multidimensional transitional interest is my own interest in the health care of immigrants, which arose from the needs of health care systems dealing with this population and the need for a broader knowledge base to support the provision of culturally competent care. It concerns immigrants in sociocultural transition, and it considers the effect of transition on clients' biological, psychological, sociological, and cultural needs and the effect of transitions on health behavior, illness behavior, illness episodes, and coping styles of any group of immigrants to the United States. The interest evolved from a nursing perspective, uses a sociologic model, and will add to the domain of nursing.

Nursing does not deal with the transition of an individual, a family, or a community in isolation from an environment (Meleis, 2015). How human beings cope with transition and how the environment affects that coping are fundamental questions for nursing. Nursing seeks to maximize clients' strengths, assets, and potentials or to contribute to the restoration of the client to optimal levels of health, function, comfort, and self-fulfillment. Coping and adapting are multidisciplinary and interdisciplinary concepts. The menopausal experience, for example, is a developmental transition and a multidomain concept. Although research in nursing considers menopause from a biopsychosociocultural perspective, the sociologist looks at it in terms of societal expectations, with the roles and status normatively accorded the menopausal woman. The psychologist views menopause from an intrapsychic perspective; the physician views it in terms of changes in cells in the endocrine system. The nurse researcher considers the subjective meaning of the entire experience, what biopsychosociocultural variables influence that meaning, what the consequences are for the person, as well as for that person's significant others, how the person is adapting to changes, and, finally, how the nurse can help the menopausal woman cope with the experience, if indeed there is a need to do so.

Although each nurse researcher considers the nursing phenomenon according to the basic premises of the field and according to a total view of the human being, the goals of research will dictate the dominant model. For example, one nurse researcher conceptualizes phenomena predominantly from a physiologic model, whereas another may use a sociologic model. Both explicate nursing phenomena and work toward the goals of enhancing healthful living, an adaptive stance, and a higher sense of well-being. Both are adding to the nursing conceptualization of an experience.

Theories are needed to describe the nature of transitions and normal patterns of responses to transitions, to explain relationships between transitions and health, and to provide guidelines for enhancing a perception of well-being.

Relationships and Interactions

Under a biomedical model, which previously guided medical and nursing practice, limited attention was placed on the health professional's relationship with the patient, so that relationship was distant at best. Medicine is beginning to adapt a biopsychosocial and a humanistic model (Gong, Diao, Pan, et al., 2015; Johnson, 2012). In the meantime, relationships between nurses and clients emerged as a defining aspect of the domain of nursing or—as described by Newman et al. (2008)—as the central focus of the discipline of nursing, or indirectly, as a unifying focus for the discipline (Willis et al., 2008). Some theorists focused on the process of building relationships and on the tools of assessment, and, therefore, viewed nursing as a relationship and an interaction process. Relationships are formed through interactions, and together they provide us with the basis for interaction theories (Dunphy, 2010). These theorists spoke of the properties of the nurse–patient dialogue, of therapeutic interaction, and of the components of interacting as being the sensing, perceiving, and validating of the patient's need for help and the sharing of information. They explicated properties of perception, thought, and feelings during health and illness situations. Together, they provided us with a framework that contains major concepts central to nursing, including trust, engagement, development of meaning, and true presence of nurses. Theories relating these concepts could come from inside or outside nursing. They could evolve from studying the work of the different theories in conjunction with either patient care situations or other interaction theories, such as those of Sullivan (1953) and Mead and Morris (1937).

Interaction is a tool for assessment, diagnosis, or intervention, and for building relationships (Hawthorne and Yurkovich, 2002). It is one of the central concepts in nursing for the following reasons:

1. A nursing client is in constant interaction with the environment (King, 1981; Nightingale, 1946; Rogers, 1970). Therefore, nursing focuses not only on individuals but also on monitoring, regulating, maintaining, and changing environments.

2. Interaction is the major tool by which nurses build trusting relationships and assess a client's needs and resources, and it is also a central tool in providing nursing therapeutics (King, 1981; Orlando, 1961; Paterson and Zderad, 1976; Travelbee, 1971; Wiedenbach, 1963).

There is some agreement that interaction is a domain concept and that interactions occur both as person–environment interactions (Flaskerud and Halloran, 1980; Forchuk, 1995) and as nurse–patient interactions (Barnum, 1994). Interaction is considered here in its broadest sense to incorporate both of these situations. Effective and authentic interactions require "presence" in the encounter and the relationship with clients (Bunkers, 2012).

In reviewing published research reports between 1999 and 2008 about nurse practitioners–patient interaction, Charlton, Dearing, Berry, et al. (2008) identified two major communication styles, a biomedical one and a biopsychosocial one. The biopsychosocial style is a more patient-centered approach to communication; it was associated with improved patient outcomes such as patient satisfaction, adherence to treatment plans, and general improvement of health. These results demonstrate the potential for advancing nursing knowledge when the domain is more specifically defined (interaction styles) to point out the potential consequences of how a nursing perspective (biopsychosocial) may influence outcomes that are central to the nursing discipline (patient satisfaction, adherence, health).

Several kinds of theories related to interactions need to be developed, including the following:

1. Theories that describe normal patterns of the interactions of human beings with significant aspects of their environments

2. Theories that describe normal patterns of interactions between clients and their environments within a context of health and illness, which should account for developmental, sociocultural, and cognitive variations

3. Theories that describe and explain interactions and the consequences of interactions that are related to assessment, diagnosis, and interventions

Kim (1987) identified four sets of variables that are related to client–nurse contacts for providing nursing care: client and nurse, a social context for the contact, a process of interaction, and outcomes. The conceptual linkages between each of these sets of variables are then amenable to theory development (Kim, 1987, p. 105).

Nurses have claimed nurse–patient interactions as central to the nursing diagnosis; however, what Kim stated in 1987 continues to hold true.

While there has been a great deal of theoretical emphasis on the importance of client–nurse interaction in the delivery of nursing care, very little has been done either in theory development or in empirical testing of these theories. More needs to be done on the meaning of therapeutic relationships and ways by which such relationships are established, nurtured, supported, discouraged, or avoided. There is a rich array of theoretical and empirical work accomplished in sociology and social psychology that is transferable to this nursing domain. There is a need to have an understanding of how the special nature of client–nurse interactions modifies sociological, social, psychological, and communication theories. Much work, therefore, needs to be done to revise and reformulate existing knowledge to explain and predict phenomena in the client–nurse domain. (Kim, 1987, p. 107)

Communication, interaction, and being present in relationships and interpersonal relationships gained a new momentum in popular literature, as well as in clinical and managerial literature, at the turn of the 21st century (Newman et al., 2008). Going back to the basics in human relationships may have been a reaction to computerization and the increasing use of gadgets and machines. Reports from the National Academy of Medicine (formerly the Institute of Medicine [IOM]) in the

United States, an independent policy analysis arm of the U.S. Congress, proposed, with ample documentation, the need for a patient-focus as well as an interaction-focus in the education of health care professionals. The discipline of nursing was the first to claim interaction and communication as the tools of professional practice. The momentum gained in developing the science of nurse–patient and patient–environment communication by nurse scientists should be continued and advanced (IOM, 2003).

Nursing Process

Another concept central to the discipline of nursing, as demonstrated in the many discourses in the literature and by many nursing theories, is that of the nursing process. The nursing process is built on communication and interaction tools and processes for nursing practice. The distinct properties of the nursing process as they differ from client–nurse or client–environment interactions have not yet been as clearly defined and distinguished. Despite some apparent overlap, it is proposed here that propositions about the nursing process, about approaches that are more effective in the process of assessing, diagnosing, or providing nursing therapeutics, and about the goals of the nursing process can be derived from the work of several theorists, namely, Abdellah, Henderson, Orem, Orlando, Travelbee, and Wiedenbach. Together, they provided nursing with a perspective on assessment, diagnosis, plan for intervention, and evaluation (Abdellah, 1969; Henderson, 1966; Orem, 1988), and on the process of defining and attaining goals (King, 1981); and placed emphasis on the patient's perception of his own condition (Wiedenbach, 1963).

The nursing process, a tool for nursing practice, was introduced to nursing by Orlando (1961) and became central to many nursing publications. It has even been considered a framework for nursing practice and nursing education (Yura and Walsh, 1978a, 1978b). Most of the theorists described and discussed the nursing process. Although some components of the process of clinical judgments are an integral part of all professional–client relationships, the process in nursing differs, just as the goals of each profession are different. It is proposed here that the nursing process is a central concept in the domain of nursing.

Many nurse metatheorists agree with this position (e.g., Torres, 1986; Walker and Avant, 1995), as demonstrated by the extensive literature on and use

of the nursing process, and by those who maintain that emerging theories and models in nursing must consider the nursing process (Thibodeau, 1983). Others question the compatibility of the holistic mission of nursing and the reductionist approach dictated by the use of the nursing process (Barnum, 1987). Barnum (1987) pointed out the potential for other processes in decision-making to be more compatible with the holistic principles of nursing, such as the problematic method described by Dewey (1966). These debates in the nursing literature demonstrate the need for further theoretical development of different processes for assessment and diagnoses and for providing nursing therapeutics. Similarly, the relationship between nursing process and processes for clinical judgment should be explored, examined, and further developed.

One significant component of the nursing process that has received the attention of the discipline throughout the 1980s is a taxonomy of nursing diagnoses. The movement toward the development of taxonomies began in the early 1970s, starting with Kristine Gebbie (a graduate of the University of California, Los Angeles [UCLA], a faculty member at UCLA, and a collaborative author with Betty Neuman and later a faculty member at Columbia University, New York). The nursing diagnoses described by participants in annual nursing-diagnoses conferences were without a binding theoretical framework to guide their development. Although these taxonomies appear to be a unifying diagnostic language for communication between nurses, they

cannot contribute to the development of scientific solutions (i.e., nursing therapeutics), [because] nursing diagnoses that are not developed within an explanatory framework have to be accepted only as descriptive "averages" to be used for the purpose of communication and documentation only. (Kim, 1987, p. 102)

Several types of theories related to the nursing process need to be developed (Frisch, 1994). These include theories to describe the actual processes that nurses use in assessing, diagnosing, and providing nursing therapeutics to different types and categories of clients; theories to describe nursing diagnoses and those that can "give order to the nomenclature" (Kim, 1987, p. 103); theories to explain diagnostic categories within the different contexts; and theories that explain nurse–patient contacts within the contexts of client variables and diagnostic categories. Processes for assessment, diagnosis, and intervention have emerged as central to nursing and its mission.

Finally, a dialogue about the congruency between a reductionist approach to viewing nursing phenomena, as assumed through using the nursing process, and the assumptions of holism, must continue. This dialogue began with effective arguments supporting the incongruity between assumptions inherent in theories of nursing process and the nature of holism in nursing (Barnum, 1987). Similarly, questions arise about the role of the nursing process in curricula and in nursing science that evolves from considering it as central to nursing. Duldt (1995) argued for better clarification of the properties inherent in the nursing process, as differentiated from the clinical inquiry process and the research processes, and proposed that such differentiation enhances the potential of using these differentiated processes to structure advanced nurse practitioner courses. Students may be better able to move easily between the different processes when they are aware of their similarities and differences in process and goals.

Environment

Ever since Florence Nightingale (1946) identified nursing in relation to a focus on optimizing an environment to promote healing and optimal health, environment has been a concept central to the nursing domain. Nightingale considered both the discomfort and the suffering that patients experience as a result of inadequacies in the environment, as well as the nurses' actions that focus on that environment. We lost track of this concept during those years when a focus on biologic systems dominated nursing and when nursing education focused on illness, medical treatment, and assistance with a medical regimen. Despite the centrality of the concept of environment, nursing theorists have not addressed it in the same depth and with the same conviction about its centrality as did Nightingale—or as they did when considering the individual. For decades, clinicians appear to have paid lip service to the importance of environment in nursing care.

More contemporary theorists see the environment as central to nursing, particularly as it relates to human beings and their responses (e.g., Paterson and Zderad, 1976; Rogers, 1970). To these theorists, environment encompasses energy fields, social systems, family, society, culture, the patient's room, the nurse, and all that surrounds the client. Rogers' theory focuses on a description of person

and environment energy fields as inseparable, and on the dynamics of human being–"environment" interactions. According to her, the process inherent in such interactions can be understood only through a careful consideration of the environment. This view assumes that the person and the environment are in constant interaction and recognizes changes in one as integral and simultaneous to changes in the other. Therefore, the aim of nursing intervention is to promote, maintain, regulate, or change the environment and/or the life processes of people to effect changes in either or in both.

Chopoorian (1986) argued for considering the environment as the central focus for nursing interventions, and warned us against continuing to develop knowledge based on the centrality of clients. She demonstrated the limited roles that nurses play in instituting policy changes when clients are considered the central focus for nursing. In reconceptualizing environment for the discipline of nursing, she suggested that "nurses develop a consciousness of environment as social, economic, and political structures; . . . as human social relations, . . . as everyday life" (Chopoorian, 1986, p. 47). She further argued that this approach has the potential to open up new opportunities for nurses to go beyond the acceptance of the status quo for patients and make contributions to resolving society's problems (p. 53). A focus on environment may prompt nurses to reconsider their goals and the mission of the discipline.

Environment, as a central domain concept, includes but is not limited to immediate client settings, family, significant others, health care professionals, and the socioeconomic and political contexts of the client's families and communities (Hedin, 1986). Stevens (1989) proposes the use of critical theory to illuminate oppressive environmental factors that influence health, hinder human potential and life possibilities, and "restrict their equal and fully conscious participation in society" (p. 63).

Both clients' and nurses' environments are undergoing tremendous changes that will drive theory development in different ways. A plausible scenario is the expansion of the environment to include outer space, with all the changes in the nature of care that will need to become more congruent with this changing environment. Other changes in environment are related to levels of risks, such as increased pollution, decreased protection offered by the ozone layer, increased aggression and decreased safety, and increased globalization. Each one of these will influence and drive the nature of theories in different ways and will require models that address the nature of healthy environments and strategies by which a healthy environment may be created and supported. Theories of the future will also have to address global issues, as well as strategies to provide care that evolve from an international perspective (Kleffel, 1996).

There have been many natural disasters (the Indian Ocean tsunami in 2004, Hurricane Katrina in 2005, and Hurricane Sandy in 2012) and human-made disasters (wars; nuclear plant explosions like the one in Chernobyl, Ukraine, in 1986; the terrorist attack on the World Trade Center in September 2001) that require not only the immediate involvement of nurses, but long-term attention while people are coping with the aftermath of these events. These situations drive the need for even more informed theories about environments and the different meanings of environments. For example, the earthquake in Kobe, Japan, in 1995, and the Loma Prieta earthquake near San Francisco in 1989 prompted a reflection on nursing and ways by which nursing could contribute to the health care of people who have experienced such devastating events. The following are some of the questions that these events raise for nurses:

- What are new definitions of environment in light of emerging knowledge about climate change and global warming, environmental hazards, and human microbiomes?
- What processes do people go through as they begin to heal from illness, surgeries, and interventions within the context of drastic internal and external environmental changes?
- What strategies do nurses use to create healing environments in spite of drastic changes in environments due to pollution, climate change and global warming, and natural and man-made disasters?
- Who gets marginalized during the disaster and during the long healing process?
- What are milestones and critical turning points in the long recovery processes, and what are the best practices at each juncture?

These are some of the questions that will drive the development of new theories to inform nursing practice.

Several types of environment-related theories need to be developed. Theories centering on environment are expected to describe those properties, components, and dimensions of environment that are healthy or that help in maintaining or in changing health care outcomes. These theories are also expected to describe the environment that promotes a client's abilities for self-care, resilience, and adaptation. In addition, they are expected to guide the development of effective interventions that may change systems that constrain access and equality in giving and receiving health care. Examples of environmental nursing theories are descriptive theories of healthy environments; theories that describe societal mechanisms that constrain the development, provision, and maintenance of healthy environments; theories that describe and explain policies for health care; and theories that guide actions for environmental changes (Salazar and Primomo, 1994). These theories also consider the work environments for nurses that affect their delivery of nursing care. Finally, with increasing attention being given to erosion of microbes due to environment changes and overmedication (e.g., antibiotics therapy), and the role of microbiomes in illness and health, nurse theorists and researchers must face the challenge of advancing knowledge about best practices that incorporate these new discoveries (Wright and Starkweather, 2015).

Nursing Therapeutics

Nursing therapeutics is defined as all nursing activities and actions deliberately designed to care for nursing clients (Barnard, 1980, 1983). Although the nursing process addresses patterns in assessing, diagnosing, and intervening, nursing therapeutics considers the content of nursing interventions and the goals of intervention. The ultimate goal of theory development in nursing is to develop theories that guide the care nurses give to patients. The existing nursing theories, as categories, provide nursing with the beginnings of nursing therapeutics. For example, interaction theorists suggest that, because we define nursing as a process and as an interaction, nursing problems reflect process and interactional problems; therefore, to these theorists, nursing therapeutics are related to making the interaction process more effective. These theorists recommend the development of empathy, the use of validation, and the use of deliberative nursing process as strategies to deal with communication and interaction problems.

The following are examples of nursing therapeutics that are being used in the nursing literature:

- Touch (stimulation and repatterning of human fields) (Krieger, Johnson, Weiss, Rogers Neuman)
- Care (Orem, Henderson, Leininger)
- Role supplementation (Meleis, Swendsen, Dracup)

- Protection (Johnson, Norris)
- Manipulation of focal, residual, and contextual stimuli (Roy)
- Comfort (Arruda, Larson, and Meleis; Morse)
- Use of self as a nursing therapeutic (Hall and Allan, 1994)
- Symptom management (Lenz, Pugh, Milligan, et al., 1997)
- Transitional care (Naylor, Brooten, Campbell, et al., 2004)

See Chapter 21 for examples of appropriate references. Each of these concepts related to nursing therapeutics could become the nucleus of a middle-range or situation-specific theory in therapeutics (see Chapters 14–17) for the different strategies to use in developing concepts and theories.

Health

Health, a goal shared by a number of health professions, emerged as a central goal in nursing in the writings of Florence Nightingale in the mid-1800s. Since then, theorists have considered health with different degrees of specificity, reductionism, and centrality. Health has been accepted as more than the absence of disease, and that concept is receiving more emphasis in nursing (Neuman, 1989; Newman, 1983, 1986; Smith, 1983).

Several different models of health were identified from the nursing literature (Meleis, 1990): health as an absence of disease (Smith, 1983), health as an internal homeostasis (Johnson, 1980), health as adaptation (Roy, 1984; Smith, 1982), health as performing roles and functions (Orem, 1988; Smith, 1982), and an existential view of health that focuses on symbolism and the place of the self in an intricate web of relations among objects and subjects (Paterson and Zderad, 1976; Travelbee, 1971). A sixth model relies on space/time/energy and consciousness expansion; health in this model is viewed in terms of awareness, personal control, personal empowerment, and mastery over body (Newman, 1986; Rogers, 1970). In this model, health and illness reflect arrhythmic fluctuations "of life processes," and, according to Newman, health is a transformation to higher levels of functioning. The last model considers the cultural, social, and political aspects of health (Allen, 1986; Jones and Meleis, 1993; Meleis, 1990; Tripp-Reimer, 1984). For further theoretical development of health as a central concept, the unity and diversity among these models need to be addressed, compared, and contrasted. Several conditions were identified

as needing to be included in further theoretical development of health. These are the need to focus on an understanding of the health care needs of underserved populations, the potential advantage in using a feminist framework, the integration between a static conception of being healthy and a process/dynamic/becoming conception of health (Meleis, 1990). A strong case could also be made for the unique contribution being made by the discipline of nursing to building the science of health promotion (Northrup and Purkis, 2001), as well as healthy work environments (Caruana, 2008).

DEFINITION OF NURSING

A discipline is also shaped, and it reflects the definition attached to it by its members and by society at large. Several definitions of nursing could drive the process and the goals of knowledge development in the discipline and, in turn, help to further define the structure of the discipline. These definitions, in turn, were shaped by the progress made in theoretical nursing. One of the most influential definitions of nursing has been the one offered by Nightingale (1859, 1946): "taking charge of the personal health" of individuals and to "put" the individual in the best possible state and "allow nature to act upon him." This definition, although old, continues to hold true, and it set the stage for nursing to claim "personal health" as part of its domain.

A second influential definition is one that was commissioned by the International Council of Nurses (ICN) for international use. Henderson offered a definition that emphasized a unique role for nursing and introduced the notion that patients have a role in caring for themselves; when patients are unable to care for themselves because of health problems, nurses provide the care they need. Once the patient is again capable, self-care can resume, and nurses are not then expected to do for patients what they are capable of doing for themselves (Henderson, 1966).

A third significant definition was offered by the ANA (1980). Nursing was defined as "the diagnosis and treatment of human responses to actual or potential health problems" (p. 9). This earlier version of the definition has been discussed and critiqued for ignoring the environment, for its inconsistency with nursing values, for its limitation to individual care instead of community care, and for its problem orientation and lack of health orientation (Allen, 1987; Field, Kritek, Christman, et al., 1983; Silva,

1983; White, 1984). However, the definition did help in further identifying the domain of the discipline and in providing boundaries that have been reflected in theory development and in research priorities. In 1995, an updated version of the definition included the affirmation that nursing is committed to caring for ill and well people as individuals, groups, or communities (ANA, 1995). That definition of professional nursing was further modified and updated in 2003. At the time of this writing, professional nursing is defined in the United States as

> *the protection, promotion, and optimization of health and abilities, prevention of illness and injury, alleviation of suffering through the diagnosis and treatment of human response, and advocacy in the care of individuals, families, communities, and populations. (ANA, 2010, p. 8)*

Currently, nursing is defined by the ICN (2015) in Geneva as:

> *encompassing autonomous and collaborative care of individuals of all ages, families, groups and communities, sick or well and in all settings. Nursing includes the promotion of health, prevention of illness, and the care of ill, disabled and dying people. Advocacy, promotion of a safe environment, research, participation in shaping health policy and in patient and health systems management, and education are also key nursing roles.*

The Royal College of Nursing (2014) defines nursing as:

> *[t]he use of clinical judgment in the provision of care to enable people to improve, maintain, or recover health, to cope with health problems, and to achieve the best possible quality of life, whatever their disease or disability until death.*

The concept of "response" that appears in the ANA's definition is yet to be fully defined; nevertheless, it reflects a more integrated approach to viewing clients' behaviors and actions. It legitimizes nurses' abilities to diagnose and treat or deal with these responses, and acknowledges the significance of giving attention to the daily lived human experiences. The taxonomy of responses provided as examples reflects the influence of theoretical nursing. Future definitions will need to reflect progress in other components of the domain, such as the emphasis on environment and its relationship to nursing care. The addition of such concepts as

prevention, protection, promotion, optimization of abilities for individuals, families, and communities, as well as advocacy on their behalf, better reflects nurses' concerns. Each of these concepts requires further analysis and development.

I have selected three other definitions to illustrate the dialectic relationship between domain definitions and progress and development in disciplines, as well as to demonstrate the systematic conversion of leading thoughts in the discipline. Based on earlier definitions of nursing, on the identification of central concepts, and on the authors' theoretical research and curricular explorations, Newman et al. (1991) defined the focus of the discipline of nursing as the "study of caring in the human health experience" (p. 3). Similarly, Meleis and Trangenstein (1994), although their definition is more specific, defined nursing as being concerned with the process and the experiences of human beings undergoing transitions; therefore, nursing is defined as "facilitating transitions to enhance a sense of well-being" (p. 257). A third definition reflects an evolving, coherent approach to defining the discipline of nursing. In searching for a unified focus of the discipline, Willis et al. (2008) engaged in a lengthy dialogue about their work for 2 years. The result is a definition of nursing as:

> *a health care discipline and healing profession, both an art and science, which facilitates and empowers human beings in envisioning and fulfilling health and healing in living and dying through the development, refinement and application of nursing knowledge for practice. (p. E33)*

They further defined the central unifying focus for the discipline as:

> *facilitating humanization, meaning, choice, quality of life and healing in living and dying. (p. E33)*

All these definitions evolved from previous definitions of nursing, from identification of central concepts, from established research traditions, and from previous theoretical work by nurse scholars. Each of these definitions drives the development of investigation at different levels, one relating to caring acts and lived experiences in health and illness, and the other focusing on the nature of transitions, responses, and consequences of transitions, and the different strategies by which nurses can enhance healthy transitions.

1. What are the key questions addressed in this chapter? What are the main points of view? What could be gained or lost by critical discourses on disciplines, perspectives, domains, and definitions?

2. Identify the implicit and explicit assumptions that the author had in formulating the ideas in this chapter. Why do you agree or disagree with them?

3. Discuss your views on the relationships between domain, perspective, science, and theory? Present your view of these relationships schematically. Now, try to identify questions that incorporate different combinations of these relationships. Discuss ways by which different combinations may or may not advance the knowledge base of nursing.

4. What inferences might you make about the discipline of nursing after reviewing this chapter? What would change these inferences?

5. What are other essential components (core) of a discipline that were not discussed in this chapter? Why do you think these components are essential or core? In what ways would each of these core components transform the discipline's quest for knowledge development?

6. In what ways is the discussion in this chapter about the core domain of nursing and the nursing perspective reflected in current dialogues about disciplines in general and about the discipline of nursing in particular?

7. Define and analyze the core and secondary components of the nursing domain within your field of nursing. Compare and contrast them with those presented in this chapter.

CONCLUSION

Disciplines are defined by the structure and substance that reflect their missions and goals. In this chapter, the nursing perspective, the domain of nursing knowledge, and the definition of nursing are provided. By identifying, acknowledging, and affirming the discipline's perspective, we could focus our knowledge development efforts on the phenomena that nurses deal with, using a perspective that best reflects nursing views and values. A nursing perspective is known by exploring nursing as a human science, with a practice orientation, caring tradition, and a health orientation. The domain of nursing deals with clients who are assumed to be in constant interaction with their environments, human beings who have unmet needs related to their health or illness status, who are not able to care for themselves or are not adapting to their environments because of interruptions or potential interruptions in health. The domain of nursing incorporates a central focus on relationships, interactions, and environments that includes sociopolitical and economic contexts for nursing clients and their significant others. The domain of nursing includes a focus on nursing therapeutics to help in meeting the needs of human beings for health and health care, to enhance adaptation capability, to develop self-care abilities,

and to maintain or promote health and well-being. Theory and research are the processes by which the domain concepts and problems are developed, validated, and communicated. Practice, education, and administration are the means by which the domain goals are implemented. Domains are redefined through theoretical and research processes, and a dialectic relationship exists between domains, definitions, and theory and research traditions. All of these are part of the structure of the discipline of nursing.

REFERENCES

Abdellah, F.G. (1969). The nature of nursing science. *Nursing Research*, 18, 390–393.

Algase, D.L. and Whall, A.F. (1993). Rosemary Ellis' views on the substantive structure of nursing. *Image: Journal of Nursing Scholarship*, 25, 69–72.

Allen, D. (1986). Using philosophical and historical methodologies to understand the concept of health. In P.L. Chinn (Ed.), *Nursing research methodology: Issues and implementation.* Rockville, MD: Aspen Systems.

Allen, D. (2014). Re-conceptualising holism in the contemporary nursing mandate: From individual to organisational relationships. *Social Science & Medicine*, 119, 131–138.

Allen, D.G. (1987). The social policy statement: A reappraisal. *Advances in Nursing Science*, 10(1), 39–48.

American Heritage Dictionary (3rd ed.). (1992). Boston, MA: Houghton-Mifflin.

American Nurses Association. (1980). *A social policy statement.* Kansas City, MO: Author.

American Nurses Association. (1995). *Nursing's social policy statement* (Publication No. NP-107). Washington, DC: Author.

American Nurses Association. (2010). *Nursing's social policy statement* (Publication No. ISBN 9781558102828) (3rd ed.). Washington, DC: Author.

Banks-Wallace, J., Despins, L., Adams-Leander, S., McBroom, L., and Tandy, L. (2008). Re/affirming and re/conceptualizing disciplinary knowledge as the foundation for doctoral education. *Advances in Nursing Science*, 31(1), 67–78.

Barnard, K. (1980). Knowledge for practice: Directions for the future. *Nursing Research*, 29, 208–212.

Barnard, K. (1983). Social policy statement can move nursing ahead. *American Nurse*, 15(1), 4–14.

Barnum, B.J. (1987). Holistic nursing and nursing process. *Holistic Nursing Practice*, 1(3), 27–35.

Barnum, B.J.S. (1994). *Nursing theory: Analysis, application, and evaluation* (4th ed.). Philadelphia, PA: J.B. Lippincott.

Benner, P. and Wrubel, J. (1989). *The primacy of caring*. Menlo Park, CA: Addison-Wesley.

Bjørk, I.T. (1995). Neglected conflicts in the discipline of nursing: Perceptions of the importance and value of practical skill. *Journal of Advanced Nursing*, 22, 6–12.

Bottorff, J.L. (1991). Nursing: A practical science of caring. *Advances in Nursing Science*, 14(1), 26–39.

Brody, J.K. (1988). Virtue ethics, caring, and nursing. *Research and Theory for Nursing Practice*, 2(2), 87–96.

Bunkers, S.S. (2012). Presence: The eye of the needle. *Nursing Science Quarterly*, 25(1), 10–14.

Caruana, E. (2008). Comprehensive systematic review of evidence on developing and sustaining nursing leadership that fosters a healthy work environment in health care. *Journal of Advanced Nursing*, 62(6), 653–654.

Charlton, C.R., Dearing, K.S., Berry, J.A., and Johnson, M.J. (2008). Nurse practitioners' communication styles and their impact on patient outcomes: An integrated literature review. *Journal of the American Academy of Nurse Practitioners*, 20(7), 382–388.

Chick, N. and Meleis, A.I. (1986). Transitions: A nursing concern. In P.L. Chinn (Ed.), *Nursing research methodology*. Boulder, CO: Aspen.

Chopoorian, T.J. (1986). Reconceptualizing the environment. In P. Moccia (Ed.), *New approaches to theory development*. New York: National League for Nursing.

Clarke, M. (1986). Action and reflection: Practice and theory in nursing. *Journal of Advanced Nursing*, 11, 3–11.

Clifford, C. (1995). Caring: Fitting the concept to nursing practice. *Journal of Clinical Nursing*, 4, 37–41.

Cohen, J.A. (1991). Two portraits of caring: A comparison of the artists, Leininger and Watson. *Journal of Advanced Nursing*, 16(8), 899–909.

Condon, E.H. (1992). Nursing and the caring metaphor: Gender and political influences on an ethics of care. *Nursing Outlook*, 40, 14–19.

Conley, Y.P. and Tinkle, M.B. (2007). The future of genomic nursing research. *Journal of Nursing Scholarship*, 39(1), 17–24.

Cook, P.R. and Cullen, J.A. (2004). Caring as an imperative for nursing education. *Nursing Education Perspective*, 24(4), 192–197.

Cowling, W.R., III and Chinn, P.L. (2001). Conversation across paradigms: Unitary-transformative and critical feminist perspectives. *Scholarly Inquiry for Nursing Practice*, 15(4), 347–365.

Crosby, L.E., Quinn, C.T., and Kalinyak, K.A. (2015). A biopsychosocial model for the management of patients with sickle-cell disease transitioning to adult medical care. *Advances in Therapy*, 32, 293–305.

Dewey, J. (1966). *Democracy and education*. New York: Macmillan.

Donaldson, S.K. and Crowley, D. (1978). The discipline of nursing. *Nursing Outlook*, 26(2), 113–120.

Duldt, B.W. (1995). Nursing process: The science of nursing in the curriculum. *Nurse Educator*, 20(1), 24–29.

Dunphy, L. (2010). *Florence Nightingale's legacy of caring and its application*. In M. Parker and M. Smith (Eds.), *Nursing theories and nursing practice* (pp. 35–51). Philadelphia, PA: F.A. Davis Company.

Fawcett, J. (1989). *Conceptual models of nursing* (2nd ed.). Philadelphia, PA: F.A. Davis.

Fawcett, J. (1995). *Analysis and evaluation of conceptual models of nursing* (3rd ed.). Philadelphia, PA: F.A. Davis.

Feldman, M.E. (1993). Uncovering clinical knowledge and caring practices. *Journal of Post Anesthesia Nursing*, 8(3), 159–162.

Field, L., Kritek, P., Christman, L., et al. (1983). Five nurse leaders discuss social policy statement. *The American Nurse*, 15(2), 4, 6, 14.

Fitzpatrick, J.J. (1983). A life-perspective rhythm model. In J.J. Fitzpatrick and A. Whall (Eds.), *Conceptual models of nursing* (pp. 295–302). Bowie, MD: Robert J. Brady.

Flaskerud, J.H. and Halloran, E.J. (1980). Areas of agreement in nursing theory development. *Advances in Nursing Science*, 3(1), 1–7.

Forchuk, C. (1995). Uniqueness within the nurse-client relationship. *Archives of Psychiatric Nursing*, 9(1), 34–39.

Friedman, M.M. and Rhinehart, E. (2000). Improving infection control in home care: From ritual to science-based practice. *Home Healthcare Nurse*, 18(2), 99–106.

Frisch, N. (1994). The nursing process revisited [editorial]. *Nursing Diagnosis*, 5(2), 51.

Gadow, S. (1985). Nurse and patient: The caring relationship. In A.A. Bishop and J.R. Scudder (Eds.), *Caring, curing, coping. Nurse-physician-patient relationships* (pp. 31–43). Birmingham, UK: University of Alabama Press.

Gelman, R. (2000). Domain specificity and variability in cognitive development. *Child Development*, 71(4), 854–856.

Gendron, D. (1988). *The expressive form of caring*. Toronto, ON: University of Toronto.

Gendron, D. (1994). The tapestry of care. *Advances in Nursing Science*, 17(1), 25–30.

Glaser, B.G. and Strauss, A.L. (1964). *Awareness of dying*. Chicago, IL: Aldine.

Glaser, B.G. and Strauss, A.L. (1967). *The discovery of grounded theory*. Chicago, IL: Aldine.

Gong, F., Diao, Y., Pan, T., Liu, M., and Sun, H. (2015). Evolution of human medical model and development course of medical humanistic spirit. *Biomedical Research*, 26(3), 407–414.

Hall, B.A. and Allan, J.D. (1994). Self in relation: A prolegomenon for holistic nursing. *Nursing Outlook*, 42(3), 110–166.

Hawthorne, D.L. and Yurkovich, N.J. (2002). Nursing as science: A critical question. *Canadian Journal of Nursing Research*, 34(2), 53–64.

Hayes, P. (2005). Communicating interdisciplinary research. *Clinical Nursing Research*, 14(3), 211–214.

Hedin, B.A. (1986). Nursing, education, and emancipation: Applying the critical theoretical approach to nursing research. In P.L. Chinn (Ed.), *Nursing research methodology: Issues and implementation*. Rockville, MD: Aspen Systems.

Heitkemper, M.M. and Bond, E.F. (2003). State of nursing science: On the edge. *Biological Research for Nursing*, 4(3), 151–162.

Henderson, V. (1966). *The nature of nursing*. New York: Macmillan.

Holmes, C.A. (1990). Alternatives to natural science foundations for nursing. *International Journal of Nursing Studies*, 27(3), 187–198.

Institute of Medicine. (2003). Health professions education: A bridge to quality. In A. Greiner and E. Knebel (Eds.), *Care services*. New York: National Academy Press.

International Council of Nurses. (2015). *Definition of professional nursing*. Retrieved from www.icn.ch/who-we-are/icn-definition-of-nursing/

Jacobs, B.B. (2001). Respect for human dignity: A central phenomenon to philosophically unite nursing theory and practice through consilience of knowledge. *Advances in Nursing Science*, 24(1), 17–35.

Jenny, J. and Logan, J. (1992). Knowing the patient: One aspect of clinical knowledge. *Image: Journal of Nursing Scholarship*, 24, 254–258.

Johnson, D.E. (1980). The behavioral system model for nursing. In J.P. Riehl and C. Roy (Eds.), *Conceptual models for nursing practice* (2nd ed.). New York: Appleton-Century-Crofts.

Johnson, J. (1994). A dialectical examination of nursing art. *Advances in Nursing Science*, 17(1), 1–14.

Johnson, S.B. (2012). Medicine's paradigm shift: An opportunity for psychology. *Monitor on Psychology*, 43(8), 5.

Jones, P.S. and Meleis, A.I. (1993). Health is empowerment. *Advances in Nursing Science*, 15(3), 1–14.

Kang, D.H. (2012). Biomarkers and boundaries to break [an editorial]. *Research in Nursing and Health*, 35, 109–111.

Kim, H.S. (1987). Structuring the nursing knowledge system: A typology of four domains. *Scholarly Inquiry for Nursing Practice*, 1(2), 99–110.

Kim, H.S. (2000). An integrative framework for conceptualizing clients: A proposal for a nursing perspective in the new century. *Nursing Science Quarterly*, 13(1), 37–40.

King, I.M. (1981). *A theory for nursing: Systems, concepts, process*. New York: John Wiley & Sons.

Kleffel, D. (1996). Environmental paradigms: Moving toward an ecocentric perspective. *Advances in Nursing Science*, 18(4), 1–10.

Klein, J.T. (1990). *Interdisciplinarity. History, theory and practice*. Detroit, MI: Wayne State University Press.

Kuhn, T.S. (1970). The structure of scientific revolutions. In O. Neurath (Ed.), *International encyclopedia of unified science* (2nd ed., Vols. 1 and 2). Chicago, IL: University of Chicago Press.

Laudan, L. (1977). *Progress and its problems: Toward a theory of scientific growth*. Berkeley, CA: University of California Press.

Laudan, L. (1981). A problem-solving approach to scientific progress. In I. Hacking (Ed.), *Scientific revolutions*. New York: Oxford University Press.

Leininger, M.M. (1978). *Transcultural nursing: Concepts, theories and practices*. New York: Wiley and Sons.

Leininger, M.M. (1981). The phenomenon of caring: Importance, research questions and theoretical considerations. In M.M. Leininger (Ed.)., *Caring: An essential human need* (pp. 3–16). Thorofare, NY: Charles B. Slack.

Lenz, E., Pugh, L.C., Milligan, R.A., Gift, A., and Suppe, F. (1997). The middle-range theory of unpleasant symptoms. *Advances in Nursing Science*, 19(3), 14–27.

Litchfield, M. and Jonsdottir, H. (2008). A practice discipline that's here and now. *Advances in Nursing Science*, 31(1), 79–91.

MacPherson, K.I. (1989). A new perspective on nursing and caring in a corporate context. *Advances in Nursing Science*, 11(4), 32–39.

Malinski, V.M. (2002). Research issues: Developing a nursing perspective on spirituality and healing. *Nursing Science Quarterly*, 15(4), 281–287.

Mapanga, K.G. and Mapanga, M.B. (2003). A community health nursing perspective of home health care management and practice within the Zimbabwean health care system. *Home Health Care Management Practice*, 15(5), 429–435.

Mariano, C. (2001). Holistic ethics. *American Journal of Nursing*, 10(1), 24a–24c.

Masson, V. (1985). Nurses and doctors as healers. *Nursing Outlook*, 33(2), 70–73.

McDonald, C. and McIntyre, M. (2001). Reinstating the marginalized body in nursing science: Epistemological privilege and the lived life. *Nursing Philosophy*, 2(3), 234–239.

McIntyre, M. (1995). The focus of the discipline of nursing: A critique and extension. *Advances in Nursing Science*, 18(1), 27–35.

McWhinney, I.R. (1989). An acquaintance with particulars. . . . *Family Medicine*, 21(4), 296–298.

Mead, G.H. and Morris, C.W. (1937). Mind, self, and society. Chicago, IL: University of Chicago Press.

Meleis, A.I. (1986). Theory development and domain concepts. In P. Moccia (Ed.), *New approaches to theory development*. New York: National League for Nursing.

Meleis, A.I. (1990). Being and becoming healthy: The core of nursing knowledge. *Nursing Science Quarterly*, 3(3), 107–114.

Meleis, A.I. (1992). Nursing: A caring science with a distinct domain. *Sairaanhoitaja*, 6, 8–12.

Meleis, A.I. (2010). *Transitions theory: Middle range and situation specific theories in research and practice*. New York: Springer Publishing.

Meleis, A.I. (2015). Transitions theory. In M.C. Smith and M.E. Parker (Eds.), *Nursing Theories and Nursing Practice* (4th ed.). Philadelphia, PA: F.A. Davis.

Meleis, A.I. and Trangenstein, P.A. (1994). Facilitating transitions: Redefinition of the nursing mission. *Nursing Outlook*, 42, 255–259.

Merton, R.K. (1973). *The sociology of science: Theoretical and empirical investigation*. Chicago, IL: University of Chicago Press.

Mitchell, G.J. (1994). Discipline-specific inquiry: The hermeneutics of theory-guided nursing research. *Nursing Outlook*, 42, 224–248.

Mitchell, G.J. and Cody, W.K. (2002). Ambiguous opportunity: Toiling for truth of nursing art and science. *Nursing Science Quarterly*, 15(1), 71–79.

Moch, S.D. (1989). Health within illness: Conceptual evolution and practice possibilities. *Advances in Nursing Science*, 11(4), 23–31.

Moore, S. (1990). Thoughts on the discipline of nursing as we approach the year 2000. *Journal of Advanced Nursing*, 15, 825–828.

Morse, J.M., Bottorff, J., Neander, W., and Solberg, S. (1991). Comparative analysis of conceptualizations and theories of caring. *Image: Journal of Nursing Scholarship*, 23, 119–126.

Morse, J.M., Solberg, S.M., Neander, W.L., Bottorff, J.L., and Johnson, J.L. (1990). Concepts of caring and caring as concept. *Advances in Nursing Science*, 13(1), 1–14.

Moss, R. (1985). *How shall I live: Transforming surgery or any health crisis into greater aliveness*. Berkeley, CA: Celestial Arts.

Naylor, M.D. (2002). Transitional care of older adults. *Annual Review of Nursing Research*, 20, 127–147.

Naylor, M.D., Brooten, D.A., Campbell, R.L., Maislin, G., McCauley, K.M., and Schwartz, M.D. (2004). Transitional care of older adults hospitalized with heart failure: A randomized, controlled trial. *Journal of the American Geriatrics Society*, 52(5), 675–684.

Neuman, B. (1989). *The Neuman systems model* (2nd ed.). East Norwalk, CT: Appleton & Lange.

Neuman, B. and Fawcett, J. (2002). *The Neuman system model* (4th ed.). Upper Saddle River, NJ: Prentice Hall.

Newman, M. (1983). The continuing revolution: A history of nursing science. In N. Chaska (Ed.), *The nursing profession: A time to speak*. New York: McGraw-Hill.

Newman, M. (1986). *Health as expanding consciousness*. St. Louis, MO: C.V. Mosby.

Newman, M.A. (2002). The pattern that connects. *Advances in Nursing Science*, 24(3), 1–7.

Newman, M.A., Sime, A.M., and Corcoran-Perry, S.A. (1991). The focus of the discipline of nursing. *Advances in Nursing Science*, 14(1), 1–6.

Newman, M.A., Smith, M.C., Pharris, M.D., and Jones, D. (2008). The focus of the discipline revisited. *Advances in Nursing Science*, 31(1), E16–E27.

Nightingale, F. (1859). *Notes on nursing: What is it and what it is not*. London, UK: Harrison.

Nightingale, F. (1946). *Notes on nursing* [Originally Published in 1859]. Philadelphia, PA: Lippincott.

Northrup, D.T. and Purkis, M.E. (2001). Building the science of health promotion practice from a human science perspective. *Nursing Philosophy*, 2(1), 62–71.

Northrup, D.T., Tschanz, C.L., Olynyk, V.G., Makaroff, K.L.S., Szabo, J., and Biasio, H.A. (2004). Nursing: Whose discipline is it anyway? *Nursing Science Quarterly*, 17(1), 55–62.

Olson, T.C. (1993). Laying claim to caring: Nursing and the language of training, 1915 1937. *Nursing Outlook*, 41(2), 68–72.

Orem, D.E. (1988). *Nursing: Concepts of practice* (3rd ed.). New York: McGraw-Hill.

Orlando, I.J. (1961). *The dynamic nurse-patient relationship*. New York: G.P. Putnam's Sons.

Owen, M.J. and Holmes, C.A. (1993). 'Holism' in the discourse of nursing. *Journal of Advanced Nursing*, 18(11), 1688–1695.

Parsons, T. (1968). *Sociological theory and modern society* (2nd ed.). New York: Free Press.

Paterson, J.G. and Zderad, L.T. (1976). *Humanistic nursing*. New York: John Wiley & Sons.

Pilkington, F.B. (2002). Book reviews and new media: Where is the human science in nursing texts? *Nursing Science Quarterly*, 15(1), 85–89.

Rawnsley, M.M. (2003). Theoretical concerns. Dimensions of scholarship and the advancement of nursing science: Articulating a vision. *Nursing Science Quarterly*, 16(1), 6–13.

Reed, P.G. (1995). A treatise on nursing knowledge development for the 21st century: Beyond postmodernism. *Advances in Nursing Science*, 17(3), 70–84.

Reynolds, C. (1988). The measurement of health in nursing research. *Advances in Nursing Science*, 10(4), 23–31.

Rogers, M.E. (1970). *An introduction to the theoretical basis of nursing*. Philadelphia, PA: F.A. Davis.

Rolfe, G. (2015). Foundations for a human science of nursing: Gadamer, Laing, and the hermeneutics of caring. *Nursing Philosophy*, 16, 141–152.

Roy, C. (1984). *Introduction to nursing: An adaptation model* (2nd ed.). Englewood Cliffs, NJ: Prentice-Hall.

Royal College of Nurses. (2014). *Defining nursing*. Retrieved from www.rcn.org.uk/__data/assets/pdf_file/0003/604038/Defining_Nursing_Web.pdf

Salazar, M.K. and Primomo, J. (1994). Taking the lead in environmental health. *AAOHN Journal*, 42(7), 317–324.

Sanford, R.C. (2000). Caring through relation and dialogue: A nursing perspective for patient education. *Advances in Nursing Science*, 22(3), 1–15.

Sarvimaki, A. and Lutzen, K. (2004). The theoretical and methodological development of the nursing discipline in Sweden. Vard I Norden. *Nursing Science and Research in the Nordic Countries*, 24(3), 31–37.

Schultz, P. (1987). When client means more than one: Extending the foundational concept of person. *Advances in Nursing Science*, 10(1), 71–86.

Schumacher, K. and Meleis, A.I. (1994). Transitions: A central concept in nursing. *Image: Journal of Nursing Scholarship*, 26(2), 119–127.

Silva, M. (1983). The American Nurses' Association's position statement on nursing and social policy: Philosophical and ethical dimensions. *Journal of Advanced Nursing*, 8, 147–151.

Smith, J.A. (1981). The idea of health: A philosophical inquiry. *Advances in Nursing Science*, 3, 43–50.

Smith, J.A. (1982). Letters to the editor. *Advances in Nursing Science*, 4(3), xi.

Smith, J.A. (1983). *The idea of health: Implications for the nursing professional*. New York: Teachers College, Columbia University.

Stevens, B. (1989). A critical social reconceptualization of environment in nursing: Implications and methodology. *Advances in Nursing Science*, 11(4), 56–68.

Stiles, K.A. (2011). Advancing nursing knowledge through complex holism. *Advances in Nursing Science*, 34(1), 39–50.

Sullivan, H. (1953). *The interpersonal theory of psychiatry*. New York: W.W. Norton.

Swoboda, W. (1979). *Disciplines and interdisciplinarity: A historical perspective. Interdisciplinarity and higher education* (p. 53). University Park, PA: Pennsylvania State University Press.

Thibodeau, J.A. (1983). *Nursing models: Analysis and evaluation*. Monterey, CA: Wadsworth.

Titler, M.G., Buckwalter, K.C., and Maas, M.L. (1993). Critical issues for the development of clinical nursing knowledge. *Advances in Clinical Nursing Research*, 28(2), 475–477.

Tornberg, M.J., McGrath, B.B., and Benoliel, J.Q. (1984, April). Oncology transition services: Partnerships of nurses and families. *Cancer Nursing*, 7(2), 131–137.

Torres, G. (1986). *Theoretical foundations of nursing*. East Norwalk, CT: Appleton-Century-Crofts.

Toulmin, S. (1972a). *The variety of rational enterprises. Human understanding* (pp. 364–411). Princeton, NJ: Princeton University Press.

Toulmin, S. (1972b). *Human understanding: The collective use and evolution of concepts* (2nd ed.). Princeton, NJ: Princeton University Press.

Travelbee, J. (1966). *Interpersonal aspects of nursing*. Philadelphia, PA: F.A. Davis.

Travelbee, J. (1971). *Interpersonal aspects of nursing* (2nd ed.). Philadelphia, PA: F.A. Davis.

Tripp-Reimer, T. (1984). Reconceptualizing the construct of health: Integrating emic and etic perspectives. *Research in Nursing and Health*, 7, 101–109.

Turner, B.S. (2006). Discipline. *Theory, Culture & Society*, 23(2–3), 183–186.

Walker, L.O. and Avant, K.C. (1995). *Strategies for theory construction in nursing* (3rd ed.). East Norwalk, CT: Appleton & Lange.

Watson, J. (1985). *Nursing: Human science and human care, a theory of nursing*. East Norwalk, CT: Appleton–Century–Crofts.

Watson, J. (1988). New dimensions of human caring theory. *Nursing Science Quarterly*, 1, 175–181.

Watson, J. (1990). Caring knowledge and informed moral passion. *Advances in Nursing Science*, 13(1), 15–24.

Weinberg, D.D. (2006). When little things are big things. In S. Nelson and S. Gordon (Eds.). *The complexities of care: Nursing reconsidered* (pp. 30–43). Ithaca, NY: ILR Cornell University Press.

White, C. (1984). A critique of the ANA social policy statement. *Nursing Outlook*, 32(6), 328–331.

Wiedenbach, E. (1963). The helping art of nursing. *American Journal of Nursing*, 63(11) 54–57.

Willetts, G. and Clarke, D. (2014). Constructing nurses' professional identity through social identity theory. *International Journal of Nursing Practice*, 20, 164–169.

Williams, J.K., Prows, C.A., Conley, Y.P., et al. (2011). Strategies to prepare faculty to integrate genomics into nursing education programs. *Journal of Nursing Scholarship*, 43(3), 231–238.

Willis, D.G., Grace, P.J., and Roy, C. (2008). A central unifying focus for the discipline: Facilitating humanization, meaning, choice, quality of life, and healing in living and dying. *Advances in Nursing Science*, 31(1), E28–E40.

Wright, M.L. and Starkweather, A.R. (2015). Antenatal microbiome: Potential contributor to fetal programming and establishment of the microbiome in offspring. *Nursing Research*, 64(4), 306–319.

Yura, H. and Torres, G. (1975). *Today's conceptual frameworks with the baccalaureate nursing programs*. New York: National League for Nursing.

Yura, H. and Walsh, M.B. (1978a). *The nursing process: Assessing, planning, implementing, evaluating*. New York: Appleton-Century-Crofts.

Yura, H. and Walsh, M.B. (1978b). *Human needs and the nursing process*. New York: Appleton-Century-Crofts.

7

Sources, Resources, and Paradoxes for Theory

Where do the ideas for theories come from? What does it mean to advance knowledge, and what are the reasons for developing theories? Are there particular conditions that support the development of theories?

In this chapter, the sources and resources of theory essential to theory development are discussed and analyzed. It is assumed that to engage, in some form or another, in the theoretical development of the discipline, members of the discipline should be aware of the sources and resources for theory, and use and promote them. The conditions that are proposed to facilitate the sources and the resources for theory development are necessary but not sufficient for theory development. Other conditions include the identification and resolution of paradoxes that may influence the processes of developing theories. Two paradoxes are identified and discussed herein. Additional conditions, such as knowledge of strategies for the development and evaluation of concepts and theories are discussed in Chapters 14 to 17. These conditions provide the contexts that enhance the processes needed for knowledge development and support the development of abilities and expertise in developing theories.

SPINOZA ON KNOWLEDGE DEVELOPMENT

To Benedict de Spinoza, a 17th-century Dutch philosopher, one of the most significant goals a human being can pursue is knowledge development because knowledge represents power and freedom for humanity. Spinoza considered the pursuit of knowledge and the pleasures of understanding to be precursors to permanent happiness, which in turn leads to healthful living. His philosophy integrates mind, body, and nature in articulating the sources and resources of knowledge: he asserted that knowledge of the body and the nature of the body are first and foremost essential for understanding the union between the body and mind (Grey, 2014; Wider, 2013). In addition, he considered some conditions essential for knowledge development, two of which are of concern to us here. He proposed that a high level of understanding of the sources of knowledge and the availability of human beings who are interested and committed to activities related to the processes of development are two essential criteria for knowledge development.

On the sources of knowledge, Spinoza distinguished among four forms of knowledge. The first is "hearsay knowledge," knowing one's birthday because we were told of the day, the time, the circumstances, and who one's parents are; the source of that knowledge is not personal experience. The second type of knowledge is perceived through the source of "vague or confused experience." Here, "general impressions" that something has "usually worked" is the source of a great deal of our knowledge, such as knowing that dogs bark, that we will die, and that water extinguishes flame. The third type of knowledge is achieved through "immediate deduction, or by reasoning, one thing is inferred from the essence of another." Specific relationships are absent; therefore, part of the reality is out there to be observed, and the other part is logically deduced. Experience may refute this type of knowledge. Hence, Spinoza called the fourth form (which is the highest, and which incorporates deduction and perception, and combines reality, perception, intuition, and feelings) intuitive knowledge (*scientia intuitiva*). It is not totally unlike the third form of knowledge. It is the kind of knowing that proceeds from "an adequate idea" to the "adequate knowledge of the essence of things" (Copleston, 1963; Durant, 1953).

Of human beings in pursuit of knowledge development, Spinoza said a person who is

---

in pursuit of knowledge should be able 1. To speak in a manner comprehensible to the people and to do for them all things that do not prevent us from attaining our ends. . . . 2. To enjoy only such pleasures as are necessary for the preservation of health. 3. Finally, to seek only enough money . . . to comply with such customs as are not opposed to what we seek. (Spinoza, cited in Durant, 1953, p. 128)

SOURCES FOR THEORY DEVELOPMENT

Ideas, questions, and phenomena are sources for theory development. Ideas originate in the mind, which is integral to a whole human being, and it is through the power of the mind that they are analyzed, separated, and sorted into mere passing thoughts or intellectual ideas worth pausing to examine and further pursue. Early philosophers differed in their discussions of where ideas come from. John Locke (cited in Nidditch, 1975) used the image of the *tabula rasa*, the "blank slate," to describe the meaning of ideas. To Locke, experience is the source of all ideas, reason, and knowledge. Knowledge is founded in experience and is derived from experience. Locke spoke of observations and reflections as mechanisms for experiences to be translated into ideas. Experience is not limited to the external senses, although these sensations are extremely important for knowledge development, but also include internal senses, reflections of the mind. It is the combination of the discourse between external and internal senses, between observations and reflections, and between the internal and external dialogue that creates ideas. The conscious experience, according to Locke, is significant but inseparable from the internal experience.

Although the *tabula rasa* idea has long since died, the inseparability of internal and external sensations is the essence of theory development in nursing. It is through the connection between experience and thinking that ideas may be formed. The mind is ultimately the vehicle through which ideas evolve, yet one question may be: What mechanisms could be used that may promote noticing and observing? Nurses have many rich sources for ideas. These sources have gone through five different eras:

1. *During the first era* nurses were almost totally dependent on other disciplines and paradigms for ideas that advanced nursing knowledge. When it continues to be dependent on other disciplines and paradigms for its sources of ideas, a scholarly discipline cannot have its needed autonomy to pursue ideas that are fundamental to the discipline or a sense of accountability. Such dependence dictates the significant phenomena or problems, instead of allowing the discipline itself to drive the generation of its areas of phenomena and problems. A focus emanating from educational paradigms promoted the development of theories that explained and predicted phenomena that better answered questions in the educational field, such as theories regarding modularized instruction or teaching and learning strategies. A medical model allowed for observations related to signs, symptoms, illness, and observations. A sociologic framework focuses on behaviors of collectivities and patterns of social order. These other disciplines do not adequately address the development of knowledge about responses to health and illness, and they do not help to elucidate patterns of behavior in daily lives as individuals attempt to respond to and live with health and illness episodes.

2. *During the second era*, methodology and functions dominated the idea reservoirs of the discipline of nursing. Ideas related to what nurses do and how nurses conduct research led to conceptualizations of nurses' roles and of methods of research (Gortner and Nahm, 1977). The few dissatisfied scholars who continued to consider sources of ideas such as patients and patient care were rejected. They were thought to advocate a single paradigm in nursing—one single explanation of the world, one system of thought and action that would cover everything. That was perceived to be the route to discipline development. The ideas of these scholars were rejected by the majority, and decades went by in which ideas were methodological and functional—research and theory methodologies—rather than substantive. Some perceived the approach of one paradigm for the entire field to be a method of mind control, a stifling approach conducive to insignificant work.

3. *During the third era*, the acknowledgment of multiple sources of ideas predominated.

clinical responses related to these phenomena, such as responses to health/illness situations.

Examples of theories deductively evolving from other paradigms but attempting to address nursing phenomena and nursing problems are Johnson's theory (based on a systems paradigm), Roy's theory (based on adaptation, systems, and interaction theory), and Rogers' theory (using systems and developmental paradigms) (see Chapters 11–13).

Developing interventions and care programs that reflect progress in scientific discoveries requires knowledge and attention to genetic biomarkers, neuroscience, and advances in the studies of brain functioning. Theories about patients' experiences and responses to health and illness episodes, prevention of disease, and transition in care systems will need to be informed by biomedical sciences; this further provides the rationale for interdisciplinary teams to continue to advance nursing knowledge (e.g., O'Connor, Doorenbos, and Voss, 2014). A prominent example of such interdisciplinary efforts that also reflects recent advances in research findings can be seen in the dialogues about the human microbiome—defined as "the composite of microorganisms that live inside and on humans along with their genomes" (Taggart and Bergstrom, 2014; Turnbaugh, Ley, Hamady, et al., 2007). This area of knowledge provides a fertile field for theoretical development of patients' experiences and responses to interventions (e.g., antibiotics, chemotherapy) as well as to assessment and diagnosis (e.g., chronic illness) (Kelly, Lyon, Yoon, et al., 2016).

Ideal Nursing Practice

One other source of ideas for nursing theories has been what Barnum (1998) called the "ought-to-be" nursing practice, as opposed to the as-is or extant nursing practice. Some theorists who have developed theories based on ideal or ought-to-be nursing practice did not use a discovery method—that is, by observing, experiencing, categorizing, and analyzing reality. Instead, they reconstructed reality; they invented what reality should be and how nurses ought to deal with it. When Johnson (1968a) conceptualized a person as a system of behavior and conceptualized assessment as a process for identifying behaviors, sets, and goals of subsystems, no nurses were actually assessing patients' systems of behaviors. It was her mental image of what nursing could and should be. A person as an energy field was not a focus of nursing action, and a nurse was not a temporary self-care agent.

However, the conceptual images of nursing dealing with a person as an energy field and a nurse as a temporary self-care agent were created by Rogers and Orem, respectively. These nurses combined non-nursing theories, not with nursing care as it was actually broadly provided at the time, but with concepts of what nursing care should be, or perhaps with nursing care as practiced by the few.

Because they were visionaries, incorporating their conceptualization into nursing practice proved to be problematical for two decades and may have slowed the further development and refinement of existing theories. It is of note that theories developed in the late 1950s and early 1960s were not fully acknowledged for discussion and refinement until the 1980s. Nurses in practice could not reconcile the images of the few with the practice of the many. Theorizing was linked with ideal (albeit nonexisting) practice, and the usefulness of a theory for practice was severely questioned. Both areas, practice and theory, were pushed further and further apart.

There are multiple opportunities to capture innovative nurses' images of how practice ought to be in the face of more contemporary challenges that nurses and patients face. For instance, questions abound regarding how nurses can make effective use of technology while still caring, interacting, building relationships, and maintaining and honoring nursing perspective and the domain of holism. (See Chapter 6 for discussions about perspective and domain.) More specifically, conceptualizations about best practices in providing patient- and family-centered care while using telehealth techniques or computer-assisted care will need to be developed, tested, and evaluated.

The Nursing Process

The nursing process, which consists of assessment, diagnosis, intervention, and evaluation, is another source of ideas for nursing theory. Interest in the nursing process has resulted in numerous conceptualizations of process in nurse–patient relationships and in decision-making in patient care. Examples are Peplau's, Orlando's, Wiedenbach's, and Travelbee's conceptualizations of components of the nurse–patient interaction process. Other early examples are the Harms and McDonald (1966) and Abdellah, Beland, Martin, et al. (1961) conceptualizations of the decision-making process. Ideas related to problem solving, priority setting, and decision-making evolved from a focus on the nursing process and from questions such as: What are the best approaches to identify needs of patients and to deliver nursing therapeutics? What are the similarities and differences between nursing process, clinical judgment process, and other decision-making processes (Duldt, 1995; Gordon, Murphy, Candee, et al., 1994)? Frisch (1994) asked the question of whether we need the nursing process, and answered by proposing it as the foundation for practice and teaching to explain and document care.

The processes of assessment and clinical judgment are impacted, in both positive and negative ways, by the current realities of health care, by short hospital stays, by the increase in home care for acute and chronic conditions, and by the use of technology and digital communication. While these processes in the nursing past assumed face-to-face interactions and longer care episodes, new assumptions must guide assessment and clinical judgment. Practicing nurses have been developing innovative strategies for their clinical judgments; describing these strategies and the outcomes could drive the development of conceptualization schemas that may guide research in this area. (See, e.g., Rodgers, Krance, Street, et al., [2014] on mobile phone use.)

CLASSIFICATIONS OF NURSING DIAGNOSIS, NURSING INTERVENTIONS, NURSING OUTCOMES, AND DECISION-MAKING

Ideas for theory may emanate from classification systems such as those developed for nursing diagnosis, nursing interventions, and nursing outcomes. *Nursing diagnoses* are defined as labels given to problems that fall within the domain of nursing. "It is a concise summary, a conceptual statement of the client's health status" (Kim and Moritz, 1982, p. 84). A diagnosis states a conclusion that is based on some order and pattern that the diagnostician arrived at through nursing investigation (Durand and Prince, 1966). It incorporates a nurse's judgment. The process of developing theories through the use of nursing diagnosis is in agreement with stages in theory development, beginning from concepts.

Jacox identified the first step in theory development as a period of specifying, defining, and classifying concepts used in describing the phenomena of the field (Jacox, 1974, p. 5). Therefore, if there is agreement that a first step in theory development is a period of specifying and classifying, and if practice is the arena for theory development, then indeed nursing diagnosis provides a springboard for theory development. Dickoff, James, and Wiedenbach (1968) would classify the result of the process of classifying diagnosis as a step toward a first-level theory. However, labeling without description of what is labeled and without propositions for testing is in itself not a theory; it is only a step toward building theories.

A classification system for nursing diagnosis began with the efforts of the St. Louis University School of Nursing, which sponsored the first conference on diagnosis in 1976 (Gebbie, 1976). The nurses who participated made a decision that theory development in nursing could not begin without the development of an agreement on its terminology. The work of nurses who participated in several of these nursing diagnosis conferences is inspiring and should continue to be the impetus for ideas that could be developed further into theories (Moorhead, Head, Johnson, et al., 1998).

A warning, however, is in order. The taxonomy that evolved out of these three decades of work resulted in a list of diagnoses that some may consider esoteric in language and nonrepresentative of the complexity of human beings. They are nontheoretical or do not emanate from a coherent theoretical perspective, and there is no evidence that they have contributed to clarifying the nursing mission or to improving communication among nurses and with the rest of the health care team (Gordon, Sweeny, and McKeehan, 1980; Shamansky and Yanni, 1983). Nursing diagnoses are only meaningful if we look at diagnosis as a concept denoting a phenomenon (Kritek, 1978). Then, questions arise such as:

- When does the phenomenon occur?
- Why does it occur?
- How do we deal with it?
- How do we prevent it?
- What other conditions occur at the same time?

These questions help in developing theories based on nursing diagnoses. In addition, the extensive reviews of research related to nursing diagnosis (e.g., Gordon, 1985; Kim, 1989) can be the impetus for the development and validation of concepts, as well as for furthering theoretical synthesis (e.g., Burns, Archbold, Stewart, et al., 1993; Dougherty, Jankin, Lunney, et al., 1993; Grant, Kinney, and Guzzetta, 1990). How nursing diagnosis and nursing theory are related should continue to be the subject of exploration (Frisch and Kelley, 2002). For instance, questions have arisen regarding the

They represent a global view of a field—its main concepts and propositions—and therefore provide the blueprint for practice, education, and research (Johnson, 1968a).

Whether conceptual frameworks are necessary steps in the process of developing theories has also been debated. Some contend that the conceptual framework is a stepping stone toward theory development (Hill and Hansen, 1960; Nye and Berardo, 1966), a view that has been adopted by some in nursing (Fawcett, 2013). Others question the necessity of conceptual frameworks for development of theory and argue that conceptual frameworks are neither necessary steps nor likely to promote or hinder theory development (Rodman, 1980).

The interchangeable use of the different concepts such as conceptual frameworks, models, and theories to describe the same thing has been a problem to the pure semanticists in the field. The attempt to differentiate between them has frequently taken on the dimension of splitting hairs and has only added to the confusion. It is just such confusion that may have contributed to the slow progress and, at times, stilted theory development in nursing and has led to an almost exclusive preoccupation with method and process rather than content and consequences. Instead of addressing the central issues in providing quality care to clients, we have had to debate and defend the methodology for theory development. Theorizing is a painstakingly long process, the results of which may be minimized by relegating them to the level of "it is only a conceptual framework." This, in itself, may decrease the impact of the conceptualizations and may make the framework (or the theoretical model) less significant. The discipline using only conceptual frameworks tends to be regarded as pretheoretical and, as a result, nursing's contribution to knowledge about patient care processes and outcomes are minimized.

There are other disadvantages to the preference of using conceptual frameworks and models when the use of theory would have been much clearer. One such disadvantage could be understood by examining analogous situations—one in which conceptual frameworks and models were used before the use of theory, and one in which theories were used from the outset.

Sociology, particularly family sociology, has been unique in believing that conceptual models are distinct from theories. Sociologists have maintained, and nursing scholars have begun to agree, that conceptual models provide a step in the development of theory. However, modern sociologists have since questioned the wisdom of using a conceptual framework to denote the results of theorizing. The skeptics in sociology have pointed out numerous examples in which conceptual frameworks have resulted in theorizing that lacked specification and definition and the slow process of developing propositions for testing (Rodman, 1980).

Conversely, physical and natural sciences do not use conceptual frameworks and models as steps toward development of theory. Instead, they may use the term *developing theory* versus *tested theory*. Notice that many theories (e.g., genetic fat theory of obesity; cholesterol theory of cardiovascular diseases; psychoanalytical theory of neurosis; microbiome, antibiotics, and offspring microbiome theories) are at different levels of abstraction and different levels of sophistication and have different scopes, different levels of clarity, and varying degrees of understandable definitions; however, they are all called theories.

To be sure, some differences exist between models, conceptual frameworks, and theory. A model has to model another entity, whereas a theory may or may not model other properties, structures, or functions. Conceptual frameworks may present a set of discrete concepts that are not as interrelated and linked in sets of propositions as we expect from theory. However, this varies, based on the level of development of the theory. Models tend to evoke the idea of empirical positivism mixed with rationalism as a guiding philosophy or a goal, rather than the tool it ought to be. Functions attributed to models as frameworks or directives for the development of research, frameworks for the generation of a hypothesis, guides for data collection, or depositories for research findings or the further development of theory are the same functions attributed to theory.

It is not entirely clear that nursing theorists, in using different labels for their conceptualizations, have done so in any systematic way. For example, in a 1983 text, eight theorists used four different labels when referring to their conceptualizations: theory, model, science, and paradigm (Clements and Roberts, 1983). Others used *theory* to describe their conceptualizations, and then developed and/ or isolated one part of these conceptualizations and defined it as conceptual frameworks and another part that was labeled a theory (King, 1995a, 1995b). The similarities and the differences in degree of specificity, level of abstraction, and number of concepts and propositions are not always consistent with the labels. One option for using these conceptualizations is to attach the label preferred by the theorist; another option is to use whatever label the user prefers, as long as a definition and rationale are given. Some literature could always be found to document any of the uses.

The perspective of this text is to minimize the differences between conceptual models, frameworks, and theories, and to relegate most of these differences to semantics and the confusion created by the many nursing scientists and theoreticians who have been educated in a multitude of fields. The rationale for taking this perspective is not to argue for a new position or to initiate a debate, but rather to cast some doubt on the significance of the differences between theories and conceptual models.

"Theory" is sufficient to describe the conceptualizations that have been proposed by our theorists. The three related aspects claimed to differentiate between theory and conceptual model are definitions, interrelationships, and level of abstraction. The first two, which state that concepts should be defined and interrelated, are considered in the present perspective as a necessity for both theory and conceptual models. The third aspect, level of abstraction, remains an important consideration. Because theories could be classified as grand, middle-range, or single domain, based on the number of phenomena that the theory addresses, the number of propositions, and the operational level of the definitions, the present perspective proposes this schema to classify nursing theory, rather than to relegate the classification system to such different labels as conceptual model, framework, metaparadigm, paradigm, and theory.

Although this perspective is proposed to enhance a common language across disciplines and to divert energy into development and progress in theoretical nursing rather than into circular debates, the final choice of a label is a personal matter and depends on the purpose for which the label is applied. Just as role theory has been proposed and used as a concept, a framework, a model, or a theory in research, practice, and administration in a number of disciplines, and just as the user may consider role theory from a cultural, structural, or intra-actionist perspective, nursing theories could also be used in the same way. The manner and the goal of the utilization may help determine the appropriate label.

On the basis of the perspective proposed here, *nursing theory* is defined as an articulated and communicated conceptualization of invented or discovered reality pertaining to nursing for the purpose of describing, explaining, predicting, or prescribing nursing care. Nursing theory is developed to answer central domain questions.

Nursing Theory Versus Borrowed Theory

Some old debates endure. Among them are the concerns and meaning of borrowed theories (Fawcett, 2000). For some time now, nurses have been involved in a debate over the types of theory that ought to be developed. They have taken either practice or basic theory positions. Each side has developed a good case as to why one or the other type is possible. The significance of taking one or the other position lies in the idea that the practice theory position encourages forging ahead with theory development, and the borrowed theory position discourages nurses from participating in the seemingly futile attempt to develop theories, when theories that exist in other disciplines could easily be borrowed and used to explicate nursing phenomena.

The proponents and supporters of the development of practice theory in nursing (Dickoff et al., 1968; Jacox, 1974; Johnson, 1968a; Wald and Leonard, 1964) view nursing theory as a conceptual framework invented by the theorist for the ultimate purpose of creating situations to meet desired, preferred end results. Therefore, the ultimate goal for theory development in nursing is to produce a change in a nursing client or a nursing situation that is desired by the nurse or the client. Dickoff and James (1968, p. 200) called this a *situation-producing theory*.

This is a fourth-level theory; theories at other levels are invented and articulated with the purpose of ultimately leading to this level. The first level is factor isolating, a level where theories help delineate and describe a phenomenon. The second level is a correlating theory, where factors or concepts are related to depict theories, and the third level is a situation in which theories permit prediction and allow the promotion or inhibition of nursing care. Each of these levels brings the theorist closer to the goals of nursing that are demonstrated in prescriptive theories, or by the situation-producing level of theory, the fourth level. The development of fourth-level theory is congruent with the purpose of the profession, which ought to be action-oriented, as opposed to only academically oriented. Nurses are shapers, not just observers, of reality.

The first-level theory, the factor-isolating theory, helps to articulate and label concepts. The significance of this kind of theory is to enable one to refer back to those concepts that are invented. Without a label, we have no concepts; without concepts, we have no relationships. Labeling allows for the creation of conceptual entities that become the cornerstones for each subsequent theory level. What Dickoff and James helped nurses to see was the significance of this level of theory, in which they had been engaged long before they began to speak of theory development.

Norris (1975), a "curious nurse clinician," observed numerous incidents of restlessness and noted that, although the term was frequently used in charting, it was not clear how restlessness was identified, when it was identified, why it occurred, and what its consequences were. More importantly, it was not clear what the nursing intervention should be. Norris' conceptual work to describe the phenomena and to label it as "Restlessness" is an excellent example of first-level theory, according to Dickoff and James (1968). Other examples are Norbeck's (1981) social support concept, Norris' (1982) classification of 15 concepts related to basic physiologic protection mechanisms, and my own (Meleis, 1975) work on role supplementation and role insufficiency.

Other nurses have proposed that nursing be organizing around concepts and, in so doing, have provided nursing with numerous identified and labeled concepts (Carlson, 1970; Meltzer, Abdellah, and Kitchell, 1969; Mitchell, 1973). Still others researched labeled concepts in search of validity and reliability (Kim, 1980; Norbeck, 1981; Weiss, 1979). All these are considered first-level theories, an end in their own right, and a beginning of other theory levels when considering the definitions of Dickoff et al. (1968). (For a review of concept and theory development, see Chapters 14 and 15.)

Once concepts are delineated and labeled, a theorist is ready to develop relationships. Correlating theories result when theorists invent relationships between labeled concepts. These theories are second-level, factor-relating theories. Relating preoperative teaching to postoperative behavior, restless and muscular tension under different conditions, social support and health, or role insufficiency and role supplementation could result in a factor-relating theory.

To predict postoperative behavior by varying preoperative teaching is an instance of third-level, predictive theory. Third-level theory depicts and predicts, using a time reference. It is not only relational—as is second-level theory—it is causal, as the theorist discovers that certain conditions lead to others. In fact, all three levels incorporate a discovery of reality but not an invention of reality. None of these three levels purports to change or influence reality. Rather, all lead to the development of the most powerful of theories for a professional

practice discipline, the situation-producing theory, which is a fourth-level theory.

One of the significant differences between third- and fourth-level theories is in commitment to a goal. A predictive theory describes what happens, such as postoperative behavior with different strategies of preoperative teaching. In a fourth-level theory, there is a commitment to finding out how it happened. An example could be that certain postoperative behavior is conceived as appropriate behavior to bring about. The theory then proceeds to describe what to do preoperatively to bring about that desired behavior. This level of theory, therefore, has several essential components: (1) an aim or goal specified by the theorist as desirable; (2) a prescription to bring about the desired aim; and (3) a "survey list" to use in future prescriptions.

The survey list is designed to respond to six crucial questions for prescriptive theory:

1. Who or what performs the activity? (Agency)
2. Who or what is the recipient of the activity? (Patiency)
3. In what context is the activity performed? (Framework)
4. What is the end point of the activity? (Terminus)
5. What is the guiding procedure, technique, or protocol of the activity? (Procedure)
6. What is the energy source for the activity? (Dynamics) (Dickoff et al., 1968, p. 422)

The activities in a prescriptive theory expected to correspond to these questions are agency, patiency, framework, terminus, procedure, and dynamics. Each incorporates internal and external resources, as well as the potential for using theories from other disciplines if deemed useful.

All survey questions are asked from the viewpoint of the goal of the activity and take the prescription into consideration. It is assumed, and practice supports such assumption, that the agent who is expected to perform the prescription does not always hold full jurisdiction over the prescription. A combination of internal resources, such as certain skills, experiences, and techniques, and external resources, such as policies and environment, specifies the agent. In some instances, prescription may be delegated; in others, it may be relegated. A fourth-level theory should include the kinds of agents who are expected to perform the prescription to bring about the desired end result. The authors (Dickoff et al., 1968) proposed a broad concept of *agency* to include all those who have the internal and external resources; they proposed a similar one about patiency. Nurses, physicians, family members, visitors, and so on may be agents performing nursing activities toward nursing goals. Therefore, a theory should specify all possible agents.

Patiency specifies the recipients of the prescriptions with whom agency interfaces for the purpose of bringing about the desired goal. Patiency may designate sick or well people, interacting or noninteracting things or people, animate or inanimate objects, recipients of activities done by registered nurses, and activities done by people other than nurses, but all are bound together by the goal of the activity. Patients are "interactors" with agency and others geared toward the "activity of a desired kind and as possessed of a repertoire of capacities and limitations (much as is the agent) to see a great range of latitude as to ways of producing desired outcomes" (Dickoff et al., 1968).

The agent and the patient in a theory have to be specific in terms of the context within which both occur. The context, called the *framework* by Dickoff and colleagues, requires that the situation-producing theory specify all variables that should be considered to bring about the desired goals through an activity produced by an agent and received by a patient. The end product of the activity is the *terminus*, the situation to be produced.

A situation-producing theory also includes the pattern by which the activity is performed. *Procedure* includes the steps to be taken to bring about the desired goal. Procedure, then, includes the arena, the equipment, the type of charting, the type of follow-up, policies to govern it, timing, and the rules-of-thumb governing activity. Although procedures could be detailed, most often they are guidelines and safeguards.

Finally, a nursing theory of the situation-producing type should consider the aesthetic satisfaction of performing the activity and the desire for self-esteem. These are motivating factors in performing and sustaining activities to realize a nursing goal. The more developed the theory, the more likely these two factors are considered. These factors are grouped under what Dickoff and colleagues called the *dynamics* of the theory. When the dynamics are conceptualized adequately, all factors that relate to the agent, such as education, reputation of institution, and rewards, or to patients, such as insurance, will have to be considered in a situation-producing theory.

To understand, explain, predict, and prescribe nursing phenomena and nursing care, nurses should develop practice theories that emanate from the discipline and guide the discipline's actions. There is one significant feature of theory in a practice discipline. Although descriptive, relating, and predictive theories are equally important, nursing practice theory needs to strive for prescriptive theory. Nurses may develop basic theories that describe discovered concepts, relationships related to human beings, nursing situations, nurse–patient interactions, environments, or health, but the ultimate goal is to develop theories to change situations. Therefore, theories that stress change as their goal are practice theories.

Discovery charts a more probable process for the development of basic theories; conversely, invention is a more probable goal of practice theory. Properties or dimensions of transitions, for example, lend themselves to basic theory that describes and explains when transitions are healthy, under what circumstances transitions in health and illness occur, what the consequences of various types and levels of transitions are, and why the variability of consequences exists. What to do to enhance smooth transitions for nursing clients, how to maintain the person–environment harmony in transition, and how to maintain homeostasis and enhance adjustment are questions that lend themselves to practice theories.

Even when theories developed in other disciplines are used to explain nursing phenomena and nursing problems, the new derivations and new syntheses make them nursing theories. The concept "nursing" does not denote who developed it or where it is used; rather, it reflects the phenomenon that the theory addresses. Nursing theories evolve out of the practice arena or anything that pertains to the practice arena. They are then tested in research. Until the time-consuming job of research is accomplished, the face validity of a theory, as it pertains to practice, should be enough to allow the theory to be a blueprint for action.

Some challenge the notion that nursing should develop its theoretical base. Their arguments are based on the premise that nursing is a practice discipline and that practice disciplines depend on other disciplines for their theoretical underpinnings. Beckstrand (1978a, 1978b, 1980), for example, contends that nursing is concerned with practice theory. For practice theory to be meaningful, practice knowledge should be different from scientific and ethical knowledge. Beckstrand then examined two aspects of practice knowledge, the knowledge of how to control and how to make changes and the knowledge of what is morally good. She examined these aspects with the question in mind of whether it is possible for practice theory to exist as distinct from science and ethics. The first part of the question needs knowledge of science and the second needs knowledge of what is morally good.

Science, to Beckstrand, seeks to develop the knowledge necessary to change and control. This knowledge, containing lawlike relationships, is synonymous with scientific knowledge. Controls are possible in practice situations; however, practice methodology proceeds by valid deductions from scientific laws. Beckstrand then showed that the field of philosophy known as ethics provides the other body of knowledge that is necessary for practice but substitutes for practice theory. Both normative ethics and metaethics have relevance to practice, and we can easily borrow and co-opt theories to explain moral obligations and moral values in the discipline. The method of obtaining such knowledge and using it is that of logical reasoning, also a borrowed concept. Nursing uses scientific knowledge and logic to meet its ethical goals—all that constitutes the knowledge base of nursing. So, in essence, there is no need for practice theory (Beckstrand, 1978a, 1978b).

Others who agreed that nursing does not need its own theory made a case for borrowed theories to describe, explain, and predict phenomena significant to nursing. Family theory, systems theory, and psychological theory are examples of theories that could be borrowed. Johnson, who was the first to use the concept of borrowing (1968a, 1974), defined borrowed theory as "that knowledge which is developed in the main by other disciplines and is drawn upon by nursing" and defined unique theory as "that knowledge derived from the observation of phenomena and the asking of questions unlike those which characterize other disciplines" (Johnson, 1968b, p. 3). However, she warned that any attempts at differentiation are hazardous, first of all because the man-made, more or less arbitrary, divisions between the sciences are neither firm nor constant. It appears a special unity exists in knowledge, corresponding to a unity in nature, which defies established boundaries and continuously presses for the larger, more cohesive view. Moreover, knowledge does not innately "belong" to any field of science. It is not exactly happenstance that a given bit of knowledge is discovered by one discipline rather than another, but the fact of discovery does not confer the right of ownership. Viewed in this light, borrowed and unique have no real permanence, or any meaning (Johnson, 1968b, p. 206).

Johnson (1968a), however, differentiated between them to make a case for the development of a unique theory of nursing that addresses knowledge of order, disorder, and control and that focuses on phenomena and research questions in a way that is not characteristic of any other discipline.

Some may agree that applied theory could evolve out of these borrowed theories to describe and explain prediction and prescribe nursing action. These critics make a distinction between basic theory, emanating from other disciplines, and applied theory, based on basic theory, with the exclusive purpose of defining nursing care and patterning interventions with predictable responses. The latter continues to be called *borrowed theory* by some, which could be considered a fallacy because if we begin with the premise that knowledge is not the exclusive property of any one field and that, eventually, knowledge is for all, "knowledge which we share in common" (Johnson, 1959, p. 199), then knowledge organized into theories in one discipline could freely be used by members of other disciplines. Therefore "borrowing" is really "adapting" or "deriving." Even if we agree that there is such a thing as the borrowing of theories to help in describing, explaining, and predicting phenomena that are significant to nursing, the mere fact that the questions and problems under consideration are nursing questions and problems changes the nature of the so-called borrowed theories. Johnson (1968b) made the point in this way:

> *If we continue to observe behavior from the perspective of sociology, anthropology, or psychology; or if we continue to study disease with the aim of elucidating etiologies, properties, or life cycle; or if we continue to inquire into biological functioning or malfunctioning, we will be serving the cause of science but not necessarily the cause of nursing. (p. 209)*

Therefore, the nursing perspective guides the reconceptualization of existing theories (Donaldson and Crowley, 1978). Synthesis of so-called borrowed theory with a nursing perspective is essential; otherwise, the focus of nursing will continue to remain within other disciplines, and, therefore, nursing problems will not be addressed (Phillips, 1977). Barnum (1994) supported this position. She stated that theories from other disciplines must be adapted to the nursing milieu and to the nursing image of a human being to be meaningful for nursing.

The so-called borrowed theories, then, are given new meaning within a perspective appropriate for nursing. Barnum supported Johnson's stand and called knowledge used in different disciplines "shared";

perhaps we should also have shared theories. To say that nursing theories are applied theories based on basic theories borrowed from other disciplines is therefore a myth that only serves to further obfuscate nursing theory. Nursing uses "borrowed theories" originating in other disciplines to describe phenomena belonging to those disciplines, when propositions remain in the context of the borrowed theory. Borrowed theories become "shared theories" when used within a nursing context. Nursing theories describe, explain, and predict domain phenomena.

Nursing needs theories to describe and explain phenomena that are significant in the act and process of nursing, to prescribe effective strategies of care, and to predict outcomes. Continuing to use borrowed theories may delay the ongoing activities in developing nursing knowledge (Walker and Alligood, 2001). Theories that were developed in other disciplines are also useful for derivation, integration, and synthesis with the nursing perspective. This process yields nursing theories or theories for nursing practice.

Interdisciplinary Theories Versus Nursing Theories

A potential paradox that may evolve during the third decade of the 21st century reflects the progress made toward interdisciplinarity and interprofessionalism. As teams of professionals work together to identify health care issues and solutions, and as research team members combine efforts in studying phenomena, will the nature and goals of theories change? Will theories informed by members of interdisciplinary teams become theories about phenomenon rather than be designated and attributed to a particular discipline? Why would pain management, or interaction, or symptom management theories be designated or presented as nursing, medical, or psychological theories? As knowledge becomes more integrated and as it becomes translated to provide care for human beings, who are whole, theories may become shared theories. The question that warrants careful dialogue is how to ensure that nursing perspective and the domain concepts are well reflected in guiding the development of these phenomenon-based (rather than discipline-driven) theories. This is a paradox that is still in its developmental stage, so it could be influenced and redirected by nurse scholars (see Chapter 19).

CONCLUSION

The sources of ideas for theory development are numerous and varied, with each inspiring different questions and providing different components to theoretical nursing. Some sources (such as biomedical models) have received more attention from nurses than others (such as nurses' daily experiences). Awareness and knowledge of the various sources may drive the development of theories that address the multidimensional and dynamic nature of nursing care.

In this chapter, I have suggested some ways by which an environment could be developed to nurture critical and theoretical thinking in nurses. Such a dialogic and affirming environment could nurture and support nurses' abilities to capture their experiences and to reflect their clinical wisdom in theoretical nursing. Once again in this chapter, support is provided for the extent to which clinical nurses are a most significant resource for theory development.

Finally, two major historical debates and one potential future paradox are discussed. The historical discourses revolve around whether nursing conceptualizations are theories or conceptual frameworks and whether nurse scholars should be engaged in developing theories or adapting borrowed theories from other disciplines. Although students of theory should be aware of the nature of these debates, I do not believe that resolving either of them is a crucial step toward continuing to advance knowledge development. The potential future paradox, presented here to stimulate dialogue, centers on the effects of becoming a member of interdisciplinary research and practice teams and the consequence of having interprofessional education on developing nursing theories. Progress in knowledge and in developing theoretical nursing can and must proceed despite historical or future paradoxes.

REFLECTIVE QUESTIONS

1. A number of sources were proposed to drive theory development. Critically consider which of these sources could promote or constrain the generation of ideas that could be evolved into theories.

2. What aspects of your own education prepared you for theoretical thinking? Why? Similarly, as you think back on your experiences, which experiences, educational or clinical, helped or hindered in forming your identity as a theoretician?

3. Discuss the dialectic relationship between sources of theory and the agents in theory development.

4. In this chapter, two historical paradoxes were discussed that have shaped our more contemporary thinking on theory. Identify and critically analyze other paradoxes that will shape the future of theory development.

5. In what ways will the move toward outcomes-based nursing or evidence-based nursing advance or constrain nursing theory development? Give examples to support your arguments to defend them.

6. Allocate time and find colleagues who think differently about the answers to previous questions and debate your positions.

REFERENCES

Abdellah, F.G., Beland, I.L., Martin, A., and Matheney, R.V. (1961). *Patient-centered approaches to nursing.* New York: Macmillan.

Agan, R.D. (1987). Intuitive knowing as a dimension of nursing. *Advances in Nursing Science*, 10(1), 63–70.

Allen, J. and Hall, B. (1988). Challenging the focus on technology: A critique of the medical model in a changing health care system. *Advances in Nursing Science*, 10, 22–34.

Arietti, S. (1976). *Creativity: The magic synthesis.* New York: Basic Books.

Armiger, B. (1974). Scholarship in nursing. *Nursing Outlook*, 22(3), 162–163.

Barnard, K. (1980). Knowledge for practice: Directions for the future. *Nursing Research*, 29(4), 208–212.

Barnum, B.J.S. (1994). *Nursing theory: Analysis, application, and evaluation* (4th ed.). Philadelphia, PA: Lippincott Williams & Wilkins.

Barnum, B.J.S. (1998). *Nursing theory: Analysis, application, and evaluation* (4th ed.). Philadelphia, PA: Lippincott Williams & Wilkins.

Beckstrand, J. (1978a). The notion of a practice theory and the relationship of scientific and ethical knowledge to practice. *Research in Nursing and Health*, 1(3), 131–136.

Beckstrand, J. (1978b). The need for a practice theory as indicated by the knowledge used in conduct of practice. *Research in Nursing and Health*, 1(4), 175–179.

Beckstrand, J. (1980). A critique of several conceptions of practice theory in nursing. *Research in Nursing and Health*, 3(2), 69–80.

Benner, P. (1983). Uncovering the knowledge embedded in clinical practice. *Image*, 15, 36–44.

Buckingham, C.D. and Adams, A. (2000). Classifying clinical decision making: Interpreting nursing intuition, heuristics and medical diagnosis. *Journal of Advanced Nursing*, 32(4), 990–998.

Burns, C., Archbold, P., Stewart, B., and Shelton, K. (1993). New diagnosis: Caregiver role strain. *Nursing Diagnosis*, 4(2), 70–76.

Byrne, M.L. and Thompson, L.F. (1978). *Key concepts for the study and practice of nursing.* St. Louis, MO: C.V. Mosby.

Canales, M.K. (2010). Othering: Difference understood? A 10-year analysis and critique of the nursing literature. *Advances in Nursing Science*, 33(1), 15–34.

Carlson, C.E. (Ed.). (1970). *Behavioral concepts and nursing intervention.* Philadelphia, PA: J.B. Lippincott Williams & Wilkins.

Carlson, C.E. and Blackwell, B. (Eds.). (1978). *Behavioral concepts and nursing intervention* (2nd ed.). Philadelphia, PA: J.B. Lippincott.

Carper, B. (1978). Fundamental patterns of knowing in nursing. *Advances in Nursing Science*, 11, 13–23.

Chin, R. (1961). The utility of system models and developmental models for practitioners. In W. Bennis, K. Benne, and R. Chin (Eds.), *The planning of change.* New York: Holt, Rinehart & Winston.

Clements, I.W. and Roberts, F.B. (1983). *Family health: A theoretical approach to nursing care.* New York: John Wiley & Sons.

Copleston, F. (1963). *A history of philosophy* (Vol. 4) *Modern philosophy: Descartes to Leibniz.* Garden City, NY: Image Books.

Dickoff, J. and James, P. (1968). A theory of theories: A position paper. *Nursing Research*, 17(3), 197–203.

Dickoff, J., James, P., and Wiedenbach, E. (1968). Theory in practice discipline: Part 1. Practice oriented theory. *Nursing Research*, 17(5), 415–435.

Donaldson, S.K. and Crowley, D. (1978). The discipline of nursing. *Nursing Outlook*, 26(2), 113–120.

Dougherty, C.M., Jankin, J.K., Lunney, M.R., and Whitley, G.G. (1993). Conceptual and research based validation of nursing diagnoses: 1950 to 1993. *Nursing Diagnosis*, 4(4), 156–165.

Duldt, B.W. (1995). Nursing process: The science of nursing in the curriculum. *Nurse Educator*, 20(1), 24–29.

Durand, M. and Prince, R. (1966). Nursing diagnostics: Process and decision. *Nursing Forum*, 5(4), 50–64.

Durant, W. (1953). *The story of philosophy: The lives and opinions of the greater philosophers*. New York: Simon & Schuster.

Eisenhauer, L.A. (1994). A typology of nursing therapeutics. *Image: Journal of Nursing Scholarship*, 26(4), 261–264.

Estabrooks, C.A., Rutakumwa, W., O'Leary, K.A., Profetto–McGrath, J., et al. (2005). Sources of practice knowledge among nurses. *Qualitative Health Research*, 15(4), 460–476.

Evers, G. (2003). Developing nursing science in Europe. *Journal of Nursing Scholarship*, 35(1), 9–13.

Fagerstrom, L., Rainio, A.K., Rauhala, A., and Nojonen, K. (2000). Validation of a new method for patient classification, the Oulu Patient Classification. *Journal of Advanced Nursing*, 31(2), 481–490.

Fawcett, J. (1989). *Analysis and evaluation of conceptual models of nursing* (2nd ed.). Philadelphia, PA: F.A. Davis.

Fawcett, J. (1995). *Analysis and evaluation of conceptual models of nursing* (3rd ed.). Philadelphia, PA: F.A. Davis.

Fawcett, J. (2000). The state of nursing science: Where is the nursing in the science? *Journal of Nursing Theory*, 9(3), 3–10.

Fawcett, J. (2013). *Contemporary nursing knowledge: Analysis and evaluation of nursing models and theories* (3rd ed.). Philadelphia, PA: F.A. Davis.

Fawcett, J., Watson, J., Neuman, B., Walker, P.H., and Fitzpatrick, J.J. (2001). On nursing theories and evidence. *Image: Journal of Nursing Scholarship*, 33(2), 115–119.

Fitzpatrick, J. and Whall, A. (1989). *Conceptual models of nursing: Analysis and application* (2nd ed.). Bowie, MD: Robert J. Brady.

Frisch, N. (1994). The nursing process revisited [editorial]. *Nursing Diagnosis*, 5(2), 51.

Frisch, N.C. and Kelley, J.H. (2002). Nursing diagnosis and nursing theory: Exploration of factors inhibiting and supporting simultaneous use. *Nursing Diagnosis*, 13(2), 53–61.

Gebbie, K. (Ed.). (1976, March 4–7). *Summary of the second national conference: Classification of nursing diagnosis*. St. Louis, MO: C.V. Mosby.

Gordon, M. (1985). Nursing diagnosis. *Annual Review of Nursing Research*, 3, 127–147.

Gordon, M., Murphy, C.P., Candee, D., and Hiltunen, E. (1994). Clinical judgment: An integrated model. *Advances in Nursing Science*, 16(4), 55–70.

Gordon, M., Sweeny, M.A., and McKeehan, K. (1980). Nursing diagnosis: Looking at its use in the clinical area. *American Journal of Nursing*, 80, 672–674.

Gortner, S.R. and Nahm, H. (1977). An overview of nursing research in the United States. *Nursing Research*, 26(1), 10–33.

Grant, J., Kinney, M., and Guzzetta, C. (1990). A methodology for validating nursing diagnoses. *Advances in Nursing Science*, 12(3), 65–74.

Grey, J. (2014). Spinoza on composition, causation, and the mind's eternity. *British Journal for the History of Philosophy*, 22(3), 446–467.

Grobe, S.J. (1990). Nursing intervention lexicon and taxonomy study: Language classification methods. *Advances in Nursing Science*, 13(2), 22–33.

Harms, M. and McDonald, F.J. (1966). A new curriculum design: Part III. *Nursing Outlook*, 14(9), 50–53.

Hill, R. and Hansen, D.A. (1960). The identification of conceptual frameworks utilized in family study. *Marriage and Family Living*, 22, 299–311.

Holmes, C.A. (2002). Academics and practitioners: Nurses as intellectuals. *Nursing Inquiry*, 9(2), 73–83.

Hunt, C.K. (2002). Concepts in care giver research. *Journal of Nursing Scholarship*, 35(1), 27–32.

International Council of Nurses (ICN). (2015). *International Classification for Nursing Practice (ICNP)*. Geneva, Switzerland: Author.

Iowa Intervention Project. (1993). The NIC taxonomy structure. *Image: Journal of Nursing Scholarship*, 25(3), 187–192.

Iowa Intervention Project. (1995). Validation and coding of the NIC taxonomy structure. *Image: Journal of Nursing Scholarship*, 27(1), 43–49.

Jacox, A. (1974). Theory construction in nursing: An overview. *Nursing Research*, 23(1), 4–13.

Jennings, B. and Meleis, A.I. (1988). Nursing theory and administrative practice: Agenda for the 1990s. *Advanced Nursing Science*, 10(3), 56–69.

Johnson, D.E. (1959). A philosophy of nursing. *Nursing Outlook*, 7(4), 198–200.

Johnson, D.E. (1968a, April). *One conceptual model of nursing*. Paper presented at Vanderbilt University, Nashville, TN.

Johnson, D.E. (1968b). Theory in nursing: Borrowed and unique. *Nursing Research*, 17(3), 206–209.

Johnson, D.E. (1974). Development of theory: A requisite for nursing as a primary health profession. *Nursing Research*, 23(5), 372–377.

Johnson, J.E. (1972). Effects of structuring patients' expectations on their reactions to threatening events. *Nursing Research*, 21(6), 499–504.

Kaplan, A. (1964). *The conduct of inquiry: Methodology of behavioral science*. San Francisco, CA: Chandler.

Kelly, D. L., Lyon, D. E., Yoon, S. L., and Horgas, A. L. (2016). The microbiome and cancer: Implications for oncology nursing science. *Cancer nursing*, 39(3), E56–E62.

Kerlinger, F.N. (1964). *Foundations of behavioral research*. New York: Holt, Rinehart & Winston.

Kim, H.S. (1980). Pain theory: Research and nursing practice. *Advances in Nursing Science*, 2, 43–59.

Kim, M.J. (1989). Nursing diagnosis. *Annual Review of Nursing Research*, 7, 117–142.

Kim, M.J. and Moritz, D.A. (Eds.). (1982). *Classification of nursing diagnosis: Proceedings of the third and fourth national conferences*. New York: McGraw–Hill.

King, I. (1995a). A systems framework for nursing. In M.A. Frey and C.L. Sieloff (Eds.), *Advancing King's systems framework and theory of nursing* (pp. 14–22). Los Angeles, CA: Sage Publications.

King, I. (1995b). The theory of goal attainment. In M.A. Frey and C.L. Sieloff (Eds.), *Advancing King's systems framework and theory of nursing* (pp. 23–32). Los Angeles, CA: Sage Publications.

Kintzel, K.C. (1971). *Advanced concepts in clinical nursing*. Philadelphia, PA: J.B. Lippincott.

Kritek, P. (1978). The generation and classification of nursing diagnosis: Toward a theory of nursing. *Image*, 10(2), 33–40.

Lee, B. (2007). Identifying outcomes from the nursing outcomes classification as indicators of quality care in Korea: A modified delphi study. *International Journal of Nursing Studies*, 44(6), 1021–1028.

Lindeman, C.A. (1980). The challenge of nursing research in the 1980s. In *Communicating nursing research: Directions for the 1980s*. Boulder, CO: Western Interstate Commission for Higher Education.

Lindsay, G.M. and Smith, F. (2003). Narrative inquiry in a nursing practicum. *Nursing Inquiry*, 10(2), 121–129.

Lopes de Lima, J., Leite de Barros, A.L, and Michel, J.L. (2009). A pilot study to validate the priority nursing interventions classification interventions and nursing outcomes classification outcomes for the nursing diagnosis "excess fluid volume" in cardiac patients. *International Journal of Nursing Terminologies and Classifications*, 20(2), 76–88.

Maier, H.W. (1969). *Three theories of child development*. New York: Harper & Row.

Mantzoukas S. and Jasper, M. (2008). Types of nursing knowledge used to guide care of hospitalized patients. *Journal of Advanced Nursing*, 62(3), 318–326.

Meleis, A.I. (1975). Role insufficiency and role supplementation: A conceptual framework. *Nursing Research*, 24(4), 264–271.

Meleis, A.I. (1985). *Theoretical nursing: Development and progress* (2nd ed.). Philadelphia, PA: J.B. Lippincott.

Meleis, A.I. and Jennings, B.M. (1989). Theoretical nursing administration: Today's challenges, tomorrow's bridges. In H.C. Arndt and M. DiVincenti (Eds.), *Dimensions and issues in nursing administration*. Oxford, UK: Blackwell Scientific Publications.

Meleis, A.I. and May, K.M. (1981). Nursing theory and scholarliness in the doctoral program. *Advances in Nursing Science*, 4(1), 31–41.

Meleis, A.I. and Price, M. (1988). Strategies and conditions for teaching theoretical nursing: An international perspective. *Journal of Advanced Nursing*, 13, 592–604.

Meltzer, L.E., Abdellah, F.G., and Kitchell, R. (Eds.). (1969). *Concepts and practice of intensive care for nurse specialists*. Philadelphia, PA: Charles Press Publishers.

Mitchell, P.H. (1973). *Concepts basic to nursing*. New York: McGraw-Hill.

Moch, S.D. (1990). Personal knowing: Evolving research and practice. *Scholarly Inquiry for Nursing Practice: An International Journal*, 4(2), 155–170.

Moorhead, S. (2009). The nursing outcomes classification. *Acta Paulista de Enfermagem*, 22, 868–871.

Moorhead, S., Head, B., Johnson, M., and Maas, M. (1998). The nursing outcomes taxonomy: Developing and coding. *Journal of Nursing Care Quality*, 12(6), 56–63.

Muller-Staub, M., Lavin, M.A., Needham, I., and van Achterberg, T. (2006). Nursing diagnoses, interventions and outcomes—application and impact on nursing practice: Systematic review. *Journal of Advanced Nursing*, 56(5), 514–531.

Nelson, S., Gordon, S., and McGillian, M. (2002). Saving the practice—top 10 unfinished issues to inform the nursing debate in the new millennium [editorial]. *Nursing Inquiry*, 9(2), 63–64.

Nidditch, P. (Ed.). (1975). *An essay concerning human understanding*. New York: Oxford University Press.

Nightingale, F. (1859). *Notes on nursing: What it is and what it is not*. London, UK: Harrison.

Noh, H.K. and Lee, E. (2015). Relationships among NANDA-1 diagnoses, nursing outcomes classification, and nursing interventions classification by nursing students for patients in medical-surgical units in Korea. *International Journal of Nursing Knowledge*, 26(1), 43–51.

Norbeck, J. (1981). Social support: A model for clinical research and application. *Advances in Nursing Science*, 3, 43–59.

Norris, C.M. (1975). Restlessness: A nursing phenomenon in search of meaning. *Nursing Outlook*, 23(2), 103–107.

Norris, C.M. (Ed.). (1982). *Concept clarification in nursing*. Germantown, MD: Aspen Systems.

Nye, F. and Berardo, F. (Eds.). (1966). *Emerging conceptual frameworks in family analysis*. New York: Macmillan.

O'Connor, M.R., Doorenbos, A., and Voss, J. (2014). Clinical update on genetic and autoimmune biomarkers in pediatric diabetes. *Biological Research for Nursing*, 16(2), 218–227.

Peplau, H.E. (1952). *Interpersonal relations in nursing*. New York: G.P. Putnam's Sons.

Phillips, J.R. (1977). Nursing systems and nursing models. *Image*, 9(1), 4–7.

Piaget, H. (1971). *Biology and knowledge*. Edinburgh, UK: Edinburgh University Press.

Register, M.E. and Herman, J. (2010). Quality of life revisited: The concept of connectedness in older adults. *Advances in Nursing Science*, 33(1), 53–63.

Rew, L. (1988). Nurses' intuition. *Applied Nursing Research*, 1(1), 27–31.

Reynolds, P.D. (1971). *Primer in theory construction*. Indianapolis, IN: Bobbs-Merrill.

Riehl, J.P. and Roy, C. (Eds.). (1974). *Conceptual models for nursing practice*. New York: Appleton-Century-Crofts.

Rodgers, C.C., Krance, R., Street, R.L., and Hockenberry, M.J. (2014). Symptom prevalence and physiologic biomarkers among adolescents using a mobile phone intervention following hematopoietic stem cell transplantation. *Oncology Nursing Forum*, 41(3), 229–236.

Rodman, H. (1980). Are conceptual frameworks necessary for theory building: The case of family sociology. *The Sociological Quarterly*, 21, 429–441.

Roe, A. (1951). A psychological study of eminent biologists. *Psychological Monographs*, 65, 1–67.

Roe, A. (1963). *The making of a scientist*. New York: Dodd Mead.

Shamansky, S.L. and Yanni, C.R. (1983). In opposition to nursing diagnosis: A minority opinion. *Image*, 15, 47–50.

Spear, H. (2007). Nursing theory and knowledge development: A descriptive review of doctoral dissertations, 2000–2004. *Advances in Nursing Science*, 30(1), E1–E14.

Taggart, H. and Bergstrom, L. (2014). An overview of the microbiome and the effects of antibiotics. *The Journal for Nurse Practitioners*, 10(7), 445–450.

Thompson, C. (1999). A conceptual treadmill: The need for 'middle ground' in clinical decision making theory in nursing. *Journal of Advanced Nursing*, 30(5), 1222–1229.

Thorne, S. (2013). The evolving nature of nursing ideas. *Nursing Inquiry*, 20(1), 1–4.

Travelbee, J. (1966). *Interpersonal aspects of nursing*. Philadelphia, PA: F.A. Davis.

Turnbaugh, P.J., Ley, R.E., Hamady, M., Fraser-Liggett, C.M., et al. (2007). The human microbiome project. *Nature*, 449(7164), 804–810.

Wald, F.S. and Leonard, R.C. (1964). Towards development of nursing practice theory. *Nursing Research*, 13(4), 309–313.

Walker, K.M. and Alligood, M.R. (2001). Empathy from a nursing perspective: Moving beyond borrowed theory. *Archives of Psychiatric Nursing*, 15(3), 140–147.

Weiss, S.J. (1979). The language of touch. *Nursing Research*, 28(2), 76–80.

Wider, K. (2013). Sartre and Spinoza on the nature of mind. *Continental Philosophy Review*, 46(4), 555–575.

Zderad, L.T. and Belcher, H.C. (1968). *Developing behavioral concepts in nursing*. Atlanta, GA: Southern Regional Education Board.

8

Our Syntax: An Epistemological Analysis

Disciplines are characterized by a perspective, a domain, sources for the development of knowledge, and ways by which knowledge is characterized and developed. In this chapter, I discuss the different patterns of knowing and the prevailing perspectives on theory development. I argue for epistemic diversity, for inclusive epistemology, and for a serious consideration to using a critical approach to ways of knowing and to truth.

Epistemology is the branch of philosophy that considers the history of knowledge. It raises and answers questions related to the kinds, origin, nature, structure, scope, trustworthiness, methods, and limitations of knowledge development. It outlines the various criteria by which knowledge is accepted. Understanding how knowledge evolves, how it is accumulated, and how knowledge is accepted is essential for development and progress in any field. Such understanding helps to further define goals to be pursued, either by the individual scientist or the discipline as a whole (Andreoli and Thompson, 1977; Baer, 1979; Carper, 1978; Silva, 1977). For nurses, a study of epistemological issues helps us to accomplish the following:

- Increase our awareness of the complexity and diversity of the perspectives, views, and theories (sometimes conflicting) of scientific progress, truth, and the methodology of truth
- Distinguish between different kinds of problems in knowledge and development and therefore deliberately pursue those that seem most germane to the theoretical progress of the nursing discipline
- Deal with potential epistemological constraints, however inappropriate, that evolve from de facto acceptance of one view, one theory, or one perspective without careful study of alternatives
- Develop and use methodologies that are innovative and more congruent with the nature of nursing science

- Utilize, acknowledge, and evaluate different forms of evidence, such as practice evidence, research evidence, and theoretical evidence

Although this book is concerned primarily with the role of theory in the development of nursing knowledge, knowledge encompasses far more than theory—it includes research, common sense, and philosophy, as well as extant and ought-to-be nursing practice. During the last few decades, we have accumulated much nursing knowledge about caring, interacting, promoting healthy environments, supplementing roles, enhancing recovery, and supporting healing. If we allow our knowledge to develop haphazardly, disconnectedly, or aimlessly, it may not progress as expediently as we wish or in the direction we choose. By reflecting on the course of the development of nursing's knowledge base and where it is located at the end of the second decade of the 21st century, particularly its theoretical progress, we can deliberately chart our future progress. More importantly, we can also better organize our approach to the future acquisition, development, and advancement of nursing knowledge.

In this chapter, I discuss two central components in our epistemology of the discipline:

- Knowing from the received view to postmodernism view
- Truth from correspondence to integrative view of truth

KNOWING FROM THE RECEIVED VIEW TO POSTMODERNISM VIEW

Knowing is not static, but dynamic and changeable, and patterns of knowing in a discipline are not discrete; they reflect the progress and maturity of the discipline as well as the agents of knowing in a discipline. Patterns of knowing in a discipline are constantly evolving, multidimensional, and may be transformed and transforming. They reflect societal trends in defining acceptable patterns, and these definitions may change over time. We still remember when knowing in nursing emanated only from traditions, history, and experiences, when all alternative complementary theories were completely ignored and rejected, and when only scientific methods were the methods of choice. We also saw new concepts such as practice theories, personal knowing, expert knowing, and interpretive knowing become mainstream in the knowledge development arenas. To understand and appreciate the framework for our most contemporary syntax in nursing, one that is likely to endure long into the future, I will present it within the context of our history. In many ways, that history has shaped our current level of tolerance of the epistemic diversity we are experiencing and in the different ways by which we claim "to know" in our discipline.

Knowing includes knowledge based on observations, research findings, clinical manifestations, and scientific approaches. Although knowing has been viewed to be more dependent on sense data, it also includes other types of data. To understand is to connect bits of knowledge in a relational form to other broader statements. For example, we know that women who work outside the household tend to work a double shift: one shift outside their home, and the other taking care of their home. We also know that women who work outside the home tend to have better mental health than do women who work only inside the home. On the basis of this knowledge, inferences could be made about the types of support and health care resources that women who work inside the home may need. Housework is an activity that was not acknowledged as work or leisure, an activity with no set hours, wages, rewards, or retirement benefits (Harding, 1988, p. 87). Considering the findings within this context of meanings may prompt a consideration of the forces and constraints in using resources that are developed especially for the promotion of health in women who are engaged primarily in housework. Similarly, we have always known that menopause was a "deficiency disease" from a biomedical perspective until feminist scholars enhanced our knowledge by demonstrating its transformation from a disease to a normal process that is experienced differently in different cultures (Andrist and MacPherson, 2001). These examples illustrate the need for developing understanding beyond sense data. Understanding,

therefore, includes putting the experiences and situations of women within historical, gender, and social contexts. It includes a consideration of the norms, values, and the meanings of housework and the barriers that societies impose on women and their work. That, then, requires epistemological diversity.

Knowing results from careful systematic research or from repeated experiences in clinical practice. Reflecting on that knowledge and interpreting the meanings of relationships, as seen and experienced by all parties concerned, and putting that which is known within a context of feelings, values, and different perspectives, is what brings us closer to an understanding of that which is known. One pattern of knowing by itself will not uncover all the knowledge needed for a human and practice-oriented science.

In a classical analysis that represented a turning point in our epistemological past, and a departure from equating reliable knowledge with objective empirical findings, Carper (1978) identified four patterns of knowing in nursing:

1. Empirical (the science of nursing)
2. Personal knowledge (concerned with the quality of interpersonal contacts, promoting therapeutic relationships, and individualized care)
3. Aesthetic (the art of nursing)
4. Ethics (moral component of nursing)

These patterns, which transcend time, but are neither complete nor static (Fry, 1988), received a great deal of attention and were instrumental in alerting nurses that science alone will not answer the significant questions in our discipline (Johnson, 1994).

The *first pattern* developed by Carper (1978) and used to guide the development of nursing knowledge is the empirics, requiring scientific competence leading to explanations and structure, requiring replication and validation, and resulting in theories and models. The *second pattern* is personal knowing, requiring therapeutic use of self, which requires openness and centering and can be achieved through the use of stories and genuine use of the self. These are organized as responses and reflections. The *third pattern* of knowing is the aesthetic pattern, manifested in critical analysis of works of art that result in transformative expressions of art or acts. The *fourth pattern* is ethics, knowing manifested in principles and codes that could evolve through processes of dialogues and justification. These could be developed by valuing and clarifying discourses and acts of caring (Chinn and Kramer, 2014).

White (1995) supported Carper's four patterns but added a fifth one, sociopolitical knowing, which is considered an essential pattern for the understanding that may evolve from all other patterns of knowing. This pattern focuses on the broader context for the caring process; it allows and drives inquiry to critically question the status quo of the participants in the caring process. It includes organizational, cultural, and political processes that influence the person, the nurse, and other health care providers; the profession; and other structures involved in the caring process. This pattern of knowing allows for the construction of alternative structures of reality and is expressed through critiques and transformations. It is a pattern predicated on collaboration and on a movement toward more equity in knowledge development.

Similarly, Chinn and Kramer (2014) expanded on Carper by developing a model that includes a fifth pattern, emancipatory knowing, which they defined as "the human capacity to be aware of and critically reflect on the social, cultural and political status quo and to determine how and why it came to be that way" (p. 5). They proposed that this pattern embody awareness and critical reflection about all aspects of nursing to uncover inequities, to identify the sociopolitical context that frames knowledge, and to influence processes of knowing. Dimensions leading to all patterns of knowing are assessment and credibility within sociopolitical context.

Although theorists have described these different types of knowing, it is possible that knowing cannot truly be fragmented into different sources or components. Consider, for instance, personal knowing, which has been explained as the nurse knowing both the self and the patient. Tanner, Benner, Chesla, et al. (1993) further explicated knowing the patient through knowing the patient's patterns of responses and knowing the patient as a person. As Mantzorou and Mastrogiannis (2011) explain, the process of knowing the patient requires the integration of all patterns of knowing. In other words, each pattern contributes to a more complete knowing (Chinn and Kramer, 2014). These classifications may have evolved and gained wide acknowledgment and use as a reaction against empirically valued sources for knowledge development that prevailed in the 1970s and 1980s. The debate that resulted from the articulation of the subjective ways of knowing has been healthy for our discipline as evidenced in the many subsequent global critical philosophical dialogues (an example is Garrett and Cutting, 2015). They counter these ways of knowing by proposing alternative ways of knowing including empirical knowing, knowing through sacred texts, knowing

beyond comprehension, knowing simply by coming to know things, visionary dreaming knowing, knowing through mental illness, as well as many other ways of knowing.

There are many ways to organize epistemic diversity, which is shaping the next phase of knowledge development in nursing. I chose to build on previous classifications (Allen, Benner, and Dickelman, 1986; Carper, 1978; Chinn and Kramer, 2014; Mantzoukas and Jasper, 2008; Stevenson and Woods, 1986) and the many subsequent debates by presenting here four views of knowing:

- The received view
- The perceived view
- The interpretive view
- The postmodernism, poststructuralism, and postcolonialism views

The Received View

Several philosophers in nursing have been concerned that nurses may have adopted a limited view of science that directly contradicts nursing's philosophy, heritage, and goals. Their view could be summarized under the rubric of "the received view," which others may call the scientific method (Suppe, 1977). It is largely a product of the scientific revolution of the 17th century, and its focus on objective and measurable criteria supports a biomedical model that may have advocated a body/mind separation and independence, a la Descartes (Ferreira, Prado, Carvalho, et al., 2015). The received view is philosophically old and outdated, but its effects lingered longer in nursing than in the field of philosophy of science (Suppe and Jacox, 1985).

The *received view* in any discipline usually denotes a set of ideas that are not to be challenged—the philosophical equivalent of being engraved in stone. It is the same premise that declares that holy books were received and therefore should not be challenged. The received view is also a label given to "empirical positivism" or "logical positivism," a 19th-century philosophical movement closely aligned with Rudolph Carnap and rooted in the celebrated Vienna circle of philosophers. This circle advocated an amalgamation of logic, with the goals of empiricism in the development of scientific theories (Runggaldier, 1984). Eventually, the concept of "positivism" was dropped from "logical positivism" and replaced with "empiricism" to avoid the connection with Auguste Comte, whose ideas were coming into disfavor at that time. When Carnap joined The University of Chicago in 1936, he introduced logical empiricism to the United States (White, 1955, pp. 203–225).

The following are the tenets of logical empiricism:

1. Theoretical statements that cannot be confirmed by sensory data and sensory experiences are not considered worthy of pursuit. As a result, they are disqualified as common sense statements. Predictive statements that have no corroboration from sensory data are not scientific. A direct relationship has to exist between experience and a meaningful theory.

2. True statements are only those that are a posteriori. That is, they are based on experience and are known from experience.

3. Positivists regard most traditional metaphysics and ethical considerations as meaningless. They regard such questions as possessing "emotive" meaning and as being "cognitively meaningless" (White, 1955).

4. Analyses of theories are based on analyses of completed theories, and completed theories are based on empirical data (Suppe, 1977, p. 125). The context of justification—that is, the verification and falsification of complete theory propositions—is the only significant context for consideration by scientists and philosophers alike. Conversely, the contexts of discovery, such as conceptual ideas, contexts within which theories are developed, logic in theory development, and usefulness, should be within the province of the sociologists of knowledge: the psychologist and historian (Reichenback, 1968).

5. Because the received view considers theories to reflect the a posteriori depiction of reality, documented by sensory experiences, it therefore follows that propositions of theories are presented symbolically, formally, and axiomatically. There is room for a priori analysis, although it is only mathematical in nature.

6. Science is value-free, and there is only one method for science, which is the scientific method.

The "ghost of the received view" loomed over nursing in its quest for a scientific base, according to Webster, Jacox, and Baldwin (1981). Others, such as Watson (1981) and Winstead-Fry (1980), also blamed nursing's slow scientific progress on the insistence of its leaders to using the outdated scientific method as its model and to strive for one scientific method.

The scientific method that they were speaking of is one based on the received view, one that espouses "reductionism, quantifiability, objectivity, and operationalization" (Watson, 1981, p. 414). As a result, the critics maintained that significant holistic problems in nursing have been ignored because they are not reducible, quantifiable, or objective. The scientific method adopted by nursing reduced a problem to its smallest unit or its most significant form and stripped it of the rich context from which it emanated (Newman, 1981). The scientific method, oriented toward quantitative methods, and highly accepted and respected, could not address theory and developing theory; therefore, it has not helped nursing to develop meaningful theories, nor has it advanced nursing to its projected goal of a scientific discipline.

Historically, some justification existed in blaming the received view for nursing's slow progress and development. Many examples support the view that an outmoded and ineffective philosophical view of science has somewhat disillusioned nurses (Newman, 1994). One example is the many theoretically disconnected but methodologically immaculate research projects that nurses have produced, a view that is shared by Batey (1977). Nevertheless, more evidence than what we have been led to believe supports the view that nursing has, in fact, considered and followed a scientific path broader in scope and more integrative in approach than the received view.

Logical empiricism succeeded from logical positivism, and it is how the received view is expressed. After many transformations, it has come to be accepted as an essential approach to knowing; it is not, however, the only approach. Although there are variations to how empiricism may be utilized, it has some common properties.

A theory for empiricists is a product of research findings that is used as a framework for further research. The empiricists' observations are not contextual and usually focus on single behaviors, events, or situations. Theorizing for empiricists is based on inductive logic, sense data supported by a set of value-free assumptions. Empiricists develop theories by providing precise, well-defined, operationalized concepts—measurable variables. Empiricists are objective, separated, and distanced from their theories; they treat theories as objects and are reluctant to share insights related to findings or evolving ideas with their clients or research subjects. The language they use is research-specific and their approach is inductive. Statistical model building is a significant tool for empiricist theory development.

Empirical theories are based on careful and methodologically impeccable research studies geared to finding relationships between different variables and finding support for a multitude of statements—all geared to answering a set of well-defined questions, hypotheses, and null hypotheses that produce prediction and verification (Table 8-1). Empiricists' theories are well understood by colleagues from other disciplines, and when theory development is discussed, it is more likely to be understood in relationship to the development of empirical theories (Dzurec, 2003). The discourse about evidence-based practice emanates and reflects a focus on a limited view of empiricism (Porter, 2010). Many narrow interpretations of evidence may exist; however, the prevailing, dominant interpretation is one that is most limited in focus (Fawcett, Watson, Neuman, et al., 2001; Chinn and Kramer, 2014) (Table 8-1). Developing theories from large data sets requires a conceptual match and consideration to how the data was obtained (Magee, Lee, Giuliano, et al., 2006; Smaldone and Connor, 2003), as well as to how the data meaning and interpretation were perceived by the participants in the data collection. Doing otherwise is considered a persistent mechanistic view advocated and supported by the received view. It is imperative that investigators who use large data sets understand and acknowledge the limitation in interpretations and in generalizing theories (Lacey and Hughes, 2007).

The Perceived View

Knowing through the more subjective view of those who are experiencing the situation and those agents who are uncovering the situation reflects another view of knowing. Knowing is not only based on sense data. Proponents of the perceived view of knowing discuss different patterns and dimensions.

Nursing theorists who have worked diligently to give us their conception of the discipline have not followed a received view approach. They have offered several conceptualizations that encompass the whole of nursing—a perceived view—based on their experiences and theory-incorporated ideas that are subjective, intuitive, humanistic, integrative, and, in many instances, not based on sense-oriented

TABLE 8-1	Comparison of the Received, Perceived, Interpretive, and Postmodern Views of Science*		
Received View	**Perceived View**	**Interpretive View**	**Postmodernism, Poststructuralism, & Postcolonialism**
Objectivity	Subjectivity	Analysis within context finding meaning	Narration
Deduction	Induction	Contextual analysis	Political and structural analysis
One truth	Multiple truths	Patterns Themes	Different views
Validation and replication	Trends and patterns	Authenticity	Uncovering opposing views
Justification	Discovery	Uncovering meaning	Uncovering inequity Marginalization
Prediction and control	Description and understanding	Narrative descriptions	Metanarrative analysis
Particulars	Patterns	Patterns within a structure and history	Stories
Reductionism	Holism	Uncover weakness and flaws	Macro-relationship with micro structures
Generalization	Individuation	Knowing about context	Knowing about structures
Logical positivism	Historicism	Historicism	Macro-analysis
Logical empiricism		Structure	

*Based on Meleis, A.I. (1985). Theoretical nursing., Philadelphia: Lippincott; and Stevenson, J.S., and Woods, N.F. (1986). Nursing science and contemporary science: Emerging paradigms. In G. Sorenson (Ed.), Setting the agenda for the year 2000: Knowledge development in nursing. Kansas City, MO: American Academy of Nursing.

data. (See Chapter 21 for citations reflecting this statement.)

The discovery of field concepts, theory development, and processes of theorizing in nursing has not been based on the received view or on a structured and strictly scientific approach. Traditionally, the context of discovery for these ideas has been case studies, personal anecdotes, and group insights. The acceptance of those visions then emanating from our nurse theorists has been slow because some have branded the theories as unscientific. Therein lies the problem.

To generalize, saying that nursing has followed a positivistic path is akin to saying that physics has followed an intuitive one. The theoreticians in nursing, those who have developed conceptualizations encompassing the field as a whole, have used the *perceived view*, which combines the phenomenological and philosophical approaches as alternate methods of theory development. The scholars in the field who believe that knowledge emanates from the context of justification may have helped to orient nursing toward considering concepts such as sensory data, verification, and falsification as ways to accept or reject nursing conceptualizations. These scholars have therefore precipitated the early mass rejection of nursing theory, as well as the continuous rejection by many in the field who are skeptical about the use or effectiveness of nursing theories.

In the perceived view, patterns of knowing include both theoretical and practical knowing. Sarvimaki (1994) makes a distinction between theoretical and practical knowledge, although she acknowledges their equal significance. Theoretical knowledge includes and reflects the basic values, guiding principles, elements, and phases of a conception of nursing. Its goals are to drive and promote thinking and understanding of that which is the nursing discipline. Its base is intellectual, and it is organized into assumptions, concepts, propositions, and models. Practical knowledge, however, does not have to be organized in the same way because many parts of this knowledge are not yet articulated and because the artistic side of practice may not be amenable to total articulation. The channel of communication for theoretical knowledge may be theories and science, whereas the channel of communication for practical knowledge may be tradition, according to Sarvimaki (1994). Practical knowledge may be achieved through personal and collective means and reflections (Winstead-Fry, 1979) and through integrating and blending evidence with clinical judgment (Paley,

2006). Personal knowing, which may be arrived at through one's own practice, reflection, synthesis, and integration of artistic, scientific, and practice components is, according to Moch (1990), essential to the development of nursing knowledge. She identifies three components in personal knowing: experiential, interpersonal, and intuitive knowing. Experiential knowing is achieved through being part of the world of nursing and becoming increasingly aware of the experiences inherent in this participation. (See powerful examples of one aspect of personal knowing through an illness experience [Hall, 2003].) Interpersonal knowing results from enhanced awareness about situations resulting from extensive, in-depth interactions with others. These interactions, which should be based on empathy, are another source of knowing, and they promote the development of knowledge. Personal knowing means knowledge of another as well as of oneself (Mantzorou and Mastrogiannis, 2011).

When a person knows without the explicit use of scientifically accepted forms of reasoning, it is said that the person achieved the knowing through intuition. It is knowing a whole without resorting to linear reasoning (Polanyi, 1962). It is knowing without knowing how (Benner and Wrubel, 1982; Rew, 1988; Rew and Barrow, 1987). When nurses use intuition to know, they open themselves up to allow sensing and understanding of the patient's responses and situations to occur, which leads to a better knowledge of the patient's situation (Agan, 1987; Paul and Heaslip, 1995). Intuitive knowing was a neglected pattern of knowing, but it has been gaining more attention as a component in "clinical knowing," as essential in a more holistic understanding of clinical situations, and as significant in making more effective therapeutic decisions, as evidenced from the many descriptive studies that affirm its significance (Rew, 1990; Rew and Barrow, 2007).

Intuition by experts is based on rapidly perceiving a whole situation without having to pause to construct the different processes or steps (Benner, Tanner, and Chesla, 1996). Many discourses in nursing have established intuition as a source of knowing to be carefully explored, and different theories about intuitive learning also should be explored (Gobet and Chassy, 2008).

Intuition has increasingly become a more valid form of knowledge in nursing. Green (2012) argues that knowledge for a nurse is the awareness of objects and realities encountered in the nurse's daily practice and that intuition includes embodied knowledge, sensing and perceiving, a vast store of conceptual knowledge and many experiences of previous actions that brought positive outcomes. Intuitive knowing is the integration of these components that result in practical knowledge. Equal to the increase in acknowledgment of intuitive knowing, there have been distractors who claimed that it is conceptual knowledge that is mistakenly considered intuition (English, 1993; Luntley, 2010).

Knowing a patient through perception or intuition, as well as through forms of knowing, allows for more particular and individualistic approaches that may be based on more general knowledge related to that patient's situations. Knowing the patient leads to more appropriately selecting nursing therapeutics, based on knowing the patient's resources, readiness, and current understanding related to his or her responses. Several processes have been identified to elucidate the meaning of "knowing the patient." These were defined by Jenny and Logan (1992) as perceiving/ envisioning, communication, self-preservation, and showing concern. Perceiving and envisioning involve identifying the meaning and significance of the patient's responses. Knowing the patient also involves communication and interaction with or about the patient. It includes having the nurse be present for the patient and being trusted by the patient and family. Knowing the patient is assumed to be connected to the extent to which a nurse shows and demonstrates concern. To be able to know a patient or a situation is to be open to know what is unknown about this individual. Munhall (1993) made a cogent argument for "unknowing" as another pattern of knowing that requires reflection on oneself—about whom we have a certain degree of knowledge—and the other (patient) about whom we have a very limited knowledge. Unknowing is another dimension of knowing; without realizing and understanding the degree, extent, and nature of what one does not know, knowing is not fully realized (Table 8-2).

Nursing phenomena reflect human conditions and situations, and, therefore, these phenomena could be developed through different patterns of discovery. Uncovering and describing the art component of nursing is predicated on developing the aesthetic pattern of knowing. Sorrell (1994) described this pattern as embodying the "unique pattern of knowing that offers enrichment to our understanding of [the] nursing experience that is not accessible through other ways of knowing" (p. 61). Aesthetic knowing depends on processes that are imaginative and creative. It allows the knower to be engaged and interpretive, and it allows for envisioning. It is also expressed through some creative means such as art, music, and expressive writing. Writing to reflect aesthetic knowing is not bound by scientific reporting; it may include poetry, narratives, stories, fiction, letters, and journals (O'Brien and Pearson, 1993; Sorrell, 1994). The knowing that results from these modes of expression integrates sensory perceptions with experiences and acts. Aesthetic knowing requires engagement and distancing from experiences, particularizing and generalizing, abstraction and concretization, objectivity and subjectivity, and separate and united components and experiences.

Experiences such as compassion, suffering, and mourning may best be uncovered through metaphors, and may be understood more fully if scientific methods are used in combination with aesthetic approaches. Younger (1990) provides an example by using the Book of Job in the Bible, analyzing it as a "literary work" to uncover knowledge of, and the meaning for, suffering. The art of nursing is closely tied to the realities of the practice situation (Timpson, 1996). These aspects of nursing can be somewhat articulated by nurses who value the uniqueness of individual experiences and who can communicate through aesthetic pathways that may fully capture the connection between the different components (Boykin, Parker, and Schoenhofer, 1994). Clinical expertise and its dimensions represent one aspect of nursing art (Hampton, 1994).

The art of clinical expertise is always evolving and multidimensional, and may be transformed or transforming. It is not always possible to classify knowledge using only one of these patterns. Knowing can and does occur through "nonlinear, meditative thinking that moves in all directions." Therefore, Silva, Sorrell, and Sorrell (1995) called this type of knowing "*the in-between*" (p. 3). There is also the knowing through "*the beyond*," which is knowledge that concerns "those aspects of reality, meaning, and being that persons only come to know with difficulty or that they cannot articulate or ever know" (p. 3). Accepting the inexplicable and the unknowable in clients, nurses, relationships, and health and illness may allow an exploration of meanings and ways by which some lived experiences cannot be felt or explained by those who never had those experiences. These patterns of knowing bring a nurse closer to a more profound understanding of the complex multidimensional aspects of reality that characterize human experiences related to health and illness.

TABLE 8-2 Perspectives on Knowing

			Interpretation			
Component	Empiricist Knowing	Feminist Knowing	Critical Knowing	Postmodernism Knowing	Poststructuralism Knowing	Postcolonialism Knowing
Units of observation	Acontextual; behavior; event; situation	Human beings; gender; experience; totality; uniqueness; perception of meanings	Social structure; power; political structure; history; relationships with structure	Multiple understanding of phenomena	Structures; positions; hierarchies	Oppressions; inequality; context of relationships that are within large structure
Strategies for theory development	Multiple research findings	Experience of participants; analysis of situation and context; advocacy	Experience of participants and nonparticipants; analysis of context	Multiple methods of analysis	Experience of groups within a structure	Meta-narratives; historically contexted; traditional values
Assumptions	Axiomatic facts; value-free	Personal; disciplinary; societal values critiqued	Action; societal values critiqued and selected; not essential	Lack of structure to constrain theoretical formulations	Structures; constrain; responses	Colonialization; unequal treatment
Concepts	Precise; operationalized; not acontextual; provide a framework; unit of analysis	Considered within gender orientation; analytical statements; patterns	Considered within sociopolitical context	Deconstruct concepts	Not taken for granted; meanings	Complex web of relationships, of situations within race, gender, class, economics, power
Goals/uses	Theory development; truth-finding for discipline	Theory development; consciousness-raising; awareness of participants; illumination	Emancipation; structural; awareness structure; understanding; knowledge is not marginalizing	Awareness; multiple truths; challenge structures; no structured theory	Transform situations; empowerment	Awareness of historical context to understand the present; challenging history
Theorist	Objective; separated; distanced; secretive	Engaged; connected	Observer of social structure and proactive participant	Interpreter	Observer; interpreter; empowering agent	
Approach	Inductive	Inductive; deductive; retroductive; philosophical analysis	Creation of new structures	Narrative analysis; critique of structures	Deconstruction of dominance and of normal structures	Meta-narration analysis
Use	Know	Understand; gender	Change	Uncover limitations of structures	Illuminate; change	Illuminate; advocate
Starting point	Research question	Experience; response; challenge of attitudes toward gender	Structure; organization; political; challenge of structures	Analysis; deconstruction	Allocations based on identity; power structures	History; inequality; dominance; relationships
Language	Research-specific	Gender-specific	Philosophical; political	Synthesis; integration of structures; tentative language; nontheoretical	Structures; positions; status	Historical colonialism

The Interpretive View

Understanding goes beyond knowing and beyond uncovering a perceived view of a situation and experience. It includes interpretation, a total comprehension of other human beings' responses based on their "feelings, ideas, choices, and purposes" as they experience the situation and as they express their own meanings and understanding of the situation through their own words and through their own responses (Schwartz and Wiggins, 1988, p. 143). The degree to which we need to develop that understanding depends on the extent to which we want to, and how significant our attempt to achieve that level of understanding is. It also depends on the degree to which clients are willing to have their responses and their situations fully uncovered and understood. True understanding not only illuminates the situation, it also uncovers weaknesses and flaws, as well as strengths and abilities. In some ways, true understanding may uncover the individual's power as well as areas of vulnerability (Tables 8-1 and 8-2).

Health and illness situations require a level of understanding that is not required from other situations in which two strangers might come in contact with each other. However, a true understanding of how individuals experience and respond to health and illness mandates an understanding of what a group of people value in life, what priorities they have, how they usually respond to disruptions in their lives, how they prefer to express their discomfort, and what are the most comfortable ways by which they usually prefer to express their feelings.

Knowing about specific groups' perceptions of health and illness, patterns of help-seeking behaviors, and patterns of responses to uncomfortable situations is essential for the level of understanding required to develop an intervention plan, whether that intervention plan is as specific as postoperative deep breathing or maintaining prenatal appointments. Knowing about the extent to which an immigrant is connected to individuals and events in his country of origin may help a nurse clinician understand the out-of-pattern expressions of pain and discomfort to a seemingly minimally painful experience. Knowing about normal patterns of touch between members of the opposite sex in different social classes may help a health care provider understand when (and when not) to communicate this way.

Understanding includes making connections and achieving syntheses that may go beyond the perception and knowledge of the client or the provider (Habermas, 1971; Schutz, 1967). Understanding has been advocated by interpretive scientists (Allen, 1988, p. 98) as the hallmark for knowledge development in nursing. This understanding includes specific research findings, the experience that evolves from the practice arena, and knowledge awareness from primary theoretical formulations. It includes all these and goes beyond them.

Understanding is predicated on knowing about phenomena, knowing about the contexts in which certain phenomena occur, and knowing about patterns of presentation of these phenomena. Knowing about the different roles women enact; knowing about the stresses, strains, and satisfactions in these roles; knowing role theory; and knowing the relationships between levels of role involvement and number of roles and health status are all important and significant for developing an understanding of why and when women tend to seek care for themselves or for their children and how they choose to maintain or enhance their health. That level of understanding is also achieved through a deliberate effort to reflect theoretically on some of these concepts and put them together in an organized way to describe and explain some central problems in nursing, such as maintaining and developing health and patterns of seeking health care.

Jaspers, a physician and a philosopher, addressed the laws of understanding as follows (Jaspers, 1963; Schwartz and Wiggins, 1988, pp. 153–155):

1. Empirical understanding is an interpretation. The data provide the impetus for interpretation, and therefore interpretation is not absolute but is subject to other interpretations—and therefore may be theoretical.

2. Understanding opens up unlimited interpretations. To have understanding as a goal frees the researcher to consider many different interpretations. These different interpretations should be subjected to more data to gain support or refutation.

3. Understanding moves in deepening spirals. To understand a certain behavior, one starts at the part, goes to the whole to put the behavior in context, and then comes back to the part for better understanding. This process increases understanding.

4. Opposites are equally meaningful. The same evidence can be interpreted in two opposite ways. In doing that, we attempt to understand the synthesis between the opposites and not settle for preconceived notions. Schwartz and Wiggins (1988, p. 154) give an example: "We can understand

the stoicism of a patient as stemming from bravery and nobility. But we can also understand this same stoicism as motivated by profound fears and a complete inability to face up to a difficult predicament."

5. Understanding is inconclusive. Not all feelings, meanings, and values can be expressed in understandable ways, and not all interpretations are willingly shared.

6. To understand is to illustrate and expose. To really comprehend, both the positive and negative aspects of any group or person have to be exposed. Ethical considerations of the balance between exposure and illumination need to be considered.

Should nursing knowledge help us to know, to understand, or to care? Does each require different approaches to knowledge development? Can these approaches substitute for each other, or do they complement each other to enhance knowledge development? I believe that the predominant goals for research are to know and that the predominant goals for theoretical development of the discipline are to understand. I am not saying that one leads exclusively to knowing and one leads exclusively to understanding. I am using the concept "predominant" to differentiate between goals. Imagine knowing and understanding on two continuums. Imagine each going from none to high. Research findings and theorizing could be plotted on the two continuums. Research findings tend to be toward the higher end of the continuum of knowing and may be the middle of the understanding pole, whereas theorizing tends to be on the higher pole of understanding and may be the middle of the knowing pole.

Two frameworks for interpretation inform knowledge development in nursing: a *feminist* and a *critical* interpretation. There are many variations in both, and there are many different ways by which they intersect.

Feminist Knowing

The history of nursing attests to how the concept of gender permeates and pervades every aspect of the discipline. Nursing has been predominantly a female profession and still continues to be so, as female nurses continue to claim about 91% membership in the profession (Landivar, 2013). Despite the many efforts to open the profession more to men and despite the many contributions men have made to nursing, nursing remains a woman's profession and continues to be saddled with all the accompanying issues related to the value of women's work, women's contributions, and the relationship between nursing and other predominately male professions.

This history could be used to the advantage of the discipline and its clients by utilizing it as a perspective for the development of gender-sensitive theories. Understanding the constraints inherent in these experiences and the lack of participation in shaping the structure and the goals of inquiry may sensitize nurses to similar experiences in clients.

Gender-sensitive theories are those based on connections between the theorist and the subject matter, the involvement of the theorist with the subjects of the theory in the development and interpretation of the theory (MacPherson, 1983; Sherwin, 1987; Stacy and Thorne, 1985). These theories are also based on the acknowledgment and affirmation of gender equity, on the premise that women should be affirmed for their contributions in a patriarchal society, on the assumption that women should have options and control over their own bodies (Sampselle, 1990), and on the assumption that nursing is also a field of study and a profession for men. The goal of gender-sensitive theories is understanding rather than just knowing; the goal is based on uncovering and including personal experiences of the nurse and client, and it evolves from considering the totality of the experiences, responses, and events described theoretically, as well as from giving similar consideration to the experience and the context of the theorist (Hagell, 1989) (Table 8-2).

A feminist perspective could be used not only in understanding issues related to women as clients or women as providers, but as a perspective for developing an understanding of all nursing clients, regardless of sex, gender, race, or culture. It could be used to understand, to explain, to raise consciousness, and to develop theories that will bring about needed changes for nursing clients (Cloyes, 2002; Cowling and Chinn, 2001; Duffy and Hedin, 1988; Jagger, 1988).

Whereas the assumptions of the empiricists may lean toward value-free axioms and facts and from truths derived from previous research findings, assumptions evolving from feminist perspectives are acknowledged as value-laden and include personal, disciplinary, and societal values (Harding, 1986, 1987).

Gender-sensitive theories (Table 8-2) could be based on similar principles that have been discussed in conjunction with gender-sensitive research. Cook and Fonow (1986) and Im and Meleis (2001) defined some guidelines for conducting gender-sensitive research. These guidelines are modified and offered for guiding the development of theories related to recipients of care in nursing. Therefore, gender-sensitive theories are theories that:

- Consider gender as a basic feature and a central agenda in the theory
- Provide guidelines for raising consciousness about the experiences described within the theory, thus heightening understanding of the role of a social system or organization in relationship to these experiences
- Challenge any norms or objectivity that create distances between participants or between theory subject matter and participants in the theory development
- Provide a critique of situations and circumstances that may interfere with healthful living
- Enhance empowerment for options, for understanding, for decision-making, or for self-care
- Decrease any potential of exploitation
- Enhance advocacy and provide guidelines for advocacy
- Provide guidelines for changes, including institutional and organizational changes

In caring for patients or clients, nurses knowingly or unknowingly have adhered to some of these principles. In fact, during the 1960s and 1970s, some nurse theorists described nursing using the very principles that reflect a gender-sensitive perspective (Paterson and Zderad, 1976; Travelbee, 1963). However, these principles may have been overshadowed by a quest for empiricalization of theories to render the nursing discipline theoretical and scientific. By considering their caring mission, nurses—whether theoreticians or researchers—may be able to synthesize their goals for caring and knowing and thus develop theories that enhance understanding of the situation, the daily experience, and responses of clients.

Gender-sensitive perspective is not to be construed as a substitute for nursing theories. It is a framework that guides the kind of phenomena that nursing theorists may select for development, the approach by which such theories are developed, and the interpretation of findings related to this phenomenon. A gender-sensitive perspective is a framework that guides nurses to study phenomena that represent and emanate from the lives of their clients, phenomena that are important to these clients, phenomena that reflect and are related to the quality of their lives or their health care, and that may be seen as problematic from their perspective (Harding, 1987; Im and Meleis, 2001).

Several properties characterize gender-sensitive theories. These are acknowledgment and inclusion of equity in voice and authority (Connell, 2012): that participants in practice or research must have options and control of their own bodies (Sampselle, 1990), and that a connection is made between subject matter and agent for knowledge development (Im and Meleis, 2001). Gender-sensitive knowledge includes the voices and experiences of participants, interpreted within a robust analysis of sociopolitical context, as well as within the historical roots of the experience, the voice, and the context.

Feminist theorizing "seeks to bring together subjective and objective ways of knowing the world" (Rose, 1983, p. 87). It challenges attitudes, beliefs, values, and assumptions that discredit women's sense of ownership of their own selves, and it also empowers nurses and clients (Sampselle, 1990; Sohier, 1992). A nursing theory that is developed using a feminist perspective is one that values the experiences of the developer, values her intuitions and analyses, values the client's world, and values the client's sociocultural and political perceptions. It is one that includes a sensitive understanding of the conditions that impinge on clients' responses and one that is representative of clients from different sociocultural backgrounds. Language is powerful; therefore, a theory from a feminist perspective is one that uses language that is empowering, that is gender-sensitive, that values experiences, and that denounces the status quo. For example, Wuest (1993) critically reviewed research on compliance and demonstrated how it was based on patriarchal and oppressive assumptions. Feminist principles may be better suited for enhancing understanding and developing insights about clients' responses, which might be ultimately more productive. Nursing theories, whether guided by a feminist perspective or an empirical perspective, should continue to inform members of the discipline. Therefore, these theories remain closely connected to the domain of nursing, with its focus on responses of human beings and their environments to health and illness situations.

Critical Knowing

Critical knowing evolves from critical theory and research. Critical theory is a philosophical perspective that emanates from the Frankfurt school of thought and was further developed in West Germany by Habermas (1971) and Gadamer (1979). It includes principles promoted by Freire (2000).

To Habermas (1971), who joined the Frankfurt school in 1950, there are three distinct but connected approaches to scientific inquiry. These approaches are empirical/analytical, historical hermeneutic, and critical-oriented. The three approaches include the technical, practical, and emancipatory interests. All three types of knowledge and approaches to knowledge development are essential for the development of knowledge for human sciences. Habermas (1971) further proposed that technical problems are best understood through an empirical/ analytical approach, practical problems through a historical hermeneutic approach, and problems that include issues critical to human beings through emancipatory approaches. The latter incorporates both the empirical/analytical and the historical hermeneutic approaches in a higher-order synthesis. The goal of the critical-oriented inquiry is an active, reflective stand that includes changes that are emancipatory (Allen, 1985, 1988; Habermas, 1974; Holter, 1987).

The feminist theorists focus on gender inasmuch as the critical theorists focus on power and emancipation through reflection and action (Table 8-2). Theories developed through this perspective provide ways of understanding the sociopolitical structure and patterns of power inequities and client oppression within such a structure and domination; they also provide guidelines for a reflective approach that is critical of the situation and ways by which the subjects of theory are transformed and emancipated from unequal power structures (Bernstein, 1978; Habermas, 1979; Reutter and Kushner, 2010). The goal of a theorist here is to develop some means by which the participants can be put on the road toward emancipation from oppressive social structures. The goal is not only to understand, but to change and to do so drastically. Reflection, understanding, communication, and action are the hallmarks of a nursing theory developed within this perspective. Critical feminist knowledge includes awareness of gender inequity as well as other samples of inequity, such as race and cultural inequities (Kushner and Morrow, 2003). It examines all power relations, with a focus on social control in addition to gender control (George and McGuire, 2004). Emancipation deals with the long-standing history of social oppression for women and vulnerable populations. Attributes of emancipation are empowerment, personal knowledge, awareness of social norms, using reflection to articulate the personal knowledge and social norms, and a flexible environment (Whittman-Price, 2004).

Developing knowledge that is not marginalizing should be an aim of enhancing critical knowing in nursing (Meleis and Im, 1999). A critical nursing theory should be developed through the involvement of all constituents and have the aim of informing marginalized and oppressed populations about ways to enhance their empowerment and emancipation. It is a theory then that challenges the status quo, actions, power relations, and patterns of thought (Fontana, 2004). To the critical theorist, reality should be deconstructed to expose true actions, but the theory should also provide a framework for constructing situations based on principles of emancipation (Habermas, 1971). Critical theory is context-laden; it abhors oppression, promotes empowerment, gives voice to the silenced, and uncovers what may have been invisible (Pitre, Kushner, Raine, et al., 2013).

A nursing theory or a research program developed within this perspective offers a focus on social structure, power, and political structure as units of analyses, a "critique of power and ideology" in existing societal structures in which the nursing client interacts (Allen et al., 1986). The theory or the research findings that emanate from this context incorporate an understanding of a phenomenon or a situation by all involved parties, and provide insights about the health/illness situation and a framework of what is to be done about it. Therefore, an equal partnership between the subject matter of a theory and the developer of the theory must be maintained.

Critical theory is not a substitute for nursing theory; rather, it is a framework or a perspective that informs the phenomena to be considered theoretically, guides the approaches for developing them, provides ways by which the phenomena are to be interpreted, and suggests approaches for handling these phenomena.

Postmodernism, Poststructuralism, and Postcolonialism Views

A number of other approaches to knowing have been discussed and utilized in the nursing literature. Among them are postmodernism, poststructuralism and postcolonialism. These reflect different aspects of critical approaches to knowing and involve the deconstruction of realities within a framework of oppression and control, and reconstructing the meaning of responses and experiences within a framework of emancipation and empowerment (Table 8-1).

Postmodernism, which has been the dominant theoretical paradigm in the late 20th century (Matthewman and Hoey, 2006), goes beyond modernist arguments that separated science from fiction, myth, religion, and superstitions (Fraser and Nicholson, 1989). Postmodernism is a critique of modernism. Both are idealistic concepts, and neither may exist in purist form. Postmodernism is based in the Enlightenment era, one that promised science as a path leading to better understanding of human nature (Table 8-2). It allows the use of multiple methods and lack of support for developing structured theories, for continuous tentativeness, arbitrariness, and relativism in theoretical thinking (Closs and Draper, 1998), and it informs the marginalized discourse in our literature (Georges, 2003; Hall, Stevens, and Meleis, 1994; Hall, 1999). However, there are those who argue that there was never a coherent view of postmodernism, that it never existed beyond the 20th century (Matthewman and Hoey, 2006; Osborne, 1998), and that it failed to have practical relevance for health problems within the field of medical sociology (Cockerham, 2007). Similar assumptions could be made about its utility for nursing science.

Viewing phenomena and situations from the perspectives of *poststructuralism* raises critical questions and situations, and provides a framework to transform these situations (Table 8-2). For example, Drevdahl (1999) raised questions about the taken-for-granted concepts of holism and uniqueness that are used in nursing to describe both clients and framed interventions. She demonstrated that the manner in which these are used in nursing leaves out the intricate interactions between race, class, and gender, and their structural effects on experiences and responses. The use of these concepts in nursing to describe static variables leaves the structural effects on experiences and responses unexplained and unchallenged.

Poststructural frameworks offer an approach to viewing hierarchies in nursing practice, as well as in areas of knowledge, that have been taken for granted as important or unimportant. It provides the lens by which to examine power influences and how nurses and clients may be positioned for empowerment (Bradbury-Jones, Sambrook, et al., 2008). Bradbury-Jones and her colleagues (2008) argue that, to illuminate the dialogue about power oppression and empowerment that have been viewed from the perspectives of critical, organizational, and management theories, as well as of social psychological theories, a fourth approach—poststructuralism—is essential to understanding the

dynamic nature of power in nursing. They utilize Foucault's (1995) ideas about knowledge and power as a springboard in proposing the primacy of the poststructural approach as a means to exploring power and empowerment in nursing. The poststructural approach provides a framework to examine beliefs and relationships, including power differential, that exist within organizations, cultures, and societies (Aston, Price, Kirk, et al., 2011).

Conversely, some arguments question the use of poststructuralism to inform nursing knowledge. These arguments maintain that although poststructuralism helps in deconstructing structures, existing discourses, and practices that are detrimental to equity, it does not provide adequate guidelines for constructing transformative discourses or practices (Francis, 2000). Poststructuralism also does not illuminate the essence and properties of the phenomena. Rather, it "historicizes" a phenomenon and uncovers what it is about this particular phenomenon, situation, or sets of relationships that may have evolved within the context of sociopolitical, cultural, and scientific context. It forces an analysis of rules that govern behaviors within and outside a discipline (Dzurec, 2003), and an analysis of gender historically (Arslanian-Engoren, 2002).

Postcolonialism is an epistemic system that is critical of colonial relationships and their aftereffects (Table 8-2). It links self, responses, and experiences with societal oppressions that result from the colonial powers of those nations within the "first world," mainly the West. Said (1999) developed and promoted the notion of colonialism and orientalism, and thus inaugurated a new era of inquiry. The dominant voices of the North in shaping what is important, valued, and worth pursuing in knowledge development is questioned when viewed through a postcolonialism lens (Ali, 2007). Postcolonialism is influenced by critical theory, postmodernism, and poststructuralism. Kirkham and Anderson (2001) identified several properties of postcolonialism knowing. It is knowing and understanding that intersects race, ethnicity, nation, and subjectivity. Each of these is intricately connected with the other, as well as with power differentials and identity of the person. Postcolonial critique uncovers resistance to changes and preferences for maintaining the status quo through ideological processes. It allows for including ways by which people, their responses, and their behaviors are maintained within boundaries imposed on them either by biology, culture, or gender. It allows a critique of the legitimacy afforded to those hierarchies created and maintained by sociopolitical forces. These forces tend to create the notion of "other" or "othering," in which identity is categorized, assigned, homogenized, and universalized. The "other" assigned by colonialism denotes inferiority and abnormality. To colonialism, the dominance of "white," "Europeanism," "westernism" promotes images of superiority and normality (Kirkham and Anderson, 2001).

Postcolonialism knowing is a critique of the definitions and allocations of participants—based on an identity shaped by colonialization, power inequities, and oppression—that interfere in accessing resources. It provides understanding of human responses within a context of a complex web of relationships of gender, race, culture, economics, and power. It also provides a framework that ensures that all people are treated equally (Anderson, Perry, Blue, et al., 2003).

A link exists between feminist and postcolonialist theories, as well as between feminism and postmodernism. A feminist approach to advancing knowledge utilizes the situation of gender and power. When combined with postcolonialism, it also engages the politics of positioning in relationship to ethnicity, race, and nationality and encourages an analysis of factors that influence activism and complacency. Thus, the emergent integrated feminist postcolonialism or postcolonial feminism could produce more integrated answers to pressing health and social questions (Ali, 2007; Anderson, Kirkham, Browne, et al., 2007), if and when nurses recognize their agency and use their voice to affect changes (Croft and Cash, 2012).

It is often said that all the "post" epistemologies are all for "everything goes" (Chinn and Kramer, 2014), and that they do not allow for constructing and developing theories. Critics should continue to question, inform, and challenge epistemic diversity for knowledge development in nursing.

TRUTH: FROM CORRESPONDENCE TO INTEGRATIVE VIEW OF TRUTH

There is another subject of concern to those who are inquisitive about the development of knowledge in nursing. What criteria has nursing used to accept or reject its theoretical notions? What concepts of truth should it use in the future? When do experiences become knowledge, and when does knowledge become truth? Does reality exist or appear?

Philosophers since Plato have addressed these epistemological ideas. Questions about truth have drawn on the writings of such diverse philosophers as Popper and Kaplan and spanned the gamut of empiricists, rationalists, pragmatists, existentialists, feminists, and critical theorists. Some questioned the received view as a guiding framework; others proposed the incorporation of intuitive thinking, combining it with the more traditional Baconian approach to nursing science. Silva (1977) and Benoliel (1977) supported the idea that nursing should not lose sight of the significant notion that truths gained from intuition are as important as truths gained through more traditional research methods. From this examination of truth, three views have emerged: correspondence, coherence, and pragmatism (Armour, 1969; Kaplan, 1964).

Correspondence Theory

Correspondence, with its careful rules, calls for sensory data, very small variables, and operational definitions. For generations, this view has dominated science, research, and theory construction in the physical and natural sciences. It is the method of truth on which the received or scientific view is based. Indeed, many philosophers of science consider truth by correspondence and the received view one and the same (Table 8-3). Nevertheless, the received view and truth represent two different processes. The received view addresses the process of research, the methodology by which data are collected and theories are developed; truth attends to examining realities, the results of the findings. Whereas the received view asks what to do to know, truth asks how to know (see Tables 8-1 and 8-3).

Empiricists, such as Bertrand Russell, and rationalists, such as J.E. McTaggart, preferring to view truth through correspondence, have designed a set of rules and norms against which they expect theory development and research to be analyzed. The most significant norm is that of truism of facts and their correspondence with their encompassing theories. One of the most significant correspondence norms is total objectivity; a separation of the observer from the observed world. Validation is based on congruence between propositions and reality. Reality means one reality, an existing reality, and not reality as it may appear to different viewers. The theorist's role is to match the world with assertions and match the facts with concepts.

TABLE 8-3	Comparison of Different Theories of Truth			
Analytical Unit	Correspondence	Coherence	Pragmatism	Integration
Norms	Corroboration	Logic	Experience	Experience and utility illumination
Contexts	Justification	Experience	Discovery and justification	Justification
Goals	Acceptance/rejection	Support	Understanding	Uncovering patterns
Reality	One	Pattern Clicks into a structure	Multiple	Diversity of views
Role of theorist	Match world with assertions Distance	Match with assertions Involvement	Match with users Humanness	Openness to multiplicity
Evaluation	Verification Falsification	Simplicity Beauty	Utility Problem solving	Validation Verification Logic Utility multiple
Process	End	Process	Process	
Validation	Congruence between propositions and reality	Endurance of ideas	Consensus of users Restructuring New techniques	Use patterns of understanding Number of solved problems

The positivists assert that correspondence truth is achieved through corroboration by verification. Popper (1959) modified the positivist view and developed the argument for falsification. He asserted that the central concept in scientific discovery is "marcation." *Demarcation criteria* require that we consider a proposition scientific only if it has the potential to be falsified. Verification of the opposite statement occurs with multiple incidents of falsification of the statement through experience. Once a single falsifying instance counters a proposition, the proposition should be rejected. On the other hand, a proposition is not scientific if it does not have the potential for falsification. Continuous attempts to falsify statements make the scientific process rigorous. Truth is achieved when we have exhausted all attempts at falsifying a proposition.

Although Popper warns against the potential for any entirely conclusive statement because of problems of reliability in testing, we nevertheless come closer to the truth by testing and retesting, with the objective of attempting to nullify and falsify the proposition under exploration. To the correspondence theorists, whether verification or falsification is the focus, truth is achieved through sensory data and controlled experiments. The correspondence of existing reality, of facts and propositions, is the goal. No room exists for metaphysics, conceptual truths, multiple realities, or for perceptions of reality. Other problems arise when viewing truth in mainly correspondence terms. If facts exist, are not facts already affected by the concepts introduced to explain them?

There are other ways by which we can corroborate theoretical developments that may be more congruent with epistemic diversity in our discipline. The "warrantable evidence" criteria proposed by Forbes, King, Kushner, et al. (1999) for reviews in nursing science could be utilized for the evaluation of theoretical formulations. The "warrants" common to pluralistic nursing scholarship are:

1. Critical scrutiny of rigor by a community of scientists
2. Use of intersubjectivity
3. Wider scope of the evidence

One approach to establishing corroboration is to use critical reflection among scholars or among participants (e.g., Gibson, 1999).

Coherence Theory

Truth through *coherence* differs considerably from truth through correspondence. Truth through coherence is manifested by the logical way in which relationships and judgments relate. Whereas the norms for correspondence are verification and falsification using sensory data, the norms for coherence are an integration of relationships, simplicity of presentation, and a certain beauty of propositions (Table 8-3). When separate components of a phenomenon "suddenly fall into a pattern of relatedness, when they click into position," then truth has been achieved (Kaplan, 1964, p. 314). Truth according to this theory endures, but perhaps in a more transitory fashion or in ways that may not be reproducible but are no less recognizable. If the proposition is sufficient for today, there is truth in it.

The coherence norms of logic, simplicity, and aesthetic presentation appear to be norms to be used in both the context of discovery and the context of justification. They are most suitable, however, for the discovery of apparent realities. They lend themselves more to the evaluation of concepts that are in the process of development than to those in the process of testing. Although norms of correspondence and coherence may appear contradictory, it is nonetheless possible to consider them as complementary. While using the coherence norms to judge and evaluate theories, we can also use correspondence norms to judge propositions that evolve out of research.

Pragmatism Theory

It is possible that the newness of nursing as a discipline makes it easier to reject both competing views of correspondence and coherence to the detriment of solving the pressing disciplinary problems and advancing knowledge. Neither correspondence nor coherence criteria could establish evidence and truth in the discipline; it may be best to use a pragmatic approach to truth.

In the 1930s, a group of American philosophers, called pragmatists, advanced a third type of theory about truth. In fact, according to Armour (1969), there are two types of *pragmatic* theories of truth. *First*, an assertion is true if it produces the right type of influence on its followers. In other words, a proposition is declared to be true when its users determine its usefulness. Experience and the ability to solve problems are two of the norms considered in this view of truth. *Second*, a proposition or any theorized relationship is true if it receives confirmation from a person or persons who have conducted the right investigations or who are designated as significant by the community of scholars. Pierce (cited in Kaplan, 1964) suggests that, according to this theory, a consensus between significant theoreticians or investigators is what constitutes truth.

Pragmatic truth depends less on evidence than on observations—on a declaration of effectiveness by whatever methods the significant members of a community of scholars use. These measures of effectiveness may be subjective, political, social, or objective. To the proponents of this view, "a theory is validated, not by showing it to be invulnerable to criticism, but by putting it to good use, in one's own problems or in those problems of coworkers" (Kaplan, 1964).

A pragmatic theory of truth allows for the validation of theories through restructuring, use of new techniques, or even better awareness and realizations of the meanings of old relationships. The value of these new relationships lies not in the answers they may provide as much as in the new questions they may ask and the consequences that result from their use (Kaplan, 1964). Humanity, tentativeness, subjectivity, collectivity, and usefulness are all qualities attached to this concept of pragmatic truth, which evolved out of the Chicago school of thought (Table 8-3).

Integrative Theory

A tension continues to exist between using a single paradigm, a pluralistic approach to paradigms, or no paradigm to guide the development of nursing knowledge. Weaver and Olson (2006) examined a number of paradigms in terms of their philosophical underpinnings and effectiveness and concluded that no single paradigm emerged as superior for nursing research. The complexity of human health experience and illness responses may require the use of all of them, or on a more integrative approach as proposed by others (Ali, 2007; Aranda 2006), and in offering integrative theory as an approach to discerning "truth" in the knowledge that is developed.

Furthermore, some conceptual problems are not as well addressed by any one of the theories of truth in isolation. Laudan (1977, p. 54) identified three. The first of these problems is an intrascientific problem, which results from two theories representing two inconsistent domains. An example is Rogers' (1970) view of a unitary human being as an energy field and of behavior as the manifestation of the pattern and organization of the energy field. This view presupposes a methodological approach to the study of a human being and his or her energy field as a whole. Conversely, Johnson (1974) views a social behavioral system, with seven subsystems revolving around subsystem goals and manifested in observable behavior. Johnson presupposes a study of humans by reducing humans to their behaviors (Table 8-3).

Because of the theoretical incompatibility between these two fundamental views of the nursing client, the nursing community may attempt (perhaps prematurely) to accept one in favor of the other. The theorist's commitment to adequacy and effectiveness may also prompt one to concede to the other. Either of these alternatives to resolving the problem may fail because of the level of conceptual and methodological knowledge. To reject Rogers' conception of a unitary human being as an energy field and behavior as a manifestation of pattern and organization of the energy field because of lack of methods to study it, could be premature, and may not allow Rogers' theory followers to be creative in developing congruent methods. Rejecting these conceptions may impede progress and creativity.

Nursing, historically, has also been beset by other philosophical inconsistencies (Munhall, 1982). Existential and pragmatic philosophies have dominated clinical nursing, and positivistic, empirical philosophies have attempted to dominate the academic discipline. This theoretical confusion has managed only to temporarily impede nursing's theoretical development. Laudan refers to such conflict between emerging conflicting theoretical and methodological paradigms as *normative difficulties*. Those who believe that the correspondence norm has dominated nursing would attribute the early rejection of nursing theories to this paradox.

It was once believed that the only credible theories in nursing were those inferred from observable data. Others asserted that a nursing philosophy that espoused holism, integration, and health was in direct conflict with its methodology of reductionism, objectivity, logic, measurement, verification, and falsification. Where does the truth lie? Which of the two options should nursing follow—the methodological view or the philosophical premise? Who determines the truth—the methodologists or the theoreticians? None of the norms in isolation would provide us with the truth. A combination of all may bring us closer.

A third difficulty that confronts theorists, and one that cannot be resolved by any one of the theories, Laudan calls "prevalent world view difficulties" (Laudan, 1977, p. 61). This phenomenon is observed when myths, beliefs, history, and practice are in opposition with developing theories. The prevalent nursing view ascribed to by clinicians is that nursing is practical and skill-oriented and that its principles, as well as its skills, are derived from other disciplines. Nursing is neither theoretical, says this worldview, nor academic.

Tension also exists between the researchers, who hold the belief that theories develop only from research, and the theoreticians, who believe that theories are culminations of experience, history, and intuition, as well as research findings. There have been many "world views" in nursing, with very few ascribing to a theoretical worldview. Because nurses deal with complex phenomena, with human beings, with behaviors, cognitions, and perceptions, the discipline cannot use one meaning of truth to the exclusion of others. Because of the consideration of the relationship between science and humanity during the 1980s, and because of the close relationships between philosophy and science and between science and ethics, nurses realized that a singular theory of truth was inadequate and would defy the essence and purpose of nursing as a human science.

The scope of meanings of responses, sense data, and findings is wide, and requires heterogeneity for different evolving "truths." Judgment about the "truth" can depend not only on one source of legitimacy (Clarke, 1999). In the face of relativism, subjectivism, postmodernism, and deconstructionism and their ideas, truth still matters (Lynch, 2005). However:

People never think there is no truth of the matter; rather they think the other side is wrong. (Gottlieb, 2005)

Therefore, there are diverse ways to establish truth, and one is by offering alternatives to correspondence norms and to the received view. Suppe (1977) suggested that what is needed is a different way to analyze theories. He called this new way *Weltanschauung* and defined it as "a comprehensive world view, especially from a specified standpoint." It addresses the many problems that none of the standalone truth theories (i.e., correspondence, coherence, and pragmatism) can address. According to Suppe, Weltanschauung is:

[an] analysis of theories which concerns itself with the epistemic factors governing the discovery, development, and acceptance or rejecting of theories; such an analysis must give serious attention to the idea that science is done from within a conceptual perspective which determines in large part which questions are worth investigating and what sorts of answers are acceptable; the perspective provides a way of thinking about a class of phenomena which define[s] the class of legitimate problems and delimits the standards for their acceptable solution. Such a perspective is intimately tied to one's language which conceptually shapes the way one experiences the world. (p. 126)

A *Weltanschauung*, an integrative worldview, of truth in theoretical nursing includes an integration of norms emanating from different theories of truth. It combines rigor and intuition, sensory data as they exist and as they appear, perceptions of the subject and of the theoretician, and logic with observable clinical data. What different theorists and researchers have advocated merely as norms for the acceptance of propositions are not contradictory, because in some situations, events, and experiences, one set of norms is more appropriate than another. Some research in nursing has been guided by the positivists' views and by correspondence. Some theory development has been guided by these norms as well. For example, Orlando and Johnson focused on observable, verifiable behavior in developing theories (Johnson, 1974; Orlando, 1961). Rogers spoke of experiences beyond the five senses (1970).

Nursing theoreticians, however, would not have developed their theories if they adhered to correspondence norms. Numerous examples have shown that nursing has used a pragmatic theory of truth. Johnson (1974) spoke about criteria for acceptance of knowledge as based on social responsibility and about how knowledge and nursing action should make a valuable difference in the people's lives. Whether the model guiding nursing is right or wrong is a social decision and not exclusively a theorist's or researcher's decision. Rogers (1970), in conceptualizing a unitary man as an energy field, spoke of experiences beyond the five senses and therefore could not use correspondence norms to verify her conceptualization, but instead used coherence norms. Many others supported the necessity of considering coherence norms in conceptualizing nursing and suggested that truth emanated from logic (Batey, 1977; Beckstrand, 1978a, 1978b; Dickoff, James, and Wiedenbach, 1968).

The integrative truth in nursing theory utilizes a diversity of views about truth. It uses validation, verification, simplicity, logic, consequences, clients, theorists, and actual or potential experiences as norms against which to compare the truth of the theory. It reflects a broader notion of evidence that relates to multiple sources of knowledge, particularly knowledge that has been marginalized because of its softness (Kirkham, Baumbusch, Schultz, et al., 2007). It accepts multiple realities and "a composite of realities" (Oiler, 1982). It accepts different expressions, different sources, and criteria such as the number of solved problems within a discipline (Laudan, 1977; Silva and Rothbart, 1984), rather than confirmation and verification only. The number and nature of the questions asked and answered become the units of analysis to determine the level of progress in the discipline (see Chapter 18 for discussion about progress in the discipline).

CONCLUSION

Our syntax includes ways of knowing in nursing and approaches by which truth has been defined. The received, perceived, interpretive, and critical patterns of knowing are more congruent with the nature of nursing as a human science. The received view provided the canons for acceptance and rejection of the road that nurses have taken in theory development. However, it is a more acceptable approach to analysis and evolution of knowing within the context of justification. The perceived view of knowing that guided nursing practice, nursing theory, and nursing education historically has been more open, variable, relativistic, and subject to experience and personal interpretations. It is holistic in approach and based on the perceptions of both the client and the theoretician. The perceived view is more appropriate to the context of discovery. The interpretive approach to knowing honors diversity and socioeconomic variations and provides a view that is critical of gender inequity, as well as of power differentials due to social class, race, and colonialism.

So, the question that this discourse produces is how is truth determined through this epistemic diversity? This diversity has created issues of acceptance and rejection of nursing knowledge. One important component that determines acceptance or rejection of knowledge in a field is how "truth" is perceived and defined. What counts as truth? How do we find it? What criteria do we have for the acceptance of nursing's major questions, assumptions, and answers? These questions guide a discussion about truth. Three competing theories of truth—correspondence, coherence, and pragmatism—were discussed in this chapter, as were the limitations they present. As we increasingly accepted the shifts from received to perceived views, we began to acknowledge that existing theories of truth were unsuited to the uniqueness of our progress; for that reason the chapter also discussed the integrative approach to truth finding that has emerged in nursing.

Progress in nursing has been unique, and phenomenal in acceleration during the end of the 20th century and the beginning of the 21st century. In the late 1980s, theorists and researchers in nursing began to accept the differences between nursing and

REFLECTIVE QUESTIONS

1. Discuss epistemic diversity and its potential outcomes on practice that is based on evidence (mostly defined from a received view and correspondence theory of truth).

2. Critically analyze the progress in the discipline of nursing within the different views of knowing. What criteria are you using to arrive at your conclusion?

3. Identify ways of knowing within your field of interest. Compare and contrast ways of knowing in your field of interest with those discussed in this chapter. In what ways are they different or similar, and why?

4. Which one of our discipline's epistemological traditions is likely to produce the evidence needed for quality care outcomes? Identify and define nursing discipline-driven quality care outcomes.

5. Compare and contrast the strengths of the different ways of knowing discussed in this chapter. What other approaches to knowing would you add to those discussed in this chapter?

6. Select one pattern of knowing and discuss how you would go about developing a theoretical framework for a research question within your field of practice. What are the most significant properties that distinguish the process you have selected?

7. What are the weaknesses and strengths of each approach to truth discussed in this chapter?

8. Discuss some of the values nurse scientists hold that may support or negate each of the ways of knowing and models of truth discussed in this chapter.

9. In what ways do values about knowing in the United States, as well as in other parts of the world, correspond or negate each way of knowing discussed in this chapter?

10. In what ways do major funding sources for nursing research shape patterns of knowing and models of truths in the discipline of nursing? Take a pro or con stand and defend it with evidence.

11. Discuss an Eastern philosophical way of knowing (e.g., Buddhism) and critically consider how it could enrich or constrain knowledge development in nursing.

other sciences, the uniqueness of nursing, and the capabilities of its scholars to develop knowledge. Nursing deals with wholeness, perceptions, experiences, multiple realities, appearances of phenomena, and the existence of phenomena. Whether it needs to or should use any of the theories of truth discussed in this chapter is up to you and future theoreticians in nursing to decide. This chapter is intended to introduce you to current discussions and to encourage you to go beyond this limited discussion to explore theories of probabilities and theories that espouse the use of the criteria of a number of solved problems within a discipline rather than truth theories.

REFERENCES

Agan, R.D. (1987). Intuitive knowing as a dimension of nursing. *Advances in Nursing Science*, 10(1), 63–70.

Ali, S. (2007). Feminism and postcolonialism: Knowledge/politics. *Ethnic and Racial Studies*, 30(2), 191–212.

Allen, D. (1985). Nursing research and social control: Alternative models of science that emphasize understanding and emancipation. *Image: The Journal of Nursing Scholarship*, 17(2), 58–64.

Allen, D. (1988). The challenge of gender for the development of nursing science. In V.C. Bridges and N. Wells (Eds.), *Proceedings of the fifth nursing science colloquium: Strategies for theory development in nursing: V.* Boston, MA: Boston University.

Allen, D., Benner, P., and Diekelmann, N. (1986). Three paradigms for methodologies to understand the concept of health. In P. Chinn (Ed.), *Nursing research methodology: Issues and implementation*. Rockville, MD: Aspen Publications.

Anderson, J., Kirkham, S.R., Browne, A.J., and Lynam, M.J. (2007). Continuing the dialogue: Postcolonial feminist scholarship and Bourdieu–discourses of culture and points of connection. *Nursing Inquiry*, 14(3), 178–188.

Anderson, J., Perry, J., Blue, C., Browne, A., Henderson, A., Khan, K.B., Kirkham, S.R., Lynam, J., Semeniuk, P., and Smye, V. (2003). 'Riting' cultural safety within the post-colonial and post-national feminist project: Toward new epistemologies of healing. *Advances in Nursing Science*, 26(3), 196–214.

Andreoli, K.G. and Thompson, C.E. (1977). The nature of science in nursing. *Image*, 9(2), 32–37.

Andrist, L.C. and MacPherson, K.I. (2001). Conceptual models for women's health research: Reclaiming menopause as an exemplar of nursing's contributions to feminist scholarship. *Annual Review of Nursing Research*, 19, 29–60.

Aranda, K. (2006). Postmodern feminist perspectives and nursing research: A passionately interested form of inquiry. *Nursing Inquiry*, 13(2), 135–143.

Armour, L. (1969). *The concept of truth*. Assen, Netherlands: Van Gorcum and Co.

Arslanian-Engoren, C. (2002). Feminist poststructuralism: A methodological paradigm for examining clinical decision-making. *Journal of Advanced Nursing*, 37(6), 512–517.

Aston, M., Price, S., Kirk, S.F., and Penney, T. (2011). More than meets the eye. Feminist poststructuralism as a lens toward understanding obesity. *Journal of Advanced Nursing*, 68(5), 1187–1194.

Baer, E.D. (1979). Philosophy provides the rationale for nursing's multiple research directions. *Image*, 11(3), 72–74.

Batey, M.V. (1977). Conceptualization: Knowledge and logic guiding empirical research. *Nursing Research*, 26(5), 324–329.

Beckstrand, J. (1978a). The notion of practice theory and the relationship of scientific and ethical knowledge to practice. *Research in Nursing and Health*, 1(3), 131–136.

Beckstrand, J. (1978b). The need for a practice theory as indicated by the knowledge used in conduct of practice. *Research in Nursing and Health*, 1(4), 175–179.

Benner, P., Tanner, C., and Chesla, C. (1996). *Expertise in nursing practice: Caring, clinical judgement, and ethics*. New York: Springer Publishing.

Benner, P. and Wrubel, J. (1982). Skilled clinical knowledge: The value of perceptual awareness. *Nurse Educator*, 12(5), 11–17.

Benoliel, J.Q. (1977). The interaction between theory and research. *Nursing Outlook*, 25(2), 108–113.

Bernstein, R.J. (1978). *The restructuring of social and political theory*. Philadelphia, PA: University of Pennsylvania Press.

Boykin, A., Parker, M.E., and Schoenhofer, S.O. (1994). Aesthetic knowing grounded in an explicit conception of nursing. *Nursing Science Quarterly*, 7(4), 158–161.

Bradbury-Jones, C., Sambrook, S., and Irvine, F. (2008). Power and empowerment in nursing: A fourth theoretical approach. *Journal of Advanced Nursing*, 62(2), 258–266.

Carper, B.A. (1978). Practice oriented theory: Part 1. Fundamental patterns of knowing in nursing. *Advances in Nursing Science*, 1(1), 13–23.

Chinn, P.L. and Kramer, M.K. (2014). *Knowledge development in nursing: Theory and process* (9th ed.). St. Louis, MO: Elsevier.

Clarke, J.B. (1999). Evidence-based practice: A retrograde step? The importance of pluralism in evidence generation for the practice of health care. *Journal of Clinical Nursing*, 8(1), 89–94.

Closs, S.J. and Draper, P. (1998). Writing ourselves: Creating knowledge in a postmodern world. *Nurse Education Today*, 18(4), 337–341.

Cloyes, K.G. (2002). Agonizing care: Care ethics, agonistic feminism and a political theory of care. *Nursing Inquiry*, 9(3), 203–214.

Cockerham, W. (2007). A note on the fate of postmodern theory and its failure to meet the basic requirements for success in medical sociology. *Social Theory and Health*, 5, 285–296.

Connell, R. (2012). Gender, health and theory: Conceptualizing the issue, in local and world perspective. *Social Science and Medicine*, 74(11), 1675–1683.

Cook, J.A. and Fonow, M.M. (1986). Knowledge and women's interests: Issues of epistemology and methodology in feminist sociological research. *Sociological Inquiry*, 56(1), 2–29.

Cowling, W.R. and Chinn, P.L. (2001). Conversations across paradigms: Unitary-transformative and critical feminist perspectives. *Scholarly Inquiry for Nursing Practice*, 15(4), 347–365.

Croft, R.K. and Cash, P.A. (2012). Deconstructing contributing factors to bullying and lateral violence in nursing using a postcolonial feminist lens. *Contemporary Nurse*, 42(2), 226–242.

Dickoff, J., James, P., and Wiedenbach, E. (1968). Theory in a practice discipline: Part 1. Practice oriented theory. *Nursing Research*, 17(5), 415–435.

Drevdahl, D. (1999). Sailing beyond: Nursing theory and the person. *Advances in Nursing Science*, 21(4), 1–13.

Duffy, M.E. and Hedin, B.A. (1988). New directions for nursing research. In N.F. Woods and M. Catanzaro (Eds.), *Nursing research: Theory and practice*. St. Louis, MO: C.V. Mosby.

Dzurec, L.C. (2003). Poststructuralist nursings on the mind/body question in health care. *Advances in Nursing Science*, 26(1), 63–76.

English, I. (1993). Intuition a function of the expert nurse: A critique of Benners' novice to expert model. *Journal of Advanced Nursing*, 18(3), 387–393.

Fawcett, J., Watson, J., Neuman, B., Hinton-Walker, P., and Fitzpatrick, J.J. (2001). On nursing theories and evidence. *Journal of Nursing Scholarship*, 33(2), 115–119.

Ferreira, F.R., Prado, S.D., Carvalho, M.C, and Kraemer, F.B. (2015). Biopower and biopolitics in the field of food and nutrition. *Revista de Nutrição*, 28(1), 109–119.

Fontana, J.S. (2004). A methodology for critical science in nursing. *Advances in Nursing Science*, 27(2), 93–101.

Forbes, D.A., King, K.M., Kushner, K.E., Letourneau, N.L., Myrick, A.F., and Profetto-McGrath, J. (1999). Warrantable evidence in nursing science. *Journal of Advanced Nursing*, 29(2), 373–379.

Foucault, M. (1995). *Discipline and punish: The birth of the prison*. Translated by A. Sheridan. New York: Vintage Books.

Francis, B. (2000). Poststructuralism and nursing: Uncomfortable bedfellows? *Nursing Inquiry*, 7(1), 20–28.

Fraser, N. and Nicholson, L.J. (1989). Social criticism without philosophy: An encounter between feminism and postmodernism. In L.J. Nicholson (Ed.), *Feminism/postmodernism* (pp. 39–62). New York: Routledge.

Freire, P. (2000). *Pedagogy of the oppressed*. New York: Continuum Publishing Corporation.

Fry, S.T. (1988). The nature of knowledge. In V.C. Bridges and N. Wells (Eds.), *Proceedings of the fifth nursing science colloquium: Strategies for theory development in nursing: V*. Boston, MA: Boston University.

Gadamer, H. (1979). The problem of historical consciousness. In P. Robinson and J. Sullivan (Eds.), *Interpretive social science—A reader*. Berkeley, CA: University of California.

Garrett, B.M. and Cutting, R.L. (2015). Ways of knowing: Realism, non-realism, nominalism and a typology revisited with a counter perspective for nursing science. *Nursing Inquiry*, 22(2), 95–105.

Georges, J.M. (2003). An emerging discourse: Toward epistemic diversity in nursing. *Advances in Nursing Science*, 26(1), 44–52.

George, J.M. and McGuire, S. (2004). Deconstructing clinical pathways: Mapping the landscape of health care. *Advances in Nursing Science*, 27(1), 2–11.

Gibson, C.H. (1999). Facilitating critical reflection in mothers of chronically ill children. *Journal of Clinical Nursing*, 8(3), 305–312.

Gobet, F. and Chassy, P. (2008). Towards an alternative to Benner's theory of expert intuition in nursing: A discussion paper. *International Journal of Nursing Studies*, 45, 129–139.

Gottlieb, A. (2005). The truth wars. *New York Times*, July 24, 2005, p. 20.

Green, C. (2012). Nursing intuition: A valid form of knowledge. *Nursing Philosophy*, 13(2), 98–111.

Habermas, J. (1971). *Knowledge and human interests*. Boston, MA: Beacon Press.

Habermas, J. (1974). *Theory and practice*. Boston, MA: Beacon Press (original work published in 1971).

Habermas, J. (1979). *Communication and the evolution of society*. Boston, MA: Beacon Press.

Hagell, E.I. (1989). Nursing knowledge: A sociological perspective. *Journal of Advanced Nursing*, 14(3), 226–233.

Hall, B.A. (2003). An essay on an authentic meaning of medicalization: The patient's perspective. *Advances in Nursing Science*, 26(1), 53–62.

Hall, J.M. (1999). Marginalization revisited: Critical, postmodern and liberation perspectives. *Advances in Nursing Science*, 22(2), 88–102.

Hall, J., Stevens, P., and Meleis, A.I. (1994). Marginalization: A guiding concept for valuing diversity in nursing knowledge development. *Advances in Nursing Science*, 16(4), 23–41.

Hampton, D.C. (1994). Expertise: The true essence of nursing art. *Advances in Nursing Science*, 17(1), 15–24.

Harding, S. (1986). *The science question in feminism*. Ithaca, NY: Cornell University Press.

Harding, S. (1987). Introduction: Is there a feminist method? In S. Harding (Ed.), *Feminism and methodology*. Bloomington, IN: Indiana University Press.

Harding, S. (1988). Feminism confronts the sciences: Reform and transformation. In V.C. Bridges and N. Wells (Eds.), *Proceedings of the fifth nursing science colloquium: Strategies for theory development in nursing: V*. Boston, MA: Boston University.

Holter, I.M. (1987). *Critical theory*. Oslo, Norway: Unpublished Master's thesis.

Im, E-O. and Meleis, A.I. (2001). An international imperative for gender sensitive theories in women's health. *Journal of Nursing Scholarship*, 33(4), 309–314.

Jagger, A.M. (1988). *Feminist politics and human nature*. Sussex, UK: Rowman & Littlefield.

Jaspers, K. (1963). *General psychopathology*. J. Hoenig and M.W. Hamilton (Trans.). Chicago, IL: University of Chicago Press.

Jenny, J. and Logan, J. (1992). Knowing the patient: One aspect of clinical knowledge. *Image: Journal of Nursing Scholarship*, 24(4), 254–258.

Johnson, D.E. (1974). Development of theory: A requisite for nursing as a primary health profession. *Nursing Research*, 23(5), 372–377.

Johnson, J.L. (1994). A dialectical examination of nursing art. *Advances in Nursing Science*, 17(1), 1–14.

Kaplan, A. (1964). *The conduct of inquiry: Methodology of behavioral science*. San Francisco, CA: Chandler Publishing Company.

Kirkham, S.R. and Anderson, J.M. (2001). Postcolonial nursing scholarship: From epistemology to method. *Advances in Nursing Science*, 25(1), 1–17.

Kirkham, S.R., Baumbusch, J.L., Schultz, A.S.H., and Anderson, J.M. (2007). Knowledge development and evidence-based practice: Insights and opportunities from a postcolonial feminist perspective for transformative nursing practice. *Advances in Nursing Science*, 30(1), 26–40.

Kushner, K.E. and Morrow, R. (2003). Grounded theory, feminist theory, critical theory: Toward theoretical triangulation. *Advances in Nursing Science*, 26(1), 30–43.

Lacey, S. and Hughes, R.G. (2007). Is power everything? What can we learn from large data sets? *Applied Nursing Research*, 20(1), 50–53.

Landivar, L.C. (2013). *Men in nursing occupations: American community survey highlight report*. Washington, DC: U.S. Census Bureau, Industry and Occupational Statistics Branch. Retrieved from www.census.gov/people/io.files/Men_in_Nursing_Occupations

Laudan, L. (1977). *Progress and its problems: Toward a theory of scientific growth*. Berkeley, CA: University of California Press.

Luntley, M. (2010). What do nurses know? *Nursing Philosophy*, 12(1), 22–33.

Lynch, M.P. (2005). *True to life: Why truth matters*. Boston, MA: MIT Press.

MacPherson, K.I. (1983). Feminist methods: A new paradigm for nursing research. *Advances in Nursing Science*, 5(2), 17–25.

Magee, T., Lee, S.M., Giuliano, K.K., and Munro, B. (2006). Generating new knowledge from existing data: The use of large data sets for nursing research. *Nursing Research*, 55(2S), S50–S56.

Mantzorou, M. and Mastrogiannis, D. (2011). The value and significance of knowing the patient for professional practice, according to the Carper's patterns of knowing. *Health Science Journal*, 5(4), 251–261

Mantzoukas, S. and Jasper, M. (2008). Types of nursing knowledge used to guide care of hospitalized patients. *Journal of Advanced Nursing*, 62(3), 318–326.

Matthewman, S. and Hoey, D. (2006). What happened to postmodernism? *Sociology*, 40(3), 529–547.

Meleis, A.I. and Im, E-O. (1999). Transcending marginalization in knowledge development. *Nursing Inquiry*, 6, 94–102.

Moch, S.D. (1990). Personal knowing: Evolving research and practice. *Scholarly Inquiry for Nursing Practice: An International Journal*, 4(2), 155–170.

Munhall, P.L. (1982). In opposition or apposition. *Nursing Research*, 31(3), 175–177.

Munhall, P.L. (1993). 'Unknowing': Toward another pattern of knowing in nursing. *Nursing Outlook*, 41, 125–128.

Newman, M. (1981, October). *Methodology of pattern*. Paper presented at the Nursing Theory Think Tank, Denver.

Newman, M.A. (1994). Theory for nursing practice. *Nursing Science Quarterly*, 7(4), 153–157.

O'Brien, B. and Pearson, A. (1993). Unwritten knowledge in nursing: Consider the spoken as well as the written word. *Scholarly Inquiry for Nursing Practice: An International Journal*, 7(2), 111–127.

Oiler, C. (1982). The phenomenological approach in nursing research. *Nursing Research*, 31(3), 178–181.

Orlando, I.J. (1961). *The dynamic nurse-patient relationship*. New York: G.P. Putman's Sons.

Osborne, T. (1998). *Aspects of enlightenment: Social theory and the ethics of truth*. London, UK: UCL Press.

Paley, J. (2006). Evidence and expertise. *Nursing Inquiry*, 13(2), 82–93.

Paterson, J.G. and Zderad, L.T. (1976). *Humanistic nursing*. New York: John Wiley & Sons.

Paul, R.W. and Heaslip, P. (1995). Critical thinking involving nursing practice. *Journal of Advanced Nursing*, 22, 40–47.

Pitre, N.Y., Kushner, K.E., Raine, K.D., and Hegadoren, K.M. (2013). Critical feminist narrative inquiry: Advancing knowledge through double-hermeneutic narrative analysis. *Advances in Nursing Science,* 36(2), 118–132.

Polanyi, M. (1962). *Personal knowledge*. New York: Harper & Row.

Popper, K. (1959). *The logic of scientific discovery*. London, UK: Hutchinson.

Porter, S. (2010). Fundamental patterns of knowing in nursing: The challenge of evidence-based practice. *Advances in Nursing Science*, 33(1), 3–14.

Reichenback, H. (1968). *The rise of scientific philosophy*. Berkeley, CA: University of California Press.

Reutter, L. and Kushner, K.E. (2010). Health equity through action on the social determinants of health: Taking up the challenge in nursing. *Nursing Inquiry,* 17(3), 269–280.

Rew, L. (1988). Nurses' intuition. *Applied Nursing Research*, 1(1), 27–31.

Rew, L. (1990). Intuition in critical care nursing practice. *Dimensions of Critical Care Nursing*, 9(1), 30–37.

Rew, L. and Barrow, E. (1987). Intuition: A neglected hallmark of nursing knowledge. *Advances in Nursing Science*, 10(1), 49–62.

Rew, L. and Barrow, E. (2007). State of the science: Intuition in nursing, a generation of studying the phenomenon. *Advances in Nursing Science,* 30(1), 15–25.

Rogers, M. (1970). *An introduction to the theoretical basis of nursing*. Philadelphia, PA: F.A. Davis.

Rose, H. (1983). Hand, brain, and heart: A feminist epistemology for the natural sciences. *Signs: Journal of Women in Culture and Society*, 9(1), 73–89.

Runggaldier, E. (1984). *Carnap's early conventionalism: An inquiry into the historical background of the Vienna circle*. Amsterdam, Netherland: Rodopi.

Said, E.W. (1999). *Out of place: A memoir*. New York: Knopf.

Sampselle, C.M. (1990). The influence of feminist philosophy on nursing practice. *Image: Journal of Nursing Scholarship*, 22(4), 243–246.

Sarvimaki A. (1994). Science and tradition in the nursing discipline. *Scandinavian Journal of Caring Sciences*, 8(3), 137–142.

Schutz, A. (1967). *The phenomenology of the social world*. G. Walsh and F. Lehnert (Trans.). Evanston, IL: Northwestern University Press.

Schwartz, M.A. and Wiggins, O.P. (1988). Scientific and humanistic medicine: A theory of clinical methods. In K.L. White (Ed.), *The task of medicine: Dialogue at Wickenburg*. Menlo Park, CA: The Henry J. Kaiser Family Foundation.

Sherwin, S. (1987). Concluding remarks: A feminist perspective. *Health Care for Women International*, 8(4), 293–304.

Silva, M.C. (1977). Philosophy, science, theory: Interrelationships and implications for nursing research. *Image*, 9(3), 59–63.

Silva, M.C. and Rothbart, D. (1984). An analysis of changing trends in philosophies of science on nursing theory development and testing. *Advances in Nursing Science,* 6(2), 1–13.

Silva, M.C., Sorrell, J.M., and Sorrell, C.D. (1995). From Carper's patterns of knowing to ways of being: An ontological philosophical shift in nursing. *Advances in Nursing Science*, 18(1), 1–13.

Smaldone, A.M. and Connor, J.A. (2003). The use of large administrative data sets in nursing research. *Applied Nursing Research*, 16(3), 205–207.

Sohier, R. (1992). Feminism and nursing knowledge: The power of the weak. *Nursing Outlook*, 40(2), 62–93.

Sorrell, J.M. (1994). Remembrance of things past through writing: Esthetic patterns of knowing in nursing. *Advances in Nursing Science*, 17(1), 60–70.

Stacy, J. and Thorne, B. (1985). The feminist revolution in sociology. *Social Problems*, 32(4), 301–315.

Stevenson, J.S. and Woods, N.F. (1986). Nursing science and contemporary science: Emerging paradigms. In G. Sorenson (Ed.), *Setting the agenda for the year 2000: Knowledge development in nursing*. Kansas City, MO: American Academy of Nursing.

Suppe, F. (Ed.). (1977). *The structure of scientific theories* (2nd ed.). Champaign, IL: University of Illinois Press.

Suppe, F. and Jacox, A.K. (1985). Philosophy of science and the development of nursing theory. *Annual Review of Nursing Research*, 3, 241–267.

Tanner, C.A., Benner, P., Chesla, C., and Gordon, D.R. (1993). The phenomenology of knowing the patient. *Image—Journal on Nursing Scholarship*, 25(4), 273–280.

Timpson, J. (1996). Nursing theory: Everything the artist spits is art? *Journal of Advanced Nursing*, 23, 1030–1036.

Travelbee, J. (1963). What do we mean by "rapport"? *American Journal of Nursing*, 63(2), 70–72.

Watson, J. (1981). Nursing's scientific quest. *Nursing Outlook*, 29(7), 413–416.

Weaver, K. and Olson, J.K. (2006). Understanding paradigms used for nursing research. *Journal of Advanced Nursing*, 53(4), 459–469.

Webster, G., Jacox, A., and Baldwin, B. (1981). Nursing theory and the ghost of the received view. In J.C. McClosky and H.K. Grace (Eds.), *Current issues in nursing*. Oxford, UK: Blackwell Scientific Publications.

White, J. (1995). Patterns of knowing: Review, critique, and update. *Advances in Nursing Science*, 17(4), 73–86.

White, M. (1955). *The age of analysis: 20th century philosophers*. Boston, MA: Houghton Mifflin.

Whittman-Price, R.A. (2004). Emancipation in decision-making in women's health care. *Journal of Advanced Nursing*, 47(4), 437–445.

Winstead-Fry, P. (1979, June). Defining clinical content of nursing. In *Proceedings of the 1979 forum on doctoral education in nursing*. San Francisco, CA: University of California.

Winstead-Fry, P. (1980). The scientific method and its impact on holistic health. *Advances in Nursing Science*, 2(6), 1–7.

Wuest, J. (1993). Removing the shackles: A feminist critique of non-compliance. *Nursing Outlook*, 41(5), 217–224.

Younger, J.B. (1990). Literary works as a mode of knowing. *Image: Journal of Nursing Scholarship*, 22(1), 39–43.

Part Four

REVIEWING AND EVALUATING: PIONEERING THEORIES

Part Four is devoted to a discussion of nursing theories in relation to current nursing research, practice, and education. This part emphasizes several themes introduced in other parts and develops them further by providing interpretive examples. A **first theme** is that nursing theories can be reviewed and evaluated through many different lenses and for different purposes. As you will see, Chapter 9 provides a framework for a gestalt categorization of theories, which was used as a framework to classify nursing theories in Chapters 11 to 13. The **second theme** is that nursing theories have evolved from a sociocultural context, were influenced by the educational and experiential background of the theorists, and cannot be understood or adequately analyzed without considering these influences. The **third theme** is that existing theories are not competitive but are complementary and may be used by the same person for different purposes or by different people for different purposes. The **fourth theme** is that theories can be viewed, interpreted, and used in many different ways and are not restricted to the purposes for which they were developed; theory users and their interpretations of theories are significant to the progress of the discipline. A **final theme**, one that is not directly or explicitly presented in this part but that could be indirectly derived, is that progress in the discipline of nursing is measured by the utilization and continuous development of theories, by the engagement in coherent research programs, by the number of theorists and researchers within the discipline, by the breadth and depth in answering the discipline's central and fundamental questions, and by the extent to which new questions are uncovered and answered.

A **model for evaluating** theories is presented in Chapter 10. The model is used in Chapters 11 through 13 to describe, analyze, critique, and provide examples of tests used in examining the theories selected in this book. Several central domain concepts are defined within each theory; however, I also encourage you to consider other domain concepts, as well as other nursing theories, that may have been influenced by the theories examined in this book. Although the selected theories are organized to reflect a particular classification system (Chapter 9), the description is general and encompasses as much of the theorists' conceptualizations as possible.

9

Nursing Theories Through Mirrors, Microscopes, or Telescopes

Pioneering nursing theories are reviewed integratively in this chapter. They are exposed to a different lens as a group. This approach allows us to categorize them in terms of their broader epistemic origins and in terms of the broad questions the theorists attempted to address. In some ways, the more contemporary multidimensional analysis proposed by Beckstead and Beckstead (2006) may lead to a more objective categorization of theories that reflects the intellectual heritage of theories based on patterns in the citations used. However, even with such objective and quantifiable analysis, the use of nonmetric and nominal data (theorist cited or not cited) needs to be complemented by systematic content analysis to determine how the citation of a paradigmatic origin is utilized, and whether or not the paradigm citation was positively or negatively used. They contend, and I agree, that multiple methods of analysis help in understanding phenomena.

The phenomena in this chapter are the theories themselves as a whole, responding to such questions as: What do they reflect? What are their goals? What are the similarities and differences between them? Can we classify and categorize them to provide some generalization? And, more importantly, are there some common themes and patterns to describe them?

I have chosen to subject the theories collectively to mirrors, microscopes, and telescopes. Mirrors reflect all or parts of reality, depending on the type of mirror, and give the parts of reality different shapes; microscopes zero in on yet another part of reality and magnify it within or without context, and telescopes bring faraway objects and events within reach for observations, careful study, and better understanding. Nursing theories reflect different realities as seen through mirrors, microscopes, or telescopes.

Throughout their development, these theories reflected the interests of nurses of the time, the dominant issues confronting nurses, the sociocultural context, and the theorists' educational and experiential backgrounds. When we consider all the theories together and hold them up to the realities of nursing practice, a number of other images are then formulated. The images are not always distinct, well-formulated, or true mirror images; however, they are not mirages or figments of the theorists' imaginations either. They reflect some realities of nursing at the time of development, and they help to shape the realities of nursing care over time.

This chapter provides several ways in which theories, which are an integral part of our history, can be viewed. These ways are neither mutually exclusive nor inclusive. They are presented to stimulate other innovative ways in which to view and classify nursing theories. The purpose of these different views and classifications is twofold. *First*, the more ways in which we can analyze any phenomenon, the more potential we have for seeing different images and details that are not readily apparent when only viewed from one perspective. The *second* purpose is related to the first: using theories for different purposes is enhanced by the many different perspectives from which we view the theories. It is like seeing the image of a garden in a mirror, showing many flowers, many colors, and many beds, and then moving the mirror closer to a bed of California poppies and seeing the rich orange-yellow cups swaying in the fine breeze, then keeping the mirror in position and stepping back a few feet to get another look, to discover the different shades of color blending with the green of the stems. Each image depends on the position of the mirror in relation to the garden and the location of the viewer in relation to the mirror and the garden. Similarly, using microscopes or telescopes will provide different highlights and details.

The *first section* of this chapter provides an analysis of nursing theories that were developed between 1950 and 1980 (see Fig. 9-1), according to the images of nursing of that time. In the *second section*, theories are classified according to their primary focus and according to how they will be evaluated in this book. In the third section, theories are classified according to images of nurses and the roles that nurses may play. Roles played by nurses are to a large extent determined by the theoretical perspective guiding their practice. In the *fourth section*, areas of agreement among and between theories are presented. Whether these are the same images or the same classifications that the theorists saw when they developed their theories is neither discussed nor debated here. What becomes apparent is that the theories together offer a number of images translated into concepts, that both the images and the concepts are reflected in the theories, and that they reflect nursing practice simultaneously. The classification systems sometimes reflect the hindsight of critics rather than of the theorists themselves. One of the earliest classifications of theories was done in 1960 by Johnson, which she used in teaching nursing theory for master students at the University of California, Los Angeles. She classified them by their paradigmatic origins as:

. . . models based on the developmental theories of Erikson (1963), Freud (1949), Maslow (1954), Peplau (1952), C. Rogers (1959), and Sullivan (1953), and based on the behaviorist school (Bijou and Baer, 1961). Among the systems models are found the adaptation system model of Roy (1970), the triad system of Howland and McDowell (1964), the life process system of M. Rogers (1970), and Johnson's behavioral system model (1968). . . . Then, in addition, there is another type of model for nursing practice, called an interaction model, since its conceptual system is dependent on symbolic interaction theory. The most well-known models in this group are those of Orlando (1961) and Wiedenbach (1964). (Johnson, 1974, p. 376)

Other ways of classifying theories include the chronologic context for the development of theory, temporal dimensions focusing on different sociocultural contexts, central theory questions, and central concepts. Once again let me emphasize that the purposes of these proposed analyses along the different dimensions are twofold: to provide opportunities for critical thinking about theoretical nursing and to stimulate the development and

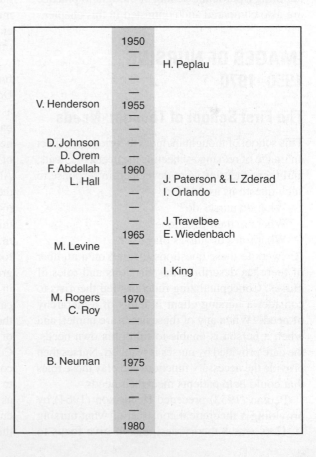

Figure 9-1 Chronology of nursing theories.

TABLE 9-1	Schools of Thought in Nursing Theories—1950–1970		
Needs Theorists	**Interaction Theorists**	**Outcomes Theorists**	
Abdellah	King	Johnson	
Henderson	Orlando	Levine	
Orem	Paterson and Zderad	Rogers	
	Peplau	Roy	
	Travelbee		
	Wiedenbach		

use of a variety of analytical frameworks. Each analysis uncovers different aspects and different explanations within and about the theories, and each different analysis and explanation could drive and further the development of theoretical nursing. The analyses of theories using these dimensions resulted in three distinct patterns or schools of thought (Table 9-1). Each school of thought is presented and discussed in this chapter and in the following chapters. Members of each school of thought are compared in terms of their views of nursing, focus of nursing, goals of nursing, nursing problems, and nursing therapeutics. The images of nurses and the central roles that nurses are expected to play when adopting a particular school of thought to practice are also compared and contrasted in this chapter.

IMAGES OF NURSING, 1950–1970

The First School of Thought: Needs

This school of thought includes theories that reflect an image of nursing as meeting the needs of clients, and these theories were developed in response to such questions as:

What do nurses do?

What are their functions?

What roles do nurses play?

Answers to these questions focused on a number of theorists describing the functions and roles of nurses. Conceptualizing functions led theorists to consider a nursing client in terms of a hierarchy of needs. When any of these needs are unmet, and when a person is unable to fulfill his own needs, the care provided by nurses is required. Nurses then provide the necessary functions and play those roles that could help patients meet their needs.

Peplau (1952) preceded Henderson (1964) by providing a theoretical construct of what nursing is. Hers was a theory designed to give focus to psychiatric nursing. Therefore, although intrapsychic needs play a major role in her theory, her interest and experience in psychiatric nursing prompted her introduction of nurse–patient interpersonal relationships as a focus in nursing. Henderson's theory, in keeping with the intrapersonal focus of the time and not deviating completely from medical science, was conceived to describe all nursing care goals in terms of the needs of patients and in terms of activities that are motivated and driven by patients' hierarchy of needs. The needs and associated actions are determined during three phases: the orientation phase, in which a nurse establishes a relationship with the patient; the working phase, during which the focus is on the work the patient must accomplish; and the termination phase, which encompasses discharge planning and the beginning of the patient's independence (Senn, 2013).

This school of thought, of need deficits or nurse functions, also included Faye Abdellah (1969) and Dorothea Orem (1995). One may refer to this group as the *need* or *deficit school of thought*, which is based on Abraham Maslow's (1954) hierarchy of needs and influenced by Erikson's (1978) stages of development (with a neo-Freudian orientation). Although proponents of this school of thought were the first to promote nursing functions as distinct from medical functions, the theories developed within this school were still greatly influenced by the biomedical model. Because most of the theorists who focused on needs and need deficits in patients either graduated from or worked at Columbia University in New York, this school of thought could also be called the *Columbia school of thought*. Although the theorists may not attribute the development of their theories to their work or association with Columbia University, by noting that they have a common educational background, we may be able to consider themes of shared assumptions as well as shared goals, and therefore explore the influence of Columbia Teachers College on nursing theory development and the development of early scholars. Judging from the number and caliber of international students who graduated from that institution, Columbia Teachers College may have had a significant influence on the development of theoretical nursing in other countries as well. The extent of the influence of this university on the development of schools of thought, and on the development of nursing education and practice nationally and internationally, is yet to be examined.

As Tables 9-2 through 9-6 indicate, "Needs Theorists" provided us with a view of a human being that was slightly different but close to the view provided by the biomedical model. The hierarchy of needs begins with physiologic and safety needs and

TABLE 9-2	Needs Theorists—A View of Nursing
Theorists	**Definition of Nursing**
Abdellah	Use of problem-solving approach to deal with 21 problems related to needs of patients
Henderson	Helping with 14 activities contributing to health or recovery, helping the individual become independent of assistance
Orem	Self-care agency to meet individual's need for self-care action to sustain life and health, recover from disease or injury, and cope with the effects

TABLE 9-3	Needs Theorists—Focus of Nursing
Theorists	**Focus of Nursing**
Abdellah	Problem-solving approach to 21 nursing activities, sustenal, remedial, restorative, preventive, self-help, need deficit or excess
Henderson	Assistance with 14 daily activities or needs
Orem	Deficit between self-care capabilities and self-care demands of patients

TABLE 9-4	Needs Theorists—Goals of Nursing
Theorists	**Goals of Nursing**
Abdellah	Help individual meet health needs and adjust to health problems
Henderson	Completeness or wholeness and independence of patient to perform daily activities
Orem	Eliminate deficit between self-care capabilities and demand

TABLE 9-5	Needs Theorists—Nursing Problems
Theorists	**Nursing Problems**
Abdellah	Condition faced by patient for which a nurse can assist, overtly and covertly (21 problems)
Henderson	Patient's lack of knowledge, strength, or will to carry out 14 activities
Orem	Deficiency in eight universal, two developmental, and six health deviation requisites/needs

TABLE 9-6	Needs Theorists—Nursing Therapeutics
Theorists	**Nursing Therapeutics**
Abdellah	Preventive care (hygiene, safety, exercise, rest, sleep, body mechanics)
	Sustenal care (psychosocial care)
	Remedial care (provision of oxygen, fluid, nutrition, elimination)
	Restorative care (coping with illness and life adjustment)
Henderson	Complementing and supplementing knowledge, will, and strength of patient to perform 14 daily activities and to carry out his medical prescriptions
Orem	Wholly compensatory system (nurse performs all self-care for patient)
	Partly compensatory system (nurse and patient perform patient self-care)
	Supportive-educative system (nurse helps in overcoming any self-care limitations)

TABLE 9-7	Needs Theorists— A Summary
Concepts	**Defining Properties**
Focus	Problems
	Nurses' function
Human being	A set of needs or problems
	A developmental being
Patient	Needs deficit
Orientation	Illness, disease
Role of nurse	Dependent on medical practice
	Beginnings of independent functions
	Fulfill needs requisites
Decision-making	Primarily health care professional

progresses to include other higher-level needs, such as belonging, love, and esteem. Neither Henderson nor Abdellah considered self-actualization needs as within the province of the nurse (as manifested in the omission rather than the commission); Orem added the development of self-care requisites as she continued to develop her theory. Peplau went further, creating a bridge from a focus on only needs to one on establishing relationships, which are essential for meeting the needs of patients (Deane and Fain, 2015).

A summary of the needs theorists' conceptualization of nursing is presented in Table 9-7. The focus of this school of thought, then, is on problems and needs of patients as seen by health care providers and on the role of nurses to assess these needs and to fulfill the need requisites. When lower needs are met, more mature needs may emerge (Peplau, 1952), and therapeutic communication and relationships may actually help in meeting those needs and influencing outcomes (Zarea, Maghsoudi, Dashtebozorgi, et al., 2014). Perceptions of clients, a focus on environment, and the role of nurse–patient interactions in dialogues and intervention are not fully developed in this school of thought. Identifying needs of patients and communicating them during handoffs continue to be used as a framework for primary care nursing (Carabetta, Lombardo, and Kline, 2013).

A Second School of Thought: Interaction

A second set of questions was then beginning to be formulated, based on a view of nursing as supporting and promoting interactions with patients. The theorists in this group, including Peplau who built communication and interaction on a needs approach to patient care, did not totally ignore the first set of questions. Rather, the new sets of questions about interaction complemented the first. Whereas the first questions that guided earlier theorists were related to the central ones—"What do nurses do?" and "What are the needs of patients?"—the second set of questions evolved from the Yale University School of Nursing and was related to another central question—"How do nurses do whatever it is they do?" Answers to the "how" question focused on the interaction process. Peplau, who considered nurse–patient relationships to be fundamental to nursing practice, was the pioneer in that group (1952); however, her answer was more congruent with the prevailing interest at the time in psychoanalytic theory and closer to a hierarchy of needs and related nursing functions. It is significant when studying the history of ideas to note the connection between the first school of thought at Teachers College and the second one at Yale. The Yale or *interactionist school of thought* grew out of the needs approach, with some of the concepts still prevailing in both; this will be demonstrated in the following discussion. The conceptualization of Imogene King (1968), also a graduate of Teachers College, evolved out of interest in the "hows" of making decisions about nursing care.

Interaction theories were conceived in the late 1950s and early 1960s by theorists who viewed nursing as an interaction process with a focus on the development of a relationship between patients and nurses. These theories grew out of a social milieu in the United States that included the following:

- This was the post-Sputnik era.
- There was a focus on such values as human integrity, as promoted by President Kennedy.
- The Cuban missile crisis may have promoted a return to focus on humanity and relationships against the fear of outside invasion.
- The beginning formation of hippie groups, communal living, and the flower children indicated a definite need for intimacy and human relations.
- Technologic advances continued, but with a growing distaste for mechanization and dehumanization.

Interaction theories also reflected several changes that were ongoing within the profession of nursing. Among them were two that had a direct impact on the development of interactional theories:

- Federal grant support was designated to improve the curricula and education of nurse researchers.

- A pioneering effort to develop an integrated curriculam arose, freeing psychiatric nurses to identify core concepts and to integrate these concepts throughout nursing curricula, and allowing them to observe and reflect on the processes of utilizing mental health concepts in all nursing subspecialties.

Tables 9-8 through 9-12 present theories that focused on interaction. Although some of the interaction theorists continued to address the needs of the

TABLE 9-8	Interaction Theorists—A View of Nursing
Theorists	**Definitions**
King	A process of action, reaction, and interaction whereby nurse and client share information about their perceptions of the nursing situation and agree on goals
Orlando	Interaction with patients who have a need or response to suffering individuals or those anticipating helplessness
	Assistance to individual to avoid, relieve, diminish, or cure sense of helplessness
Paterson and Zderad	A human dialogue, intersubjective transaction, a shared situation, a transactional process, a presence of both patient and nurse
Peplau	Therapeutic interpersonal, serial, goal-oriented process
	A health-focused human relationship
Travelbee	An interpersonal process, an assistance to prevent, cope with experiences of illness and suffering, and to find meaning in these experiences
Wiedenbach	Sensing, perceiving, validating patients need for help, ministering help needed in a deliberate, goal-oriented way

TABLE 9-9	Interaction Theorists—Focus of Nursing
Theorists	**Focus of Nursing**
King	Nurse–patient interactions that lead to goal attainment in a natural environment
Orlando	Care for the needs of the patients who are distressed, with consideration for perception, thought, and feeling through deliberate action
Paterson and Zderad	Patient is a unique being
	Patient's perception of events
	Both patient and nurse are the focus
Peplau	Nurse–patient relationship and its phases
	Orientation, identification, exploitation, and resolution
	Harnessing energy from anxiety and tension to positively defining understanding, and meeting productively the problem at hand
Travelbee	Interpersonal relations, finding meaning in suffering, pain, and illness
	Self-actualization
Wiedenbach	Patient's perception of condition, care, action

TABLE 9-10	Interaction Theorists—Goals of Nursing
Theorists	**Goals of Nursing**
King	Help individuals maintain their health so they can function in their role
Orlando	Relieve distress, physical and mental discomfort
	Improve sense of well-being
Paterson and Zderad	Develop human potential, more well-being for both patient and nurse
Peplau	Develop personality, making illness an eventful experience
	Forward movement of personality and other ongoing human processes in the direction of creative, constructive, productive personal and community living
Travelbee	Cope with an illness situation and find meaning in the experience
	Assist patient to accept humanness
Wiedenbach	Meet the needs of an individual experiencing need for help

TABLE 9-11	Interaction Theorists—Nursing Problems
Theorists	**Nursing Problems**
King	When nurse and patient do not perceive each other, the situation, or communicate information, transactions are not made, goals are not attained
Orlando	Distress due to unmet needs
Paterson and Zderad	Persons with perceived needs related to the health/illness quality of living
Peplau	Unsuccessful or incomplete learning of life tasks
	Energy used in tensions and frustrations due to unmet needs, opposing goals—giving rise to conflict, aggression, anxiety
	Discomfort, anxiety, doubt, guilt, obsession, compulsion
Travelbee	Lack of support in nurse–patient relationship
	Not finding meaning in illness, transitory discomfort, anguish, malignant despair, apathetic indifference
Wiedenbach	Person with need for help (unmet needs due to physical or inadequate environment)

TABLE 9-12	Interaction Theorists—Nursing Therapeutics
Theorists	**Nursing Therapeutics**
King	Goal attainment, transaction, perceptual validation
Orlando	Deliberate nursing process not automatic
Paterson and Zderad	Humanness—use of nurse's self, existential nurturing, being, relating, meeting, maximum participation
Peplau	Development of problem-solving skills through the interpersonal process (educational, therapeutic, and collaborative)
Travelbee	Use of nurse's self, original encounter, emerging identities, empathy, sympathy, rapport
Wiedenbach	Ministration of help, validation, rational, reactional, and deliberate

patient, all the interactionist theorists focused on the processes of care and on the various interaction episodes between nurses and clients. Their theories were based on interactionism, phenomenology, and existentialist philosophy. See Table 9-13 for a summary of the major components of the interaction theories.

What did we learn from the interactionists?

- Nurse–patient interaction is fundamental to providing care.
- Nursing is a deliberate process that can be elucidated.
- Nursing encompasses help and assistance.
- Nursing is an interpersonal process occurring between a person in need of help and a person capable of giving help.
- The nurse, to be able to give help, should clarify her own values, use the self in a therapeutic way, and be involved in the care.
- Care is not a mechanistic act but a humanistic act.
- The humanistic interactionist nurses used existential philosophy, symbolic interaction, and developmental theories to develop their conceptions of nursing.

TABLE 9-13	Interaction Theorists—A Summary
Concepts	**Defining Properties**
Focus	Nurse–patient interactions
	Illness as an experience
Human being	Interacting being
	A set of needs
	Can validate needs
	Human experience with meanings
Patient	Helpless being
	A human experience with meaning
Orientation	Illness/disease
Role of nurse	Deliberate helping process
	Self as a therapeutic agent
	Use of the nursing process
Decision-making	Primarily health care professional
	Validated by clients

- Patient-centered care is based on developing a relationship with patients.
- Illness is defined as an inevitable human experience; if one learns to find meaning in it, it will become a growing experience. In this, these theorists differ from the previous group of theorists who defined illness as a deviation that must be corrected.
- Nursing is defined as caring, assisting (all other health care professionals), and helping patients to find meaning and actions that increase human potential and improve well-being.
- Nurses need systematic knowledge to help them in assessing, diagnosing, and intervening.
- The nursing process is well developed by these theorists.
- Properties, antecedents, and consequences of interactions are advanced by this group of theorists, and all the theories reflect the relationships that are formed to relieve distress, as well as those formed to enhance trust.
- These theories mark the beginning of a movement that led toward the patient becoming an equal partner in the nursing process.
- The interactionist nurse considers uniqueness, dignity, and worth values of patients as important in the development of wellness. The view of an autonomous individual with individually established norms was beginning to emerge. Help, it was emphasized, was to be tailored to individual needs.
- Properties of interaction as validation (Wiedenbach), as meeting the needs of patients (Orlando), as being totally present (Parse), as relating to others (Paterson and Zderad), and as human to human (Travelbee) are delineated and defined by this group of theorists.
- The theories concede that perceptions of the patient are important in assessing illness and its meaning.
- The major nurse–patient interaction relationship goal is derived from their observation that the person in need of help becomes distressed; the purpose is to prevent or deal with this distress.
- The interactionist theorists remind us that nurses are human beings who need to participate in self-reflection to understand their own values. Without such understanding, nurses will not be able to care, give care, establish connections, and help patients relieve their distress.
- The interactionist theorists tentatively introduced the notion of effect of environment on

patients. To them, unmet needs of the patient develop because of:
- ○ Physical limitations (from incomplete development, temporary or permanent disability, or restrictions in environment)
- ○ Adverse reactions to inadequate environment (Orlando)
- This group of theorists reintroduced the significance of nurses' intuition and subjectivity in the nursing act.
- Some common assumptions guided the development of the interactionist theories. These are:
- ○ The integrity of an individual has to be maintained.
- ○ Individuals have self-awareness and are therefore able to identify their needs.
- ○ Individuals strive toward actualization.
- ○ Events in life are human experiences inevitable and essential in helping to move to the next stage in development.
- ○ The nurse cannot separate herself as an individual from the act of care—the nurse is an integral part of care.
- ○ Within the historical context of the discipline's development, interaction theorists provided nursing with a new perspective on viewing the nursing care act:
  - ○ There is a *reciprocal* assessment process.
  - ○ Patient *perspective* is significant in health care.
  - ○ *Situation* determines needs and care.
  - ○ Patients are *helpless* and *suffer* due to illness.

A number of concepts were identified by the interaction theorists as central to nursing. These concepts continue to be significant components of the discipline of nursing. These concepts are integral to nurses' roles and actions in planning, providing, and evaluating care:

Sensing

Perceiving

Validating

Existential transactions

Goal orientation of interaction

Nurses' self-development

Interaction theories neither addressed nor focused on:

A more complete view of a human being (human beings are interacting beings with a minimal focus on biopsychocultural focus) as a biophysiologic and a genetic being

A view of the environment, although the centrality of environment was tangential in some of the theories

The Third School of Thought: Outcomes

The third set of questions that nurse theorists asked was related to the central question—the "whys" of nursing care. Although not ignoring the "what" and "how" questions, this group of theorists attempted to conceptualize the outcomes of nursing care and then described the recipient of care. The image of nursing as portrayed by this group of theorists is that of concern over the outcomes and end results of the caring processes. Two of the most influential theorists in this group are Dorothy Johnson (1968) and Martha Rogers (1970). They graduated from Harvard and Johns Hopkins, respectively, but did most of their work at opposite ends of the North American continent—Los Angeles and New York, respectively. This East/West school of thought is referred to in this book as the *outcomes school of thought*. (Other theorists who belong to this school of thought are Levine and Roy, and their theories are discussed at length in Chapter 13.)

Johnson influenced theoretical thinking in nursing, and her theory will influence nursing more so in the future than it did in the past as the goals of nursing become more congruent with stability than with change (Hall, 1983). Rogers, on the other hand, has helped to shape nursing research based on theoretical thinking. Neither theory is as developed as that of Sister Callista Roy who, as nursing director of Mount St. Mary's (Los Angeles, California) had the faculty resources to implement her theory into courses and content, thereby helping in turn to operationalize the theory further. Both Johnson and Rogers, with faculty members of the University of California, Los Angeles, and New York University, respectively, have also partially operationalized their theories, but not to the same extent. Roy's publications on the uses of theory in practice have enhanced the use of her theory in several schools of nursing. Myra Levine, who views the goals of nursing as conservation of energy, also belongs in this group.

This group of theorists (Tables 9-14 through 9-18) conceptualized the goal of nursing care as bringing back some balance, stability, and preservation of energy, or enhancing harmony between the individual and the environment. They based their conceptualizations on system, adaptation, and developmental theories. They directed their focus

TABLE 9-14	Outcomes Theorists—A View of Nursing
Theorists	**Definitions of Nursing**
Johnson	External regulatory force acting to preserve the organization and integration of patient's behavior at an optimal level when behavior is a threat to social, physical health, or illness
Levine	Patient advocacy, devotion to humanity and self-respect of patient, perception and support for personal and individualized needs, compassion, commitment, and protection
Rogers	Humanistic science for maintaining and promoting health, preventing illness, caring for and rehabilitating the sick and disabled
Roy	Theoretical system of knowledge viewing client as biopsychosocial being (ill or potentially so) who adapts to changing environment
	Nurse acts through nursing process to promote adaptation

TABLE 9-15	Outcomes Theorists—Focus on Nursing
Theorists	**Focus of Nursing**
Johnson	Man as a behavioral system with subsystems, each having a structure, a function, and functional imperatives (drive, set, behavior) and each requiring protection, stimulation, and nurturance
Levine	Four principles guide conception of human being (energy, personal, structural, and social integrities) and their organismic responses (fear, inflammation, stress, sensory)
	Nursing is conservation of energy and integrities
Rogers	Life processes of human beings, unitary person–environment energy fields, complementarity, resonance, and helicy
Roy	Focal, contextual, and residual stimuli and their effect on the cognator and regulator mechanisms, in turn affecting four adaptive modes: physiologic, self-concept, role function, and interdependence

TABLE 9-16	Outcomes Theorists—Goals of Nursing
Theorists	*Goals of Nursing*
Johnson	Behavioral system balance, subsystems that function efficiently and effectively
Levine	Conservation of energy and integrities (personal, structural, social), restoration of well-being, and independent activity
	Nursing is conservation of energy and integrities
Rogers	Promote symphonic interaction and harmony between man and environment
	Strengthen coherence and integrity of human field
Roy	Promote person's adaptation in physiologic needs, self-concept, role function, and interdependence

TABLE 9-17	Outcomes Theorists—Nursing Problems
Theorists	*Nursing Problems*
Johnson	Structural functional stress in one subsystem (insufficiency, discrepancy) and between subsystems (incompatibility, dominance)
Levine	Response to fear, response to stress, inflammatory response, sensory response
Rogers	Disruptions in organization and structure of interacting human–environment fields
Roy	Ineffective coping mechanisms causing ineffective responses that disrupt the integrity of the person

TABLE 9-18	Outcomes Theorists—Nursing Therapeutics
Theorists	*Nursing Therapeutics*
Johnson	Inhibition, constriction, supplementation, protection, nurturing (supportive/maintenance, teaching, counseling, and behavior modification)
Levine	Therapeutic—alter course of adaptation
	Supportive—maintain course of adaptation
Rogers	Repatterning of human environment fields or assistance in mobilizing inner resources
Roy	Manipulation of focal, residual, and contextual stimuli with patient's zone of positive coping

on the outcomes of care. Their view of a human being and the nursing client incorporated the need theorists' conceptualization of the human being experiencing need deficit, having problems, and needing nursing care. (The goals of subsystems of behavior in Johnson's theory and adaptive modes by Roy have parallels in the hierarchy of needs by Henderson, nursing functions by Abdellah, and universal needs by Orem.) Although they spoke of harmony with the environment, stability, conservation of energy, and homeostasis as potential outcomes, the consequences are at a high level of abstraction, limiting the utility of these theories in outcomes measures. The outcome theories provide nursing with a well-articulated conception of a human being as a nursing client and of nursing as an external regulatory mechanism (Table 9-19).

TABLE 9-19	Outcomes Theorists—A Summary
Concepts	*Defining Properties*
Focus	Energy
	Balance, stability, homeostasis presentation
	Outcomes of care
Human being	Adaptive and developmental being
Patient	Lack of adaptation
	Systems deficiency
Orientation	Illness, disease
Role of nurse	External regulatory mechanism
Decision-making	Primarily health care provider

A Fourth School of Thought: Caring/Becoming

Caring theories emerged in the 1980s and were influenced by existential philosophy and by principles of equity in relationships. The questions that guided the development of caring theories are "What do nurses do?" (care for patients), and "How do nurses do what they do?" (by caring for patients). These are somewhat similar to those questions that prompted the development of interaction theories. (Theories that are central to this school of thought are not analyzed in this volume.)

Therefore, caring/becoming theories have many similarities to interaction theories. However, caring theories elucidate the act of caring in interactive situations, based on values that honor and respect human capacity, spirituality and dignity, hope, trust, and altruism in giving and receiving care. According to Jean Watson (1979, 1988, 1999, 2002), the very act of caring for others is considered caring for the self. Rosemarie Parse's (1981, 1995, 1998) central conception of nursing is the transformation of the nurse and the client during the act of providing and receiving care (Cody, 2000; Cowling, 1989). The process of care is defined as a process of becoming for both clients and nurses; however, transformation is only possible if each is open to it (Baldursdottir and Jonsdottir, 2002). Patients and nurses are human beings who are coexisting and coconstituting rhythmic patterns with their environments, and choosing meaning and bearing responsibilities for their actions. They are actors and reactors simultaneously, and every caring act transforms both to different levels of being.

Caring theories, although evolved from interaction theories, Parse's in particular, are based on Rogerian views of uniting human beings and on the ideas of energy and connection between people and their environments (Watson and Smith, 2002). They are grounded in true presence manifested by structuring meaning, configuring rhythmic patterns, and transforming the nurse and client (Bunkers, 2012).

Tables 9-20 through 9-25 present theories of caring. Although these theories address nurse–patient interactions, the process of caring occurs between two independent human beings who are fully present to each other and who connect equally in a relationship that transforms them both.

Caring theories have taught us that:
- The fundamental act of caring is central in processes that bring patients and nurses into each other's lives.
- Caring is central to the discipline of nursing.

TABLE 9-20	Caring Theorists—A View of Nursing
Theorists	**View of Nursing**
Watson	Nursing is a human science consisting of knowledge, thought, values, philosophy, commitment, and action with passion in human care transactions.
Parse	Nursing helps human beings toward becoming through choosing ways of cocreating their own health and finding meanings in situations.

TABLE 9-21	Caring Theorists—Focus of Nursing
Theorists	**Focus of Nursing**
Watson	Transpersonal caring relationship. A moral commitment to protect and enhance human dignity. Allow human beings to determine and find their own meaning.
Parse	Unitary being with freedom to choose and decide. Nursing guides unitary human beings in finding meaning in situations, in choosing ways to cocreate their health and to deal with illness. Nursing guides in authentic living in the "day and dayness" of a human being's life.

TABLE 9-22	Caring Theorists—Goals of Nursing
Theorists	**Goals of Nursing**
Watson	Mental and spiritual growth for human beings (nurses and clients), finding meaning in one's own existence and experience.
Parse	Cocreating meaning and finding ways of being. Transforming through coconstituting new ways in deliberate ways through the human universe process.

TABLE 9-23	Caring Theorists—Nursing Problems
Theorists	**Nursing Problem**
Watson	Imbalance caused by deficit in human transcending; disharmony among the mind, body and soul, between person and world.
Parse	A pattern of human–universe rather than a disease or a problem, process related to man-living-health tied to meaning, rhythmicity and contranscendence. Discontinuity and interruption.

TABLE 9-24	Caring Theorists—Nursing Therapeutics
Theorists	**Nursing Therapeutics**
Watson	Use of entire self in affirming the subjective significance of a person. Detecting and responding to true feelings of human beings.
Parse	Practice methodology: illuminating meaning, synchronizing rhythms and mobilizing transcendence through being truly present with a person or a group.

TABLE 9-25	Caring Theorists—A Summary
Focus	Human–universe health process, meaning, mutual relations, unity of body, mind and spirit, humanity.
Human being	Man-living-health; continuously becoming and continuously in relationship with their environment.
Patient	Unique human being with ability toward transformation and transcendence, disharmony between spirit, body, mind, soul. Felt and experienced a sense of incongruence.
Orientation	Health, human becoming for both the patient and nurse.
Role of nurse	Connect with clients, be present, extract meaning.
Decision-making	Mutual between health care provider and client.

- Nurses giving the care, if care is truly provided, emerge from the relationship transformed because caring for another human being affects them profoundly.
- Meanings of health–illness situations are determined individually and modified collectively.
- Choices, values, interpretations, and meanings are rights of both patients and nurses. Understanding each other's perspectives is part of the caring act.
- The moment of nurse–patient encounter involves connection and dialogue on how the relationship is formed and what the consequences are.
- Although the nurse and patient have a historical context, it is the current moment that shapes their interaction and the consequences of their interaction.
- Nurses and persons/communities are transformed by their encounters.

THEORIES' PRIMARY FOCUS

Nursing theories are further classified in this text according to their *primary focus*. In classifying theories for analysis, it is assumed that each classification system adds more understanding to each theory. Correspondence between each of the classification systems is neither presented nor discussed in this text. You, as a theory student, may wish to consider the relationship between the different classification systems and critically consider how classification systems may enhance understanding of each of the theories.

In reviewing the theories for classification, I have included in the analysis central domain concepts, the central questions the theory addresses, and those areas that seem to be most developed. Each of these was used to guide the theory classification. *Four central foci* appear to reflect the theories: clients, person–environment interactions, interactions, and nursing therapeutics. Although theories may appear to have more than one focus, my decision to place a theory within a particular focus in this text was based on my decision to select a primary focus for the sake of analysis and discussion.

Johnson, Roy, and Neuman focused their theoretical development on the *client* or the client system. These theories provide a comprehensive analysis of the client as seen from a nursing perspective. Although each of these theorists also discussed how health is defined within their theories, these concepts do not appear to be as central in these theories. Hence, Johnson's, Roy's, and Neuman's works were classified as client-focused theories, and also as outcome theories, and they appear in Chapter 13 as such. These theories have been instrumental in changing the definition of human beings from biomedical beings to psychosocial beings.

Rogers' central focus is on the relationship between clients and their environment. In fact, clients in Rogers' theory are the environment, and one cannot be assessed in isolation from the other. Rogers' theory is one of the most supportive of the centrality of environment in the mission of the discipline of nursing; however, because its focus is on the outcome of promoting harmony with the environment, it could also be classified as an outcome theory.

The properties, components, and nature of the interactions between clients and nurses were the focus of several theoretical formulations. King, Orlando, Paterson and Zderad, Travelbee, and Wiedenbach concentrated on nurse–patient interactions and considered them the focus of nursing. These theories are evaluated in Chapter 12.

What nurses should do and under what circumstances these actions should be delivered were the focus of theoretical formulations in Levine's and Orem's theories. These theories are therefore evaluated as theories that could provide nurses with frameworks for *intervention*. However, because Orem's theory's dominant focus is on hierarchy of needs, I have placed her in Chapter 11 as a needs theorist. Unlike client-oriented theories, which are more effective in providing nurses with a framework for assessment, intervention theories provide nurses with guidelines for intervention. However, it is important to note that each of the theorists provided recommended points of entry for interventions.

IMAGES, METAPHORS, AND ROLES

The preceding analyses suggest that nurses focus on different aspects of care at different times or for different purposes (see Table 9-26). Nursing is not exemplified by one group of theories more than

another at all times. Rather, the situation may dictate when nursing should focus on needs, interaction, or outcomes. Similarly, focus on clients, interactions, environment, or interventions may require different theories. Newman (1983) makes the following point:

> *One of the factors determining the applicability of a theory is the temporal frame of reference. For example, if one is viewing a relatively short time-frame, the adaptation model might apply, whereas in a longer time-frame, phenomena would be apparent that could not be explained by adaptation alone. (p. 391)*

Nurses play different roles at different times and project different images, and nursing theories have helped to suggest these different images and roles that nurses play. *Need-oriented nurses* are actively doing and functioning; they rely on problem solving, they carefully plan their interventions, and they evaluate their work mainly (but not only) by the activities performed.

Interaction-oriented nurses rely on the process of interaction and include themselves in the sphere of other actions; they use themselves therapeutically, and evaluate their actions primarily in terms of interactions. *Interaction-oriented nurses* rely more on counseling, guiding, and teaching—helping clients find meanings in their situations—and less on doing and functioning. Among the interactionists are the existentialists, who focus on the support and development of the human potential. That potential includes, for both the nurse and the client, the goal of authentic being, the process of creating options, and an openness to present and future experiences.

Outcomes-oriented nurses focus on the goals of maintaining and promoting energy and harmony with the environment and on enhancing the development of healthy environments. Outcomes nurses do not include themselves as therapeutic agents; they enact the healing roles but do not necessarily consider authentic being as essential in the healing processes. The roles and images of nurses as reflected in the different groups of nursing theories are summarized in Table 9-26.

Care-oriented theorists focus on the personal development or transformation of both the nurse and the patient (Parse, 1995; Watson, 2002). Care theorists include equally the self-reflections of patients and nurses as they transform each other into different and more self-examined human beings.

TABLE 9-26	Roles and Images of Nurses in Different Categories of Theories	
Theorists	*Roles Nurses Play*	*Image*
Needs Theorists		
Abdellah Henderson Orem	Problem solver and performer of 21 physiologic and psychosocial activities for the patient Complementing, supplementing knowledge The will to perform daily activities Temporary self-care agent for universal health deviation and development of self-care needs	They provide an image of a nurse who is active and busy working and a patient who is striving for independence. The nurse's work is focused on doing a deliberate and well-planned activity.
Interaction Theorists		
King Orlando Paterson and Zderad Peplau Travelbee Wiedenbach	Goal attainer or else! Teach, counsel, guide, give care, gather information, set mutual goals Deliberate, repetitive, and situational interactions Existentialist and phenomenological nurturer of the human potential (self and patient) Freudian helper Stranger who works hard to become a surrogate Meaning finder (more than a dictionary meaning) and existentialist Deliberate helper who focuses on extrasensory perception and does not forget to validate the process	They provide an image of a nurse as a present-oriented, situational, a humanist, a process-oriented professional whose interest is the interaction and, for some, also the person. The nurse, to some, is also important in the interaction.
Outcomes Theorists		
Johnson Levine Rogers Roy	The external manipulator: external regulatory force to preserve organization and integration of patient's behavior Controller Conservator of all The environmental nurse, the symphony player: promotion of person–environment interaction The healer without touch The pace setter: external regulatory force to modify stimuli affecting adaptation to create four modes of adaptation	They provide an image of the nurse as goal setter, a futurist, environmentalist, who has extrasensory and energy preservation powers.
Caring/Human Becoming Theorists		
Watson	Coparticipant and time investment with embodiment of caring. Spiritual person helping people gain. Self-knowledge. A person with self-control and ability to self-heal (Baldursdottir and Jonsdottir, 2002; Watson and Smith, 2002).	Centered healing person, aware, reflective and humanist caring.
Parse	Understands patient's lived experience, brings out the best in patients to be able to make choices (Cody, 2000; Cowling, 1989).	A present-oriented, situational, process-oriented and interactive individual.

AREAS OF AGREEMENT AMONG AND BETWEEN THEORISTS AND SCHOOLS OF THOUGHT

Nursing theories have been considered in terms of their contrasting and competitive views. In the first section of this chapter, an attempt was made to address how these views may complement each other as theories and as different schools of thought. In this section, areas of agreement among the various schools of thought are identified.

- Nursing theories offer a beginning articulation of what nursing is and what roles nurses play.
- Nursing theories offer a view of the philosophical underpinnings in nursing (e.g., interaction, phenomenology, and existentialism).

REFLECTIVE QUESTIONS

1. What are the advantages and disadvantages of classifying nursing theories?

2. What categories do you consider as more productive in creating a critical discourse about the theoretical heritage of nursing?

3. As you assess the current climate and structure of health care systems, what group of theories may provide frameworks for better quality care? Which group of theories may be antithetical or complementary to the needs of patients in the 21st century?

4. Compare and contrast the societal and professional contexts for any two of the four sets of theory categories.

5. How else would you categorize the theories presented in this chapter and why?

6. Identify and discuss metaphors about nurses that reflect the different theories. In what ways do these metaphors stereotype or enhance nurses' roles?

- Nursing theories provide descriptions of how to help patients become comfortable, how to deliver treatment with the least damage, and how to enhance high-level wellness.
- Nursing theories offer a beginning common language and a beginning agreement about who nursing care recipients are.
- It is obvious that we should not view the recipients only through biologic glasses (as biologic systems) or psychological glasses (as id, ego, and superego), but rather through holistic glasses. Nursing clients are more than the sum total of their psychological, sociological, cultural, or biologic parts.
- Recipients of care respond to events in a holistic way.
- The recipient is a member of a reference group set, and interventions are only meaningful if the whole unit is considered.
- Recipients have needs, and nursing assists them in meeting those needs.

The theories have other themes in common. These emerge when one considers images evolving from the theories when compared with nursing realities. In this process, several concepts emerge as central to nursing. These are identified in the following conclusion.

CONCLUSION

The discipline of nursing deals with people who are assumed to be in constant interaction with their environment and yet have unmet needs, are not able to care for themselves, or are not adapting to the environment because of interruptions or potential interruptions in health. Nursing focuses on therapeutics to help in meeting the needs of the person and to enhance adaptation capability, self-care ability, health, and well-being. Nursing theories capture and reflect different visions of this domain; they mirror different aspects of nursing realities as they are and as they ought to be. The mission of nursing, the processes by which nursing care is provided, and the images of nursing portrayed in these theories continue to be shared by nurses around the globe. Considering the theories in the categories presented in this chapter may lead to many productive explorations and explanations of the processes of clinical judgment and clinical decision-making.

REFERENCES

Abdellah, F. (1969). The nature of nursing science. *Nursing Research*, 18(5), 390–393.

Baldursdottir, G. and Jonsdottir, H. (2002). The importance of nurse caring behaviors as perceived by patients receiving care at an emergency department. *Heart & Lung: Journal of Acute & Critical Care*, 31(1), 67–75.

Beckstead, J.W. and Beckstead, L.G. (2006). A multidimensional analysis of the epistemic origins of nursing theories, models, and frameworks. *International Journal of Nursing Studies*, 43(1), 113–122.

Bijou, J.W. and Baer, D.M. (1961). *Child development: A systematic and empirical theory*. New York: Appleton-Century-Crofts.

Bunkers, S.S. (2012). Presence: The eye of the needle. *Nursing Science Quarterly*, 25(1), 10–14.

Carabetta, M., Lombardo, K., and Kline, N.E. (2013). Implementing primary care in the perianesthesia setting using a relationship-based care model. *Journal of PeriAnesthesia Nursing*, 28(1), 16–20.

Cody, W.K. (2000). Parse's human becoming school of thought and families. *Nursing Science Quarterly*, 13(4), 281–284.

Cowling, W.R. (1989). Parse's theory of nursing. In J. Fitzpatrick and A. Whall (Eds.). *Conceptual models of nursing: Analysis and application*. New Jersey: Appleton & Lange.

Deane, W.H. and Fain, J.A. (2015, April 8). Incorporating Peplau's theory of interpersonal relations to promote holistic communication between older adults and nursing students. *Journal of Holistic Nursing,* 34(1), 35–41.

Erikson, E.H. (1963). *Childhood and society* (2nd ed.). New York: W.W. Norton.

Freud, S. (1949). *An outline of psychoanalysis.* New York: W.W. Norton.

Hall, B. (1983). Toward an understanding of stability in nursing phenomena. *Advances in Nursing Science,* 5(3), 15–20.

Henderson, V. (1964). The nature of nursing. *American Journal of Nursing,* 64(8), 62–68.

Howland, D. and McDowell, W.E. (1964). Measurement of patient care: A conceptual framework. *Nursing Research,* 13(1), 4–7.

Johnson, D.E. (1968). *One conceptual model of nursing.* Paper presented at Vanderbilt University, Nashville, TN.

Johnson, D.E. (1974). Development of theory: A requisite for nursing as a primary health profession. *Nursing Research,* 23(5), 372–377.

King, I. (1968). A conceptual framework of reference for nursing. *Nursing Research,* 17(1), 27–31.

Maslow, A.H. (1954). *Motivation and personality.* New York: Harper & Row.

Newman, M. (1983). The continuing revolution: A history of nursing science. In N. Chaska (Ed.). *The nursing profession: A time to speak.* New York: McGraw-Hill.

Orem, D. (1995). *Nursing: Concepts of practice* (5th ed.). St. Louis, MO: C.V. Mosby.

Orlando, I.J. (1961). *The dynamic nurse-patient relationship.* New York: G.P. Putnam's Sons.

Parse, R.R. (1981). *Man-living-health: A theory of nursing.* New York: John Wiley & Sons.

Parse, R.R. (1995). The human becoming practice methodology. In R.R. Parse (Ed.). *Illuminations: The human becoming theory in practice and research.* New York: National League for Nursing Press.

Parse, R.R. (1998). *The human becoming school of thought: A perspective for nurses and other health professionals.* Thousand Oaks, CA: Sage.

Peplau, H. (1952). *Interpersonal relations in nursing.* New York: G.P. Putnam's Sons.

Rogers, C. (1959). A theory of therapy, personality, interpersonal relations as developed in a client-centered framework. In J. Koch (Ed.). *Psychology: A study of a science* (Vol. 3). New York: McGraw-Hill.

Rogers, M.E. (1970). *An introduction to the theoretical basis of nursing.* Philadelphia, PA: F.A. Davis.

Roy, C. (1970, March). Adaptation: A conceptual framework for nursing. *Nursing Outlook,* 18, 42–48.

Senn, J.F. (2013). Peplau's theory of interpersonal relations: Application in emergency and rural nursing. *Nursing Science Quarterly,* 26(1), 31–35.

Sullivan, H. (1953). *The interpersonal theory of psychiatry.* New York: W.W. Norton.

Watson, J. (1979). *The philosophy and science of caring.* Boston, MA: Little, Brown and Company.

Watson, J. (1988). *Nursing: Human science and human care, a theory of nursing.* New York: National League for Nursing Press.

Watson, J. (1999). *Post modern nursing and beyond.* London, UK: Churchill Livingstone.

Watson, J. (2002). Intentionality and caring-healing consciousness: A practice of transpersonal nursing. *Holistic Nursing Practice,* 16(4), 12–19.

Watson, J. and Smith, M.C. (2002). Caring science and the science of unitary human beings: A trans-theoretical discourse for nursing knowledge development. *Journal of Advanced Nursing,* 37(5), 452–461.

Wiedenbach, E. (1964). *Clinical nursing: A helping art.* New York: Springer-Verlag.

Zarea, K., Maghsoudi, S., Dashtebozorgi, B., Hghighizadeh, M.H., and Javadi, M. (2014). The impact of Peplau's therapeutic communication model on anxiety and depression in patients candidate for coronary artery bypass. *Clinical Practice and Epidemiology in Mental Health,* 10, 159–165.

10

A Model for Evaluation of Theories: Description, Analysis, Critique, Testing, and Support*

A critical review of evidence before and while translating it into practice, and a critical assessment and evaluation of theories before and while utilizing them in practice or research are activities that nurses have always engaged in. Quality care, as well as coherent research programs, requires critical analyses and judgment of theories. Nurses evaluate theories to apply to practice, to develop curricula, to operationalize for research, or to use in daily decision-making. These evaluations may be deliberate, systematic, criteria-based, objective, conscious, and elaborate, or they may be subjective, experiential, quick, and based on a limited set of criteria. Both types of evaluations are essential; neither type is sufficient by itself.

Evaluation of theory is an essential component of nursing practice and of knowledge development to:

1. Decide which theory is more appropriate to use as a framework for research, teaching, administration, or consultation
2. Identify effective theories in exploring some aspect of practice or in guiding a research project
3. Compare and contrast different explanations of the same phenomenon
4. Enhance the potential of constructive changes and further theory development
5. Identify epistemological approaches of a discipline through attention to the sociocultural context of the theorist and the theory
6. Critically examine and question the ontological beliefs in a discipline

7. Identify competing and complementary schools of thought in a discipline
8. Effect changes in clinical practice, define research priorities, and identify content for teaching and guidelines for nursing administration
9. Utilize coherent and integrative frameworks to communicate to the public the rationales and goals of nursing practice
10. Identify strategies that could be used to advance the development of theories
11. Define and articulate the discipline's demand and perspective
12. Be a critical consumer of theories, as well as a critical consumer of evidence-based practice

To date, utilizers of theory have not consistently subjected theories to systematic, criteria-based evaluation (Im, 2015). This lack of rigor may have hindered revision of existing theories as well as the development of new nursing theories.

Before going any further in reading this chapter, you should take a few minutes to identify one or two theories (nursing or non-nursing) that you have used in your work or personal life. Whether you are a critical care nurse, a primary care provider, or a researcher who may be studying biomarkers of pain responses, you can reflect on frameworks from which your care or questions emanate. For example, you may identify role theory as a framework for your research on women's daily activities in a nursing home and their health; endorphin theory linking stress with exercise; or Maslow's theory in understanding a patient's needs. The next set of questions to ask and reflect on are: Why did you select these theories to apply in your work? Why not other theories that may provide a different set

---

*This chapter is adapted, with considerable changes, from an earlier manuscript written by A.I. Meleis and published in Chaska, N. (1982). *The nursing profession: Time to speak.* New York: McGraw-Hill, 1982.

BOX 10-1	CRITERIA USED FOR SELECTING THEORIES

Personal: Individuals who use this criterion discuss their personal comfort in using the theory, their intuitive choices, and the theory's congruency with their philosophical view of life.

Mentor: There are those who use a theory because they were mentored by a theorist, or they were exposed to the teaching of a theorist who profoundly influenced and transformed them. They spoke of personal influence, respect, personal contact, and educational experience.

Theorist: Many select and utilize a theory as a framework for their research or practice based on who the theorists are, their standing in the field, their status, and how well they are recognized.

Literature support: Others identified the availability of extensive writings about the theory that gave them assurance of the level of significance of the theory and the status it holds.

Sociopolitical congruency: Another criterion used for selecting theory is the congruency between the theory implementation process and the sociopolitical as well as economic climate at the time of the choice. These people spoke of a climate that supports one theory over another because, for example, there was no need to institute structural changes in the organization, or the theory required minimal preparation of members of an organization. Within this category are those who indicated that the theory was imposed by administration.

Utility: The ease by which a theory was understood and applied prompted this group of users to indicate that utility was the prime factor.

of equally plausible explanations? To complete this exercise, you should be able to identify the criteria you used in making a decision about what theory to use. You may also want to review and discuss with your peers the reflective questions presented at the end of this chapter.

Over a 30-year span of teaching, I have asked students, faculty, clinicians, and administrators in the United States, as well as in many other countries, the questions outlined in the preceding text. In reviewing the answers and analyzing their content, I noticed the emergence of a number of criteria for selection and use of theory. Now, compare your criteria with those identified in Box 10-1.

SELECTING THEORIES FOR UTILIZATION

Although these criteria are neither all-inclusive nor representative of all nurses, definite themes evolve that are consistently supported by much anecdotal evidence. The decision to use one theory and not another involves both subjective and objective processes. The decision process could be considered as falling on two continua, each ranging from low to high. Therefore, a decision could be both highly objective and highly subjective, low on subjectivity

and on objectivity, or could be one of numerous other combinations of levels of objectivity and subjectivity.

The subjectivity in the selection of a theory is as important as is the objectivity in the selection. Although we can select a theory by using a number of well-defined criteria, and through a systematic evaluation process, using well-defined and agreed-upon criteria, make the process highly objective, if the theory's assumptions are not congruent with our own, if we have concerns with the theorist's level of experience, or if we are not comfortable with other work done by the theorist, the decision process becomes subjective. Conversely, a selection may be based on one's having worked with the theorist or her disciples and that in itself becomes the deciding factor in continuing to use the theory. Neither of these processes of decision-making is sufficient. Another set of questions are related. The first one is: How did you use that particular theory and framework? A highly objective decision with low subjectivity could result in theory use that is not as true to the theory's premises and propositions, and the converse is also true. Using a particular theory to describe components of care or to provide an explanation of the use of a particular variable in research is different from testing, refuting, or supporting theories (Norman, 2004). All these processes are important for theory evaluation and contribute to advancing knowledge related to the theory.

The objective evaluation and critique of theories is as complex as the subjective evaluation. To simplify any evaluation, we must break it down into components. For example, when a research project is critiqued, the analysis is done along structural criteria, such as the introduction, conceptual framework, research questions and hypotheses, methodology, results, discussion, conclusions, and limitations. The critique is then completed by looking for clarity, significance, timeliness, and documentation, among other criteria. To analyze and critique theories objectively, numerous criteria have been recommended by a number of authors. In fact, analysis and critique of theories have preoccupied many nurse metatheorists over a period that even preceded diligent theory development efforts.

Two disciplines have profoundly influenced the evaluation of nursing theory: sociology and psychology. The result has been a synthesis of criteria from these disciplines—at times too empirically based and at other times too critical of the theories that were developed by nurses—and those driven by our own nursing phenomena. When we adhered to some of these criteria, we tended to discount nursing theories, relegating them to the category of individual subjective philosophical expositions. Although some of these criteria are appropriate for the discipline of nursing, many were not and did not reflect the nature of nursing and the goals of our discipline. Others have emerged that directly relate to and represent nursing. The rationale for developing a different set of criteria is embedded in the nature of nursing care, the assumptions on which the discipline of nursing is built, and the quality of its scientific and humanistic bases. The domain of nursing encompasses human experiences and interactions, and deals with complex sets of contextual variables; therefore, the criteria for theory evaluation must consider ways by which its theories reflect and represent these contexts.

Each one of the evaluation models offered in nursing literature addressed one aspect of a theory to the exclusion of others. For example, Johnson (1974) focused on a congruence of theory mission with goals relegated by society to nurses (social congruence, utility, and significance). Earlier, in an unpublished manuscript on requirements of an effective model, Johnson (1970) offered a set of requirements that focused on the mission of nursing practice: goals of action, patience, the actor's place and role, source of difficulty, intervention focus, and mode and consequences of care. Although Johnson also addressed the necessity of explicit and consistent structure (assumption and values) and content (nursing's unique goal, ability to be generalized, restrictiveness, continuity, and specificity), other utility criteria were not included, such as research utility and potential for developing and testing theoretical propositions. Johnson pioneered the development of a set of objective requirements for effective models in nursing and the use of internal and external requirements. Her evaluation model was not published, however, and was therefore limited in exposure and refinement.

Barnum (1998) suggested that passing judgment on theories happens both subjectively and objectively. Judgment may be "simply a matter of personal taste" (p. 171), just as is judgment of art that is based on personal taste, and/or it could be based on clear criteria. The criteria selected by Barnum (1998) are both internal and external. These evaluative criteria are appropriate for internal criticism (internal construction of theory) and external criticism (which considers theory in its relationships to human beings, nursing, and health). The criteria for internal criticism are clarity, consistency, adequacy, logical development, and level of theory development. The criteria for external criticism are reality conversion, utility, significance, discrimination, scope of theory, and complexity (Barnum, 1998, pp. 171–185). These criteria represent one framework for critiquing theories that could be used independently or in conjunction with the descriptive and analytical criteria offered in the model proposed in this chapter.

A similar framework was offered by Ellis (1968), whose insights endure and transcend time, and who delineated seven criteria for what she considered significant theories. Significant theories, according to Ellis, have a broad scope, are sufficiently complex to consider different propositions reflecting the wide scope, and contain propositions that are testable and useful. Significant theories are also those that have explicit values and in which implicit values are carefully delineated. These theories must have well-defined and meaningful terminology, and they provide opportunities for further generation of information (Ellis, 1968). Hardy (1974) borrowed heavily from the discipline of sociology, organizing her criteria around the concept of "adequacy": meaning, logic, operationalization, empirical evidence, and pragmatism. She also believed that adequate theories should have the ability to be generalized, should contribute to understanding, and should be able to predict. It is indeed a challenge to find theories in any discipline to meet all these criteria simultaneously; however, these criteria provide serious theory developers with milestones toward which they should strive.

Lest theory developers become discouraged by the rigorous criteria, Duffey and Muhlenkamp (1974, p. 571) offered the following modest set of questions by which theories can be evaluated:

- Does the theory generate testable hypotheses?
- Does the theory guide practice?
- How complete is its subject matter?
- Did the theorist make her biases explicit?
- Does the theory have propositions, and are relationships explicit?
- Is the theory parsimonious?

Chinn and Kramer (2010, pp. 185–205) offer a set of questions that should guide the evaluation of integrated knowledge that incorporates theories. These sets of questions are driven by their definition of theory as "a creative and rigorous structuring of ideas that projects a tentative, purposeful, and systematic view of phenomena" (p. 185). They use a series of questions to guide the reviewer toward describing a theory, and then another set of questions to guide the reviewer on a journey of critical reflection of theory. To review and describe a theory, they propose these questions:

- What is the purpose of this theory?
- What are the concepts of this theory?
- What are the definitions in this theory?
- What are the relationships in this theory?
- What is the structure of this theory?
- What are the assumptions of this theory?

To reflect and critique the theory, they pose a series of *whys*? In each of the preceding points, the major ideas to consider are clarity, simplicity, generalizability, and accessibility.

Fawcett and DeSanto-Madeya, dissatisfied with previously developed evaluation criteria because of the seeming overlap between criteria for evaluating theories and those more appropriate for evaluating conceptual frameworks, offered, and continued to update, one analytical and evaluative framework for conceptual models, and a separate one for theories (Fawcett, 2005; Fawcett and DeSanto-Madeya, 2013). Their framework for conceptual models separates questions for analysis from those intended for evaluation. For analysis, Fawcett and DeSanto-Madeya proposed a consideration of the historical evolution of the model, of the unique focus of the nursing model, and of the content of the model. For the evaluation, they proposed evaluation (judgment based on criteria) of the origins of the model; the comprehensiveness of content; the logical congruence

of the model's internal structure; the ability of the model to generate and test theories; the degree to which the model is credible (their old concept) as demonstrated in its social utility (use, implementation), social congruency, and significance to society; and, finally, the model's contributions to the discipline of nursing (Fawcett and DeSanto-Madeya, 2013, pp. 45–54). They speak, however, of legitimacy rather than credibility to avoid the confusion of its use for qualitative research data. Legitimacy refers to the extent that a model guides nursing actions.

Although these same criteria could be used in analyzing and evaluating theories, Fawcett and DeSanto-Madeya (2013, pp. 309–319) proposed a distinct set of criteria for theory critique that they believed to be more congruent with their definition of theory. As they did with models, Fawcett and DeSanto-Madeya divided critique of theories into analysis and evaluation. For theory analysis, they proposed criteria similar to those of other metatheorists, such as consideration of the scope of the theory, the context of theory, and the attention and consideration the theorists give to the content of the theory, its concepts and propositions. Fawcett and DeSanto-Madeya also propose an evaluation of theories to complement the analysis described in the preceding text. The content of theories, they say, could be evaluated in terms of its significance to the discipline of nursing, to society and to advancing knowledge, its internal consistency, the extent to which the theory is stated clearly and concisely (parsimony), and the potential testability of its propositions. Theories must also be evaluated through the adequacy of their empirical evidence and their utility for practice (pragmatic adequacy) (Fawcett and DeSanto-Madeya, 2013, pp. 309–319).

Fawcett also differentiates between the evaluation of grand and middle-range theories and provides similarities and differences in the types and level of questions to ask of the two levels of theories. The levels of theories may be differentiated by the kind of methods used, tests performed, measurements utilized, and their empirical adequacy. For grand theories, Fawcett (2005) believes that questions should focus on congruency between methods and philosophical claims, and on the adequacy of the inductive descriptions of data and its congruency with the concepts and propositions of the theory. For middle-range theories, the questions focus more on the observability of concepts, potential for measurement, and the congruency between the theoretical assertions and the empirical evidence. Fawcett (2005) provides a strong convincing argument against differentiating criteria that are based on whether theories used quantitative or qualitative data. I would further propose that theories that withstand the tests of time and repeated research findings could neither be classified based on the type of data nor differentiated only by research data. This argument will become even more apparent as you review the evaluations of the theories offered in the next few chapters and as you review and study strategies for theory development in Part Five.

Whall (2005) defines theory as a "group of concepts interrelated via propositional statements which are based upon a group of underlying assumptions" (p. 5). As such, she proposes that analysis and evaluation use three major criteria: (1) critical review of basic considerations of theory, in which adequacy is examined; (2) internal analysis and evaluation, in which review of completeness, consistency, and assumptions are examined; and (3) external analysis and evaluation, in which the connection between theory, research, practice, and education are carefully examined and reviewed (pp. 11–13). Whall also differentiates between the separate review and analysis of each theory level (micropractice, middle-range, and grand nursing models). Each level drives a different set of questions that the reviewer must use. However, analysis and evaluation of all levels of theory must address basic structure, internal analysis and evaluation, and external analysis (Whall, 2005, pp. 5–20).

Table 10-1 compares and contrasts the criteria for evaluating theories, as proposed by four metatheorists. I encourage you to review as many of these proposals for evaluation as possible. As you can see in Table 10-1, there are some similarities and some differences in how each metatheorist conceptualized the criteria of analysis and evaluation of theories. The criteria reflect the level and sophistication of our knowledge at different stages of the development of nursing as a scientific discipline. In reviewing the different criteria, several trends emerge:

- Theories are described, analyzed, and tested.
- Internal and external criteria exist for evaluating theories.
- The internal descriptive criteria include assumptions, concepts, relationships, and definitions.
- The internal critical criteria include some areas of agreement, such as consistency, clarity, and logical development.
- Evaluation criteria consider the fit between the theory and external criteria (human beings, society, prevailing paradigms) and not only the intrinsic criteria.

- A more accepting attitude has evolved, shifting away from the rigor of empiricism to the more realistic rigor of potential for testability.
- There is wider acknowledgment of the complexity of evaluation criteria (the two sides of simplicity, the many meanings of complexity, etc.) and, therefore, wider acceptance of multiple criteria.
- There is less prejudice toward descriptive theories.

Common themes in description and analysis are presented in Table 10-2.

FRAMEWORK FOR EVALUATING THEORIES

The model proposed here considers these trends, draws on many of the previously delineated criteria, and further acknowledges that even when systematic criteria are advanced to ensure objective analysis and critique, objectivity is not guaranteed or required in critiquing theories for one's use in research or practice. Furthermore, individuals may differ on how they use the critique criteria, and the perceptions of the meaning of each of these criteria may be influenced by individual variations and by context variations. It is also acknowledged here that some criteria may be conflicting; that to enhance simplicity, complexity may suffer; and that to advocate a wider scope, accuracy for deviant cases or opposing situations may be jeopardized and generalization may not be as desirable as it once was.

The proposed model defines *evaluation* as encompassing description, analyses, critique, testing, and support. By using this model, a reviewer acknowledges extant evaluations that have been completed by nurse theorists, researchers, and clinicians, among others. The model is also based philosophically more on a historical view of science than on an empirical view. Therefore, the model proposes to analyze the central questions that are solved by the theory. It considers the background of the theorist in the development of the theory and the sociocultural context of the theory (the theorist's education, previous work, etc.), the evaluator as an agent for knowledge development, and the discipline's level of development. In other words, human processes are considered an integral part of theory description, analysis, critique, testing (Laudan, 1977), and support (Meleis, 1995).

The framework for theory evaluation proposed in this chapter is to be used as a guideline for systematic

TABLE 10-1	Comparison of Criteria for Evaluating Theory		
Barnum (1998)	**Chinn and Kramer (2010)**	**Fawcett and DeSanto-Madeya (2013)**	**Whall (2005)**
Internal Criticism	*Description of Theory*	*Analysis & Evaluation of Nursing Models*	*Criteria for Practice Theory*
• Clarity • Consistency • Adequacy • Logic development • Level of theory development	• Purpose • Concepts • Definitions • Relationships • Structure • Assumptions	*Analysis* • Origins • Focus • Content *Evaluation* • Origins • Content • Logical congruence • Generation • Legitimacy	*Basic consideration:* definition adequacy; empirical adequacy; statement/prepositional adequacy. *Internal analysis and evaluation:* completeness and consistency; assumptions of theory. *External analysis and evaluation:* analysis of existing standards; analysis of nursing practice and education; analysis of research.
External Criticism	*Critical Reflection*	*Analysis & Evaluation of Nursing Theories*	*Criteria for Middle-Range Theory*
• Reality convergence • Utility • Significance discrimination • Scope of theory • Complexity	• Clarity • Simplicity • Generalizability • Accessibility • Importance	*Analysis* • Scope • Context • Content *Evaluation* • Significance • Internal consistency • Parsimony • Testability • Empirical adequacy • Pragmatic adequacy	*Basic consideration:* definitions and relative importance of major concepts; the type and relative importance of major theoretical statements and/or propositions. *Internal analysis and evaluation:* assumptions, science positions; concepts; internal consistency and congruency; empirical adequacy. *External analysis:* congruence with related theory and research internal and external to nursing; congruence with the perspective of nursing, the domains, and the persistent questions; ethical, cultural, and social policy issues.
			Criteria for Conceptual Models
			Basic paradigm concepts included in the model: person, nursing, health, and environment (definitions, additional understandings, and interrelationships); descriptions of other concepts in the model. *Internal analysis:* assumptions, definitions of any other components of the model; relative importance of basic concepts or other components of the model; internal and external consistency; adequacy. *External analysis:* relationship to nursing research, nursing education, nursing practice, to the existing nursing diagnoses and interventions systems.

TABLE 10-2	Common Themes in Description and Analysis
Common Themes	**Metatheorists**
Adequacy	Barnum, Whall
Clarity	Barnum, Chinn, & Kramer
Consistency	Barnum, Chinn, & Kramer, Whall
Complexity/simplicity	Barnum, Chinn, & Kramer, Whall
Generality/scope of theory	Barnum, Chinn, & Kramer
Significance	Barnum, Chinn, & Kramer; Fawcett, Whall
Internal & external evaluation/criticism	Barnum, Whall

TABLE 10-3	Theory Description
Criteria	**Unit of Analysis**
Structural components	Assumptions
	Concepts
	Propositions
Functional components	Focus
	Client
	Nursing
	Health
	Nurse–patient interactions
	Environment
	Nursing problem
	Nursing therapeutics

evaluation of theory prior to using the theory in practice, research, education, or administration. It is proposed for all types of theories—grand, middle-range, or situation-specific. With the increase in middle-range and situation-specific theories, it is imperative to ensure that the use of a particular theory is subjected to objective scrutiny. However, it is also important to note that it is not possible to subject every theory to all the proposed criteria. The goal for theory utilization should be used as a guideline for theory evaluation.

Before embarking on theory evaluation, the reviewer should recognize and identify the boundaries of the review. Boundaries include degree of exposure to theory, length of time devoted to understanding theory, and type of work done with theory (e.g., having taught theory, used it in practice, used it in research, worked with the theoretician). In doing so, the reviewer attempts to separate objective and subjective rationales and may thus be able to make implicit assumptions more explicit.

Theory Description

Description is the first phase in evaluating theory. Readers of a theory must thoroughly review it by identifying its structural components as well as its functional components. A thorough initial reading of the theory helps to identify the fundamental questions the theorist is attempting to answer. For example, central questions for developmental theorists are "How do human beings mature?" and "What is the nature of maturity?" More often than not, at the onset of reviewing a nursing theory, it is not entirely clear what questions the theorist is attempting to answer; therefore, identification of

the theory's structure and function could facilitate understanding before moving to other phases of evaluation. (Table 10-3 offers a summary of theory descriptions.)

Structural Components

A theory begins with a set of "givens" that have been either empirically tested or accepted by a number of other theories or previous research. These givens are the *theory assumptions*. They could evolve from a philosophical standpoint, from ideologic positions, from ethical considerations, from cultural heritage, from social structure, or from previously tested and supported hypotheses. Assumptions also represent one's values. Assumptions of a theory are not subject to testing by the same theory; rather, they lead to a set of propositions that are to be tested. They are the basis from which we can determine the viewpoint of the theorist. In nursing theories, assumptions are made about nursing, human behavior, life, death, health, and illness.

Early writing in theory provides *implicit assumptions*; these are statements not identified as *explicit assumptions* by the theorist. Explicit assumptions are identified by authors as their assumptions. Implicit assumptions are embedded in the writings; they are statements not identified as assumptions, yet they are central for the development of theory propositions or answers to questions. They are statements considered by the reviewer to be significant in the development of the theory. Assumptions may reflect the values of a person or a culture. These assumptions then have attached to them a level of valuation that needs to be carefully examined. For example, ensuring that patients do their own care is based on the assumption that people want to take care of themselves, an assumption imbedded in a Western value of individualism. Another example of an implicit assumption based on values of Western society is that a patient has the right to learn about the gravity of his illness; this contrasts with an implicit assumption in Middle Eastern cultures that a patient does not want to know the details about his illness, particularly if it is grave or terminal. A proposition built on this assumption responds to the question of what is the most effective way to impart the information about a grave diagnosis to the patient. Another proposition would question whether a relationship exists, for example, between certain strategies for giving information about diagnosis and rate of recovery. The rationale for the proposition is understood only when the assumptions underlying it are delineated.

As theorists in nursing become more systematic in their theory development efforts, more explicit assumptions are stated, and fewer assumptions are left implicit. The plethora of literature that has discussed theory critique and theory development should be credited with the constructive changes demonstrated in the updated, further developed, or new theories evolving in nursing. Roy, for example, in further developing her theory, followed a more systematic approach in which she identified assumptions and carefully related many of the concepts to the assumptions, thereby providing her theoretical propositions with better potential for testability (Roy and Roberts, 1981).

When identifying the internal structure of a theory, one should use a description that involves a careful search of the inherent assumptions; at the same time, one should not overlook the implicit ones. The more effective theories are those in which authors explicitly state the assumptions that guide their thinking. The more explicit the premises of the theory, the less ambiguity arises when interpreting its conditions and goals.

The internal structure of a theory could be further described by delineating the concepts on which it is built. Descriptive properties used in relation to concepts are clarity, conceptual definitions, observable properties, and boundaries; concepts are also described as being *primitive* (i.e., concepts that originated in this particular theory) or *derived* (i.e., concepts that were derived from other theories). Hage (1972) provided criteria to help determine whether concepts in a theory are primitive or derived. The introduction in a theory of a concept with no definition—because the concept has an agreed-on meaning, has simple definitions, has an intuitively obvious definition, or has been defined elsewhere—designates a primitive concept. The definition of the derived concept is that it occurs within the theory and is based on primitive terms that are taken for granted for their shared meaning. The definitions of primitive terms are outside the theory (Hage, 1972, pp. 111–115).

The usage of primitive and derived concepts in this book differs from Hage's usage. *Primitive concepts* are those concepts introduced in the theory as new and therefore defined within the theory. *Derived concepts* are concepts from outside the theory that have taken on a different meaning within the theory. For example, in Meleis (1975), role is a derived concept, and role supplementation is a primitive concept—that is, it is a new concept with a new definition (see Chapter 16). Fawcett (2012) warns against using concepts defined within a theory and applying the concept across populations with exactly the same meaning and considering this use similar to using the concept but redefining its meaning for each different population. The former is application; the latter should be a new concept. Said differently, the first use is considered the concept, a primitive, and the latter should be considered a new concept, hence a derived one.

Concepts are also evaluated along the abstract–concrete dimension. The degree of generality of a concept determines its abstract–concrete level. The more general a concept is, the more it transcends time and geography, and the higher its level of abstraction. Concepts have also been classified along the general variable–nonvariable dimension (Hage, 1972). Nonvariable concepts in nursing are sex, ethnic background, religion, and marital status. Examples of variable concepts (general variables) are sex-role orientation, level of well-being, degree of cultural identity, and level of sick role. It becomes apparent that each nonvariable could be converted into a general variable.

There are several advantages to having general variables (Hage, 1972). General variables allow more precise classification and allow for variations that are more congruent with variations occurring in reality. Classification of a patient as male or female yields some significant data and a certain degree of predictability of the structure and function of the biologic systems as well as some of the health–illness responses. However, sex-role orientation and/or gender may help us to more precisely describe clients and predict their patterns of rehabilitation. General variables are more complex and more nuanced.

Just as assumptions and concepts are delineated, sometimes simultaneously and at other times cyclically, theory propositions also should be delineated and described. A *proposition* is a descriptive statement of the properties and dimensions of a concept or a statement that links two or more concepts together. Propositions are the crux of the theory, answering its central questions and providing it with the powers of description, explanation, or prediction. Identifying propositions at the outset helps make the job of delineating assumptions and concepts easier. This is not a linear process, but a cyclical one, in which concepts may be identified, followed by pertinent propositions, followed by more concepts and pertinent assumptions, and so on. A theory that has more assumptions than propositions is a theory with limited power. It indicates that we have to agree to too many conditions for a few descriptions or predictions. If we consider the relationship of assumptions and propositions in a ratio form, an inverse relationship (with the number of propositions being higher than the number of assumptions) allows for more explanatory power.

There are different types of propositions, with each having a different purpose. *Existence propositions* are constructed around one phenomenon and therefore describe and assert the existence of only this one phenomenon. Propositions with the power of explanation, on the other hand, link concepts; therefore, they are expected to have two or more concepts. They are formulated to explain and assert something pertaining to the reality embodied in the theory. These are *relational propositions*, which encompass many types of propositions, such as those that simply describe the existence of a relationship, those that describe the direction of such a relationship, and those that can predict the relationship, the direction of the relationship, and the conditions under which that relationship may or may not occur.

Further description of a proposition could be done along dimensions specified by Zetterberg (1963, pp. 69–71). This is best illustrated by using an example of a two-concept proposition derived from Johnson's subsystem theory:

The higher the level of met functional requirements of the affiliative subsystem of behaviors of Middle Eastern immigrants, the greater the recovery rate.

A *reversible proposition* would have "and vice versa" at the end of the statement, thus, requiring two testings—one with the condition of "met functional requirements" and prospectively considering recovery rate, and the other beginning with different levels of the recovery rate and then retrospectively considering levels of "met functional requirements."

A second dimension is whether the proposition *is deterministic* or *stochastic*. Nursing has a predisposition toward more stochastic propositions that incorporate a probability condition, rather than "if X then always Y," which is deterministic and improbable in a humanistic science. A stochastic proposition, albeit a probabilistic one, would be:

The higher the level of met functional requirements of the affiliative subsystem of behaviors, the more probable is a greater recovery rate.

A third dimension is whether the proposition is *sequential* or *coexisting*. A sequential proposition assumes that one variable occurred before the other variable. Propositions in nursing lend themselves more to coexisting propositions when describing existing relationships and to sequential propositions when engaged in theorizing about interventions and the consequences of intervention. This dimension characterizes theorizing that is central and essential to nursing.

A fourth dimension is demonstrated in the relationships between concepts. This relationship may be sufficient (if X, then Y, regardless of anything else) or contingent (if X, then Y, but only if Z) (Zetterberg, 1963, p. 71). Humanistic sciences cannot strive to produce sufficient propositions. Propositions in nursing theory include numerous variables and probabilistic relationships.

The last dimension identifies whether the relationship is necessary or can be substituted. A necessary relationship is "if X, and only if X, then Y." A substitutable relationship is "if X, then Y; but if Z, then also Y." Like other concepts in nursing, greater recovery rate is contingent on a number of variables and not only on "met functional requirements of one subsystem"; therefore, a substitutable proposition is more appropriate. To increase the explanatory power of such a proposition and then the predictive power, all other concepts related to recovery rate could be identified. For example:

The higher the level of met functional requirements of the affiliative subsystem of behaviors of Middle Eastern immigrants, the greater the recovery rate. The higher the level of met functional requirements of the aggressive subsystem of behaviors, the greater the recovery rate.

Therefore, propositions in nursing may be reversible, stochastic, coexisting, contingent, and substitutable. Attention to each dimension provides a way to describe the propositions and to deliberately develop propositions along these dimensions; this may help in enhancing the power of contextual explanations, if that is what the theorist wishes to do. This labeling also allows appropriate assessment of the propositions and their power of explanation and predictability. The clarity and systematization of propositions are also considered when we analyze the selected ordering and sequencing of propositions.

This first level of description is structural. The next level involves a description of a theory in terms of its function. This level considers whether the theory addresses the central concepts of the domain of nursing.

Functional Components

Unlike a structural analysis of a theory, a functional assessment of a theory carefully considers the anticipated consequences and purpose of the theory by examining its major agreed-upon concepts within the context of the nursing domain. (Again, refer to Table 10-3 for a summary of theory description.) Questions used to identify the functional components are these related to the focus of the theory as well as to the definitions of client, nursing, health, interaction, environment, nursing problems, and therapeutics. Examples of questions to help in describing the functions of a theory include the following:

- Who is acted on? This is the major question that begins to address the function of theory. Does the theory identify its focus as the client, family, community, or society, or does the theory consider the target as being one to the exclusion of others? The target of action here denotes both the target of assessment and the target of intervention; the target in nursing should be the client (in the broadest sense) in health or illness.
- What definitions does the theory offer for nursing, client, health, nursing problems, environment, and nurse–patient interactions? Are definitions explicit and clear?
- Does the theory offer a clear idea of what the sources of the nursing problem are, whether the sources lie within or outside of the individual?
- Does the theory provide any insights in the form of intervention for nursing? Are the variables to be manipulated well delineated? Is

it clear what the points of entry are for a nursing intervention? Is the focus of intervention justifiable within the theory? Points of entry could vary from manipulating outside stimuli (Johnson, 1968) to interactions and transactions between client and nurse (King, 1971), to behaviors within systems (Auger, 1976).
- Are there guidelines for intervention modalities? Are they specified? Is there potential for the evolution of such intervention modalities?
- As a nursing theory, does it provide guidelines for the role of the nurse?
- Are the consequences of nurses' actions articulated in the theory? Are they intended or unintended, positive or negative, anticipated and delineated? Is there a plan for dealing with such consequences?

Analysis

Analysis is defined as a process of identifying parts and components and examining them against a number of identified criteria. Analysis includes concept and theory analysis.

Concept Analysis

Concept analysis is a useful process in the cycle of theory development, as well as in theory evaluation. Concept analysis may occur at many different points in the process of evaluation and development. Wilson (1969) proposed several steps and techniques in analyzing concepts. These steps do not necessarily have to be completed in this order.

1. Definition, identification, and description of the different dimensions and components of the concept. For example, we proposed "transitions" as a central concept in nursing; we have defined the concept as "those periods in between fairly stable states, a passage from one life phase, condition, or status to another" (Chick and Meleis, 1986, pp. 238–239). We have identified some of its components and dimensions as process, disconnectedness, perception of transition, and patterns of response.

2. Comparison of the concept to others with similar properties and dimensions to establish its boundaries (Norris, 1982; Walker and Avant, 1995). Transition, for example, can be differentiated sufficiently from the general concept of change to make it useful in alerting nurses to relevant aspects

of the life contexts of clients. In this case, transition is seen as a special case of the general phenomenon of change (Chick and Meleis, 1986).

3. Description of some of the antecedents to the concept and of some of the consequences (Lindsey, Piper, and Stotts, 1982), and matching some of these descriptions with what occurs in nursing practice. Examples of antecedents of transition are illness, recovery, loss, and birthing; examples of consequences are distress, role performance changes, and disorientation.

4. Development, description, and analysis of exemplars or model cases. This step may include empirical results that are related to the concept.

5. Development, description, and analysis of contrary cases and their comparison with normative cases. Situations in which the concept appears only occasionally or appears under a new set of conditions are called *borderline cases* and are also useful in analyzing concepts. (See Chapter 14 for a more comprehensive discussion of concept analysis as a strategy for concept development.)

The process of concept analysis may include *semantic analysis*, which is analysis of linguistic meanings of the label given to the concept; analysis of *logical derivation*, which is the logical progression of identifying, supporting, and labeling a concept; and *context analysis* of the concept, which includes the conditions under which the concept is manifested. Any inferences about the concept should be analyzed for their sources, whether they are logically or empirically derived.

Each one of these steps is a test of the occurrence of the concept. These tests are both conceptual and clinical, but they are not tests as defined by empiricists. They are, however, equally necessary tests and equally important steps in the process of testing concepts that involve the development of empirically valid and reliable research instruments.

Theory Analysis

Whereas concept analysis is a process that could occur early in the process and cycle of theory development and theory testing, theory analysis is a later process. Table 10-4 compares theory analysis and concept analysis. Theory analysis involves considering important variables that may have

TABLE 10-4	Analysis	
Analysis	*Criteria*	*Units of Analysis*
Concepts	Differentiation from others	Definitions
		Semantic
		Logic
		Context
		Antecedents
		Consequences
		Exemplars
Theories	The theorist	Educational background
		Experiential background
		Professional network
		Sociocultural context
	Paradigmatic origins	References, citations
		Assumptions
		Concepts
		Propositions
		Hypotheses
		Laws
	Internal dimensions	Rationale
		System of relations
		Content
		Beginnings
		Scope
		Goal
		Context
		Abstractness
		Method

influenced the development of the theory and its current structure. In analyzing theories, consider several criteria: the theorist, paradigmatic origins, and internal dimensions. These criteria provide a better understanding of choices of central theory questions, goals of theory, the theory phenomena, and the strategy of theory development; these criteria also set the stage for the critique.

The Theorist. A comprehensive analysis of theories includes a careful consideration of the theory's author. Areas for exploration include experiential background, educational background, employment, and reconstruction of the professional and academic networks that surrounded the theorist while the theory was evolving. Such an analysis may include mentors, students, and sponsors when appropriate. This analysis helps in identifying influencing factors on the theory's inception and on its further development. Often, clarification in a theory, redefinitions, or extensions are directly or indirectly related to a new mentor relationship, a new degree, an employment move, or other variables that contribute to shifts in orientation. Analysis helps to uncover the external and internal factors influencing a theorist, such as beliefs held by the theorist, and the patterns of reasoning and the origins of these patterns. This may lead to a better understanding of the human parameters involved in theory development, an essential component of a historically contexted conception of science (Silva and Rothbart, 1984).

This segment of analysis could be done in a number of different ways, including a thorough review of all that has been written by the theorist and all that has been written by others about the theorist, direct communication with the theorist, and communication with mentors and students. A review may also focus on only one (or more) aspect of the theorist (Fulton, 1987). Analyzing the theorist's background will help to clarify internal dimensions, which follows as the next order of business in analyzing theories.

Consideration of who the theorists are as people, as nurses, educators, clinicians, and theorists has been the subject of analyses for many decades. These analyses range from short reviews (for example, Alligood, 2013; Smith and Parker, 2015) to elaborate videos (see Chapter 21). These analyses are indications of the value the discipline places on the contributions of these theorists, the significance of knowing the theorist behind the theory for further understanding of the theory and for enhancing the potential for others to model the theorist's thought processes and strategies in developing the theory.

Paradigmatic Origins of Theory. Theoretical thinking in nursing either evolves from a prototype theory or can be traced to theories used in other fields. Examples of such theories are those of Johnson, who derived her theory from the premises of the systems paradigm (Parsons, 1949; Riehl and Roy, 1980, pp. 207–216), and Paterson and Zderad (1988), who based their work on the existentialist philosophy. Therefore, for a careful consideration of this component, the theory analyst should become conversant with the paradigmatic origins of the theory under consideration and address those origins in the analysis.

To identify the paradigm from which the theory may have evolved or other theories that may have

influenced its development, the review considers the following:

- References, bibliography provided
- Background of theorist, educationally and experientially
- Sociocultural context that may have influenced the theory's development.

Analysis of the theory in relationship to these components provides answers to three major questions:

1. Is the theory derived from and built on a specific paradigm?
2. What are the origins of the paradigm?
3. Why was this particular paradigm used?

More specifically, on what prototype theory or paradigm did the theorist build the conceptual structures? How extensively is the original paradigm or theory used?

Beckstead and Beckstead (2006) offer another approach for determining the epistemic origins of nursing theories and models of framework. They used the multidimensional scaling (MDS) approach in an attempt to systematically and objectively determine the nature of paradigms that influenced nursing theorists from various fields such as psychology, biology, or philosophy. By identifying the scholars from other fields cited by 20 nurse theorists, they tentatively concluded that the themes of adaptation and wholeness may be traced to the field of biology and specifically to general systems theory, and the themes of humanism to Abraham Maslow and Carl Rogers. More importantly, by experimenting with this evaluative technique, they propose that nursing science is derived from both *a priori* (philosophical) and *posteriori* knowledge (sense experiences). Thus, theorists may utilize wider ranges of scholars from different disciplines, to provide a wider scope of influence; or they may use a smaller and more homogeneous set of scholars, to provide a more focused influence. Evaluating theories by the MDS approach may shed light on the intellectual inspiration of theorists; however, the nature of this inspiration must be uncovered by the content analysis of the explicit and implicit assumptions used in the theory.

Other content questions to consider are the following: Is the use of paradigm obvious to the reviewer, made explicit or implicit by the writer? Does the theorist present the rationale for selection of the theory or parts of the theory used? From where do theory inadequacies originate: prototype theory or nursing theory? Do the problems detected reflect those of borrowed theory, or are they the result of translation? Does nursing theory improve on prototype theory? How congruent or incongruent is the use of components of prototype theory with nursing theory? How different or similar are the definitions to prototype theory definitions? Are goals the same? Is justification for variance included? Are other nursing theories derived from the prototype theory? What are they?

Internal Dimensions. The components of the internal structure act as guidelines to describe a theory, as discussed in the section, Theory Description. Dimensions described in this section help in analyzing a theory to enhance understanding of the approaches used to develop it, in delineating gaps in the theory, and in giving perspective to why some omissions are not necessarily gaps in the theory but in some instances are merely what the theory intended. This will soon become clear. The dimensions described next provide the necessary lexicon to describe a theory.

The first dimension to consider is the *rationale on which the theory is built*. Questions to consider in describing the theory along this dimension include: Are components of the theory united in a chain-link fashion? Is it a theory of the factor type? Is the theory developed around concepts and thus a concatenated theory? Or, is it based on certain sets of relationships that are deduced from a small set of basic principles and are therefore hierarchical in nature? The concatenated theory has fewer explanations that converge on a central point and therefore embodies existence propositions, whereas the set of relationships theory embodies an interpretive model (Kaplan, 1964).

The second dimension to consider is that of *system of relations*. Questions to be asked are: Do relations explain elements, or do elements explain relations? A monadic approach in theory construction considers single irreducible units, as opposed to a field approach, which considers its unit of analysis in terms of a number of other miniunits. An example of the monadic approach is cell theory, and an example of the field approach is a theory of personality in terms of roles. A monadic approach is one in which the attributes and properties of the phenomenon are the focus of the theory. A field approach focuses on the relationships between the phenomena and thus explains the phenomena through these relationships. Therefore, a theory of a human being as a subsystem of behavior would be monadic, and a theory of human environmental interaction would be a field theory.

Content of the theory is a third descriptive dimension (Kaplan, 1964). Content is distinguished by the range of laws and group of individuals to which the theory refers. A theory could be classified as molar or macrotheory, or as molecular or microtheory. Organizational theories in sociology are macro in content, whereas rule theory is micro. This dimension considers the range of relationships in the theory and the set of individuals to which the relationships refer. When a theory considers the human being in totality, it is macrotheory. When the theory addresses needs during illness, it is a microtheory. Therefore, Rogers' work (1970) is an example of macrotheory, whereas that of Orem (1985) is an example of microtheory.

The point at which a theorist begins articulating ideas and addresses either a theory of extant nursing practice or one of ideal nursing practice specifies another dimension, namely, that of *theory beginnings* (Kaplan, 1964). A constructive beginning is hypothetical and is intended to build up a picture of more complex phenomena, whereas a principle theory beginning is more empirically grounded (discovered). A theory with a constructive beginning tends to be more complete, clear, and adaptable and tends to consider relationships hypothetically; the latter is more analytical and addresses the "is" rather that the "ought to be." It is more perfect and better substantiated.

A theory with a constructive beginning is also called a *deductive theory* because it emphasizes a conceptual structure deduced from another conceptual structure (Duffey and Muhlenkamp, 1974). Its laws are logically interrelated. It is through such deductive logic that some theories are derived. The major criticism of deductive theories is the lack of empirical support until they are tested in research. An example of a deductive theory in nursing is Rogers' (1970) theoretical conceptualization of man in his symphonic harmony with the environment. Her theory evolved from principles of physics, thermodynamics, and evolution, among others.

The principle theory beginning is also called the *inductive beginning*. It, on the other hand, consists essentially of summary statements or empirical relations. An example of an inductive theory is a conceptualization of issues surrounding dying, evolving from Glaser and Strauss' (1965) and Benoliel's (1967) work, even though these have not been formally labeled nursing theories.

Many theorists have addressed the *scope of theory* and its significance in describing the capability of the theory. The basic question that considers a theory's scope is: How many of the basic problems in nursing or any of its specialties could be addressed by the same theory? The significance of scope stems from the notion that theories having wider scope tend to be more general and last longer (Kuhn, 1970). In addition, the significance of a theory increases as its scope broadens (Ellis, 1968). Therefore, to answer questions related to scope, we also address generality. Theories with a wide scope are also called "grand theories," as opposed to "single-domain theories," which could be placed at the other end of a scope continuum.

The major criticism associated with both ends of the scope continuum (i.e., grand theories and single-domain theories) involves the attempts of grand theories to explain everything surrounding a set of phenomena, which is also why they may be limited in their power to explain (a major criticism of Parsons' [1949] attempts at a theory of sociology). *Single-domain theories* address only simple, abstract, isolated factors and principles. The empiricist and methodologist Robert Merton (1964) is credited with advocating middle-range theories, thus avoiding those criticisms. *Middle-range theories* consider a limited number of variables, have a particular substantive focus, focus on a limited aspect of relationship, are more susceptible to empirical testing, and could be consolidated into more wide-ranging theories (see Chapters 15 and 16).

In nursing, Jacox (1974), following Merton's ideas, urged the development of middle-range theories for limited aspects within the discipline of nursing, such as pain alleviation or promotion of sleep. A major criticism of middle-range theories is that they lead to fragmentation of a discipline when the discipline has no agreed-on phenomenon. Middle-range theories are more appropriate now in nursing, particularly after we have identified and broadly agreed on the boundaries of nursing knowledge and nursing domain concepts. Situation-specific theories are evolving to reflect specific contexts, limited scope, and more conditions that limit generalization. There are more indications that the level of maturity of the nursing discipline allows for more specificity in the theories. Currently, I urge the development of situation-specific theories as they are more congruent with the nature of nursing as a practice-based human science in which context is essential. (See Chapter 17 for situation-specific theories. Also see Lee, Fawcett, Yang, et al., 2012.)

Questions to ask when considering the *goal of a theory* are: Why was the theory developed? What is its aim and intent? Theories are constructed to describe, explain, predict, or prescribe. A descriptive theory gives information related to phenomena under consideration but does not make a claim beyond that, nor does it tell us what to expect in the future. When a beginning linkage and description of relationships between derived concepts are provided, the theory becomes an explanatory theory. Correlative studies to test explanatory theories provide empirical evidence in support of these theories. Another goal explicated in some theories is that of prediction. A predictive theory encompasses propositions of an "if . . . then" nature in a consequential manner. The ultimate goal in nursing is to prescribe; therefore, prescription is another theory goal. Theories might have all of these goals, or they may explicate only one goal or another. At this time in the developmental history of nursing theory, it is essential that a theory represent each of the goals.

The *context of a theory* in which the central phenomenon is addressed is yet another dimension for theory evaluation. Johnson (1959) called attention to the need in nursing for theories addressing knowledge of order, knowledge of disorder, and knowledge of control. The knowledge of order addresses phenomena that are central to objects, events, and interactions in a healthy context. They describe regularities in such phenomena. They describe the normal state and natural scheme of things. They provide baseline data. An example of such knowledge is provided by Auger (1976) in her explication of Johnson's (1968) normal patterns of a person's behavior within systems of behavior. Knowledge of disorder recognizes a context or disorder within which nurses deal. An attempt to develop such knowledge, not yet bound together in a theoretical schema, was manifested in the first conference on classification of nursing diagnosis (Gebbie, 1976) and in subsequent conferences. To prescribe a course of action that, when implemented, could change the sequence of events in a desired way is to have knowledge of control. Examples of theories addressing such knowledge are Orem's self-care theory (1985) and Meleis (1975) and Meleis, Swendsen, and Jones' role-supplementation (1980) theories, among others. Theories could also address knowledge of process, which included the nursing process and nurse–patient interactions (Paterson and Zderad, 1988).

Abstractness, another theory dimension, is evaluated by length of reduction and deduction between its propositions. A highly abstract theory requires more steps to reduce the chain "connecting the theoretical terms with the observable ones" (Kaplan, 1964, p. 301). It is a theory with wide spaces between its proposition and conceptual schema that is highly removed from reality but still pertains to it. If abstractness is put on a continuum from high to low abstractness, Rogers and Johnson would be at the high end and Orem at the low end.

Finally, the *method of theory development* should be carefully assessed. Barnum (1998) proposed that four methods are used in developing theories. One can assess these methods by considering the reasoning on which the theory is built, the system of action, and the plan for progression. A dialectical method is exemplified by Rogers' work (Barnum, 1998) and is based on Hegel's dialectical process. It speaks to the fusion of opposites (Newman, 1979). It emphasizes relationship with a whole and, in fact, each whole explains parts and each part is a whole explaining other parts. A dialectical method encompasses contradictions, apposition, and dilemmas, but order evolves from the interaction among all of them. Erikson's developmental theory (1963) is an example of resolution of conflict and crisis in the process of moving into the next level of development. A dialectical method defies Aristotelian logic, which is another method of theory development—the logical method. This is a method in which the parts are organized to describe the whole systematically and categorically. Nursing process is organized in a logical sequence. A theory of this nature offers a description of each part, and the whole is more than and different from the sum total of all parts. Barnum (1998) also warns of the misuse of "systems" as a subject matter to classify a theory as system theory. There are many different ways to use systems theories to develop the substance of a theory. It is important to differentiate the different foci. Barnum (1998) considers the theories of Johnson and Roy in this category.

The other two methods of theory development, according to Barnum (1998), are problematic method and operational method. Both appeal more to common sense, use persuasion in supporting ideas, and use their experiences in theory development, and in both the agent is part of the method. Problem theories (Henderson, 1966; Nursing Theories Conference Group, 1980) are organized around nursing problems, whereas operational theories (Orem, 1985) are organized around methods of intervention and differential diagnosis.

Critique of Theory

Critique is defined by *Webster's Third New International Dictionary* as "critical examination or estimate of a thing or situation with the view

to determining its nature and limitations or its conformity to standards."[1] Several criteria are essential in critiquing theory. These are relationships between structure and function, diagram of theory, circle of contagiousness, usefulness, and external components. Each is defined and presented in the following sections.

Relationship Between Structure and Function

In critiquing a theory according to the criteria listed next, the critic considers the relationship between structure and function (Table 10-5). This is accomplished by making a critical assessment and judgment of the relationship between the different components of the theory, such as assumptions, concepts, propositions, and domain concepts. In doing so, the critic cannot judge the logic inherent in the development of a dialectic theory by the same criteria used when judging a logical theory; rather, the method used dictates the critique. Several criteria could be considered, such as clarity, consistency, simplicity/complexity, and tautology/teleology.

Clarity. Clarity is defined on a continuum ranging from high to low. It denotes precision of boundaries, a communication of a sense of orderliness, vividness of meaning, and consistency through the theory. Clarity is also defined by Chinn and Kramer (2010) as "how well the theory can be understood and how consistently the ideas are conceptualized" (p. 198). Clarity is demonstrated in assumptions, concepts, and propositions, as well as in domain concepts. To have clarity in concepts is to have theoretical and operational definitions that are consistent throughout the theory, are presented in a parsimonious way, and are consistent with theory assumptions and propositions. Questions such as the following help to determine concept clarity: Are concepts operationally defined? Do they seem to have content and construct validity? Propositional clarity is manifested in a coherent and logical presentation of propositions and systematic linkages between the theory concepts. The criterion of clarity varies within a range from high to low clarity.

Consistency. The boundaries between clarity and consistency are not easily determined. The degree to which a congruency exists between the different components of a theory describes its consistency.

---

[1]By permission. From Webster's Third New International Dictionary. (1986). Springfield, MA: Merriam-Webster, Inc.

TABLE 10-5	Theory Critique—Relationship Between Structure and Function, Diagram of Theory, and Circle of Contagiousness
Criteria	*Units of Analysis*
Relationship between structure and function	Clarity
	Consistency
	Simplicity/Complexity
	Tautology/Teleology
Diagram of theory	Visual and graphic presentation
	Logical representation
	Clarity
Circle of contagiousness	Geographical origin of theory and geographical spread

The fit between the different components of a theory describes its consistency. The fit between assumptions and concept definitions, between concepts as defined and their use in propositions, and between concepts and clinical exemplars can all be considered determinants of consistency.

Simplicity/Complexity. Another criterion with which to critique a theory is its level of simplicity/complexity. The more phenomena the theory considers, the more potential relationships it could generate, and the more complex the theory is (Ellis, 1968). Simplicity of a theory is more desirable if it focuses on fewer concepts and few relationships that may enhance its utility. Complexity of a theory may be a desirable criterion if the complexity enhances the number of explanations and predictions that the theory offers. Therefore, simplicity in the face of complex contextual reality is as unadvisable as complexity in theory would be when the theory explains a limited number of relationships. Chinn and Kramer (2010) advocate simplicity in a theory that has been tested and as a means for generating ideas and hypotheses. Levels of theory simplicity and complexity correspond with the stage of theory development. Some nursing situations require a higher degree of complexity and less empirical accessibility. Other situations require a limited number of elements and thus reflect simplicity.

Tautology/Teleology. The clarity, consistency, and simplicity/complexity of a theory could also be described through tautology and teleology. A general assessment of *tautology* is done by considering the needless repetition of an idea in different parts of the theory. Tautology decreases a theory's clarity. A careful consideration of the extent and the care by which causes and consequences are kept separate ensures that the theorist avoids teleology. *Teleology* occurs when the definition of concepts, conditions, and events uses consequences rather than properties and dimensions. When defining concepts by consequences only, the theorist introduces new concepts to define existing ones. This practice leaves the original concept undefined. Teleology is another dimension in the relationship between structure and function. The critic, therefore, should consider questions such as: Does the theory have logical coherence? Are definitions of nursing phenomena concise? Is it a teleologic theory?

Diagram of Theory

The clarity of theories and models is further enhanced by visual representation of the theory. Major questions to be addressed in relation to this component are: Was the theory visually and graphically presented? Did the graphic presentation enhance understanding of different components of the theory? More specifically: How clear is the visual representation? Is it an accurate representation of the text? Does it include major concepts? Are linkages clear? Are linkage directions indicated? Is representation logical? Are there overlaps? Are there gaps? Is representation a substitute for words and explanation or is it a supplementation? Is the diagram clear and well defined? Is there a correspondence between diagram and concepts and propositions in the text? Do the diagrams enhance understanding of the text?

Circle of Contagiousness

The final test of any theory is whether it is adopted by others (see Table 10-5). The units of analysis here are geographical location and type of institution. Theories in nursing have been used within the geographical areas from which they emanated. Rogers' theory is used at New York University and tested by Rogers' students; Johnson's is used in Los Angeles and tested by her students. Therefore, when a theory begins to cross several concentric circles from its origin, its circle of contagiousness increases, and we can infer that the theory is receiving more acceptability, uninfluenced by the theorist.

The critic should review the literature, indexes, and citations for answers to questions such as: Where has the theory been developed and used? Where is it being used both geographically and institutionally? What is it used for (research, education, administration, clinical practice, etc.)? How influential was the theorist in prompting the implementation of the theory? Where was it first introduced? What happened in the interim? Has the theory been considered and used cross-culturally and transculturally? Can the critic differentiate between the influence of the theory and the influence of the theorist? What is the difference? What are the consequences? A critique of the circle of contagiousness of a theory is made in conjunction with the usefulness of theory.

Usefulness

A critique of the usefulness of a theory encompasses four areas: its potential for usefulness in practice, research, education, and administration (Roper, Logan, and Tierney, 1996) (Table 10-6).

Usefulness in Practice. A thorough review and assessment of theory has to consider its potential for operationalization and utilization in nursing practice. A practitioner who is considering using a theory in some practice area should assess the theory in terms of its function: its goals, consequences, and potential for practice. Therefore, the theory should be able to respond to these questions or have a framework to help the clinician respond to them: Does the theory provide enough direction to affect practice? Does it have a framework for prescription? Does the theory include abstract notions that are not applicable to practice? Does the level of abstraction or understandability render it applicable or inapplicable? Does the theory cover all areas of nursing? Should it? Does the theory currently apply to practice? Who pays for use of the theory in practice? Is it cost-effective? Is it a timely nursing practice theory? Does it have relevance for the way nursing is practiced today? Where does the theory fit in terms of nursing process? Is the theory understandable to the practitioner? What is the assessment of practitioners of the theory as to its

TABLE 10-6	Theory Critique— Usefulness
Criteria	*Unit of Analysis*
Practice	Direction
	Applicability
	Generalizability
	Cost-effectiveness
	Relevance
Research	Consistency
	Testability
	Predictability
Education	Philosophical statement
	Objectives
	Concepts
Administration	Structure of care
	Organization of care
	Guidelines for patient care
	Patient classification system

uniqueness and its esoteric language? How does it relate to diagnosis-related groups? In what ways is the theory translatable to an existing or a proposed informational technology or system?

Finally, a different question is proposed by Reed (2008) as one test of the pragmatic adequacy of nursing theories. It is related to the extent to which the theory is able to inform nurses about the human health experience of well-being or adversity. Reed proposes that developing theories may be influenced by adverse circumstances, depending on how science is defined at the time of the theory's development. In addition, considering how the theory deals with patients' experiences with any misfortune, as well as how it provides guidelines for restoring theory, would be an important evaluative point.

Usefulness in Research. The *raison d'être* of theories is to guide and be guided by research; therefore, a critique of a theory should include questions related to the assessment of a theory's potential for testability. The concepts and propositions should eventually be related in a consistent manner to a systematic set of observable or testable data. Otherwise, if a theory remains untested, its usefulness is in question. Schrag (1967) emphasizes the significance of a theory's potential for research, which he calls "the empirical adequacy" of a theory, and this potential is realized through congruence between "theoretical claims and empirical evidence." He asserts that credibility refers to the "goodness of fit between claims and existing evidence, while predictability estimates how well the claims will hold true in the future" (Schrag, 1967, p. 250).

Theories are established on current information; it usually is up to utilizers of theories to provide evidence that corroborates them. Although the aim of research is not to establish the absolute truth of the theoretical propositions, it is essential that it begins to indicate a degree of confidence based on empirical evidence. It is noteworthy that, to the unsophisticated reviewer, any supportive corroboration between theory and data uncovered through research may be interpreted as giving support to the entire theory structure. However, corroboration may be confined to a particular proposition of a theory containing multiple propositions. Therefore, the type and extent of empirical corroboration should be skeptically considered by answering several questions, including: What specific theory propositions did the research consider? Were these central or peripheral propositions? Was the research undertaken to provide validity to concepts or relationships? Was theory used to test propositions or to interpret findings? Were explicit theory assumptions considered in designing methodology?

Although it is significant to the theory critic to note that theories are tested on a piecemeal basis, the critic should still consider finding responses to the following questions: Does the theory build on previous research? Was research done using the theory? What propositions were being tested? How reproducible is the research? Can the findings be generalized? What research designs have been used? Why? How appropriate are they? Can proscriptive and predictive (experimental and quasi-experimental) studies be designed? Are the research results relevant to other fields? Is the research used appropriately? Do the theories state what research is to be completed to support central theory propositions? Has there been empirical verification of its properties? How consistent are its propositions with other theories and laws? Is there evidence for corroboration (Schrag, 1967)? Finally, one can detect any spuriousness in the theory's components as manifested in a logical or research determination of whether or not dependent variables are potentially related to other, independent variables.

The research potential or testability of a theory should not be critiqued lightly. As Berthold (1968) and Ellis (1968) stressed, the ultimate criteria for evaluating a theory's usefulness are whether it generates predictions or propositions concerning relevant components of the theory and whether it stimulates new observations, insights, and questions that could subsequently be corroborated. Units of analysis for testability are theoretical and operational definitions, theoretical propositions, ongoing research, and completed research.

Usefulness in Education. The beginning evaluation of nursing theories for their potential to offer guidelines for nursing curricula and programs coincided almost completely with the development of most of the theories that we now consider to be nursing theories. In fact, as we analyze the rationales and the goals of a good number of the nursing theories, we find that nursing education invariably prompted their development through the search for a coherent presentation of what nursing is about, and to guide and structure the curriculum, the biomedical model that dominated nursing curricula. Invariably, a growing uneasiness prompted a shift to a needs orientation, such as that offered by Henderson (1966) and Abdellah (1969), and with it a rejection of biologic systems and disease orientation as frameworks. Unfortunately, the shift to a nursing conceptualization was premature because it occurred simultaneously with the theory being developed, and, therefore, many faculty members suffered from the pitfalls of attempting to operationalize a theory while still developing it.

The National League for Nursing criteria in the 1960s for accrediting and adopting a conceptual framework to guide curricula was both a blessing and a menace to nursing curricula and to theory development. The blessing was the reorientation of faculty to nursing theory; the menace emanated from the prematurity of the use of nursing theories in nursing education. Nursing theories could provide the major premises on which a curriculum is built, yet I believe that it is not feasible to develop an entire program on just one conceptualization of nursing. For example, theories about teaching and learning, about the learner, and about the environment are complementary to nursing conceptualizations in defining and structuring curricula.

It is possible that this premature translation has contributed to recent educational trends in which utilization of nursing theory plays a smaller role in guiding curricula. In several trends that emerged in the second decade of the 21st century, curricula are not based on a particular nursing theory; students may not be asked to identify the theoretical framework that guides their studies, and graduate students may tend to view theory more for guiding practice and less for guiding their education. These trends may also be driven by changes in accreditation criteria and by advanced practice guidelines, neither of which provide explicit requirements for the use of theory (Donohue-Porter, Forbes, and White, 2011).

Usefulness in Administration. Use of nursing theory in administration is considered in terms of the structure and organization of care. Theories ought to provide the potential for guiding and describing nursing care. Nursing theories are expected to guide the care of clients and are not expected to provide the administrator with guidelines for administration or for leadership style. Analysis shows how useful theory can be in providing guidelines in patient care on a large scale. Some questions to consider are: Does it help the patient classification system? How congruent is the mission of nursing as articulated by theory with the mission as articulated by the particular organization that is utilizing the theory? Does the theory provide any specific guidelines for theory implementation on an organizational scale? Does it provide assistance in determining criteria for quality control?

Other criteria for the evaluation of theories for nursing administration were identified by Buchanan (1987). These include the congruency of theory with professional standards, such as licensing requirements, as well as standards stipulated by such accrediting bodies as the American Nurses Association and the American Hospital Association. Theories selected by administrators should also be congruent with the legal structure governing nursing functions in different countries.

External Components

Finally, the theory should be critiqued by assessing it against several external criteria. These are: personal values, other professional values, social values, and social significance (Table 10-7).

Personal Values. Ellis (1968) and Johnson (1987) emphasized the importance of recognizing values inherent in theories and in making them explicit. Review of values occurs as the assumptions of a theory are uncovered and described. A critical consideration of values should account for those values of the theorist and the critic. In the latter, the fit between the theorist's and critic's personal and professional values should be considered. It is through such careful assessment that biases can be delineated.

Congruence with Other Professional Values. A similar assessment of the values espoused in the theory should be made of the values of other

TABLE 10-7	Theory Critique—External Components of Theory
Criteria	*Units of Analysis*
Personal values	Theorist implicit/explicit values
	Critic implicit/explicit values
Congruence with other professional values	Complementarity
	Esotericism
	Competition
Congruence with social values	Beliefs
	Values
	Customs
Social significance	Value to humanity

professions. Health care professionals will be able to enhance patient care through collaboration and complementarity of value systems. Awareness of such complementarity or competition in professional values enhances the potential of the development of a collaborative working schema to close the professional value gaps (Johnson, 1974).

Congruence with Social Values. Beliefs, values, and expectations of different societies and cultures within societies shape and direct the type of theory that is most useful. Although self-help, self-care (at its different levels), and individuality are goals congruent with some cultures' value systems, they are the antithesis of those espoused in others. Therefore, theories with such goals and consequences would be incongruent and inappropriate to some societies and should be avoided. Careful critical assessment of societal values and theory values is an integral part of a thorough theory critique. Questions should be addressed such as: Is the role of the nurse within the model congruent with the role of the nurse as perceived by society? Are actions and outcomes congruent with societal expectations of nursing (Johnson, 1974, 1987)?

Social Significance. In our attempt to enhance nursing science and articulate the discipline of nursing, we must not neglect the significance of its practice to humanity and society. The philanthropic Bacon's profound words of the 18th century still hold true today:

Lastly, I would address one general admonition to all; that they consider what are the true ends of knowledge, and that they seek it not either for pleasure of mind, or for contention, or for superiority to others, or for profit, or fame, or power, or any of these inferior things, but for the benefit and use of life; and that they perfect and govern it in charity. For it was from lust of power that the angels fell, from lust of knowledge that man fell; but of charity there can be no excess, neither did angel or man ever come in danger by it. (Bacon, in Ravetz, 1971, p. 436)

A critic should ask philosophically whether the goals and consequences of theory make a substantial and valued difference in the lives of people. (Consider questions from the perspective of clients and from the perspective of other health professionals.) The critic should also ask whether intended and unintended consequences are carefully considered (Johnson, 1974, 1987).

Theory Testing

The development of theory and the continuance and advancement of a theory for the purpose of providing evidence in practice requires theory testing, as well as a replication of that testing. The definition of theory testing has been the subject of many discussions and dialogues in nursing (Chinn, 1984, 1986; Clift and Barrett, 1998; Silva and Sorrell, 1992). It has also been equated with the evaluation of theories and considered the most significant goal in developing, accepting, and using theories. Theory testing is different from theory-based research. Theory testing provides evidence, advances predictions, and adds substantially to theory building (Norman, 2004); theory-based research affirms its utility in conceptualizing the research questions and variables. Both provide different types of support for theories. Theory testing is considered here as only one component of a comprehensive evaluation of theories in the discipline. To equate testing with evaluation and to consider it the only significant goal for theory development is to ignore all the descriptive, analytical, and critical commentaries on theories that have been published and that have added to our understanding of theories and are significant for knowledge development. (Refer to *Advances in Nursing Science*, *Nursing Outlook*, *American Journal of Nursing*, and *Journal of Advanced Nursing* during 1970–1990 for extensive examples of writings describing, analyzing, and critiquing theories and theoretical thoughts.) To equate testing with evaluation is also to reduce theoretical knowledge to the context of justification and to exclude the context of discovery with its process orientation.

Theory testing is a systematic process of subjecting theoretical propositions to the rigor of research in all its forms and approaches, and consequently, the use of the results to modify or refine the research propositions. Theory testing presumes the complete cyclical relationship between theory, research, and theory. Theory testing is neither a static process nor an end result. The dynamic testing process begins with theory development and continues with testing and more development of theory, pausing long enough to reflect and go through the cycle again.

Theory testing is not a single entity. It has many dimensions, needing many different approaches. Silva and Sorrell (1992) reviewed tests of nursing theories and identified three alternative approaches:

- Tests to verify theories through critical reasoning
- Tests to verify theories through the description of personal experiences
- Tests to verify theories through application to nursing practice

Earlier, in a review of 62 studies in which the use of theories by Johnson, Roy, Orem, and Rogers guided the studies, Silva (1986) found three ways in which theory testing was used. In 24 studies, there was a *minimal* use of the theory other than in identifying it as a framework for the study. She labeled 29 of the studies as *insufficient*, simply using the theories as a way to organize their review of literature or to select their instruments. Only 9 of the 62 studies qualified in the third category of *adequate* use of theories. These were studies in which the hypothesis testing and findings were integral to the theory and actually provided evidence to modify, accept, or reject theory propositions.

Silva proposed that this third category, which she labeled *adequate* use of the theory, is an integral part of problem identification, analysis, and interpretation. It is the type of test that should be the goal of nurse scientists in the development of knowledge in the discipline. She further attributed the lack of empirical testing to the pressure on nurse investigators to use a conceptual framework for their studies without clear guidelines on what is involved in testing, to the use of highly abstract theories, to the lack of precise measures, to the subsequent "lack of tolerance to methodological imperfections," and finally to an inability to systematically retrieve theory-based research (Silva, 1986).

Testing of theory in nursing is more complex than mere proposition testing. Considering the types of theories nurses have and will develop—that is, theories that attempt to explain responses of clients, environments, and nursing therapeutics to enhance the health of clients—it would be inadvisable to limit the investigative processes and goals to a limited definition of testing. Meleis (1995) proposed the consideration of theory testing through six principles. Each of these six principles could be used to judge the appropriateness of the tests used for the theory. The principles are gender sensitivity of the testing, the extent to which a diverse population was used, whether or not the theory was tested on populations that are considered vulnerable and marginalized, whether the questions and the methods reflect cultural competence, whether the theory testing was done nationally or internationally, and finally, what philosophy of health care provided a framework for the testing (curative care or primary health care). Throughout the history of theory testing in nursing, at least six approaches are utilized. These are:

1. *Testing the utility of nursing theory*: Research developed to evaluate the use of theory in practice, teaching, or administration falls under this category. Units of analysis for this category are the individual nurse, teacher, student, or administrator. The intent of this type of research is to determine the feasibility of the use of theory by the group of individuals using that theory. These individuals may not be limited to nurses; they may also be patients who are tested for their intention to comply with healthy behaviors such as breast-feeding (Giles, McClenahan, Armour, et al., 2014). This research tests the learner's ability to recall, comprehend, evaluate, and use the theory. Results of such tests relate to and enhance adult learning theories or cognitive theories rather than nursing practice theories (e.g., Jacobson, 1984). A variation of this category is testing the difference between the use of the different existing theories. Jacobson (1984), for example, used a semantic differential scale to define some of the differences among the King, Orem, Rogers, Roy, and Wiedenbach theories as perceived by users. Eight factors emerged to account for 49% to 56% of the variation between the theories as perceived by users. The factors are sophistication, dynamism, clarity, usefulness, focus, utility, scope, and scientific rigor. This approach to testing a model was critiqued conceptually and methodologically (e.g., Nicoll, Meyer, and Abraham, 1985). In their view, nursing models are to be evaluated individually in terms of their

content. An external evaluation, from their perspective, is incongruent with the nature of models as specific to a certain context and thus ineffectual in advancing nursing knowledge. Tests designed to compare the feasibility of implementing different theories are useful if they are problem- and context-specific. For example, using Johnson's theory and King's theory to assess and diagnose the nursing care needs of an immigrant patient undergoing a kidney transplant, and then comparing the processes and contents of assessment, could help in understanding learners' abilities to use the theories and to compare the efficiency and effectiveness of the theories in defining the priority needs of the patient.

2. *Testing propositions from other disciplines*: Research in this category is designed to test propositions from theories that were developed in other disciplines. Nursing literature has numerous examples of this type of research. Tests related to theory utilization also fall under this category because they are designed to address propositions related to educational theory. Other examples are research to test propositions evolving from systems theory, adaptation theory, role theory, and stress theory. Maslow's theory (Davis-Sharts, 1986) is an example of a theory derived from other disciplines.

3. *Testing propositions from other disciplines as they relate to nursing*: Research in this category involves, more specifically, testing propositions as they relate to a nursing phenomenon or testing propositions that are of interest to nursing. Examples of this research include studies designed to test role strain in nursing faculty (Meter and Agronow, 1982; O'Shea, 1982) and in women (Woods, 1985a, 1985b), based on role theory, and studies to test concepts from other disciplines (Wewers and Lenz, 1987).

4. *Testing nursing concepts*: Research in this category is designed to develop a measurable concept by identifying corresponding variables. The objective of testing in this category is to develop a valid and reliable means by which the concept is tested. Validity means that the instrument, the tool, or the means by which the concept is measured indeed measures that concept, and the extent to which it is used provides data compatible

with other relevant evidence (Diers, 1979). Fawcett (2013) consistently advocated for measurement validity of a concept, not only with appropriate instruments but through the conceptual meaning that emanates from the conceptual or theoretical model. Reliability means that these instruments consistently measure the same concept. The development of valid and reliable instruments, tools, or means by which concepts could be measured is one of the priorities in the development and testing of nursing theories. Examples include Lush, Janson-Bjerklie, Carrieri, et al. (1988); Nield, Kim, and Patel (1989); Carrieri, Janson-Bjerklie, and Jacobs (1984); and Derdiarian and Forsythe (1983).

5. *Testing nursing propositions*: Empirical theory testing is vital for developing, modifying, extending, or verifying theories. This requires a deliberate orderly and systematic process (Kaariainen, Kanste, Elo, et al., 2011). Research in this category is designed to test theoretical propositions that are derived from nursing theories. There are three major types of propositions tested in nursing, each of which may benefit from factor analyses processes:

   • *Existence propositions*: These relate two or more concepts to demonstrate their existence. Research designed to test existence propositions merely demonstrates that the two concepts exist concurrently. Descriptive studies of levels of self-care of oncology patients are one example; others may relate levels of self-care to degree of anxiety. Correlational tests are the most suitable analytical models for this type of research.

   • *Predictive propositions*: Tests designed to explore predictive propositions demonstrate the effect of one concept on another. Such propositions are modeled after the question: What will happen if . . . ? For example, studies designed to test interactional theory propositions asked: What will happen if patients are given an opportunity to express their feelings of anxiety before surgery (Dumas and Leonard, 1963)?

   • *Prescriptive propositions*: Research designed to test nursing interventions use principles from evaluation research. The objective is to find out how effective is the intervention in bringing about the desired goals. Examples are Smith (1986), who tested Rogers' principle of integrality, and Mentzer and Schorr (1986), who tested Newman's proposition linking situational control and perception of duration of time.

6. *Testing through interpretation*: Theory may also be tested by using it as a framework for discussion or interpretation of research findings, even when the theory may not have guided the research process used to obtain those findings. This may support, refine, or extend a theory.

Theory Support

One other evaluative component for theories is the extent to which the theory is supported. This component of evaluation addresses the extent to which the theory has garnered support, has attracted a dedicated and loyal audience, and for which there is an identifiable community of scholars who are using the theory in their own work and in a variety of situations.

Theory support is a broader concept than testing, more friendly to alternative ways of theory validation, and more congruent with the nature of the discipline (Meleis, 1995). It is not only the validation of a theory that should be considered in evaluating theory—we need to think of support and affirmation of parts of theories, and we need to think of components of theories. Even if we cannot generalize from a theory about individuals' health and illness situations and experiences, it is still extremely useful to understand the experience of the few who experience health and illness in certain unique ways, particularly in sciences that deal with human experiences and with practice-oriented issues. What other criteria can affirm or support a theory? Accounts, exemplars, and stories can be used as tests of a theory's credibility and could bolster a theory's validity. Theory support includes increased advocacy for central statements, goodness of fit with some central problems in the discipline, and new insights about nursing phenomena. Support for a theory could also be obtained through networks formed to evaluate the theory's potential and capability, and by determining what other criteria can affirm or support a theory. Scholars in the discipline of nursing—and I mean by scholars both scientists and clinicians—can provide support for theories through a number of approaches. The following are different ways by which the extent of support for a theory could be determined:

1. Supporting nursing theory through philosophical analyses
2. Supporting nursing theory through conceptual analysis
3. Supporting nursing theory through existing data
   - Analytical synthesis of single utilization studies
   - Component-based meta-analyses
   - National and regional databases
4. Supporting nursing theory through new data
   - Narrative studies based on clinicians' experiences, assessment of clients' situations, and therapeutics used
   - Interpretive studies based on clients' experiences
   - Predictive studies of stress and wellness
   - Studies to support the utility of nursing therapeutics and through further development of predictive theory studies

CONCLUSION

Theory development and evaluation are cyclical, continuous, and dynamic processes. One cannot exist without the other. Theory evaluation includes description, concept analysis, theory critique, theory testing, and theory support. These processes are based on the view that science is a human process that includes not only valid findings but also observations, agreements, and useful solutions to problems. It is also important to consider the experiences, the lens, and the level of credibility that the theorists were able to garner.

Theory evaluation is central to the development of theory; it is the responsibility of every clinician, academician, and administrator. If each does her share, we are then assured of the continuous growth of a body of knowledge to guide research and practice (see fig. 10-1).

The theory evaluation model provided here is not designated to be used as a whole for every theory the evaluator wishes or plans to use. Different parts of it could be used for different evaluation purposes. One evaluator could not complete a full theory evaluation by using all components of the model. An evaluator may choose to focus on description, analysis, critique, or testing, or on one part of any of these components. Teaming nurses, faculty, and clinicians for a more thorough evaluation may enhance

the results (Dean and Mountford, 1998). A careful analysis of the theorist and her contributions is also as valuable in advancing knowledge as is testing one proposition of a theory. Each offers members of the discipline different findings. Analyses focused on the theorist provide strategies for the development of theories and theorists, as well as forces and constraints that promote scholarship. Tests focused on accepting or rejecting propositions or generating propositions help in explaining, describing, and predicting substantive content of the field.

Despite the many critics who have been skeptical of Kuhn's attempts to delineate criteria that govern choices of good theory and have labeled them as futile, and because "the decision of a scientific group to adopt a new paradigm cannot be based on good reasons of any kind, factual or otherwise" (Shapere, 1966), Kuhn continued to assert that, indeed, we can delineate such criteria and that accuracy, consistency, broad scope, simplicity, and fruitfulness in research are essential as objective criteria for judging competing theories (Kuhn, 1977, p. 321). However, Kuhn also maintained that "every individual's choice between competing theories depends on a mixture of objective and subjective factors, or of shared and individual criteria" (p. 325). The subjective factors are based on idiosyncratic factors and are therefore dependent on individuals' preferences and personalities. Both subjective and objective factors have a place in our understanding of the philosophy of science.

The discussion provided here acknowledged subjective criteria and emphasized objective criteria. It provided criteria for theory description, analysis, critique, testing, and support, in an attempt to decrease the margin of subjectivity and to enhance that of objectivity. The goal is not to avoid subjectivity altogether, but to continue in the attempts to develop and refine components of theory evaluation and of the criteria used in these evaluations. The model of theory critique (Fig. 10-1) is designed not only to provide the basis for understanding the internal structure of theory but also the social, intellectual, and structural context that surrounds its development. It delineates a comprehensive framework for all the norms and parameters against which theories ought to be analyzed and critiqued.

When using the delineated criteria for evaluating theories, it is important to note that theories may be superior in some points and evolving in other aspects. No one theory will satisfy or be able to address all criteria. Styles of inquiry and personal preferences for theory design affect the configuration

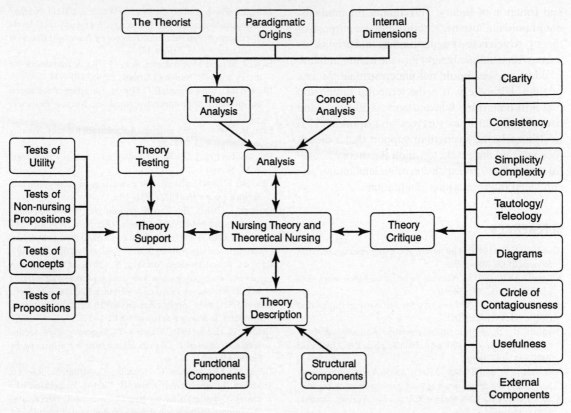

Figure 10-1   A model of theory evaluation.

REFLECTIVE QUESTIONS

1. For what reasons should members of the discipline evaluate and critique theories?

2. What might be three critical outcomes that could result from evaluating theories and three critical outcomes of not evaluating theories? Give specific examples of both approaches.

3. Can you identify and describe two or three theories that you have used in your work? Now, write down and present to your colleagues why you selected each of the theories, and ways by which you evaluated them prior to or while using them. Step back from all three and describe themes in the selection and utilization process.

4. Compare and contrast your selection criteria with the criteria discussed in this chapter.

5. Select one theory to evaluate. Identify implicit or explicit values that may create ethical dilemmas for nurses and/or for patients and their families. Would you use this theory in spite of, or because of, these values?

6. Compare and contrast the different evaluation elements of theories, description, analysis, critique, support, and testing. Which of these illuminate your understanding of theory? Which are essential for further development?

7. Select and define the most essential criteria for theory evaluation. Indicate why these particular criteria are the most essential.

8. Identify and discuss theory evaluation criteria proposed and utilized in one other discipline of your choice.

and function of theory. Throughout the analysis, one should not lose track of the ultimate purpose of theory, which is to systematize data and provide its users with a unique insight into the matter at hand. In addition, we should not underestimate the test of time. Ultimately, it is the temporal dimension that will determine which theory is adequate and useful and therefore survives and dominates. It is ultimately the strength of support that a theory receives and the extent to which the theory is useful that leads to an expansion of understanding and enhanced interpretations of situations.

REFERENCES

Abdellah, F.G. (1969). The nature of nursing science. *Nursing Research*, 18, 390–393.

Alligood, M.R. (2013). *Nursing theorists and their work* (8th ed.). St. Louis, MO: Mosby

Auger, J.R. (1976). *Behavioral systems and nursing*. Englewood Cliffs, NJ: Prentice-Hall.

Barnum, B.J.S. (1998). *Nursing theory: Analysis, application, and evaluation* (5th ed.). Philadelphia, PA: Lippincott Williams & Wilkins.

Beckstead, J.W. and Beckstead, L.G. (2006). A multidimensional analysis of the epistemic origins of nursing theories, models, and frameworks. *International Journal of Nursing Studies*, 43(1), 113–122.

Benoliel, J.Q. (1967). *The nurse and the dying patient*. New York: Macmillan.

Berthold, F.S. (1968). Symposium on theory development in nursing. *Nursing Research*, 17(3), 196–197.

Buchanan, B.F. (1987). Conceptual models: An assessment framework. *Journal of Nursing Administration*, 17(10), 22–26.

Carrieri, V.K., Janson-Bjerklie, S.J., and Jacobs, S. (1984). The sensation of dyspnea: A review. *Heart Lung*, 13(4), 436–447.

Chick, N. and Meleis, A.I. (1986). Transitions: A nursing concern. In P.L. Chinn (Ed.), *Nursing research methodology* (pp. 237–257). Boulder, CO: Aspen.

Chinn, P.L. (1984). From the editor. *Advances in Nursing Science*, 6(2), ix.

Chinn, P.L. (1986). From the editor. *Advances in Nursing Science*, 6(2), viii.

Chinn, P.L. and Kramer, M.K. (2010). *Integrated theory and knowledge development in nursing* (8th ed.). St. Louis, MO: C.V. Mosby.

Clift, J. and Barrett, E. (1998). Testing nursing theory cross culturally. *International Nursing Review*, 45(4), 123–126.

Davis-Sharts, J. (1986). An empirical test of Maslow's theory of need hierarchy using hologeistic comparison by statistical sampling. *Advances in Nursing Science*, 9(1), 58–72.

Dean, J.M. and Mountford, B. (1998). Innovation in the assessment of nursing theory and its evaluation: A team approach. *Journal of Advanced Nursing*, 28(2), 409–418.

Derdiarian, A.K. and Forsythe, A.B. (1983). An instrument for theory and research development using the behavioral systems model for nursing: The cancer patient. Part 2. *Nursing Research*, 32(5), 260–266.

Diers, D. (1979). *Research in nursing practice*. Philadelphia, PA: J.B. Lippincott.

Donohue-Porter, P., Forbes, M., and White, J. (2011). Nursing theory in curricula today: Challenges for faculty at all levels of education. *International Journal of Nursing Education Scholarship*, 8(1), Article 14.

Duffey, M. and Muhlenkamp, A.F. (1974). A framework for theory analysis. *Nursing Outlook*, 22(9), 570–574.

Dumas, R.G. and Leonard, R.C. (1963). The effect of nursing on the incidence of postoperative vomiting. *Nursing Research*, 12(1), 12–15.

Ellis, R. (1968). Characteristics of significant theories. *Nursing Research*, 17(3), 217–222.

Erikson, E. (1963). *Childhood and society* (2nd ed.). New York: W.W. Norton.

Fawcett, J. (2005). Criteria for evaluation of theory. *Nursing Science Quarterly*, 18(2), 131–135.

Fawcett, J. (2012). Thoughts on concept analysis: Multiple approaches, one result. *Nursing Science Quarterly*, 25(3), 285–287.

Fawcett, J. (2013). Thoughts about conceptual models and measurement validity. *Nursing Science Quarterly*, 26(2), 189–191.

Fawcett, J. and Desanto-Madeya, S. (2013). *Contemporary nursing knowledge: Analysis and evaluation of nursing models and theories* (3rd ed.). Philadelphia, PA: F.A. Davis

Fulton, J.S. (1987). Virginia Henderson: Theorist, prophet, poet. *Advances in Nursing Science*, 10(1), 1–17.

Gebbie, K. (Ed.). (1976, March 4–7). *Summary of the second national conference: Classification of nursing diagnosis*. St. Louis, MO: C.V. Mosby.

Giles, M., McClenahan, C., Armour, C., Millar, S., Rae, G., Mallet, J., and Stewart-Knox, B. (2014). Evaluation of a theory of planned behavior-based breastfeeding intervention in Northern Irish schools using a randomized cluster design. *British Journal of Health Psychology*, 19(1), 16–35.

Glaser, B.G. and Strauss, A.L. (1965). *Awareness of dying*. Chicago, IL: Aldine.

Hage, J. (1972). *Techniques of problems of theory construction in sociology*. New York: John Wiley & Sons.

Hardy, M.E. (1974). Theories: Components, development, evaluation. *Nursing Research*, 23(2), 100–107.

Henderson, V. (1966). *The nature of nursing*. New York: Macmillan.

Im, E-O. (2015). The current status of theory evaluation in nursing. *Journal of Advanced Nursing*, 71(10), 2268–2278.

Jacobson, S.F. (1984). A semantic differential for external comparison of conceptual nursing models. *Advances in Nursing Science*, 6(2), 58–70.

Jacox, A. (1974). Theory construction in nursing: An overview. *Nursing Research*, 23(1), 4–13.

Johnson, D.E. (1959). The nature of a science of nursing. *Nursing Outlook*, 7(5), 291–294.

Johnson, D.E. (1968). *One conceptual model of nursing*. Paper presented at Vanderbilt University, Nashville, TN.

Johnson, D.E. (1970, Winter). *Requirements of an effective model* [For N203, Class in Theory]. Unpublished manuscript. Los Angeles, CA: University of California.

Johnson, D.E. (1974). Development of theory: A requisite for nursing as a primary health profession. *Nursing Research*, 23(5), 372–377.

Johnson, D.E. (1987). Evaluating conceptual models for use in critical care nursing practice. *Dimensions of Critical Nursing Care*, 6(4), 195–197.

Kaariainen, M., Kanste, O., Elo, S., Polkki, T., Miettunen, J., and Kyngas, H. (2011). Testing and verifying nursing theory by confirmatory factor analysis. *Journal of Advanced Nursing*, 67(5), 1163–1172.

Kaplan, A. (1964). *The conduct of inquiry: Methodology of behavioral science*. San Francisco, CA: Chandler.

King, I. (1971). *Toward a theory for nursing*. New York: John Wiley & Sons.

Kuhn, T.S. (1970). The structure of scientific revolutions. In O. Neurath (Ed.), *International encyclopedia of unified science* (2nd ed., Vol. 2). Chicago, IL: University of Chicago Press.

Kuhn, T.S. (1977). *The essential tension*. Chicago, IL: University of Chicago Press.

Laudan, L. (1977). *Progress and its problems: Toward a theory of scientific growth*. Berkeley, CA: University of California Press.

Lee, H., Fawcett, J., Yang, J., and Hann, H. (2012). Correlates of hepatitis B virus health-related behaviors of Korean Americans: A situation-specific nursing theory. *Journal of Nursing Scholarship, 44*(4), 315–322.

Lindsey, A.M., Piper, B.F., and Stotts, N.A. (1982). The phenomenon of cancer cachexia: A review. *Oncology Nursing Forum, 9*(2), 38–42.

Lush, M.T., Janson-Bjerklie, S., Carrieri, V.K., and Lovejoy, N. (1988). Dyspnea in the ventilator-assisted patient. *Heart Lung, 17*(5), 528–535.

Meleis, A.I. (1975). Role insufficiency and role supplementation: A conceptual framework. *Nursing Research, 24*(4), 264–271.

Meleis, A.I. (1995). Theory testing and theory support: Principles, challenges, and a sojourn into the future. In Betty Neuman (Ed.), *The Neuman systems model* (pp. 447–457). East Norwalk, CT: Appleton & Lange.

Meleis, A.I., Swendsen, L., and Jones, D. (1980). Preventive role supplementation: A grounded conceptual framework. In M.H. Miller and B. Flynn (Eds.), *Current perspectives in nursing: Social issues and trends*. St. Louis, MO: C.V. Mosby.

Merton, R. (1964). *Social theory and social structure* (Rev. ed.). London, UK: Free Press of Glencoe.

Mentzer, C.A. and Schorr, J.A. (1986). Perceived situational control and perceived duration of time: Expressions of life patterns. *Advances in Nursing Science, 9*(1), 12–20.

Meter, M.J. and Agronow, S.J. (1982). The stress of multiple roles: The case for role strain among married college women. *Family Relations, 31*(1), 131–138.

Newman, M.A. (1979). *Theory development in nursing*. Philadelphia, PA: F.A. Davis.

Nicoll, L.H., Meyer, P.A., and Abraham, I.L. (1985). Critique: External comparison of conceptual nursing models. *Advances in Nursing Science, 7*(4), 1–9.

Nield, M., Kim, M.J., and Patel, M. (1989). Use of magnitude estimation for estimating the parameters of dyspnea. *Nursing Research, 38*(2), 77–80.

Norman, G. (2004). Editorial – Theory testing research versus theory–based research. *Advances in Health Sciences Education, 9*, 175–178.

Norris, C.M. (1982). *Concept clarification in nursing*. Rockville, MD: Aspen Systems.

The Nursing Theories Conference Group. (1980). *Nursing theories: The base for professional nursing practice*. Englewood Cliffs, NJ: Prentice-Hall.

Orem, D.E. (1985). *Nursing: Concepts of practice* (3rd ed.). New York: McGraw-Hill.

O'Shea, H.S. (1982). Role orientation and role strain of clinical nurse faculty in baccalaureate programs. *Nursing Research, 31*(5), 306–310.

Parsons, T. (1949). *The structure of social action*. New York: Free Press.

Paterson, J.G. and Zderad, L.T. (1988). *Humanistic nursing*. New York: National League for Nursing, Publication No. 41–2218.

Ravetz, J. (1971). *Scientific knowledge and its social problems*. New York: Oxford University Press.

Reed, P.G. (2008). Adversity and advancing nursing knowledge. *Nursing Science Quarterly, 21*(2), 133–139.

Riehl, J.P. and Roy, C. (Eds.). (1980). *Conceptual models for nursing practice* (2nd ed.). New York: Appleton-Century-Crofts.

Rogers, M. (1970). *An introduction to the theoretical basis of nursing*. Philadelphia, PA: F.A. Davis.

Roper, N., Logan, W., and Tierney, A. (1996). The Roper-Logan-Tierney Model: A model in nursing practice. In P.H. Walker (Ed.), *Blueprint for use of nursing models: Education, research, practice, and administration* (pp. 289–314). New York: National League for Nursing.

Roy, C. and Roberts, S.L. (1981). *Theory construction in nursing*. Englewood Cliffs, NJ: Prentice-Hall.

Schrag, C. (1967). Elements of theoretical analysis in sociology. In L. Gross (Ed.), *Sociological theory: Inquiries and paradigms*. New York: Harper & Row.

Shapere, D. (1966). Meaning and scientific change. In R.G. Colodny (Ed.), *Mind and cosmos: Essays in contemporary science and philosophy*. University of Pittsburgh Series in the Philosophy of Science (Vol. 3). Pittsburgh, PA: University of Pittsburgh Press.

Silva, M.C. (1986). Research testing nursing theory: State of the art. *Advances in Nursing Science, 9*(1), 1–11.

Silva, M.C. and Rothbart, D. (1984). An analysis of changing trends in philosophies of science on nursing theory development and testing. *Advances in Nursing Science, 6*(2), 1–13.

Silva, M.C. and Sorrell, J.M. (1992). Testing of nursing theory: Critique and philosophical expansion. *Advances in Nursing Science, 14*(4), 12–23.

Smith, M.C. and Parker M.E. (2015). *Nursing theories and nursing practice* (4th ed.). Philadelphia, PA: F.A. Davis Company.

Smith, M.J. (1986). Human-environment process: A test of Rogers' principle of integrality. *Advances in Nursing Science, 9*(1), 21–28.

Walker, L.O. and Avant, K.C. (1995). *Strategies for theory construction in nursing* (3rd ed.). East Norwalk, CT: Appleton & Lange.

Wewers, M.E. and Lenz, E.R. (1987). Relapse among ex-smokers: An example of theory derivation. *Advances in Nursing Science, 9*(2), 44–53.

Whall, A.L. (2005). Conceptual models of nursing. In J.J. Fitzpatrick and A.L. Whall (Eds.), *Conceptual models of nursing: Analysis and application* (4th ed.). New York: Lippincott Williams & Wilkins.

Wilson, J. (1969). *Thinking with concepts*. London, UK: Cambridge University Press.

Woods, N.F. (1985a). Employment, family roles, and mental ill health in young married women. *Nursing Research, 34*(1), 4–10.

Woods, N.F. (1985b). Relationship of socialization and stress to perimenstrual symptoms, disability, and menstrual attitudes. *Nursing Research, 34*(3), 145–149.

Zetterberg, H.L. (1963). *On theory and verification in sociology* (Rev. ed.). Totowa, NJ: Bedminster Press.

11

On Needs and Self-Care

The needs theorists were the first group of nurse theorists who thought of giving nursing care a conceptual order. Virginia Henderson is a historical figure and a pioneer in addressing patients' needs. Dorothea Orem is a contemporary figure. Her ideas about a hierarchy of needs for patients and the activities that nurses perform provided an organizing framework that built on Henderson's work, though she herself does not acknowledge Henderson's influence on her theory (Orem and Taylor, 1986). Her central thesis is a framework that facilitates the assessment of needs, as well as the provision of care that enhances self-care. Orem's theory is reviewed and evaluated in this chapter as a premiere example of needs theories. It is also an example of nursing therapeutics. Fawcett and DeSanto-Madeya (2013) classified her in a developmental category of knowledge based on its focus on growth and development and progression in self-care requisites and self-agency.

DOROTHEA OREM

Theory Description

Orem's theory continues to be one of the most widely discussed and nationally and internationally used theories in nursing. Self-care, although an ambiguous concept with many different meanings, is invariably credited to her. The impetus of Orem's ideas, as is the case for a number of other theorists, was to define content for nursing curricula; this required her to first understand the proper focus of nursing. The seeds of her theory were first published in 1959, in a guide for developing a curriculum for practical nurses (Orem, 1959). As a member of a curriculum subcommittee at Catholic University (1965–1968), Orem recognized that work needed to continue in developing a conceptualization of nursing. Five of the subcommittee members continued to work with another six colleagues for about a decade (1968–1979) to formalize a theory of the process of nursing. In the process, Orem published the first

formal articulation of her ideas (1971), and the group articulated the process of nursing theory development and identified universal elements in nursing that are congruent with Orem's theory (Nursing Development Conference Group [NDCG], 1973, 1979). The second edition of Orem's book appeared in 1980, in which she refined and extended the theory that appeared in the first edition (Orem, 1980). She continued to develop her theoretical framework in subsequent editions to her major book (Orem, 1985, 1991, 1995, 2001a). The major changes in her theory are the advancement in the development of the conceptual components of the three theories, and more specificity in proposing substantive areas in the practical science of self-care. In addition, Orem reformulated the nature of self-care requisites and provided a practice guide to reflect each of the requisites (Denyes, Orem, and SozWiss, 2001).

In her major book at the beginning of the 21st century, in which she provides structure and content not only for the theory of self-care deficit, but for her vision of nursing as a "direct human service," she outlined six themes as a framework. The major one from which she developed the Self-Care Deficit Theory of Nursing (SCDTN) is "why persons need and can be helped through nursing." The second is that there is a "tridimensional relationship" between a person needing nursing care, a relationship with society, an interpersonal relationship, and a relationship with technology. The third theme is that human beings are of a "unitary nature," functioning as persons in their own situations. The fourth theme is very central to her theory: it is that actions are all deliberate, and they are performed to achieve desired ends. The fifth theme is that "methods of helping or assisting" are the foundation for uncovering and developing nursing systems. The sixth very important theme for Orem's thinking is that nursing has both practical and theoretical science components with each having a structure and substance (Orem, 2001a, pp. vi–ix). There is also a theme of intentionality in Orem's work and theoretical development of nursing (Burks, 2001).

The original set of questions that prompted the development of Orem's self-care theory is very similar to most other theorists' questions. What is nursing? How is it differentiated from medicine? What knowledge base should be included in nursing? More specifically, Orem's questions, which she progressively refined over many publications, include (Orem and Taylor, 1986, 2011):

- What is nursing?
- When and why do persons need nursing?
- Do people vary in their needs?
- What types of valid assistance are given?
- What is the proper objective of nursing?
- Why do nurses do what they do?
- What is the structure of what they do?
- What are the outcomes of their care?
- What human and environmental conditions exist calling for the specific actions of nurses?

These questions and Orem's answers to them over the years classified her work as a theory of nursing therapeutics, in addition to classifying it as a "needs" theory. Orem's theory provides a framework for intervention. Orem herself believed that:

. . . self-care deficit theory of nursing will fit into any nursing situation because it is a general theory, that is, an explanation of what is common to all nursing situations, not just an explanation of an individual situation. (Orem, in Fawcett, 2001)

Orem extended SCDTN by specifying three separate theories of self-care, self-care deficit, and nursing systems. The connection among the three theories forms the whole of the self-care deficit theory. Orem indicated that "the general theory [SCDTN] brings together and unifies a theory of self-care and a theory of self-care deficits with the subsuming theory of nursing systems" (Orem and Taylor, 2011, p. 38). Orem identified four themes (postulated entities) in all the theories. These are the person within a particular space/time, attributes of persons, motion or change, and products in each. These entities differentiate among the three theories (Orem, 1991, p. 68). Central to all three theories is that people function and maintain life, health, and well-being by caring for themselves. Implicit in self-care theory is the view of patients as empowered human beings who have self-agency, who are active participants, and who are voiced in their own care (Brown, 2015).

The first theory—the theory of self-care—is based on the fundamental idea of Orem's theory of self-care deficit. Self-care is a human regulatory function that is performed by individuals or is performed for them by others (dependent care). The purpose of self-care is to maintain life, to keep the essential physical and psychic functions going, and to maintain the integrity of a person's functions and development within the framework of conditions that are essential for life (Orem, 2001a). This central focus is based on the presumption that individuals learn self-care practices through experience, education, culture, scientific knowledge, growth, and development. A relationship exists between deliberate self-care actions and the development and functioning of individuals and groups.

The second theory, the essential constituent of self-care deficit nursing theory is "self-care deficit." It is the most comprehensive element, and is the core of her ideas. The central idea of this theory is a conceptual image of individuals who are completely or partially unable to know or to engage in providing care that ensures functioning and development for themselves or for their dependents. This theory is based on two sets of presuppositions. The first revolves around the person's ability to manage and engage in providing self-care and dependent care and to take actions to maintain and manage health and functioning. The second revolves around what societies are capable of offering to help with services for individuals who are in a state of dependency.

The third theory, the theory of nursing system(s), describes therapeutic self-care requisites and the actions or systems involved in self-care within the context of their contractual and interpersonal relations in human beings with self-care deficits (Orem and Taylor, 1986, p. 44). It presupposes that experienced nurses provide intentional care for individuals whose care needs exceed their ability to provide such care for themselves. All three theories together become a general theory of nursing, the SCDTN (Orem, 1995).

Advancing knowledge in nursing requires a focus on the three theories of *self-care*, which is defined as "the practice of activities that individuals initiate and perform on their own behalf in maintaining life, health, and well-being" (Orem, 1985, p. 84). Self-care is not limited to a person providing care for himself; it includes care offered by others on behalf of the person (dependent care). Care may be offered by members of the family or outsiders until a person is able to perform self-care. Self-care is purposeful and contributes to human structural integrity, functioning, and development (Orem, 1985, p. 86). As such, Orem negated some who criticized this theory's applicability to other cultures that are more family- and community-focused, and she indicated that the knowledge needed for self-care requisites must incorporate variations by cultural groups (Orem and Taylor, 2011). Developing the theoretical and practical knowledge about self-care requisites is in essence considered as the fundamental science for self-care. It requires qualitative and quantitative standards for the content and regulation of the requisites, identification of barriers to meeting the self-care requisites, availability of what self-care agents should know and be aware of, and evidence and exemplars of effective experiences in meeting the requisites (Denyes et al., 2001). The purposes to be attained are universal, developmental, and health-deviation self-care requisites. Self-care deficit is the relationship between the action capabilities of an individual and the demands for self-care. Deficit, which should be considered a relationship rather than a disorder, is a relationship between the actions an individual takes or should take, and his capability to do so (Orem, 2001a).

The three types of self-care requisites are universal, developmental, and health deviation. The universal self-care requisites are found in all human beings and are associated with their life processes and general well-being. There are eight universal self-care requisites, which in other theories may be considered human needs: (1) maintenance of sufficient intake of care, (2) water, (3) food, (4) care associated with elimination, (5) maintenance of balance between activity and rest, (6) prevention of hazards, (7) promotion of functioning, and (8) development and maintenance with social groups (Orem, 2001a). Developmental requisites are related to the different stages that human beings undergo, such as adolescence, pregnancy, and aging, among other stages in the life cycle. Examples of developmental self-care requisites are those related to needs for understanding of habits of introspection and reflection about self; meaningful engagement in productive work; understanding values, emotions, actions, and impulses; and the promotion of positive mental health (Orem, 2001a). The third set of requisites result from or are attached to deviations in the structural or functional aspects of human beings (Orem, 1991, p. 125). The health deviation self-care requisites arise from disease, genetic and constitutional defects, and human structural and functional deviation. Actions for treatment require seeking medical assistance, being cognizant of deleterious effects of disease, medical care, learning to live with conditions and complying with prescribed medical regimes, and therapeutic and rehabilitative

measures (Orem, 2001a). Orem operationalized each one of these requisites. The focus of nursing is on the identification of self-care requisites (Box 11-1), the designing of methods and actions to meet the requisites, and "the totality of the demands for self-care action" (Orem, 1985, p. 88).

The totality of self-care actions that are to be performed for some duration to meet human self-care requisites by using valid methods and related sets of operations or actions is termed the *therapeutic self-care demand* (Orem, 1985, p. 88). Therapeutic self-care demand is based on deliberate action (Orem, 2001a, p. 150). "Deliberate actions of persons are based on their judgments about what is appropriate under existent conditions or circumstances" (Orem, 1991, p. 79). Nurses use "compound actions," meaning that their actions need to be coordinated, performed simultaneously, or related. The agent who performs the action must have "sensory knowledge" and an "awareness" of the situation; the agent "reflects" on that knowledge and "makes decisions." Actions are performed in phases (Orem, 1991, pp. 79–86).

The provider of self-care, whether self or other, is considered a *self-care agent*. It is an entity to be described in terms of development and operability—which are influenced by such variables as genetics, and cultural or experiential backgrounds—and in terms of adequacy. The latter could be evaluated by considering self-care capabilities and self-care demand (Orem, 1987). The agent is a person who takes action, whether this person is the patient or the nurse (Orem, 2001a). If the nurse is the agent, then the care provided is based on the nurse's abilities to diagnose self-care deficits through cumulated levels of cognitive processes that include level of presentation (sensory data taken and organized), level of intelligence (questioning data), level of reflection (forming hypotheses), and reasoning (forming judgments) (Renpenning, SozWiss, Denyes, et al., 2011).

Nursing care is therapeutic self-care designed to supplement self-care requisites in the absence of capabilities to do so. There are three fundamental nursing sciences:

- **Wholly compensatory:** The nurse is expected to accomplish all the patient's therapeutic self-care or to compensate for the patient's inability to engage in self-care, or when the patient needs continuous guidance in self-care. This is the science of self-care (Fawcett, 2001, p. 35).
- **Partly compensatory:** Both nurse and patient engage in meeting self-care needs. This is

BOX 11-1	SELF-CARE REQUISITES—OREM

Universal Self-Care Requisites

- The maintenance of a sufficient intake of air.
- The maintenance of a sufficient intake of water.
- The maintenance of a sufficient intake of food.
- The provision of care associated with elimination processes and excrements.
- The maintenance of a balance between activity and rest.
- The maintenance of a balance between solitude and social interaction.
- The prevention of hazards to human life, human functioning, and human well-being.
- The promotion of human functioning and development within social groups in accord with human potential, known human limitations, and the human desire to be normal (Orem, 1985, pp. 90–91).

Developmental Self-Care Requisites

- The bringing about and maintenance of living conditions that support life processes and promote the processes of development; that is, human progress toward higher levels of the organization of human structures and toward maturation.
- Provision of care either to prevent the occurrence of deleterious effects of conditions that can affect human development or so as to mitigate or overcome these effects from various conditions (1985, p. 96).

Health-Deviation Self-Care Requisites

- Seeking and securing appropriate medical assistance in the event of exposure to specific physical or biologic agents or environmental conditions associated with human pathologic events and states, or when there is evidence of genetic, physiologic, or psychological conditions known to produce or be associated with human pathology.
- Being aware of and attending to the effects and results of pathologic conditions and states
- Effectively carrying out medically prescribed diagnostic, therapeutic, and rehabilitative measures directed to the prevention of specific types of pathology, to the pathology itself, to the resolution of human integrated functioning, to the correction of deformities or abnormalities, or to compensation for disabilities.
- Being aware of and attending to or regulating the discomforting or deleterious effects of medical care measures performed or prescribed by the physician.
- Modifying the self-concept (and self-image) in accepting oneself as being in a particular state of health and in need of specific forms of health care.
- Learning to live with the effects of pathologic conditions and states and the effects of medical diagnostic and treatment measures in a lifestyle that promotes continued personal development (1985, pp. 99–100).

the science of development and exercise of self-care agency (SCA).

- **Supportive developmental system:** The system requires assistance in decision-making, behavior control, and acquisition of knowledge and skills. Under this system, patients are able to perform self-care with assistance (Orem, 1985, pp. 152–156). This is the science of human assistance for persons who have self-care deficits.

Orem's theory is based on explicit and implicit premises (Orem, 1983, 1987, 2001a) (Box 11-2) that "do not express a singular belief in a clear way at either the philosophical or more general level of discourse" (Smith, 1987, p. 93).

Orem provides nursing with a number of primitive concepts (Box 11-3) that are defined theoretically and operationally, the esoteric nature of the

terminology being one of the obstacles that may have influenced the initially slow use of the theory in practice (Anna, Christensen, Hohn, et al., 1978). The theory includes both abstract (health, SCA) and concrete (universal self-care needs) variables (Box 11-4).

When concepts are defined, their relationships are not entirely clear as, for example, with health and self-care or illness and self-care deficit. The primitiveness, the overlap, and the undefined boundaries between concepts create multiple interpretations, particularly for those who are new to operationalizing the theory. The SCA is an example of an undefined or primitive concept with multiple meanings. When should an agent be identified? What is the extent of self-care performed by an agent to make it self-care by self or by others? How do you determine the agent? By whose perception? (Anna

BOX 11-2	ASSUMPTIONS—OREM

Explicit Assumptions

- Nursing is a deliberate, purposeful helping service performed by nurses for the sake of others over a period of time.
- Persons (human agency) are capable and willing to perform self-care for self or for dependent members of the family.
- Self-care is part of life that is necessary for health, human development, and well-being.
- Education and culture influence individuals.
- Self-care is learned through human interaction and communication.
- Self-care includes deliberate and systematic actions performed to meet known needs for care (Orem, 1980, pp. 34–38).
- "Human agency is exercised in discovering, developing, and transmitting to others ways and means to identify needs for and make inputs to self and others" (1987, p. 73).
- Each person possesses "powers and capabilities, personal dispositions, talents, interests, and values" (Orem, 2001a, vii).

Implicit Assumptions

- People should be self-reliant and responsible for their own care needs, as well as for others in the family who are not able to care for themselves.
- People are individuals with entities that are distinct from others and from their environment.
- "Nursing is a form of *action-in-interaction* between two or more persons. The person is an essential substantial unity" (Taylor, Geden, Isaramalai, et al., 2000, p. 105).
- "Successfully meeting universal and developmental self-care requisites is an important component of primary prevention of disease and ill health" (Ailinger, Lasus, and Braun, 2003, p. 198).
- "A person's knowledge of potential health problem is a prerequisite for promoting healthy self-care behaviors to prevent disease" (Ailinger et al., 2003, p. 198).
- "Self-care and dependent care are both behaviors learned within the context of the group and within a sociocultural context" (Taylor, Renpenning, Geden, et al., 2001).
- "The culture and class can influence professional judgments" (Lauder, 2001, p. 550).

BOX 11-3	CONCEPTS—OREM

Self-care
  Deficits
  Capabilities
  Demands
  Dependent care
  Dependent-care deficit
Nursing systems
  Wholly compensatory
  Partly compensatory
  Supportive educative
Self-care requisites
  Universal self-care
  Developmental self-care
  Health-deviation self-care
Therapeutic self-care demands
Self-care agency
Nursing agency
Dependent-care agency
Human and environment
BCFS
  Internal
  External

et al., 1978; Smith, 1979). These are examples of what an adequate theoretical and operational definition could do to decrease ambiguity and enhance clarity. Some of the variables are nonvariables (e.g., self-care), thereby limiting their propositional power (Table 11-1).

Limitations of the theory are also demonstrated in other ways, as when definitions are considered in relationship to health care systems. As the world of health care is shifting from predominately acute/hospital care to chronic/community/home care, how self-care is conceptualized and used must also be modified to reflect how society and health care systems define, support, and pay for nurses who modify and enhance self-care. According to Wilkinson and Whitehead (2009), the ambiguity of the definition of the self-care concept becomes more acute when health care delivery systems and political structures are not supportive of self-care management by individuals, families, and communities. A more congruent consensual definition is needed before self-care can be fully utilized.

BOX 11-4	THEORIES—OREM

Self-care deficit theory of nursing: "A general theory descriptive and explanatory of what nursing is and should be."

1. A theory of self-care
   A. Self-care
   B. SCA
      1. Foundational capabilities and dispositions (FCD)
      2. Power components (PC) of SCA
      3. Self-care operations: the phases of deliberate actions
   C. Self-care requisites (see Table 11-1: Denyes, Orem, and SozWiss, 2001, p. 50)
      1. Essential enduring requisites: regulatory of human functioning and development
         • Universal self-care requisites
         • Developmental self-care requisites
      2. Situation-specific requisites: existent or predicted internal or external conditions of functioning and development
         • Health deviation self-care requisites: regulation or control of human structural or functional disorders
         • Developmental self-care requisites: mitigating or overcoming deleterious effects of developmental disorders and disabilities
2. A theory of self-care deficit
3. A theory of nursing system

A theory of dependent-care (Taylor, Renpenning, Geden, et al., 2001)
Dependency, Dependent-care agency, Dependent-care agent, Dependent-care demand, Dependent-care deficit, Dependent-care system, Dependent-care unit, Social dependency

Orem's propositions are summarized in Box 11-5 Propositions developed by Orem (1985, 2001a) correspond to her three proposed theories and their central ideas. These have progressed from existence propositions, to relational and predictive propositions, attesting to the stage of development of the theory (Orem, 1995). Despite the complexity of the construct of self-care, Orem's theory has become part of the lexicon of health care and is beginning to be adopted by patients and health care professionals alike.

Theory Analysis

The Theorist

The late Dorothea Orem, born in Maryland, in 1914, earned her Diploma and Bachelor of Science degree in the 1930s, and her Master of Science degree in 1945, from the Catholic University of America, Washington, DC. She earned honorary doctorates in 1976 from Georgetown University, Washington, DC, and in 1980, from Incarnate Word College, San Antonio, Texas. She established a private consulting company, Orem and Shields, Inc., in Chevy Chase, Maryland, perhaps to accommodate the diverse practice arenas that are using

her theory and that need her assistance. She was involved in nursing practice, nursing service, and nursing education at different levels of education (practical, diploma, baccalaureate, and graduate). She taught at two schools of nursing: the Catholic University of America and the Medical College of Virginia, Richmond (Foster and Janssens, 1980). Dorothea Orem passed away in June 2007, after a long life (93 years) of dedication to articulating the essence and meaning of nursing.

The impetus of Orem's theory was an attempt to conceptualize a curriculum for a diploma program by isolating and specifying nursing actions. In this work, she introduced the ideas related to self-care (1959). She continued her theory development activities as a member of two crucial overlapping groups, the Nursing Model Committee of the Catholic University nursing faculty and the NDCG (1973, 1979). She incorporated the ideas evolving from these two collaborative groups into her own text in different forms until 1991, when she integrated and acknowledged their work in her own major book on self-care.

Orem's work benefited from these collaborations, and she continued in the same collaborative tradition with other groups who worked on the further development of self-care requisites. Among these

TABLE 11-1	Definition of Domain Concepts—Orem
Nursing	Nursing is art, a helping service, and a technology (Orem, 1985, pp. 144–146).
	Actions are deliberately selected and performed by nurses to help individuals or groups under their care to maintain or change conditions in themselves or their environments (p. 5).
	Encompasses the patient's perspective of health condition, the physician's perspective, and the nursing perspective. Universal, developmental, and health deviation self-care requisites.
Goal of nursing	To render the patient or members of his family capable of meeting the patient's self-care needs (1985, p. 54).
	"1. To maintain a state of health; 2. To regain normal or near normal state of health in the event of disease or injury; 3. To stabilize, control, or minimize the effects of chronic poor health or disability" (1980, p. 124).
Health	"Health and healthy are terms used to describe living things . . . [it is when] they are structurally and functionally whole or sound . . . wholeness or integrity . . . includes that which makes a person human, . . . operating in conjunction with physiological and psychophysiological mechanisms and a material structure (biologic life) and in relation to and interacting with other human beings (interpersonal and social life)" (1980, pp. 118–119).
	"A state of being whole and sound" (1985, p. 176).
	Well-being is a perception of contentment, happiness, and pleasure, by spiritual experiences and through a sense of personalization (1985, p. 179).
Environment	Environment components are environmental factors, environmental elements, environmental conditions, and developmental environment (1985, pp. 140–141).
	Limited view of environment to its usefulness as a helping method. Therefore, defined under Nursing Therapeutics. Although environment is mentioned in a diagram (1985, p. 85) and in the definition of nursing (1985, p. 53), it is not defined.
Human being	Has the capacity to reflect, symbolize, and use symbols (1985, p. 174).
	Conceptualized as a total being with universal, developmental needs and capable of continuous self-care (1985).
	A unity that can function biologically, symbolically, and socially (1985, p. 175).
Nursing client	A human being who has "health-related or health-derived limitations that render him incapable of continuous self-care or dependent care or limitations that result in ineffective or incomplete care" (1985, pp. 34–35). A person who is deficient in universal, developmental, or health-related self-care requisites. . . . A human being is the focus of nursing only when a self-care requisite exceeds self-care capabilities (1985, p. 35).
Nursing problem	Deficits in universal, developmental, and health-derived or health-related conditions.
Nursing process	A system to determine (1) why a person is under care, (2) a plan for care, (3) the implementation of care.
Nurse–patient relations	Not defined.
Nursing therapeutics	Deliberate, systematic, and purposeful action.
	Total compensatory, partly compensatory, or educative supportive care in universal, developmental, and health-deviation self-care deficits, using several helping methods; acting or doing for others, guiding, supporting, providing a developmental environment, teaching (1985, pp. 88–90).
Focus	"The special concern of nursing is the individual's need for self-care action and the provision and management of it on a continuous basis in order to sustain life and health, recover from disease or injury, and cope with their effects" (Orem, 1985, p. 54).
	Dependency or incapacities due to health/illness situation (1983, p. 208).

various groups are the International Orem Society for Nursing Science and Scholarship, which was founded at the beginning of the 1990s and which started by publishing newsletters that further developed into a journal, *Self-Care, Dependent Care and Nursing*. Faculty from the University of Missouri, Columbia, under the leadership of Susan Taylor, have continued to extend and refine her theory, seeking Dorothea Orem's consultation and guidance (Cox and Taylor, 2005; Denyes et al.,

BOX 11-5 | PROPOSITIONS—OREM

Person and Nursing Client

- Human beings are capable of providing their own self-care or care for dependents to meet universal, developmental, and health-deviation self-care requisites. These capabilities are learned and recalled.
- Self-care abilities are influenced by age, developmental state, experiences, and sociocultural background, as well as by other variables.
- Self-care deficits are to balance between self-care demands and self-care capabilities and are an indication of a state of social dependency.
- Self-care or dependent care is mediated by age, developmental stage, life experience, sociocultural orientation, health, and available resources.
- Human beings are persons/selves, agents, organisms, users of symbols, and objects (Orem, 1997).
- "Mature and maturing individuals have requirements and responsibilities for self-maintenance, self-management, care of dependents, and the fulfillment of their human potential" (Orem, 2001a, viii).
- "The formulation of a requisite requires evidence of persons' states of human functioning and human development and factors that condition these states. Within the framework of the self-care deficit nursing theory these factors are named basic conditioning factors (e.g., age, health state, and the developmental state)" (Denyes, Orem, and SozWiss, 2001, p. 49).
- "Five areas of a science of self-care are self-care, self-care agency, self-care requisites, therapeutic self-care demand, and self-care practices/self-care systems" (Denyes et al., 2001, p. 50).
- "Self-care requisites are principles to guide the selection, choice, and conduct of regulatory actions in the care of self" (Denyes et al., 2001, p. 51).
- "Self-care requisites that are unique to an individual because of a life situation or prevailing internal or external conditions and circumstances are specific and not generalizable" (Denyes et al., 2001, p. 51).
- "Self-care systems and dependent-care systems are produced by individuals through the exercise of human powers and capabilities named self-care agency and dependent-care agency" (Denyes et al., 2001, p. 54) (Orem, 2001a, viii).

Nursing Therapeutics

- Therapeutic self-care includes actions of nurses, patients, and others who regulate self-care capabilities and meet self-care needs.
- Nurses assess the abilities of patients to meet their self-care needs and their potential for refraining from performing their self-care.
- Nurses engage in selecting valid and reliable processes or technologies or actions for meeting self-care demands.
- Components of therapeutic self-care are wholly compensatory, partly compensatory, and supportive–educative.

Based on Orem (1985), Orem and Taylor (1986), and Orem (2001a).

2001; Taylor, 2001; Taylor, Renpenning, Geden, et al., 2001). In addition, the establishment of the Institute for Self-Care at George Mason University promoted a more general concept of self-care as central in nursing and made a contribution to the measurements of Orem's basic condition factors (Moore and Pichler, 2000). Another important milestone related to Orem's conceptualization is the federal support given by Wayne State University for predoctoral and postdoctoral fellows promoting studies in self-care (Artinian, Magnan, Sloan, et al., 2002). Orem continued to refine her ideas through the Orem Study Group (Fawcett

and DeSanto-Madeya, 2013), and Orem scholars continue to publish their work in *Self-Care, Dependent Care and Nursing*, the official journal of the International Orem Society (Clarke, Allison, Berbiglia, et al., 2009). In her honor, Susan Taylor published a paper that Dorothea Orem had, prior to her death, drafted for a conference held in 2004 in Ulm, Germany (Orem and Taylor, 2011).

Paradigmatic Origins

Orem's theory has been classified as a systems theory by Riehl-Sisca and Roy (1980), as an interaction model by Riehl-Sisca (1989), as developmental by Fawcett (1995), and as a needs theory in this book. Orem used concepts from all these paradigms, a process that may lead to the conclusion that the theory evolved over time from a synthesis and integration of all of them. Her definition of health as a state of wholeness, her conception of the integrity of the person, and the use of systems of nursing may have evolved from systems theory. These, however, are isolated concepts, more like terms, not derived conceptually or defined in terms of the original paradigm. A system model implies a feedback mechanism between nurse and patient, and such bidirectional movement is not congruent with this theory, in which the nurse–patient relationship is predicated by the one-way transfer of agency (Melnyk, 1983, p. 173).

Similarly, Orem views a person with self-care deficits as socially dependent; the capability to engage in self-care and to meet universal self-care needs appears to characterize a more integrated development. These are concepts reflecting a developmental view of human beings, yet their lack of centrality in the theory, lack of definition, and absence of developmental stages and deliberate progression to more complex entities deny the theory a developmental origin. In fact, classifying the theory as either a systems or a developmental theory would highlight gaps in defining concepts and propositions central to the two paradigms but tangential to Orem's theory.

Through my analysis, I have concluded that the paradigmatic origin of the theory is more appropriately the needs theory of Henderson (1991) or the functional theory of Abdellah, Beland, Martin, et al. (1961). Henderson (1991) identified 14 needs (Pearson, 2008). Universal self-care needs are similar to the needs identified by Henderson, although the uniqueness of Orem's theory lies more in the expectation of that person's capability to engage in his own self-care. Health-deviation requisites are an extension and not a refinement of Henderson's concept of nursing. Orem offers a fine example of the process inherent in theory development, based on other theories in which new concepts evolve and others are derived. It is an example to be emulated as nurses refine and extend other theories.

Orem's theory has been designated as being based on "moderate realism" by Banfield (1997, 2001) in doctoral dissertation research from Wayne State University (Biggs, 2008; Taylor, Geden, Isaramalai, et al., 2000). This view of the philosophical underpinnings has been endorsed by Orem (Fawcett, 2001) and further explicated by others (Taylor et al., 2000). Tenets of moderate realism are that human beings are powerful agents to act on their own behalf, that there is an objective world outside an individual, that knowing is partial but constantly evolving, and that there is a tendency toward determinism and causability. However, according to Wallace (1996), a realistic philosopher, even with a focus on determinism and causability, there is room for probability and tendencies toward alternative and chance outcomes. Orem acknowledged Wallace as influencing her thinking about science in nursing as intellectual knowledge as opposed to sense knowledge. Intellectual knowledge is concerned with the nature, meanings, and content of knowledge achieved through intellectual processes (Orem and Taylor, 2011).

Beyond discussing the origins in their analysis of the philosophic foundation of Orem's theory, Taylor et al. (2000) concluded that Orem's proposed nursing science is a practical science with both speculative and practical knowledge. The focus is on action, hence my classification of this theory as a nursing therapeutic theory as well as a needs and self-care theory. Both nurses and patients engage in deliberate actions, and these actions form the bases of the practical science of nursing (Orem, 2001a). The actions of both nurses and patients have been linked with Bandura's (1997, 2000) theory and research on self-efficacy and self-agency. The idea of linking them stemmed from the assumptions that perception of capacity to act and self-manage is predicated on the skills, knowledge, abilities, and beliefs in the ability to manage and care for self. An example of such integration is in the analysis provided by Timmins (2008), in which the author argued that, in reviewing the effectiveness of conceptual models, the notion of self-care for clients with cardiovascular problems tends to surface as important, but equally or even more significant is the relationship between clients and nurses.

Internal Dimensions

Orem's theories are interrelated and centered around self-care. Their level of development and interrelationship suggest that they are concepts and part of one theory, a nursing therapeutic theory of self-care. Orem's theory of self-care is a descriptive theory developed around an attempt to clarify the components of care offered by nurses and a conceptualization of the nursing client. It is a deductive theory with a hypothetical constructive beginning (Orem, 1985,

1991, 1997, 2001a) that is based on support from clinical experiences. Fawcett and DeSanto-Madeya (2013) makes the point that Orem made extensive use of inductive reasoning because Orem used her clinical experiences as examples to support the notion that self-care limitation is the need for nursing care. However, the theory evolved deductively from other theories, with support from collaborators in the NDCG (1973, 1979) and from questions that Orem posited in her writing, *Guides for Developing Curricula for the Education of Practical Nurses* in 1959 (Orem, 1959). The genesis of the ideas did not come from practice situations (inductive reasoning); they evolved from thinking, other theories, group discussions, and the logical and formal development of ideas (deductive reasoning) supported by clinical exemplars. Orem herself credits her own practice and reflections on others' practice for her theory's beginnings, making it an inductive theory. Perhaps this theory origin is an example of how induction and deduction are synergistically connected, as there is rationale to classify it as both inductive and deductive. It is a concatenated theory with more potential for existence propositions to describe the properties of the various concepts and to delineate the elements of such complex constructs as the exercise of self-care. It uses a field approach to theory construction. The units are understood in terms of other smaller units, and the theory of self-care is subsumed by the theory of self-care deficit, and that, in turn, subsumed by the theory of nursing system.

The theory of self-care deficit is focused on and limited to dealing with individual self-care deficits, rather than with the entire human being. It deals essentially in what Orem calls the *practical science* of nursing, with one of the domain concepts—clinical therapeutics—and the actions contained in that therapeutic, and it offers one modality for care—the development of self-care abilities to meet the deficit and to meet the requirements and demands for self-care. The theory focuses on actions and deals with knowledge of control. It is a theory developed using an operational method; alternative methods of action are dependent on the nurse's discrimination and decision about the needs and the action (Barnum, 1994, pp. 143–144). It is the agent's perspective that decides on alternative action. All actions are deliberate, and they depend on the power and capabilities of an individual who is a nurse or a patient. Power has two components, self-care or nursing-care agency. She identified 10 SCA power components that make it possible to

perform in self-care. These range from awareness of self as self-care agent to use of physical energy, body position, and movements to the importance of being motivated, communicating, and integrating self-care in personal, family, and community living. There are also eight nursing agency power components that include managing the self as a professional; having the necessary knowledge, skills, motives, and willingness to provide nursing; possessing the ability to direct action toward outcomes; and having the ability to be flexible and consistent.

Orem's theory of self-care provides a comprehensive view and framework for simplistic nursing therapeutics and components that can be operationalized in different practice areas, including the community (Aponte and Nickitas, 2007; Hines, Sampselle, Ronis, et al., 2007), and for dealing with different types of problems (Gast and Montgomery, 2005).

Theory Critique

Orem's theory has been operationalized and used in research, practice, and administration. It lends itself to research for a number of reasons. Orem herself developed propositions linking the theory concepts and addressing at least two of the central concepts in nursing—patient–nurse interaction and self-care. Both are used for diagnosis and intervention. Orem also continued to revise and refine her theory with her mentees and collaborators. However, because the theory provides a framework to organize practice and interventions, it therefore appeals to nurses for its high relevance to their daily care and is used more to guide practice than for research. It is a theory about practice and a theory that is for practice, even though it was developed initially to guide curricula. It provides a framework in which appropriate parts of each of the theories can be used in isolation or together, depending on the situation. There are several reasons for the rather speedy adoption of the theory by nursing practice. The language of the theory extends concepts advanced by Henderson, Abdellah, and, to some extent, Nightingale, using language that is familiar to nurses. As nursing care shifted from a medical model, curricula and practice used a needs and functional approach, a shift that was gentle and gradual, the kind of progress that is integral to Orem's theory. Orem also delineated the technical and professional aspects of nursing practice in both the Nursing Development Conference publications (1973, 1979) and in her first book (Orem, 1971). This differentiation resonated well with those who were developing curricula, although, according to Orem, her theory could be used, is used, and should be used as a framework for diploma, associate degree, baccalaureate, and continuing-education programs (Berbiglia and Banfield, 2014; Fawcett, 2001; Fawcett and DeSanto-Madeya, 2013).

Orem's theory also incorporates rather than rejects the medical perspective (Johnston, 1983) and purports to build nursing practice on it. Furthermore, the theory uses medical science language, with which most nurses are familiar and which many prefer. It presumes a list of needs that evolve out of a pathophysiologic or medical focus, which explains its utility to hospital care. It establishes a relationship between a sick person and a nurse, but not enough of a relationship between a well person and a nurse. It also provides limited utility for nurses who care for patients who refuse to achieve their maximum level of independence (Easton, 1993). The theory is developed around the ill person and conveys the centrality of individual and institutional care, perhaps the most appealing feature for the majority of nurses who care for the sick (Taylor, 1990). However, it has been used for all ages and in all settings. Orem extended the use of the theory to the care of families (Orem, 1983; Taylor, 2001), and it was further extended by her colleagues to multiperson and community situations (Taylor and Renpenning, 2001). It also appeals to those who wish to model Kinlein (1977), who "hung her own shingle" when she went into private practice. It is perhaps because of all these reasons, and the operational method in theory development, that we see more literature documenting the utility of this theory for practice than is true for other theories.

The theory has broad application across care settings. It has wide appeal for use in critical care (Hurlock-Chorostecki, 1999), with chronically ill patients (Burks, 1999), with patients with diabetes (Allison, 1973; Backscheider, 1971, 1974; Berhe, Demissie, Kahsay, et al., 2012; Fitzgerald, 1980), in caring for patients with amyotrophic lateral sclerosis (Taylor, 1988), in psychiatry (Buckwalter and Kerfoot, 1982; Caley, Dirksen, Engalla, et al., 1980; Underwood, 1980), in critical and acute-care settings (Budinger, 2007; Coyle and Martin, 2007; Mullin, 1980; Noone, 1995), in preoperative and postoperative care (Bromley, 1980; Campuzano, 1982; Dropkin, 1981), in hospice care (Murphy, 1981; Walborn, 1980), and with adult and geriatric patients, as well as with children (Anna et al., 1978; Cox and Taylor, 2005; Mosher and Moore, 1998).

Researchers and clinicians have adapted it to older people living at home (Westerbotn, Fahlström, Agüero-Torres, et al., 2008), and with hypertensive patients in the community (Akyol, Cetinkaya, Bakan, et al., 2007). The theory was used to individualize care for cancer patients (Morse and Werner, 1988), for patients with end-stage renal disease (Greenfield and Pace, 1985), for patients on dialysis (Simmons, 2009), for patients with drug problems (Compton, 1989), and in managing anxiety in HIV-infected patients (Phillips and Morrow, 1998).

Although the theory has generally been considered more appropriate for use with adults (Kumar, 2007; Melnyk, 1983), some extended its use to the care of children and adolescents (Baker and Denyes, 2008; Michael and Sewall, 1980; Moore and Beckwitt, 2006; Norris, 1991; Slusher, 1999). In applying an asthma action plan based on developing self-care skills in adolescents who live in Turkey, the investigators observed significant improvements in the adolescents' abilities to manage their asthma (Altay and Cavusoglu, 2013).

It is important to note that developing and enhancing self-care requires a certain level of health literacy. There is evidence that health literacy has positive effects on knowledge about health and illness conditions. However, this relationship is not always supported. For example, Chen, Yehle, Albert, et al. (2014) found out that there was an independent effect for health literacy on knowledge of heart failure and for self-efficacy on self-care, but there was no indirect effect for health literacy on self-care or self-efficacy. They conclude that there may be other factors that could better explain the relationship between knowledge, self-efficacy, and self-care.

The theory appeals to global scholars as a framework for research. Researchers found that training nurses to provide patient-centered care and testing their level of SCA was related to increased activity level in patients with hypertension; that is, the higher the SCA of the nurses, the more the patients increased their physical activity (Drevenhorn, Bengtson, Nyberg, et al., 2015). It was the basis for the development and validation of a research instrument to measure self-care requisites in Spanish-speaking populations with schizophrenia (Roldan-Merino, Lluch-Canut, Menarguez-Alcaina, et al., 2013; Roldan-Merino, Miguel-Ruiz, Lluch-Canut, et al., 2015). It was used in Scandinavia to develop caring strategies to alleviate suffering in patients with chronic pain by confirming the patient's humanity, by providing sympathy and compassion, and by helping patients recognize and deal with their own needs (Arman and Hok, 2015). Similarly, it was used to test level of adherence to self-care practices, particularly in monitoring blood glucose and diet management practices of patients in Ethiopia (Berhe et al., 2012).Using the theory, researchers studying how socioeconomic status and health literacy affect the ability of South African patients to be effective as self-care agents concluded that providing professional nursing care can help patients achieve better symptom management, fewer visits to hospital, and prevention of self-neglect (Rabie, Klopper, and Watson, 2015). In a randomized clinical trial in Iran, the quality of life of patients hospitalized with burns significantly improved when a self-care model was used (Hashemi, Dolatabad, Yektatalab, et al., 2014).

The theory was also used in caring for gerontologic patients in community health nursing settings (Clark, 1986). It has been used as a framework for community health care (Taylor and McLaughlin, 1991; Taylor and Renpenning, 2001) and for identifying the best ways to communicate information to parents about children's vaccinations, thus increasing knowledge and empowering self-care for parents (Wilson, Baker, Nordstrom, et al., 2008) and demonstrating its utility for community care. The theory also has institutional utility (Bonamy, Schultz, Graham, et al., 1995). The clarity of the theory is questionable in light of its complexity, but the diversity of its utility, as demonstrated in a variety of subspecialties, has made it appealing to clinicians and, more recently, to researchers as well. It provides nurses with collegial visibility (Bennett, 1980), and once nurses acquire the language of the theory through staff development programs, they tend to use it (McLaughlin, 1993; Walker, 1993).

Nurse administrators have found the theory amenable to implementation in a number of institutions, and a great number of chief nurses (16 of 24) of Department of Veterans Affairs medical centers reported using either Orem's theory alone or in combination with the work of other theorists (Bonamy et al., 1995). Orem (1989) herself proposed a framework for nursing administration (Orem, 2001a). Miller (1980) challenged nursing administrators to create a climate that would enhance the use of theory, although she did not give much guidance or exemplars for implementation on a large scale involving nursing administrators. She offered a model for nursing practice based on Orem's theory, demonstrating its utility for care in acute illness, convalescence, and restored health.

The model was based more on a developmental, health–illness continuum than on Orem's theory. Others have described the utility of the theory as "a guide for the nursing activities within a hospital nursing service" (Coleman, 1980, p. 323); in organizing nursing care in independent practice (Backscheider, 1974); in psychiatric units (Underwood, 1980); particularly, in nurse-run clinics (Allison, 1973); in five pilot units at the Toronto General Hospital (Reid, Allen, Gauthier, et al., 1989); and in a Veterans Affairs medical center (Bonamy et al., 1995). It was also used effectively as a framework for a hospital-based utilization review process (Harrison-Raines, 1993). It is used in clinical practice internationally in Canada (Lanigan, 2000), the United Kingdom, and Australia, among other countries (Fawcett and DeSanto-Madeya, 2013; Walker, 1993).

The theory evolved from interest in curricula for diploma and baccalaureate programs and the need to differentiate between technical and professional education. Therefore, its utility to nursing education is enhanced by the theorist's interest. The curriculum subcommittee of the School of Nursing, Georgetown University, of which Orem, Backscheider, and Kinlein were members, developed a curriculum based on ideas that later informed the development of the theory. Not surprisingly, the theory has been used as a conceptual framework in associate-degree programs (Fenner, 1979). The framework is also used in the schools of nursing at the University of Southern Mississippi in Hattiesburg and the University of Missouri at Columbia (Fawcett, 1995), and partially for specific courses in a number of other universities (Fawcett, 2001). In 2001, Orem identified two types of knowledge, the foundational and the practice nursing sciences, which inspired faculty members at some schools in the United States to utilize the SCDTN as an educational model for their baccalaureate program curricula (Berbiglia, 2011). It is of note that Orem's theory was also used to support the revised German Nursing Act by providing a framework for integrated curriculum for general nursing knowledge prior to specialization (Hintze, 2011). While these examples provide evidence for the use of Orem's theory as a framework for curricula, they also provide a strong support for the significance and utility of using a conceptual framework to guide the development, implementation, and evaluation of nursing curricula (Berbiglia, 2011). Similarly, the theory could be used as a framework for assessing self-care activities in students (Ashcraft and Gatto, 2015).

External Components of Theory

Orem's theory is congruent with the prevailing era of nursing practice that focuses on the sick and the institutionalized, which has increasingly become the core of health (illness) care at the turn of the 21st century. As we shift focus to well individuals and to the community, extensions and refinements will need to be made. The focus on health deficits due to illness creating self-care deficits will need to be supplemented with a focus on health benefit/assets, centering resources, and potential (Melnyk, 1983), thereby allowing prevention and health promotion care. Its congruence with prevailing social values is paradoxical. Although the theory promotes the patient as being responsible for his own self-care and a partner in all decisions pertaining to his care (prevailing values in nursing, specifically, and in Western society, in general), the theory is based on values that see the patient as dependent, expecting goals to be set for him, goals that involve him in developing the highest potential for self-care. Furthermore, what if a patient prefers that others take care of him? Orem herself has a response to this question: Nurses must help the patient to reconceptualize himself or herself as a self-care agent (Orem, 2001a). Patients need to be aware of the need and learn to care for self.

The theory enjoys a wide circle of contagiousness that extends to practice, research, and administration, and includes many geographical areas such as Asia, Europe, and the Americas. There are indications and testimonials to its cross-cultural utility (Wang, 1997). However, some have determined that a fundamental constraint in using the theory is related to the values of the individualism principle, which is more prevalent in U.S. cultures (Behi, 1986) as compared to other cultures that expect families and communities to continue to provide care for patients until healing and recovery are complete. In spite of these concerns, researchers and clinicians from different countries used Orem theories as is or modified them to reflect the practices of a particular country. Examples include descriptions of management strategies for medications among older people in Sweden (Westerbotn et al., 2008). The findings demonstrated that older people are capable of medication self-management, provided they have good cognitive ability and are able to get help from some close individuals. In a Taiwanese study, Yun-Fang Tsai (2007) found that institutionalized older people used some creative strategies to manage their depressive systems. Orem's ideas

also were formed as a framework for studies in Turkey (Akyol et al., 2007), the United Kingdom (Lauder, Kroll, and Jones, 2007), the Netherlands (Moser, van der Bruggen, Widdershoven, et al., 2008), Scandinavia (Arman and Hok, 2015), Ethiopia (Berhe et al., 2012), South Africa (Rabie et al., 2015), and other countries.

Therefore, while used in many countries, it continues to need adaptation for use in practice in other cultures; for example, values of patients in Japan include group care and the inseparability of the environment and the individual. Conversely, the theory is usable in some societies in which, although hospital patients are not expected to be self-care agents, family members are expected to and actually do become the self-care agents, as in many Middle Eastern countries. The nurse's role in these countries is to educate and support family members who assume the care. When these patients come to the United States alone, without their families or other self-care agents, they are unreceptive to nurses' attempts to promote self-care skills. However, the theory still has global practice utility. It has been used in Sweden to determine the effectiveness of using a nurse-led clinic to promote self-care for home dialysis patients and to compare the results with a comparison group receiving regular care. Self-care in the nurse-led clinic included reflective listening, timed exchange information, individualized care, motivational dialogues, information giving, education about kidney function, providing test results, and communicating about the effects of medications and other aspects of self-care. The results demonstrated that the nurse-led group had more instances of self-care dialysis as compared with those receiving traditional care (Pagels, Wang, and Wergström, 2008). The theory was also used in China to determine the level of self-care behaviors of school-aged children who were diagnosed with heart disease (Fan, 2008), in Germany to describe its utility in developing a nurse-led education program for patients with leg ulcers to meet their therapeutic self-care demands (Herber, Schnepp, and Rieger, 2008), and in Taiwan to define self-care strategies to manage sleep disturbances among older residents in nursing homes (Tsai, Wong, and Ku, 2008).

Orem's proposed theory may indeed make a substantial and valued difference in the lives of people whose self-care abilities are curtailed because of acute or chronic conditions, but it may not make the same difference in enhancing prevention and promoting health and well-being.

Theory Testing

Orem herself did not believe that nursing research should be focused on testing her theory as much as on developing knowledge related to the different components of the theories of self-care, self-care deficit, and systems of care. Taylor et al. (2000) reviewed six published research reports that used self-care deficit theory or components of it and performed an analysis of these reports, concluding that the studies demonstrated five stages in theory development. The framework of theory development that they used for the analysis was proposed by Orem (1985, 1987, 1995, 2001a). *The first stage* is description, as exemplified by the further development of the theory of dependent-care (Taylor et al., 2001), as well as descriptions related to other components and theories in self-care deficit theory.

Several descriptive studies focused on self-care practices. Allan (1988) examined the use and interpretation of health information in the practice of self-care activities of women as related to their weight. She found that women in her study were more concerned about their self-image than risk factors, and she was able to describe the self-care activities that they used to protect that image in the face of the reality of failure to maintain their weight. Hsieh, Wang, McCubbin, et al. (2008) found that self-efficacy, as reflected in self-care theory, was a better predictor for engaging in osteoporosis preventive behaviors than other behaviors. Miller (1982) used the theory to identify categories of self-care needs for patients with diabetes, and Storm and Baumgartner (1987) illustrated through a research case study method the use of self-care theory in the successful discharge of ventilator-dependent patients. Kubricht (1984) described the self-care needs of radiation patients, and Sandman, Norberg, Adolfsson, et al. (1986) described the needs and actions of Alzheimer-type dementia patients and nurses. Maunz and Woods (1988) described self-care actions by women. The theory was used to assess the perceived demands or changes in universal and self-care activities, and the degree of perceived difficulty in attempting to meet these demands among English- and Spanish-speaking women with HIV infection. For these women, the universal self-care tasks with the highest burden were caring for their children, engaging in physical activity, and attempting to fulfill the demands of their work responsibilities (Anastasio, McMahan, Daniels, et al., 1995). Others found that the higher the level of disability in Turkish patients suffering from rheumatoid arthritis, the lower their SCA (Tokem, Akyol, and Argon, 2007). Infant birth weight was significantly and directly related to SCA and prenatal care actions (Hart, 1995). The theory was also tested with patients experiencing taste changes after chemotherapy. Although the sample was small, patients were provided with strategies to enhance their self-care in managing the effects of taste change. The majority reported that they tried the provided strategies but also added to the strategies by suggesting more strategies. The authors conclude that providing strategies helped patients anticipate taste change and thus activated their own self-help strategies (Rehwaldt, Wickham, Purl, et al., 2009).

Homeless adolescents were studied to explore their self-care attitudes and behaviors (Rew, 2003). The results supported the utility of SCA in caring for self in a vulnerable situation. These homeless adolescents took care and protected themselves by becoming aware of their situation, by gaining self-respect, and by increasing self-reliance. They learned how to stay alive with limited resources, and handled their own health through interactions with others they met and by confronting obstacles.

The theory was effective as a framework to examine the relationship among several conditioning factors, self-agency, and self-care behaviors among adolescent girls who have been diagnosed with dysmenorrhea. The authors concluded that finding the relationship between the different factors and the adolescent girls' abilities of self-care could drive the development of more effective interventions to promote self-care and reduce suffering from dysmenorrhea (Wong, Ip, Choi, et al., 2015).

A second stage is "discrimination and verification of variations in person properties," as exemplified by a study by Söderhamn and Cliffordson (2001), in which they investigated the structure of self-care in elderly populations in Sweden. One component of this stage is instrumentation, as exemplified by the many studies conducted to develop research and health assessment instruments. Orem's theory has been used as the basis for the development of research instruments to assist researchers in using the theory (Clinton, Denyes, Goodwin, et al., 1977; Denyes, 1982; Kearney and Fleischer, 1979; Kuriansky, Gurland, Fleiss, et al., 1976). Kearney and Fleischer (1979) described the development of a valid and reliable instrument to measure the exercise of SCA (McBride, 1987). The instrument can be used to measure the level of involvement of patients in self-care, and eventually measurements could be developed to determine outcomes of the increase in self-care abilities. Hanson and Bickel (1985) and Weaver (1987) developed, described, and critiqued an instrument to measure patients' perceptions of SCA. A self-care practice questionnaire was developed and tested by Moore (1995) for the special purpose of measuring the self-care practice of children and adolescents. The Danger Assessment Instrument (Campbell, 1986) was developed to measure the danger level of homicide for battered women. Along the same lines, the Performance Test of Activities of Daily Living is another tool developed to measure SCA (Kuriansky et al., 1976).

Several others instruments were developed based on Orem theories. Among them is the Appraisal of Self-Care Agency Scale, containing a single substantive dimension. This instrument has adequate construct validity and reliability (Sousa, Zauszniewski, Zeller, et al., 2008). Another instrument, the European Heart Failure Self-care Behavior Scale was developed from attempts to quantify patient strategies in managing their heart failure. This scale was tested, and although it demonstrated reliability, its internal consistency was only moderate (Shuldham, Theaker, Jaarsma, et al., 2007). An updated and revised instrument based on self-care theory was designed to measure knowledge of facts about osteoporosis, and was retested, validated, and proved reliable (Ailinger, Lasus, and Braun, 2003).

Another component of this stage is the extension of the theory. Some researchers proposed extending the theory by incorporating a "sense of coherence" to strengthen prediction of outcomes for self-care (Baker and Denyes, 2008; Söderhamn, Bachrach-Lindström, and Ek, 2008). Continuity in the development of instruments is an indication of a potentially cumulative knowledge base.

Another component of the discrimination and verification studies are those focused on basic conditioning factors (BCFS). BCFS include age, gender, developmental state, health state, socioeconomic orientation, health care, family systems, and environmental factors, as well as patterns of living and resource availability (Orem, 2001a, p. 245). Wang (2001) compared two models of health-promoting lifestyles in rural elderly Taiwanese women and concluded that a number of the basic conditioning variables affect the outcome of self-care and that SCA is a strong variable in predicting the use of health-promoting lifestyles.

Despite these studies elucidating the various relationships between Orem's BCFS, there is an apparent lack of consensus in the operational definitions, as well as measurements, and this continues to need much work. For example, in family systems, Moore and Pichler (2000) determined a lack of consensus among the studies they reviewed. One of the authors' recommendations was that factors and measurements need to become more specific. There is also a lack of clarity in what constitutes adequate self-care (Ricka, Vanrenterghem, and Evers, 2002). Another component of this stage is human action. Examples are Orem and Vardiman (1995), as well as a study of self-care requisites by Pickens (1999).

The third stage is nursing cases and their natural history, as exemplified by the publication of case studies. The fourth stage is concerned with integrating practice knowledge; this is called "models and rules of nursing practice." Taylor et al. (2000) gave Hagopian (1996) as an example. In addition, other studies that were published later, such as those designed to describe self-care behaviors, would fit in this category (Artinian et al., 2002). The fifth stage is designing care for specific populations and describing that care and its outcomes. An example of this stage is the development and evaluation of appropriate self-care materials that fit patients' BCFS (Wilson, Mood, Risk, et al., 2003). Another example of this stage is using the theory to clarify similar concepts, such as activity and rest (Allison, 2007).

Other tests of interventions lend further support to the utility of Orem's theories. The relationship between self-care as a nursing therapeutic and nursing outcomes was examined in a number of studies. For example, Toth (1980) examined the relationship of a structured transfer preparation on patients' anxiety; Watkins (1995) tested patients' comprehension of discharge instructions based on Orem; Rothlis (1984) explored the effect of self-help groups on perceptions of hopelessness and helplessness; and Moore (1987) described the effects of various learning strategies on the development of autonomy and SCA among school-aged children. Using Orem as a framework, it was demonstrated that patients tended to accept responsibility for self-infusion at home, which increased their independence and sense of freedom (Gardulf, Bjorvell, Andersen, et al., 1995), and that adolescents are better able to take responsibility for managing their asthma (Altay and Cavusoglu, 2013). Dashiff (1988) reviewed research and clinical literature in psychiatric nursing based on Orem's self-care deficit theory. She compared the contributions of this literature to the development of theory for use in psychiatric nursing with other nursing specialties, and concluded that psychiatric nurses are using Orem's theory, although with limited indications of research productivity. Hanucharurnkui and Vinya-nguag (1991) tested the use of Orem's and King's theories on expediting the rate of recovery from surgery and increasing satisfaction of adult patients undergoing surgery. Interventions derived from Orem's and King's theories were related to less pain sensation and distress, using fewer analgesics, more ambulation, and higher satisfaction of patients than with those who did not receive the theory-driven care. Arman and Hok (2015) demonstrated that self-care is more than advice, education, and training, and that the care provided to enhance the ability of patients for self-care must include creating a caring culture and developing a compassionate relationship with self and others. They reflected on Orem's ideas, indicating perhaps that these goals are components of Orem's notion that health is promoted through self-care. The theory was used as a framework for a community-based intervention study in a smoking cessation program, with results pointing to the need for "tailored" self-care strategies (Williams, Shuster, Merwin, et al., 1994), and in the design, selection, and evaluation of appropriate patient education materials for patients with low literacy skills (Wilson et al., 2003). As the foundation for an intervention plan based on self-care, it helped children with type 1 diabetes improve, and the intervention changed their care from wholly compensatory or partly compensatory to educative/supportive (Ali, Sayej, and Fashafsheh, 2014).

Other studies tested relationships between propositions. One example is Denyes (1988), who provided partial support for the relationship between SCA and self-care in determining health outcomes. Hartley (1988) tested the relationship between nursing system and self-care behavior by examining the congruence between teaching strategies and learning styles of women and their effect on the accuracy and frequency of breast self-examination performance. The study demonstrated that SCA could evolve through the recall of observations or actions of others: "Knowledge of self-care breast self-examination developed through the use of supportive-educative nursing system, a system through which efficient and effective learning occurred" (Hartley, 1988, p. 166). Hart (1995) provided support for the significant relationship between basic prenatal care actions and SCA, which, in turn, was directly related to infants' birth weight. The relationship among health-promoting

self-care behaviors, self-care efficacy, and SCA was investigated using the canonical correlation model (Callaghan, 2003). The only variable that influenced SCA was the variable of spiritual growth.

A self-care model of women's responses to battering was constructed by Campbell and Weber (2000). The model included a number of BCFS that would directly relate to relational conflict and negatively relate to SCA. These would then be indirectly related to health and well-being. Although the results are congruent with Orem's proposition of the efficacy of SCA on health, the women's relationship problems had a stronger effect on them than did their ability to take care of themselves. Conversely, self-care was found to explain 30% of the variance in well-being in a population of adult homeless participants in a research study by Anderson (2001). These studies offer support for the category of self-care and its relationship to health.

An indirect effect of focusing on a nursing theory was reported by Denyes, O'Connor, Oakley, et al. (1989). A collaborative research project was initiated between nursing service and nursing education, focusing on contraceptive nursing care and self-care of women using primary care facilities. The results of the research—that women are their own self-care agents—gave impetus "for revising the clinic's family planning standards so that they would more fully operationalize the concepts" (1989, p. 144).

Theory-driven research is most effective and productive when a program of research is established, versus a single study approach. Williams and Ramos (1993) demonstrated this in a series of four studies based on Orem's theory to describe the self-care needs of people with symptomatic mitral valve prolapse. The approach resulted in more focused questions that built on each other, which contributed to building systematic knowledge about the experience of patients suffering from this disease. The phases of the research included a review of medical records, analysis of health perception and body image, and a survey of cardiovascular nurses; and it led to the construction and validation of a research instrument.

Biggs (2008) provided a synthesis of the state of the art and science related to Orem's theory, and concluded that, in the period between 1999 and 2007, there have been many impressive contributions to the discipline made by researchers, clinicians, and educators pertaining to all areas of practice. However, Susan Taylor, an important Orem scholar, in an interview conducted by Pamela

Clarke (Clarke et al., 2009) voiced a concern that, in the 50 years since Orem started to write about her theory, many of the issues in practice and education still remain the same. She goes further to indicate that if views of theory, practice, and education do not change drastically, Orem will be relegated to other similar historical figures such as Florence Nightingale. Pearson (2008) considers Orem an important figure in what he hopes will become a "Dead Nursing Theorists" Society (in the footsteps of "Dead Poets"), affirming the widespread use of self-care as evidenced by the extensive use of her theory to support improvements in health outcomes and enhancing the satisfaction of nurses and patients.

As with all other theories, Orem's theory could be used more broadly as a schematic to analyze the focus of research conducted in nursing and to set a direction for future research in nursing (Smith, 1979). Hoy, Wagner, and Hall (2007) reviewed the literature related to self-care in elders, with particular focus on health promotion, and concluded that elders' SCA is composed of actions, capabilities, and processes for health. These included fundamental, power, and performance capabilities, a process of life experience, and learning process. They also determined that the interaction between all of these leads to the understanding of the nature of self-care. On the whole, the theory has been used productively as a guide for practice; however, there is still a paucity of its outcomes on patient care outcomes (Chang, 1980; Roberts, 1982). In general, theory testing has been problematic, because of the different levels of its utilization in research (Silva, 1986; Timmins, 2008). In 2000, one study was designated as experimental, only two as replication, and few explicitly linked theory variables to practice (Taylor et al., 2000). However, in 2016 there appears to be an increasing number of studies designed as clinical trials to test nursing therapeutics based on Orem and the resulting health care outcomes (e.g., Altay and Cavusoglu, 2013; Berhe et al., 2012).

Research driven by Orem's theory, published in 1986–1991, was evaluated by Spearman, Duldt, and Brown (1993). They concluded that 32% of the studies used Orem's theory minimally, and 55% used it insufficiently; that is, the researchers used the theory superficially as a framework but the theory was not used in the discussion of the results. Only 13% of the studies used the theory adequately. Among these are studies that tested propositions relevant to health and health promotion among adolescents with diabetes (Frey and Fox, 1990), and relevance of the effects of computer-assisted instruction on avoidance of dust in adult asthmatics (Huss, Salerno, and Huss, 1991).

A test of the potential productivity of a theory is in its potential to stimulate theoretical discourses in the literature. Few dialogues in the literature of theory stimulate critical responses from a theorist or a metatheorist; however, one example would be a publication about how self-care theory could be used to understand self-inflicted health neglect, or "self-neglect" (Lauder, 2001). The author proposed that self-care theory is useful in offering insight into how some conditions are implicated in the development of self-neglect. Orem, while not critiquing the extension, questioned the misrepresentation of aspects of self-care and implicitly disagreed that self-care illuminates self-neglect. Instead, she proposed that self-care theory, as well as models of deliberate action and SCA, could explain self-neglect (Orem, 2001b). The ultimate test of the utility of her theory is in the ability to build on it by extending it or developing other theories. An example is Riegel's situation-specific theory of self-care for patients with heart failure (Riegel and Dickson, 2008). Several propositions of this theory were tested and supported, providing evidence that symptom recognition information and confidence enhanced self-care in patients with heart failure. Other examples are the theory of keeping vigil over the patient (Schreiber and MacDonald, 2010) and the theory of taking care of oneself in a high-risk environment (Rew, 2003). The next generation of theories, such as these, provide explanation and prediction for desired outcomes in nursing.

CONCLUSION

Nursing therapeutics are those deliberate actions provided by nurses to prevent illness and to maintain or promote health. Although every developed nursing theory may be used as a framework to develop a model of intervention, Orem's theory is categorized as a theory whose primary focus provides a framework for assessing needs of clients and developing intervention in enhancing peoples' abilities to manage daily care of themselves and their dependents, and conserve their energy, and structural, personal, and social integrity. Nurses intentionally use principles of self-care and conservation to provide supportive and therapeutic care. Her theory, as well as Henderson's, generated many dialogues in the literature, reflecting on clinical utility as well as their accessibility to operational definitions in research programs.

REFLECTIVE QUESTIONS

1. Why do you agree or do not agree with the identification of nursing needs as a category for nursing theories? Critically discuss the rationale for the inclusion of Orem's theories under this category.

2. Compare and contrast three major outcomes of nursing care intervention that are informed by Orem's theory.

3. Compare and contrast the conceptual attributes of "conservation" and "self-care" and critically describe the differences and similarities of their external components.

4. Review the most recent research studies in which Orem's theory was identified as a framework. In what ways do the results support or refute central theory propositions?

5. Identify, describe, and critically discuss research findings related to nursing therapeutics used in your field of practice. What are the theories that inform these nursing therapeutics?

6. In what ways do the theories of self-care, self-care deficit, and theory of nursing system reflect the current goals of health care reform in your country of residence? In what ways do they not?

7. Critically analyze the different uses of self-care in nursing literature. Compare these uses with those informed by policies in your work system.

8. Discuss and contrast the use of self-care deficit theory for patients at different points in the developmental life cycle.

9. Discuss and analyze the effective or ineffective utilization of any or all Orem theories while patients are on palliative care, hospice care, or end-of-life care.

REFERENCES

Abdellah, G.F., Beland, I.L., Martin, A., and Matheney, R.V. (1961). *Patient-centered approaches to nursing*. New York: Macmillan.

Ailinger, R.L., Lasus, H., and Braun, M.A. (2003). Revision of the facts on osteoporosis quiz. *Nursing Research*, 52(3), 198–201.

Akyol, A.D., Cetinkaya, Y., Bakan, G., et al. (2007). Self-care agency and factors related to this agency among patients with hypertension. *Journal of Clinical Nursing*, 16(4), 679–687.

Ali, A.J.I, Sayej, S., and Fashafsheh, I.H. (2014). Evaluating self-care practices of children with type 1 diabetes mellitus in Northern West Bank: A controlled randomized study utilizing Orem Self-Care theory. *Journal of Education and Practice*, 5(11), 53–63.

Allan, J.D. (1988). Knowing what to weigh: Woman self-care activities related to weight. *Advances in Nursing Science*, 11(1), 47–60.

Allison, S.E. (1973). A framework for nursing action in a nurse-conducted diabetic management clinic. *Journal of Nursing Administration*, 3(4), 53–60.

Allison, S.E. (2007). Self-care requirements for activity and rest: An Orem nursing focus. *Nursing Science Quarterly*, 20(1), 68–76.

Altay, N. and Cavusoglu, H. (2013). Using Orem's self-care model for asthmatic adolescents. *Journal for Specialists in Pediatric Nursing*, 18(3), 233–242.

Anastasio, C., McMahan, T., Daniels, A., Nicholas, P.K., and Paul-Simon, A. (1995). Self-care burden in women with human immunodeficiency virus. *Journal of the Association of Nurses in AIDS Care*, 6(3), 31–42.

Anderson, J.A. (2001). Understanding homeless adults by testing the theory of self-care. *Nursing Science Quarterly*, 14(1), 59–67.

Anna, D.J., Christensen, D.G., Hohn, S.A., Ord, L., and Wells, S.R. (1978). Implementing Orem's conceptual framework. *Journal of Nursing Administration*, 8(11), 8–11.

Aponte, J. and Nickitas, D.M. (2007). Community as client: Reaching an underserved urban community and meeting unmet primary health care needs. *Journal of Community Health Nursing*, 24(3), 177–190.

Arman, M. and Hok, J. (2015, September 22). Self-care follows from compassionate care – Chronic pain patients' experience of integrative rehabilitation. *Scandinavian Journal of Caring Sciences*, 30(2), 374–381.

Artinian, N.T., Magnan, M., Sloan, M., and Lange, M.P. (2002). Self-care behaviors among patients with heart failure. *Heart and Lung*, 31(3), 161–172.

Ashcraft, P.F. and Gatto, S.L. (2015). Care-of-self in undergraduate nursing students: A pilot study. *Nursing Education Perspectives*, 36(4), 255–256.

Backscheider, J.E. (1971). The use of self as the essence of clinical supervision in ambulatory patient care. *Nursing Clinics of North America*, 6(4), 785–794.

Backscheider, J.E. (1974). Self-care requirements, self-care capabilities, and nursing systems in the diabetic nurse management clinic. *American Journal of Public Health*, 64(12), 1138–1146.

Baker, L.K. and Denyes, M.J. (2008). Predictors of self-care in adolescents with cystic fibrosis: A test of Orem's theories of self-care and self-care deficit. *Journal of Pediatric Nursing*, 23(1), 37–48.

Bandura, A. (1997). *Self-efficacy: The exercise of control*. New York: Freeman.

Bandura, A. (2000). Cultivate self-efficacy for personal and organizational effectiveness. In E.A. Lock (Ed.), *Handbook of Principles of Organization Behavior* (pp. 120–136). Oxford, UK: Blackwell.

Banfield, B.E. (1997). A philosophical inquiry of Orem's self-care deficit theory. Unpublished doctoral dissertation. Ann Arbor, MI: Wayne State University.

Banfield, B.E. (2001). Philosophic foundations of Orem's work. In D. Orem (Ed.), *Nursing: Concepts of Practice* (pp. xi–xvi). St. Louis, MO: Mosby.

Barnum, B.J.S. (1994). *Nursing theory: Analysis, application, and evaluation*. Philadelphia, PA: Lippincott.

Behi, R. (1986). Look after yourself. *Nursing Times*, 82(37), 35–37.

Bennett, J.G. (1980). Foreword to the symposium on the self-care concept in nursing. *Nursing Clinics of North America*, 15(1), 129–130.

Berbiglia, V.A. (2011). The self-care deficit nursing theory as a curriculum conceptual framework in baccalaureate education. *Nursing Science Quarterly*, 24(2), 137–145.

Berbiglia, V.A. and Banfield, B. (2014). Self-care deficit theory of nursing. In M.R. Alligood (Ed.), *Nursing theorists and their work*. St. Louis, MO: Mosby.

Berhe, K.K., Demissie, A., Kahsay, A.B., and Gebru, H.B. (2012). Diabetes self-care practices and associated factors among type 2 diabetic patients in Tikur Anbessa Specialized Hospital, Addis Ababa, Ethiopia – A cross-sectional study. *International Journal of Pharmaceutical Sciences and Research*, 3(11), 4219–4229.

Biggs, A. (2008). Orem's self-care deficit nursing theory: Update on the state of the art and science. *Nursing Science Quarterly*, 21(3), 200–206.

Bonamy, C., Schultz, P., Graham, K., and Hampton, M. (1995). The use of theory-based nursing practice in the Department of Veterans' Affairs Medical Centers. *Journal of Nursing Staff Development*, 11(1), 27–30.

Bromley, B. (1980). Applying Orem's self-care theory in enterostomal therapy. *American Journal of Nursing*, 80(2), 245–249.

Brown, B. (2015). Towards a critical understanding of mutuality in mental healthcare: Relationships, power and social capital. *Journal of Psychiatric and Mental Health Nursing*, 22(10), 829–835.

Buckwalter, K.C. and Kerfoot, K.M. (1982). Teaching patients self-care: A critical aspect of psychiatric discharge planning. *Journal of Psychiatric Nursing and Mental Health Services*, 20(5), 15–20.

Budinger, J.M. (2007). A patient education tool for nonoperative management of blunt abdominal trauma. *Journal of Trauma Nursing*, 14(1), 19–23.

Burks, K.J. (1999). A nursing practice model for chronic illness. *Rehabilitation Nursing*, 24(5), 197–200.

Burks, K.J. (2001). Intentional action. *Journal of Advanced Nursing*, 34(5), 668–675.

Caley, J.M., Dirksen, M., Engalla, M., and Hennrich, M. (1980). The Orem self-care nursing model. In J.P. Riehl and C. Roy (Eds.), *Conceptual models for nursing practice* (2nd ed.). New York: Appleton-Century-Crofts.

Callaghan, D.M. (2003). Health-promoting self-care behaviors, self-care self-efficacy, and self-care agency. *Nursing Science Quarterly*, 16(3), 247–254.

Campbell, J.C. (1986). Nursing assessment for risk of homicide with battered women. *Advances in Nursing Science*, 8(4), 36–51.

Campbell, J.C. and Weber, N. (2000). An empirical test of a self-care model of women's responses to battering. *Nursing Science Quarterly*, 13(1), 45–53.

Campuzano, M. (1982, April/May). Self-care following coronary artery bypass surgery. *Focus*, 9(2), 55–56.

Chang, B.L. (1980). Evaluation of health care professionals in facilitating self-care: Review of the literature and a conceptual model. *Advances in Nursing Science*, 3(1), 43–58.

Chen, A.M.H., Yehle, K.S., Albert, N.M., Ferraro, K.F., et al. (2014). Relationships between health literacy and heart failure knowledge, self-efficacy, and self-care adherence. *Research in Social and Administrative Pharmacy*, 10(2), 378–386.

Clark, M.D. (1986). Application of Orem's theory of self-care: A case study. *Journal of Community Health Nursing*, 3(3), 127–135.

Clarke, P.N., Allison, S.E., Berbiglia, V.A., and Taylor, S.G. (2009). The impact of Dorothea E. Orem's life and work. *Nursing Science Quarterly*, 22(1), 41–46.

Clinton, J.F., Denyes, M.J., Goodwin, J.O., and Koto, E.M. (1977). Developing criterion measures of nursing care: Case study of a process. *Journal of Nursing Administration*, 7(7), 41–45.

Coleman, L.J. (1980). Orem's self-care concept of nursing. In J.P. Riehl and C. Roy (Eds.), *Conceptual models for nursing practice* (2nd ed.). New York: Appleton-Century-Crofts.

Compton, P. (1989). Drug abuse, a self-care deficit. *Journal of Psychosocial Nursing*, 27(3), 22–26.

Cox, K.R. and Taylor, S.G. (2005). Orem's self-care deficit nursing theory: Pediatric asthma as exemplar. *Nursing Science Quarterly*, 18(3), 249–257.

Coyle, M.K. and Martin, E.M. (2007). Reflecting on a self-care process in the home setting for traumatic brain injury survivors. *Journal of Neuroscience Nursing*, 39(5), 274–277.

Dashiff, C.J. (1988). Theory development in psychiatric-mental health nursing: An analysis of Orem's theory. *Archives of Psychiatric Nursing*, 2(6), 366–372.

Denyes, M.J. (1982). Measurement of self-care agency in adolescents [Abstract]. *Nursing Research*, 31(1), 63.

Denyes, M.J. (1988). Orem's model used for health promotion: Directions from research. *Advances in Nursing Science*, 11(1), 13–21.

Denyes, M.J., O'Connor, N.A., Oakley, D., and Ferguson, S. (1989). Integrating nursing theory, practice and research through collaborative research. *Journal of Advanced Nursing*, 14, 141–145.

Denyes, M.J., Orem, D.E., and SozWiss, G.B. (2001). Self-care: A foundational science. *Nursing Science Quarterly*, 14(1), 48–54.

Drevenhorn, E., Bengtson, A., Nyberg, P., and Kjellgren, K.I. (2015). Assessment of hypertensive patients' self-care agency after counseling training of nurses. *Journal of the American Association of Nurse Practitioners*, 27(11), 624–630.

Dropkin, M.J. (1981). Development of a self-care teaching program for postoperative head and neck patients. *Cancer Nursing*, 4(2), 103–106.

Easton, K.L. (1993). Defining the concept of self-care. *Rehabilitation Nursing*, 18(6), 384–387.

Fan, L. (2008). Self-care behaviors of school-age children with heart disease. *Pediatric Nursing*, 34(2), 131–138.

Fawcett, J. (1995). *Analysis and evaluation of conceptual models of nursing* (3rd ed.). Philadelphia, PA: F.A. Davis.

Fawcett, J. (2001). The nurse theorists: 21st-century updates–Dorothea E. Orem. *Nursing Science Quarterly*, 14(1), 34–38.

Fawcett, J. and DeSanto-Madeya, S. (2013). *Contemporary nursing knowledge: Analysis and evaluation of nursing models and theories* (3rd ed.). Philadelphia, PA: F.A. Davis.

Fenner, K. (1979). Developing a conceptual framework. *Nursing Outlook*, 27, 122–126.

Fitzgerald, S. (1980). Utilizing Orem's self-care nursing model in designing an educational program for the diabetic. *Topics in Clinical Nursing*, 2(2), 57–65.

Foster, P.C. and Janssens, N.P. (1980). Dorothea E. Orem. In The Nursing Theories Conference Group (Eds.), *Nursing theories:*

The base for professional nursing practice. Englewood Cliffs, NJ: Prentice-Hall.

Frey, M.A. and Fox, M.A. (1990). Assessing and teaching self-care to youths with diabetes mellitus. *Pediatric Nursing*, 16, 597–800.

Gardulf, A., Bjorvell, H., Andersen, V., Bjorkander, J., Ericson, D., Froland, S.S., et al. (1995). Lifelong treatment with gammaglobulin for primary antibody deficiencies: The patients' experiences of subcutaneous self-infusions and home therapy. *Journal of Advanced Nursing*, 21(5), 917–927.

Gast, H. and Montgomery, K.S. (2005). Orem model of self-care. In J. Fitzpatrick and A. Whall (Eds.), *Conceptual models of nursing: Analysis and application* (pp. 104–145). New York: Pearson-Prentice Hall.

Greenfield, E. and Pace, J. (1985). Orem's self-care theory of nursing: Practical application to the end stage renal disease (ESRD) patient. *Journal of Nephrology Nursing*, 2(4), 187–193.

Hagopian, G.A. (1996). The effects of informational audiotapes on knowledge and self-care behaviors of patients undergoing radiation therapy. *Oncology Nursing Forum*, 23(4), 697–700.

Hanson, B.R. and Bickel, L. (1985). Development and testing of the questionnaire on perception of self-care agency. In J. Riehl-Sisca (Ed.), *The science and art of self-care*. Norwalk, CT: Appleton-Century-Crofts.

Hanucharurnkui, S. and Vinya-nguag P. (1991). Effects of promoting patients' participation in self-care on postoperative recovery and satisfaction with care. *Nursing Science Quarterly*, 4(1), 14–20.

Harrison-Raines, K. (1993). Nursing and self-care theory applied to utilization review: Concepts and cases. *American Journal of Medical Quality*, 8(4), 197–199.

Hart, M.A. (1995). Orem's self-care deficit theory: Research with pregnant women. *Nursing Science Quarterly*, 8(3), 120–126.

Hartley, L.A. (1988). Congruence between teaching and learning self-care: A pilot study. *Nursing Science Quarterly*, 1(4), 161–167.

Hashemi, F., Dolatabad, F.R., Yektatalab, S., Ayaz, M., Zare, N., and Mansouri, P. (2014). Effect of Orem self-care program on the life quality of burn patients referred to Ghotb-al-Din-e-Shirazi Burn Center, Shiraz, Iran: A randomized controlled trial. *International Journal of Community Based Nursing and Midwifery*, 2(1), 40–50.

Henderson, V. (1991). *The nature of nursing* (2nd ed). New York: Harry N. Abrams.

Herber, O.R., Schnepp, W., and Rieger, M.A. (2008). Developing a nurse-led education program to enhance self-care agency in leg ulcer patients. *Nursing Science Quarterly*, 21(2), 150–155.

Hines, S.H., Sampselle, C.M., Ronis, D.L., Yeo, S., et al. (2007). Women's self-care agency to manage urinary incontinence: The impact of nursing agency and body experience. *Advances in Nursing Science*, 30(2), 175–188.

Hintze, A. (2011). Orem-based nursing education in Germany. *Nursing Science Quarterly*, 24(1), 66–70.

Hoy, B., Wagner, L., and Hall, E.O.C. (2007). Self-care as a health source of elders: An integrative review of the concept. *Scandinavian Journal of Caring Science*, 21(4), 456–466.

Hsieh, C.H., Wang, C.Y., McCubbin, M., Zhang, S., and Inouye, J. (2008). Factors influencing osteoporosis preventive behaviours: Testing a path model. *Journal of Advanced Nursing*, 62(3), 336–345.

Hurlock-Chorostecki, C. (1999). Holistic care in the critical care setting: Application of a concept through Watson's and Orem's theories of nursing. *Official Journal of the Canadian Association of Critical Care Nurses*, 10(4), 20–25.

Huss, K., Salerno, M., and Huss, R.W. (1991). Computer-assisted reinforcement of instruction: Effects on adherence in adult atopic asthmatics. *Research in Nursing and Health*, 14(4), 259–267.

Johnston, R.L. (1983). Orem self-care model of nursing. In J.J. Fitzpatrick and A.L. Whall (Eds.), *Conceptual models of nursing: Analysis and application*. Bowie, MD: Robert J. Brady Co.

Kearney, B.Y. and Fleischer, B.J. (1979). Development of an instrument to measure exercise of self-care agency. *Research in Nursing and Health*, 2(1), 25–34.

Kinlein, M.L. (1977). Self-care concept. *American Journal of Nursing*, 77, 598–601.

Kubricht, D. (1984). Therapeutic self-care demands expressed by outpatients receiving external radiation therapy. *Cancer Nursing*, 7, 43–52.

Kumar, C.P. (2007). Application of Orem's self-care deficit theory and standardized nursing languages in a case study of a woman with diabetes. *International Journal of Nursing Terminologies and Classifications*, 18(3), 103–110.

Kuriansky, J., Gurland, B., Fleiss, J., and Cowan, D. (1976). The assessment of self-care capacity in geriatric psychiatric patients by objective and subjective methods. *Journal of Clinical Psychology*, 32, 95–102.

Lanigan, T.L. (2000). The patient-family learning centre. *Canadian Nurse*, 96(3), 18–21.

Lauder, W. (2001). The utility of self-care theory as a theoretical basis for self-neglect. *Journal of Advanced Nursing*, 34(4), 545–553.

Lauder, W., Kroll, T., and Jones M. (2007). Social determinants of mental health: The missing dimensions of mental health nursing? *Journal of Psychiatric and Mental Health Nursing*, 14(7), 661–669.

Maunz, E.R. and Woods, N.F. (1988). Self-care practices among young adult women: Influence of symptoms, employment, and sex-role orientation. *Health Care for Women International*, 9, 29–41.

McBride, S. (1987). Validation of an instrument to measure exercise of self-care agency. *Research in Nursing and Health*, 10, 311–316.

McLaughlin, K. (1993). Implementing self-care deficit nursing theory: A process of staff development. In M.E. Parker (Ed.), *Patterns of nursing theories in practice* (pp. 241–251). New York: National League for Nursing.

Melnyk, K.A.M. (1983). The process of theory analysis: An examination of the nursing theory of Dorothea E. Orem. *Nursing Research*, 32(3), 170–174.

Michael, M.M. and Sewall, K.S. (1980). Use of the adolescent peer group to increase the self-care agency of adolescent alcohol abusers. *Nursing Clinics of North America*, 15, 157–176.

Miller, J.F. (1980). The dynamic focus of nursing: A challenge to nursing administration. *The Journal of Nursing Administration*, 10(1), 13–18.

Miller, J.F. (1982). Categories of self-care needs of ambulatory patients with diabetes. *Journal of Advanced Nursing*, 7, 25–31.

Moore, J.B. (1987). Effects of assertion training and first aid instruction on children's autonomy and self-care agency. *Research in Nursing and Health*, 10, 101–109.

Moore, J.B. (1995). Measuring self-care practice of children and adolescents: Instrument development. *Maternal-child Nursing Journal*, 23(3), 101–108.

Moore, J.B and Beckwitt, A.E. (2006). Self-care operations and nursing interventions for children with cancer and their parents. *Nursing Science Quarterly*, 19(2), 147–156.

Moore, J.B. and Pichler, V.H. (2000). Measurement of Orem's basic conditioning factors: A review of published research. *Nursing Science Quarterly*, 13(2), 137–142.

Morse, W. and Werner, J.S. (1988). Individualization of patient care using Orem's theory. *Cancer Nursing*, 11(3), 195–202.

Moser, A., van der Bruggen, H., Widdershoven, G., and Spreeuwenberg, C. (2008). Self-management of type 2 diabetes mellitus: A qualitative investigation from the perspective of participants in a nurse-led, shared-care program in the Netherlands. *BMC Public Health*, 8, 91.

Mosher, R.B. and Moore, J.B. (1998). The relationship of self-concept and self-care in children with cancer. *Nursing Science Quarterly*, 11(3), 116–122.

Mullin, V.I. (1980). Implementing the self-care concept in the acute care setting. *Nursing Clinics of North America*, 15(4), 177–190.

Murphy, P.P. (1981). A hospice model and self-care theory. *Oncology Nursing Forum*, 8(2), 19–21.

Noone, J. (1995). Acute pancreatitis: An Orem approach to nursing assessment and care. *Critical Care Nurse*, 15(4), 27–35.

Norris, M.K. (1991). Applying Orem's theory to the long-term care of adolescent transplant recipients. *American Nephrology Nurses' Association Journal*, 18(1), 45–47, 53.

Nursing Development Conference Group. (1973). *Concept formalization in nursing: Process and product*. Boston, MA: Little, Brown.

Nursing Development Conference Group. (1979). *Concept formalization in nursing: Process and product* (2nd ed.). Boston, MA: Little, Brown.

Orem, D.E. (1959). *Guides for developing curricula for the education of practical nurses*. Washington, DC: U.S. Department of Health, Education, & Welfare, Office of Education.

Orem, D.E. (1971). *Nursing: Concepts of practice*. New York: McGraw-Hill.

Orem, D.E. (1980). *Nursing: Concepts of practice* (2nd ed.). New York: McGraw Hill.

Orem, D.E. (1983). The self-care deficit theory of nursing: A general theory. In I.W. Clements and F.B. Roberts (Eds.), *Family health: A theoretical approach to nursing care*. New York: John Wiley & Sons.

Orem, D.E. (1985). *Nursing: Concepts of practice* (3rd ed.). New York: McGraw-Hill.

Orem, D.E. (1987). Orem's general theory of nursing. In R. Parse (Ed.), *Nursing science: Major paradigms, theories, and critiques*. Philadelphia, PA: W.B. Saunders.

Orem, D.E. (1989). Theories and hypotheses for nursing administration. In B. Henry, M. Di Vincenti, C. Arndt, and A. Marriner (Eds.), *Dimensions of nursing administration. Theory, research, education, and practice*. Boston, MA: Blackwell Scientific Publications.

Orem, D.E. (1991). *Nursing: Concepts of practice* (4th ed.). St. Louis, MO: C.V. Mosby.

Orem, D.E. (1995). *Nursing: Concepts of practice* (5th ed.). St. Louis, MO: C.V. Mosby.

Orem, D.E. (1997). Views of human beings specific to nursing. *Nursing Science Quarterly*, 10(1), 26–31.

Orem, D.E. (2001a). *Nursing: Concepts of practice* (6th ed.). St. Louis, MO: Mosby.

Orem, D.E. (2001b). Response to: Lauder, W. (2001). Comment: The utility of self-care theory as a theoretical basis for self-neglect. *Journal of Advanced Nursing*, 34(4), 552–553.

Orem, D.E. and Taylor, S.G. (1986). Orem's general theory of nursing. In P. Winstead-Fry (Ed.), *Case studies in nursing theory*. New York: National League for Nursing.

Orem, D.E. and Taylor, S.G. (2011). Reflections on nursing practice science: The nature, the structure, and the foundation of nursing science. *Nursing Science Quarterly*, 24(1), 35–41.

Orem, D.E. and Vardiman, E.M. (1995). Orem's nursing theory and positive mental health: Practical considerations. *Nursing Science Quarterly*, 8(4), 165–173.

Pagels, A.A., Wang, M., and Wengström, Y. (2008). The impact of a nurse-led clinic on self-care ability, disease-specific knowledge, and home dialysis modality. *Nephrology Nursing Journal*, 35(3), 242–248.

Pearson, A. (2008). Dead poets, nursing theorists and contemporary nursing practice. *International Journal of Nursing Practice*, 14, 1–2.

Phillips, K.D. and Morrow, J.H. (1998). Nursing management of anxiety in HIV infection. *Issues in Mental Health Nursing*, 19(4), 375–397.

Pickens, J.M. (1999). Living with serious mental illness: The desire for normalcy. *Nursing Science Quarterly*, 12(3), 233–239.

Rabie, T., Klopper, H.C., and Watson, M.J. (2015). Effect of socioeconomic status on self-care of the older person in the Potchefstroom district, South Africa. *Health SA Gesondheid*. doi: 10:1016/j.hsag.2015.02.007

Rehwaldt, M., Wickham, R., Purl, S., Tariman, J., et al. (2009). Self-care strategies to cope with taste changes after chemotherapy. *Oncology Nursing Forum*, 36(2), E47–E56.

Reid, B., Allen, A., Gauthier, T., and Campbell, H. (1989). Solving the Orem mystery: An educational strategy. *Journal of Continuing Education in Nursing*, 20(3), 108–111.

Renpenning, K.M., SozWiss, G.B., Denyes, M.J., Orem, D.E., and Taylor, S.G. (2011). Explication of the nature and meaning of nursing diagnosis. *Nursing Science Quarterly*, 24(2), 130–136.

Rew, L. (2003). A theory of taking care of oneself grounded in experiences of homeless youth. *Nursing Research*, 52(4), 234–241.

Ricka, R., Vanrenterghem, Y., and Evers, G.C.M. (2002). Adequate self-care of dialysed patients: A review of the literature. *International Journal of Nursing Studies*, 39(3), 329–339.

Riegel, B. and Dickson, V.V. (2008). A situation-specific theory of heart failure self-care. *Journal of Cardiovascular Nursing*, 23(3), 190–196.

Riehl-Sisca, J.P. (1989). *Conceptual models for nursing practice* (3rd ed.). East Norwalk, CT: Appleton & Lange.

Riehl-Sisca, J.P. and Roy, C. (Eds.). (1980). *Conceptual models for nursing practice* (2nd ed.). New York: Appleton-Century-Crofts.

Roberts, C.S. (1982). Identifying the real patient problems. *Nursing Clinics of North America*, 17(3), 481–489.

Roldan-Merino, J., Lluch-Canut, T., Menarguez-Alcaina, M., Foix-Sanjuan, A., Abad, J.M., and QuestERA Working Group. (2013). Psychometric evaluation of a new instrument in Spanish to measure self-care requisites in patients with schizophrenia. *Perspectives in Psychiatric Care*, 50(2), 93–101.

Roldan-Merino, J., Miguel-Ruiz, D., Lluch-Canut, M.T., Puig-Llobet, M., Feria-Raposo, I., and QuestERA Working Group. (2015, August 13). Psychometric properties of self-care requisites scale (SCRS-h) in hospitalized patients diagnosed with schizophrenia. *Perspectives in Psychiatric Care*. doi: 10.1111/ppc.12133.

Rothlis, J. (1984). The effect of a self-help group on feelings of hopelessness and helplessness. *Western Journal of Nursing Research*, 6, 157–173.

Sandman, P.O., Norberg, A., Adolfsson, R., Axelsson, K., and Hedly, V. (1986). Morning care of patients with Alzheimer-type dementia. A theoretical model based on direct observations. *Journal of Advanced Nursing*, 11, 369–378.

Schreiber, R. and MacDonald, M. (2010). Keeping vigil over the patient: A grounded theory of nurse anesthesia practice. *Journal of Advanced Nursing*, 66(3), 552–561.

Shuldham, C., Theaker, C., Jaarsma, T., and Cowie, M.R. (2007). Evaluation of the European heart failure self-care behaviour scale in a United Kingdom population. *Journal of Advanced Nursing*, 60(1), 87–95.

Silva, M.C. (1986). Research testing nursing theory: State of the art. *Advances in Nursing Science*, 9(1), 1–11.

Simmons, L. (2009). Dorthea Orem's self care theory as related to nursing practice in hemodialysis. *Nephrology Nursing Journal*, 36(4), 419–421.

Slusher, I.L. (1999). Self-care agency and self-care practice of adolescents. *Issues in Comprehensive Pediatric Nursing*, 22(1), 49–58.

Smith, M.C. (1979). Proposed metaparadigm for nursing research and theory development. *Image*, 11(3), 75–79.

Smith, M.C. (1987). A critique of Orem's theory. In R.R. Parse (Ed.), *Nursing science. Major paradigms, theories, and critiques*. Philadelphia, PA: W.B. Saunders.

Söderhamn, O. and Cliffordson, C. (2001). The structure of self-care in a group of elderly people. *Nursing Science Quarterly*, 14(1), 55–58.

Söderhamn, U., Bachrach-Lindström, M., and Ek, A-C. (2008). Self-care ability and sense of coherence in older nutritional at-risk patients. *European Journal of Clinical Nutrition*, 62, 96–103.

Sousa, V.D., Zauszniewski, J.A., Zeller, R.A., and Neese, J.B. (2008). Factor analysis of the appraisal of self-care agency scale in American adults with diabetes. *The Diabetes Educator*, 34(1), 98–108.

Spearman, S.A., Duldt, B.W., and Brown, S. (1993). Research testing theory: A selective review of Orem's self-care theory, 1986–1991. *Journal of Advanced Nursing*, 18, 1626–1631.

Storm, D.S. and Baumgartner, R.G. (1987). Achieving self-care in the ventilator-dependent patient: A critical analysis of a case study. *International Journal of Nursing Studies*, 24, 95–96.

Taylor, S.G. (1988). Nursing theory and nursing process: Orem's theory in practice. *Nursing Science Quarterly*, 1(3), 111–119.

Taylor, S.G. (1990). Practical applications of Orem's theory of self-care deficit nursing theory. In M.E. Parker (Ed.), *Nursing theories in practice* (pp. 61–70). New York: National League for Nursing.

Taylor, S.G. (2001). Orem's general theory of nursing and families. *Nursing Science Quarterly*, 14(1), 7–9.

Taylor, S.G. and McLaughlin, K. (1991). Orem's general theory of nursing and community nursing. *Nursing Science Quarterly*, 4, 153–160.

Taylor, S.G. and Renpenning, K.M. (2001). The practice of nursing in multiperson situations, family and community. In D. Orem (Ed.), *Nursing: Concepts of practice* (pp. 394–433). St. Louis, MO: Mosby.

Taylor, S.G., Geden, E., Isaramalai, S., and Wongvatunyu, S. (2000). Orem's self-care deficit nursing theory: Its philosophic foundation and the state of the science. *Nursing Science Quarterly*, 13(2), 104–110.

Taylor, S.G., Renpenning, K.E., Geden, E.A., Neuman, B.M., and Hart, M.A. (2001). A theory of dependent-care: A corollary theory to Orem's theory of self-care. *Nursing Science Quarterly*, 14(1), 39–47.

Timmins, F. (2008). A critical review of appropriate conceptual models for use by coronary care nurses. *International Nursing Review*, 55(1), 117–124.

Tokem, Y., Akyol, A.D., and Argon, G. (2007). The relationship between disability and self-care agency of Turkish people with rheumatoid arthritis. *Journal of Nursing and Healthcare of Chronic Illness*, 16(3a), 44–50.

Toth, J.C. (1980). Effect of structured preparation for transfer on patient anxiety on leaving coronary care unit. *Nursing Research*, 29(1), 28–34.

Tsai, Y.F. (2007). Self-care management and risk factors for depressive symptoms among Taiwanese institutionalized older persons. *Nursing Research*, 56(2), 124–131.

Tsai, Y.-F., Wong, T.K.S., and Ku, Y-C. (2008). Self-care management of sleep disturbances and risk factors for poor sleep among older residents of Taiwanese nursing homes. *Journal of Clinical Nursing*, 17(9), 1219–1226.

Underwood, P.R. (1980). Facilitating self-care. In P. Pothier (Ed.), *Psychiatric Nursing*. Boston, MA: Little, Brown.

Walborn, K.A. (1980). A nursing model for hospice: Primary and self-care. *Nursing Clinics of North America*, 15(1), 205–217.

Walker, D.M. (1993). A nursing administration perspective on use of Orem's self-care deficit nursing theory. In M.E. Parker (Ed.), *Patterns of nursing theories in practice* (pp. 252–264). New York: National League for Nursing.

Wallace, W.A. (1996). *The modeling of nature: Philosophy of science and philosophy of nature in synthesis*. Washington, DC: The Catholic University of America Press.

Wang, C.Y. (1997). The cross-cultural applicability of Orem's conceptual framework. *Journal of Cultural Diversity*, 4(2), 44–48.

Wang, H.H. (2001). A comparison of two models of health-promoting lifestyle in rural elderly Taiwanese women. *Public Health Nursing*, 18(3), 204–211.

Watkins, G.R. (1995). Patient comprehension of gastroenterology (GI) educational materials. *Gastroenterology Nursing*, 18(4), 123–127.

Weaver, M.T. (1987). Perceived self-care agency: A LISREL, factor analysis of Bickel and Hanson's questionnaire. *Nursing Research*, 36, 381–387.

Westerbotn, M., Fahlström, J., Agüero-Torres, H., and Hilleras, P. (2008). How do older people experience their management of medicines? *Journal of Clinical Nursing*, 17(5a), 106–115.

Wilkinson, A. and Whitehead, L. (2009). Evolution of the concept of self-care and implications for nurses: A literature review. *International Journal of Nursing Studies*, 48(8), 1143–1147.

Williams S. and Ramos, M.C. (1993). Mitral valve prolapse and its effects: A program of inquiry within Orem's self-care deficit theory of nursing. *Journal of Advanced Nursing*, 18, 242–251.

Williams, S., Shuster, G.F., III, Merwin, E., and Williams, B. (1994). A community-based smoking cessation program: Self-care behaviors and success. *Public Health Nursing*, 11(5), 291–299.

Wilson, F.L., Baker, L.M., Nordstrom, C.K., and Legwand, C. (2008). Using the teach-back and Orem's self-care deficit nursing theory to increase childhood immunization communication among low-income mothers. *Issues in Comprehensive Pediatric Nursing*, 31, 7–22.

Wilson, F.L., Mood, D.W., Risk, J., and Kershaw, T. (2003). Evaluation of education materials using Orem's self-care deficit theory. *Nursing Science Quarterly*, 16(1), 68–76.

Wong, C.L., Ip, W.Y., Choi, K.C., and Lam, L.W. (2015). Examining self-care behaviors and their associated factors among adolescent girls with dysmenorrhea: An application of Orem's self-care deficit nursing theory. *Journal of Nursing Scholarship*, 47(3), 219–227.

12

On Interactions

Several nurse theorists addressed nursing as a process of interaction and nursing care as a human relationship. I selected the following theorists to represent the central domain concepts related to human interactions: Imogene King, Ida Orlando (Pelletier), Josephine G. Paterson and Loretta T. Zderad, Joyce Travelbee, and Ernestine Wiedenbach. The theories of King, Orlando, Travelbee, and Wiedenbach may also be used as the frameworks to describe and explain significant questions and the knowledge base related to the processes essential in decision-making and clinical judgment.

IMOGENE KING—A THEORY OF GOAL ATTAINMENT

Theory Description

King's theory evolved in the mid-1960s, when she raised questions about how nurses make decisions in their daily practice and how to define the nursing act, leading her to focus and develop the concept of the "human act" (King, 1997a). King also attempted to describe the essence of nursing and the interactional patterns and goals that govern the nurse–patient relationship. Like other nurse theorists of her generation, she asked fundamental questions to explain what nursing is (King, 1981, 1990a); to differentiate it from other disciplines; and to identify the curricular components that differentiate the educational levels in preparing nurses (diploma, associate degree, and BS programs) (King, 1986a, 1986b). The development of her conceptualization progressed from the idea that nursing could be provided through a framework that contains a synthesis of ideas (a frame of reference that she entitled, in 1971, "Toward a Theory for Nursing") to the development of King's Theory of Goal Attainment (prompting her to rename her conceptualization "A Theory for Nursing" [1981 and 1996b]). In a curious way, the difference between

the first tentative title and the second is analogous to nursing's tentativeness about theory in the 1970s and the determination to theorize in the 1980s. The difference between King's two books can be found in the last chapter of the second book, where she articulated her theory "for" nursing. Her theory is that nursing is a process that is interactional in nature between two human beings engaged in a human act. These interactions lead to transactions resulting in goal attainment (King, 1990a, 1992a).

At the beginning of the 1990s, King also entitled her work, "general systems framework" and then derived from it a "theory of goal attainment" (King, 1992a, 1992b, 1996a, 1996b, 1997b, 1997c). King provided nursing with four sets of concepts as part of her conceptual framework for nursing (King, 1988a). These concepts continue to be central to the field of nursing and provide the basis on which she developed her theory of goal attainment, beginning with an assumption that nurses as human beings interact with patients as human beings, and both are open systems that also interact with the environment. Therefore, the personal systems (nurse and patient) interact with each other in an interpersonal system (small and large groups) and with the environment, which she called the social systems (institutional organizations). The relationships between these systems led to the development of the theory of goal attainment, with a distinct set of concepts, some of which were derived from the conceptual framework. Other theories have evolved from the conceptual framework. To understand her theory fully, it should be read in conjunction with the conceptual framework. The goal of the development of the conceptual system of relations was to delineate major concepts for our discipline, to derive theories, to provide a structure for educational programs, to use as a framework for nursing practice, and to deliver care to individuals, families, and communities (King, 1997c).

The theory deals with the central questions of interaction between nurses and clients (King,

BOX 12-1   ASSUMPTIONS—KING

Explicit Assumptions

- The central focus of nursing is the interaction of human beings and environment, with the goal being health for human beings (King, 1982, p. 143).
- Individuals are social, sentient, rational, reacting, perceiving, controlling, purposeful, action-oriented, and time-oriented beings (King, 1981, p. 143).
- The interaction process is influenced by perceptions, goals, needs, and values of both the client and the nurse (1981, 1992b).
- Human beings as patients have rights to obtain information; to participate in decisions that may influence their life, health, and community services; and to accept or reject care (1981).
- It is the responsibility of health care members to inform individuals of all aspects of health care to help them in making "informed decisions" (1981).
- Incongruities may exist between the goals of health caregivers and recipients. Persons have the right to either accept or reject any aspect of health care (1981, pp. 143–144).
- Human beings are in continuous transaction with their internal and external environments (1997d, p. 21).
- Individuals are spiritual (1997b, p. 16).

Implicit Assumptions

- Patients want to participate actively in the care process.
- Patients are conscious, active, and cognitively capable to participate in decision-making (Austin and Champion, 1983, p. 56).
- All individuals should be respected as human beings of equal worth and who have their own set of values (King, 1999, p. 296).

1996b) and the processes of decision-making, and it extends arguments and guidelines for ethical decision-making (King, 1999). King considered questions related to the nature of the process of interaction that lead to the achievement of goals and the significance of mutual goal setting in achieving nursing care goals. By emphasizing the collaborative role of the patient in decision-making and in making and providing choices, she acknowledges the importance of empowering patients (Whelton, 2008). The theory evolved from several explicit assumptions to provide the basis for action (Box 12-1). One of the modifications in her assumptions is that individuals are spiritual (King, 1997b). The explicit assumptions are congruent with the contemporary and future-oriented views that nursing holds and aspires to maintain, particularly as she explicitly stated an assumption about the continuous transaction of individuals with internal and external environments (King, 1997d). All King's assumptions speak to the significance of patient involvement in their care, as well as in the decision-making process; the importance of collaboration; the humanity of the nurse–patient encounter; and the dynamic changes in environments (King, 1999). The theory provides guidelines for ways to decrease the confusion occurring in the health care system as patients try to deal

with a myriad of options, as they exercise their right to having choices and making informed decisions.

It is important to note, too, that King's assumptions encompass the nurse's perceptions, goals, needs, and values—not only those of the patient—and these are expected to influence the interaction process and, indeed, the outcomes. Although King designated the nurse as a central concept in nursing theory, she did not go as far as Paterson and Zderad did in focusing on the significance of the consideration of the continuous growth of the nurse in every interaction. The theory assumptions explicitly address the rationality of human beings, and King's theory proceeds to develop consistent concepts related to clients who can perceive, interpret, and solve problems. Austin and Champion (1983) argued that, as such, the theory is not useful to some situations in nursing (e.g., when patients are comatose or psychotic), and I might add, as options increase and/or as evidence of the particular decision is yet to be conclusive. How decisions are made during times of uncertainty remains problematic. However, Whelton (2008) makes the case of its utility for patients who are in palliative care.

There are inconsistencies in the different lists of concepts provided by King (Box 12-2). In one instance, she listed human being, environment,

BOX 12-2	CONCEPTS: A CONCEPTUAL FRAMEWORK FOR NURSING—KING

Personal Systems

Perception	Growth and development
Self	Time
Body image	Space

Interpersonal Systems

Role	Transactions
Human interaction	Stress
Communication	Coping
Coping (1997b, p. 16)	

Social Systems

Organization	Decision-making
Power, authority, status	Control
Goal attainment	

Concepts: A Theory of Goal Attainment

Interaction	Growth and development
Perception	Time
Communication	Space (Personal)
Transaction	Goal attainment
Self	Effective nursing care
Role	Appropriate information
Stress (stressors)	Satisfaction

Concepts: A Theory of Administration

Organization	Decision-making
Power	Perception
Authority	Communication
Status	Interaction
Role	Transaction
Control	
Conceptual system (instead of conceptual frame-work, conceptual model, or paradigm) (King, 1997b, p. 162; 2001, p. 281)	

health, and society as the abstract concepts. She also identified personal, interpersonal, and social systems as the major concepts (King, 1981, p. 142, 1997b, 2001). She defined interaction, perception, communication, transaction, role, stress, growth and development, time, and space as they represent the theory of goal attainment. Although King clarified the relationship between the latter set of concepts in the interpersonal system, it is not clear how these "major concepts in the theory" relate to human beings, environment, health, and society (King, 1988a). Perception appears to be a central concept in her theory (Bunting, 1988), including perceptions of patients, which must be honored and accepted, and the importance of nurses' perceptions (Clarke, Killeen, Messmer, et al., 2009). This was further developed by Alligood and May

(2000) into a theory of personal system empathy. King and Whelton (2001), however, criticized this theory for its inaccurate reflection of King's ideas, for lack of support for the need of another theory without the use of King's entire theory, and for its lack of expansion of her theory. I highly recommend reviewing this exchange of ideas and subsequent related publications by others.

King offered, in the conceptual framework, almost every concept that nurses may have historically used in nursing care (see Box 12-2). It is not entirely clear how the goal-attainment theory evolved from the myriad concepts that appear in the conceptual framework; however, King indicated that the selection was based on those she believed represented "a broad conceptualization of knowledge" (King, 1997b). In the goal-attainment theory,

King restricted concepts to the interaction system central to the nursing act. Most of her concepts are derived, except for goal attainment, health transaction, effective nursing, appropriate information, and satisfaction. She also added the concept of coping to the personal system (King, 1997b). Although the derived concepts are defined conceptually and have the potential for operational definition, they have not been delineated as central concepts, nor were they defined theoretically or operationally. However, the theory purports to have as a goal nurse–patient interactions that enhance goal setting and lead to goal attainments of outcomes, which are a measure of effective nursing care (King, 1996b).

Other concepts not defined are satisfaction and effective nursing care, and although these are seemingly central to patient outcomes, they are defined neither conceptually nor operationally. Much later, Plummer and Molzahn (2009) explicated how quality of life and life satisfaction are interconnected and explained by one's ability to set and attain goals. To attain goals, appropriate information should be given; what is "appropriate," what is considered "information," and who decides what is appropriate or what is considered information are only a few of the questions that point out the lack of theoretical definitions and lack of boundaries between concepts (Table 12-1), and the incongruence between assumptions, concepts, and statements (Uys, 1987). King updates concepts to reflect more contemporary health care language. For example, as she indicated, she changed quality nursing care to effective nursing care, to quality assurance, to continuous quality care, to outcomes, and now to evidence-based practice (King, in Fawcett, 2001).

The focus of King's theory is on the nurse–client dyads and on interaction for decision-making toward health. Health is defined in terms of the ability to function in a social role (King, 1986a), and it includes genetic, subjective, relative, dynamic, environmental, functional, cultural, and perceptual components (King, 1990b). However, Magan (1987) questioned ways by which the levels and quality of functioning could be assessed, a critique that could inspire a more effective and productive conceptualization of health. Explication of health in terms of morbidity and mortality data and accidents is more congruent with a disease orientation than with a role-functioning orientation. King's views of health and illness are problematic. As Magan puts it:

The difficulty with a consistent understanding of health in King's framework is further complicated by her assertion that health and disease do not constitute polarities, while she also maintained that illness is an interference or disturbance in health. (Magan, 1987, p. 119)

The inconsistencies in King's definition of health are manifest in viewing health and illness as nonpolar and not dichotomies, and illness as an interference or disturbance, and at the same time viewing health in terms of a dynamic life experience. Doornbos (2000), using King's theory to develop and test a derivative theory of family health, defined King's driven family health as adaptability, cohesion, satisfaction, and conflict using instruments to test adaptability, cohesion, and satisfaction with the level of functioning. By doing that, she helped to advance an explication of health à la King. Quality of life, implicitly considered in King's theory to be imbedded in well-being and life satisfaction, is similarly not well defined (Plummer and Molzahn, 2009).

King offers strategies to measure health (King, 1988b) and examples of how her theory can be tested through a set of propositions that link perceptions, transactions, goal attainment, satisfaction, and effective nursing care; these are more congruent with educational goals rather than research goals. The propositions are relative and tend to be deterministic (Zetterberg, 1963). They are based on a cause-and-effect approach and are designed for prediction, not description, which could be equally effective in further development of theory. Propositions link some of the defined concepts (transactions, interactions, role performance), but they also link the undefined concepts, such as health and outcomes.

Theory Analysis

The Theorist

Imogene King is well known for more than her theory; she is one of the pioneers who promoted a theoretical base for nursing (King, 1964, 1975, 1976). She is, like a number of other theorists, a graduate (EdD, 1961) of Teachers College of Columbia University. In 1945, she graduated from St. John's Hospital School of Nursing in St. Louis and received a Bachelor's Degree in Nursing Education in 1948 and a Master of Science in Nursing in 1957 from St. Louis University. She completed a postdoctoral study in systems research, advanced statistics, research design, and computers (King, 1986a, 2001). She considered her life in terms of many opportunities. In one of her last essays,

TABLE 12-1	Definition of Domain Concepts—King
Nursing	"A process of human interaction between nurse and client whereby each perceives the other in the situation and, through communication, they set goals, explore means, and agree on means to achieve goals" (King, 1981, p. 144), "and their actions indicate movement toward goal achievement" (1987a, p. 113). "A process of action, reaction, interaction and transaction" (1971, p. 89 and 1981, p. 2). Nursing services are called on when individuals cannot function in their roles.
Goal of nursing	"To help individuals to maintain their health so they can function in their roles" (1981, p. 3).
	"To help individuals to attain and restore health or die in dignity" (1981, p. 13). The goal of nursing is then to maintain, restore, and promote health (1992b). The goal of nursing is "to help individuals and groups attain, maintain, and regain a healthy state" (King, 2001, p. 283). Or, to help individuals die with dignity (King, 1971).
Health	"A dynamic life experience of a human being, which implies continuous adjustment to stressors in the internal and external environment through optimum use of one's resources to achieve maximum potential for daily living" (1981, p. 5 and 1983b, p. 186).
	Ability to function in social role.
	Process of growth and development (King, 1990b, 1992b).
Environment	The internal environment of human beings transforms energy to enable them to adjust to continuous external environmental changes (1981, p. 5). The external environment is the formal and informal organization. "A social system is defined as an organized boundary system of social roles, behaviors, and practices developed to maintain values and the mechanisms to regulate practice and rules" (1981, p. 115). The nurse is part of the patient's environment.
Human being	Rational, sentient, social being, perceiving, thinking, feeling, able to choose between alternative actions, able to set goals, to select means toward goals, to make decisions, and to have a symbolic way of communicating thoughts, actions, customs, and beliefs. Is time oriented and reacting. Reactions are based on perceptions, expectations, and needs (1981, p. 19).
Nursing client	A unique, total, open system with perception, self, body image, time, space, growth, and development throughout the life span and with experiences of changes in structure and function of body influencing perception of self (1981, pp. 19–20).
	Person as open system exhibits permeable boundaries permitting an exchange of matter, energy, and information (1981, p. 69).
	A person who cannot perform daily activities and cannot carry the responsibilities of their roles (1976).
Nursing problem	Inability to meet needs for daily living (1981, p. 5).
	Inability to function in their roles (1981, p. 3).
	The central problem is nonmutual goal setting and lack of agreement on goals and means leading to unattained goals (1981, p. 144). "Felt needs" as perceived by patient or real needs as perceived by nurse (1968, p. 29).
Nursing process	A focal concept in King's theory called transactional process. The goal of nursing is to help patients attain their goals. The mechanism for that is the nursing process. Through this process, nurses interact purposefully with clients (1981, p. 176). The purpose is information sharing, setting of mutual goals, participation in decisions about goals and means, implementing plans and evaluations. It is based on a knowledge base.
Nurse–patient relations	"A process of perception and communication between person and environment and between person and person, represented by verbal and nonverbal behaviors that are goal-oriented" (1981, p. 145).
	Variables affecting interactions are knowledge, needs, goals, past experiences, and perceptions of nurse and patient. The interaction process also includes reaction and transaction (1981, p. 145).
Nursing therapeutics	Transactions: informing, sharing, setting of mutual goals, participation in decisions about goals and means (1981, p. 176).
	Goal-oriented nursing record (1983b, pp. 183–186).

published after she passed away (King, 2008), she was asked whether "adversity" played a role in her life or her theory. Her answer was a resounding "no," and she concluded by suggesting that this "concept of adversity" should be replaced with challenges and opportunities. She acknowledged that her theory evolved as a result of many opportunities, giving the example of how a chance meeting with Dr. Hildegard Peplau (another early giant theorist) led to Peplau reading and providing a constructive critique of King's early draft of a manuscript of her theory. This led to revisions and publication in 1971. In many ways, King's theoretical tenets did not waver far from this early manuscript.

A clinician, an administrator, but primarily an educator with multiple honors and awards, including the Jessie Scott Award for Leadership, which was presented by the American Nurses Association at the 100th anniversary convention in 1996 and an honorary doctor of science in 1998 (King, 2001), she was inducted to the American Nurses Association Hall of Fame and the Teacher's College, Columbia University Hall of Fame. She was also named a Living Legend by the American Academy of Nursing. She has been a professor at the College of Nursing, University of South Florida at Tampa, the dean of the School of Nursing at Ohio State University, Columbus, and professor of nursing at Loyola University in Chicago. Besides being an author, she was an effective speaker whose joy in presenting and describing her theory was readily apparent to her audiences. Her commitment to students was continuously demonstrated whenever they sought her council. Dr. King passed away on December 24, 2007 (Clarke et al., 2009; Stevens and Messmer, 2008).

Paradigmatic Origins

King used the language of systems theory to introduce her ideas, and she credits von Bertalanffy (1968) and his science of wholeness and system elements in mutual interaction to the beginnings of her ideas (King, 1990a). Fawcett and DeSanto-Madeya classified her as a systems theorist (2013, Chapter 5) with a reciprocal interaction worldview. King classifies her ideas as emerging from systems theory (King, 1990a), and George classified her as an adaptation theorist (1980, p. 186). Her conceptual framework evolves from all paradigms that have been used in nursing; for example, the developmental (growth and development), systems (structural–functional view of role, open systems, social systems, and

energy), adaptation (continuous adjustment to stressors), psychoanalytical (self), and stress (energy response to environment) paradigms. The theory of goal attainment derives a great deal from symbolic interactionism, and what King offers helps in the understanding of the nursing process and the process of interaction; this prompts a classification of her theory as an interactionist theory.

Although King personally stated that she never used the symbolic interactionist school of thought (Fawcett, 1995), the influence of interactionism is marked. Several indications of parallelism between King's theory and symbolic interactionism are the descriptions of a person as a social being, actor, and reactor, who is constantly structuring and restructuring his perception of the world, thereby communicating through symbols. Nurse–patient interactions occur within the perceptual repertoire of both. The present meaning of any situation and the perceptions of time and situations of both nurse and patient are significant to the interaction, to the choices, options, and discussions (King, 1981, p. 148). In addition, King's use of roles (although more congruent with a structural–functional approach) and the personal element of perception and interpretation, are also indications of an interactionist approach. King recognized that a functionalist view of role is related to the study of social systems, but . . .

[t]he interactionist view of role is basic to understanding individuals in organizations when role is thought of as a relationship with another person or group of individuals, it is related to interpersonal systems. . . . The interactionist view relates to social interaction. (1981, p. 90)

Therefore, the entire focus of theory, and the central question around process, interaction, and goal attainment, makes it more congruent with a symbolic interactionist approach. However, whether or not the refinement of the theory may be more enhanced if the backdrop is interaction, rather than the inconsistent and mixed use of both system and interaction paradigms, is a question that continues to require an answer (Burney, 1992). Finally, both the paradigmatic origin and the theory suffer from the limitation of viewing a person as a social being rather than as a biopsychosocial being, or a holistic being.

These limitations may be an artifact of claimed paradigmatic origins as systems (von Bertalanffy, 1968) or even a limitation of the concepts of Dewey, who King, in 1992a, credited as providing the philosophical underpinnings for "transaction," which is a key concept in her theory. Whelton (1999) provided the most comprehensive analysis of a possible different philosophical core of King's theory. She indicated that King's framework is consistent with the philosophical assumptions of the Greek philosopher Aristotle (Whelton, 1999, 2008). Such a view is congruent with King's initial question of what it means to be human and what the properties of the human act are. Whelton (1999, 2008) provides a new major insight on King's theory by isolating "human nature" as the core of her theory and intimating that, by considering Aristotle's teachings, there is far more complexity and richness in making King's view of human capacity more dynamic and encompassing of personal, interpersonal, and social interactions. By providing a critical analysis of a different paradigmatic origin of King's theory, Whelton (1999) provides an answer to the question that may have prompted King to develop her theory, which was "what is human nature?" (King, 1997b), and she also shifts the emphasis from interaction to a focus on the person and his or her human acts.

Internal Dimensions

The microtheory of goal attainment was developed from a field approach centering on concepts rather than on propositions, and is therefore concatenated in structure. It is a mental image, with a constructive beginning deduced from a conceptual framework, the concepts of which were also deduced from other paradigms, systems, symbolic interactionism, or Aristotelian logic. Its scope is limited to the process of interaction, focusing on the perceptions of clients for the purpose of goal attainment. It deals with the interactions of one nurse with one patient. Despite the fact that King extensively discusses the social system, her theory, evolving from the interpersonal system, is limited to nurse–patient interactions, as it ought to be. She later expanded it to incorporate the family and their perceptions (King, 1983a, 1983b, 1990b) and discussed the use of the theory in the community (King, 2001). Others have also expanded it to include families (Doornbos, 2000; Temple and Fawdry, 1992) and the community (Sowell and Lowenstein, 1994).

The microtheory of goal attainment purports to predict processes inherent in goal attainment and provides descriptions of the concepts and properties of the interpersonal system. The theory was classified as providing a description of the nursing process (nursing transaction); it mainly explains how and when to use transactions to achieve mutually agreed-on goals. It is a single-domain theory about decision-making processes, with an average level of abstractness for the different concepts. King developed her theory using a logical method of development. The parts of the interactional system (interaction, transaction) lead to goal attainment.

Theory Critique

The literature provides numerous examples of the utility of King's theory for practice, research, education, and administration. Theory development progressed from a conceptual framework using a variety of unrelated concepts to a theory of nursing in the interpersonal system. King herself completed one research project and operationalized her theory for practice (King, 1981, 1986a) as well as for educational programs (King, 1986b). Propositions emanating from the theory are presented in Box 12-3. In an analysis of her theory, Caceres (2015) demonstrated that King's theory of goal attainment could be the vehicle that is useful in assessing and in facilitating client-family–centered care and achieving a health functional status.

King's theory is parsimonious, with distinct concepts and limited relationships, but teleological because interaction is defined by interaction and transaction (King, 1981, p. 145). Goal attainment appears to be a process of transaction toward effective nursing care, and it is a product equated with effective nursing care and satisfaction (King, 1981, pp. 147 and 153).

Considering that interaction has emerged as one of the central concepts in nursing, King's contribution is substantial to nursing knowledge (King, 1987b). The theory's clarity is enhanced when considered as a theory to describe and answer questions related to nurse–patient interactions for the purpose of setting goals. The nursing care process has been conceived by other theorists as a process involving assessment, diagnosis, intervention, and evaluation (King, 1986a). She called it a method only in 2001. Her transaction process, on the other hand, provides theoretical knowledge as a base for this process that she considers a transaction. Therefore, in making assessments and diagnoses, nurses must use perceptions, communication, and interaction to be able to make judgments.

A transaction is made when the nurse and the patient decide mutually on the goals to be attained, agree on the means to attain the goals that

BOX 12-3	PROPOSITIONS—KING

1. If perceptual accuracy is present in nurse–patient interactions, transactions will occur.
2. If nurse and patient transact, goals will be attained.
3. If goals are attained, satisfactions will occur.
4. If goals are attained, effective nursing will occur.
5. If transactions are made in nurse–patient interactions, growth and development will be enhanced.
6. If role expectation and role performance, as perceived by nurse and patients, are congruent, transactions will occur.
7. If role conflict is experienced by nurse or patient or both, stress in nurse–patient interactions will occur.
8. Nurses with special knowledge and skills communicate appropriate information to patients; mutual goal setting and goal attainment will occur.
9. Knowledge of oneself will bring about a helping relationship with patients.
10. Accurate perceptions of time and space in nurse–patient interactions lead to transactions.

From King, I.M. (1981). *A theory for nursing: Systems, concepts, process* (p. 149). New York: John Wiley & Sons; and King, I. M. (1986a). King's theory of goal attainment. In P. Winstead-Fry (Ed.), *Case studies in nursing theory*. New York: National League for Nursing.

represent the plan of care, and then implement the plan. Evaluation determines whether or not goals were attained. If not, you ask why not, and the process begins again. (King, 2001, p. 280)

For King, the process is dynamic; it is differentiated from other disciplines by its knowledge base. She further extended her use of the transaction process model (perception, communication, interaction, and transaction) to incorporate moral and ethical reasoning. To her, entering a nurse–patient relationship should be based on the assumption that every human being is of equal worth and value, that the relationship is based on justice, and that the nurse maintains a responsibility to continuously enhance competence and skills. In addition to the concepts of respect for equality and justice, the nurse should observe beneficence, which occurs when nurses use a knowledge base to help patients maintain or regain their health (King, 1999). The transaction process depends on three significant clinical tools: observation, interaction, and documentation. According to King (2001), the transaction process should be used by every student, staff nurse, and administrator.

King offers the nursing profession a description of the properties of interaction that is essential to the nursing act; indeed, it is the nursing act, and one of its cornerstones is the attainment of mutually agreed-on goals. King also offers it as a unique variation of the nursing process. The goal-oriented nursing record (GONR), developed as a tool analogous to the problem-oriented medical record developed by Weed (1969), includes both "process and outcomes in nursing situations" and a record of the goals, the means to achieve those agreed-on goals, and the process used to achieve them. It consists of five components: a database, a problem list, a goal list, a plan, and progress notes (King, 1981, pp. 164–165).

The GONR is similar to the nursing process used by other theorists, but it offers a more dynamic dimension that addresses the process, not only the goals. GONR has the potential of offering organized nursing care, and it could facilitate nursing audits, enhance abilities in making nursing diagnoses, increase focus on patients' participation, and validate the perceptions of patients during the process (King, 1981, p. 172). Although George (2002) critiqued the theory for its limitation in applicability to caring for groups, families, and communities, King expanded her methods to incorporate the family as a client in 1983 (Gonot, 1983, 1986), and the theory has been used by others as a framework for caring for families and communities.

The numerous examples of use of King's theory in clinical practice (Smith, 1988) include:

- An elderly patient with a cerebral vascular accident (King, 1983a)
- A patient with renal disease (King, 1984)
- Caring for families (Doornbos, 1995; King, 1983b; Moreira, Araujo, and Pagliuca, 2001)
- Providing care for critically ill infants (Norris and Frey, 2002)
- Providing care for women with hospitalized preterm infants (Viera and Rossi, 2000)
- As a problem-solving tool to facilitate the development of a healthy work environment

and to decrease the incidence of diseases of the computer age, such as carpal tunnel syndrome (Norgan, Ettipio, and Lasome, 1995)

- Providing community health nursing care (Asay and Ossler, 1984; Sowell and Lowenstein, 1994)
- Developing alcohol use/dependency care for adult females (McKinney and Dean, 2000)
- Providing psychiatric care (Gonot, 1983)
- Caring for comatose patients (King, 1986a)
- Caring for adults with diabetes (Husband, 1988)
- As a framework for managed care (Hampton, 1994), and for hospital care (Messmer, 1995)

The theory was extended for testing under King's guidelines in Japan, Sweden, Portugal, Denmark, Germany, and the United States (Bauer, 1998, 1999; Franca and Pagliuca, 2002; Frey, Rooke, Sieloff, et al., 1995; King, 2000; Zoffmann, Harder, and Kirkevold, 2008), thus providing a forward-looking approach to decision-making and collaboration in chronic illness care, which is a hallmark for knowledge development in the future (Meleis, 1985). Woods (1994) used the theory to demonstrate how mutual identification and achievement of goals were facilitated between nurses and a group of elderly people with chronic health problems. The theory has been used with attention to newly evolving concepts, such as quality of care (Sowell and Lowenstein, 1994) and quality of life (King, 1994). The theory has been used to develop a framework for neonatal care that is built less on medical models and medicalization and more on a process of interaction between parents and nurses (Norris and Hoyer, 1993). Such examples of the theory–practice link support its utility in and potential for transcending the boundaries of time, geography, and specializations; they also demonstrate that the theory has been used innovatively and with a trend-setting approach.

With the increasing need for decision-making related to "advanced directives," in which individuals make known their wishes for their own care during crises, King's theory may provide the definitive decision-making transactional framework. The Patient Self-Determination Act (PSDA) provides individuals with a legal means to accept or reject care even if they may not be able to make such a decision cognitively or physically. Goodwin, Kiehl, and Peterson (2002) developed a model for decision-making, the Advanced Directive Decision Making Model (ADDM), based on King's theory and using seven components: perception and time (personal system), interaction and role (interpersonal systems), power, status, and decision-making

(social systems). This model guides interactions, addresses complex end-of-life issues, and facilitates the process of achieving mutual goal attainment for clinicians and clients. It is one of the best examples of developing a situation-specific theory, derived from an existing theory, to address an important health care phenomenon. It is also an example of why theories need to be and are reflective of certain historical moments. The situation-specific ADDM was not needed prior to the imperative development of the PSDA (Omnibus Budget Reconciliation Act of 1990).

To determine the risks of bleeding and complications for clients who cease to use anticoagulants when undergoing endoscopic procedures, Ryle (2008) used King's theory to integrate evidence related to personal, interpersonal, and social systems, as well as her theory of goal attainment, with an emphasis on the role of the nurse and the perceptions of nurses and patients. By utilizing the theory to guide the integration and analyses of ten research studies, the author concluded that there was no evidence of an increase in complications.

Despite these examples of the clinical utility of the theory, it appears to be more useful for assessing active, autonomous, collaborative, and individual (fewer examples of group or aggregate utility) relationships with nurses. It is more useful for long-term nurse–patient relationships, to evaluate "satisfaction, goal attainment, and effective nursing care." The utility of GONR for care of infants, children, comatose patients, some psychiatric patients, dementia patients, or some mentally retarded patients is still in question (Austin and Champion, 1983; Barnum, 1994). King's theory is also limited to use only in some health care settings.

The theory would have limited application in settings where clients are unable to interact competently. In addition, it is not clear how the theory could be utilized with groups. Utilizing transactions with groups of individuals who had different goals is not addressed by King. (Austin and Champion, 1983, p. 60)

There are a number of other limitations to clinical utility. The theory does not give explicit guidelines for assessment, diagnosis, or intervention. The theoretical boundaries to help a practitioner in assessing problems and potential problems and in deciding on clinical therapeutics are not identified. It analyzes problems, but does not offer guidelines for interventions. Interaction is a process in all helping relationships; its uniqueness to nursing stems from its relationship to other phenomena. This is lacking in King's theory. Carter and Dufour (1994) disagree with these criticisms and offer compelling arguments for the theory's flexibility and utility, and George (2002) questions its use for groups, families, and communities.

Although King's theory focused on the client–nurse relationship, it was also used as a framework to identify barriers to achieving goals for interdisciplinary collaborations of health care professionals. Barriers identified are patriarchal relationships, time, lack of role clarification, gender, and culture. Research findings on the outcomes for lack of collaboration were integrated by Fewster-Thuente and Velsor-Friedrich (2008), who concluded that lack of collaboration puts patients at high risk for readmission to intensive care units, death, error, and longer length of stay. The authors conclude that, by using the theory, they were able to provide a coherent account of barriers, with negative and positive attainment of goals.

Nursing administration could also use the theory in developing a recording system for nursing care plans with refinement and modifications related to patient care outcomes. King promised that, if nurses use goal-attainment theory and GONR to enhance accurate documentation and recording of the goals identified and attained in interactions, effective nursing care could be measured (King, 1981, p. 155, 1989, pp. 42–45). King discussed the development of a theory of administration following the same principles used in developing a theory of goal attainment. King believed that when such theory is communicated in the literature, it will be useful for both nursing science administration and nursing education administration (King, 1989). Elberson (1989) presented a description of the utility of King's theory in nursing administration, and Byrne-Coker and Schreiber (1990) provided an analysis of the effective use of the theory as a framework for nursing practice in an agency. It was also used in Canada for developing and implementing a system for care delivery (Fawcett, Vaillancourt, and Watson, 1995), and for transforming nursing practice in neonatal intensive care units (Norris and Hoyer, 1993) and in the homes of the elderly (Woods, 1994). Further, the theory—with its focus on perceptions of human beings and their patterns of interactions, functional roles, and physical well-being—proved useful as a framework to study the experiences of administrators dealing with nurses who have been rehabilitated from chemical dependency developed in the clinical setting (Miller, Kanai, Kebritchi, et al., 2015).

King's theory is suitable for use in nursing education as a basis for learning, which is one significant phase and component of the nursing process. Evidence suggests that the theory provides a conceptual framework for curricula (Daubenmire and King, 1973; King, 1978, 1996c), and it is used to guide a curriculum in continuing education (Brown and Lee, 1980). King provided guidelines for implementing her theory in an educational setting (1968, p. 30), and in 1986, she published a book on curriculum development in which she carefully demonstrated how her theory could be used as a curricular framework (King, 1986b). She also summarized the potential utility of theory in curricula (Gulitz and King, 1988; King, 1988a). King's theory has been used as a conceptual framework for a baccalaureate program at Ohio State University School of Nursing in Columbus (Daubenmire and King, 1973; King, 1986b) and in models for improved patient care (Rooke, 1995). The graduate program at Loyola University in Chicago used her theory as a framework (Fawcett, 2001). Other schools also used her theory or components of it as a framework for curriculum development, as well as for teaching (Fawcett, 1995).

Diagrams depicting relationships between central concepts of the theory, central concepts in nursing, and major propositions would have enhanced the clarity of the theory and may have contributed even more to the extensive utilization of King's theory in educational and practice settings.

External Components of Theory

King's theory is congruent with the values and beliefs about nursing, humanity, autonomy, patient advocacy, self-reliance, and planning that are espoused by Western societies. Because it pertains to the conscious, self-directed patient, it is more suited to U.S. values. The focus of the theory on mutual goal setting and attainment, on interacting with individuals, and on helping individuals become sufficiently healthy to function in roles is congruent with Western philosophy and mores of pragmatism and the usefulness of adult members of society. Many other societies that consider patients helpless, that espouse the sick role as an abandonment of social roles and responsibilities, and that support the rights of patients to be sheltered from prognosis and health care goals (as in some Middle Eastern cultures) would consider this theory culturally limited (Meleis and Jones, 1983). Patients in these societies prefer to relinquish all decisions and goal setting to the expertise of health care professionals.

This claim of the theory's apparent ethnocentrism is refuted by Husting (1997), Carter and Dufour (1994), and by King as cited in Fawcett and DeSanto-Madeya (2013, Chapter 5). The bases for such refutation are examples of the successful implementation of King's theory in Japan and Sweden (Rooke, 1995) and that her books have been translated into Spanish and Japanese. More support for the theory's cross-cultural applicability was provided by Rooda (1992). King (1997c) cites a Sigma Theta Tau International Conference in Madrid, at which presenters demonstrated her theory's relevance, appropriateness, and utility for diverse cultures. Portuguese-speaking scholars used her theory to describe the perceptions of patients, compliance, and treatment decisions (Franca and Pagliuca, 2002; Moreira and Araujo, 2002). Many Western theories, in many disciplines, enjoy international utilization by certain proponents. These select few scholars are, in most cases, Western educated; many others regard U.S.-generated theories as the answer to all issues. I continue to offer and encourage skepticism about the use of U.S.-generated theories in providing frameworks to uncover, explain, and understand health care issues in different cultures and societies. Until equal and reciprocal development and utilization of theories occurs internationally, my warning remains—international utilizers use our U.S.-generated theories carefully, critically, and skeptically. And, at best, be critical about the fundamental assumptions upon which theories are developed. As to you, the reader, my hope is that you contribute your critical, supportive, or refuting ideas to keep a healthy dialogue going.

Theory Development and Testing

King outlined hypotheses for testing her theoretical propositions (King, 1987a), and she proposed future studies to test these hypotheses (King, 1986a; Uys, 1987). Fawcett (1995) reports that, in February 1988, a conference held at the University of South Florida, College of Nursing, focused on research designed to test King's theory. As Fawcett indicates, this is a reflection of a growing body of knowledge related to King. King also developed a criterion-referenced instrument designed to assess physical and behavioral functional abilities, goal setting with clients, and goal attainment (King, 1986a).

Several studies testing various properties derived from King's theory are reported in the literature.

Brower (1981) described nurses' attitudes toward the elderly; Rosendahl and Ross (1982) described the relationship between attending behaviors on mental status; and Frey (1989) described the development and initial testing of parent support, child support, family health, and child health in families coping with insulin-dependent diabetes mellitus. Frey used King's theory as the basis for defining concepts, selecting indicators, and developing propositions for testing. Although Frey questioned the availability of appropriate instruments to use in testing King's theory (Frey, 1989, p. 146), these findings lend support to the relationship between interaction and health as proposed by King, as well as to the relationship between the perceptions of nurses and the perceptions of patients regarding the patients' information needs (Isac, Ezhilarau, and Chacko, 2012). There are also indications of the international utility of King's theory in research (Rooke and Norberg, 1988). The theory was used to describe awareness and perceptions of prostate and testicular cancers and an intervention to enhance such awareness (Martin, 1990). It was tested and supported for its cultural relevance by Frey et al. (1995) and Rooda (1992). The theory was used as a framework for testing postoperative recovery and satisfaction of patients (Hanucharurnkui and Vinya-nguag, 1991).

Several studies support the relationship between central concepts in King's theories. Human-to-human interaction adds to the perceptual accuracy of nurses of their patients' expectations, which in turn contribute to goal attainment (Daniel, 2002). Sieloff's (2003) study on the assessment of a departmental power instrument that she developed demonstrated initial support. Walker and Alligood (2001) compared and contrasted two theories of empathy and concluded that using King's theory is more suited for nursing care. Doornbos (2000) developed and tested a theory of family caregiving of young adults with mental illness based on King's theory. This is an example of situation-specific theory that could prove to be more effective in predicting outcomes as well as dictating nurses' actions.

King also tested her theory and reported the results in her 1981 book. The study was designed to answer three questions:

1. What elements in nurse–patient interactions lead to transactions?
2. What are the relationships between the elements in the interactions that lead to transactions?
3. What are the essential variables in nurse–patient interactions that result in transactions? (King, 1981, p. 151)

The results of this descriptive study supported the components of the interpersonal system and lent construct validity. The study limitations are numerous, but the study could be considered a pilot for further research. The study was based on data generated by nonparticipant observations of the verbal and nonverbal behaviors of nurses and patients. The sample consisted of 17 cases. The results of this descriptive study support the components of the interpersonal system and provide construct validity. Specifically, King's study indicated that interaction was verbal and nonverbal, and that nurse–patient interactions led to transactions and identification of problems, concerns, or disturbances in the patient's environment. Variables that helped in the achievement of goals were "accurate perceptions of nurse and patient, adequate communication, and mutual goal setting" (King, 1981, p. 155). Despite several limitations of the study (sample size, biases of the researchers, and limited analysis), this pilot study indicates the potential testability of the theory (King, 1996b).

In an extensive research review of King's theory-driven projects, the authors provide several seminal conclusions. Among these conclusions is that, although there has been ongoing discussion and clarification of the theory, only a few changes have occurred, including adding the concepts of coping and spirituality (Frey, Sieloff, and Norris, 2002). There have been over 576 publications related to King's theory between 1978 and 2000 (Frey et al., 2002), 33 descriptive studies, 14 correlational studies, and 9 experimental (Fawcett and DeSanto-Madeya, 2013). Despite this volume of utilization as a framework for research, the validity of its propositions remains limited, and its contribution to advancing knowledge remains limited. It is not enough to claim the theory's use as a framework or to publish the research. It is imperative to develop a trajectory of related findings, develop a program of sustained research, develop conceptually based interventions, interpret the data with the theory, and complete the cycle by refining and extending the theory (Fawcett and DeSanto-Madeya, 2013). In one example of such a study, Ehrenberger, Alligood, Thomas, et al. (2002) related uncertainty, role functioning, and social support to emotional health and to treatment decision-making; their findings provide some support for understanding the human emotional state on treatment decisions. In another study, researchers found that using a nurse–client contractual agreement and mutual decision-making based on King's theory of goal attainment promoted

improvement in self-care in renal dialysis patients in Korea (Cho, 2013). Similarly, a third study found that improvements in rehabilitation from spinal cord injury relied on utilizing patients' perceptions and collaborating with them in setting goals (Draaistra, Singh, Ireland, et al., 2012). However, the authors add that understanding the meaning the patients attribute to the process of goal setting is vital for enhancing a collaborative process of goal setting.

In sum, I share the conclusions by Frey and her colleagues (2002):

King's contribution to nursing science is long-standing and universally recognized . . . Continued work in developing and testing middle-range theories derived from the conceptual system and validating the theory of goal attainment will increase as the number of nurse scholars who work to advance and extend her perspective of nursing increases. (p. 111)

These contributions are evident in the number of theories that were inspired by, influenced by, or derived from King's theories. Among them is a theory of group outcome attainment that Sieloff (2007, 2010) developed based on her work in measuring power in work environments (2003). Another is a theory of empathy (Alligood and May, 2000; Alligood, 2014) based on King's focus on perceptions and empathy. A list of theories that were directly derived from King's conceptual system is listed in Fawcett and DeSanto-Madeya (2013, pp. 95–96).

The support of the King International Nursing Group, founded in 1998, will undoubtedly sustain the development of more research studies, additional testing of the theory's evolving propositions (Frey et al., 2002), and further development of King's theories as well as the development of other related theories and perhaps situation-specific theories. The publication of collected papers on the use of King's theory in developing middle-range theory may stimulate research beyond using the theory only as a framework to integrate findings from other research (Sieloff, 2007). This group is increasing in number and visibility, and it produces a newsletter with opportunities for meetings and dialogues to extend King's theory and to contribute to its development.

King's vision for the future extension of her theory is contained in the following:

The conceptual system of 3 interacting personal systems, interpersonal systems & social systems has identified 15 concepts (perception,

communication, interaction & transaction, etc.)
that represent basic theoretical knowledge that
should be taught with the Nursing Process method
of assess, plan, implement & evaluate. The transac-
tion process in King's theory of goal attainment
leads to mutual goal setting (the critical variable),
and when goals are achieved this represents out-
comes which provide for evidence based practice.
(King, 2005, personal communication)

IDA ORLANDO

Theory Description

In the mid- to late-1950s, the Yale School of Nursing
shifted from undergraduate to graduate education
and integrated psychiatric concepts into the entire
curriculum. Orlando's theory grew out of processes
inherent in these curricular changes and out of dissatisfaction with the possibility that nursing care
was being prompted by organizational rules rather
than by attention to patients' needs. Orlando's theory
is based on two central questions: What prompts
nursing actions? What are the properties of dynamic
nurse–patient relationships that may lead to knowing patients' needs and providing effective care?

When Orlando began formulating her conceptualization of nursing, the answer to the first question
was that nurses were prompted in their actions by
physician's prescriptions, organizational needs, and
personal repertoire of experiences rather than by
patient needs—in other words, for reasons other than
the patients' immediate experiences and immediate
needs for help (1961, p. 60). This answer did not
satisfy Orlando and may have prompted the ideas
for the development of her theory. When Orlando
revisited the terms she used in her theory and the
goal of the theory, she redefined it as a "nursing
process theory" rather than a theory of "effective
nursing care" (Orlando-Pelletier, 1990a).

The focus of Orlando's theory is on identifying and clarifying the nurse–patient interpersonal
process during health and illness situations. To her,
basically, nurses' reactions or responses to patients
may be automatic, "disciplined professional," (1972)
or "deliberative" (1961, 1990a). In each situation,
the reaction is based on observation of the patient's
verbal or nonverbal behavior and is influenced by
perceptions, thoughts, and feelings related to the
patient's action that prompted the nurse's reaction,
or vice versa. The automatic response is guided by
"secretiveness," during which neither the meaning
of the behavior nor the perceptions of the nurse or

the patient are validated. The "disciplined professional response" is guided by "explicitness" of
perceptions, thoughts, and feelings, indicating that
the patient's needs are validated, and ambivalence
and distress are explored. The disciplined professional response also indicates that the nurse has
validated the effectiveness of nursing actions in
helping the patient.

The nursing disciplined process requires the
following conditions:

- What the nurse says to the individual in the
  contact must match (be consistent with) any
  or all of the items contained in the immediate reaction.
- What the nurse does nonverbally must be
  verbally expressed, and the expression must
  match one or all of the items contained in the
  immediate reaction.
- The nurse must clearly communicate to the
  individual that the item being expressed belongs to herself.
- The nurse must ask the individual about the item
  expressed to obtain correction or verification
  from that same individual (1972, pp. 29–30).

Conversely, not all interactions are based on a
nursing process discipline. Nurses may give automatic nursing care, exemplified in routine care
(Orlando, 1961, 1972). Automatic nursing care does
not encompass perception, thoughts, and feelings.
These also deal less with finding out and meeting
the patients' needs for help. There are two types
of automatic responses. One is stimulated by the
patients' needs, and, insofar as nurses respond to
needs that patients cannot take care of by themselves, automatic response is expected to be effective. This is deliberative, automatic response. The
other automatic responses are those that result from
reasons other than the patients' immediate needs
for help. Automatic responses neither acknowledge
nor consider patients' perceptions and thoughts of
the problem.

A nurse's professional identity is exemplified
by her offering disciplined professional actions
that are stimulated by knowledge of patient needs
and that are validated by patient responses. These
actions involve a continuous process of reflection
as the nurse attempts to explore the meaning of
the patient's behavior. The nurse perceives the
behavior and its meaning, shares these perceptions,
and explores and validates the meanings of these
perceptions with the patient. By sharing, exploring, and validating perceptions, misinterpretations
are minimized. Modeling for interpretation and

validation would enhance further use of this process and would enhance understanding of our own and others' reactions and actions (Schmieding, 1987).

When nurses provide these actions, the result is a patient who experiences improvement in behavior, who has needs met, who feels comfortable, who has a sense of adequacy, and who does not manifest helplessness or distress. Nurses deal with "immediate needs" in "immediate experiences" of a patient in an illness situation by engaging in "immediate exploration" of the patient's perceptions, thoughts, and feelings (Orlando, 1961, p. 65). If nurses provide effective nursing care, they will see immediate behavioral changes for the better, they will see increased ability and adequacy in better care of self, and, eventually, they will see an increased sense of well-being. Need "is situationally defined as a requirement of the patient that, if supplied, relieves or diminishes his immediate distress or improves his immediate sense of adequacy or well-being" (Orlando, 1961, p. 5). Orlando based her conceptualization of nursing as dynamic interaction on several implicit assumptions (Box 12-4). It is also based on acknowledgment of feelings and emotions.

There are three problems with the assumptions. First, it is not clear how Orlando derived her assumptions; no documentation exists. Second, the nature of some of her assumptions limits nursing to administering only to patients who are under the care of medicine and who cannot meet their own needs comfortably. Neither of these assumptions is acceptable in nursing today; nurses may care for patients who are not receiving medical care, and may help to more effectively meet the needs of patients who are able to meet their own needs. Third, the ratio of assumptions to propositions is high, necessitating too many conditions for the number of propositions and placing a severe limitation on the exploratory power of the theory. Fourth, a mechanistic and reductionist view of human beings appears to be implicit in her theory (Sellers, 1991). However, Orlando was one of the early thinkers in nursing who proposed that patients have their own meanings and interpretations of situations, and, therefore, nurses must validate their inferences and analyses with patients before drawing conclusions about patients' experiences or needs (Forchuk, 1991; Orlando, 1961).

Orlando's theory contains more primitive concepts that are unique to her theory (deliberative, automatic, disciplined professional, dynamic nurse–patient relationship) than derived concepts that have been

---

BOX 12-4   ASSUMPTIONS—ORLANDO

Implicit Assumptions

- When patients cannot cope with their needs without help, they become distressed with feelings of helplessness (Orlando, 1961, p. 11).
- Nursing, in its professional character, does not add to the distress of the patient (1961, p. 9).
- Patients are unique and individual in their responses (1961, p. 59).
- Patients' distress reactions are based on lack of understanding of their experience (1961, p. 17).
- Nursing offers mothering and nurturing analogous to an adult mothering and nurturing a child (1961, p. 4).
- Nursing deals with people, environment, and health.
- Patients need help in communicating needs; they are uncomfortable and ambivalent about dependency needs (1961, p. 24).
- Human beings (nurses and patients) are able to be "secretive" or explicit about their needs, perceptions, thoughts, and feelings (1972, p. 26).
- The nurse–patient situation is dynamic; actions and reactions are influenced by both nurse and patient (1961).
- Human beings attach meanings to situations and actions that are not apparent to others.
- Patient entry into nursing care is through medicine (1961, p. 5).
- The patient cannot state the "nature and meaning of his distress for his need without the nurse's help or without her first having established a helpful relationship with him" (1961, p. 23).
- "Any observation shared and explored with the patient is immediately useful in ascertaining and meeting his need or finding out that he is not in need at that time" (1961, p. 36).
- Nurses are concerned with needs that patients cannot meet on their own (1961, p. 5).
- Nurses concern themselves with patient's distress (1961, p. 22).
- Nurses should not add to patient's distress (1961, p. 9).

BOX 12-5	CONCEPTS—ORLANDO

Need for help
Distress
Immediate
  Need
  Experience
  Exploration
  Behavioral changes
Sense of adequacy
Helplessness
Situational conflict
Nursing process discipline
Deliberative nursing process
Disciplined professional response
Visual manifestations
  Need for help or improvement
  Motor activities
    Eating, walking, twitching, and trembling
  Physiological activities
    Urinating, defecating, temperature, blood
      pressure reading, respiratory rate, skin color

Vocal manifestations
  Behavior heard
    Crying, moaning, laughing, coughing,
      sneezing, sighing, yelling, screaming,
      singing
  Patients may complain, request, question, re-
    fuse, demand, comment, provide statements
Reaction
  Perception
  Thought
  Feeling
Actions
  Secret
    Automatic response
  Explicit
    Personal response
Improvement
Reactions
  Explicit
  Secret

discussed in other theories (needs, helplessness, environment), which gives the theory its own unique focus and enhances its contribution to nursing theory (Box 12-5). Many of the central concepts are not defined (environment, health) or, when defined (e.g., interaction), they are nonvariables (Hage, 1972) (Table 12-2). Because the concepts evolved from her conceptual image of nursing's potential reality, they have empirical references, and, therefore, have the potential to be operationalized (Andrews, 1983).

Properties of action and reaction are well explicated, but outcomes are not defined—such as improvement, distress, need for help, helplessness—thus making it difficult not only to ascertain conceptually the need for help but also to ascertain the consequences of either automatic or deliberate nursing actions. The most significant variable—effective nursing care—is equated with either the disciplined professional process or lack of helplessness, distress, and even, at times, meeting the needs of patients, making the theory both tautological and teleological.

Theory Analysis

The Theorist

Ida Jean Orlando-Pelletier was an associate professor and the director of the graduate program in mental health and psychiatric nursing (1958–1961) at Yale University School of Nursing when her 1961 book was published. The book was the product of a 1954–1959 National Institute of Mental Health grant, initiated to integrate mental health concepts in nursing programs (Crane, 1980). Her second book, in 1972, was a result of another supported research project (by the National Institute of Mental Health, Public Health Service) and a general research grant. She was, at that time, a clinical nurse consultant at McLean Hospital, Belmont, Massachusetts (1962–1972).

Orlando has held numerous other positions, including consultant to nursing service administration and nursing education to schools, to health departments, and to the many students who called her from across the United States. She was appointed consultant to the New England Board of Higher Education and the board of the Harvard Community Health Plan. Orlando's most recent position was director of nursing at the Tri-City Unit of Metropolitan State Hospital in Waltham, Massachusetts.

According to Schmieding (1986), (Orlando's 1961) book has been translated into five languages. Orlando worked closely with and was influenced by Wiedenbach; she, in turn, influenced Travelbee's theoretical notions of nursing. Orlando's book was reissued with new introductions by the National League for Nursing (1990a, 1990b); this republication of her work acknowledges the significance of her contributions and the timelessness of her ideas.

TABLE 12-2	Definition of Domain Concepts—Orlando
Nursing	"Is responsive to individuals who suffer or anticipate a sense of helplessness." "Process of care in an immediate experience . . . for avoiding, relieving, diminishing, or curing the individual's sense of helplessness" (Orlando, 1972, p. 13). "Finding out and meeting the patient's immediate need for help" (1972, p. 20). Nurse's reaction encompasses perception, thought and feeling (1972, p. 59).
Goal of nursing	Increased sense of well-being; increase in ability, adequacy in better care of self and improvement in patient's behavior (1961).
Health	Sense of adequacy or well-being Fulfilled needs. Sense of comfort (1961, p. 9)
Environment	Not defined directly but implicitly in the immediate context for a patient (Orlando, 1972).
Human being	Developmental beings with needs; individuals have their own subjective perceptions and feelings that may not be observable directly.
Nursing client	Patients who are under medical care and who cannot deal with their needs or who cannot carry out medical treatment alone. There are two dimensions to their behavior: need for help and improvement expressed verbally and nonverbally.
Nursing problem	Distress due to unmet needs due to "physical limitations," "adverse reactions to the setting," or "experiences which prevent the patient from communicating his needs (1961, p. 11). Ineffective nursing activities: acting in a way not helpful to patient or not achieving professional purpose (1961, p. 72). Ineffective patient behavior such as uncooperative, unreasonable, demanding, or commanding behaviors that prevent the nurse from carrying out her care of maintaining a satisfactory relationship with the patient.
Nursing process	The interaction of "(1) the behavior of the patient, (2) the reaction of the nurse, and (3) the nursing actions which are assigned for the patient's benefit" (1961, p. 36). Process by which a nurse acts (1972, p. 29).
Nurse–patient relations	Central in theory and not differentiated from nursing therapeutics or nursing process.
Nursing therapeutics	Direct function: "(1) Initiates a process of helping the patient express the specific meaning of his behavior in order to ascertain his distress and (2) helps the patient explore the distress in order to ascertain the help he requires so that his distress may be relieved." Indirect function: Calling for the help of others (1961, p. 29). "Whatever help the patient may require for his need to be met" (i.e., for his physical and mental comfort to be assured as far as possible while he is undergoing some form of medical treatment or supervision [(1961, p. 5]). Automatic or deliberative instructing, suggesting, directing, explaining, informing, requesting, questioning, making decisions for the patient, handling the body of the patient, administering medications or treatments, or changing the patient's immediate environment. Automatic activities: (1) routines of patient care such as serving food, evening care, (2) routines to protect the interests and safety of patient, such as locking doors, adjusting side rails, (3) routine practices of organization, such as signatures for consent forms and releases (1961, p. 84). Automatic activities redefined in 1972: (1) perception by five senses, (2) automatic thoughts, (3) automatic feelings, (4) action (p. 25). Disciplined and professional activities: automatic activities plus matching of verbal and nonverbal responses, validation of perceptions, matching of thoughts and feelings with action (1972, pp. 25–32).

Paradigmatic Origins

Although Orlando's theory evolved from extant practice through the analysis of some 2,000 nurse–patient interactions to discern what is good and bad practice, Orlando's writing appears to be influenced by Peplau's (1952, 1991) focus on interpersonal relationships in nursing. Peplau defined nursing in terms of relationships between a person in need of help and the nurse who is able to recognize such a need. Definitions by Orlando and Peplau have some common properties and, considering that Peplau's ideas were published in 1952 and Orlando began to formulate hers in 1954 (Yale received a grant for the purpose of developing an integrated program and, later, a faculty research development grant that facilitated testing some of Orlando's theoretical propositions), one can make an assumption of Peplau's influence on Orlando. Peplau acknowledged the influence of Harry Stack Sullivan on the development of her ideas; therefore, one may deduce that Orlando's theory has also used some of Sullivan's concepts and assumptions (dynamic relations, inadequate communication).

Perceptions, meaning, and evaluation of meaning are central concepts in the theory and are also central to symbolic interactionism. Considering that Orlando used a method of research that grew out of the Chicago school of symbolic interactionism in the 1950s, understanding of her theory could be enhanced by studying the assumptions and major concepts of symbolic interactionism. Orlando used field methodology before it became a worldview in research.

Schmieding (1987) suggested that by studying established theories in other disciplines, nursing theories could be better clarified and developed. She, therefore, proposed to analyze Orlando's theory by using John Dewey's theory of inquiry. She described the similarities and the differences between Orlando's and Dewey's organizing principles around the meaning of experience, habit, and functions in acting and reacting. She demonstrated that Orlando used experiences, the meaning of experience, and the immediacy of nurse–patient situations as the basis for her theory and that these same principles are central to Dewey's theory. Orlando herself did not acknowledge the paradigmatic origins of her theory, and no references appeared in her original writings.

Internal Dimensions

Orlando analyzed some 2,000 nurse–patient interactions to identify the properties, dimensions, and goals of interaction. The theory that evolved inductively from these analyses focused on the nature and dynamics of nurse–patient interactions. All statements in the theory relate to interactions; therefore, it is a concatenated theory. She used a field approach in developing the theory. Orlando's background in psychiatric nursing (her academic objectives were to identify psychiatric content that should be integrated in nursing curricula) has most probably influenced the focus of the theory on

describing the psychosocial aspects of the nurse–patient interactions.

As a single-domain theory that is also a microtheory of nurse–patient interactions, it is limited to immediate exploration and responses to a given situation. The nurse is an integral part of this theory; nurses' perceptions, thoughts, and feelings affect their actions and the patients' reactions. The entire theory is built on nurse–patient encounters; therefore, using Barnum's (1994, 1998) classification method of theory development, Orlando used a mixture of operational and problematic methods—more of the former than of the latter—and her theory is based on a reciprocal principle. Forchuk (1991) compared Peplau's and Orlando's theories and determined that Orlando has an interaction paradigmatic perspective, whereas Sellers (1991) proposed that Orlando's theory is predicated on a stimulus–response approach. The stimulus is comfort maintenance and the response is tension reduction. The nurse and patient provide the stimulus and response approach.

Orlando identified a number of problems (helplessness, distress) and what nurses should do to handle these problems. The concepts in the problems are not operationally defined, and this limits the development of research hypotheses. Orlando's theory is focused on the delivery of nursing care through a disciplined nursing process. However, her focus is on how to deliver care and not on what care to give. Therefore, her theory provided an early attempt to conceptualize knowledge of process. It is a nursing process theory of medium- to low-level abstraction, leaning more toward low-level abstraction. This analysis of the theory was confirmed by Orlando in introducing her book for republication in (1990a, 1990b). She described her theory as a "nursing process theory."

Theory Critique

The early 1960s marked a milestone shift in the way the nursing perspective was viewed. The interaction theorists, epitomized by Orlando, marked a shift in the perspective of nursing from phenomena dealing with nurses, functions of nurses, and needs of patients to a focus on the process of interaction and the potential consequences for the patient. Orlando's theory—with its major proposition being a deliberative nursing process (or the nursing process discipline, as it was relabeled in 1972, and then relabeled nursing process theory in 1990)—is a more effective process for identifying patient needs and evaluating patient care. Providing effective

BOX 12-6	PROPOSITIONS—ORLANDO

- There will be greater improvement in patient behavior and more effective nursing care when nurses use the disciplined professional response than when they use automatic personal response.
- The nursing reactions include perceptions, thoughts, feelings, and actions.
- When a nurse assesses a patient's immediate needs, immediate experiences, and immediate resultant behaviors, nursing care is more effective in decreasing distress and helplessness and increasing comfort.
- When nurse–patient dynamics and an "explicit" relationship are established, the patient is able to communicate his needs more clearly.
- Effective nursing interactions and processes enhance patients' comfort and decrease their stress.
- Patient's and nurse's reactions are the outcome of a situation.

care was the focus of many research projects and provided the framework for numerous Yale studies and published research (Diers, 1970).

Systematic explorations of relationships between each of the theory's concepts and patient outcomes is possible when patient outcomes (improvement, met needs) are articulated, defined, and operationalized. Explorations could also focus on the effect of the "nursing process discipline" on the assessment process and on implementation of other clinical therapeutics (Orlando, 1972, p. 4). Examples of potential propositions are presented in Box 12-6.

Although Orlando considered the theory to be a theoretical framework for the practice of professional nursing (Orlando, 1972, p. 1), it is more congruent in guiding nurse–patient interactions for the purpose of assessing needs and in providing the nursing therapeutics deemed necessary to patient care. The process is in fact considered a universal process of interactions between patients and all health professionals (Marriner-Tomey, Mills, and Sauter, 1989). What may make it more unique to nursing is the addition of such dimensions as space (hospital) and length of encounters (number of hours nurses interact with patients).

This theory is used to explicate nurse–nurse relations as well as nurse–patient relations. For example, it was used in acute psychiatric hospitals and was combined with professional values of caring for both patients and nurses, and with the use of evidence-based practice, as a foundation of nursing practice. The result was a relationship-based framework in which reflections and respectful interactions between providers and clients resulted in excellent practice (Allen, Bockenhauer, Egan, et al., 2006).

There is evidence that it has been creatively utilized to identify the elements of effective nurse–client interactions among postsurgical nursing home residents (England, 2005). The use of this deliberative

communication process provided the framework for identifying patients' concerns. Similarly, Williamson (2007) found that using Orlando's theory in home health care helped nurses' effective communication styles, led to better observation and identification of patient's needs, and empowered nurses in their professional practice.

Orlando's theory has also been used in nurse–patient interactions with patients who have been diagnosed with a chronic illness (Zoffmann et al., 2008). Zoffmann et al. (2008) used it in a research study to determine how patterns of interaction between providers and diabetic patients may lead to shared decision-making. The assumption is that shared decision-making will be more accurately based on knowing what patients need, thus leading to more quality care that results in better compliance.

The theory has several limitations, among them the seeming focus on ill people in acute care or psychiatric hospitals; on individuals, particularly those who are aware and conscious; on immediate time and situations; on short- rather than long-term care and planning; and on the virtual absence of a reference group or family members. There are other limitations in the theory, such as the lack of definition of environment, health, patient outcomes, physiologic aspects of needs, and the nonvariable nature of the central concepts of the theory (e.g., improvement, immediacy, effectiveness). When we limit the theory goals to only describing the nurse–patient interaction process for assessment of needs and for evaluation of care, then its limitations diminish, as is manifested by the numerous publications related to this aspect of the theory.

Nurses always have used focused interactions and deliberative processes, whether they have been aware of it or not. Even when aware of this use, whether they always credit Orlando remains debatable. Increasingly, however, there are publications on the importance of storytelling as an educational strategy (Hunter and Hunter, 2006), and on the use of relational conversation, such as "Self-Care TALK," as methods for creating partnerships in practice (Leenerts and Teel, 2006). In this literature, Orlando, as well as other interaction nursing theorists, is credited. Concepts and linkage from the theory, such as validation of observation and nurse–patient discussion of feelings, thoughts, perceptions, and reactions, are used as the bases for these strategies, which are designed to enhance quality interaction and the care it provides. Further use would be enhanced by refinements, extensions, and proposition testing.

Orlando's theory evolved from the need for curricular changes, and it is therefore logical that her first test of ideas occurred in an educational setting (Yale University). The first book (1961) identified teaching and learning strategies and some of the content that could be used in teaching students how to use the deliberative nursing process.

In her second book (1972), Orlando relayed the results of a training program over a 3-month period. The training was for 28 staff nurses (as opposed to students in an educational system) in the use of the nursing process discipline. The purpose was to change their responsiveness from one that was "personal and automatic" to one that was "disciplined and professional" (Orlando, 1972, p. 4). Outcome variables were observed in nurses, and the study results indicated effective use of nursing process discipline in nurse–patient encounters by nurses who were in the training program (Orlando, 1972).

Although there has been relatively limited use of Orlando's theory as a complete theory in practice, educational, or administrative settings, the concepts permeate our educational and practice settings. Since Schmieding (1986) provided the most comprehensive use of Orlando's theory in nursing practice and nursing administration, others have used only some components of it either to illustrate the importance of nurse–patient interactions or for processes to identify the needs of patients (Williamson, 2007). Sheafor (1991) provides an analysis that supports the need to incorporate the deliberative Orlando approach in graduate programs. Each situation presented focuses on problematic situations with patients, nurses, physicians, or other colleagues. Nurses' immediate responses and deliberate process responses are then described, illustrating Orlando's propositions. In each one of the vignettes offered, the deliberative process clarified assumptions, cleared misconceptions, checked judgmental thoughts, and enhanced expressions and interpretations.

External Components of Theory

The theory represents a shift from a view of nursing that was task- and function-oriented—with goals that stemmed from organizational needs, and with therapeutics that were offered and based on physicians' prescriptions—to nursing as an interactive process. Values of nursing shifted because of, or as a product of, interaction theories. These theories proposed that nursing is a process, patients are the focus, patients should be consulted in their own care, and patients should be spared the distress and discomfort associated with misconceptions, misinterpretations, and noninvolvement in their own care. Patients' behaviors and participation in interpreting meaning and validating perceptions should be significant factors in nurses' reactions. Although the patient was still viewed as helpless and the deliberative process appeared to be always initiated by the nurse, many of the assumptions of the theory are congruent with the social and professional values of the 1980s and 1990s. The uniqueness of individuals assumed by the theory could counteract automatic responses of nurses because even a nursing process discipline or deliberative nursing process could turn into an automatic response if the nurse forgets the basic assumptions guiding the theory.

The theory is useful in assessing patients, but utilizers must be trained for its appropriate use (Schmieding, 2002). It is used effectively for caring for elderly people (Faust, 2002). Laurent (2000) developed a leadership theory for the management of patient care, emphasizing that existing theories borrowed from other disciplines (e.g., Deming Management method, Managers as Developers model, and Shared Governance and Transaction Leadership) are not as productive for nursing goals of leadership. Orlando's theory was used as a road map for nurses providing care in a mental health setting, to develop a research instrument for testing immediate distress, and for a study, the results of which demonstrated that the care provided significantly decreased distress (Potter and Bockenhauer, 2000; Potter and Tinker, 2000). Study of the relationship between nurse-expressed empathy and patient distress and between patient-perceived empathy and patient distress was significantly negative. Although a moderately positive relationship was found between nurse-expressed empathy and patient-perceived empathy, the findings supported some of Orlando's propositions (Olson and Hanchett, 1997).

The theory appeared initially to be culturally bound because it was perceived by nurses that patients in other parts of the world and from other cultures may not want to participate in identifying their needs, and may not feel free to engage in interpretations of meanings. It was also assumed that patients may prefer to rely on their significant others and health care professionals to do that for them, and that they may misinterpret the continuous validation proposed in this theory as lack of knowledge, lack of expertise, or lack of accountability in the care process (Lipson and Meleis, 1983). It should be noted, however, that her theory has been used in Brazil, where the author analyzed its use in Brazilian journals (Toniolli and Pagliuca, 2002), and in Denmark to develop a model of care based on communication and reflection to enhance shared decision-making (Zoffmann et al., 2008).

Theory Testing

The theory evolved from Orlando's observations of nurse–patient interactions. Although the findings were not reported in a research report, her 1961 book is based on that research. The research was done in various patient settings to explore the effect of the deliberative process, which includes the perceptions, thoughts, and feelings of the patient and the nurse regarding patient needs and the care given. Validation of perceptions, thoughts, and feelings is essential for enhancing the congruence between patient needs and the care given. Results indicate unique nursing process is more effective than other approaches in dealing with pain (Barron, 1966; Bochnak, 1963), in reducing stress (Mertz, 1962), in understanding patient needs (Cameron, 1963), in decreasing postoperative vomiting (Dumas and Leonard, 1963), in relieving distress experienced by patients during the process of admission to a hospital (Elms and Leonard, 1966), and in enhancing the use of an ambulatory program for patients with bipolar disorder (Shea, McBride, Gavin, et al., 1997). In addition, nursing process is also more effective than other approaches on the outcomes of implicit and explicit verbal acceptance of a nursing procedure, as well as on the degree of effectiveness of enemas and progress in labor (Tryon, 1963), with the indicators being higher retention rate, more fecal return, and higher ratio of fluid intake and return (Tryon and Leonard, 1964).

A number of studies focused on explicating the properties and components of nurse–patient interactions (Diers, 1966; Gowan and Morris, 1964; Pienschke, 1973; Rhymes, 1964; Wolfer and Visintainer, 1975) and relational conversations (Leenerts

and Teel, 2006). The latter study uncovered several properties for conversations used to create partnerships to promote health. These include listening with intent, affirming emotions, creating relational images, and planning enactments. Others explored the relationship between the nurses' social approval of patients and postoperative recovery behavior as an outcome, finding a significant but weak inverse relationship between physical status (self-report) and social desirability (Eisler, Wolfer, and Diers, 1972). These authors question the process and intent of validating experiences with patients (central to Orlando and Wiedenbach), suspecting that some patients may respond to validation on the basis of social expectation rather than from "the patient's inner experience" (Eisler et al., 1972, p. 524). A recent Ethiopian study (Aseratie, Murugan, and Molla, 2014) that utilized Orlando's theory concluded that nurses were significantly less likely to utilize a deliberative nursing process in work environments exhibiting low satisfaction and high stress (e.g., high workload or staff turnover, disorganized structure). Orlando's theory for interaction as well as Paterson and Zderad (also discussed in this chapter) inspire nurse researchers in developing research projects as well as developing theoretical formulations. An example is the Understanding-oriented Interaction framework that explicates the relationship between the social circumstances in the health care practice arena as important context for effective nurse–patient communication (Sieger, Fritz, and Them, 2012).

A significant central concept in Orlando's theory—perceptions—was used as a framework to describe the needs of grieving spouses. A study of the grieving spouses' perceptions of their own needs before and after the death event revealed high reliability in the ability to identify needs and a consistency in the identified needs (Hampe, 1975). However, when identified needs were compared with met needs, a discrepancy became apparent. Implicitly, if the nurses had asked the grieving spouses to identify their own needs, perhaps the nurses would have planned to meet each of those needs in a more systematic and effective manner. A deliberative interaction process can elicit perceptions of needs even when patients cannot communicate their needs (Gowan and Morris, 1964). When nurses used the previously identified needs of grieving spouses as specific targets in their nursing interventions, grieving spouses experienced more met needs (Dracup and Breu, 1978). In this latter study, the greater satisfaction in nursing care was attributed to the systematic approach in needs identification.

Gilliss (1976) undertook another study that supports Orlando's differentiation between presenting problems as perceived by nurses and those as perceived and validated by patients. Gilliss demonstrated that fewer patients with sleeplessness required sleep medication in an experimental group in which Orlando's deliberative process was implemented. In this group, patients' specific needs were identified, defined, validated, and met.

Orlando's theory was used as a framework to research nursing administration. Schmieding (1988, 1990a, 1990b, 1990c) demonstrated that nursing administrators did not explore the reaction of their staff to problematic situations; the majority of administrators handled by themselves problematic situations that did not involve their staff, or they told nurses what to do rather than solicit from them their thoughts or action plans. Using Schmieding's application of Orlando, Sheafor (1991) provided recommendations on how to enhance productivity in hospitals.

The processes of interaction, action, and decision-making in nursing administration are similar to these processes involved in nurse–patient interactions. Schmieding (1983) systematically explored the nature of interaction, decision-making, and action processes in problematic situations in nursing administration and discovered that Orlando's theory could provide the needed nursing focus in nursing service administration. An instrument was developed to describe the action process of different members of nursing service personnel (Schmieding, 1987). Orlando's theory was also used in describing the responses of nursing students to distressed patients (Haggerty, 1987).

The findings lend support to consideration of the interaction process in achieving effective patient and nursing care outcomes. However, numerous methodological issues are related to need identification and increasing patterns of interaction in the nursing process discipline. One such problem is the paucity of research tools to identify patient needs. Williamson (1978), in attempting to identify patient needs, questioned the existence of mutually exclusive variables such as physical and emotional needs and the contextuality of needs and socioeconomic cultural variables.

Orlando's books have been translated into Japanese, Portuguese, and Hebrew, among other languages, thus attesting to its international appeal and utility (Orlando-Pelletier, 1990b). As with other international uses of a Western theory, the extent of actually using the theory in practice or in research should be carefully assessed.

JOSEPHINE PATERSON AND LORETTA ZDERAD

Theory Description

Paterson and Zderad (1988) addressed three central questions: What is the meaning of nursing? How do nurses and patients interact? How can nurses develop the knowledge base for the act of nursing? The humanistic-practice nursing theory proposes that the nurse and the patient are significant components in the nurse–patient situation and that the act of caring increases the humanness of both. They both approach the situation with their own lived experiences that influence the process and outcomes of their encounter. Nurses, therefore, should consider such encounters as existential experiences and should describe them from observing "the thing itself," the phenomena of nursing as they occur in the world. They use a phenomenological perspective as the basis for a dialogue about lived experiences to uncover answers to the questions. The sum total of all these experiences will enhance the development of the science of nursing.

In selecting existentialism and phenomenology as context and method for the development of nursing knowledge, Paterson and Zderad operate from several premises. The progress of nursing as a human science is hampered by the mechanistic, deterministic, cause-and-effect methods that have dominated it; in other words, they rejected the received view, the logical positivist view of theory development (Paterson, 1971, p. 143). Paterson and Zderad were a decade ahead of the literature in nursing that later advocated such a move. They have also developed their ideas on the premise that the experiences of nurses in practice supply the impetus for any useful theory for nurses. However, they also warned us that preconceived notions influence what is significant and determinately affect the development of knowledge.

Nursing is a lived dialogue that incorporates an intersubjective transaction in which a nurse and a patient meet, relate, and are totally present in the experience in an existential way that includes intimacy and mutuality (Paterson and Zderad, 1970–1971). Nursing brings a person together with a nurse because of the call of that person for help and the response of the nurse. The encounter is influenced by all other human beings in the patient's and nurse's lives and by other things, whether ordinary objects (such as utensils, clothes, furniture) or special

---

BOX 12-7 | **ASSUMPTIONS—PATERSON AND ZDERAD**

Implicit Assumptions

- Nursing involves two human beings who are willing to enter into an existential relationship with each other.
- Nurses and patients as human beings are unique and total biopsychosocial beings with the potential for becoming through choice and intersubjectivity.
- The present experiences are more than the sum total of the past, present, and the future, and are influenced by the past, present, and future. In their totality, they are less than the future.
- Every encounter with another human being is an open and profound one, with a great deal of intimacy that deeply and humanistically influences members in the encounter.
- Human beings are free and are expected to be involved in their own care and in decisions involving them.
- All nursing acts influence the quality of a person's living and dying.
- Nurses and patients coexist; they are independent and interdependent.
- A nurse has to "accept and believe in the chaos of existence as lived and experienced by each man despite the shadows he casts, interpreted as poise, control, order, and joy" (Paterson and Zderad, 1988, p. 56).
- Human beings have an innate force that moves them to know their angular views and other's angular views of the world (Paterson and Zderad, 1976; Zderad, 1969).

From Paterson J.G. and Zderad, L.T. (1976). *Humanistic nursing*. New York: John Wiley & Sons; Zderad, L.T. (1969). Empathetic nursing: Realization of a human capacity. *Nursing Clinics of North America*, 4, 655–662; and Paterson, J.G. and Zderad, L.T. (1988). *Humanistic nursing*. NLN Publication, March (41–2218).

objects (such as life-sustaining equipment). The dialogue during these encounters occurs in a time frame as experienced by both partners. When there is synchronization in timing, the intersubjective dialogue is enhanced. Dialogue occurs in a certain space that is objective, the physical setting, or subjective, personal space. In their theory, the nurse is expected to know "the nurse's unique perspective and responses, the others' knowable responses, and the reciprocal call and responses, the in-between, as they occur in a nursing situation" (Paterson and Zderad, 1988, p. 7).

Paterson and Zderad's theory is based on a number of implicit assumptions (Box 12-7). The theory has the potential for highly abstract propositions related to nurse–patient interactions (Box 12-8). The level of abstraction does not render propositions ready for testing. Concepts of the theory are well delineated (Box 12-9); however, some conceptual definitions are not complete in the theory (I/thou, I/it, we, all at once), whereas others provide useful conceptual definitions, such as empathy (Zderad, 1969) and nursology (Paterson, 1971). The theorists did not offer operational definitions; however, the theory provides opportunities for others to continue to explicate and further develop concepts. Central nursing phenomena, such as environment or well-being, are neither defined nor are they central concepts of the theory. Others, such as nurturance, comfort, and empathy, are primitive to the theory and are better related to clinical process. Derived concepts, such as the nursing dialogue, as "meeting, relating, and presence" is more comprehensively defined than any of the primitive concepts (Table 12-3).

BOX 12-8 | **PROPOSITIONS—PATERSON AND ZDERAD**

- Nursing's existential involvement in patient care is manifested in the active presence of the whole nurse in time and space as viewed by the patient.
- Nursing's goal of more well-being is enhanced by both nurse and patient as they experience the process of making responsible choices.
- Because nursing is involved with human beings, its phenomena are a person needing help and a person helping in his own situation.
- Intimacy and mutuality in relationships enhance more well-being.

BOX 12-9	CONCEPTS—PATERSON AND ZDERAD

Between	Becoming
Nurturing	I/Thou
Comfort	I/it
Being and doing	We
Lived dialogue	All at once
Nurturing	Well-being
Intersubjective transaction	More-being
Meeting	Choices
Relating	Authenticity with one's self
Presence	Intellectual awareness
Intimacy	Community
Mutuality	Concepts for research
Call and response	Authenticity with self
Other human beings	Nursology
Things	
Time	
Synchronicity	
Space	

TABLE 12-3	Definition of Domain Concepts—Paterson and Zderad
Nursing	A human discipline involving one human being helping another in an interhuman and intersubjective transaction "containing all the human potentials and limitations of each unique participant" (Paterson and Zderad, 1988, p. 3). Incorporates all human responses of a person needing another. "The ability to struggle with other man through peak experiences related to health and suffering in which the participants in the nursing situation are and become in accordance with their human potential" (1988, p. 7).
Goals of nursing	1. Humanistic nursing itself is a goal. 2. Help patients and self to develop their human potential and to come toward, through choice and intersubjectivity, well-being or more well-being. To help patients and self to increase possibility of making responsible choices (1988, pp. 14–17).
Health	More than absence of disease: equated with more well-being, as much as humanly possible (1988, p. 12).
Environment	Objective world as manifested in "other human beings" and things. The subjective meaning of the people and things. Refers to nurses' and patient's environment (1988, pp. 31–33, 37).
Human being	A unique and "incarnate being always becoming in relation with men and things in a world of time and space" (1988, p. 18). Has the capacity to reflect, value, experience to become more. One who asks for help and one who gives help.
Nursing client	Both nurse and patient are the nursing clients (incarnate men), who are unique, when they "meet in a goal-directed (nurturing well-being and more well-being) intersubjective transaction (being with and doing with) occurring in time and space (as measured and as lived by patient and nurse)" (1988, p. 21).
Nursing problem	Seeming discomfort that prompts a call for help. "A person with perceived needs related to the health/illness quality of living" (1988, p. 18).
Nursing process	"Deliberate, responsible, conscious, aware, nonjudgmental existence of the nurse in the nursing situation, followed by disciplined, authentic reflection and description" (1988, pp. 7–8). Based on awareness on the part of the nurse, continuous assessment (p. 16), and developing the human potential of the patient for responsible choosing between alternatives.
Nurse–patient Relations	The human dialogue is the essence of nursing, interaction is nursing. Experience is an intersubjective transaction with empathy.
Nursing therapeutics	A human dialogue involves being and doing, nurturing, well-being or more well-being, and comforting. Existential involvement that is an active presence besides the doing, to provide nurturing and comfort and involves experiencing, reflecting, and conceptualizing (1988, pp. 12–23). Nurses offer alternatives and support responsible choosing, share self, knowledge, and experience.
Focus of nursing	On the person's unique being and becoming (1988, p. 19).

Theory Analysis

The Theorists

Josephine G. Paterson, DNS, and Loretta T. Zderad, PhD, were nurse researchers at the Veterans Administration Hospital in Northport, New York. Paterson (Diploma from Lenox Hill Hospital, BSNE from St. Johns University, MPH from Johns Hopkins University) received her DNS from the Boston University School of Nursing. Zderad (Diploma from St. Bernard's Hospital, BSNE from Loyola University, MSNE from Catholic University) received her PhD from Georgetown University. Their interest in public health and psychiatric nursing, respectively, is complementary and well represented in their theory. Their ideas evolved in 1960, while collaboratively teaching graduate students. After completing their respective doctorates, they developed a course on humanistic nursing at the Veterans Administration Hospital in 1972. In the process of teaching the course, their theory evolved. Their 1976 collaborative book is a result of their teaching and observing clinicians in practice. Their book was republished by the National League for Nursing in 1988, an indication of the contemporary nature of their ideas and the demand for their theory. After their retirement, the book was made available as an e-text and may be freely copied for academic purposes with copyright clearly indicated. Based on their work, Susan Kleiman published her own book on human-centered nursing (Kleiman, 2008a) and an instructor's guide for integration of their theory in practice (Kleiman, 2008b).

Paradigmatic Origins

It is easy to determine the paradigmatic origins of Paterson and Zderad's theory. The origins are explicitly identified as being existential philosophy for theory development and phenomenology for research. Existentialism considers a person as a unique being and the sum of all her life experiences. It does not purport to find out the "why" of human experience, but just describes the "is" of it. It views human existence as inexplicable and emphasizes the freedom of human choice and responsibility for one's acts. Existential philosophy projects that a person exists but lacks a fixed nature and is always in a state of becoming.

The theory is based on several sets of ideas: that the person possesses autonomy, free will, and many opportunities for choosing among available options. However, the options and choices are considered relative and are perceived subjectively. An absolute reality does not exist for those who follow the existentialist school of thought. This theory allows nurses to use knowledge processed through their own lenses and experiences. There is total freedom to create, enhance, determine, and act. Existential philosophy emphasizes a complete sense of responsibility for all actions, and Paterson and Zderad based their theory on this stance.

Their theory also has roots in phenomenology. Phenomenology is the study of all aspects of a phenomenon in all its richness, in all its dimensions, in its entirety—without attempting to separate the human experiences of any partners in the study (Kant, 1953, pp. 80–90). The focus is on the here-and-now. Nursing deals with more than that; therefore, any limitations in the theory are limitations of its paradigmatic origins.

Paterson and Zderad relied heavily on such existentialist philosophers as Teilhard de Chardin, Martin Buber, Gabriel Marcel, and Frederick Nietzsche to develop their theory of nursing, and they also relied on such phenomenologists as James Agee. Both existentialism and phenomenology are compatible paradigms, allowing the humanistic nursing theory to integrate their assumptions and concepts and to evolve from both traditions. Barnum identified several advantages in the use of these paradigms to develop the nursing domain. A person could be considered in totality, experience could be viewed as a whole, and knowledge for nursing could be viewed as more than the sum total of diverse views from a variety of disciplines. Indeed, these paradigmatic origins give nursing its *raison d'être* (Barnum, 1994, p. 275). Existential nursing furthers a better understanding of the environment of one's self. To use the accepting nature of existentialism is antithetical to the advocacy needed to make changes in intolerable and oppressive situations that are mitigated by illness or by other social or political conditions. Existential nursing may provide the rationale for accepting an unhealthy and noneffective status quo. And it provides no guidelines for releasing patients from suffering (Barnum, 1998).

Internal Dimensions

The purpose of the theory is to describe the authentic dialogue between nurses and patients and their lived experiences for the purpose of changing the situation. It is to describe humanistic nursing practice theory and its components and the human method of *nursology*—the study of nursing aimed toward the development of nursing theory. Paterson and Zderad used a method to develop theory, and the theory is the method. They aimed to develop a theory, using methodology and proposing research, congruent with the nature of nursing as a human science (Kleiman, 1986, 2010). The theory evolved deductively from a philosophical view—existentialism—but they used a phenomenological approach to inductively develop a theoretical conception of nursing. Because most of the concepts are derived from existentialism, one can deduce that the theory is more deductive than inductive.

This is a highly abstract theory developed around an interest in exploring authentic interaction and the experience of unique people (nurse–patient) as concepts. The theory focuses on properties of the human encounter—the human situation that exists between nurses and patients; therefore, it is classified as a microtheory, with more derived than primitive concepts. Its scope is narrow, describing one aspect of nursing therapeutics or the nursing process—interaction—and one aspect of interaction, that is, human encounter. Therefore, it is a single-domain theory. It deals with the knowledge of process: How do people interact, particularly when one needs help and one is willing to give help?

Paterson and Zderad used a dialogue form to describe the "nursing dialogue." Therefore, McKeon (as cited in Stevens, 1984, p. 51) would consider their approach to theory development a dialectical one. They present a whole, explaining the whole (humanistic nursing) through the parts (the various concepts) and the parts through the whole. The uniqueness of this theory lies in the lack of boundaries between the experience of the authors as nurses, theoreticians, methodologists, and writers. Concepts in the theory describe all that, and all experiences describe concepts.

Theory Critique

The theorists, in proposing their humanistic theory of nursing, have also proposed a methodology congruent with the assumptions of the theory to develop nursing knowledge (Paterson, 1971). They use the logic of phenomenological methodology and call it *phenomenological nursology*. The method is aimed at the reality as experienced by the nurse and the patient, subjectively and objectively. They propose the method for research and nursing practice. Existentialism is the context of nursing, and concepts are used to develop theory. Phenomenology is the process for clinical nursing and for research in nursing. Phenomenological nursology evolved from nursing practice and is usable for nursing research.

The theorists proposed five phases of phenomenological nursology (Paterson, 1971, pp. 144–146):

1. "Preparation of the nurse knower for coming to know." This could be accomplished by total immersion in selected and related literary work. Immersion includes reflecting, contemplating, and discussing.
2. "Nurse knowing of the other intuitively" by seeing the world through the eyes of the subject or the patient, becoming an insider rather than an outsider.
3. "Nurse knowing the other scientifically" by replaying the subjective experiences, reflecting on them, and transcribing the amalgamated view. The nurse considers relationships and analyzes, synthesizes, and then conceptualizes.
4. "Nurse complementarity synthesizing known others" by comparing and contrasting the differences of like nursing situations to arrive at an expanded view.
5. "Succession within the nurse from the many to the paradoxical one," evolving from the multiple realities to an inclusive conception of the whole that incorporates the multiplicities and contradictions.

This is a method to find truths related to everyday practice in nursing or as evolving out of nursing research.

The theory depicts a way of life, an attitude toward humanity, a goal of actualization worth striving for on all levels of personal and professional lives. However, it is limited in the form of guidelines for nursing practice. The only indication of the use of this theory as a framework for practice has been offered by Paterson and Zderad as occurring in the Veterans Administration Hospital in Northport, New York. However, the theory is used in discussions of research findings related to a person's relationship to time and space, such as hospital rooms or the meaning of waiting for particular procedures (Hall and Brinchmann, 2009). Another example demonstrating its selection as a framework for discussion was undertaken by Chan, Lou, Arthur, et al. (2008), who used it to describe how nurses' attitudes toward perinatal bereavement may render bereaving parents powerless when the focus is not the whole person. Focusing on a disease, a limb, or one aspect of a situation may be an indication of lack of consideration of the context and the wholeness of the person and experience.

The theory is a philosophy and a methodology that purports to improve not only quality of care but also the quality of life for the nurse, the teacher, and the administrator. Objective criteria to measure outcomes are antithetical to the theory and the methodology proposed. Therefore, the subjective/objective assessment of each individual nurse is expected and accepted; there are no valid or reliable criteria to measure concepts, nor are they warranted within the philosophical view that guides the theory.

This is a tautological theory; the process of humanistic nursing is described by the goal of humanistic nursing, and the complexity of the phenomenon it addresses stems from abstractness and lack of boundaries between its concepts. It appears to focus on the nurse rather than on the patient as becoming and actualizing in the course of nursing care. Barnum (1994, pp. 104–109) asked if what we need is really a holistic nurse, in which case the proper subject matter of existential nursing theory would appropriately be the nurse rather than the patient. If that is one of the focuses of nursing, and Donaldson (1983) would agree, then Paterson and Zderad have offered a theory that appropriately describes one of the nursing phenomena.

External Components of Theory

The theory may be incongruent with some prevailing values of practice that address outcome over process, but it is congruent with values surrounding the research and knowledge development in nursing that emerged in the mid-1980s in the United States. Humanistic theory proposes understanding human beings and their experiences as they exist, rather than how they ought to be or rather than changing them. The goals of humanistic nursing—of understanding, supporting, and maintaining—may be in direct conflict with other professional values and goals, such as intervention goals for changes in pain responses or for alleviation of suffering. The notion of total autonomy may also be in conflict in the nurse's role to plan and provide care for those who have diminished capacities (cognitive or otherwise) who are not able to make their own decisions (Risjord, 2014). As illustrated by Barnum (1998, pp. 209–217),

it is a common existential position that suffering brings about a state of heightened self-awareness, thereby creating an openness to authentic experience that the patient might not otherwise experience and express. Suffering creates a state in which the person is brought face to face with his own being. Most nurses, however, seek to remove (alleviate) suffering. It might be difficult for a nurse who is adhering to this theory to justify nursing acts that remove a patient from the authentic experience of suffering. Neither Travelbee nor Paterson and Zderad would advocate the removal of suffering. Nursing to them is to help the patients articulate their perceptions of the situation and the meaning of the suffering and to grow through this suffering.

According to this theory, a nurse–patient encounter involves an open human dialogue that incorporates high degrees of autonomy and intimacy to enhance understanding of the subjective world of the patient (Barnum, 1998, pp. 209–217). In how many such meetings can a nurse be involved in the course of her working day, and is there potential for emotional drainage leading to burnout? Do all patients seek and approve of such genuine encounters? Paterson and Zderad would argue that the higher levels of experience gleaned from each encounter indicate rejuvenation rather than burnout.

The theory is congruent with that segment of society that espouses subjectivity and being, but patients may want to experience and evolve their being in genuine encounters within their own circle rather than with the nursing staff. It is also congruent with caring encounters that involve profound health illness experiences, such a palliative, hospice, and end-of-life care (Wu and Volker, 2012). It is also responsive to those who support the use of poetry and reflection in providing care (Wagner, 2000).

When, in 1960, Paterson and Zderad were developing the seeds of their theory, they may or may not have anticipated the supportive literature of the 1980s that advocated phenomenology as the methodology most compatible with nursing. The 1980s witnessed an emerging worldview in nursing, denouncing the empirical positivist view (see Chapters 4 and 8) and supporting a phenomenological view (Menke, 1978; Munhall, 1982; Oiler, 1982). Paterson and Zderad advocated respecting nursing experiences as sources of knowledge and, indeed, of wisdom, providing nursing with nonmechanistic and nonpositivistic strategies for theory development and research (Paterson, 1978; Zderad, 1978). Nursing would do well to adopt their views.

Theory Testing

Patients' perceptions of hospice day care were explored using a phenomenological methodology derived from Paterson and Zderad's humanistic nursing theory. The authors concluded that patients expressed satisfaction with the service because the nursing care was based on humanistic care. The staff responded to individuals' opinions and feelings, and their needs for a sense of well-being. They gave patients time, and responded to their individual concerns in a flexible way (Hopkinson and Hallett, 2001).

The theory was also used as a framework to describe nurse practitioners' interactions with patients. Their lived experiences of interacting with patients were the focus of the study to uncover the nature and the meaning of the interaction. Results demonstrated that there are eight essential meanings that characterize the interactions: openness, connection, concern, respect, reciprocity, competence, time, and professional identity. These meanings contributed to valuation of the relationships, which in turn was inferred to contribute to personal and professional growth (Kleiman, 2004).

Numerous other research findings have used grounded theory, modified phenomenological approaches, and qualitative approaches to nursing research and are congruent with the assumptions of this theory. Researchers have used these concepts interchangeably to describe methodologies depicting parts of each (Stern, 1980; Wilson, 1977). Paterson and Zderad have used the approach to articulate concepts of empathy (Zderad, 1968, 1969, 1970) and comfort (Paterson and Zderad, 1976), but these reports appear to be for teaching and clinical insights, as a prelude to systematic research findings, and require more clarification (Cutcliffe and Cassedy, 1999; Tutton and Seers, 2003). These reports inspired others to explore the same or similar concepts (Kolcaba and Kolcaba, 1991), and to use them as a means to develop a generation of nurses respectful of changing demographics and globalization (Dariel, 2009). Kleiman (2009) used the theory, as well as Heideggerian's work, to explore the concepts of thinking and learning in the nursing experience. She offered humanistic learning experiences, an inquiry that is based on generative processes of reflection and self-discovery (personal communication, May 26, 2010).

However, the theory appears to be incongruent with forensic psychiatry, which requires a focus on the well-being of patients while simultaneously providing a framework to respond to the possibility of putting the providers at risk of violent action (Jacob, Holmes, and Buus, 2008). Humanistic theory does not allow for understanding and coping with these opposite responses.

The theory lends itself to utilization by nurses from different countries. Several international studies were conducted based on Paterson and Zderad's theory, to describe the nature of interactions and relationship between nurses and patients (Muniz, Santana, and Serqueira, 2000; Souza and Padilha, 2000), to describe families' responses to patients undergoing chemotherapy (Azevedo, Kantorski, and Ornellas, 2000), to expand and elucidate the concept of presence (Silva, 2013), and to develop a psychometric assessment of presence (Kostovich, 2012). Others used the theory and tested its effect as an intervention in critical care (Souza and Padilha, 2000) and in the care of patients who had undergone surgeries (Medina and Backes, 2002).

Research to explore other theory propositions has potential after the concepts have been operationalized. For example, the concepts of authenticity, the "between," more well-being, and all-at-once are abstract and lack definition to render them researchable. The potential of the theory to generate research is exemplified in the use of the self (the nurse) and different patterns of presence in the patient's "time–space spheres." However, expansion and extension of this and other similar humanistic theories may be constrained with the quest for objectivity and the academic support for traditional forms of scholarship (Merryfeather, 2015).

JOYCE TRAVELBEE

Theory Description

Nursing to Travelbee is an interpersonal process between two human beings, one of whom needs assistance because of an illness and another who is able to give such assistance. The goal of the assistance is to help a human being cope with an illness situation, learn from the experience, find meaning in the experience, and grow from the experience. For a nurse to be able to achieve that goal, she also has to find meaning in each encounter. Because illness brings with it suffering and pain, the role of the nurse is to deal with suffering and pain. If the nurse experienced personal suffering, she would be far better able to understand the patient's suffering. Nurses should not shy away from becoming emotionally, interpersonally, and existentially involved with their patients because it is through such involvement that empathy, sympathy, trust, and eventually, rapport, are established.

The central questions that Travelbee's theory answers are: How do nurse–patient, human-to-human relationships get established? For what purpose? Travelbee (personal communication, 1970) further asked: What is it that enables some individuals to cope with stress over a prolonged period of time? In attempting to answer these questions, Travelbee theorized that suffering is a common life experience that every person encounters at some point, that particularly occurs around illness, and that is divided into phases.

Human relationships help people cope with suffering, and Travelbee conceptualized relationships as progressing in stages, beginning with the phase of original encounter and progressing through the phases of emerging identities, empathy, sympathy, and, finally, rapport. A person's attitude toward suffering ultimately determines how effectively he copes with illness. The nurse's role is focused on helping patients find different meanings for suffering, meanings that are of particular importance to them.

Travelbee provides us with an exhaustive conceptualization of sympathy, rapport, and suffering as fine examples of a factor-isolating theory. Suffering is defined as:

> . . . a feeling of displeasure that ranges from simple transitory mental, physical, or spiritual discomfort to extreme anguish and to those phases beyond anguish; namely, the malignant phase of despair, the feeling of "not caring," and the terminal phase of apathetic, indifference. (Travelbee, 1966, p. 70)

Therefore, suffering is an experience that is variable in its intensity, duration, and depth. Beyond the beginning feelings of suffering, and when suffering becomes extremely intense physically, mentally, and spiritually, suffering progresses to the malignant phase, in which a person experiences anger, helplessness, and bitterness. If suffering persists, a person ceases to complain or express feelings related to anger and helplessness and instead displays apathetic indifference.

Although reactions to suffering are individualistic, there are some common responses. These are "nonacceptance, blaming self or others, bafflement, anger, self-pity, depression, anguish" during a "why me?" stage (Travelbee, 1966, p. 88). Or, human beings may respond to suffering through no protest

or even with an affirmative reaction, thereby accepting the suffering. Acceptance may occur because of personal philosophy, perception of the nature of humanity, or religious convictions. Pain and suffering are related. "To suffer is to be immersed in a black ocean of pain" (Travelbee, 1966, p. 89).

To deal with pain and suffering, a nurse has to establish nurse–patient interactions by getting to know the patient, by becoming involved, by ascertaining needs, and by fulfilling the purpose of nursing, which is to alleviate suffering and to help people find meaning in a situation. Communication is the key tool for the nurse. Nurses use various clinical therapeutics to keep channels of communication open, such as validating perceptions, reflecting by self or with patient, and using open-ended comments to solicit more information. Nurses can deliberately prevent communication breakdown by perceiving patients as human beings, recognizing levels of meaning when communicating, listening with reflection, and avoiding clichés, automatic responses, and undue interruptions (Travelbee, 1966, pp. 91–117).

Communication is the vehicle through which nurse–patient relationships are established. Such a relationship is defined as "an experience or series of experiences between a nurse and a patient . . . [or] a family member . . . in need of the service of the nurse." The relationship has two characteristics: it is a "mutually significant meaningful experience" and, through it, the nursing needs of the individual (or family member) are met (Travelbee, 1966, p. 125). Nurses and patients go through several stages to achieve the goal of established nurse–patient relationships. Each stage has certain tasks, and a healthy development of the relationship is accomplished by mastering each task. The stages are:

1. **Phase of the original encounter:** Emotional knowledge colors impressions and perceptions of both nurse and patient during initial encounters. The task is "to break the bond of categorization in order to perceive the human being in the patient" and vice versa (Travelbee, 1966, p. 133).

2. **Phase of emerging identities:** Both nurse and patient begin to transcend their respective roles and perceive uniqueness in each other. Tasks include separating oneself and one's experiences from others and avoiding "using oneself as a yardstick" by which to evaluate others. Barriers to such tasks may be because of role envy, lack of interest in others, inability to transcend the self, or refusal to initiate emotional investment.

3. **Phase of empathy:** This phase involves sharing another's psychological state but standing apart and not sharing feelings. It is characterized "by the ability to predict the behavior of another" (Travelbee, 1966, p. 143).

4. **Phase of sympathy:** Sharing, feeling, and experiencing what others are feeling and experiencing is accomplished. This phase demonstrates emotional involvement and discredits objectivity as dehumanizing. The task of the nurse is to translate sympathy into helpful nursing actions (Travelbee, 1964).

5. **Phase of rapport:** All previous phases culminate into rapport, defined as all those experiences, thoughts, feelings, and attitudes that both nurse and patient undergo and are able to perceive, share, and communicate (Travelbee, 1963, 1966, pp. 133–162).

When relationships are established, the nurse can help patients to accept and find meaning in their experiences or to accept their humanness through either circuitous or indirect methods (avoiding direct confrontation by using parables or by the nurse opening herself and sharing similar personal experiences) or direct methods (asking pertinent questions or logically explaining the situation). Establishment of rapport in nurse–patient relationships and finding meaning in suffering eventually lead to the development of hope in patients (Travelbee, 1971).

Travelbee based her theory on numerous assumptions that are interspersed throughout her book. These assumptions are presented in Box 12-10. Travelbee's assumptions are explicit and congruent with selected concepts and theory propositions. The concepts are abstract and have face validity, but the boundaries are not clear or operationally defined (What is hope and how can it be measured?) (Box 12-11). Travelbee is consistent in her views of humanity, uniqueness, existential encounters, and nursing. The theorist's definitions of health, nursing, relationships, nursing problems, and nursing therapeutics are conceptually clear, with the integrity of the assumptions preserved throughout the definitions (Table 12-4). Rapport is a phase toward the nurse–patient relationship; the phases overlap. Further operationalization will help determine which behaviors belong in which phase of the process of establishing nurse–patient relationships. Travelbee often relied on dictionary definitions. Research relating to different concepts was not cited. The theory lends itself to numerous propositions central to the practice of nursing. Examples are offered in Box 12-12.

BOX 12-10	**ASSUMPTIONS—TRAVELBEE**

- The nurse–patient relationship is the essence of the purpose of nursing (Travelbee, 1966, p. 13).
- Human beings are rational, social, and unique beings and are more different than alike (1966, p. 29).
- All human beings undergo certain experiences and will search for meaning in them during the process of living. These experiences could be considered as coherent wholes and could be understood (e.g., illness, anxiety, joy, harm). Therefore, likeness and similarities between human beings are in the nature of their experiences (1966, p. 30).
- Labels tend to evoke stereotypical categories. Nurses should remember that patients are human beings who differ from other human beings only in "requesting the assistance of other human beings believed capable of helping them solve health problems" (1966, p. 34).
- Relationships are established when both partners perceive each other's uniqueness. Then, such human relationships transcend roles and are true, meaningful, and effective relationships based on perceptions of uniqueness (1966, p. 36).
- Nurse–patient relationships are based on perceiving the patient as an illness or nursing as a task. Illness is only understood in the context of perceptions of the patient and the nurse.
- Illness, suffering, and pain experiences could be self-actualizing if individuals find meaning in them.
- Human beings are motivated to search for and understand the meaning of all life experiences.
- Illness and suffering are not only physical encounters for human beings, they are emotional and spiritual encounters as well (1966, p. 69).
- Nurse–patient interaction, when purposeful, fulfills the goals of nursing (1966, p. 93).
- "Communication is a process that can enable the nurse to establish a nurse–patient relationship and thereby fulfill the purpose of nursing—namely to assist individuals and families, to prevent and cope with the experience of illness and suffering and, if necessary, to assist them to find meaning in these experiences" (1966, p. 94).
- Nurses are expected to ascertain the meaning of exchanged messages.

BOX 12-11	CONCEPTS—TRAVELBEE

Perception
Pain
Suffering
Communication
Therapeutic self
Hope
Self-actualization
Transcend self
Therapeutic self
Nurse–patient relationship/human to human
  relationship
  Phase of original encounter
  Phase of emerging identities
  Phase of empathy
  Phase of sympathy
  Phase of rapport

Finding meaning in illness and suffering
  Circuitous
    Parable approach
    Veiled
    Personal experience
  Direct
    Questioning
    Explanation
Transitory discomfort
Anguish
Malignant despair
  Not caring
Apathetic indifference
Love

TABLE 12-4	Definition of Domain Concepts—Travelbee
Nursing	An interpersonal process and service vitally concerned with change and influence of others.
	An interpersonal process whereby the professional nurse practitioner assists an individual or family to prevent or cope with the experience of illness and suffering and, if necessary, to assist the individual or family to find meaning in these experiences (Travelbee, 1966, pp. 5–6).
Goal of nursing	To assist an individual or family to prevent or cope with the experience or illness and suffering and, if necessary, to assist the individual or family to find meaning in these experiences (1966, pp. 10–12, 20), with the ultimate goal being the presence of hope (1971).
Health	World Health Organization (WHO) definition: "Health is a state of complete physical, mental, and social well-being and not merely the absence of disease or infirmity. The enjoyment of the highest attainable standard of health is one of the fundamental rights of every human being without distinction of race, religion, political, economic, or social condition" (1966, p. 7).
Environment	Not defined.
Human being	A unique thinking, biologic, and social organism, an irreplaceable individual who is unlike any other person, who is influenced by heredity, environment, culture, and experiences. Always in the process of becoming and capable of choosing (1966, pp. 26–34).
	Understanding of a human being is through his perception of himself.
Nursing client	A patient is a human being who requests assistance from another human being who he believes is capable of helping and will help in solving his health problems.
Nursing problem	Communication breakdown and distortion:
	"1. Failure to perceive patient as a human being
	2. Failure to recognize levels of meaning in communication
	3. Failure to listen, using value statements without reflection
	4. Clichés and automatic responses
	5. Failure to interrupt" (1966, pp. 106–117)
Nursing process	Process to ascertain needs, validate inferences, decide who should meet needs, plan a course of action, and validate.
	"Disciplined intellectual approach," a logical method of approaching nursing problems, using knowledge and understanding of concepts from all other sciences and nursing in caring for patients (1966, p. 15).

(continued)

TABLE 12-4	Definition of Domain Concepts—Travelbee (*continued*)
Nurse–patient relations	An experience between an individual in need of the services of a nurse, and a nurse for the purpose of meeting the needs of the individual.
Nursing therapeutics	Therapeutic use of self (nurse). Disciplined intellectual approach to patient problems.
	Everything the nurse does for and with the patient is designed to help the individual or family in coping with or bearing the stress of illness and suffering in the event the individual or family encounters these experiences (1966, p. 8).
	Help patients find meaning in their experiences (1966, p. 10).
	Methods to find meaning are: (1) Circuitous (indirect) method, which includes (a) parable method (tell analogous story), (b) veiled problem approach (use indefinite pronouns), or (c) personal experience approach (shared experience); (2) Direct method, which includes questioning in jest and explaining (1966, pp. 16–19, 173–179).
	"Communication techniques:
	Use of open-ended comments or questions
	Use of reflecting technique
	Use of sharing perceptions
	Deliberate use of clichés" (1966, pp. 106–110).

BOX 12-12	PROPOSITIONS—TRAVELBEE

- Knowing and understanding perceptions of time and life experiences increases the nurse's abilities to meet the needs of patients.
- "The nurse's perception of patients is a major factor in determining the quality and quantity of nursing care she will render each patient" (Travelbee, 1966, p. 34).
- If nurses perceive patients as illnesses, tasks, or sets of stereotype characteristics, their focus in care is (institutional) rather than person-centered (1966, pp. 36–41).
- As patients become a "chore and a task, the nurse withdraws and directs her energy toward meeting institutional needs" and patients experience anger, irritability, tension, restlessness, sadness, depression, hopelessness, apathy, and transient somatic symptoms (1966, pp. 38–40).
- An individual's socioeconomic status affects the level of dehumanization a person is subjected to.
- "The quality of nursing care given any patient is determined by the nurses' beliefs about illness, suffering, and death" (1966, p. 55).
- "The spiritual values of the nurse or her philosophical beliefs about illness and suffering will determine the extent to which she will be able to help patients find meaning (or no meaning) in these situations" (1966, p. 55).
- Nurses are able to empathize with patients who are similar to themselves (1966, p. 142).
- Experience of illness affects, to a varying degree, all those associated with the patient, and subsequently affects the patient's perception of the experience (1966, p. 66).
- There is a direct relationship between caring and suffering; the more a person cares and is attached to an object or a person, the more the person suffers when that object or person is lost (1966, p. 72).
- Responses to pain are influenced by cultural background of the person, philosophical premises, spirituality, level of anxiety, and responses of others to the person in pain (1966, p. 81).
- Identify the properties of hope, determinants of hope and hopelessness (1971).
- There is a direct relationship between the extent to which the individual's need for cognitive clarity and security are met and the individual's anxiety level (1971, p. 190).

Theory Analysis

The Theorist

The late Joyce Travelbee was a faculty member at several schools of nursing. She worked as an assistant professor in the Department of Nursing, Louisiana State University, New Orleans, then as an instructor in psychiatric and mental health nursing in the Department of Nursing Education at New York University, then as a professor at the University of Mississippi School of Nursing in Jackson, and finally at Hotel Dieu School of Nursing in New Orleans. She received a Diploma in Nursing from Charity

Hospital, New Orleans, Bachelor of Science from Louisiana State University, and graduated Yale with a Master of Science in Nursing. She acknowledged Ida Orlando's influence on her work.

Paradigmatic Origins

Travelbee based her theoretical formulations on existentialist philosophy, from which she drew many of the theory's assumptions. A developmental approach is somewhat demonstrated in her writing, as she used the concepts of stages of development of the nurse–patient relationship, stages of suffering, tasks to be mastered, constant change and development, and the becoming nature (Chin, 1974), after going through each of the stages. The continuous sense of becoming is both a developmental and an existential concept.

The incongruence perhaps lies in the assumptions of developmental theory of an orderly progression, and the lack of orderliness inherent in the existentialist philosophy. Despite this shortcoming, Travelbee has effectively and usefully synthesized assumptions and concepts of both developmental theory and existential philosophy by depicting the complexity of humanity through significant milestones (Sarlore, 1966). Her conception of empathy could be clearer if cast within the framework of role theory, particularly role taking.

Travelbee herself credited Victor Frankel (1963) (with whom she corresponded and met) and Rollo May (1953) with influencing her theories.

Internal Dimensions

Travelbee's theory is a hierarchical one, developed around the concepts of nurse–patient relationship, suffering, and pain to explore the relationships among them. It is both a concatenated theory, isolating and conceptualizing the central theory concepts, and a hierarchical one, as it interprets the relationship among these variables. Travelbee used the field approach in developing her theory, as is demonstrated in conceptualizing rapport in terms of other phases leading to and incorporating rapport. It is a descriptive and prescriptive microtheory that is also considered a single-domain theory.

The theory addresses one of the major concepts in nursing—interaction—but is limited to interaction surrounding illness. The theory focuses on those components of illness that are considered of concern to nursing; these are suffering and pain. It adds mainly to knowledge of the process of providing nursing care and provides significant existence propositions (nurse–patient interactions proceed through phases) and relational propositions (rapport increases patient's acceptance of illness).

Travelbee uses an operational method to develop highly abstract relationships. She incorporates the nurses' perceptions and acceptance with components of the nursing problem areas and nursing therapeutics. The nurse perceives, understands, and assigns meaning to behavior and is therefore part of the theory. The nurse's communication is one of the nursing problems, and the self could be used as the intervention through empathy and sympathy.

An operational method of theory development allows choices between alternate theories and actions. An example can be seen in the alternatives that Travelbee provides to dealing with suffering. She proposes using the direct method of confronting the patient with his suffering or the indirect method of having the nurse sharing her own experiences to prompt mutuality in sharing. Operational methods tend to be more acceptable to nurses because of their preferences for well-identified choices.

The theory's explanatory power is low (higher ratio of assumptions to explicitly stated propositions) and is limited to knowledge of disorder (suffering) and knowledge of process (relationships).

Travelbee used a deductive approach to develop her theory (Duffey and Muhlenkamp, 1974). Although she explicitly stated the sources that influenced the theory deductively (existentialist philosophy), the inductive approach is more assumed than explicit. It is assumed that she observed nurse–patient relationships in acute and suffering incidents. Such observations are not an integral part of her theory, and it is not clear whether she developed her theory based on extant or ought-to-be practice. One can deduce that it was the former rather than the latter.

Theory Critique

The theory is teleological. The process of establishing relationships is achieved after several stages in nurse–patient encounters, including rapport; however, rapport is considered the nurse–patient interaction. It is both goal and process; it is both process and product. The theory is tautological and parsimonious; assumptions and relationships could be presented without the numerous repetitions, and more attention needs to be given to the propositions. Finding meaning is analogous to coping but leads to coping, and vice versa.

The complexity of the theory is demonstrated in the abstractness of the concepts, limited operational definitions, and potential multiplicity of relationships. Therefore, its use in research, practice, education, and administration appears to be limited.

Although many of the central concepts in Travelbee's theory are derived from other theories (empathy, sympathy), she does not appear to have developed her propositions using the findings of other researchers. Some of Travelbee's ideas are common practice in nursing. The nursing process as we have come to teach it and use it involves several of the steps outlined by Travelbee. Observations are carried out to validate the needs of patients, to validate inferences made, to make decisions about personally taking action or not, and to then plan a course of action; then, the action is evaluated. The patient is the final authority.

Doona (1979), in preparing a second edition of an earlier Travelbee book (1969), used Travelbee's intervention theory as a guideline for the field of psychiatric nursing. Beyond this publication, no published evidence was found that directly develops, implements, or refines Travelbee's ideas. The theory has the potential for use in practice within the limitations of its scope and its microtheory nature, both of which refer only to individual patients who are ill and suffering, who are conscious, who are willing to invest in the development of rapport, and who participate in finding meaning in and making decisions about their care.

Cook (1989) demonstrated the utility of the theory in assessing suffering of nurses because of job distress at the height of the nursing shortage that forced their hospital to adopt a new system of patient care. The theory was used to define the nature and degree of suffering, the nature of each phase in the development of meaningful interactions between members of a group of nurses who met regularly to deal with their job stress. The rapport described by Travelbee was achieved prior to planning interventions. The intervention plan based on Travelbee (1971) included alleviating suffering, redefining the situation, and finding meaning in their experiences through disciplined and intellectual approaches and the use of the self (Cook, 1989, p. 205). The process of rapport development and the interventions helped the group members to feel less victimized and to gain control over their professional lives. The result was improved self-esteem, better problem solving, a more supportive environment, and rediscovery that a new system was providing them with greater autonomy and more challenging roles.

While her theory is not used in its totality as a framework for research, curriculum, or practice, it is often cited in support of the nurse's role in interpersonal relationships with patients to understand their suffering (Tranvag and Kristoffersen, 2008), in exploring the definitions and meanings in the concept of "hope" (O'Baugh, Wilkes, Luke, et al., 2008; Haugan, 2013a, 2013b; Tutton, Seers, and Langstaff, 2009), and in the therapeutic use of self (Wadensten, Engholm, Fahlström, et al., 2009). While interpersonal processes in nurse–patient relations and patient-centered care continue to gain momentum, some authors continue to attribute these concepts to Travelbee's writings (Weaver, Morse, and Mitcham, 2008; Wiklund, 2008). Similarly, as more questions arise about the role of spirituality in health and illness, Travelbee's concepts of meaning and purpose in life lend credibility and support to the primacy of establishing a strong rapport with patients (Timmins and Kelly, 2008).

Her existentially based ideas about the interpersonal relationship have also been used as providing a humane perspective in developing models for electronic patient records (von Krogh and Naden, 2008) or in strategies for treating adults with depression (Parrish, Peden, and Staten, 2008). It is notable that her ideas about hope, suffering, relationship, and interpersonal rapport continue to inform the writings of nurse researchers in different parts of the world; for example, Norway (von Krogh and Naden, 2008), Australia (O'Baugh et al., 2008), Ireland (Timmins and Kelly, 2008), Sweden (Tutton et al., 2009; Wiklund, 2008; Wadensten et al., 2009), and other countries.

No other published material uses Travelbee's theory in education or administration, despite favorable review of her 1966 book (Sloane, 1966; Wolff, 1966). Travelbee indicated that the University of Mississippi School of Nursing in Jackson was beginning to modify its curriculum to use her theory (personal communication, 1970). However, the limited scope of the theory restricts its utility for all aspects of nursing.

External Components of Theory

The focus of the theory on the uniqueness and dignity of the human being, on humanity, on autonomy, and on acceptance of others' values makes its assumptions congruent with Western values. The more recent emphasis on the role of hope—the ultimate goal of finding meaning in suffering—in healing and recovery tends to give more theoretical credence to Travelbee's propositions pertaining to the meaning of an illness and attitudes toward suffering. However, illness is viewed by society as an aberration, an abnormality, or a condition to be avoided and eliminated. This value is antithetical to Travelbee's basic assumption that illness is a part of life, and finding meaning in illness and suffering is a growing experience. Therefore, professional values could clash with the theory's values (used here as an assumption). Many patients could consider the assumption of shared nurse–patient relationships to find meaning problematic and may even go so far as questioning the cost-effectiveness of such emphasis on relationships. The lack of a biologic view of the patient and the limited positivistic orientation of the theory undoubtedly limit the utility and the acceptance of the theory by nurses.

Relationships are significant in the helping fields; they are an integral part of assessment for care, and they are focal in delivering care. Travelbee articulated for nursing how such relationships are formed and for what purpose. Hers is a theory to describe one of the central domain concepts in nursing.

Theory Testing

Central relationships in Travelbee's theory—effects of nurse–patient relationship on suffering and coping—have not been researched. However, the concept of empathy has been the center of numerous research studies. Various tools have been developed to measure degrees of empathy (Barrett-Leonard, 1962; Cartwright and Lerner, 1963; Truax and Carkhuff, 1967). Most of the studies of the 1960s and 1970s concluded that existing tools lacked construct and predictive validity and that their reliability was low (Chinsky and Rappaport, 1970; Kurtz and Grummon, 1972).

Other studies using Travelbee's theory explore differences between perceptions of high and low empathizers in effective communication (Stetler, 1977) and properties of interaction surrounding pain (McBride, 1967). Results have been inconclusive. Freihofer and Felton (1976) explored the nature of nursing actions perceived to offer support, comfort, and ease the suffering of a terminally ill patient and of significant others of terminally ill patients. More descriptive studies of this type will lend data to explore the construct validity of nurses' actions and options for suffering patients.

The theory was cited widely by authors and researchers in the United States and Japan in the late 1990s and at the turn of the century (Hisama,

2001; Moses, 1994) as a framework to describe suffering (Morse, 2001, 2005), and spirituality and spiritual care (Hawley, 1998; Narayanasamy, 1999; Tuck, Wallace, and Pullen, 2001). It has been used in some research studies (Begat and Severinsson, 2001; Landmark, Strandmark, and Wahl, 2001; McCann and Baker, 2001) as a framework for intervention to increase hope (Rustoen and Hanestad, 1998a, 1998b).

Several researchers have made use of the theory in studies related to the care of the older adult patient. It has been used as a framework for sharing of the self for the elderly (Nowak and Wandel, 1998), for supporting the process of aging (Wadensten and Carlsson, 2003), and for considering a reconceptualization of aging (Topaz, Troutman-Jordan, and MacKenzie, 2014). In a study involving cognitively intact nursing home patients, Haugan (2013a, 2013b) concluded that nurse–patient interactions influence hope, meaning in life, and self-transcendence among such populations, which in turn helps support health and general well-being. With the global increase in the aged population, particularly those who are 80 years and older, who may live alone or reside in nursing homes, nurse–patient interactions become even more vital in decreasing anxiety and depression (Haugan, Innstrand, and Moksnes, 2013) and in promoting interpersonal and intrapersonal self-transcendence, which translates to emotional and physical well-being (Haugan, Rannestad, Hanssen, et al., 2012).

Studies are mostly single episodes and do not provide systematically for theory refinement, extension, or further development. Travelbee's theory remains significant in providing a framework to describe the human encounter between nurses and patients who are suffering from life-threatening illness or a long, debilitating disease course, as well as for the cognitively intact nursing home dwellers. To establish these relationships, Travelbee envisioned extended encounters, which can be established in nursing homes, in long-term facilities, in rehabilitation centers, and, to a lesser degree, in the newly instituted short-stay hospital.

ERNESTINE WIEDENBACH

Theory Description

Ernestine Wiedenbach developed a concept of nursing that was congruent with the prevailing ideas at Yale in the late 1950s and early 1960s, and that shifted nursing focus from the medical model to a patient model. She introduced the notion of caring into nursing. In her early work, "The helping art of nursing" (1963), she attempted to develop a concept that encompassed all nursing; this evolved into a prescriptive theory. The theory addresses the central question: How do nurses help patients meet their needs? Help, to Wiedenbach, is an integral part of nursing, and it is composed of all actions that enable individuals to overcome whatever hampers their ability to function. Help came in different ways, one of which is in the form of intentional caring, as differentiated from help without caring. According to Wiedenbach's theory, the nurse's central purpose has three components: to motivate the patient; to facilitate efforts to overcome obstacles; and to develop a helping prescription, which is a deliberate action based on the realities of the immediate situation (Wiedenbach, 1964, 1970a, 1970b).

Needs and functions that dominated nursing thought at the time continued to be a dominant theme. However, Wiedenbach added to it concern for patients, in focusing on ways to allow them to express their fears. Needs can be ascertained only if the nurse validates her perceptions, feelings, and thoughts with those of the patient. Therefore, nurses' actions should abide by the following parameters: actions should be mutually understood and agreed on with full knowledge of implications, and they should be either patient-directed or nurse-directed or both. When they are nurse-directed, they must be deliberate and based on patient needs. To Wiedenbach, nurses develop a helping prescription with the reality of the situation (physical, physiological, psychological, emotional, and spiritual) by exploring nurses' philosophies of nursing (central purpose and assessment of the situation). Throughout a continuous process of observation and validation, nurses' observations are focused on determining inconsistencies (deviations from normal) and perseverance in ensuring that the patients realize their needs. Nurses make plans for action to "minister help needed." The plan has to be validated by patients before implementation. Nurses use themselves, patients, or appropriate others as therapeutic agents.

Wiedenbach (1970a) identified several assumptions that guided her theory, and there are other implicit assumptions (Box 12-13). There are some

---

BOX 12-13 | ASSUMPTIONS—WIEDENBACH

Explicit Assumptions

- "Each human being is endowed with a unique potential to develop within himself the resources that enable him to maintain and sustain himself" (Wiedenbach, 1970b, p. 1058).
- "The human being basically strives toward self-direction and relative independence and desires not only to make best use of his capabilities and potentialities, but desires to fulfill his responsibilities as well" (1970b, p. 1058).
- "The human being needs stimulation in order to make best use of his capabilities and realize his self-worth" (1970b, p. 1058).
- "Whatever the individual does represents his best judgment at the moment of doing it" (1970b, p. 1058).
- "The helping art of clinical nursing is a deliberate blending of thoughts, feelings, and overt actions" (1964, p. 11).
- "There are three more basic premises in nursing: 'reverence for the gift of life,' 'respect for dignity, worth, autonomy, and individuality of each human being,' and 'resolution to act dynamically in relation to one's beliefs'" (1964, p. 16).
- Characteristics of professionalism and being theoretical: clarity of purpose, mastery of skills and knowledge, sustaining purposeful working relationships with others, interest in advancing knowledge and dedication to furthering the goal of mankind (Dickoff, James, and Wiedenbach, 1968a, 1968b).

Implicit Assumptions

- Patients are dependent beings normally willing to utilize help (Wiedenbach, 1970b, p. 1060).
- Patients can use their sensitivities to frustrate health caregivers and "thwart their efforts to obtain the results they desire" (1970b, p. 1060).
- Individuals like to live an orderly life, and life is an orderly process.
- Factors such as physical, physiological, psychological, and spiritual influence the nursing situation.
- Individuals want and have the resources to be healthy, comfortable, and capable (1964).
- Professional nursing respects dignity, worth, autonomy, and individuality of each human being.

BOX 12-14	CONCEPTS— WIEDENBACH

Need for help
Help
   Inconsistency/consistency
   Purposeful perseverance
   Self-extension
   Preconception
   Interpretation
Actions
   Rational
   Reactionary
   Deliberate
Ministration
Realities
Central purpose
Prescription
Skills
   Procedural
   Communication

inconsistencies in the assumptions, such as unique-ness and orderliness, self-directed and dependent, but on the whole, Wiedenbach made a deliberate effort to identify the philosophical premises on which she developed her theory. A student of her theory may be confused by the numerous premises appearing at different points throughout her work. Inconsistencies also exist in using principles, phi-losophy, and assumptions interchangeably, when, at times, any one of these also were used to mean propositions.

Assumptions and concepts are congruent (Box 12-14). Concepts in the theory are mostly derived (needs, interaction, perception), and because Orlando, Wiedenbach, Dickoff, and James all worked together closely in developing their ideas, despite some of their perceptions of differences (Wiedenbach, 1970b), it is not easy to discern which concepts are primitive and which are derived. All these theories are extensions of each other; although Wiedenbach developed the concept of validation, validation is an integral part of Orlando's nursing process discipline. For Wiedenbach, one of nursing's goals is to promote comfort; for Orlando, a goal is to alleviate distress. Wiedenbach focused on perceptions of people in need of help, and Orlando focused on perceptions as a significant concept in interaction. Wiedenbach provided interpretation of the invisible act of "caring" and proposed its significance in successful nursing care. The helping art of nursing depends, in theory,

on the importance the nurse attaches to her thoughts and feelings and how deliberately she uses them (Wiedenbach, 1963). Barnum (1998) equated the concept of concern described by Wiedenbach with what later was called caring.

The major concepts in this theory tend to be concrete and nonvariable (comfort, validation, need for help), and they are not operationally defined, perhaps by design, because whether a patient is comfortable or not depends on the patient's per-ception and the meaning he or she attributes to the event and situation (Table 12-5). The definitions tend to be contextual, and this has the advantage of allowing variable definitions (comfort is in the eye of the beholder), but it also decreases utility in practice and research. Health and environment are not defined; a nursing client is defined in terms of hospital care and is contingent on awareness of needs. Relationships between concepts in Wiedenbach's early and later writing are not always clear (i.e., prescription, validation). The explanatory power of the theory is hampered by a lack of clarity.

The theory lacks propositions and linkages between concepts, but one can derive propositions related to the process of assessment and intervention. The principles of help are amenable to the develop-ment of existence propositions and, subsequently, relational propositions (Box 12-15).

Theory Analysis

The Theorist

The late Ernestine Wiedenbach earned a Bachelor of Arts from Wellesley College in Wellesley, Mas-sachusetts, in 1922 and a Diploma in Nursing from Johns Hopkins School of Nursing in Baltimore in 1952. She received her Master's Degree and a Certificate in Public Health Nursing from Teachers College, Columbia University. She practiced as a nurse midwife after completing a training program at the School of Nurse-Midwives of the Maternity Center Association of New York (VandeVusse, 1997). At the time of her theory's development, she was an Associate Professor of Maternity Nursing at the School of Nursing, Yale University, where she had begun working around 1952 (Bennett and Foster, 1980). She worked closely with two philosophers, Patricia James and James Dickoff, who were teaching a course in philosophy for nurses. She also worked closely with Ida Orlando and was an Associate Professor Emeritus at Yale. Wiedenbach died in 1998 (Burst, 1998), but her legacy in midwifery

TABLE 12-5	Definition of Domain Concepts—Wiedenbach
Nursing	A helping art with knowledge and theories. A goal-directed and deliberate blending of thoughts, feelings, perceptions, and actions to understand the patient and his condition, situation, and needs, to enhance his capability, improve his care, prevent recurrence of problem, and deal with anxiety, disability, or distress (Wiedenbach, 1964).
Goal of nursing	"To facilitate the efforts of the individual to overcome the obstacles which currently interfere (or maybe later interfere [(1970b, p. 1058]) with his ability to respond capably to demands made of him by his condition, environment, situation, and time" (1963, p. 55). "To meet the need the individual is experiencing as a need for help" (1963, p. 55).
Health	Not defined.
Environment	Conglomerate of objects, policies, setting, atmosphere, time, human beings, happenings past, current, or anticipated that are dynamic, unpredictable, exhilarating, baffling, and disruptive (1970, p. 1061).
Human being	Possesses self-direction and relative independence, makes best use of capabilities, fulfills responsibilities, has resources to maintain self; in other words, is a functioning being (1964).
Nursing client	A person who is under the care of some member of health care personnel, who is in a vulnerable position, with a perceived need for help.
Nursing problem	Inability or impaired ability of an individual to cope with situational demands due to interferences (1963, p. 56). Discomfort.
Nursing process	Deliberative, to identify need for help and interferences with ability to cope. Through observation, understanding, and clarification of the meaning of cues, determination of causes of discomfort (through inspection, palpation, temperature, etc.) and determination of whether or not patient is able to meet his own needs. Ministration of help needed and, the last step in the process, validation that help given was indeed help needed (1963, pp. 56–57).
Nurse–patient relations	The deliberate use of nurses' perceptions, thoughts, feelings, and actions.
Nursing therapeutics	Deliberate action that is either nurse directed, patient directed, or mutually understood and agreed on (1970b, p. 1059). (These are the nurse's options, and the choice is hers.) It is designed to deal with a person who is in need of help by "any measure or action required and desired by the individual that has the potential for restoring or extending his ability to cope with the demands implicit in his situation" (1963, p. 56). Help, which is any measure or action that enables the individual to overcome whatever interferes with his ability to function capably in relation to his situation (1963, p. 56). Giving advice, information, referral, ministering or applying a comfort measure. Deliberate actions are mutually understood and agreed on, patient directed, and nurse directed. Communication is an important tool. Helping is based on three principles: inconsistency or consistency, purposeful perseverance, and self-extension (1970b).
Focus of nursing	Goal-directed activities focused on identifying "the patient's perception of his condition" and his need for help (1963, p. 55).

endures (Nickel, Gesse, and MacLaren, 1992). She was the second recipient of the American College of Nurse-Midwives' Hattie Hemschemeyer Award and is considered a theoretical leader in nursing midwifery (Barger, Faucher, and Murphy, 2015).

Paradigmatic Origins

Basically, Wiedenbach's view of a human being and her view of a nurse are functional. She views patients in terms of their capabilities to function and carry out their responsibilities. Wiedenbach

was influenced by Ida Orlando, James Dickoff, and Patricia James (and perhaps the reverse is also true). Such influence is seen in her explication of nurses' actions and reactions and the focus on interpretation and validation of perceptions, feelings, thoughts, and actions. Therefore, it would be useful for the reader to also review the discussion of paradigmatic origins found under Orlando.

Some of Wiedenbach's assumptions and concepts regarding the motivation of human beings and nurses' impulsive responses appear at times to reflect conditions or stimulus–response types of

BOX 12-15	PROPOSITIONS—WIEDENBACH[1]

- When nurses observe inconsistencies in patients' actions, they use their perseverance in identifying the need for help and in offering help.
- Exploration and validation of nurses' and patients' perceptions, thoughts, and feelings increase the effectiveness of help offered to patients in need of help.
- Deliberate nursing action is an overt act consisting of several components: the need for help, validation, and ministration of help.
- Congruent nurse and patient perceptions of the need for help and evaluation of help enhance effective care and decrease discomfort.
- Mutually understood and agreed-on nursing actions will have a positive effect on the patient.
- Help given to individuals in need of help is categorized as: identification of variance from normal (principle of inconsistency/consistency); identification of an individual's need for help (principle of purposeful perseverance); utilizing self or others for help, advice, information, referral, or comfort (principle of self-extension).

[1]Propositions delineated under Orlando could also be propositions derived from this theory.

actions and reactions (Wiedenbach, 1968). Careful analysis of the theory may identify developmental themes or parallel themes with a psychoanalytical orientation, such as internal needs, frustrations, and motivations. However, the meaning of the situation or the event as perceived and expressed by an individual demonstrates a departure from psychoanalytical concepts to a phenomenological approach. These are speculations on paradigmatic origins. One origin is clear and documented; this theory evolved out of 40 years of clinical and teaching experiences (Wiedenbach, 1964, p. vii, 1968), and later developments supported the process nature of the theory (Wiedenbach and Falls, 1978).

Internal Dimensions

Wiedenbach's theory was developed around the need for help; the ministration for the needed help, and the validation of such need through patient perceptions. It is therefore a concatenated theory that lends itself first and foremost to existence propositions. It is an inductive theory evolving from observations of clinical practice and patients' needs for help after many years of practice in the maternal and child nursing subspecialty. It is a microtheory, explicating a component of the interaction process focused on validating perceptions, thoughts, and feelings before a deliberate action is planned. It is a theory with narrow scope—the deliberative nurse–patient interactive process used in a clinical situation to identify needs and verify actions. It addresses one component of one of the central concepts in nursing: nurse–patient interaction. It deals with knowledge

of process and with describing a component of the process inherent in assessing and providing care.

Wiedenbach used a field approach in identifying dimensions of interaction and validation, and used a combination of operational and problem approaches to theory development. She focused her conceptualization around problems of discomfort and the need for help, and around the function of the nurse in observing, assessing, and exploring and validating feelings, thoughts, and fears. She used persuasion and personal beliefs to drive these concepts home to nurses.

Perhaps because of the concreteness of the theory, the circle of contagiousness of ideas was wide and reached diverse geographical locations and settings, particularly in the midwifery circle. Although nurses may not articulate the concepts and linkages emanating from Wiedenbach, the central ideas of her theory are used widely. Hers is a good example of theory with tautology, lack of parsimoniousness in presenting ideas (presented in philosophical dialogue), and teleology (identifying the need for help is both a process and an outcome). The ratio of assumptions to existing propositions decreases its current power of explanation.

Theory Critique

The patient's perspective has become an integral part of the lexicon of nursing since the 1980s. Whether these concepts infiltrated nursing thought as a result of Orlando and Wiedenbach can only be determined through extensive analysis of nursing literature and through comparison of writings in the decades prior to 1960 and the decades following the publications of Orlando, Wiedenbach, Travelbee, Paterson, Zderad, and other interactionist theorists. An analysis of networking of ideas and people and the development of conceptual genealogical trees may enable us to ascertain the influence of the different theorists on the development of nursing knowledge.

It is apparent that the circle of contagiousness for research was limited to research in or surrounding Yale, but the circle of contagiousness for practice was much wider and engulfed the United States and foreign countries. Concepts such as patient-centered care, perceptions, validation, and exploration of thoughts, feelings, and actions are used in many practice settings, and concepts such as comfort are credited to Wiedenbach and Orlando (Griffiths and Andres, 2007; Williams, 2008). Some considered Wiedenbach instrumental in focusing on comfort and give her credit for the subsequent development of Kolcaba's theory of comfort (Kolcaba, 2003). The theory provides guidelines for implementing the nursing process and has stimulated many attempts at conceptualizing the interaction process, but it is limited in its power for prescription (Rickleman, 1971). The scope of the theory remains limited to individuals who are conscious in a hospital setting, who are basically motivated to participate in their own care, who are inconsistent (in a state of disharmony with their surroundings, situation, or expectations) (Wiedenbach, 1965), and who are able to perceive their need for help. Patients who are consistent (do not deviate from normalcy), who are noncompliant, and who do not perceive a need for help are not nursing clients. It has inspired nurse midwives by providing a framework that explicates a midwifery perspective (Burst, 2000; Sharp, 1998; VandeVusse, 1997). It was also used as a framework for studying nursing care of cancer patients (Andersen and Adamsen, 2001). However, its use in practice continues to be limited.

Administration literature in nursing may be considered an extension of Wiedenbach's theory; however, deliberate action, perceptual clarification, and validation could be claimed by any effective and efficient organizational theory.

External Components of Theory

The external components of Wiedenbach's theory are the same as those for Orlando's theory.

Theory Testing

As with Orlando's theory and perhaps in combination with it, numerous research studies were launched to test the what and how of a deliberative process and validation of interaction in assessing and intervening with patients in need of help. A review of the research and publications based on Wiedenbach's theory revealed two findings: first, both Orlando and Wiedenbach are cited in most research related to concepts of either theory; and second, Wiedenbach's ideas still appear in the literature as researchers continue to test propositions emanating from her theory.

One type of research using Wiedenbach's theory focused more on the prescriptive propositions of effect of deliberate nursing process (validation) on several patient outcomes. Such research was hospital-oriented (preoperative preparation, admission procedures, obstetric preparation, and patients in need of pain relief). (See discussion under Ida Orlando.) Experimental groups usually received care that included an identification of patient's needs focused on verbal and nonverbal behavior (Shields, 1978), nurses' perceptions compared and contrasted with patients' perceptions, and actions to provide help to restore the patient's functional ability based on a continuous process of validation.

Conversely, nonexperimental care given to the control group was personal, automatic, technique oriented, organizationally focused, and more authoritarian or friendly, but not deliberate and goal-oriented. Patient outcomes generally were significantly better in the first than in the second group. Outcomes considered included physiologic measures, such as emesis during postoperative or postdelivery recovery, and degree of change in heart and respiration rates. Other outcomes were psychological, and included subjective patient reports of alleviation of distress (Elms and Leonard, 1966; Leonard, Skipper, and Woolridge, 1967; Wolfer and Visintainer, 1975).

Other research was related to the exploration of an implicit assumption that the client is truthful in validating the nurse's perception of his condition. Eisler et al. (1972) found that a slight correlation existed between social approval needs of patients (but not the patients' inner experience) and their reports of physical well-being, thereby casting doubt on previously unchallenged assumptions that validation indeed gets at patients' true perceptions of the situation.

REFLECTIVE QUESTIONS

1. Interactions between patients and nurses are considered central to the nursing encounter and act. Discuss the place of "interactions" in contemporary nursing.

2. Which of the theories presented in this chapter reflects current values and goals in the practice of nursing?

3. In what ways could utilizing the theories of interaction contribute to quality care? Select one of the theories discussed in this chapter and identify three research questions derived from the theoretical propositions in the theory. Briefly describe how you may go about developing a research study to answer the questions.

4. Compare and contrast how communication, interaction, and interpersonal relations are conceptualized and defined in the theories discussed in this chapter.

5. The paradigmatic roots for Paterson and Zderad's theory appear to be substantively different from Orlando's and Weidenbach's theories. Can you discuss the truth of this statement and speculate on the "whys?"

6. Discuss ways by which you may or may not use any of the theories discussed in this chapter to advance knowledge in your field of nursing.

7. Select one proposition in each theory that you consider critical for testing to advance and build theory.

Numerous other research reports could be related to the theory, providing further validation or invalidation of its concepts. For example, Larson (1977) found that a client's socioeconomic status and social desirability of the diagnosis affected the nurse's perceptions of the patient's characteristics. The "should" advice in Wiedenbach's theory is therefore expanded to include the "realities" of the nurse–patient situation. There is no indication that Wiedenbach made any substantial changes in her conceptualization based on the results of these research studies. A set of propositions for using change as an outcome variable is presented in Box 12-15.

CONCLUSION

The theorists presented in this chapter transformed how nurses thought about their practice and changed the nature of research questions investigated in the discipline of nursing. They provided the rationale to study processes of care and relationships between nurses and patients, as well as the organization and structure of interpersonal relationships. They provided the language, concepts, and outcomes that characterize care, as well as define the nature of the discipline. It is through the theories articulated by the interaction theorists that such concepts as process, validation, interpretation, lived experiences, interaction, interpersonal relations, trust building, forming bonds, and advocacy, among many others, became an integral part of our lexicon. Although these ideas were pioneering when these theorists took the risk to introduce them, they now serve as integral parts of our discipline and drive changes in interactions and relationships in the increasingly client-centered health care system.

REFERENCES

King

Alligood, M.R. (2014). Philosophies, models, and theories: Critical thinking structure. In M.A. Alligood (Ed.), *Nursing theory utilization and application* (5th ed., pp. 40–62). St Louis, MO: Mosby Company.

Alligood, M.R. and May, B.A. (2000). A nursing theory of personal system empathy: Interpreting a conceptualizing of empathy in King's interacting systems. *Nursing Science Quarterly*, 13(3), 243–247.

Asay, M.K. and Ossler, C.C. (Eds.). (1984). *Conceptual models of nursing. Applications in community health nursing*. In Proceedings of the Eighth Annual Community Health Nursing Conference. Chapel Hill, NC: Department of Public Health Nursing, School of Public Health, University of North Carolina.

Austin, J.K. and Champion, V.L. (1983). King's theory for nursing: Explication and evaluation. In P. Chinn (Ed.), *Advances in nursing theory development*. Germantown, MD: Aspen.

Barnum, B.J.S. (1994). *Nursing theory: Analysis, application, and evaluation* (4th ed.). Philadelphia, PA: Lippincott Williams & Wilkins.

Bauer, R. (1998). A dialectic reflection on the psychotherapeutic efficacy of nursing interventions [German]. *Pflege*, 11(6), 305–311.

Bauer, R. (1999). A dialectic view of the efficacy of nursing interventions. Connections between interventions and effects of psychotherapy [German]. *Pflege*, 12(1), 5–10.

Brower, H.T. (1981). Social organization and nurses' attitudes toward older persons. *Journal of Gerontological Nursing*, 7, 293–298.

Brown, S.T. and Lee, B.T. (1980). Imogene King's conceptual framework: A proposed model for continuing nursing education. *Journal of Advanced Nursing*, 5(5), 467–473.

Bunting, S. (1988). The concept of perception in selected nursing theories. *Nursing Science Quarterly*, 1(4), 168–174.

Burney, M.A. (1992). King and Neuman: In search of the nursing paradigm. *Journal of Advanced Nursing*, 17, 601–603.

Byrne-Coker, E. and Schreiber, R. (1990). King at the bedside. *Canadian Nurse*, 86(11), 24–26.

Caceres, B.A. (2015). King's theory of goal attainment: Exploring functional status. *Nursing Science Quarterly*, 28(2), 151–155.

Carter, K.F. and Dufour, L.T. (1994). King's theory: A critique of the critiques. *Nursing Science Quarterly*, 7(3), 128–133.

Cho, M.K. (2013). Effect of health contract intervention on renal dialysis patients in Korea. *Nursing and Health Sciences*, 15(1), 86–93.

Clarke, P.N., Killeen, M.B, Messmer, P.R., and Sieloff, C.L. (2009). Imogene M. King's scholars reflect on her wisdom and influence on nursing science. *Nursing Science Quarterly*, 22(2), 128–133.

Daniel, J.M. (2002). Young adults' perceptions of living with chronic inflammatory bowel disease *Gastroenterology Nursing*, 25(3), 83–94.

Daubenmire, M.J. and King, I.M. (1973). Nursing process models: A systems approach. *Nursing Outlook*, 2(8), 512–517.

Doornbos, M.M. (1995). Using King's systems framework to explore family health in the families of the young chronically mentally ill. In M.A. Frey and C.L. Sieloff (Eds.), *Advancing King's systems framework and theory of nursing* (pp. 192–205). Thousand Oaks, CA: Sage.

Doornbos, M.M. (2000). King's systems framework and family health: The derivation and testing of a theory. *Journal of Theory Construction and Testing*, 4(1), 20–26.

Draaistra, H., Singh, M.D., Ireland, S, and Harper, T. (2012). Patients' perceptions of their roles in goal setting in a spinal cord injury regional rehabilitation program. *Canadian Journal of Neuroscience Nursing*, 34(3), 22–30.

Ehrenberger, H.E., Alligood, M.R., Thomas, S.P., Wallace, D.C., and Licavoli, C.M. (2002). Testing a theory of decision-making derived from King's systems framework in women eligible for a cancer clinical trial. *Nursing Science Quarterly*, 15(2), 156–163.

Elberson, K. (1989). Applying King's model to nursing administration. In B. Henry, C. Arndt, M. Di Vincenti, and A. Marriner-Tomey (Eds.), *Dimensions of nursing administration*. London, UK: Blackwell Scientific Publications.

Fawcett, J. (1995). *Analysis and evaluation of conceptual models of nursing* (3rd ed.). Philadelphia, PA: F.A. Davis.

Fawcett, J. (2001). The nurse theorists: 21st-century updates— Imogene M. King. *Nursing Science Quarterly*, 14(4), 311–315.

Fawcett, J.M. and DeSanto-Madeya, S. (2013). *Contemporary nursing knowledge: Analysis and evaluation of nursing models and theories* (3rd ed.). Philadelphia, PA: F.A. Davis.

Fawcett, J.M., Vaillancourt, V.H., and Watson, C.A. (1995). Integration of King's framework into nursing practice. In M.A. Frey and C.L. Sieloff (Eds.), *Advancing King's system framework and theory of goal attainment* (p. 176). Thousand Oaks, CA: Sage Publications.

Fewster-Thuente, L. and Velsor-Friedrich B.(2008). Interdisciplinary collaboration for health care professionals. *Nursing Administration Quarterly*, 32(1), 40–48.

Franca, I.S.X. and Pagliuca, L.M.F. (2002). Usefulness and the social significance of the theory of goal attainment by King [Portuguese]. *Revista Brasileira De Enfermagem*, 55(1), 44–51.

Frey, M. (1989). Social support and health: A theoretical formulation derived from King's conceptual framework. *Nursing Science Quarterly*, 2(3), 138–148.

Frey, M.A., Rooke, L., Sieloff, C., Messmer, P.R., and Kameoka, T. (1995). King's framework theory in Japan, Sweden, and the United States. *Image: Journal of Nursing Scholarship*, 27, 127–130.

Frey, M.A., Sieloff, C.L., and Norris, D.M. (2002). King's conceptual system and theory of goal attainment: Past, present, and future. *Nursing Science Quarterly*, 15(2), 107–112.

George, J.B. (1980). Imogene King. In The Nursing Theories Conference Group, *Nursing theories: The base for professional nursing practice*. Englewood Cliffs, NJ: Prentice-Hall.

George, J.B. (2002). Systems framework and theory of goal attainment—Imogene M. King. In J.B. George (Ed.), *Nursing theories: The base for professional nursing practice* (5th ed., pp. 241–267). Upper Saddle River, NJ: Prentice Hall.

Gonot, P.J. (1983). Imogene M. King: A theory for nursing. In J.J. Fitzpatrick and A.L. Whall (Eds.), *Conceptual models of nursing: Analysis and application*. Bowie, MD: Brady.

Gonot, P.J. (1986). Family therapy as derived from King's conceptual model. In A.L. Whall (Ed.), *Family therapy for nursing: Four approaches*. Norwalk, CT: Appleton-Century-Crofts.

Goodwin, Z., Kiehl, E.M., and Peterson, J.Z. (2002). King's theory as foundation for an advance directive decision-making model. *Nursing Science Quarterly*, 15(3), 237–241.

Gulitz, E.A. and King, I.M. (1988). King's general systems model: Application to curriculum development. *Nursing Science Quarterly*, 1(3), 128–132.

Hampton, D.C. (1994). King's theory of goal attainment as a framework for managed care implementation in a hospital setting. *Nursing Science Quarterly*, 7(4), 170–173.

Hanucharurnkui, S. and Vinya-nguag P. (1991). Effects of promoting patients' participation in self-care on postoperative recovery and satisfaction with care. *Nursing Science Quarterly*, 4(1), 14–20.

Husband, A. (1988). Application of King's theory of nursing to the care of the adult with diabetes. *Journal of Advanced Nursing*, 13, 484–488.

Husting, P.M. (1997). A transcultural critique of Imogene King's theory of global attainment. *Journal of Multicultural Nursing and Health*, 3(3), 15–20.

Isac, C., Ezhilarau, P., and Chacko, R.T. (2012). Information: A priceless gift in chronic care management of cancer patients. *International Journal of BioSciences*, 2(1), 80–85.

King, I.M. (1964). Nursing theory: Problems and prospects. *Nursing Science*, 2, 394–403.

King, I.M. (1968). A conceptual frame of reference for nursing. *Nursing Research*, 17(1), 27–31.

King, I.M. (1971). *Toward a theory for nursing*. New York: John Wiley & Sons.

King, I.M. (1975). A process for developing concepts for nursing through research. In P.J. Verhonick (Ed.), *Nursing research* (Vol. 1). Boston, MA: Little, Brown.

King, I.M. (1976). The health care system: Nursing intervention subsystem. In W.H. Werley, A. Zuzich, M. Zajkowski, and

A.D. Zagornik (Eds.), *Health research: The systems approach* (pp. 51–60). New York: Springer-Verlag.

King, I.M. (1978). USA: Loyola University of Chicago, School of Nursing. *Journal of Advanced Nursing*, 3, 390.

King, I.M. (1981). *A theory for nursing: Systems, concepts, process*. New York: John Wiley & Sons.

King, I.M. (1983a). The family coping with a medical illness. Analysis and application of King's theory of goal attainment. In I.W. Clements and F.B. Roberts (Eds.), *Family health: A theoretical approach to nursing*. New York: John Wiley & Sons.

King, I.M. (1983b). King's theory of nursing. In I.W. Clements and F.B. Roberts (Eds.), *Family health: A theoretical approach to nursing*. New York: John Wiley & Sons.

King, I.M. (1984). Effectiveness of nursing care: Use of a goal oriented nursing record in end stage renal disease. *American Association of Nephrology Nurses and Technicians Journal*, 11(2), 11–17, 60.

King, I.M. (1986a). King's theory of goal attainment. In P. Winstead-Fry (Ed.), *Case studies in nursing theory* (Chapter 7, pp. 197–213). New York: National League for Nursing.

King, I.M. (1986b). *Curriculum and instruction in nursing*. Norwalk, CT: Appleton-Century-Crofts.

King, I.M. (1987a). King's theory of goal attainment. In R. Parse (Ed.), *Nursing science: Major paradigms, theories, and critiques*. Philadelphia, PA: W.B. Saunders.

King, I.M. (1987b). Translating research into practice. *Journal of Neuroscience Nursing*, 19(1), 44–48.

King, I.M. (1988a). Concepts: Essential elements of theories. *Nursing Science Quarterly*, 1(1), 22–25.

King, I.M. (1988b). Measuring health goal attainment in patients. In C.F. Waltz and O. Strickland (Eds.), *Measurement of nursing outcomes: Measuring client outcomes*. New York: Springer.

King, I.M. (1989). King's systems framework for nursing administration. In B. Henry, C. Arndt, M. Di Vincenti, and A. Marriner-Tomey (Eds.), *Dimensions of nursing administration*. London, UK: Blackwell Scientific Publications.

King, I.M. (1990a). King's conceptual framework and theory of goal attainment. In M.E. Parker (Ed.), *Nursing theories in practice* (pp. 73–84). New York: National League for Nursing.

King, I.M. (1990b). Health as the goal for nursing. *Nursing Science Quarterly*, 3(3), 123–128.

King, I.M. (1992a). Window on general systems framework and theory of goal attainment. In M. O'Toole (Ed.), *Miller Keane encyclopedia and dictionary of medicine, nursing, and allied health* (p. 604). Philadelphia, PA: W.B. Saunders.

King, I.M. (1992b). King's theory of goal attainment. *Nursing Science Quarterly*, 5, 19–26.

King, I.M. (1994). Quality of life and goal attainment. *Nursing Science Quarterly*, 7(1), 29–32.

King, I.M. (1996a). A systems framework for nursing. In M.A. Frey and C.L. Sieloff (Eds.), *Advancing King's systems framework and theory of nursing* (pp. 14–22). Los Angeles, CA: Sage Publications.

King, I.M. (1996b). The theory of goal attainment. In M.A. Frey and C.L. Sieloff (Eds.), *Advancing King's systems framework and theory of nursing* (pp. 23–32). Los Angeles, CA: Sage Publications.

King, I.M. (1996c). The theory of goal attainment in research and practice. *Nursing Science Quarterly*, 9(2), 61–66.

King, I.M. (1997a). King's theory of goal attainment in practice. *Nursing Science Quarterly*, 10(4), 180–185.

King, I.M. (1997b). Reflections of the past and a vision for the future. *Nursing Science Quarterly*, 10(1), 15–17.

King, I.M. (1997c). King's theory of goal attainment in practice. *Nursing Science Quarterly*, 10(4), 180–185.

King, I.M. (1997d). Knowledge development for nursing: A process. In I.M. King and J. Fawcett (Eds.), *The language of nursing theory and metatheory* (pp. 19–25). Indianapolis, IN: Sigma Theta Tau International Center Nursing Press.

King, I.M. (1999). A theory of goal attainment: Philosophical and ethical implications. *Nursing Science Quarterly*, 12(4), 292–296.

King, I.M. (2000). Evidence-based nursing practice. *Theoria: Journal of Nursing Theory*, 9(2), 4–9.

King, I.M. (2001). Imogene M. King: Theory of goal attainment. In M.E. Parker (Ed.), *Nursing theories and nursing practice* (pp. 275–286). Philadelphia, PA: F.A. Davis.

King, I.M. (2008). Adversity and theory development. *Nursing Science Quarterly*, 21(2), 137–138.

King, I.M. and Whelton, B.J.B. (2001). Letters to the editor . . . "A nursing theory of personal system empathy: Interpreting a conceptualization of empathy in King's interaction systems." *Nursing Science Quarterly*, 14(1), 80–82.

Magan, S. (1987). A critique of King's theory. In R. Parse (Ed.), *Nursing science: Major paradigms, theories, and critiques*. Philadelphia, PA: W.B. Saunders.

Martin, J.P. (1990). Male cancer awareness: Impact of an employee education program. *Oncology Nursing Forum*, 17, 59–64.

McKinney, N.L. and Dean, P.R. (2000). Application of King's theory of dynamic interacting systems to the study of child abuse and the development of alcohol use/dependence in adult females. *Journal of Addictions Nursing*, 12(2), 73–82.

Meleis, A.I. (1985). International nursing for knowledge development. *Nursing Outlook*, 33(3), 144–147.

Meleis, A.I. and Jones, A. (1983). Ethical crises and cultural differences. *Western Journal of Medicine*, 138(6), 889–893.

Messmer, P. (1995). Implementation of theory-based nursing practice. In M.A. Frey and C.L. Sieloff (Eds.), *Advancing King's systems framework and theory of nursing* (p. 294). Thousand Oaks, CA: Sage Publications.

Miller, T., Kanai, T., Kebritchi, M., Grendell, R., and Howard, T. (2015). Hiring nurses re-entering the workforce after chemical dependence. *Journal of Nursing Education and Practice*, 5(11), 65–72.

Moreira, T.M.M. and Araujo, T.L. (2002). Interpersonal system of Imogene King: The relationships among patients with no-compliance to the treatment of the hypertension and professionals of health [Portuguese]. *Acta Paulista de Enfermagem*, 15(3), 35–43.

Moreira, T.M.M., Araujo, T.L., and Pagliuca, L.M.F. (2001). King's theory reach to families of persons with systemic arterial hypertension [Portuguese]. *Revista Gaucha de Enfermagem*, 22(2), 74–89.

Norgan, G.H., Ettipio, A.M., and Lasome, C.E.M. (1995). A program plan addressing carpal tunnel syndrome: The utility of King's goal attainment theory. *American Association of Occupational Health Nursing*, 43, 407–411.

Norris, D.M. and Frey, M.A. (2002). King's interacting systems framework and theory in nursing practice. In M.R. Alligood and A. Mariner-Tomey (Eds.), *Nursing theory utilization and application* (2nd ed., pp. 173–196). St. Louis, MO: Mosby.

Norris, D.M. and Hoyer, P.J. (1993). Dynamism in practice: Parenting within King's framework. *Nursing Science Quarterly*, 6(2), 79–85.

Omnibus Budget Reconciliation Act. (1990). Pub. L. No. 101–508 and 4206, 4751 (From Goodwin, Kiehl, and Patterson, 2002).

Plummer, M. and Molzahn, A.E. (2009). Quality of life in contemporary nursing theory: A concept analysis. *Nursing Science Quarterly*, 22(2), 134–140.

Rooda, L.A. (1992). The development of a conceptual model for multicultural nursing. *Journal of Holistic Nursing*, 10(4), 337–347.

Rooke, L. (1995). Focusing on King's theory and systems framework in education by using an experiential learning model: A challenge to improve the quality of nursing care. In M.A. Frey and C.L. Sieloff (Eds.), *Advancing King's framework and theory for nursing* (pp. 278–293). Newbury Park, CA: Sage Publications.

Rooke, L. and Norberg, A. (1988). Problematic and meaningful situations in nursing interpreted by concepts from King's nursing theory and four additional concepts. *Scandinavian Journal of Caring Sciences*, 2(2), 80–87.

Rosendahl, P.B. and Ross, V. (1982). Does your behavior affect your patient's response? *Journal of Gerontological Nursing*, 8, 572–575.

Ryle, S. (2008). Current evidence on anticoagulant management and outcomes for postpolypectomy. *Gastroenterology Nursing*, 31(5), 354–364.

Sieloff, C.L. (2003). Measuring nursing power within organizations. *Journal of Nursing Scholarship*, 35(2), 183–187.

Sieloff, C.L. (2007). The theory of group power within organizations evaluating conceptualization within King's conceptual system. In C.L. Sieloff and M.A. Frey (Eds.), *Middle-range theory development using King's conceptual system* (pp. 196–214). New York: Springer Publishing Company.

Sieloff, C.L. (2010). Improving work environment through the use of research instrument: An example. *Nursing Administration Quarterly*, 34(1), 56–60.

Smith, M.C. (1988). King's theory in practice. *Nursing Science Quarterly*, 1(4), 145–146.

Sowell, R.L. and Lowenstein, A. (1994). King's theory as a framework for quality: Linking theory to practice. *Nursing-connections*, 7(2), 19–31.

Stevens, K.R. and Messmer, P.R. (2008). In remembrance of Imogene M. King, January 30, 1923–December 24, 2007: Imogene, a pioneer and dear colleague. *Nursing Outlook*, 56(3), 100–101.

Temple, A. and Fawdry, K. (1992). King's theory of goal attainment: Resolving filial caregiver role strain. *Journal of Gerontological Nursing*, 18(3), 11–15.

Uys, L.R. (1987). Foundational studies in nursing. *Journal of Advanced Nursing*, 12(3), 275–280.

Viera, C.S. and Rossi, L. (2000). Nursing diagnoses from NANDA's taxonomy in women with a hospitalized preterm child and King's conceptual system [Portuguese]. *Revista Latino-Americana de Enfermagem*, 8(6), 110–116.

Walker, K.M. and Alligood, M.R. (2001). Empathy from a nursing perspective: Moving beyond borrowed theory. *Archives of Psychiatric Nursing*, 15(3), 140–147.

Weed, L.L. (1969). *Medical records, medical education, and patient care*. Cleveland, OH: Case Western Reserve University Press.

Whelton, B.J.B. (1999). The philosophical core of King's conceptual system. *Nursing Science Quarterly*, 12(2), 158–163.

Whelton, B.J.B. (2008). Human nature: A foundation for palliative care. *Nursing Philosophy*, 9(2), 77–88.

Woods, E.C. (1994). King's theory in practice with elders. *Nursing Science Quarterly*, 7(2), 65–69.

Zetterberg, H.L. (1963). *On theory and verification in sociology* (Rev. ed.). Totowa, NJ: Bedminster Press.

Zoffmann, V., Harder, I., and Kirkevold, M. (2008). A person-centered communication and reflection model: Sharing decision-making in chronic care. *Qualitative Health Research*, 18(5), 670–685.

Orlando

Allen, D.E., Bockenhauer, B., Egan, C., and Kinnaird, L.S. (2006). Relating outcomes to excellent nursing practice. *Journal of Nursing Administration*, 36(3), 140–147.

Andrews, C.M. (1983). Ida Orlando's model for nursing. In J. Fitzpatrick and A. Whall (Eds.), *Conceptual models of nursing: Analysis and application*. Bowie, MD: Robert J. Brady Company.

Aseratie, M., Murugan, R., and Molla, M. (2014). Assessment of factors affecting implementation of nursing process among nurses in selected governmental hospitals, Adis Ababa, Ethiopia; Cross-sectional study. *Journal of Nursing Care*, 3(3), 1–8.

Barnum, B.J.S. (1994). *Nursing theory: Analysis, application, and evaluation* (4th ed.). Philadelphia, PA: Lippincott Williams & Wilkins.

Barnum, B.J.S. (1998). *Nursing theory: Analysis, application, evaluation* (5th ed.). Philadelphia, PA: Lippincott Williams & Wilkins.

Barron, M.A. (1966). The effects varied nursing approaches have on patients' complaints of pain [Abstract]. *Nursing Research*, 15(1), 90–91.

Bochnak, M.A. (1963). The effect of an automatic and deliberative process of nursing activity on the relief of patients' pain: A clinical experiment. *Nursing Research*, 12(3), 191–192.

Cameron, J. (1963). An exploratory study of the verbal responses of the nurse-patient interactions. *Nursing Research*, 12(3), 192.

Crane, M.D. (1980). Ida Jean Orlando: In Nursing Theories Conference Group, *Nursing theories: The base for professional nursing practice*. Englewood Cliffs, NJ: Prentice-Hall.

Diers, D. (1970). Faculty research development at Yale. *Nursing Research*, 19(1), 64–71.

Diers, D.K. (1966). The nurse orientation system: A method for analyzing the nurse-patient interactions [Abstract]. *Nursing Research*, 15(1), 91.

Dracup, K.A. and Breu, C.S. (1978). Using nursing research findings to meet the needs of grieving spouses. *Nursing Research*, 27(4), 212.

Dumas, R.G. and Leonard, R.C. (1963). The effect of nursing on the incidence of postoperative vomiting. *Nursing Research*, 12(1), 12–15.

Eisler, J., Wolfer, J., and Diers, D. (1972). Relationship between the need for social approval and postoperative recovery and welfare. *Nursing Research*, 21(5), 520–525.

Elms, R.R. and Leonard, R.C. (1966). The effects of nursing approaches during admission. *Nursing Research*, 15(1), 39–48.

England, M. (2005). Analysis of nurse conversation: methodology of the process recording. *Journal of Psychiatric and Mental Health Nursing*, 12(6), 661–671.

Faust, C. (2002). Orlando's deliberative nursing process theory: A practice application in an extended care facility. *Journal of Gerontological Nursing*, 28(7), 14–18.

Forchuk, C. (1991). A comparison of the works of Peplau and Orlando. *Archives of Psychiatric Nursing*, 5, 38–45.

Gilliss, L. (1976). Sleeplessness: Can you help? *The Canadian Nurse*, 72(7), 32–34.

Gowan, N.I. and Morris, M. (1964). Nurses' responses to expressed patient needs. *Nursing Research*, 13(1), 68–71.

Hage, J. (1972). *Techniques and problems of theory construction in sociology*. New York: John Wiley & Sons.

Haggerty, L.A. (1987). An analysis of senior nursing students' immediate responses to distressed patients. *Journal of Advanced Nursing*, 12, 451–461.

Hampe, S.O. (1975). Needs of grieving spouses in a hospital setting. *Nursing Research*, 24(2), 113.

Hunter, L.P. and Hunter, L.A. (2006). Storytelling as an educational strategy for midwifery students. *Journal of Midwifery & Women's Health*, 51(4), 273–278.

Laurent, C.L. (2000). A nursing theory for nursing leadership. *Journal of Nursing Management*, 8(2), 83–87.

Leenerts, M.H. and Teel, C.S. (2006). Relational conversation as method for creating partnerships: Pilot study. *Journal of Advanced Nursing*, 54(4), 467–476.

Lipson, J. and Meleis, A.I. (1983). Issues in health care of Middle-Eastern patients. *The Western Journal of Medicine*, 139, 854–861.

Marriner-Tomey, A., Mills, D., and Sauter, M. (1989). Ida Jean Orlando (Pelletier): Nursing process theory. In A. Marriner-Tomey (Ed.), *Nursing theorists and their work*. St. Louis, MO: C.V. Mosby.

Mertz, H. (1962). Nurse actions that reduce stress in patients. In *Emergency intervention by the nurse* (Monograph 1, pp. 10–14). New York: American Nurses Association.

Olson, J. and Hanchett, E. (1997). Nurse-expressed empathy, patient outcomes, and development of a middle-range theory. *Image: The Journal of Nursing Scholarship*, 29(1), 71–76.

Orlando, I.J. (1961). *The dynamic nurse-patient relationship*. New York: G.P. Putnam's Sons.

Orlando, I.J. (1972). *The discipline and teaching of nursing process*. New York: G.P. Putnam's Sons.

Orlando-Pelletier, I.J. (1990a). Preface to the NLN edition. In I.J. Orlando (Ed.), *The dynamic nurse patient relationship: Function, process, and principles* (pp. vii–viii). New York: National League for Nursing.

Orlando-Pelletier, I.J. (1990b). *The dynamic nurse patient relationship: Function, process, and principles*. New York: National League for Nursing.

Peplau, H. (1952). *Interpersonal relations in nursing*. New York: G.P. Putnam's Sons.

Peplau, H.E. (1991). *Interpersonal relations in nursing: A conceptual frame of reference for psychodynamic nursing*. New York: Springer. (Original work published 1952.)

Pienschke, D. (1973). Guardedness or openness on the cancer unit. *Nursing Research*, 22(6), 484–490.

Potter, M.L. and Bockenhauer, B.J. (2000). Implementing Orlando's nursing theory: A pilot study. *Journal of Psychosocial Nursing and Mental Health Services*, 38(3), 14–21.

Potter, M. and Tinker, S. (2000). Put power in nurses' hands: Orlando's nursing theory supports nurses—Simply. *Nursing Management*, 31(7 Part 1), 40–41.

Rhymes, J. (1964). A description of nurse-patient interaction in effective nursing activity. *Nursing Research*, 13(4), 365.

Schmieding, N.J. (1983). An analysis of Orlando's theory based on Kuhn's theory of science. In P.L. Chinn (Ed.), *Advances in nursing theory development*. Rockville, MD: Aspen Systems.

Schmieding, N.J. (1986). Orlando's theory. In P. Winstead-Fry (Ed.), *Case studies in nursing theory*. New York: National League for Nursing.

Schmieding, N.J. (1987). Problematic situations in nursing: Analysis of Orlando's theory based on Dewey's theory of inquiry. *Journal of Advanced Nursing*, 12, 431–440.

Schmieding, N.J. (1988). Action process of nurse administrators to problematic situations based on Orlando's theory. *Journal of Advanced Nursing*, 13, 99–107.

Schmieding, N.J. (1990a). Do head nurses include staff nurses in problem-solving? *Nursing Management*, 21(3), 58–60.

Schmieding, N.J. (1990b). A model for assessing nurse administrators' actions. *Western Journal of Nursing Research*, 12(3), 293–306.

Schmieding, N.J. (1990c). An integrative nursing theoretical framework. *Journal of Advanced Nursing*, 15(4), 463–467.

Schmieding, N.J. (2002). Ida Jean Orlando (Pelletier): Nursing process theory. In A.M. Tomey and M.R. Alligood (Eds.), *Nurse theorists and their work* (5th ed., pp. 399–417). St. Louis, MO: Mosby.

Sellers, S.C. (1991). A philosophical analysis of conceptual models of nursing. Dissertation Abstracts International, 52, 1937B. (University Microfilms No. AAC91–26248).

Sheafor, M. (1991). Productive work groups in complex hospital units: Proposed contributions of the nurse-executive. *Journal of Nursing Administration*, 21(5), 25–30.

Shea, N., McBride, L., Gavin, C., and Bauer, M.S. (1997). The effects of an ambulatory collaborative practice model on process outcomes of care for bipolar disorder. *Journal of the American Psychiatric Nurses Association*, 3(2), 49–57.

Sieger, M., Fritz, E., and Them, C. (2012). In discourse: Bourdieu's theory of practice and habitus in the context of a communication-oriented nursing interaction model. *Journal of Advanced Nursing*, 68(2), 480–489.

Toniolli, A.C. and Pagliuca, L.M. (2002). Analysis of the applicability of Orlando's theory in Brazilian nursing journals [Portuguese]. *Revista Brasileira de Enfermagem*, 55(5), 489–494.

Tryon, P.A. (1963). An experiment of the effect of patients' participation in planning the administration of a nursing procedure. *Nursing Research*, 12(4), 262–265.

Tryon, P.A. and Leonard, R.C. (1964). The effect of patients' participation on the outcome of a nursing procedure. *Nursing Forum*, 3(2), 79–89.

Williamson, K.M. (2007). Home health care nurses' perceptions of empowerment. *Journal of Community Health Nursing*, 24(3), 133–153.

Williamson, Y. (1978). Methodologic dilemmas in tapping the concept of patient needs. *Nursing Research*, 27(3), 172.

Wolfer, J.A. and Visintainer, M.A. (1975). Pediatric surgical patients' and parents' stress responses and adjustment. *Nursing Research*, 24(4), 244–255.

Zoffmann, V., Harder, I., and Kirkevold, M. (2008). A person-centered communication and reflection model: Sharing decision-making in chronic care. *Qualitative Health Research*, 18(5), 670–685.

Paterson and Zderad

Azevedo, N.A., Kantorski, L.P., and Ornellas, C.P. (2000). Families of patients undergoing chemotherapy, based on Paterson and Zderad's theory [Portuguese]. *Texto & Contexto Enfermagem*, 9(2 Part 1), 17–27.

Barnum, B.J.S. (1994). *Nursing theory: Analysis, application, and evaluation* (4th ed.). Philadelphia, PA: Lippincott.

Barnum, B.J.S. (1998). *Nursing theory: Analysis, application, evaluation* (5th ed.). Philadelphia, PA: Lippincott Williams & Wilkins.

Chan, M.F., Lou, F.L., Arthur, D.G., Cao, F.L., Wu, L.H, Li, P., et al. (2008). Investigating factors associate to nurses' attitudes towards perinatal bereavement care. *Journal of Clinical Nursing*, 17(4), 509–518.

Cutcliffe, J.R. and Cassedy, P. (1999). The development of empathy in students on a short, skills based counselling course: A pilot study. *Nurse Education Today*, 19(3), 250–257.

Dariel, O.P.D. (2009). Nursing education: In pursuit of cosmopolitanism. *Nurse Education Today*, 29(5), 566–569.

Donaldson, S.K. (1983). Let us not abandon the humanities. *Nursing Outlook*, 31(1), 40–43.

Hall, E.O.C. and Brinchmann, B.S. (2009). Mothers of preterm infants: Experiences of space, tone and transfer in the neonatal care unit. *Journal of Neonatal Nursing*, 15(4), 129–136.

Hopkinson, J.B. and Hallett, C.E. (2001). Patients' perceptions of hospice day care: A phenomenological study. *International Journal of Nursing Studies*, 38(1), 117–125.

Jacob, J.D., Holmes, D., and Buus, N. (2008). Humanism in forensic psychiatry: the use of the tidal nursing model. *Nursing Inquiry*, 15(3), 224–230.

Kant, I. (1953). *Prolegomena to any future metaphysics* (P.G. Lucas, Trans.). Manchester, England: University of Manchester Press.

Kleiman, S. (1986). Humanistic nursing: The phenomenological theory of Paterson and Zderad. In P. Winstead-Fry (Ed.), *Case studies in nursing theory*. New York: National League for Nursing.

Kleiman, S. (2004). What is the nature of nurse practitioners' lived experiences interacting with patients? *Journal of the American Academy of Nurse Practitioners*, 16(6), 263–269.

Kleiman, S. (2008a). *Human centered nursing: The foundation of quality care*. Philadelphia, PA: F.A. Davis.

Kleiman, S. (2008b). *Instructor's guide for human centered nursing: The foundation of quality care*. New York: Institute for Human Centered Caring.

Kleiman, S. (2009). On the way to learning. *MEDSURG Nursing*, 18(1), 33–37.

Kleiman, S. (2010, May 26). Humanistic nursing inquiry: A humanistic learning experience. Personal communication.

Kleiman, S. (2010). Josephine Paterson and Loretta Zderad's humanistic nursing theory. In M.E. Parker and M.C. Smith (Eds), *Nursing theories and nursing practice* (3rd ed., pp. 337–350). Philadelphia, PA: F.A. Davis Company.

Kolcaba, K.Y. and Kolcaba, R.J. (1991). An analysis of the concept of comfort. *Journal of Advanced Nursing*, 16(11), 1301–1310.

Kostovich, C.T. (2012). Development and psychometric assessment of the presence of nursing scale. *Nursing Science Quarterly*, 25(2), 167–175.

Medina, R.F. and Backes, V.M. (2002). Humanism in the care of surgery patients [Portuguese]. *Revista Brasileira de Enfermagem*, 55(5), 522–527.

Menke, E.M. (1978). Theory development: A challenge for nursing. In N.L. Chaska (Ed.), *The nursing profession: Views through the mist*. New York: McGraw-Hill.

Merryfeather, L. (2015). Passionate scholarship or academic safety: An ethical issue. *Journal of Holistic Nursing*, 33(1), 60–67.

Munhall, P.L. (1982). Nursing philosophy and nursing research: In apposition or opposition? *Nursing Research*, 31(3), 776–786.

Muniz, R.M., Santana, M.G., and Serqueira, H.C. (2000). Nursing care tuned to the young adult human being who is the carrier of a chronic disease, under the light of Paterson and Zderad's humanistic nursing theory [Portuguese]. *Texto & Contexto Enfermagem*, 9(2 Part 1), 158–168.

Oiler, C. (1982). The phenomenological approach in nursing research. *Nursing Research*, 31(3), 178–181.

Paterson, J.G. (1971). From a philosophy of clinical nursing to a method of nursology. *Nursing Research*, 20(2), 143–146.

Paterson, J.G. (1978). The tortuous way toward nursing theory. In *Theory development: What, why, how?* (NLN Publication No. 15-1708, pp. 49–65). New York: National League for Nursing.

Paterson, J.G. and Zderad, L.T. (1970–1971). All together through complementary syntheses are the worlds of the many. *Image: Journal of Nursing Scholarship*, 4(3), 13–16.

Paterson, J.G. and Zderad, L.T. (1976). *Humanistic nursing*. New York: John Wiley & Sons.

Paterson, J.G. and Zderad, L.T. (1988). *Humanistic nursing* (2nd ed.). New York: National League of Nursing.

Risjord, M. (2014). Nursing and human freedom. *Nursing Philosophy*, 15(1), 35–45.

Silva, T.N. (2013). Paterson and Zderad's humanistic theory: Entering the between through being when called upon. *Nursing Science Quarterly*, 26(2), 132–135.

Souza, L.N.A. and Padilha, M.I.C. (2000). Humanization in critical care: A way under construction [Portuguese]. *Texto & Contexto Enfermagem*, 9(2 Part 1), 324–335.

Stern, P.N. (1980). Grounded theory methodology: Its uses and processes. *Image*, 12, 20–23.

Stevens, B.J.S. (1984). *Nursing theory: Analysis, application, and evaluation* (2nd ed.). Boston, MA: Little, Brown.

Tutton, E. and Seers, K. (2003). An exploration of the concept of comfort. *Journal of Clinical Nursing*, 12(5), 689–696.

Wagner, A.L. (2000). Connecting to nurse-self through reflective poetic story. *International Journal for Human Caring*, 4(2), 7–12.

Wilson, H.S. (1977). Limiting intrusion: Social control of outsiders in a healing community. *Nursing Research*, 26(2), 103–111.

Wu, H.L. and Volker, D.L. (2012). Humanistic nursing theory: Application to hospice and palliative care. *Journal of Advanced Nursing*, 68(2), 471–479.

Zderad, L.T. (1968). *A concept of empathy*. Doctoral dissertation, Washington, DC: Georgetown University.

Zderad, L.T. (1969). Empathetic nursing: Realization of a human capacity. *Nursing Clinics of North America*, 4, 655–662.

Zderad, L.T. (1970). *Empathy: From cliche to construct*. In Proceedings of the Third Nursing Theory Conference. Lawrence, KS: University of Kansas Medical Center Department of Nursing.

Zderad, L.T. (1978). *From here and now to theory: Reflections on "how." In Theory development: What, why, how?* (NLN Publication No. 15-1708, pp. 35–48.) New York: National League for Nursing.

Travelbee

Barrett-Leonard, G.T. (1962). Dimensions of therapist responses as causal factors in therapeutic change. *Psychological Monographs*, 76(43, Whole No. 562).

Begat, I.B.E. and Severinsson, E.I. (2001). Nurses' reflections on episodes occurring during their provision of care—An interview study. *International Journal of Nursing Studies*, 38(1), 71–77.

Cartwright, R.D. and Lerner, B. (1963). Empathy, need to change, and improvement with psychotherapy. *Journal of Consulting Psychology*, 27, 138–144.

Chin, R. (1974). The utility of system models and developmental models for practitioners. In J. Riehl and C. Roy (Eds.), *Conceptual models in nursing practice*. New York: Appleton-Century-Crofts.

Chinsky, J.M. and Rappaport, J. (1970). Brief critique of the meaning and reliability of "accurate empathy" ratings. *Psychological Bulletin*, 73, 379–382.

Cook, L. (1989). Nurses in crisis: A support group based on Travelbee's nursing theory. *Nursing and Health Care*, 10(4), 203–205.

Doona, M.E. (1979). *Travelbee's intervention in psychiatric nursing* (2nd ed.). Philadelphia, PA: F.A. Davis.

Duffey, M. and Muhlenkamp, A.F. (1974). A framework for theory analysis. *Nursing Outlook*, 22(9), 570–574.

Frankel, V. (1963). *Man's search for meaning: An introduction to logotherapy*. New York: Washington Square Press.

Freihofer, P. and Felton, G. (1976). Nursing behaviors in bereavement: An exploratory study. *Nursing Research*, 25(5), 332–337.

Haugan, G. (2013a). Nurse-patient interaction is a resource for hope, meaning in life and self-transcendence in nursing home patients. *Scandinavian Journal of Caring Sciences*, 28(1), 74–88.

Haugan, G. (2013b). The relationship between nurse-patient interaction and meaning-in-life in cognitively intact nursing home patients. *Journal of Advanced Nursing*, 70(1), 107–120.

Haugan, G., Innstrand, S.T., and Moksnes, U.K. (2013). The effect of nurse-patient interaction on anxiety and depression in cognitively intact nursing home patients. *Journal of Clinical Nursing*, 22, 2192–2205.

Haugan, G., Rannestad, T., Hanssen, B., and Espnes, G.A. (2012). Self-transcendence and nurse-patient interaction in cognitively intact nursing home patients. *Journal of Clinical Nursing*, 21, 3429–3441.

Hawley, G. (1998). Facing uncertainty and possible death: The Christian patients' experience. *Journal of Advanced Nursing*, 26(2), 295–303.

Hisama, K.K. (2001). The acceptance of nursing theory in Japan: A cultural perspective. *Nursing Science Quarterly*, 14(3), 255–259.

Kurtz, R.R. and Grummon, D.L. (1972). Different approaches to the measurement of therapist empathy and their relationship to therapy outcomes. *Journal of Consulting and Clinical Psychology*, 30, 106–115.

Landmark, B.T., Strandmark, M., and Wahl, A.K. (2001). Living with newly diagnosed breast cancer—The meaning of existential issues—A qualitative study of 10 women with newly diagnosed breast cancer, based on grounded theory. *Cancer Nursing*, 24(3), 220–226.

May, R. (1953). *Man's search for himself*. New York: W.W. Norton.

McBride, M.A. (1967). Nursing approach, pain, and relief: An exploratory experiment. *Nursing Research*, 16(4), 337–341.

McCann, T.V. and Baker, H. (2001). Mutual relating: Developing interpersonal relationships in the community. *Journal of Advanced Nursing*, 34(4), 530–537.

Morse, J.M. (2001). Toward a praxis theory of suffering. *Advances in Nursing Science*, 24(1), 47–59.

Morse, J.M. (2005). Towards a praxis theory of suffering. In J.R. Cutliff and H.P. McKenna (Eds.), *The essential concepts of nursing* (pp. 257–272). London, UK: Elsevier, Churchill Livingstone.

Moses, M.M. (1994). Caring incidents: A gift to the present. *Journal of Holistic Nursing*, 12(2), 193–203.

Narayanasamy, A. (1999). Learning spiritual dimensions of care from a historical perspective. *Nurse Education Today*, 19(5), 386–395.

Nowak, K.B. and Wandel, J.C. (1998). The sharing of self in geriatric clinical practice: Case report and analysis. *Geriatric Nursing*, 19(1), 34–37.

O'Baugh, J., Wilkes, L.M., Luke, S., and George, A. (2008). Positive attitude in cancer: The nurse's perspective. *International Journal of Nursing Practice*, 14, 109–114.

Parrish, E., Peden, A., and Staten, R.T. (2008). Strategies used by advanced practice psychiatric nurses in treating adults with depression. *Perspectives in Psychiatric Care*, 44(4), 232–240.

Rustoen, T. and Hanestad, B.R. (1998a). Nursing intervention to increase hope and quality of life in newly diagnosed cancer patients. *Cancer Nursing*, 21(4), 235–245.

Rustoen, T. and Hanestad, B.R. (1998b). Nursing intervention to increase hope in cancer patients. *Journal of Clinical Nursing*, 7(1), 19–27.

Sarlore, J.P. (1966). Existentialism. In W.V. Spanos (Ed.), *A casebook on existentialism*. New York: Thomas V. Crowell.

Sloane, A. (1966). Review of "Interpersonal aspects of nursing" by J. Travelbee. *American Journal of Nursing*, 66(6), 77.

Stetler, C. (1977). Relationship of perceived empathy of nurses' communication. *Nursing Research*, 26(6), 432–438.

Timmins, F. and Kelly, J. (2008). Spiritual assessment in intensive and cardiac care nursing. *Nursing in Critical Care*, 13(3), 124–131.

Topaz, M., Troutman-Jordan, M., and MacKenzie, M. (2014). Construction, deconstruction, and reconstruction: The roots of successful aging theories. *Nursing Science Quarterly*, 27(3), 226–233.

Tranvag, O. and Kristoffersen, K. (2008). Experience of being the spouse/cohabitant of a person with bipolar affective disorder: A cumulative process over time. *Scandinavian Journal of Caring Sciences*, 22(1), 5–18.

Travelbee, J. (1963). What do we mean by "rapport?" *American Journal of Nursing*, 63(2), 70–72.

Travelbee, J. 1964). What's wrong with sympathy? *American Journal of Nursing*, 64(1), 68–71.

Travelbee, J. (1966). *Interpersonal aspects of nursing*. Philadelphia, PA: F.A. Davis.

Travelbee, J. (1969). *Intervention in psychiatric nursing*. Philadelphia, PA: F.A. Davis.

Travelbee, J. (1971). *Interpersonal aspects of nursing* (2nd ed.). Philadelphia, PA: F.A. Davis.

Truax, C. and Carkhuff, R.R. (1967). *Toward effective counseling and psychotherapy*. Chicago, IL: Aldine.

Tuck, I., Wallace, D., and Pullen, L. (2001). Spirituality and spiritual care provided by parish nurses. *Western Journal of Nursing Research*, 23(5), 441–453.

Tutton, E., Seers, K., and Langstaff, D. (2009). An exploration of hope as a concept for nursing. *Journal of Orthopaedic Nursing*, 13, 119–127.

von Bertalanffy, L. (1968). *General systems theory: Foundations, development, application*. New York: George Braziller.

von Krogh, G. and Naden, D. (2008). A nursing-specific model of EPR documentation: Organizational and professional requirements. *Journal of Nursing Scholarship*, 40(1), 68–75.

Wadensten, B. and Carlsson, M. (2003). Nursing theory views on how to support the process of ageing. *Journal of Advanced Nursing*, 42(2), 118–124.

Wadensten, B., Engholm, R., Fahlström, G., and Hägglund, D. (2009). Nursing staff's description of a good encounter in nursing homes. *International Journal of Older People Nursing*, 4, 203–210.

Weaver, K., Morse, J., and Mitcham, C. (2008). Ethical sensitivity in professional practice: Concept analysis. *Journal of Advanced Nursing*, 62(5), 607–618.

Wiklund, L. (2008). Existential aspects of living with addiction – Part II: Caring needs. A hermeneutic expansion of qualitative findings. *Journal of Clinical Nursing*, 17, 2435–2443.

Wolff, I.S. (1966). Review of "Interpersonal aspects of nursing" by J. Travelbee. *American Journal of Nursing*, 66(7), 1504–1506.

Wiedenbach

Andersen, C. and Adamsen, L. (2001). Continuous video recording: A new clinical research tool for studying the nursing care of cancer patients. *Journal of Advanced Nursing*, 35(2), 257–267.

Barger, M., Faucher, M.A., and Murphy, P.A. (2015). Theorists and historical influences. *Journal of Midwifery and Women's Health*, 60(1), 89–98.

Barnum, B.J.S. (1998). *Nursing theory: Analysis, application, evaluation* (5th ed.). Philadelphia, PA: Lippincott Williams & Wilkins.

Bennett, A.M. and Foster, P.C. (1980). Ernestine Wiedenbach. In The Nursing Theories Conference Group, *Nursing theories: The base for professional nursing practice*. Englewood Cliffs, NJ: Prentice-Hall.

Burst, H.V. (1998). In memoriam: Ernestine Wiedenbach, CNM, MA, FACNM. *Journal of Nurse-Midwifery*, 43(5), 361–362.

Burst, H.V. (2000). The circle of safety: A tool for clinical preceptors. *Journal of Midwifery and Women's Health*, 45(5), 408–410.

Dickoff, J., James, P., & Wiedenbach, E. (1968a). Theory in a practice discipline: Part 1. Practice oriented theory. *Nursing research*, 17(5), 415–434.

Dickoff, J., James, P., & Wiedenbach, E. (1968b). Theory in a practice discipline: Part II. Practice oriented theory. *Nursing research*, 17(6), 545–554.

Eisler, J., Wolfer, J.A., and Diers, D. (1972). Relationship between the need for social approval and postoperative recovery welfare. *Nursing Research*, 21(5), 520–525.

Elms, R.R. and Leonard, R.C. (1966). Effects of nursing approaches during admission. *Nursing Research*, 15(1), 37–48.

Griffiths, B. and Andres, C.M. (2007). Putting nursing theory into practice. *Gastroenterology Nursing*, 30(6), 440–442.

Kolcaba, K. (2003). *Comfort theory and practice: A vision for holistic health care and research*. New York: Springer Publishing Company.

Larson, P.A. (1977). Nurse perception of client illness. *Nursing Research*, 26(6), 416–421.

Leonard, R.C., Skipper, J.K., and Woolridge, P.J. (1967). Small sample field experiments for evaluating patient care. *Health Services Research*, 2(1), 47–50.

Nickel, S, Gesse, T., and MacLaren, A. (1992). Ernestine Wiedenbach: Her professional legacy. *Journal of Nurse-Midwifery*, 37(3), 161–167.

Rickleman, B.L. (1971). Bio-psychosocial linguistics: A conceptual approach to nurse-patient interaction. *Nursing Research*, 20(5), 398–403.

Sharp, E.S. (1998). Ethics in reproductive health care: A midwifery perspective. *Journal of Nurse-Midwifery*, 43(3), 235–245.

Shields, D. (1978). Nursing care in labor and patient satisfaction. A descriptive study. *Journal of Advances in Nursing*, 3, 535–550.

VandeVusse, L. (1997). Sculpting a nurse midwifery philosophy. Ernestine Wiedenbach's influence. *Journal of Nurse-Midwifery*, 42(1), 43–48.

Wiedenbach, E. (1963). The helping art of nursing. *American Journal of Nursing*, 63(11), 54–57.

Wiedenbach, E. (1964). *Clinical nursing: A helping art*. New York: Springer-Verlag.

Wiedenbach, E. (1965). Family nurse practitioner for maternal and child care. *Nursing Outlook*, 13, 50–52.

Wiedenbach, E. (1968). Nurse's role in family planning: A conceptual base for practice. *Nursing Clinics of North America*, 3(2), 355–365.

Wiedenbach, E. (1970a). Comment on beliefs and values: Basis for curriculum design. *Nursing Research*, 19(5), 427.

Wiedenbach, E. (1970b). Nurses' wisdom in nursing theory. *American Journal of Nursing*, 70(5), 1057–1062.

Wiedenbach, E. and Falls, C.E. (1978). *Communication: Key to effective nursing*. New York: Tiresias Press.

Williams, D.L. (2008). Safeguarding attitudes. *Journal of Forensic Nursing*, 4(1), 47–48.

Wolfer, J. and Visintainer, M. (1975). Pediatric surgical patients' and parents' stress responses and adjustment. *Nursing Research*, 24(4), 244–255.

13

On Outcomes

In this chapter, ideas of five theorists have been presented. All five theorists are focused primarily on the outcomes of nursing care, facilitating and promoting harmony with the environment, balancing and stabilizing internal and external systems, conserving energy, and mobilizing resources to meet the challenges of stressors and/or adaptation. Although grouped together because of the ultimate goals for nursing for each of the theorists, they differ in their paradigmatic origins and the central questions they ask.

Among the theories discussed in this chapter is Martha Rogers' theory, which provides a unique focus on the conceptualization of the irreducible nature of the connection of person and environment. When Martha Rogers asked the central question of her theory, What is the focus of nursing? the answer was readily human being–environmental fields, "people and their world" (Rogers, 1992). Human beings and the environment are both unitary, irreducible, pandimensional, negentropic energy fields that are identifiable by pattern. Neither unitary human being nor unitary environment can be discussed, considered, or understood in isolation from the other. They are interrelated in an irreducible way. This innovative and visionary approach on human being–environment, unique to nursing and different from other theorists' views of human being–environment, made it easy to consider Rogers as a significant force in our conceptual understanding not only of the centrality of environment in nursing thoughts and actions, but also of the inseparability of human being–environment relationships and the significance of harmony between them as a consequence of nursing care. Rogers' theory is described, analyzed, and critiqued in this chapter. Rogers' science of unitary human beings (SUHB) also provides many insights about "environment" from a nursing perspective. I also encourage you to look at Florence Nightingale's work for a conceptualization of environment, as well as at other theorists' conceptualizations of environment. As of this writing, I believe that Rogers' theory is the only one that integrated human being–environment interactions into a coherent whole and proposed it as a unit of analysis. Hers is a prototype theory.

The works of the four other theorists—Levine, Johnson, Neuman, and Roy—emerge as significant developments in the conceptualization of the nursing client and the goals and outcomes of nursing care. Central questions for these theorists are: Who is the nursing client? In what ways does a nursing client benefit from nursing care? What is the outcome of care? Three theorists, Dorothy Johnson, Sister Callista Roy (a mentee and student of Johnson's), and Betty Neuman focused on defining client systems. Johnson asserted in all her metatheory, as well as in theory publications, that what differentiates nursing from medicine and other health sciences is its perspective of a nursing client as a behavioral system. To Roy, a client is an adaptive being with two subsystems for adapting—the regulator and cognator mechanisms—and four adaptive modes. According to Neuman, the human being—as represented by central structure, lines of defense, and resistance—becomes a client when threatened or attacked by environmental stressors. The nursing activities and actions that are deliberately destined for caring for patients, potential patients, or people at risk (or families and communities) are the rationale for grouping these theorists under nursing outcomes. The theorists have described and discussed nursing therapeutics with various degrees of emphasis that lead to different outcomes. Many images emerge when the concept "nursing therapeutics" is considered. One is Levine's proposed actions for conservation of energy (outcome theorist); a second is Orem's proposed strategies to enhance self-care (need theorist), and others may be delineated from the writings of different theorists (see Chapter 9, Tables 9-6, 9-12, and 9-18).

DOROTHY JOHNSON

Theory Description

The early questions addressed by Dorothy Johnson pertained to the knowledge base nurses needed for nursing care (Johnson, 1959a). To Johnson, nursing care did not depend on medical care, nor was its goal recovery from illness or adoption of more desirable health practices. She labeled nursing's responsibilities that are related to medical care and better health as "delegated medical care" and "health care," respectively (Johnson, 1961). Although nurses also performed functions related to "delegated medical care," the essence of nursing, its central mission, should lie in "nursing care," which Johnson considered ill-defined, with no delineated theoretical framework. When the latter is defined, when the specific goals are articulated, then we will be able to speak of a science of nursing (Johnson, 1959b). She even went further to declare that it is imperative to develop nursing theoretical heritage as a requisite both for establishing nursing science as well as nursing practice (Johnson, 1974). To be a professional is to continue to develop knowledge. Her words and writings continue to echo in contemporary analyses of the philosophical bases of nursing science (Bluhm, 2014).

Johnson's conceptualization of nursing, then, is based on the premise that nursing makes a unique, independent contribution to health care that is distinct from its delegated dependent contributions (Johnson, 1964). All contributions delegated to nurses, and unique to patient care and cure, are significant, but, as professionals, nurses are obligated to articulate and communicate to the public their primary mission and their nursing goals, as well as their secondary mission, which is delegated from medicine. The public is aware of the latter but less aware of the former. A client, to Johnson, behaves in an integrated, systematic, patterned, ordered, and predictable way. Behavior is goal oriented, and goals are an organizing framework for all behavior. Behavior is the sum total of biologic, social, cultural, and psychological behaviors. Nurses deal with the integrated responses of clients.

One of the major contributions of Johnson (1980) is her conceptualization of a nursing client as a behavioral system, a notion that served as the basis for her grand theory of the person (Alligood, 2014). The behaviors of interest to nursing in the client are organized into seven subsystems of behavior (Box 13-1). Each one of the subsystems is analogous to the anatomy of a biologic subsystem. It has similar components, a structure, and a function. Each of these has subcomponents that distinguish the subsystem of behavior and make it identifiable (Johnson, 1990). The structural components are a drive or a goal, a set, a choice, and an action or behavior.

- First is the *drive* or the *goal* of the subsystem, which is also the reason or motivation for behaviors in the subsystem. Goals or drives are universal; however, the strength of the goal may differ and, in fact, may fluctuate in the same person from strong to weak. Goals have different meanings in different people or at different times in the same person, and goals are not observable. Another parameter on which goals may differ is their objects. For example, when observing the eating behavior of a Middle Eastern immigrant, an inference may be made that the goal of eating is to achieve appetite pleasure or to internalize an external environment (universal drive). The variety of the food and the total absorption into the act of eating (to the exclusion of external environment) may demonstrate the strength and the meaning of the eating behaviors. The object is the type of food preferred by Middle Eastern immigrants (who are Muslim), usually highly salty, high in protein, and free of pork and alcohol.

- A second structural component is the *set*, which is the ordinary, regular, normal behavior a client prefers to use to meet the goal of the subsystem. For example, pureed vegetable soup is a type of food (preferred for healing properties) normally eaten by Middle Eastern immigrants during an illness. Another example of set is a Middle Eastern immigrant's preference to have a room full of visitors during a hospitalization to meet his or her affiliative needs and to handle the stress of hospitalization. Therefore, expecting and maintaining a large group of family members at the bedside is a structural imperative acquired through previous experiences of this particular person.

- *Choices* represent another component in the structure of a subsystem. Choices represent the available repertoire of options that a person has to meet particular goals. Choices are regulated by gender, age, cultural background, and socioeconomic status, among other variables. To meet the needs of procreation without a commitment to a partner—for example,

BOX 13-1	THE SUBSYSTEMS OF BEHAVIOR—JOHNSON[1]

Achievement Subsystem

The function is mastery or control either of some parts of environment or of self in such areas as physical, creative, mechanical, social, and intellectual skills. These are measured against some acceptable yardsticks.

Affiliative Subsystem

Inclusion into relations, intimacy, relating, bonding with the ultimate function of survival.

Aggressive Subsystem

Modes used to protect and preserve oneself from dangers, whether real or imaginary.

Dependence Subsystem

Used interchangeably with attachment; the ultimate function being approval, attention, or recognition and physical assistance through assistance from a repertoire of others.

Eliminative Subsystem

Difficult to differentiate from the biologic elimination system. It incorporates modes of behavior in the excretion of wastes, addresses when, how, why, and under what conditions a person externalizes what is internal and what needs to be expelled.

Ingestive Subsystem

Similar to digestive biologic system but incorporates when, why, how, and under what normative conditions the internalizing of external environment takes place. Its function is "appetitive satisfaction."

Sexual Subsystem

Recognizes strong similarity to biologic system but considers all other behaviors that are related to subsystem (e.g., gender–role identity, courting, mating). The function is procreation and gratification.

[1]Based on Grubbs, J. (1980). An interpretation of the Johnson behavioral system model. In J. P. Riehl and C. Roy (Eds.), *Conceptual models for nursing practice* (2nd ed., pp. 217–254). New York: Appleton-Century-Crofts; and based on Johnson, D. E. (1980). The behavioral system model for nursing. In J. P. Riehl and C. Roy (Eds.), *Conceptual models for nursing practice* (2nd ed., pp. 207–216). New York: Appleton-Century-Crofts.

through artificial insemination—is an option within the repertoire of some women and not of others, based on their perceptions of their own choices. Choices are not readily observed, but they could be inferred.

- Finally, the goal, set, and choice are complemented by directly *observing* the *behavior* of the client or his or her actions. The behaviors that bring about desired goals, and whether or not the normal patterns of behavior are appropriate under the circumstances of the health or illness situation, are examples of observations and analyses that may be useful. Behaviors are also compared and contrasted with available options for the individual.

In addition to having structural components, each of the subsystems also has a *function* that is analogous to the physiology of biologic systems. The goals of the subsystem, which are part of the structure, are not entirely distinct from its function. The functional requirements of the subsystems, and indeed the client system, continue to grow, develop, and remain viable. Therefore, Johnson questioned

what assistance subsystems may need to be able to survive, and her answer was "certain functional requirements" (1980, p. 212) that can be met by the individual or by others when the individual cannot meet such requirements. These functional requirements are:

1. Protection from unwanted, disturbing stimuli
2. Nurturance through giving input from environment (food, friendship, caring)
3. Stimulation by experiences, events, and behavior that would "enhance growth and prevent stagnation" (Johnson, 1980, p. 212)

Johnson also spoke of the relationship between the human being and the environment. This relationship was not as well explicated in her theory, although its importance is strongly inferred; she referred to environments as internal or external. Subsystems continue to maintain themselves as long as both the internal and external environments are orderly, organized, and predictable, and as long as each of the goals is met. When a disturbance occurs in structure, in function, or even in the functional requirements (even though the structure and function may not have

TABLE 13-1	Definition of Domain Concepts—Johnson
Nursing	An external regulatory force that acts to preserve the organization and integration of the patient's behavior at an optimal level under those conditions in which the behavior constitutes a threat to physical or social health or in which illness is found (Johnson, 1980, p. 214).
Goal of nursing	Restore, maintain or attain behavioral integrity, system stability, adjustment and adaptation, efficient and effective functioning of system (Johnson, 1980, p. 214).
Health	Efficient and effective functioning of system; behavioral system balance and stability.
Environment	Identified internal and external environments, but provided no specific definition.
Human being	A biopsychosocial being who is a behavioral system with seven subsystems of behavior.
Nursing client	A biopsychosocial being as a behavioral system threatened by loss of order, predictability, or stability due to illness or potential illness. "All patterned, repetitive, purposeful ways of behaving that characterize each man's life are considered to comprise his behavioral system" (Johnson, 1980, p. 209).
Nursing problem	Instability in the system or one of the subsystems due to functional or structural stress: (1) inadequate drive satisfaction; (2) inadequate fulfillment of the functional requirements; (3) changes in environmental conditions (Grubbs, 1980, p. 224).
Nursing process	Not addressed.
Nurse–patient relations	Not addressed.
Nursing therapeutics	Regulate and control: (1) providing protection, nurturance, or stimulation to subsystems; (2) by external mechanisms restricting, defending, inhibiting, or facilitating (Johnson, 1961, 1980).
Focus	Responses of person to stress, the reduction of stress, and the support of natural defenses and adaptive processes (Johnson, 1961, p. 66).

been affected), nursing care is indicated. Nursing has the goal of maintaining, restoring, or attaining a balance or stability in the behavioral subsystem or the system as a whole. Nursing acts as an "external regulatory force" to modify or change the structure or to provide ways in which subsystems fulfill the structure's functional requirement (Johnson, 1980, p. 214; 1990). According to Holaday (2015), who not only worked closely with Dorothy Johnson but also continued to use her theory in research and pediatric nursing, Johnson's theory is based on five core principles: wholeness and order, stabilization, reorganization, hierarchic interaction, and dialectic contradiction. Each of these core principles form the bases for each behavioral subsystem, for the interaction between the subsystems, as well as the bases for the interaction of the subsystem with the environment. The environment must provide protection, nurturance, and stimulation to each of the subsystems to allow them to develop and be stable. (See definition of concepts in Table 13-1).

Johnson based her theory on a number of explicit and implicit assumptions (Box 13-2). The theory specifies that the behavior of the person who is ill is the object of nursing care and not the disease. Therefore, nursing's specific contribution to patient welfare is fostering efficient and effective behavioral

functioning in the patient during and following illness (Johnson, 1980, p. 207). Later, Johnson added prevention as a nursing situation requiring nursing actions, although this goal was not included in her early writings (1990, 1992).

Nursing makes its major contributions through the identification of a behavioral subsystem or subsystems that are threatened or could potentially be threatened by illness or hospitalization. In Johnson's theory, the source of difficulty is clearly within the subsystem or within the functional requirements, whether or not manifested in structure, function, or functional requirements. Johnson's assumptions are explicit and clear (Johnson, 1990). The theory provides useful definitions for person, health, nursing problem, and nursing therapeutics, and no definitions for nursing process, interactions, or environment. Definitions are highly abstract; however, extensions offered by Auger (1976) and Holaday (1980, 2015) provide clear operationalization of definitions of person and of nursing therapeutics. One of the potential problem areas in clarity is the use of some concepts with different meanings, one set is more acceptable (as defined by medical science) and less esoteric than another (as defined from subsystems of behavior perspective). Ingestion and elimination definitions are more mainstream. Both, when considered from

BOX 13-2 | ASSUMPTIONS—JOHNSON

Explicit Assumptions[2]
- Behavior is the sum total of physical, biologic, and social factors/behaviors.
- "The behavior of an individual evident at any given point in time is the product of the net aggregate of consequences of these factors over time and at that point in time."
- "When these regularities and constancies are disturbed, the integrity of the person is threatened and the functions served by such order are less than adequately fulfilled."
- A person is a system of behavior characterized by repetitive, regular, predictable, and goal-directed behaviors that always strive toward balance.
- There are different levels of balance and stabilization. Levels are different at different time periods.
- Balance is essential for effective and efficient functions of the individual (a minimum of energy expenditure, maximum satisfaction, and survival).
- Balance is developed and maintained within the subsystem or the system as a whole to maintain adaptation and environment.
- Changes in structure or function of a behavioral subsystem are related to dissatisfied drive, lack of functional requirements, or changes in environmental conditions.

Implicit Assumptions
- A person could be reduced to small components to be studied.
- A person as a system is the sum total of its parts (i.e., subsystems).
- All behaviors can be observed through sensory data.

[2]This section is based on D. Johnson's class notes from the University of California, Los Angeles, 1970 and (Johnson, 1968a).

a biologic standpoint as compared to behavioral subsystems, denote different meanings (Box 13-3 and Table 13-1).

The goals of nursing are to maintain or restore a behavioral system's balance and stability. These goals are observed in those behaviors of human beings that are orderly, purposeful, systematic, and are effective in meeting the structural and functional needs of each subsystem. These behaviors, if effective, will allow human beings to benefit from their nurses' caring. Hence, the subsystems could be self-maintaining. Illness causes behavioral system imbalance and instability. The consequences of nursing care are adjustment, balance, and stability. An unintended consequence that was not discussed by Johnson is unwarranted dependence on others for meeting the needs of the subsystems. The theory does not address the potential consequences of such dependence.

Johnson did not clearly identify theoretical propositions in her published work, but she discussed the implications of her theory for nursing research in a number of theory and research conferences. Her position has been that appropriate, cumulative research in nursing is only possible when we agree on the mission and goals of nursing (Johnson, 1974). Propositions in Johnson's theory are existence

BOX 13-3 | CONCEPTS—JOHNSON

Behavior
Subsystems of behavior
  Achievement
  Affiliative/Attachment
  Aggressive
  Dependency
  Eliminative
  Ingestive
  Sexual
Structural components
  Action
  Choice
  Function
  Goal
  Set
Functional requirements
  Attain
  External regulation
  Instability
  Internal regulation
  Maintain
  Nurturance
  Protection
  Restore
  Stability
  Stimulation

BOX 13-4	POTENTIAL PROPOSITIONS—JOHNSON

Person

1. Behavior is orderly, systematic, and organized around seven subsystems of behavior. Each subsystem of behavior is identifiable by structure, goal, set, choice, behavior by function, and by a number of functional requirements.
2. Internal regulatory mechanisms affect the structure, function, and functional requirements in the subsystem of behavior of the entire system.
3. Behavioral subsystem disorders are manifested in disturbances in structure, function, or functional requirements in each subsystem. Behavioral subsystem disorders are differentiated into insufficiency in one of the subsystems, dominance in one or more of the subsystems, or incompatibility between two or more of the subsystems.

Environment

1. External regulatory mechanisms affect each subsystem of behavior, and the entire system is demonstrated by structure function and the subsystem functional requirements.

Health

1. Health, a behavioral system balance or stability, is manifested in the effective and efficient attainment of the goals and functions of each subsystem of behavior as judged by the nurse and mediated by the right of the patient.
2. Balance could be determined through manifestations of general harmony with and between the behavioral systems.

Nursing Process

1. Johnson's theory does not yield any theoretical propositions related to the nursing process. Assessing and diagnosing, using Johnson's theory, brings about efficient and effective nursing care.

Interactions

1. Johnson's theory does not yield any theoretical propositions related to the nursing process except when we consider subsystem interactions.

Nursing Therapeutics

1. Nursing is an external force that functions through control or modification of external regulatory mechanisms for the purpose of achieving balance and stability as demonstrated by efficient and effective functioning.
2. Nursing therapeutics are differentiated into nurturance, stimulation, and maintenance.
3. Nursing therapeutics deal with insufficiency, dominance, and incompatibility.

propositions. Existence propositions (Zetterberg, 1963) in this case lead to factor-isolating theories (Dickoff, James, and Wiedenbach, 1968) (Box 13-4).

Theory Analysis

The Theorist

The late Dorothy Johnson, a pediatric nurse by training, received an Associate of Arts degree from Armstrong Junior College in Savannah, Georgia, a Bachelor of Science degree from Vanderbilt University School of Nursing in Nashville, Tennessee, in 1942, and a Master of Public Health degree from Harvard University in 1948. She started her career at the Vanderbilt University School of Nursing in

Nashville, and spent the balance of her nursing career (until she retired in 1978) as a professor of pediatrics at the University of California, Los Angeles (UCLA), where she influenced the lives and theoretical identities of many faculty members, administrators, and students (and where I had the privilege to work with her). Her interest in sociology and psychology influenced the development of her theory. She also had a strong influence on the theoretical and clinical work of many of her mentees.

Johnson worked with students in the master's program. Although some wrote master's theses and many went on for further education, the focus of the program, for which she was primarily responsible, was on preparing clinical specialists in pediatrics. Perhaps that may explain the paucity of research related to her theory, as well as her strong influence on the theoretical and clinical work of many of her mentees. Dorothy Johnson was one of the pioneers in developing and teaching nursing theory. She died on February 4, 1999 in Florida.

Paradigmatic Origins

Johnson stated that her theory is a product of philosophical ideas; sound theory and research; her clinical experiences; and many years of thinking, discussing, and writing (Johnson, 1978). Her theory had several sources. First and foremost, her conception of a person as a system of behavior is analogous to the concept of a person as a biologic system, differentiated into a set of biologic systems, such as cardiovascular, skeletal, endocrine, digestive, and so on. Just as each biologic subsystem is differentiated by a structure, as demonstrated in anatomic dissection, a behavioral system has a structure when abstractly dissected. A structure has several components: a goal, a set, a choice, and behavior. Biologic subsystems have functions and so do behavioral subsystems. Physiology speaks to biologic subsystem functions. Both sets of subsystems have functional requirements.

Johnson's assumptions are congruent with general systems theory assumptions, and concepts consistently evolve from Johnson's systems assumptions. For example, functioning of systems; interdependency of subsystems; balance in subsystems; and regularity and constancy of behaviors, energy, boundaries, and disequilibrium are concepts defined by von Bertalanffy (1968). Some concepts were used by Johnson with consistent meaning. Johnson considered wholeness, organization, interaction, and integration of a human being as subsystems, all of which are derived from systems theory. The impact of her writings on nursing science in general and on theory in particular underwent a revival in the 1980s. More writing in theory in the 1980s and 1990s demonstrated the profound impact of her 1950s renaissance theory ideas.

Johnson's theory is also based on a systems paradigm, as perceived from a sociologic perspective. One sees the influence of Talcott Parsons (1951) on her writing in more than one way, but especially in her attempt to conceptualize all nursing as dealing with a person as a system of behavior. Parsons attempted to conceptualize one theory to encompass all sociology. He perceived the science for Social System Analysis, with the social system representing society, as the focus of sociologic explorations.

Components of the structure of a social system—goal, set, choice, and behavior—are the same in Johnson's as in Parsons' theory.

Johnson relied on practice to provide the impetus for her theory, on sociology to provide a paradigm for her writing (Buckley, 1968; Chin, 1961; Johnson, 1992; Parsons, 1951), and on psychology (Rapaport, 1968; Sears, Maccoby, and Levin, 1957) to support the validity of the derived concepts, such as Ainsworth's (1972) on affiliation and Feshback's (1970) on aggression. She acknowledges the profound influence of Nightingale on her thinking about nursing and on the development of her theory (Johnson, 1992).

Internal Dimensions

Johnson's theory embodies an analytical model of what a nursing client is and the problems a client manifests when she or he experiences an illness. It is a theory developed to answer the questions: What is nursing? How different is nursing from medicine? When does a person become a nursing client? The answers are presented by explicating the person as a behavioral system model, and the problems are situated in the structural or functional components of each behavioral system and between systems. This model is based on a field system of relations focusing on the ill or potentially ill person, the relationships within and between the subsystems of behavior, and between the person and the environment system. The theory revolves around the human being as a behavioral system.

Johnson's theory has a constructive beginning that is a hypothetical conceptualization of a human being from a nursing perspective. It is based on a parallel conceptualization of a human being as a set of biologic subsystems. It is also analogous to the conceptualization of Parson's (1951) social system in terms of a structure, function, goals, set, choices, action, functional imperatives, and the goal of stability for the subsystems. Therefore, Johnson's is a deductive, hypothetical theory. However, Johnson grounds her theory in the care of children, and one can see her pediatric nursing expertise in the development of this theory.

Although Johnson's goal was that her ideas would describe and explain all behaviors and actions that are within the domain of nursing (therefore making it a macrotheory of nursing), her theory is useful microtheory in describing and assessing the effect of the illness experience and its consequences on human beings. It is a middle-range theory addressing normal and abnormal patterns of behavior in the nursing client. It provides guidelines for understanding an individual patient's experience but not that patient's relationship with the environment, as well as the prevention of the patient's illness or the nursing therapeutic needed. Johnson's theory has a broad scope as it describes and explains a wide range of problems related to the assessment of clients (all drives, needs, and regulators affecting behavior).

It is interesting to note that, whereas Johnson advocates that nursing should develop knowledge of control (1968a), the phenomena that she addresses and develops are related to knowledge of order in human beings and are related somewhat to the beginnings of knowledge of disorder, hence the classification of middle-range and broad scope.

Three extension theories are credited to Johnson's subsystems of behaviors. The first, according to Alligood (2014), is the theory of person as a behavioral system. The second theory is the theory of a restorative subsystem with the goal of achieving a state of equilibrium by redistributing energy between and among all subsystems of behavior (Alligood, 2014; Grubbs, 1980). The third is the theory of sustainable imperatives. Holaday (Holaday, 2002; Holaday and Turner-Henson, 1987) explicated this part of Johnson's theory through her own work with children who are chronically ill. Johnson considers restoration as a goal rather than a separate subsystem of behavior (Johnson, 1990).

Theory Critique

Johnson's theory provides nursing with a sufficiently broad scope to include a number of diverse areas of nursing. However, the theory is limited to nursing's concern for the ill, hospitalized person, and is less congruent with nursing's orientation toward health (e.g., Johnson, 1987).

Johnson offers the nursing practice a concept, broad in scope, of a person as a system of behavior. This concept helps in organizing the assessment of normal patterns of behavior and deviations from the normal workings of internal and external environmental mechanisms. These deviations may influence any one of the subsystems of behavior, which subsequently will affect other subsystems in meeting their goals. Although the theory includes concepts of nursing problems and nursing therapeutics, these concepts are highly abstract in Johnson's work. The extensions offered by Auger (1976), with the addition of the restorative subsystem, and somewhat by Grubbs (1980), of further extending

this new subsystem, help to provide a point of entry for nursing therapeutics. Despite Dorothy Johnson's close working relationship with Jeanine Auger, Judy Grubbs, and Bonnie Holaday, Johnson did not support the changes and extensions they proposed and developed. She reiterated in the 1990s that her conceptualization of human beings includes the original seven subsystems of behavior (Johnson, 1990). Johnson's theory clearly articulates a mission of nursing and differentiates it from medicine. Knowledge of order (normal patterns of behavior) and knowledge of disorder (abnormal patterns of behavior) are synthesized from social, behavioral, and natural sciences, making the patient the focus of care, rather than focusing on the disease, surgery, or malfunctioning of biologic systems. The theory provides, in abstraction, broad guidelines to knowledge of control—that is, to nursing therapeutics; the theory's complexity, however, stems from its high abstraction level.

The nursing process used by many educational and nursing service institutions was not addressed in Johnson's theory because Johnson focused on a theory of human behavior responses to the stress of illness. Grubbs (1980) demonstrated how Johnson's client assessment theory could be used in conjunction with the nursing process. Holaday (1987, 2002, 2014) provided a way to use the theory to assess a person and environment, and to plan and evaluate interventions. She built on Randell (1991), who helped in expanding the definition of environment.

Hence, their extensions added to the assessment component, which focused only on the human being. Auger and Dee (1983) used the theory as a guideline to develop a patient classification system. The system provided nursing and hospital administration with the capability to establish levels of staffing based on patients' needs. Clinicians used Johnson's theory as a basis for the development of a classification system that was helpful in providing purposeful care to patients in psychiatric units (Dee and Auger, 1983). The classification system they developed could be used effectively in other settings as well (Dee, 1986, 1990).

Several other analyses documented the theory's utility in practice (Derdiarian, 1993a, 1993b). Small (1980) used the theory to interpret her research and as a framework for caring for visually impaired children. The authors found it helpful in providing a framework for diagnosis, selecting interventions, and evaluating outcomes. Rawls (1980) described and evaluated the theory's utility in caring for patients with amputations. The theory's utility for nursing therapeutics, however, is yet to be realized, fully developed, and adequately used (Reynolds and Cormack, 1991).

Because the assessment of individual patterns of behaviors requires contiguous time in which to get to know the patient, Johnson's theory is better suited for long-term care, and the complexity of the model requires a professional nurse with sound grounding in a number of sciences. It provides an effective guide for assessment and a frame for the diagnosis and intervention of individuals, but lacks a framework for the assessment of families or communities (Lobo, 2002). However, patterns of behavior that reflect disorder and that require a nurse's care are yet to be systematically identified, defined, and developed.

Johnson has profoundly influenced theoretical thinking since 1959, but sparse publication of her theory has limited the radius of her ideas. Johnson always maintained that nursing curricula should be guided by a well-evaluated conceptualization framework of nursing (Johnson, 1989). Within that belief system, several curricula emanated from her theory. Most of the application work was done at the institution where Johnson taught—UCLA (implementation began in about 1964). However, the mobility of her colleagues and students has helped in implementing her theory in educational programs at the University of Colorado (Hadley, 1970), the University of Hawaii (Marjorie Dunlop), and Vanderbilt University. The theory was used as a framework for nursing practice at the UCLA Neuropsychiatric Institute (Dee, 1990; Dee and Poster, 1995; Dee and van Servellen, 1998) and for testing care provided to adolescents in inpatient psychiatric hospitals (Poster and Beliz, 1988, 1992).

The use of Johnson's theory in the United States was based on an operationalization of the theory into the UCLA curriculum and on the fact that Wu (1973) and Auger (1976) developed and published their books, in which they extended Johnson's ideas. The combination of these two books provided the beginning student with knowledge of order that replaced the old fundamentals of nursing. Those fundamentals were based on the medical model and were taught to beginning students. No published material is available to describe the painstaking efforts of the UCLA School of Nursing faculty in translating Johnson's ideas into a curriculum—a curriculum that was later emulated with refinements in Hawaii and Colorado. In the 1980s, Harris (1986) chronicled the utilization of Johnson's theory as a framework for the curriculum at UCLA.

External Components of Theory

Johnson diligently identified the assumptions, defined some of nursing's central domain concepts (person and health), and provided guidelines for their utilization in conjunction with the nursing process. The assumptions and conceptualizations are congruent with current professional values regarding the uniqueness of nursing, its separateness, and its interdependence. In addition, the view of stability is becoming accepted as a worldview for nursing. However, the theory's focus on the individual and disorder is incongruent with nursing's claim to health maintenance and promotion and to nursing's interest in aggregates, as seen in community health.

Johnson was one of the first nursing scholars to identify the significance of congruence between nursing goals and societal expectations (Johnson, 1974, p. 376). She continued over the years to emphasize that the client and the public are the ultimate judges of the nursing mission, which is to preserve the integrity of a patient's behavior particularly as the patient's physical or social health is threatened (Johnson, 1990). The theory grew from her conviction that improvement in care is the ultimate goal. The studies done by Grubbs (1980), Holaday (1981), and Small (1980) assume such congruence and speak to patients' satisfaction with care. However, as with all other theories, such congruence between public expectations and nurses' stated goals needs to be explored. Perhaps the public's interest in health and health care commensurate to its cost is in the best interest of nurses and will augment nurses' views of their mission with the public's view of nursing's goals. Until then, it is safe to assume that a theorist who spoke vehemently for improved patient care and for the significance of the public view in shaping the nursing mission has translated those views into her theory.

Theory Testing

Johnson, in presenting her theory, invariably spoke of the significance of theory in guiding research (1968b, 1990, 1996). She admonished that research using her theory should focus on identifying and explaining "the behavioral system disorders which arise in connection with illness, and . . . develop the rationale for and means of management" (Johnson, 1968b, p. 6). Other components of her theory that have or are yet to be the focus of research are the determinants of those behaviors or actions that are part of the structure, and the function of behavioral subsystems.

Damus (1980) explored the validity of theory in practice and collected observations related to behavioral system disorder in patients with post-transfusion hepatitis. Her study demonstrated a positive relationship between behavioral and physiologic disequilibrium, and a relationship between nursing diagnosis and nursing intervention. More important, this study lent support to the idea that, indeed, the "source of subsystem disorders can be identified and predicted" and also lent unequivocal support to the theory's usefulness in nursing practice (Damus, 1980, p. 287).

Holaday's study of achievement utilizing a study population of well and chronically ill children (1974, 1981), as well as Holaday and Turner-Henson's (1987) and Holaday, Turner-Henson, and Swan's (1996) studies of chronically ill children and family use of physical and nonphysical activities out of the school system, were designed to explicate the achievement subsystem and lend validity to the notion of integral patterns of behaviors. Alligood (2014) provided a label for a theory based on these results; the label she used is "a theory of sustenal imperative." In addition, Porter's (1972) work on stimulation of premature infants lends similar validity to notions of the subsystem, its utility, and isolation in patient care. Holaday completed two research studies related to the affiliative subsystem of behavior (1981, 1982) and the achievement subsystem (1974). In the first, the cry of the chronically ill infant received a different pattern of maternal response than the cry of the well infant. The set–goal components of the subsystems provided the interpretation for the mother's responses to the cry. Derdiarian (1990a) provided further support to the theory's utility as a framework for enhancing nurses' satisfaction. She also supported Johnson's assumptions about the interrelationships between subsystems of behavior (Derdiarian, 1990b). The theory was also used as a framework to explain the attitudes of nurse administrators toward nurses who are impaired by alcohol and drug use (Lachicotte and Alexander, 1990). In addition, the theory was used as a framework for a study about pain management in adult patients with cancer and bone metastasis (Coward and Wilkie, 2000; Wilkie, 1990). The focus of this study was the aggressive system of behavior and the role of pain in protecting patients from overdoing and enticing them to seek treatment. Johnson's theory was the first to point out the importance of organizing the observations of patients' actions and behaviors into patterns of behavioral systems. Colling, Owen, McCreedy,

et al. (2003) studied the impact of the Pattern Urge–Response Toileting (PURT) of frail elderly living in a community dwelling. The results demonstrated that PURT is useful in providing better intervention to the incontinent elderly. More importantly, their interpretations of the results indicate that, by restoring the goals of the eliminative subsystem, the goals of other subsystems could also be restored, hence achieving an outcome of balance in the total system of the human being. The consistent use of Johnson's theory in a psychiatric hospital allowed researchers to identify and evaluate the outcomes of patient care driven by a nursing perspective (Poster, Dee, and Randell, 1997). Johnson's theory was used as a framework to understand dating behaviors from a development perspective (Draucker, Martsolf, and Stephenson, 2012).

Five research tools were developed to measure perceived quality of nursing care and perceived behavioral changes of cancer patients, based on Johnson's theory. The first patient indicators of nursing care were developed to record "incidences of readily observable physiological complications acquired by institutionalized patients" and to measure quality of care (Majesky, Brester, and Nishio, 1978, p. 365). They were based on Johnson's assumption that the occurrence of a complication is a manifestation of a person's "ability to cope with stresses on the behavioral systems" (p. 365). Therefore, to monitor behavioral changes, a nurse can derive the status of a person on a health–illness continuum. The 105 items of potential complications representing infection, immobility, and fluid imbalance were subjected to validity screening and reliability testing.

The second research tool, the Derdiarian behavioral system model, resulted in 193 items categorized to represent each subsystem of the behavior, which are useful for identifying perceived changes due to cancer (Derdiarian, 1983, 1984; Derdiarian and Forsythe, 1983). Derdiarian (1990a, 1991) demonstrated that the use of theory-driven assessment tools enhances the satisfaction of nurses and patients and the quality of care. These attempts are useful beginnings for factor isolating, categorizing, and providing empirical descriptions of some central concepts in the theory.

The third research tool was a projective test developed by Lovejoy (1983, 1985) to assess family functioning as perceived by children with leukemia. The fourth instrument was developed and validated by Dee (1986) as a classification instrument for psychiatric patients. The fifth was developed by

Bruce, Hinds, Hudak, et al. (1980) to measure the quality of outcomes for patients with renal disease. Each of these tools has the potential for further support of the theory and its utility.

These tools demonstrate the theory's usefulness in the assessment of nursing problems. One of the requirements for subsystem survival is the provision of stimulation. To identify the needs of premature infants, Porter (1972) explored the relationship of sensory stimulation and growth and development of premature infants. Subsequently, others have provided evidence that marked growth and development occurred when premature infants were stroked frequently and when infants were handled frequently.

Attributions of success to internal and external variables differentiated between chronically ill and healthy children. The chronically ill children tended to attribute success and failure to outside variables, and normal children tended to attribute the same to internal variables. Holaday (1974) interpreted the results to indicate disequilibrium in the achievement subsystem. Both studies lend more empirical clarity to two of Johnson's subsystems. She built further on her previous studies by considering chronically ill children's use of out-of-school time (Holaday and Turner-Henson, 1987; Holaday et al., 1996). The dependency subsystem also received some investigative attention (Stamler and Palmer, 1971). These studies support the presence of subsystems conceptually and their relationship to other subsystems.

Other studies are based on psychiatric patients (Dee, 1986), in which those indicators in patient care central to nursing were described (Majesky et al., 1978). The potential in these studies is tremendous because the researchers are attempting to delineate patient care outcomes based on nursing interventions.

Johnson's theory was used as a framework for comparing maternal–fetal and maternal–infant attachments (dependence subsystem of behavior) in naturally impregnated women to attachments in infertility-treated women (Chen, Chen, Sung, et al., 2011). The study, which demonstrated that infertility-treated women tend to have higher fetal and infant attachment, suggests changes that could improve nursing care for the prenatal and postnatal client. Kaya (2012), by assessing achievement styles (achievement subsystem of behavior) of patients discharged from intensive care, concluded that a correlation exists between achievement style and intensive care experience; thus each individual's achievement style should be taken into account in planning and implementing nursing care. By focusing on four subsystems—attachment, dependency, achievement, and sexual—Oyedele, Wright, and Maja (2013) discovered that nurses could systematically assess the health of pregnant teenagers and plan counseling that is congruent with the drive underpinning their behavior as well as the choices they make. Following their study of the support needed by women awaiting breast cancer surgery, Dickerson, Alqaissi, Underhill, et al. (2011) concluded that their findings lent credence to Johnson's theory's focus on the patient as a subsystem of behavior in constant interaction with the environment, which helped focus the support on meeting each of the subsystem needs.

Outcomes of behavioral system stability are still complex and highly abstract. Factor-isolating studies and exemplars are needed to delineate different states of stability. The theory's clarity is demonstrated in its view of the person, and its lack of clarity is viewed in outcomes. Nursing service administrations have used the theory to develop nursing assessment forms for history, nursing admission, and discharge. The questions in the forms evolve from a behavior system framework that characterizes this theory (Dee, 1986; Dee and Auger, 1983).

Theories can be used as a framework for interpretation. A good example of this use is provided in the research of Holaday (1981, 1982, 1987), described previously. Holaday found that maternal responses to ill infants were characterized by quick response time and immediacy, mothers were in the close vicinity of infants at all times, and the mother's interventions were multiple rather than singular. In other words, mothers tended to pick up the ill infant, and rock, pat, and give a pacifier, as compared with just picking up the well infant. Mothers of the ill infants did not discriminate between different types of cries as well as did mothers of the well infants (e.g., cries due to pain or restlessness). Holaday interpreted her results using Johnson's components of the behavioral subsystems theory, that is, set–goal, which was narrow in the case of ill children. In other words, mothers of chronically ill children responded to every cry with no discrimination. With this theory-based interpretation, nursing implications according to Holaday (1981, 1987) were for helping mothers with their set–goal of the affiliative subsystem, that is, the subsystem that focuses on relationships.

It is of note that her theory has been used internationally as a framework for research in South

Africa (Oyedele et al., 2013), in Turkey (Kaya, 2012), and in Taiwan (Chen et al., 2011), and her ideas continue to resonate with those studying philosophy (e.g., Bluhm, 2014). Johnson's theory was also used internationally as a framework to describe perceived rights for disclosure of information related to each subsystem of behavior. Two factors emerged to be significantly related to perceptions of rights for disclosure. These factors correspond to the achievement, ingestion, and elimination subsystems. The findings support these subsystems' functions of the need for mastering the environment through information and the need for incorporating information regarding patients' concerns (Naguib, 1988).

MYRA LEVINE

To the late Myra Levine, nursing action was a conservation activity, and the outcome she conceptualized is the conservation of energies, which for her equals health. Myra Levine is distinguished from other theorists by her focus on conservation principles as a framework for nurses' actions. When Levine spoke of conservation, she included the need for conservation of environments as well as endangered species (Levine, 1996).

With constant changes in the world, stability through conservation is essential. The outcome of conservation is adaptation, which leads to wholeness and which includes historicity (the information transmitted through genes and survival instincts) and specificity (parameters specific to uniqueness and well-being of an individual) to enhance the individual's fit and harmony with internal and external environments. Adaptation also includes *redundancy*—wave-like adaptive responses that include activities that spread the energy cost. Redundancy is the "frugal use of energy guaranteed by fail-safe systems" (Levine, 1996, p. 39). When I think of Myra Levine, the first images that are conjured are of an integrator who was able to assimilate nursing as a "humanitarian enterprise" (Levine, 1999) with physics, from which she utilized great conservation laws (Feynman, 1965), with physiology (living organisms) (Bernard, 1957), and adaptation (homeorhesis) (Bertalanffy, 1968; Cannon, 1939). I also think of her as a critical thinker whose skepticism prompted her to write a scathing critique of nursing theory entitled "The Rhetoric of Nursing Theory" (Levine, 1995). Levine, like other pioneering theorists, provided an innovative, coherent view of nursing to differentiate it from medicine

(a differentiation that occupied nursing's thinkers in the 1960s) but went even further to suggest an alternative to the concept of medical diagnosis, proposing *trophicognosis* to better reflect nursing's focus on the art and science of nursing (Levine, 1966a, p. 57). Finally, Levine was the consummate supporter of liberal arts and humanities education in nursing (Levine, 1999).

Theory Description

The central questions that Levine addressed are:
- What are the ways in which nursing care is delivered?
- What are the goals of nursing actions?
- Why are nursing actions provided?

To answer these questions, Levine conceptualized the methods of nursing as conservation of patient resources, as alteration of environment to fit those resources, and as an extension of the patient's perceptual system until his own system is healed. These questions address nursing therapeutics and, to a lesser degree, a perspective on health. The central idea in her theory is well manifested and exemplified in the label she chose: *Energy Conservation: A Universal Concept* (Levine, 1990).

The impetus for Levine's conceptualization of nursing appears to be her attempt to separate the domains of medicine and nursing. Her first published work focused on proposing trophicognosis as a new label for nursing assessment and a "plan of action to substitute the concept of nursing diagnosis" (Levine, 1966a, p. 57). Her rationale for the proposal was her desire to differentiate between diagnoses that have the connotation of medical diagnosis and disease orientation. However, using the concept of diagnosis tends to highlight the overlap between medicine and nursing rather than highlight the differences. *Trophicognosis* is defined as "a nursing care judgment arrived at by the scientific method" (Levine, 1966a, p. 57). It denotes the knowledge of the art of nursing and is analogous to diagnosis and prognosis for the art of medicine. Labeling nursing assessment as a nursing diagnosis is only giving diagnosis a new label, but when trophicognosis is used, it emphasizes nursing care judgment based on the process of scientific method. Levine offered, then, a useful beginning for the use of the nursing process. Although the new label was not used in nursing, Levine's attempts in 1965 (published in 1966a) supported what other theorists had begun doing: delineating nursing's focus and differentiating between nursing and medicine. However, Levine later admonished nurses to simplify their language and not invent language that confuses other health care providers (Levine, 1989a), an admonition that contradicts her original proposal (to describe diagnosis as trophicognosis).

Levine then put her "intellectual energy" into conceptualizing a human being as an adaptive being, in constant interaction with the environment, whose behaviors are integrated in responses to internal and external environmental stimuli. Nurses are interested in integrated responses of whole patients to noxious stimuli, particularly when the individual is not able to adapt behavior to environmental demands. Nursing is expected to create an atmosphere (therefore, environment was beginning to reemerge as a central phenomenon in nursing) to encourage healing and to promote adaptation (1966b). Although this theory is classified as an outcome theory, it demonstrates a focus on nursing therapeutics, and some have used it as a framework for diagnosis and intervention (Taylor, 1989). Levine also provided a detailed description of environment. She described environmental dimensions as internal and external. Responses of human beings emanate from the internal environment. Both the internal and external environments influence each other, and the internal environment is constantly challenged to meet the external environment's demands. The two environments are joined through adaptive patterns, and when the interaction between them is harmonious, the wholeness of an individual manifests itself. Throughout the challenges and changes in the environments, the body maintains its integrity through some control mechanisms that lead to autoregulation of the internal environment (Levine, 1973).

Building on Bates' (1967) description of environment, Levine described the external environment as perceptual, operational, and conceptual. The *perceptual environment* is that component "which an individual responds to with sense organs" (Levine, 1973, p. 12). The *operational environment* includes all that affects an individual physically, such as microorganisms and pollutants. The *conceptual environment* includes symbols, values, culture, language, thinking, and personal styles, among others (Levine, 1973, 1989b). The interaction between the internal and the external environments is where a person's adaptation resides; it is where the fit between person and environment occurs (Levine, 1989b).

Levine (1973) identified nine models to guide assessment (the relationship between each major theory concept and every model is not entirely explicit):

1. Vital signs
2. Body movement and positioning
3. Ministration of personal hygiene needs
4. Pressure gradient systems in nursing intervention (fluids)
5. Nursing determinants in provision for nutritional needs
6. Pressure gradient system in nursing (gases)
7. Local application of heat and cold
8. Administration of medication
9. Establishing an aseptic environment

Assessment would include the organismic and environmental systems. The first allows for description of all physiologic and biologic adaptive integrative systems, such as response to fear (fight or flight), response to inflammation, and response to stress. The other systems of response are to the environment, which is more than one's immediate surroundings (Levine, 1969). It is the perceptual environment "depending on the ability of a person to receive sensory stimuli via his sense organs," the operational environment, including all those physical entities that do not need to be recorded by senses (radiation, microorganisms), and the conceptual environment "determined by the dependence of human beings on the symbolic exchange of language and ideas." It also includes cultural determinants (Levine, 1971a, p. 262).

The environment is not always "user-friendly." Successful engagement with the environment depends upon the individual's repertoire—that store of adaptations which is either built into the genes or achieved through life experience. While there are redundant or back-up systems that offer options when the initial response is insufficient, health and safety are products of a competent conservation process. The goal of conservation is health. (Levine, 1990, p. 193)

The "holistic nursing challenge" is to nurse whole patients at the interface of organism and environment to promote adaptation. Levine decided against "holistic" in 1969 in favor of "organismic" in describing human beings because holism was more a myth rather than based on science. She returned to holism in 1973 "because I realized it was too important to be abandoned to the mystics" (Levine, 1996, p. 39). She accepted Erik Erikson's (1968) definition of holism—which acknowledges mutuality between the parts, open and fluid boundaries—because it stood the test of time. Her utilization of adaptation as an outcome through energy conservation was also a constant in her writings. Conservation of energy is important to the disease process, and begins with regulation of metabolism in response to noxious forces that have instigated the disease process. It does not only mean limitation of activity, it also means "proper disbursement of energy expense, allowing for activity within the range of the individual's capability, safety, and comfort" (Levine, 1971a, p. 259). Conservation of structural integrity is accomplished through tasks that support the physiologic and anatomic positioning. Conservation of integrity is related to environmental processes. It includes conservation of personal integrity through preservation of sense of worth and integrity and conservation of social integrity through the recognition of cultural, ethnic, religious, and family relationships (Levine, 1967).

Levine defines health through the definitions of integrity and wholeness. She defines *integrity* as:

. . . having the freedom to choose; to move without constraint, as slowly or as swiftly as desired, and to exercise decisions in all matters—trivial and otherwise—without apology, indebtedness, or guilt. Integrity is the experience of life, the sensations of the body and its limbs, the sensory recording of every place and time on the mind and in the spirit. (Levine, 1990, p. 93)

Maintenance of system integrity depends on perceptual systems (basic orienting, visual, auditory, hepatic, and taste and smell). When perceptual systems are deficient, the organismic responses are altered, and the nurse uses her perceptual system in an attempt to maintain wholeness in the individual. This is how healing can proceed (Levine, 1969). Health is also a pattern of adaptive changes (Levine, 1973), with many degrees of adaptation. Health is personally defined, thereby reflecting one's life experiences (Levine, 1991). Even disease, to Levine, is a pattern of adaptive change because there is neither good nor bad adaptation nor maladaptation (Levine, 1996). Organismic responses, which are the physiologic and behavioral responses to environment, influence each other and coexist in individuals. They have four dimensions. The first is the fight-or-flight response, which is the most primitive organismic response (Levine, 1973). The second is the inflammatory immune response, which is essential for maintaining structural continuity and for promoting healing (Levine, 1989b). The third

response level is that of stress, which is cumulative over time (Levine, 1989b). And the fourth level of organismic response she calls "perceptual awareness," which is the mechanism of collecting and integrating environmental information and then converting it into meaningful experiences (Levine, 1969). Perceptual awareness encompasses five subdivisions: the basic orienting system (inner ear, which responds to balance, change in gravity, acceleration, and movement), the visual systems (for looking), the auditory systems (for listening to sounds), the hepatic system (for touch), and the taste/smell system (for information and facilitation of chemical and nutritional stimuli and needs) (Levine, 1969).

Levine's conceptualization is based on numerous implicit and explicit assumptions that were dispersed throughout her writings between 1966 and 1989. They are presented in Box 13-5. Basic to her theory are her beliefs in the wholeness of patients (Levine, 1989c, p. 126). Patients are partners in the care process, and nurses should work to develop a trusting dialogue. It is interesting to note that Levine used the term "patients" instead of "clients" because "clients" comes from a Latin root that means a follower; however, "client" does not exactly mean a follower. The derivation of client is from Latin *clinare*, to bend or incline, and *cliens*, one who has someone to lean on, which comes from Greek *klinein*, to lean, which has its roots in Sanskrit *srayate*, he leans on (*Webster's Third New International Dictionary*, 1986).

All major concepts are derived from other paradigms, except for the concepts of trophicognosis and conservation, which are primitive to this theory (Box 13-6). Both are theoretically defined; the first was also operationally defined, but because of its esoteric nature, nurses preferred "nursing diagnosis" over trophicognosis. The derived concepts are not operationally defined and have unclear boundaries. Concepts such as wholeness, social well-being, integrity, and adaptation are used interchangeably and are not well differentiated (Table 13-2).

Levine's theory offers existence propositions that are based on conceptualizing the assessment of levels of responses, internal and external environments, and focus of nursing as conservation of energy and integrity through therapy or support. It offers concepts that appear on the surface to be linked together; however, relationships between each set of these concepts are not clear (e.g., well-being and adaptation, conservation and responses). Therefore, as it stands now, this is a theory with

BOX 13-5	ASSUMPTIONS—LEVINE

Implicit Assumptions

- The nurse creates an environment in which healing could occur (Levine, 1966a).
- A human being is more than the sum of parts.
- Human beings respond in a predictable way (1966a).
- Human beings are unique in their responses (1966a).
- Human beings know and appraise objects, conditions, and situations (1973).
- Human beings sense, reflect, reason, and understand (1973).
- Human beings' actions are self-determined even when emotional (1973).
- Human beings are capable of prolonging reflection through such strategies as raising questions or redirecting attention.
- Human beings make decisions through prioritizing courses of actions.
- Human beings must be aware and able to contemplate objects, conditions, and situations to act purposively.
- Human beings are agents who act deliberately to attain goals (1973, pp. 12–13).
- Adaptive changes involve the whole individual (1967).
- Human beings are adaptive (1967).
- A human being has unity in his response to the environment. He responds in an integrated way (1966a).
- Every person possesses a unique adaptive ability based on one's life experience, which creates a unique message (1967).
- There is an order and continuity to life (1966a).
- Change is not random.
- A human being (as a whole) responds organismically in an ever-changing manner (1967).
- A theory of nursing must recognize the importance of detail of care for a single patient within an empiric framework that successfully describes the requirements of all patients (1966a).
- A human being is a social animal.
- A human being is in constant interaction with an ever-changing society.
- Change is inevitable in life (1973, p. 10).
- Nursing meets existing and emerging demands of self-care and dependent care (1985).
- Nursing is associated with conditions of regulation of exercise or development of capabilities of providing care (1973).

BOX 13-6	CONCEPTS—LEVINE

Wholeness	Environmental exchange	Auditory
Holism	Orderly synchronization = Health	Hepatic
Noxious stimuli	Desynchronization = Disease	Taste, smell
Organismic responses	Conservation	Environment
Fight or flight	Energy	Perceptual
Inflammatory responses	Integrity	Operational
Stress	Structural	Conceptual
Perceptual awareness	Personal	Perceptual systems
Homeostasis	Social	Basic orienting
Homeorhesis	Intervention	Anatomical
Adaptation	Supportive	Visual
Historicity	Therapeutic	Dynamic exchange
Specificity	Perceptual systems	Trophicognosis
Redundancy	Basic orienting	
Equilibrium	Visual	

TABLE 13-2	Definition of Domain Concepts—Levine
Nursing	Has a unique body of knowledge and is a human interaction. Its goal is to conserve energies and integrities through changes in the environment.
Goal of nursing	Restoration of individual's wholeness, integrity, well-being, and independent activity.
	Conservation of energy, social, personal, and structural (Levine, 1967).
	When necessary, maintenance of appropriate balance between patient abilities, involvement in the care, and nurses' actions.
	Maintenance and individuality.
Health	"Health and illness are patterns of adaptive change" (1966b, p. 2452).
	Is equated with successful adaptation; in fact, one criterion of successful adaptation is the attainment of social well-being (1966b, p. 2452).
	Health as integrity means being in control of one's life and having the freedom to choose (Levine, 1990).
Environment	Is both internal and external. It is a setting, a background, and the dynamic exchange that involves both the individual organism and the setting and background. Environment is perceptual, operational, and conceptual. Perceptual environment is based on a person's sense organs' interpretation. Operational environment includes the things that affect an individual physically, such as virus, and the conceptual environment evolves out of an individual's cultural patterns, values, and spirituality and is mediated by symbols of language and thought (1969, p. 94; 1973, p. 12).
Person	An ever-changing organism who is in constant interaction with his environment and who is constantly striving to maintain his integrity. Responses of a human being are a unified whole.
Nursing client	A total, whole person, a system of systems, in a state of dys-synchronization and in need of assistance to conserve energy, structural, personal, and social integrity (1969, 1973). An ill client maintains his integrity through four levels of physiologically predetermined protective responses. These are fear, inflammatory process, stress, and perceptual awareness as mediated through sense organs.
Nursing problem	The internal or external environment as it threatens the total integrity of a whole person. Organism responses to threat coexist in a single individual: (1) Response to fear by fight or flight, an instantaneous reaction, a most primitive reaction; (2) Inflammatory response, a second-level response, a response of entire resources of an individual, a systematized energy directed as exclusion and removal of intruding irritant or pathogen; (3) Response to stress produces defensive response in the form of changes that are nonspecific in a human being. Structural changes and gradual loss of adaptation energy occurs, until exhaustion is reached; (4) Sensory response producing perceptual awareness, the information and experience in life are only meaningful when perceived in an integrated whole by the individual. All are energy exchange transmissions from individual to environment and back. The result is a physiologic or behavioral activity.
Nursing process	Assessment, diagnosis, and intervention, using steps of the scientific method, with great emphasis on observation as a central tool (1973, pp. 23–29).
Nurse–patient relations	"Depend on perceptual system of both persons" (1969, p. 97).
	The nursing process and action are for conservation.
Nursing therapeutics	The nurse acts in a therapeutic way when the intervention changes the course of adaptation toward a renewed social well-being. The nurse acts in a supportive way when the intervention maintains or fails to maintain the status quo and when there is no alteration in the course of adaptation (1966a, 1967).
	Focus is on creating an atmosphere where healing could occur; therefore, the target is the environment. It is based on appreciation of the patient's responses.
	To conserve patient's resources, alter the environment to fit the resources, and act as the patient's perceptual system when his own is impaired.
Adaptation	The process of change whereby the individual retains his integrity, his wholeness within the realities of his environment (1969, p. 95).
Focus of nursing	Organism responses that are singular but integrated, maintenance of wholeness. Nurse–patient interaction.
Consequences	Adaptation process of change within which an individual maintains his integrity and his wholeness.
Illness	Dys-synchronization with outer events.
	Loss of a portion of well-being
	Loss of wholeness; "Health and illness are patterns of adaptive response" (Levine, 1966b, p. 2452).

BOX 13-7	PROPOSITIONS—LEVINE

- Awareness of an environment-influenced behavior at all times.
- Conservation of patients' energy is a consequence of nursing intervention.
- Components of nursing interventions are conservation of individual patient's structural integrity, personal integrity, and social integrity.
- Nurses are participants in every patient's environment and influence patient's adaptation.
- "Conservation insures stability and familiarity, consistency and reliability" (Levine, 1996, p. 38).
- "The internal environment and the external environment are joined through adaptive patterns, and the individual's wholeness is a function of their harmonious interaction" (Levine, 1996, pg. 38).
- "Negative feedbacks provide the mechanisms for successful adaptation by supporting the living systems with the most economic, most energy-sparing systems" (Levine, 1996, p. 39).
- "The loss of redundant systems in adapting accounts for the process of aging. A critical loss of redundancy is not compatible with health and is often life-threatening" (Levine, 1996, p. 39).
- "The humanities promise a tempering and a gentling of the relationships between patient and nurse" (Levine, 1999, p. 217).

existence propositions and no relational ones. Levine's propositions are summarized in Box 13-7.

Although Levine described the conservation principles in what may be construed as assumptions, her principles could formulate the major propositions. She proposed that the goal and the process of nursing action is the conservation of energy, the goal of conservation is health, and health is to be whole with integrity (Levine, 1990). Such propositions are supported by assumptions emanating from other paradigms about the significance of energy and integrity for a human being.

Levine, in a personal communication (cited in Fawcett, 1989, p. 157), provided further support for the classification of her theory as a theory for nursing therapeutics. She proposed a theory that she called "therapeutic interventions," in which she described seven areas for which interventions should be developed. These are therapeutic regimens to support the healing process of the body, to substitute for failure of autoregulation, to focus on restoring the integrity and well-being of individuals, to promote comfort and human concern, to decrease the threat of disease, to create functional changes, and to correct metabolic imbalances.

Theory Analysis

The Theorist

Myra Levine was a graduate of the Cook County diploma program, and she earned a non-nursing bachelor's degree from the University of Chicago and a Master of Science in Nursing from Wayne State University in Detroit. She took postgraduate

courses at the University of Chicago (Artigue, Foli, Johnson, et al., 1994). She then retired and became a professor emeritus in the Medical–Surgical Nursing graduate program at the University of Illinois, Chicago, where she taught and collaborated in teaching the theory seminars. Her writings evolved while she was a predoctoral and postgraduate student at the University of Chicago. She had an extensive clinical (private duty nurse, staff nurse), administrative (director of nursing), and teaching background (preclinical instructor in Cook County; faculty member at Loyola University, at Rush University, and at the University of Illinois) (Esposito and Leonard, 1980). Myra Levine died on March 20, 1996, in Illinois.

Paradigmatic Origins

In introducing holism in the mid-1960s, Levine was critical of the scientific approach that advocated experimentation, deductive thinking, and analysis of experiences that only led to more mechanistic and dualistic approaches to patient care. The ultimate result was the compartmentalization of human beings. She recommended an inductive approach that evolved from experience and clinical practice and incorporated the wisdom of the person. To her, a paradox existed between holism and humanism on the one hand and dualism and scientific thought on the other. Despite these admonitions, Levine used a deductive approach to develop her theory and recommended the scientific method for collecting data about nursing care.

Levine's clinical background in medical–surgical nursing and the close association of this background with medical, biologic, and pathophysiological sciences influenced the development of her theory. The theory draws on concepts and assumptions from systems theory (Bertalanffy, 1968), adaptation theory (Cannon, 1939; Dubos, 1966; Selye, 1956), developmental theory (surprisingly, Erik Erikson [1968] was cited for the definition of wholeness, totality, and system [Levine, 1969, p. 94]), existentialism (Buber, 1967; Tillich, 1961), and nursing theorists (Abdellah and Levine, 1986; Nightingale, 1969; Rogers, 1961).

Levine also drew her ideas from several concepts that, in her view, had a major impact on nursing. These are the natural healing concept, the germ theory, theory of multiple factors, and the unified theory of health and disease. Although she promoted the scientific method for nursing in both the development of nursing science (Levine, 1966b) and in the development of nursing process (Levine, 1966a), she encouraged us to consider life processes holistically by transcending the duality of mind and body. She also warned against the apparent dissociation between environment and individual as evidenced in the nature–nurture arguments. Cause-and-effect mechanistic views are dehumanizing and antiholistic. Organism responses, purposeful life, integrative approach, and adaptation are concepts that guided her view of nursing. She advocated a return to nursing as it used to be:

Nursing has always been characterized by an intensely humanistic purpose, an expression at once of the selfless giving as opposed to selfish rewards that accompany human interaction. (Levine, 1971a, p. 263)

It is, after all, in the role of patient advocate that the nurse has historically fulfilled her responsibility to bring compassion, protection, and commitment to the bedside (Levine, 1971b, p. 43).

Internal Dimensions

Levine's is a concatenated theory developed around concepts of adaptation, conservation, responses, and environment and therefore has an appropriate set of existence propositions. It is a microtheory with limited scope, addressing conservation of energy and integrity. It evolved deductively out of hypothetical beginnings, a view of what nursing ought to be. It is a descriptive theory that attempts to describe strategies of nursing care and of the nursing client. It addresses mainly phenomena of

disorder, fight-or-flight, stress responses, inflammation responses, and perceptual awareness responses.

Levine used a problematic method approach in her theory (Barnum, 1994, p. 29). Responses of people are holistic, but are differentiated into four different problems; conservation is offered separately in four different types. Whereas a person is not reduced to components, responses are limited to four problematic responses. Nurses' actions are limited to conservation. It could be argued, therefore, that there is a certain element of reductionism in Levine's theory.

Theory Critique

Levine developed her notions in the mid-1960s, when nurses were struggling with increasing mechanization, when they were beset with fragmentation caused by specialization, and when they were trying to differentiate between different types of nursing and also between nursing and medicine. She began by differentiating between medical and nursing judgment, by offering trophicognosis to replace nursing diagnosis. She saw the process of clinical judgment—the nursing process—as a means of focusing on nursing issues in patient care. Holism and humanism, and person–environment interactions are abstract concepts attached to the nursing act and not clearly defined, but Levine was among the first to redirect our attention to them. The essence of the nursing act is conservation. It is what all human beings strive for and, when not able to adapt to noxious stimuli, the nurse becomes their conservator.

Fortunately, or unfortunately, the theory drew heavily from pathophysiology and was therefore perceived as a theory oriented to acute care of ill individuals. However, Hirschfeld (1976) discussed the cognitively impaired older adult and demonstrated how Levine's four principles of conservation could be applied to give direction to nursing interventions when impairments are present. Similarly, her theory was proposed as a structure for providing care for older adults by nurse practitioners specializing in adult gerontology (Abumaria, Hastings-Tolsma, and Sakraida, 2015). Fawcett (2014) used Levine's conservation theory to develop quality improvement criteria for therapeutic interventions for postoperative wound care, demonstrating its practice utility. While these appear to be the only published indications of the utility of Levine's theory in the practice arena, they provide support for the notion that the theory can be used clinically.

Levine's use of holism, humanism, and integrative approaches to understanding response reflects the philosophical bases of nursing; however, these approaches tend to be abstract concepts and in need of operational referents. There is inconsistency in how they are used in her writing, arising from the view of human beings through a pathophysiological approach and a reduction of responses to those that are biologically bound. The inclusion of perceptual awareness amid the focus on biologic responses to fear, stress, and inflammation almost seems an additive thought and not an integrative one. The theory's major concepts—adaptation and energy—are not well defined. Yet, in a clinical sense, nurses constantly deal with and consider the energy of the patient in their plans for any therapeutic interventions.

The theory's complexity is perhaps due to its lack of clarity and the disconnectedness of its concepts—the principles of conservation, organismic responses, and adaptation—as well as to the lack of clarity about the boundaries between the concepts (Levine, 1971a, p. 258). Conservation is a goal and an intervention process in different parts of the theory, but organismic and environmental responses overlap when Levine discusses perceptual awareness. In later work, she defined the goal of conservation as health and health as integrity (Levine, 1990). The goals of conserving energy are also adaptation (Levine, 1996). It could be argued that three responses—fear, stress, and inflammation—are simply syndromes in response to stress, as defined by Selye. Complete definitions and the development of propositions connecting responses, environment, and conservation would render this theory testable.

Other functional limitations in the theory may have deterred others from using it, and this may be the reason that a literature review reveals few writings that utilized the theory. Holistic nursing appears to be limited to integrating the social and personal aspects of care in acute care individuals who are dependent on the health care professional. The theory has limited utility without extensive interpretation to long-term care and care of families or communities. (There are two exceptions: in 1991, Cox provided a compelling example of how the theory was translated for use in long-term care; and in 2015 Abumaria, Hastings-Tolsma, and Sakraida demonstrated its potential utility for advance practice nurses in gerontology.) While the theory offers guidelines for assessment of responses and environment, and guidelines for goals of nursing therapeutics, it is limited in conceptualizing the means by which the nurse can achieve these goals. Similarly, the theory does not lend itself readily to preventive and health promotion care, but the potential for extension exists. However, the theory has been used effectively as a framework to guide community nursing services for the homeless in Philadelphia, in emergency rooms, and for patients with congestive heart failure (Pond, 1990, 1991; Pond and Taney, 1991).

Some have used the theory in curricula development for educational settings (Grindley and Paradowski, 1991; Hall, 1979; Riehl, 1980). Others have used it in administration settings as a framework for identifying outcome criteria for nursing care of patients on a neurology unit (Taylor, 1974). Taylor's account of her use also substantiates the theory's utility for the use of the nursing process in assessment and diagnosis.

The theory's circle of contagiousness is limited. Its use in research, education, and administration has suffered from the problematic approach in articulating the theory, the lack of interpretation of holistic and total human beings, the limited operationalization of integrative responses, the overlap between concepts (e.g., personal and social integrity), and, most of all, the lack of propositions. That is not to say that the potential is not there; it only means that the existing literature by Levine focuses on assumptions, concepts, and definitions. Each of the conservation principles lends itself to existence propositions and each of the nine descriptive models can generate research questions.

External Components of Theory

The theory is congruent with general professional and societal views of health and patient care. Levine espoused holistic care before holism became an accepted lexicon in both nursing and societal language. The definition of patients as total individuals has a parallel in Rogers' unitary human being (Rogers, 1970). Two other of Levine's ideas are widely accepted now in nursing thought: the focus of nursing on life processes and the significance of the environment (Donaldson and Crowley, 1978; Flaskerud and Halloran, 1980), although not directly credited to her.

To use an individual's natural resources, to conserve energy, and to preserve the integrity of the individual were, at the time of its writing, values of the future that have now become more intrinsic in our discipline. Their social significance makes the theory appealing to the general public, but the challenge remains. How do we achieve these goals of nursing care? What are the outcome criteria by which we nurses know when we have and when we have not achieved these goals? Are they or are they not cost-effective in prevention and intervention?

While nursing was attempting to devise ways to measure energy and study unitary human beings and the meaning of healing, Levine demonstrated inconsistencies in ideas and displayed impatience with the lack of scientific data used to study therapeutic touch. In response to an article by Krieger, she wrote a scathing letter to the editor, admonishing nurses to stick to science in developing nursing (Levine, 1979). In this letter she warned:

The professional implications of nurses engaging in "healing" based on the spurious notion that "excesses of energy" in the human body can be transmitted to the "ill person who can be thought of as being in less than an optimal energy state" are frightening. The science is spurious, as is the explanation that this "appears to be done physiologically by a kind of electron transfer resonance." (p. 1379)

Levine charges that this type of thinking will take nursing on to a "hocus pocus" "faith healing" path and that nursing cannot afford to indulge in this kind of "charlatanism" (p. 1380).

Levine is an advocate of theoretical formulations that are based on coherence, but calls for corroboration of truth in nursing. She offered nursing in the mid-1960s a forward view of environment, holistic nursing, the total person, potential significance of perceptual apparatus in nursing, and nursing action as conservation.

Theory Testing

One research study tested a proposition that could be viewed as an extension of Levine's theory. The proposition states that mediation of stimuli through the perceptual system of the nurse could be enhanced if the nurse and patient share the same subjective time. To explore this proposition, which is closely related to Levine's notion of hepatic perceptual system (which mediates touch, thought, muscles, joints, and skeletal system), Tompkins (1980) explored the effect of restricted mobility on the perceived duration of adverse events. She found that "decreased perceived duration . . . may be a mechanism for preserving system integrity in those

whose mobility is restricted" (p. 333). This is the only published study that has tested the relationship between system integrity and perceptual systems.

Hirschfeld (1976) applied Levine's theory to the care of cognitively impaired elderly patients and found the theory useful in determining priorities. Newport (1984) used Levine's theory as a framework for a study designed to contrast temperatures of newborns who were put in warmers with those who were placed in skin-to-skin contact with mothers. Other research could evolve from the propositions described earlier in Box 13-7.

Levine's theory supports a holistic approach to caring through conservation of energy and conservation of structural integrity; this may be accomplished when there is an intensity (of nursing care) and consistency (of nursing caregivers) that require a different model of primary nursing. Mefford and Alligood (2011) demonstrated that providing intensity and consistency could improve health outcomes, increase organizational effectiveness, and enhance satisfaction of both patients and caregivers.

Levine's theory has also been used as a framework to assess the impact of value congruence between nurses and the organizations that employ them (Bao, Vedina, Moodie, et al., 2013). The findings indicate that ethical value congruence acts as a buffer against burnout and dissatisfaction, lending support to viewing the nurse holistically as having a sense of personal and social integrity that impacts workplace attrition. The theory has also been useful in studying the effect of intimate partner violence on the integrity of women (Netto, Moura, Queiroz, et al., 2014).

The principles of conservation were used with elderly study populations, with populations suffering from decubitus ulcers, and in exploring Finnish nurses' perceptions of the extent to which elderly patients' integrity is maintained in long-term institutions (Teeri, Välimäki, Katajisto, et al., 2007). Fawcett and DeSanto-Madeya (2013) indicated that, even when research was conducted utilizing Levine's theory, it was limited almost exclusively to single studies, thereby precluding its further development. There are a few exceptions, one of which is a multisite study of the effects of exercise on fatigue in patients undergoing a series of cancer treatments (Mock, Pickett, Ropka, et al., 2001; Mock, Ropka, Rhodes, et al., 1998).

Levine's theory has also been used to describe pressure ulcers, as well as in developing different nursing therapeutics to heal the wounds that result from these ulcers (Burd, Langemo, Olson, et al., 1992; Burd, Olson, Langemo, et al., 1994). Her theory has been used to guide both investigations as well as the discussion sections of research studies that focused on understanding the relationship between fatigue as an alteration in physiologic function and expenditure of energy (Mock, St. Ours, Hall, et al., 2007; Delmore, 2006; Allvin, Berg, Idvall, et al., 2007). It has proved to be a useful framework to use in describing how illness undermines the physical, structural, and social integrity of individuals, whether due to hearing changes or intrusive procedures (Irvin, 2007), and in designing theory-based interventions such as an exercise program for patients with cancer (Mock et al., 2007).

In Levine's tradition of integrating liberal arts with nursing, the use of music therapy in the acute care setting was investigated. The recommendation of the authors is to emphasize how significant the support of educators and administrators is in facilitating the use of music therapy as a helpful tool to conserve physical and emotional energy from anxiety (Gagner-Tjellesen, Yurkovich, and Gragert, 2001). (Levine would be pleased!) The theory was used to identify a nursing diagnosis of infection risk at preoperative time (Piccoli and Galvao, 2001). The theory also lends itself well to being utilized as a framework for complementary therapies (Mantle, 2001).

It is refreshing to see attempts to identify different schools of thought that inform nursing phenomena and to simultaneously uncover similarities that could lead to more refinement of theories. Energy, a major concept in Levine's theory, is also addressed by Martha Rogers (1964, 1970), as well as by Florence Nightingale (1969). Todaro-Franceschi (2001) identified two ideas of energy in nursing: energy as part of a process and energy as a phenomenon. She concluded that Levine's energy is more mechanistic, as part of casual processes, whereas Rogers' idea of energy is as a phenomenon not necessarily observable, measurable, or quantifiable. However, for both, the common thread is that change is purposeful and depicted by transformation. Nurses can assist human beings with energy transformation/interchange, and this transformation/interchange of person and environment is purposeful.

Theories are judged by the extent to which they guide subsequent work, and although the studies presented above demonstrate the utility of Levine's theory in framing research studies and interpreting data, that utilization is limited. As a result, the theory has not been refined or extended to date. Still, the stimulation of dialogues about significant phenomena in nursing, such as the one offered by Todaro-Franceschi (2001) based on Levine's theory, is encouraging and indicative of the robustness of Levine's ideas for a future that is more person-focused.

BETTY NEUMAN

Theory Description

The client open system is the focus of Neuman's systems theory (she calls it *Neuman systems model*). This system is open to environments but maintains stability and integrity through elaborate circles of protection and defenses; the goal of nursing is to prevent instability or to bring a state of stability to individuals who need or are receiving nursing care. Questions that led Neuman to develop her conceptualization in the early 1970s arose when teaching a graduate course in community mental health consultation (Neuman, 2002a, 2011a). The central questions for this theory are: How can nurses organize the vast knowledge needed to deal with complex human situations that require nursing care? How do nursing clients interact, adjust to, and react to stress? Neuman considers her theory to be wellness-oriented, and she provides a holistically focused conceptualization of clients, as well as a holistic view of nurses (Neuman, 1989a, 1995). Neuman articulated a number of basic assumptions about client systems, environmental stressors, responses to stress, lines of resistance and defense health, energy, and wellness (Neuman, 1989a, pp. 17–22; 2002b). These explicit assumptions are described in Box 13-8. Central concepts of her theory are presented in Box 13-9.

To Neuman, nurses deal with each client as a whole. Nursing clients are people who are anticipating stress or who are dealing with stress (Neuman and Young, 1972). A client, also referred to as a client system, encompasses four dimensions: an individual or a person, a family, a community, and a social issue. Whether well or ill, a client is composed of dynamic interrelated components of five variables. These are the physiologic variables, which are related to body structure and function; psychological variables, which are related to mental processes and interactive environmental responses; sociocultural variables, which are related to the integrated influences of sociocultural conditions;

BOX 13-8	ASSUMPTIONS—NEUMAN[3]

1. Nursing clients are dynamic; they have both unique and universal characteristics and are in constant energy exchange with environments.
2. The relationship between client variables—physiological, psychological, sociocultural, developmental, and spiritual—influence a client's protective mechanisms and determine a client's response.
3. Clients present normal range of responses to the environment that represent wellness and stability.
4. Stressors attack flexible lines of defense, then normal lines of defense.
5. Nurses' actions are focused on primary, secondary, and tertiary prevention.

[3]These assumptions are based on Neuman (1995).

BOX 13-9	CONCEPTS—NEUMAN

Person/client system (individual, family, community, social issue)
  Physiological
  Psychological
  Sociocultural
  Developmental
  Spiritual
Basic structure/central core
Flexible line of defense
Normal line of defense
Lines of resistance
Stressors
  Intrapersonal
  Interpersonal
  Extrapersonal

Environment
  Internal
  External
  Created
Health
  Optimal client system stability
  Wellness
  Stability
  System integrity
Prevention and interaction
  Primary
  Secondary
  Tertiary
Reconstitution
Theory of optimum client system stability
Theory of prevention

the developmental variables, which are related to age and development; and the spiritual variables, which are related to beliefs and influences that are spiritual (Neuman, 2002b). The spiritual aspects of Neuman's theory were absent in her earlier conceptualization (Neuman, 1982). They were added to other variables and developed in her conceptualizations of the composite client system (Neuman, 1989a, 1989b), and they were further developed in her subsequent writings and reinforced as essential in assessment and intervention (Neuman and Fawcett, 2012; Newman and Reed, 2007).

The client or client system is defined in terms of a core structure and a series of concentric circles, in addition to the five variables. The core structure includes basic survival factors that are universal and that characterize all species, as well as all unique features of a particular client system. The basic universal survival factors are the innate and genetic factors and natural strengths and weaknesses of

the system. Therefore, according to Neuman, this component of the universal core structure is where the innate factors that regulate temperatures, the genetic response patterns, and any innate strengths or weaknesses in all body organs are found. However, this core structure also contains those unique aspects of a client system that characterize a person, such as cognitive abilities. A client's response patterns are determined and regulated by this core structure. Both universal and unique features of a client system are described by Neuman as normal temperature range, genetic structure, response pattern, organ strength and weakness, ego structure, and "knowns" or commonalities (1989a, pp. 27–29; 2002b, 2011b).

A client system is also described through two lines of defenses: a flexible one and a normal one (Neuman, 1982, 2011b). All environmental stressors first attempt to attack the flexible line of defense. It is visually represented in Neuman's diagrams as the outermost circle surrounding the basic core structure of energy sources; the line is depicted as broken to signify its flexible nature. It is a buffer to a client's normal line of defense, also known as the "client's normal or stable state." The function of this line of defense is to fight the invasions of stressors or to fight the responses to stressors. Neuman (1989a, 2002b, 2011b) describes this line of defense as:

> . . . *accordionlike [sic] in function. As it expands away from the normal defense line, greater protection is provided; as it draws closer, less protection is available. It is dynamic rather than stable and can be rapidly altered over a relatively short time period or in a situation like a state of emergency or a condition like undernutrition, sleeplessness, or dehydration. (1989a, pp. 28–29; 2002b, p. 17; 2011b, p, 18)*

The function of the flexible line of defense as buffer to the normal line of defense is rendered ineffective by some stressors, singularly or in groups. The stressors will then attack the normal line of defense, and when that in turn becomes ineffective in warding off the effect of the stressor—allowing it to penetrate the core structure or allowing reactions to stress to occur—then a response to stress will be manifested. Responses are described as instability or illness.

The normal line of defense is another component of the client system. It is vital in protecting the basic core structure and integrity of the system. "This line represents what the client has become, the state to which the client has evolved over time or the usual wellness level" (Neuman, 1989a, p. 30; 2002b, p. 17). Although not quite as flexible as the flexible line of defense, the normal line of defense still has the capability of expanding or contracting over time. It is depicted by a solid circle surrounding the next layer of the client system, which denotes the lines of resistance. This is where system stability and integrity are manifested, and this is where the normal patterns of wellness levels for the client system are found. Its dynamic nature is apparent in its ability to remain stabilized in dealing with stressors. Levels of stability could be determined through the analyses of lines of defense, lines of resistance, basic structure, energy resources, or survival factors interacting with the five sets of variables: physiologic, psychological, sociocultural, developmental, and spiritual (Neuman, 2002b, 2011b).

Stressors singularly or in groups could continue to penetrate the client system, heading for its basic structure and energy resources. Before the stressor is allowed to influence the basic core of a client system, however, it has to penetrate what Neuman calls lines of resistance. These lines, which are involuntarily activated, are represented by three broken concentric circles surrounding the core of a client system. As a stressor succeeds in penetrating the normal lines of defense, the lines of resistance are activated. "These resistance lines contain certain known and unknown internal factors that support the clients' basic structure and normal defense line, thus protecting system integrity" (Neuman, 1989a, p. 30; 2011b, p. 18).

A question that could be posed is: Are there common stressors for all client systems? Neuman Systems Model Research Institute selected "stressors attacking client systems" as a potential focus for collaboration. An integrative study was initiated to integrate the results of studies conducted by researchers who used Neuman's theory as a framework between 1983 and 2005 (Skalski, DiGerolamo, and Gigliotti, 2006). The findings delineated five client populations as subjects of the reviewed studies: caregivers, cancer survivors, ICU patients, care receivers, and parents of children undergoing surgeries. The authors concluded that the stressors identified were dependent on context, and that middle-range theories could be developed specifically related to any one client group, such as caregiver role strain or cancer survivors. These situation-specific stressors activate and attack different lines of resistance and defense.

Neuman provides the "mobilization of white blood cells" as an example of activation of a line of resistance. If lines of resistance succeed in warding off stressors, that is, "reversing the reaction to stressors," then the client system reconstitutes its energy resources and basic structure (Neuman, 1989a, p. 31). If lines of resistance fail, then energy is depleted. The degree of energy depletion goes from minimal to death.

Each one of these concentric circles has a major function. The flexible line of defense shields the normal line of defense; the normal line of defense is a buffer to each of the lines of resistance; and all these lines combine function to prohibit the stressor from invading the core structure of a human being. All the lines combined also protect the core structure from reacting to stress. Each defense and resistance line varies according to such variables as age and development (Neuman and Fawcett, 2011).

Nurse theorists were asked to reflect on how their theory related to the stressor "adversity." Gehrling and

Memmott (2008) responded on behalf of Neuman's theory. In the face of adversity (i.e., extremely unfavorable conditions, situations, and experiences), the lines of defense are activated. However, in the process, the client (person, family, or a community) experiences a state of imbalance, which, in Neuman's terms, is a result of the adverse event. The client system faces the task of attempting to become more stable (Neuman, 2011b). Reconstitution is the process of bringing back a balanced outcome, with or without a nurse's event. Nursing action is designed to return the system to a balanced state. During reconstitution, nurses strengthen the client system through such interventions as correcting misperceptions, strengthening coping strategies, and providing support (Gehrling and Memmott, 2008).

According to Neuman, environments are internal, external, and created, and all may influence a client system in a circular fashion (Table 13-3). Client systems and environments relate reciprocally, and the outcome of this relationship is corrective or regulative for the client system. The internal environment is intrapersonal; the external environment includes the interpersonal and extrapersonal components; and the created environment is a composite of the intrapersonal, interpersonal, and extrapersonal components. Neuman described the internal and external environments in the following way:

> *The internal environment consists of all forces or interactive influences internal to or contained solely within the boundaries of the defined client/client system. It correlates with the model intrapersonal factors or stressors. The external environment consists of all forces or interactive influences external to or existing outside the defined client/client system. It correlates with both the model's inter- and extrapersonal factors or stressors. (Neuman, 1989a, p. 31)*

The created environment is dynamic and is an interface that exists and connects the internal and external environments (Neuman, 2002b, 2011b). Although the created environment may be created unconsciously by a client, it acts as a reservoir for the existence or maintenance of the integrity of the client system. The expressions related to this environment are conscious, unconscious, or both. The environment infiltrates all systems and all structures; it is purposeful, and it protects the functions of client/client systems.

TABLE 13-3	Definition of Domain Concepts—Neuman
Nursing	Is concerned with all and potential stressors. Deals with assessment of effect and potential effects of environmental stressors (Neuman, 1989a, p. 34).
Goal of nursing	To keep client's system stable. To assist clients to adjust, which is a requirement for optimum wellness level (1989a, p. 34). "Facilitate optimum wellness for the client through retention, attainment or maintenance of client system's stability" (1989a, p. 25).
Health	Health is wellness. It is a point on a continuum running from greatest negentropy to maximum entropy (1989a, p. 25). When all parts of a client are in harmony or in balance, and when all needs are met, optimal health is achieved. Health is also energy. Optimal is the best possible health state achievable.
Human being	A physiological, psychological, sociocultural, developmental, and spiritual being. Represented by central structure, lines of defense, and lines of resistance.
Nursing client	A human being, family, group, community that is threatened with, or that is attacked by, environmental stressors.
Environment	"All internal and external factors or influences surrounding the identified client or client system." Three types of environments were identified: internal, external, and created. The stressors are part of the environment. The internal environment is contained within the boundaries of the client system. The external environment contains forces outside a client system. The created environment denotes a client's unconscious mobilization of such structural components as energy factors, stability, and integrity (1989a, pp. 31–33; 1995).
Nursing problem	A whole client system threatened with or actually manifesting responses to stressors.
Nursing process	Neuman describes three central steps: nursing diagnoses, nursing goals, and outcomes (1989a, pp. 39–41).
Nurse–patient relations	Not discussed.
Nursing intervention	Prevention is the intervention identified by Neuman. There are three components in her prevention as intervention typology: primary, secondary, and tertiary. Reconstitution is part of tertiary prevention.

The insulating effect of the created-environment changes the response or possible response of the client to environmental stressors, for example, the use of denial or envy (psychological), physical rigidity or muscular constraint (physiological), life cycle continuation of survival patterns (developmental), required social space range (sociocultural), and sustaining hope (spiritual). (Neuman, 1989a, p. 32; 2002b, p. 20; 2011b, p. 21)

The goal of the created environment is the unconscious stimulation of the client's health. It includes self-esteem, values, beliefs, and energy exchanges. Therefore, caregivers should explore ideas, beliefs, and fears as much as they explore symptoms and other causal factors. Finally, we should remember that energy is continuously flowing between client and environment. The purpose of the caregiver's assessment and intervention is to bring optimal stability, which is the best possible state of wellness. Determining levels of wellness is accomplished through a consideration of client energy levels (Neuman, 1989a, p. 33). When more energy is expended than generated, the client system moves to entropy or illness. As more and more energy is expended, and less and less energy is being generated, death may result. Neuman defined entropy as "a process of energy depletion and disorganization, moving the system toward illness or possible death" (Neuman, 1989a, p. 48).

To Neuman, stressors occur within the internal and external environmental boundaries of clients and have the potential for disrupting the stability of the client system (1989a, p. 50). Stressors attempt to penetrate the flexible and normal lines of defense, and the results are positive or negative responses. How a client system responds to stress is determined by the resistance demonstrated through lines of defense and resistance, and by the dynamic relationship of the five variable areas (Neuman, 2002a) described earlier. Stressors, to Neuman, can be intrapersonal, which occur within the boundary of the client system. Or, stressors can be interpersonal, which are external environmental forces outside the boundary of the person, but within what she calls the *proximal range*, which is between one or more roles or systems of communication. The third set of stressors, the extrapersonal stressors, are external to the individual boundaries; she calls this a *distal range*, such as policies, economics, or other social concerns (Neuman, 2002b).

Nurses focus their attention on responses that are labeled stressful, and these responses are within the domain of nursing. The nurse diagnoses the ▢ of stability, internal and external environmen ▢ stressors, and the effect of stressors on a clien ▢ system stability (Neuman, 2002c).

The goal of the caregiver is to maintain or to bring about the system's stability, a process Neuman calls *reconstitution*. Reconstitution brings the system to a state of stability or wellness that is higher or lower than the previous state. Nursing actions are described in terms of prevention. Prevention is primary, secondary, or tertiary. Those preventive aspects of care that occur before the stressors invade the client system are primary. Primary prevention identifies potential stressors and augments positive coping and function. When stressors attack the client system, nurses mobilize and support internal and external responses, protect the core structure, facilitate treatment, and continue with any needed primary prevention. These actions are described by Neuman as secondary prevention (Neuman, 1989a, p. 21; 1989b, p. 56; 2002c). Tertiary prevention takes place after the system has been treated through secondary prevention strategies. Tertiary prevention provides support to the client and attempts to add energy to the system or reduce energy needed to facilitate reconstitution (Current Nursing, 2010).

Neuman (2002b, p. 30) acknowledges the development of two theories as extensions from her model. With Audrey Koertvelyessy, she identified the major theory of the model as the theory of optimal client system stability, as well as a proposed theory of prevention as intervention (cited in Neuman, 2002b, p. 31; 2011b, p, 31).

Fawcett and DeSanto-Madeya (2013, p. 157) identified a number of other theories derived from Neuman's model, including three middle-range theories based on client system stability: a theory of optimum student system stability developed by Lamb (1999), a theory of well-being by Casalenuovo (2002), and a theory of infant exposure to tobacco smoke by Stepans and Knight (2002). In Lamb's theory, student and faculty levels of interaction are related to their level of stress. In the Casalenuovo theory, the research proposes that stress, fatigue, and well-being are related in patients with diabetes. And, in their theory, Stepans and Knight focused on the relationship between stress generated by environmental tobacco smoke and the normal lines of defenses, and sudden infant death syndrome. Additionally, while Gigliotti originally argued (Gigliotti, 2003) that no explicit middle-range theories had been generated from Neuman's model, she eventually drew on Neuman to develop the theory of ernal–student role stress (Gigliotti, 2007, 2011). ...s theory is used as a framework to analyze and ...evelop the concept of resilience in nursing and ...o describe strategies to build nurses' resilience.

Theory Analysis

The Theorist

Betty Neuman, a community mental health nurse, graduated from a Diploma program in Akron, Ohio, then received her Bachelor's degree in Nursing in 1957 and Master's degree in Nursing in 1966 from UCLA. She started her teaching job in 1967 (when we became office mates at UCLA), and was charged with coordinating the community mental health consultation clinical specialist program. She received a Doctorate in Clinical Psychology in 1985 from Pacific Western University.

Although the UCLA faculty was busily operationalizing and implementing Johnson's theory at that time, Neuman was uninvolved in this process. She was concerned about the development of a framework to describe the consultation role of nurses, one that could help students describe and explain their actions and the rationale for their actions. The result of that concern was the development of her theory of a client who is in need of health care. Because the role of community mental health consultant is not necessarily exclusively a nursing role, this may explain why Neuman maintains in her writings that her theory is designed for use by any health professional (Neuman, 2002a, 2011a).

Neuman has worked as a teacher, consultant, and writer, and she has maintained a small private practice as a licensed marriage and family counselor. She taught programs in stress reduction and self-help for retarded children. Neuman received a doctorate from Ohio University in 1985. Currently, she is retired; however, she continues to lecture, write, and consult, and she is a consultant for the Neuman Systems Model implementation trustee group (Neuman, 1989c, p. 453; 2002a).

Paradigmatic Origins

Neuman's theory has several paradigmatic origins (Neuman, 2002a, 2011a). One origin explicitly identified by Neuman is systems theory, as conceptualized by Bertalanffy (1968). Neuman used Caplan's (1964) preventive functions, which she used in teaching the Master's program in Community Mental Health to define the levels of actions of nurses (Neuman, 1989c). Other origins identified by Neuman are Chardin's (1955) conceptualization of wholeness; Putt's (1972) application of systems theory in nursing; ideas about adaptation and environment (Neuman, 1989a, p. 12); Marxist ideas of synthesis of man and environment (Cornu, 1957); Gestalt psychology (Edelson, 1970), in which the interactions of people and their environments are described; and Selye's (1950) ideas about stress and bodily responses. Neuman relied heavily on these sources, which are all equally appropriate for use by mental health workers. It is the multiplicity of Neuman's sources that provides the breadth in her theory and its potential interdisciplinary nature.

Internal Dimensions

This is a highly abstract and deductive theory, constructed from hypothetical beginnings, and it was derived from a number of paradigms. The theory is hierarchical, evolving from a set of principles describing relationships between lines of defense, lines of resistance, basic structure, and energy resources. Neuman's is a field theory that explains the relationship of a client system to the environment, and it is a macrotheory that attempts to describe client system relationships with the environment and nurse actions in any situation that requires nursing care. The theory has a broad scope; it provides a framework that describes components of the domain of nursing as a whole. It is also a grand theory of the nursing client, and it explains the primary, secondary, and tertiary prevention needs of nursing clients and the nursing actions for each level of prevention.

Neuman's theory was constructed through the synthesis of different theories that she believed are essential for use by community mental health consultants in their practice. Examples of such theories are systems theory, crisis theory, Gestalt theory, and stress and adaptation theory. Neuman's theory was also developed to identify a nurse's actions and the focus of such actions. It provides a comprehensive description of nursing clients and a framework to describe nursing interventions. It describes knowledge of order; that is, it provides a descriptive account of the normal structure of client's systems, the patterns by which stress tends to attack human beings, and the layers of resistance and defenses that ward off stress. The theory lacks a framework to identify, describe, and explain the different patterns of responses to stress.

Neuman's theory is logically developed, as demonstrated in her conceptualization of a client system as having several parts, with these parts interacting and relating to form a larger whole, and the system grows more complex through the addition of new parts (Barnum, 1998). Three preventions as interventions (primary, secondary, and tertiary) are identified, leaving the question of why other intervention actions are excluded, or, if included, where they should be placed within the conceptualization of prevention as intervention. Are there interventions that are not for prevention? Caring for patients in a critical situation may prompt questions about the rationale and assumptions for including all nursing interventions within a prevention framework. There are other critical questions to consider in reviewing this theory. Neuman addresses antithetical and mutually exclusive concepts without addressing their complementarity and supplementarity. Examples are stability and dynamism, the conscious and unconscious environments, and holism and isolated responses (e.g., psychological responses of denial). The relationship between these opposites and the ways in which they are synthesized could be considered by others who are attempting to extend and develop the theory further.

This theory has many strengths, acknowledged by its scope of utilization. One of these strengths is Neuman's use of clear diagrams. These diagrams, used in all the descriptions of her theory, make it visually appealing; they enhance its clarity and provide nurses with opportunities to consider the logic and interrelationships between theory concepts.

Theory Critique

Neuman clearly identified some assumptions on which her theory is built (Fawcett and DeSanto-Madeya, 2013). However, some implicit assumptions are not well defined, such as valuing the individuality of clients (Lancaster and Whall, 1989, p. 262), which was not addressed in her later work (Neuman, 2002a). She clearly and intentionally used the term *client* instead of *patient* and thus implicitly valued autonomy of the person in health care. Although a client or a client system is defined as families and communities, Neuman does not identify assumptions related to such potential. Values inherent in nursing in relationship to the role of patients in maintaining and promoting their own health and their responsibility in seeking and utilizing health care are also not well addressed.

The central concepts of Neuman's theory have, over the years, been clarified conceptually. Utilizers of the theory have added to that clarity (e.g., Lowry

and Anderson, 1993; Neuman and Fawcett, 2002), and her theory is used as a framework for concept analysis and development.

Reed (2003) clarified the concept of grief by using Neuman's theory as a framework, finding it more suitable to uncover and identify the attributes of the concept. By using Neuman's theory, Reed defined antecedents, modifiers to grief responses, consequences, and nursing intervention strategies to help with reconstitution of client systems, and she identified ranges of normal responses that Neuman (1995) called the *wellness–illness continuum*. Various degrees of grief responses could occur depending on the balanced effect on the client system and the management of resources. Neuman's theory, from Reed's (2003) analysis, allows the outcome to be the development of new reality and new identity in the client system through interactions that occur with the environment. Turner and Kaylor (2015) used similar analysis in developing the concept of resilience.

Neuman discusses her conception of health in terms of living energy, met needs, the degree to which the five client variables are harmonious, and by the amount of energy required to seek and maintain system stability. Although she relates this conception to the World Health Organization's definition of health (Haggart, 1993), this relationship can only be inferred. Similarly, wellness and health are used interchangeably.

Neuman (1989c) describes a wide circle of contagiousness for the theory that spans the United States and other countries (also see Fawcett and DeSanto-Madeya, 2013). Use of her theory encompasses all educational and a variety of nursing programs. The literature details an impressive list of utilizers of her theory during the 1970s and 1980s (Neuman, 1989c, pp. 460–466), as well as during the 1990s and 2000s (Fawcett and DeSanto-Madeya, 2013; Neuman and Fawcett, 2002). According to the board of trustees of Neuman System Model International, many global collaborations have utilized this theory. One example is its use in Holland as a guide for the administration of nursing services (Lowry, Beckman, Gehrling, et al., 2007). The International Neuman Systems Model Association credits the widespread use of Neuman's theory in Holland to its congruence with the Dutch health care system's emphases on patient safety, innovation, and self-management for stress reduction and prevention (Merks, Verberk, de Kuiper, et al., 2012). However, a critique of the theory's use in Holland, Baumann (2012) expresses concern about the emphasis on self-management when patients may be ill-prepared to assume their own decisions.

In addition, as Fawcett (2005, pp. 166–282) described and documented, this theory is well presented but perhaps not as well refined and extended. Many books, monographs, and conferences reflect its use in many corners of the world. There are also symposia held every 2 to 3 years in which those who use the theory are stimulated, inspired, and challenged by one another's work.

The dialogues created by those who provided integrative analysis of the research generated by the theory (Breckenridge, 2002; Fawcett and Giangrande, 2001) are vital for its continuing refinement and extension. Similarly, critical reviewers of tests for middle-range theories (Gigliotti, 2003), identifying and critiquing instruments used for concepts generated from the theory (Gigliotti and Fawcett, 2002), as well as analysis of the international research based on Neuman's theory (McDowell, Chang, and Choi, 2003; Pothiban, 2002) are fostering a process of building knowledge to describe the client system and its defense mechanism against stressors. The use of this theory could enhance research program development, which in turn could advance knowledge, but only if the theory informs all aspects of the research process, including interpretation of results. This is not always the case in the utilization of Neuman's theory in research, as is illustrated in this section.

The utility of Neuman's theory has been demonstrated in the diversity of its use (Campbell and Keller, 1989). Neuman (1989b) describes patient situations in which her theory could be used in suicide counseling, and Lillis and Cora (1989) provide an analysis of its use in a case study. Neuman's theory has been used in community health nursing settings (Beddome, 1989; Benedict and Sproles, 1982; Newman, 2005), as a framework for family assessment (Reed, 1989), as a guide for assessing and intervening in dysfunctional families (Herrick and Goodykoontz, 1989), for preventing abuse in the elderly (Delunas, 1990), in caring for patients in hospital settings (Brink, Neuman, and Wynn, 1992; Burke, Capers, O'Connell, et al., 1989), as a framework for perinatal nursing (Dunn and Trepanier, 1989), for assessing renal patients (Breckenridge, 1989), for interstitial cystitis symptom control (Kubsch, Linton, Hankerson, et al., 2008), in critical care (Bergstrom, 1992; Heffline, 1991), as a framework for patients recovering at home from myocardial infarction (Ross and Bourbonnais, 1985; Smith, 1989), in the care of

patients positive for human immunodeficiency virus (Pierce and Hutton, 1992), and for nursing during the acute stage of spinal cord injury (Foote, Piazza, and Schultz, 1990; Hoeman and Winters, 1990; Sullivan, 1986). Neuman's theory also was adopted in the community to integrate services for the elderly (Neuman, Newman, and Holder, 2000).

What is distinctive about this theory is that it is used as a holistic framework (though Newman uses the term *wholistic*), and many types of interventions can be grouped together to use for patients, nurses, students, and administrators, all under the rubric of the theory (Neuman and Reed, 2007). For example, in designing an intervention for managing symptoms of interstitial cystitis, the authors proposed a variety of interventions to promote system equilibrium including centering, lived experience interview, journaling, progressive muscle relaxation, guided imagery, acupressure, reflexology, and meditation. In developing the framework for intervention, the authors contended that a holistic approach based on Neuman's theory provides opportunities for primary prevention/intervention to strengthen the patient's flexible line of defense, thus preventing stressors from entering the system (relaxation and meditation). Other modalities are for other lines of defense and for prevention (Kubsch et al., 2008). It is also used effectively to prevent delirium in intensive care patients (Gomez-Tovar, Diaz-Suarez, and Cortes-Munoz, 2016).

Buchanan (1987) offers a modification of the theory for use with aggregates, families, and communities. She clarified and added an extension to each of the central theory concepts; however, the major additional contribution appears to be the collaborative decision-making process. These additions are congruent with Neuman's rationale for the development of her ideas, which is the development of a framework to be used by different members of the health care team. The theory has been used to anticipate vulnerability to nursing education, to identify stressors on students, and to develop intervention strategies to help them cope with nursing education (Meyer and Xu, 2005; Moscaritolo, 2009). It is of note that the strategies developed to ward off the anxiety and stress that nursing students experience due to the challenges they confront during their educational years—a threat to their success—are holistic. Reflecting and being true to Neuman's framework, these strategies include humor and mindfulness, yoga, meditation, and body scan awareness exercises. The Neuman theory provided a comprehensive framework for faculty and students to increase their wellness and mobilize their normal lines of defense as they entered practice (Moscaritolo, 2009). The extensions to many populations are also congruent with the theory's assumptions and the intent of the theorist to provide a framework for clients and caregivers. The theory's potential application to the caring of people with different cultural heritages was discussed by Sohier (1989) and demonstrated in studying the caring for aged parents by African American daughters (Jones-Cannon and Davis, 2005). Fawcett (2004) demonstrated through interviews that Neuman's theory is used internationally (e.g., in Holland).

There are many accounts of the use of Neuman's theory in curriculum development. These examples were collected by Neuman and others (Clarke and Lowry, 2012; Lowry, 2002; Neuman, 1989a). These collections demonstrate the extensive utility of her theory for baccalaureate and associate-degree programs, as well as for a framework for multilevel planning. In addition, an entire section in Neuman and Fawcett's 2011 book is devoted to Neuman's model for utilization in nursing education. Fawcett and DeSanto-Madeya (2013, pp. 162–163) list two pages of practical degree, associate degree, bachelor degree, and continuing education programs that are based on Neuman's theory. In addition, Newman, Neuman, and Fawcett (2002, pp. 193–215) identified and discussed guidelines for using the theory in education for health care professions, and they provided a prototype curriculum for each educational level in nursing. How this model differentiates the goals of nursing from those of other disciplines is not entirely clear.

There are many other examples of its utility in developing nursing curricula. Louis and Koertvelyessy (1989) surveyed schools of nursing to determine the use of nursing models in curricula and research. The questionnaires contained specific information related to the use of Neuman's theory. The response rate of 38% was analyzed, and the results indicated that 92% of the responding schools used one of 26 nursing models in their graduate programs as a framework. The respondents identified 41 different models studied by graduate students, and Neuman's was one of the most cited models.

Neuman's theory is reported to have guided the development of curricula in United States (Cammuso and Wallen, 2002; Lowry, 2002) and in other countries. For example, it is used in Neuman's college (Mirenda, 1986), as well as in a framework for programs in transition from associate to baccalaureate programs (Lowry and Jopp, 1989; Sipple and Freese, 1989); as a framework for the experiences of some specific students (Dale and Savala, 1990); as a framework for cooperative (two-school) baccalaureate programs (Nelson, Hansen, and McCullagh, 1989); as a framework for interdisciplinary graduate education; and as a way to think about curricula (Lowry, 2002). The faculty and administrators in most of these programs find Neuman's theory clear; it provides a holistic vision of nursing—a clear nursing perspective; and it provides an emphasis on client's perceptions—a useful framework for the analysis of clients. One example of this evaluation is provided in Nelson et al. (1989).

A program, which integrated a Neuman theory-based associate degree with an eclectic theory-based baccalaureate program, was challenging but the authors concluded that utilizing Neuman as the guiding framework, because of its clarity, was critical to the completion of the integrative journey (Beckman, Boxley-Harges, and Kaskel, 2012). It was also demonstrated that it is an effective organizing framework for simulation debriefing to maximize learning (McClure and Gigliotti, 2012).

There are many indications of the theory's international use; examples are provided by Ross, Bourbonnais, and Carroll (1987) and Bourbonnais and Ross' (1985) descriptive accounts of the theory's utility for the fourth and final year of a baccalaureate program in Canada. Story and Ross (1986) demonstrated the theory's effective utility in the development and implementation of a framework for clinical learning experiences for nursing with families of the elderly at home. These authors also discussed the feasibility of using multiple nursing theories within the same curriculum to guide different learning experiences.

The theory has also been used in programs that have different organizational affiliations. For example, Mrkonich, Hessian, and Miller (1989) describe using Neuman's theory as a framework for three accredited baccalaureate nursing programs that are situated in private, religious, and liberal arts colleges. The authors report that the theory's use was enhanced by its common language, which facilitated communication among health care professionals (p. 93). They also credit the theory for its potential to stimulate research and further development of theory (Mrkonich, Miller, and Hessian, 1989). Mirenda (1986) describes the Neuman college nursing process tool that was developed to be used by students in assessing nursing clients. The tool is reported to help students use Neuman's theory clinically. A thorough review of the use of Neuman's model in developing educational tools is provided by Reed (2002), who concludes that there is a surprising paucity of educational tools based on Neuman's model, considering its extensive use in education. The two potential explanations for this paucity are either that utilizers of her theory are not publishing the tools they develop, or that the complexity and abstractions of theory make it difficult to translate it into the development of tools (Reed, 2002). The richness of the diagrammatic representation of the theory concepts and relationships has helped faculty members in one college devise visual representations to assist students in learning about conceptual models (Johnson, 1989) and prompted the development of slide shows, videotapes, and the Neuman Systems Model Trustee Group, Individual, which is charged with the task of seeing that Neuman's theory flourishes and continues to be used accurately.

The theory's utility in administrative practice has also been the subject of many dialogues. In an integrative analysis of such use, Sanders and Kelley (2002) demonstrated its use in a variety of health care agencies in the United States, as well as in Canada and Holland (de Munck and Murk, 2002) among other countries (Fawcett and DeSanto-Madeya, 2013, pp. 166–202 and Neuman and Fawcett, 2011, Appendix F1, pp. 359–363). Similarly, it is also used as a framework at unit or organizational level in health care systems in the United States, Canada, Iceland, England, Wales, Slovenia, Belgium, and Sweden.

As an example, it was used as a framework for community health administration (Drew, Craig, and Beynon, 1989), and it was used as a framework for the reorganization of structure and function of the nursing department at Jefferson Davis Memorial Hospital (Hinton-Walker and Raborn, 1989). Kelley, Sanders, and Pierce (1989) describe its utility in guiding nurse administrators in their management and leadership roles in educational and practice settings. They also report the development of a tool for assessing and evaluating "conditions upon which the nurse administrators' goals are established and modified" (p. 129). It is also used in developing research in clinical areas, in finding and interpreting evidence for best practices, and to implement evidence-based practice through the Research Approach in Nursing that was developed and implemented by Breckenridge (2011).

The Neuman Systems Management Tool, well described and illustrated, is tailored to provide

BOX 13-10	EXAMPLES OF PROPOSITIONS—NEUMAN

- Primary prevention prevents stressors from penetration of flexible line of defense.
- Primary prevention prevents stress responses.
- Secondary prevention enhances wellness and decreases stress.
- By supporting strengths of clients' systems and conserving their energy, nurses can increase level of wellness.

administrators with a guide for actions and decisions within 3 minutes of use. No reports of validity or reliability of the tool were provided. Others report its use in the development of nursing care plans (Capers and Kelly, 1987), as well as its use in the planning and implementation in nursing practice (Capers, O'Brien, Quinn, et al., 1985). It is also used as a framework for nursing education and to guide the care in nursing homes in the United States and internationally.

External Components of Theory

Neuman's theory is congruent with values about holism in nursing and the reciprocal relationship between environments and client systems. The theory is also highly useful for nurses who tend to speak in terms of prevention rather than treatment or intervention (Box 13-10). The theory's focus on involvement of clients and on assessment that includes defense and resistance is an acceptable nursing focus. The theory is particularly useful for nurses who believe that all health care professionals share the same goals and actions. In proposing the universality of assessment and intervention among the different health care professionals, Neuman failed to identify the unique contributions of nurses to the health care team.

Theory Testing

Several integrative review analyses were done of published research that was carried out using all or some components of Neuman's theory (Fawcett and Giangrande, 2001, 2002; Gigliotti, 2001, 2003; Louis, 1995). The latter was an extension of earlier reviews, with the goal of using that integrative review to entice future researchers to fill in gaps in the refinement and extension of the theory.

Louis and Koertvelyessy (1989) report that they were able to identify 38 research studies that used Neuman's theory. They concluded that the studies were descriptive, and that most of the concepts of Neuman's theory were studied. (The lone exception was the spiritual variable, which has since been used in research studies [Lowry, 2012].) The researchers used the theory as an outline of the phenomenon, as a framework for the methodology, and as a framework for interpretation and for implications. The report did not include information on the nature of the studies, the findings, or the implications of the findings on Neuman's theory or nursing practice. No citations were provided.

Findings from all other integrative reviews indicate that Neuman's theory, although generating increasingly more research studies (Harris, Hermiz, Meininger, et al., 1989; Louis, 1995), dissertations, and theories (Fawcett and Giangrande, 2002), either shows study results that failed to support a proposition in the theory (Ziemer, 1983) or the linkages between the theory, the methods, and the operational definitions (Fawcett and Giangrande, 2001, 2002).

The theory is useful as a framework in research studies to uncover and describe variables. For example, the theory is used to provide insight into the risk factors for coronary heart disease for Filipino Americans as well as implications for preventive strategics (Angosta, Ceria-Ulep, and Tse, 2014). It was also used in a European hospital to test team learning patterns and assess their effects on effective implementation and utilization of innovations in patient care (Timmermans, van Linge, van Petegem, et al., 2013). The findings suggest that, by identifying the exact processes by which teams learn to implement new innovations, managers can develop effective mechanisms. Although this investigation did not test the theory per se, it demonstrated another example of its practice utility. The theory was used to identify intrapersonal, interpersonal, and extrapersonal stressors in nurses' environments in Southern Brazil (Martins, Echevarria-Guanilo, Silveira, et al., 2015). Investigators studying chemotherapy-induced nausea and vomiting in patients diagnosed with breast cancer concluded that the theory lends itself to predicting and explaining chemotherapy side effects as well as to developing interventions to care for patients (Bourdeanu and Dee, 2013). Turner and Kaylor (2015) demonstrate primary and secondary interventions utilizing Neuman's theory.

To decrease restrictions on clients in a mental health practice and to increase their safety, Moore (2009) uses Neuman's and Watson's theories to identify, organize, and decrease intrapersonal, interpersonal, and extrapersonal stressors, and to enhance caring by increasing empathy, support, and transpersonal care (protect dignity). The preliminary results indicate a decrease in the average number of restrictions needed (Moore, 2009).

Despite the proliferation of the apparent use of the theory in research, there is no evidence for systematic programs of research, or of how the results are used to refine, extend, or modify the theory. Furthermore, none of the integrative reports included a meta-analysis of results due to the lack of programmatic research. As Fawcett and Giangrande (2002, p. 137) conclude, the lack of systematic and coherent programs of research precludes the potential of meta-analysis, which decreases the credibility and utility of the theory. In providing a fresh look at the Neuman Systems Model, Lowry (2009), a trustee of the Neuman Systems Model group, proposed that future challenges for the theory are the strengthening of the research agenda and publications, utilizing technology in further developing the theory, and marketing the theory to magnet hospitals (Lowry, 2009). Despite this limitation, Neuman's theory has provided a useful framework for the study of different populations and a wide range of phenomena, such as elder abuse (Kottwitz and Bowling, 2003), assessment of community health needs to implement a mini cardiovascular health fair (Wilson, 2000), and examining the reactions of the elderly with rheumatoid arthritis to stress, lines of defense, and resistance on their health (Potter and Zauszniewski, 2000).

Introducing spirituality as an innate component prompted a number of analyses and dialogues. Among them is a study to explore the meaning of spirituality by aged adults in various states of health (Lowry, 2012). Three themes were identified; connection to God, spirituality's contribution to personal wholeness and health, and the sustainability of comfort in stressful situations. The author concludes that these themes, which are congruent with Neuman's ideas, lend credibility to the importance of assessing spirituality and its meaning for clients. Another study investigated the relationship between spirituality and well-being in patients living with HIV, demonstrating that meaningfulness in life is the best predictor of health status (Cobb, 2012). The author argues that meaningfulness is a strong dimension of spirituality and, hence, these findings lend support to the centrality of variables articulated in Neuman's theory for health care. While some investigators have used the theory exclusively as a framework for research, some suggest it is congruent with other theories, such as complexity theory, which demonstrates its scope and flexible assumptions and propositions (Florczak, Poradzisz, and Hampson, 2012).

Neuman's theory provides a framework to organize information about the client system and about how such a system may interface with stress through different lines of resistance and defense. The "what," "how," and "why" of responses have yet to be described, explained, and tested.

There is no doubt that the utility of Neuman's theory in the clinical and educational spheres has been amply documented.

MARTHA ROGERS

Theory Description

Rogers, a nurse leader and significant nursing theorist, specifically identified her theory, which she called the SUHB as a conceptual system of nursing intended to stimulate the development of nursing theories. Nursing theories, Rogers maintained, could be developed only as a result of nursing research completed within the conceptual system she conceived. In later work, Rogers relabeled her conceptualization as the science of unitary man (1980a), and, even later, as a paradigm for nursing (Rogers, 1983a). She also changed the word "man" to "human beings" and "individuals." She proposed that the science of human beings is as applicable to groups as it is to individuals (Rogers, 1992). Groups may be a family, a social group, a community, a crowd, or any other combinations of individuals.

According to Rogers, examples of theories that may evolve from her paradigm are a "theory of accelerating evolution," a "theory for paranormal phenomena," and "rhythmical correlates of change" (1980a, 1987, 1992). Consistent with the premises of this book and based on the arguments developed in Chapter 3 on conceptual frameworks and theory, Rogers' conceptualization will be treated here as a theory. As has been done with each theory, the analysis and critique are provided to enhance an understanding of the theory, to explain its role in the development of nursing's domain, and to encourage the further use, refinement, and development of the theory.

The central questions that Rogers attempted to answer are:

- What is the focus of nursing?
- What knowledge gives nursing an identity?

- Who is the nursing client?
- What is the relationship between a human being and an environment?
- What are the phenomena of concern in nursing?
- What knowledge is needed to develop the science of nursing?
- What are the outcomes of people's interactions with their environment?

Rogers' conceptualization of nursing as a distinct science is based on several explicit assumptions, presented in Box 13-11, and it encompasses several major concepts, presented in Box 13-12.

Most of Rogers' concepts are unique to her conceptualization. They are innovative, and, as many of her disciples indicate, they transcend time and space and have no boundaries. The concept of a unitary human being, with which Rogers' name has become synonymous, is a primitive concept. All other concepts are derived from a general systems theory (pattern, organization, negentropy), physics (electrodynamic), an evolutionary theory (life process, helicy), and adaptation theories (homeostasis, adaptation). Her concepts are abstract, general, conceptually defined, and documented, but they are limited in their operational referents, which may explain the slow wave of utilization of this theory by nurses, but particularly by nurses who are in practice (Table 13-4). The use of her theory has not increased significantly over time, but the theory has inspired use of alternative integrative therapies (e.g., imagery and meditation) and has enabled the creation of more diverse areas of knowledge expansion. And, although there is a definite trend in differentiating her ideas (Fawcett, 2003a), there is another dialectic trend toward integrating her theory (Watson and Smith, 2002), in developing concepts (Plummer and Molzahn, 2009), and in developing and testing alternative and complementary therapies (Ring, 2009a).

To Rogers, a unitary human being is an irreducible, indivisible energy field in constant interaction with the environment, which is a unitary energy field. Energy fields are not reducible or divisible, nor are they the sum total of their parts, which may be physical, social, psychological, or biologic in nature. In fact, human beings and environments *do not have* energy fields; *they are* energy fields. They are open to exchange and extend to infinity. Energy fields are identifiable through dynamic–nonstatic wave patterns, and through organization that changes from "lower frequency, longer wave pattern to high frequency, shorter wave pattern" based on the principle of resonancy. Energy fields are pandimensional, transcend

---

BOX 13-11 | ASSUMPTIONS—ROGERS

- Nursing is concerned with the life process of a human being, which is irreversible, along a space–time continuum (Rogers, 1970, p. 59).
- The focus of the science of nursing is the unitary human being, his innovative wholeness, and his integral and continuous relationship with the environment. That relationship involves energy and matter exchange. Matter is energy (1970, pp. 47, 54).
- There is pattern and organization in the wholeness of the unitary human being, but causality cannot explain it (1970, pp. 53, 65).
- Conceptual systems are preludes to theories, and theories are tested in real life with a feedback to theories. The cycle is continuous, open, and changeable based on changes in knowledge (1970, pp. 83–88).
- Unitary human beings are characterized by the ability to use abstraction, imagery, language, thought, sensation, and emotion (1970, p. 73).
- Reality does not exist but appears to exist as expressed by human beings (1980, p. 333).
- Nursing is based on a humanistic and not a mechanistic model (1970, pp. 87, 138).
- Generalization can only occur from a study of the whole but not any of the parts in isolation.
- Human behavior demonstrates reason and feelings (1970).
- Unitary man possesses the ability to join in the process of change deliberately and with probability (1983b, p. 222, 1986).
- The human field and its environmental field are postulated to be coextensive with the universe (1983b, p. 222).

Implicit Assumptions

- Human behavior contains probabilistic and unpredictable nonrepeating elements that linear models cannot grasp. These are usually referred to as "error variance" (Winstead-Fry, 2000, p. 280).

BOX 13-12 | CONCEPTS—ROGERS

Unitary human being
  Human field
Unitary environment
  Environment field
Energy field
  Open
  Pattern and organization
  Pandimensionality
Unidirectionality
Sentience
Life process
Rhythmicity
Self-regulation
Negentropy
Evolutionary emergence
Unitary human processes
  Helicy
  Resonancy
  Integrality
  Unpredictability

---

p. 30). Four concepts are basic to Rogers in her own last writings: energy fields, pattern, openness, and pandimensionality (Barrett, 1990a). Change is one of the basic tenets of her theory. Change is innovative, probabilistic, continuous, and relative. It furthers the differentiation of human and environmental fields from lower to higher diversity. Change is based on continuous interaction between a unitary human being's energy field and the environmental energy field. Human development was cited as a goal (Rogers, 1970) and rejected later (Malinski, 1986). The end point is not balance or equilibrium; rather than an actual end point, there is a harmony that evolves and manifests in mutuality or integrality of the person–environment–energy fields. These states of integrality, if we can call them states, are identified through patterns. Field pattern, which has been a central idea for Rogers since the beginning of the formulation of her theory is:

> . . . an abstraction. It gives identity to the field. The nature of the pattern changes continuously. Each human field pattern is unique and is integral with its own unique environmental field pattern. (Rogers, 1986, p. 5)

Rogers postulated three principles to describe the patterns of human being and environment interactions

---

time and space, and therefore may have imaginary boundaries that are unique and changeable (Rogers, 1980a, 1983b, 1986, 1992). Rogers considers fields as open "unifying concepts." Energy for her "signifies the dynamic nature of the field" (Rogers, 1992,

TABLE 13-4	Definition of Domain Concepts—Rogers
Nursing	A learned profession, a science of unitary human beings, and the art of "imaginative and creative use of this knowledge in human service" (Rogers, 1980b, p. 122). It is concerned with living and dying. Fields of practice span the gamut of in and out of hospital, community, and outer space (Rogers, 1992). The central phenomenon of concern is "the study of unitary irreducible human beings and their respective environments" (Rogers, 1990, p. 108).
Goal of nursing	To bring and promote symphonic interaction between a human being and his environment through participation in a process of change. This is done to "strengthen the coherence and integrity of the human field and to direct and redirect patterning of the human and environmental fields" (1970, p. 122).
	Maximum health potential (p. 86).
	"Meaningful life and meaningful transition from life to death" (1970, p. 125).
Health	Health and illness are not dichotomous but continuous, are part of the same continuum, and are an expression of the life process; they are socially defined. Health is "characteristics and behaviors emerging out of the mutual, simultaneous interaction of the human and environment fields" (1980b). One can extrapolate that Rogers' view of health could be the greater developmental coherence that evolves from human being–environment energy fields that are novel, emerging, and more diverse in pattern and organization. Health and illness are not differentiated, nor are there any norms of health (Madrid and Winstead-Fry, 1986).
Environment	"An irreducible, pandimensional, negentropic energy field, identified by pattern and manifesting characteristics different from those of the parts and encompassing all that is other than any given human field" (1983b, p. 222; modified in (Rogers, 1992).
Human being	"An irreducible, irreversible, pandimensional, negentropic energy field identified by pattern and manifesting characteristics that are different from those of the parts and which cannot be predicted from knowledge of the parts" (1983a, glossary). Unitary human being develops through three principles: helicy, resonancy, and integrality.
Nursing client	Human being–environment energy fields relationship (1970, p. 127).
Nursing problem	Not specifically addressed because Rogers believes labels of problems and illness are tentative and based on societal definition. Problems may denote changes in wave patterns and organization and in rhythmical correlates of change (1980a, pp. 334–335). Disharmony or lack of integrity in human being–environment energy fields.
Nursing process	Not specifically addressed. However, what Rogers says about scientific process applies here: "The subjective world of human feelings must be incorporated into so-called 'objective science'" (1970, p. 87).
Nurse–patient relations	Not addressed.
Nursing therapeutics	"Repatterning of man and environment for more effective fulfillment of life's capabilities" (1970, p. 127). Beliefs in innovative therapeutic modalities such as therapeutic touch (1985).
Focus	"Activities of daily living" must be considered within the context of the opportunities for human being–environment interchange that would stimulate the "flow of repatterning commensurate with the openness of nature" (1970, p. 123).
	Unitary human being in interaction with unitary environment. Human beings and environment are energy fields.

and change (Rogers, 1986). These replaced an earlier conceptualization of the principles of reciprocity, synchrony, helicy, and resonancy (Rogers, 1970). To understand the nature, direction, and power of change, one has to consider motion and changes in energy fields through these principles, which were the cornerstones of her theory at its inception: resonancy, helicy, and integrality. *Resonancy* describes the direction of change from lower to

higher wave patterns. The principle of *helicy* postulates that change manifested in increasing diversity and nonrepeating rhythmicity is continuous and unpredictable. *Integrality* describes the nature and process of mutuality between the human and environmental energy fields that negates a separation between those fields (Fawcett and DeSanto-Madeya, 2013, p. 316). All three principles are characterized by their continuity and are manifested through patterns. Human and environmental fields are also characterized by their "pandimensionality," which replaced her earlier concepts of "four-dimensional" and "multi-dimensional" (Rogers, 1992, p. 31). The change in this concept does not reflect a change in definitions, only a change in label. Pandimensionality "is a way of perceiving reality," "it expresses the idea of a unitary whole," and it reinforces the nonlinearity and lack of spatial and temporal characteristics (Rogers, 1992, p. 32). The changes that the human and environmental fields experience are continuous; they emerge out of nonequilibrium and are continuously accelerating.

Theory Analysis

The Theorist

It is difficult to think of the New York University nursing program without thinking of the late Martha Rogers (who died in Arizona in 1994). It is equally impossible to consider environment as a central concept in nursing without immediately thinking of Florence Nightingale and Martha Rogers. Both have left their imprints on nursing in more ways than one, but certainly on theoretical nursing and, more particularly, on the meaning of environment and its centrality to nursing.

Martha Rogers is one of the pioneers who envisioned a science of nursing in the late 1950s and early 1960s and advocated for nursing to have its own body of knowledge. She maintained that the science of nursing is unique and not a synthesis of all sciences—it is more than that. Although synthesis may occur, the result is an integrated whole, as different from the parts as a unitary human being is different from the sum total of its parts. Martha Rogers began advocating that view in 1952.

Rogers received a diploma in nursing from Knoxville General Hospital School of Nursing, Knoxville, Tennessee, in 1936. She earned a Bachelor of Science degree from George Peabody College, Nashville, in 1937. From Teachers' College, she received a Master's degree in nursing in 1945, and she also received a Master's degree in Public Health from Johns Hopkins University in 1952 (Rogers, 1983b). She worked as a public health nurse in rural Michigan and Connecticut and established the first visiting nurse service in Arizona (Hektor, 1989).

Rogers completed the requirements for her doctorate degree in science at Johns Hopkins in 1954, boarded a train, and one day later, was head of the nursing program at New York University. One of

her first acts was to teach doctoral student seminars. She noted that the dissertation students in nursing were part and parcel of dissertation seminars in the education department. Rogers' belief in the uniqueness of nursing and its science prompted her to design a separate seminar for nursing students. She quickly realized that the parameters of that unique knowledge had not yet been identified. That became Rogers' mission in nursing (P. Winstead-Fry, personal communication, 1984).

As an advocate of diversity of thought, Rogers demonstrated it in her personal life through her love of music and science fiction; in her writing, which incorporated philosophy, music, futurology, and physics; and the special talent with which she combined wit, humor, science, and art in speaking about nursing. Martha Rogers was one of the few scholars in nursing who will transcend her time and the profession. John Phillips (2015) described her as a heretic, a person who never conformed to existing doctrines, and a heroine, a person who had courage and bravery to present very different ideas. On a personal note, I invited Martha on behalf of the University of Alexandria in Egypt to give a keynote address for an international nursing conference. Her love of history, cultures, people, and life was evident in this last international trip before her death in 1994. I will always treasure having shared that long and tiring trip with a great and courageous nurse scholar and having her in the house of my mother, another heretic and heroine. As in her many other public lectures and appearances, she inspired all, baffled some with her ideas, challenged many, and drove others to question and argue.

Paradigmatic Origins

Rogers developed her theory from a number of paradigms; concepts were synthesized into what is now a whole around unitary human being, unitary environment, energy fields, continuous interaction with the environment as an energy field, patterns, and change. Understanding of Rogers' theory is enhanced by the study of general systems theory (Rogers, 1985). The constant interaction between human beings and environment, the interrelationships of the energy field, and the openness of both to continuous exchange of matter and energy are based on von Bertalanffy's (1968) definition of an open system. Although Rogers uses some of the terminology of systems theory, she denies the study of subsystems and isolated behavior as representing the whole of the unitary human being.

Rogers also draws on the assumptions and concepts of the general systems theory in two other ways: the unitary human being as an organization of the whole, which is more than the sum of the parts, and the individuality and uniqueness of human beings as reflected in this pattern and organization and in their wholeness. Furthermore, Rogers uses the concept of negentropy—a general systems theory concept—to develop helicy, which is the "continuous innovative, probabilistic, increasing diversity of human and environmental field patterns characterized by nonrepeating rhythmicities" (Rogers, 1980a). Negentropy is a property of both the human being and his environment. Probabilism was later changed to unpredictability (Rogers, 1992).

Physics and electromagnetic theory provide some of the basic premises and concepts of Rogers' theory. The energy field of the unitary human being and the environment are dynamic, irreducible, unbound, extends to infinity, and is identifiable by waves and patterns. Physicists provide the rationale for the existence of such energy fields and for the understanding of resonancy as the "continuous change from lower frequency to higher frequency wave patterns" in human and environmental fields (Rogers, 1980b, p. 2).

The electrodynamic theory of life (Burr and Northrop, 1935) was used by Rogers as the link between physics and life processes in nursing. Rogers used the tenets of evolution theory to explain the increase in diversity, differentiation, complexity, and patterning in developing human and environmental behaviors. A unitary human being is always in the process of "becoming" rather than "being"; at any point, he is more than he has been because all his previous actions, experiences, interactions, and being are incorporated into his present being. Rogers saw dying as part of the rhythmical pattern of life and death as a creative process (Malinski, 2012). A unitary human being is a homeodynamic being and is not homeostatic (Rogers, 1980c, 1992). The process from an evolutionary standpoint, therefore, is toward more complexity; dynamic equilibrium, which characterizes adaptation theory, is not possible as a goal in life.

Rogers was influenced by the early Greek philosophers and by modern theory and philosophy. Her writings drew on Burr and Northrop (1935), Chardin (1961), Polanyi (1958), and Lewin (1964), among others. Hanchett (1992) pointed out the relationship between Rogers' ideas and some of Buddhist principles. In addition, she drew on her vast fiction reading, and interest in classical music and modern physics to describe her concept of nursing science. She was one of the few early thinkers in nursing who conceptualized nursing clients from a holistic perspective (Barnum, 1994), although she initially rejected the concept of holism (Rogers, 1992) because it was "ambiguous" and has "varied meanings" (Fawcett and DeSanto-Madeya, 2013, p. 319). Similarly, Rogers rejected stimulus–response theories, reductionism, mechanism, causality, the separation of person and environment, the effect of negative environmental influences on human beings, and the notion that nursing deals with health problems (Rogers, 1970, 1987, 1989).

Fawcett and DeSanto-Madeya (2013), in addition to agreeing that Rogers' theory is predominately based on systems theory, believe that it contains content related to developmental categories of knowledge, even though Rogers herself may have stopped using human development as a guiding framework. The rationale for this classification is that Rogers' principles of helicy and resonancy, which postulate that patterns in the human and environmental fields are characterized by continuous, unpredictable, and increasingly diverse change, shares characteristics with growth, development, maturation, and change, as well as with direction of change.

Internal Dimensions

Rogers used the dialectic method of reasoning in developing her theory, as manifested in the way that higher-level principles are subsumed under lower-level concepts (Barnum, 1994). The theory is basically concatenated and has a hypothetical constructive beginning, evolving from the synthesis of concepts from a number of fields, the core of which are a number of concepts that are central to nursing. These are unitary human being, unitary environment, energy field, open systems, patterns, pandimensionality, and human development. The relationships between concepts are still at a tentative stage.

Rogers' theory is a monadic, deductive theory. It has several irreducible units, but it is macro in content and wide in scope, as it purports to describe life processes that result from person–environment–energy field interactions. The theory's intent is to explain these continuous, evolving, but unpredictable patterns. It provides a framework to describe the life process of unitary human beings and could provide knowledge of order. The theory does not offer conceptual guidelines for knowledge of disorder or control. The concepts lead to the description of patterns, rhythmicities, symphonic harmony, and evaluation of change in whatever direction human beings may think they are going (Rogers, 1987), as cited in Fawcett (2005, p. 320).

Theory Critique

The discipline of nursing deals with phenomena related to the life process of unitary human beings and their environments, which are expressed in health and illness. The discipline of nursing contains science and art, and nursing is a profession learned through education. The science of nursing is basic. It is the "organized body of abstract knowledge arrived at by scientific research and logical analysis" (Rogers, 1992, p. 28). The art of nursing, on the other hand, encompasses the innovative ways by which the science is used to enhance the lives of human beings. "The aim of nursing is to assist people in achieving their maximum health potential . . . their maximum well-being within the capability of each person" (Rogers, 1970, pp. 86, 135). Rogers defined the goal of professional nursing as follows:

> *Professional practice in nursing seeks to promote symphonic interaction between man and environment, to strengthen the conference and integrity of the human field, and to direct and redirect patterning of the human and environment fields for realization of maximum health potentials. (Rogers, 1970, p. 122)*

She also proposed that the purpose of nursing "is to promote health and well-being for all persons wherever they are" (Rogers, 1992, p. 28). A nurse using Rogers' theory works on mobilizing individual or family resources, heightening her integrity, and strengthening the human being–environment or family–environment relationships (Barrett, 1990a; Rogers, 1988).

The scope of Rogers' theory is broad, and it has the potential to encompass the phenomena of the nursing domain. However, although it articulates the central phenomena, it does not define different patterns of human being–environment interactions or energy field manifestations. The theory appears too abstract; concepts—although defined theoretically—do not lend themselves readily to the practice arena or to measurable variables for research. Rogers never claimed her conceptualization to be a theory, and her thinking and ideas preceded all current attempts at theory building. This may be why she has not offered a systematic

operationalization of her concepts for use in practice and research. Nevertheless, the notion of considering the individual as a whole and of placing the focus of nursing on the human being–environment relationship is appealing to nursing and lends itself to a theory of human being–environment interaction.

Others have extended Rogers' theory and have postulated that the characteristics of a unitary human being could be related to needs and activities of daily living. Because unitary human beings can feel, exchange, be awake, move, choose, value, and relate, a group of nurses (theoreticians, clinicians, and researchers) have developed such a conception and delineated a number of nursing diagnoses according to these characteristics (Kim and Moritz, 1982) (Table 13-5).

Rogers' theory stimulated research in the use of integrative and complementary therapies and those that are grouped under the rubric of alternative types of interventions, traditional healing practices, or indigenous holistic perspectives. Using a quasi-experimental design, the use of meditation was found to facilitate the achievement of a sense of well-being, as well as of a perception of power as knowing in a sample of well Korean adults (Kim, Park, and Kim, 2008). A 6-week prenatal yoga program in second and third trimesters created functional and positive changes in patterns of optimism and sense of power and well-being (Reis and Alligood, 2014). Guided imagery for relaxation was shown to provide relief from pain and depression in patients suffering from fibromyalgia, with the implication that the practice influenced the energy fields of the patients and their environments and promoted their health (Onieva-Zafra, Garcia, and del Valle, 2015). Healing touch or therapeutic touch—developed by Dolores Krieger and based on Dr. Martha Rogers' theory of continuous exchanges between individuals and their environment—is another intervention modality with extensive literature. For example, touch therapy was used in an intervention to determine its effect on both physiologic and subjective anxiety. The results indicated that the participants experienced less stress and were more relaxed, as demonstrated by a number of physiologic measures (Maville, Bowen, and Benham, 2008). Others used her theory to propose research hypotheses related to complementary therapies. Aromas produced through essential oils that carry plant vibrations and memories may facilitate changes in life patterns and processes and may lead to the integration of human–environment relationship (Smith and Kyle, 2008). Similar hypothesis reflecting alternative and

TABLE 13-5	Characteristics of Unitary Human Being—Rogers

Factor I. Interaction

A. Exchanging
  1. Eating and drinking
  2. Eliminating
  3. Breathing
  4. Giving and receiving
B. Communicating
  1. Verbal
  2. Nonverbal
C. Relating
  1. Spacing
  2. Touching
  3. Eye contact
  4. Belonging
  5. Referencing
  6. Family response to patient illness

Factor II. Action

A. Valuing
  1. Philosophical beliefs about health, human interactions, and spirituality
B. Choosing (human beings knowingly making choices—wise, unwise, or detrimental)
  2. Judgment and decision-making capacity regarding alternatives, consequences, commitments
C. Moving
  1. Mobility (rhythm and patterns)

Factor III. Awareness

A. Waking (sleep behavior, patterns, and quality)
B. Feeling (as perceived and as manifested)
C. Knowing (health knowledge, abstractions, motor skills)

Adapted from Field, L., and Newman, M., Clinical application of the unitary man: Case study analysis. In Kim, M.J. and Moritz, D.A. (Eds.). (1982). *Classification of nursing diagnosis: Proceedings of the third and fourth national conferences.* New York: McGraw-Hill; copyright C.V. Mosby Co., St. Louis.

complementary therapies and based on Rogers' theory were formulated about the outcomes of using Reiki as well as puppetry in enhancing the capacity for health (Ring, 2009a), and in health promotion and suicide prevention (Jacono and Jacono, 2008).

Diagnoses such as noncompliance (choosing), anxiety (feeling), respiratory dysfunction (exchanging), impairment of mobility (moving), spiritual concern (valuing), alterations in sleep–rest activity (waking), and alterations in patterns of sexuality (relating) have been defined in relation to a unitary human being (Kim and Moritz, 1982; Rossi and Krekeler, 1982, pp. 276–277). These definitions enhance the theory's clarity for clinicians, decrease its level of abstraction, and render it more amenable to testing. Alternative models of care were used to enhance healing for these types of alterations, to bring about harmony between individuals and their environments.

Several writers have demonstrated some of the theory's utility in practice. Barrett (1990a) and Madrid and Winstead-Fry (1986) proposed a useful assessment framework derived from Rogers' focus on patterns. One component of this framework is living in the relative present, experiencing comfort with the past and present of the individual. Shared communication, a sense of rhythm (a flow in daily life), a connection to environment (a sense of place in a community), personal myth (a sense of self-identity), and system integrity (survival) are other components of the assessment framework. For each of the components, the authors offer a range of intervention options. Carboni (1995a) extended Rogers' ideas for practice and developed a theory of Rogerian nursing practice as an enfolding of health with wholeness and harmony as components. In this theory, nurses and clients participate knowingly in patterning the human and environmental energy fields to create health and wholeness.

Rogers is considered a pioneer in nursing by introducing the concept of energy into the nursing theoretical language. Although this concept is central to Rogers' theory, its definition and utilization to advance fundamental nursing knowledge has been limited. "Energy" is also central in many sciences; however, viewed from a nursing perspective, it is a phenomenon that may not be quantifiable and measurable (Todaro-Franceschi, 2001). This concept, once proposed as central to human science discipline, is elusive in its patterns and characteristics and may (and has) pose issues for researchers and clinicians. Analyses, critiques, and extensions of such concepts (e.g., Todaro-Franceschi, 2001) are essential for clarifying this theory and making it more user-friendly.

Whelton (1979) synthesized Rogers' theory with nursing process theory in delivering care to patients with decreased cardiac input and impaired neurologic function. Others have demonstrated the theory's principles in therapeutic touch (Krieger, 1976), its positive outcomes on injury (Herdtner, 2000), and its use in conceptualizing hyperactivity in children within the framework of synergism as being merely changes in a person's pattern of interaction with the environment (Blair, 1979).

Rogers provided the potential for understanding aging and hyperactivity (1980a), offering more positive evolutionary changes to explain outcomes through her theory. Minimal sleep needs of the hyperactive child are considered by Rogers as a normal response to the increasing complexity and diversity of wave patterns and frequencies of environmental fields. Hyperactivity, therefore, if not viewed from unitary human being–environment interactions, tends to be labeled as a disease. Mason and Patterson (1990) used Rogers' theory to assess a problematic middle-aged man with 33 previous admissions to psychiatric hospitals; although they discussed some limitations, such as their inability to use some holistic principles (such as touch), they concluded that the theory helped them break traditional practices and provided them with support to use visionary and innovative practices to help the patient.

Rogers' theory has inspired the development of assessment tools (Tettero, Jackson, and Wilson, 1993) and provided a framework to assess the perception and meaning of passage of time and the need for diversional activities for the elderly (Biley, 1992). It was used as a framework for many practices (Leddy, 2003; Bultemeier, 2002).

Despite many examples of clinical operationalization and utilization, the general sentiment in practice, education, and administration remains the same: this theory has application limitations. The potential is there, but the complex nature of its concepts and propositions, the esoteric concepts and level of abstraction, and the overlap between concepts due to lack of definition all render the use of Rogers' theory limited in practice. Not only is it difficult to operationalize and measure the characteristics and actions of unitary human beings and energy fields, to identify manifestations of patterns of energy fields, but one is also faced with the limitations of the existing English language in describing the pandimensionality of a human being field and the influence of the tremendous acceleration of change on humanity (Rogers, 1980a). However, Rogers' theory became more meaningful in the 21st century than it had been in the prior century. It is more congruent with accelerating changes, fascination with outer space, acceptance of lack of predictability, and chaos theories. It is also a theory that resonates with current thinking about family dynamics. Winstead-Fry (2000) provided compelling support of how "helicy" reflects many of the family theorists' ideas that have evolved over 40 years. She therefore suggested that Roger's visionary thought was ahead of its time and has become more mainstream in family theory. Furthermore, she proposed that extensions of Rogerian ideas by her disciples, such as Barrett's (1990b) work on power as knowing participant, could inform researchers in other fields who are interested in family research.

External Components of Theory

From the 1960s through the 1980s, Rogers' theory was unknown; it was esoteric and not reflective of nursing. The changes in prevailing views of health, developments in physics, and the movement toward holism have facilitated nurses' acceptance to further explore her theory. The view that the discipline of nursing deals with unitary human beings who are in constant interaction with the environment has gained momentum and support, particularly when it is equated erroneously with holism. There is indication that nursing practice is more positive about the potential of Rogers' theory (Garon, 1992; Rossi and Krekeler, 1982). In an article marking the 100th year since her birth, Baumann, Wright, and Settecase-Wu (2014) revisited Rogers' theory in light of globalization and digitalization. The authors proposed that her integration and synthesis of sciences toward the betterment of humankind and the universe, her focus on change of wave patterns, and her optimistic vision have become even more relevant today in the 21st century than they were in the 1980s.

Each nurse–patient interaction is an interaction of energy fields that evolves into repatterning and reorganizing waves in the direction of increasing differentiation and diversity (Bultemeier, 1997). Each encounter is unique; it moves forward and becomes more complex. Feelings, thoughts, experiences, and awareness of the nurse and patient and their environments blend together, each one emerging not entirely the same as before. Repatterning is a new pattern evolving from a previous pattern; it requires investigation into the "nature of field patterns and organization." These views are valued by nurses, consumers, and, indeed, more and more by other health professionals. Her work inspired many educators (Barrett, 1990c).

Interactions are also empowering. Using an empowerment intervention to build a person–environment relationship utilizing a nurse–patient participation model facilitated the achievement of desired outcomes in managing the care needs of patients with heart failure (Shearer, Cisar, and Greenberg, 2007). This was manifested in adherence to such treatment plans as edema checks, low salt diet, and weighing self on a daily basis. However, the use of this Rogerian-based intervention did not result in such variables as increasing awareness, choices, freedom to act, and involvement in creating change as measured by an instrument designed for these variables (Shearer et al., 2007).

Rogers' theory proposed that change is unpredictable; therefore, a nurse using this framework focuses on building a relationship, to access the unitary field by performing therapeutic touch to help patients to center and become more self-aware of their intention and role in healing. By using these principles, Farren (2009) demonstrated, in a case study of one oncology patient, how she did better in her relationship, coping, self-concept, and mood. Her overall sense of personal well-being improved. Thus, Farren (2009) concludes that the use of Rogers' framework could enhance patients' quality of life. Quality of life has been defined in many different ways in nursing. Implicit in Rogers' theory is a focus on quality care as manifested in having a dynamic life, life satisfaction, and valuation of life processes (Plummer and Molzahn, 2009; Rogers, 1970, 1990).

Theory Testing

Gill and Atwood (1981) attempted to use Rogers' theory as the basis for a study of wound healing in animals, but were legitimately criticized by Kim (1983) for reductionism, causality, and inappropriate use of the animal model. Others have successfully explained some of Rogers' propositions without resorting to reductionism or mechanistic approaches. For example, Rogers' proposition that unitary human beings and environments are dynamic fields of energy, always sending and receiving messages that change both the human and environmental fields in complexity and diversity, has been tested and has received some support (Katz, 1971). Although Katz, a graduate of New York University, did not link her findings to Rogers' theory per se, her findings lend support to this proposition. Katz's experimental subjects, premature infants who were subjected to a patterned regimen of auditory stimulation from tape recordings of the maternal voice, achieved greater motor and tactile adaptive maturation.

Porter's (1972) findings support Katz's (1971) and Rogers' proposition that environmentally imposed motions speed up infant growth and development. Goldberg and Fitzpatrick (1980) hypothesized that movement therapy for institutionalized individuals, as a holistic nursing intervention derived from Rogerian theory, would improve psychological well-being as demonstrated in morale and in attitudes toward aging. The hypothesis was supported, lending further support to Rogers' theoretical propositions. Heidt (1981), testing another intervention based on Rogerian premises, found that subjects who received nursing intervention through therapeutic touch had greater reduction in posttest anxiety scores than did those who received it through casual or no touch. Interventions using Rogers' framework have positive effects on people's lives. For example, those who are provided with interventions that enhance their rhythmic synergy with the environment through yoga (Reis and Alligood, 2014) or guided imagery relaxation (Onieva-Zafra et al., 2015) may have enhanced well-being and experience increased optimism, sense of power, and quality of life.

Other studies reformulated and deduced a theorem regarding environmental disruption and sleep–wakefulness rhythms, and tested it on a general population and a clinic population. More specifically, the theorem stated:

Persons experiencing a deviation in the rhythmic relationship with their environment will manifest greater complexity and diversity in their sleep–wakefulness patterns than persons who are not experiencing a deviation in the rhythmic relationship with their environment. (Floyd, 1983, p. 43)

Although the findings demonstrated a significant difference in "increasing diversity" (total wakefulness time was greater for rotating shift workers than for nonrotating shift workers), there was minimal support for "increasing complexity" (rotating shift workers slept less than nonrotating shift workers). The study lends support to the theorem, but raises some questions when the study used a clinical sample. Floyd's (1983) study represents an example of the potential innovation in testing Rogers' propositions and the significance of systematic study of propositions emanating from nursing theory.

Developmental stages and time orientation were the foci of another study based on Rogerian theory, which concluded that there is "support for the developmentally based nature of specific dimensions of temporality" (Johnston, Fitzpatrick, and Donovan, 1982, p. 120). These studies, together with Newman's (1979, 1994) theory of health, are based on the interrelationships between time, space, consciousness, and movement, and are fine extensions of Rogers' ideas.

Despite such progress, there are still major gaps in our methodology for unitary human beings/unitary environments and their energy fields (Butcher, 1993). Should such gaps in our present knowledge halt all research investigations using Rogers' theory? Is it possible to develop investigations accounting for all Rogers' premises and concepts using our present limited knowledge? The answer is "no" to both the questions. As demonstrated previously, researchers who have been inspired by Rogers' theory and theoretical propositions have found innovative ways to test and support some theory propositions without adhering to or accounting for all assumptions and principles of the theory. For example, well-being in Goldberg and Fitzpatrick's (1980) study was measured in terms of psychological well-being rather than in terms of the greater developmental coherence that involves human being–environment energy fields, as Rogers would emphasize. There are, however, some indications of increasing congruency between her ideas and methods used for research, either because tools have been developed based on the theory assumptions (such as the person–environment participation tool developed by Leddy [1995]), or because creative processes of inquiry are proposed and developed (Carboni, 1995b). And as Winstead-Fry (personal communication, 1984) indicated, Rogers' students, colleagues, and others continue to work on developing congruent measures related to meditation, to measure development as defined by Rogers, and to engage in studies on creativity, differentiation, and parent–child interactions. For instance, Caratao-Mojica (2015), as a creative way to think about patients, has proposed using art to elucidate and reflect Rogers' theory about human beings and environments. Because Rogers was the consummate innovator of ideas and synthesis of different disciplines, Caratao-Mojica used a painting to illustrate the wholeness and pandimensionality in the theory. She concluded that just as a painting should be seen as a whole, inseparable from its context, human beings should be understood, appreciated, and valued in the same way.

A valuable resource that contains comprehensive analyses of tests completed on Rogers' theory is edited by Malinski (1986). This compilation, in addition to a review of literature based on Rogers' theory, may indicate several conclusions about the theory, including:

- A worldview is emerging in nursing that is congruent with Rogers' principles (Malinski, 1986).

- There are some universal questions about Rogers' worldview (Meleis, 1988).
- Research work that uses Rogers' principles is increasing (Benonis, 1989; Quinn, 1989; Schodt, 1989).
- Existing methodological approaches are not entirely useful in investigating principles postulated in her theory (Moccia, 1985; Phillips, 1989; Smith, 1986, 1988), and, therefore, "there is an essential need for methodological studies aimed at development, validation, and evaluation research tools and strategies for the unitary science framework" (Cowling, 1986, p. 74).
- There is a definite evaluation in the types of studies completed to test or further develop Rogers' principles (Clarke, 1986; Ference, 1986; Fitzpatrick, 1988).

Ference (1986) describes the mid-1960s studies, which are mainly doctoral dissertations, as studies of human development; in the 1970s, the studies revolved around the principle of complementarity, which was later relabeled integrality. Concurrently, several of Rogers' students studied body image in an attempt to explain human and environmental fields. The variable of time dominated investigations in the mid-1970s; for example, Newman (1976, 1989) researched perception of time in relationship to gait tempo. According to Ference (1986, p. 38), "these studies helped future researchers to define the meaning of time in a space–time context."

According to Ference (1986), other studies during that period focused on locus of control, field independence, and differentiation. Several instruments unique to Rogers' theory have been developed. Two have been reported. These are the Human Field Motion Test (Ference, 1986) and the Human Field Power Test (Barrett, 1986).

Barrett (1990c, 2003) developed a measure of *power as knowing participation in change*. This measure has been used in many studies. For example, Caroselli (1995) demonstrated that, among female nurse executives, a weak relationship exists between power and feminism, as measured by the power as knowing participation in change instrument. A group of Korean and Korean American scholars used Rogers' theory as the framework to examine the relationship in healthy Korean adults between power defined as knowing participation in change and well-being. They found out that these two concepts are positively correlated. They concluded that Roger's theory is applicable to their culture (Kim, Kim, Park, et al., 2008). Observable manifestations of human patterning that Rogers (1986) describes as correlates were examined by Yarcheski and Mahon (1991) in a study comparing early, middle, and late adolescent boys and girls. The authors selected perceived field motion, human field rhythms, creativity, sentience, perception of time, and waking and sleeping periods. The findings, although not supporting the relationships proposed in Rogers' theory, suggest that age may be related to the correlates. This, according to the researchers, suggests some linearity that may have been deleted prematurely from Rogers' theory. Other researchers attempted to define and test the proposal of increasing frequency patterning in explaining the healing processes involved in recovery (Schneider, 1995) and patterns of perceived field motion and health status (Yarcheski and Mahon, 1995).

Another area of exploration is the degree of spirituality in health care. Rogers' theory has been used as a framework to conceptualize the relationship between spirituality and a number of outcomes. Cox (2003) provided exemplars of using spiritual intervention by advanced practice nurses, and Hardin (2003) explained spirituality as a pattern manifestation of the principle of integrality, both claiming that spirituality is an aspect of quality of life. Closely related to spirituality, but differentiated by the principle of helicy, is the meaning and role of compassion, unpredictability, and participating knowingly in mutual and reciprocal processes (Butcher, 2002).

Smith (1995) compared patterns of power and spirituality in people who have survived polio and those who never had polio. Polio survivors show similar power and more spirituality than participants who did not have polio. This finding suggests that patterns of human field change were related to surviving polio. The study suggests that nurses' awareness of spirituality as a human potential may drive more attention to enhancing the different potentials of patients, and they could facilitate the patients' ability to connect with other aspects of their energy fields. The investigators used Rogers' theory to drive the research questions and propose continuity to develop spirituality with this theory.

Another significant test of any theory is the extent to which it has stimulated theoretical published discourse. Rogers' theory inspired the development of other theories, such as Newman's theory of health as expanding consciousness (Newman, 1994).

Hills and Hanchett (2001) developed a middle-range theory of "enlightenment" based on the three principles of helicy, resonancy, and integrality. Their theory evolved from clinical observations. They proposed that awareness, wakefulness, and human field motion could result in higher levels of well-being through a process of change and individuation. The clinical exemplar the authors provide illustrate this abstract relation. They observed 250 parents who had children with the birth defect of myelomeningocele, and noted that although the parents struggled with the meaning of this birth defect, when obstacles were overcome, the parents

. . .would report deeper insights and awareness, a greater sense of harmony, and an enthusiastic commitment to actively participate in their own process of individuation. (Hills and Hanchett, 2001, p. 8)

The *enlightenment experience* was defined as:

Anything which [fosters reflection and] involves a compassionate commitment to others, or to both self and others. (Hills, 1998, p. 12, as cited in Hills and Hanchett [2001, p. 8])

Other theories inspired by Rogers include: the Theory of Emergence of Paranormal Phenomena, which provides a framework to explain and interpret intuitive recognitions, telepathy, and similar phenomena (Butcher and Malinski, 2010); the Theory of Health Empowerment (Shearer, 2009); and the Theory of Power as Knowing Participation in Change (Barrett, 1990b, 2003, 2010). In addition to inspiring theory developments by others, Rogers' theory has inspired concept developments such as "the will to thrive" in adult mental health, in some senses the opposite of the concept "failure to thrive" in babies deprived of nurturance and stimulation (Powers, Hart, Shattell, et al., 2012). The "will to thrive" is manifested in the resilience of human beings with a sense to transform, to engage deliberately in a forward motion to grow. Rogers' writings and teaching also inspired creative reflections and epiphanies about Rogers living her theory of energy field in the universe after passing (not dying) (Phillips, 2013).

Others, particularly graduate students from Wayne State University, Case Western Reserve University, the University of Rochester, and New York University are engaged in researching propositions derived from Rogers' theory, which has been operationalized for educational settings. The curriculum of nursing at New York University is not the only one based on Rogers' theory. Her theory has been used to develop curricula at Duquesne, College of Mount

St. Vincent, and Fairleigh Dickinson University (P. Winstead-Fry, personal communication, 1984).

This is a theory whose complexity of primitive concepts has undermined the clarity of the relationship between the concepts as well as the boundaries. Can energy fields of a human being be defined distinctly from that of an environment? If helicy is unpredictable (Rogers, 1990), what use is it in science, which presumes certain order and predictability? What Rogers succeeded in doing—creating a rich environment of uncertainty for intellectual discourse—has failed to attract a rich dialogue except among the select few who either studied under her guidance at New York University, or joined the Rogerian society (the believers), a community that needs no urging to use her ideas.

A critical evaluation of the fit between her theory and therapeutic touch by a number of UK scholars, became an important contribution to stimulate a discourse and a debate (O'Mathuna, Pryjmachuk, Spencer, et al., 2002).

Although many have written about touch or therapeutic touch and its outcomes, as driven by Rogerian Science of Unitary Man (Herdtner, 2000; Kelly, Sullivan, Fawcett, et al., 2004; Lowry, 2002; Smith, Kemp, Hemphill, et al., 2002; Ugarriza, 2002), O'Mathuna et al. (2002) eloquently refuted the connection of Rogerian energy fields with the mechanisms and the premises of therapeutic touch. They provided arguments demonstrating the lack of evidence of potential negative or positive effects of therapeutic touch on patients' outcomes.

Rogers' theory stimulated robust dialogues on several concepts germane to the discipline of nursing and for which, prior to Rogers, there were no productive frameworks. Examples are developing and testing energy (Todaro-Franceschi, 2001), and use of therapeutic music in enhancing coping skills in patients with psychiatric disorders (Covington, 2001). Rogers' theory inspired Barrett to develop her investigation of the principle of helicy by focusing on the relationship of human field motion and power as knowing (Barrett, 1986; Barrett and Caroselli, 1998; Caroselli and Barrett, 1998). In addition, subsequently, her operationalization of power from a Rogerian theory provided a framework to study it in relationship to pain and trust (Kim, 2001; Lewandowski, 2002; Wright, 2004), in relationship to hope and exercise (Wall, 2000), in studying people's experiences (Phillips, 2000), in relationship to humor and health (Yarcheski, Mahon, and Yarcheski, 2002), and in perception of time as an ever-evolving process (Ring, 2009b).

Finally, in another integrative review of research studies based on Rogers' SUHB, Kim (2008) concluded that Rogers' theory continues to provide a valuable theoretical framework. However, the need continues for clarification of concepts and methods and of the congruency between them. Energy, one of Rogers' core concepts, was not well defined in her work, and it continues to draw nurses into philosophical dialogues. Among them is Todaro-Franceschi (2008), who compares and contrasts a mechanistic view of energy as a part of causal process with that of Roger's humanistic and wholistic views. In the first, energy is exchanged, transmitted, lost, and/or gained through various change processes. Rogers' view of energy, as clarified by Todaro-Franceschi (2008), is a phenomenon that denotes universal life energy that is more congruent with Eastern philosophies, from which such concepts as *chi* and *prana* evolved. It is important to note that, whether Rogers would agree with this view or not, her concepts continue to inspire dialogues, clarification, and development. Rogers, however, would agree that the SUHB is subject to the dynamic and continuous process of development (Wright, 2007).

Two discourses could stimulate debates and critical consideration. The first is a published interview conducted by Jacqueline Fawcett with Ann Manhart Barrett (2002), Violet M. Malinski (1986), and John Phillips (2000) related to a 21st-century update (Fawcett, 2003b). The interview provides an effective summary of how scholars well-versed and trained within a school of thought view the tenets of the theory (with conviction), the supporters of the theory (with no skepticism), and the future of our discipline (with fear of demise for lack of theory or for attempting to integrate different schools of thought). A nonbeliever could have rendered this interview more powerful and more useful in generating a true critical intellectual discourse.

The second important discourse is provided by Watson and Smith, who described two prevailing themes in theoretical thinking in nursing: unitary direction in nursing (Rogers' SUHB) and caring science. These two schools of thought appear controversial, separate, and parallel. After a critical review, they proposed a synthesis between the unitary view of humans with relational caring ontology and ethics. They believe that the result is likely to be a "trans-theoretical, trans-disciplinary view for nursing knowledge development" (Watson and Smith, 2002, p. 452). Newman (2003), another Rogerian theorist and a theorist in her own right, would agree that we have entered an era with no disciplinary boundaries. Theorists and utilizers with a sense of theoretical purity would expect to disagree with this integrative discourse.

Rogers' theory is complex, is somewhat tautological (she acknowledges an overlap between concepts), and has an aura of coherent truth, but presents a challenge to operationalization. Although difficult for the American practitioner, it still inspires the education of new generations of nurses (Karnick, 2014). Its view of humanity and environment, and the lack of separation between mind and body, is congruent with the Eastern view; therefore, it is expected that its circle of contagiousness will increase more rapidly than ever in the decade ahead, particularly outside the United States. It is congruent with professional values in nursing and with the emerging perceptions of the vital role nurses play as humanitarians.

SISTER CALLISTA ROY

Theory Description

The central questions of Sister Callista Roy's theory, which is known as the Roy Adaptation Model (RAM),

are: What is the target of nursing care? When is nursing care indicated? And what is the ultimate goal of nursing care? As with theories that evolved early in the history of theoretical nursing, the intent was to differentiate the discipline of nursing from medicine and to provide it with it owns focus. Over the years, Roy, her colleagues, and theory utilizers have developed different aspects of the theory that specifically deal with adaptation levels at changing points that are influenced by the situation as well as by available inner resources.

Roy's first ideas appeared in 1964, in a graduate course paper written at UCLA in one of Dorothy Johnson's classes. Roy published these ideas in 1970, and subsequently, different components of her framework crystallized during the 1970s, 1980s, 1990s, and into the 21st century. Over the years, Roy identified the assumptions on which her theory is based (Box 13-13), starting with scientific assumptions, then incorporating humanistic and veritivity assumptions regarding the dignity of human beings and the role of nurses in promoting integrity in life and death. Increasingly, her theory is defining and connecting spirituality and religiosity to experiencing and coping with illness (Roy and

BOX 13-13	ASSUMPTIONS—ROY

Explicit Assumptions (Roy, 2000a, p. 7; Roy, 2000b, p. 127; Roy and Andrews, 1999, p. 35)

Scientific
- "Systems of matter and energy progress to higher levels of complex self-organization."
- "Consciousness and meaning are constitutive of person and environmental integration."
- "Awareness of self and environment is rooted in thinking and feeling."
- "Human decisions are accountable for the integration of creative processes."
- "Thinking and feeling mediate human action."
- "System relationships include acceptance, protection, and fostering of interdependence."
- "People and the earth have common patterns and integral relations."
- "Person and environment transformations are created in human consciousness."
- "Integration of human and environment meaning results in adaptation."

Philosophical
- "Persons have mutual relationships with the world and with a God figure."
- "Human meaning is rooted in an omega point convergence of the universe."
- "God is ultimately revealed in the diversity of creation and is the common destiny of creation."
- "Persons use human creative abilities of awareness, enlightenment, and faith."
- "Persons are accountable for the process of deriving, sustaining, and transforming the universe."

Implicit Assumptions
- "Individual persons, their perceptions, and their experiences are the starting point of nursing" (Whittemore and Roy, 2002).
- A person can be reduced to parts for study and care.
- Nursing is based on causality.
- Patients' values and opinions are to be considered and respected.
- "A state of adaptation frees an individual's energy to respond to other stimuli" (Roy, 1984, p. 38).

Andrews, 1999; Roy, 2000a, 2000b). One can see the integration of her religious background in her more recent writings (Roy, 2008).

Roy's assumptions in general are in agreement with current views in nursing regarding adaptations, human beings, and nursing. Her assumptions are based on humanism and veritivity (Hanna and Roy, 2001). Her implicit assumptions attest to the totality of the individual, as manifested in behavior, active participation of individuals in life, and an individual's potential for self-actualization. Humanistic values have been identified in Roy's theory (1984, 1987, 1988a); Roy and Andrews (1991, 1999), followed by values related to truth, and oneness with the truth, "also known as a creator, God" (Roy, 2000b, p. 127). The principles of humanism are creative power, holism, subjectivity, purposefulness in life, interpersonal relations, and activity. Although others have tended to view the holistic nature of the theory (Mastal and Hammond, 1980), it was not until 1984 that Roy emphasized the holistic nature of a person and the humanistic care of nurses. In 1987 and 1988, these humanistic values were described, and in 1988, the philosophical stand moving beyond rationalism and relativity toward veritivity was explicated (Roy and Andrews, 1999). Roy and Corliss (1993) presented a set of revised assumptions for Roy's theory that included attention to holism, interdependence, central processes of systems, information feedback, and the complexity inherent in living systems. These assumptions reflected a general systems theory approach to viewing her theory and clarified the philosophical origins of Roy's theory. In her revisions, theorist Roy combines scientific rationalist assumptions with those based on personal and religious convictions (Roy and Andrews, 1999, p. 35).

According to Roy's theory, a person—a biopsychosocial being, an adaptive system, a human being—is in constant interaction with a changing environment; therefore, a person is continually changing and attempting to adapt. When the person is not adapting positively and is therefore manifesting ineffective responses, he or she is of concern to nursing; however, once a person manifests effective behavior, he or she no longer needs nursing attention. A person uses both innate and acquired mechanisms to ready himself to adapt to his environment (Andrews and Roy, 1986; Roy and Andrews, 1999). A person is also defined in terms of purposefulness of existence and as reflecting the context of humankind's unity of purpose and the common good, as well as the value and meaning inherent in life (Roy, 1988a)

In addition, Roy views the innate creative powers as essential to understanding the nature of a human being. In an adaptive person, she calls these powers "veritivity," which she uses to mean the truth of human nature, and which reflects activity, creativity, unity, purposefulness, and value (Roy, 1987; Roy, 2000a; Senesac and Roy, 2015).

A person is an adaptive system with two major internal central mechanisms used for adapting. These are the regulator and the cognator subsystems, which are viewed as innate or acquired coping mechanisms. These innate or acquired mechanisms are used to deal with a constantly changing environment (Roy, 1991; Roy and Andrews, 1999). The regulator mechanism works primarily through the autonomic nervous system to organize a reflex action that prepares the individual to respond and adapt to the environment. The regulator subsystem uses physiologic processes such as chemical, neurologic, and endocrine responses. The regulator mechanism receives stimuli from the internal and external environments, both of which are basically chemical or neural, and receives all input into the central nervous system. Body responses observed by the nurse are effects of autonomic responses, responsiveness of endocrine glands, and the perception process. The latter is altered by cultural and social factors (external stimuli) and "must remain in short-term memory long enough for a psychomotor choice or response to be made" (Roy and McLeod, 1981, p. 60). The bodily responses, brought about through chemical–neural–endocrine channels, are fed back as additional stimuli to the regulator system (Roy, 1984, pp. 28–36; Senesac and Roy, 2015, pp. 155–56).

The second mechanism is the cognator subsystem, which identifies, stores, and relates stimuli so that a symbolic meaning can be attached to the behavior. The cognator mechanism is composed of several parts and corresponding processes: (1) perceptual/information processing manifested in the processes of selective attention, coding, and memory; (2) learning, manifested in imitation, reinforcement, and insight; (3) judgment, which involves the process of problem solving and decision-making; and (4) emotion, which is manifested in defenses to seek relief and affective appraisal and attachment (Roy, 1988b; Roy and Andrews, 1999). These processes are influenced by internal and external stimuli and affect the psychomotor choice of response of orientation, approach, avoidance, flight, or hiding as demonstrated in the form of spoken or unspoken words. Failure in either the regulator or the cognator mechanisms results in maladaptation (Roy, 1984).

All *input* is channeled through the processes of the regulator and the cognator and produces responses through four effector modes. Roy's theory has been expanded and extended to use in family and group relationships encompassing their coping processes, adaptive modes, and their adaptation levels (Hanna and Roy, 2001, p. 9). The four modes have also expanded to encompass groups (p. 48). Roy specifies terminology for collective human systems—physical, group identity, role function, and interdependence—to correspond with the four adaptive modes associated with the individual. The collective is regarded as a whole, and the nursing process is applied in relation to the whole, just as it is applied to individual circumstances (p. 102). Therefore, the four modes are: physiologic–physical needs, self-concept–group identity, role function, and interdependence. The two subsystems are related to each other through perception, and are related to each effector mode differently, whereas the regulator is related predominantly to the physiologic/physical mode.

[S]ince very little is known physiologically about the process of perception formation, memory, and choice of psychomotor responses, the other modes of self-concept, role function, and interdependence must relate to the meaning of a given perception for the individual human system. The meaning of the perception will, therefore, influence the body response. (Roy and McLeod, 1981, p. 67)

Conversely, the cognator subsystem is related to all adaptive modes. Processes such as selective attention, imitation, problem solving, and appraisal influence nutritional intake in the physiologic mode, role function, self-concept, and interdependence. Within each mode, all cognator processes could be manifested; for example, attachment, reinforcement, and memory are integral parts of role cues selected by a person. The physiologic–physical mode for individuals and groups is a result of the needs of individuals for physiologic integrity and the ways humans interact as physical beings with the environment. Behavior in this mode reflects physiologic processes of cells, tissues, organs, and body systems. There are five basic physiologic needs and four regulator processes in this mode. The physiologic needs are activity and rest, nutrition, elimination, oxygenation, and protection. The regulator processes are described as the senses, fluids, and electrolytes, acid–base balance, neurologic functions, and endocrine functions. The

concept "physical" is more appropriate for use for humans in groups. This is the first adaptive mode for groups. Basic needs for groups in the physical mode are resource adequacy, or wholeness, which is achieved by adapting to change in needs for physical resources (Roy and Andrews, 1999).

The self-concept mode is related to the need for psychic and spiritual integrity (Roy and Andrews, 1999). Self-concept is defined by a person through the definitions of significant others, and it includes perceptions of self and others. It also includes an integrative view of the physical and personal selves. The physical self is manifested in body sensations (feelings and experience) and image (view of self). The components of the personal self are self-consistency (continuity of self), self-ideal (expectations), and the moral–ethical–spiritual self (values) (Andrews and Roy, 1986; Roy, 1987; Roy and Andrews, 1999). Self-esteem is a component of self-concept and is defined as the extent to which individuals perceive their self-worth (Andrews, 1991). Group identity is used for the self-concept mode related to groups, and it is composed of interpersonal relations, group self-image, social milieu, and culture (Roy and Andrews, 1999). The self-concept mode operates through three processes to meet individuals' needs; the developing self, the perceiving self, and the focusing self. These, as well as the group level that Roy later incorporated in the self-concept mode as group identity, are defined through interaction with the environment.

The role function and interdependence mode for both individuals and groups is focused on the need for social integrity. Role is viewed in Roy's theory as a set of expectations of individuals toward each other. She classified roles as primary (based on age, sex, and development), secondary (acquired through relations with others and made permanent), and tertiary (activities that are more temporary) (Andrews and Roy, 1986). The interdependence between individuals is expressed in the ability to love, respect, and value, and to receive love and respect and to be valued. Roles within groups provide mechanisms for achieving social system goals (Roy and Andrews, 1999). These include functions of managers and administrators and systems for maintaining order and making decisions.

Stimuli affecting modes and mechanisms are identifiable as focal stimuli (those that are immediate in an individual's life), residual stimuli (attitudes and previous experiences), and contextual stimuli (all other stimuli, e.g., heat aggravating a rash, or noise that is irritating to a person in pain).

In early writings, Roy and McLeod (1981) proposed that a theory of the person as an adaptive system (i.e., regulator and cognator mechanisms) should be used in conjunction with the Roy adaptation model. This was later modified and synthesized, so that there was no differentiation between the model and the theory (Roy, 1984). A person is conceptualized as an adaptive system that includes input (stimuli and an adaptation level), control processes (the regulator and the cognator as coping mechanisms), effectors (four modes), and output (adaptive and ineffective responses) (Roy, 1984, p. 30) (Box 13-14).

Later developments in Roy's theory have helped to clarify her view of a person. However, some concepts remain ambiguous and overlapping. Although concepts are mainly derived from other paradigms, the primitive ones (regulator and cognator) are not as precisely identified and defined. Concept boundaries are not clear. For example, effector modes and focal stimuli overlap (overlap persists in some effector modes, such as in interdependence role, self-concept, and role function). Overlap also occurs between adaptive modes and mechanisms, and the definitions lack clarity (Mastal and Hammond, 1980), allowing utilizers of the theory to derive their own definitions, which in some ways marks the theory's strength and versatility. Environment and internal stimuli were initially operationally undifferentiated (Tiedeman, 1983) (Table 13-6). However, later Roy (2009) defined environment as "all conditions that may influence people's behavior including all those circumstances generated by human and earth resources," which made it more differentiated from internal stimuli. The definition of environment was more amenable to operational differentiation as she further modified the definition to "all conditions, circumstances and influences surrounding and affecting the development and behavior of individuals and groups" (Senesac and Roy, 2015, p. 158). It is important to note that Roy considers environment also to be a community of beings that includes complex set of interactions and rhythm.

Roy and McLeod (1981), Roy and Roberts (1981), Roy and Andrews (1991), and Roy and Corliss (1993) have provided a useful systematic presentation of all possible links between variables, resulting in a multitude of theoretical propositions. This is clearly a theory that lends itself to the development of propositions and hypotheses. The propositions provided by the theorist are theoretically sound, structurally adequate, systematic, and relational. The researcher's task

is in operationalizing propositions for research projects and in generating many research studies. The propositions tend to focus on biologic events (physiologic response, intact neural pathways) rather than nursing phenomena. These propositions evolved over the years to reflect changing global needs with more focus on group identity, group coherence, and transformations in the face of risks and the influence of internal and external environments (Roy, 2011a). The propositions are linear and bivariate, but Roy is striving for nonlinear and multivariate relationships (Roy and Roberts, 1981, p. xiv). Others have also used the theory to develop more propositions specific to particular groups of patients, such as those suffering from bulimia nervosa (Hannon-Engel, 2008), chronic obstructive pulmonary disease (Akyil and Erguney, 2013), and social support issues during perinatal and postpartum periods (Aktan, 2012).

Roy's theory has a high descriptive and explanatory power of the individual as an adaptive system amenable to descriptive studies in each of the modes, but the theory has limited predictive and prescriptive powers. The descriptive and explanatory potential has been enhanced with existence propositions that then drive qualitative, correlational, and controlled studies. Over the years many descriptive studies helped in illuminating, clarifying, and operationalizing concepts, leading to the development of middle-range theories. Although Roy has systematically continued to work on establishing theoretical validity of each coping system and effector mode, establishing their empirical validity has yet to be achieved. However, several research studies demonstrated and supported the relationships proposed by Roy's theory of environment and adaptive modes (Shyu, Liang, Lu, et al., 2004; Yeh, 2003). She herself has analyzed and integrated 25 years of her research program, driven by the Roy theory, which resulted in a middle-range theory of coping and adaptation processing (Roy, 2011b).

Theory Analysis

The Theorist

After receiving a Master of Science degree in pediatric nursing, Sister Callista Roy, who was a pediatric nurse by training, studied sociology at UCLA, where she received her doctorate in 1976. The impetus of her theory was inspired by her

BOX 13-14	CONCEPTS—ROY

Adaptation
　Adaptation level
　Adaptation zone
　Adaptive response
Client: An Adaptive System
　Biologic
　　Anatomy
　　Physiology
　Psychological
　　Perceiving
　　Learning
　　Acting
　Social
　　Family
　　Community
　　Work group
　　Society
Adaptive System
　Cognator
　Regulator
Adaptive Stimuli
　Focal
　Contextual
　Residual
　Physical, personal, moral–ethical–spiritual self
　　Self-consistency
　　Self-ideal/self-expectancy
　　Learning
　　Inner self and self-concept
　　Self-esteem
Veritivity "pertains to the principle of human nature that affirms a common purposefulness of human existence" (Hanna and Roy, 2001, p. 10).
　Components
　1. Purposefulness of human existence
　2. Unity of purpose of humankind
　3. Activity and creativity for the common good
　4. Value and meaning of life
Humans: adaptive systems
Behavior: output of human systems
　Adaptive responses
　Ineffective responses
Environment: stimuli
　Focal
　Contextual
　Residual
Stimuli: provoking a response
　External
　Internal
Adaptation level: the condition of the life processes
　Integrated
　Compensatory
　Compromised

Adaptive modes
　Physiologic–physical mode (pp. 103–104)
　　Physiologic
　　　Five needs: oxygenation, nutrition, elimination, activity and rest, protection
　　　Four complex processes: senses, fluid (electrolyte and acid–base balance), neurologic function, endocrine function
　　Physical
　　　Basic need: operating integrity
　　　Components: participants, capacities, physical facilities
　Self-concept–group identity mode (pp. 107–108, 383–385)
　　Self-concept—individual
　　　Basic need: psychic and spiritual integrity
　　　Components: physical self (body sensation, body image), personal self (self-consistency, self-ideal, moral–ethical–spiritual self)
　　Group identity
　　　Basic need: identity integrity
　　　Components: shared relations, goals and values, social milieu and culture, group self-image and co-responsibility for goal achievement
　Role function mode (pp. 109–110, 432–433)
　　Basic need: social integrity (individual level), role clarity (group level)
　　Components: role set and aggregate role set, structural approach (instrumental behavior, expressive behavior), interactional approach (role-taking), developing roles (primary, secondary, tertiary), integrating roles (collective patterns)
　Interdependence mode (pp. 111–112, 475–480)
　　Basic need: relational integrity
　　Components (individual level): affectional adequacy, developmental adequacy, resource adequacy
　　Components (group level): context, infrastructure, participants
　　Focus: relationship with significant others, support systems
Coping processes: innate or acquired ways
　Individual
　　Regulatory subsystem
　　Cognator subsystem
　Group
　　Stabilizer subsystem
　　Innovator subsystem

TABLE 13-6	Definition of Domain Concepts—Roy
When nursing is needed	The adaptive system of a person who is ill or has the potential of illness "when unusual stresses or weakened coping mechanisms make the person's usual attempts to cope ineffective."
Goal of nursing	To enhance the adaptation of the patient in the four modes to free energy to respond to other stimuli. Freed energy promotes healing abilities and wellness (Roy and Roberts, 1981). "To promote adaptation" (Roy, 1984, p. 36) and "to decrease ineffective responses" (Roy, 1984, pp. 37–38).
	• Goal of nursing is defined "as the promotion of adaptation in each for the four modes, thereby contributing to health, quality of life, or dying with dignity" Roy and Andrews (1999, p. 55).
Nursing client	A person, family, group, or community. Biopsychosocial adaptive systems with two processor subsystems that are mechanisms for adapting or coping—the regulator and the cognator. The system has four affecters of adaptation, or the adaptive modes: physiologic needs, self-concept, role function, and interdependence (Roy and Roberts, 1981, p. 43). A holistic, adaptive system (Roy, 1984, p. 36).
Human being	Functions holistically (Roy, 1984, p. 36), highest possible fulfillment of human potential (Andrews and Roy, 1986).
	• "Humans (1) are individuals and groups share in creative power; (2) behave purposefully, (3) possess intrinsic holism, and (4) strive to maintain integrity and to realize the need for relationships" (Hanna and Roy [2001]).
	• "Persons as individuals and members of families also are interrelated with all of creation and are accountable for deriving, sustaining, and transforming the universe" (Hanna and Roy [2001]).
Nursing process	A "particular format" used in nursing that uses the problem-solving approach. It comprises the six steps of assessment of behaviors, assessment of influencing factors, nursing diagnosis, goal setting, intervention, and evaluation (Roy and Andrews, 1991; Roy, 1984, pp. 42–62).
	• "Nursing process consists of six steps, assessment of behavior, of stimuli, nursing diagnosis, goal setting, intervention and evaluation" (Roy and Andrews [1999, pp. 63–96]).
	• "The nursing process involves an active search by the nurse to identify, interpret, and respond to human coping processes" (Roy and Andrews [1999, pp. 63–96]).
Nursing problem	The source of difficulty is the coping activity that is inadequate to maintain integrity in the face of a need deficit or excess (Roy, 1980, p. 184).
Nurse–patient relations	Acknowledged in 1984 as important, but not defined. Defined in 1987 through nursing process.
Nursing diagnosis	"Changes in internal or external environment can trigger need deficits or excesses. Within the appropriate adaptive mode, coping activation is stimulated. When the coping mechanism is ineffective in meeting the demand, ineffective behavior results" (Roy and Roberts, 1981, p. 47).
	"The behavior with its predominant stimulus" (Roy and Roberts, 1981, p. 47).
	• Nursing diagnosis is a "judgment process resulting in statements conveying the adaptation status of the human adaptive system" Roy and Andrews (1999, p. 77).
Nursing therapeutics	Traditional techniques such as comfort measures or health teaching, or entirely new activities that have not been discovered, all with the goal of promoting adaptation (Roy and Roberts, 1981, pp. 47–48).
	• "Nursing intervention is described as the selection of nursing approaches to promote adaptation by changing stimuli or strengthening adaptive processes" Roy and Andrews (1999, p. 86).
	• "The response of the nurse has been either to provide or support adaptive behaviors, or to compensate for behaviors that may lead to compromised adaptation, often using interpersonal strategies such as teaching" (Roy and Andrews [1999, p. 87]).
Health	A state of adaptation that is manifested in free energy to deal with other stimuli. A process of promoting integrity and wholeness (Roy, 1984, p. 39). A continuous process of being and becoming integrated (Roy and Gliss, 1993).
	• "Coping processes are primary in terms of understanding individual people and relational people, their adaptation, and the nurse's role in enhancing adaptation" (Roy and Andrews [1999, p.87]).

(continued)

TABLE 13-6	Definition of Domain Concepts—Roy (*continued*)
Environment	Internal and external stimuli. There are three classes of stimuli: the focal stimuli (immediately confronting a patient); contextual (all stimuli); residual (pertinent stimuli), but cannot validate effect on current situation. In other words, it is "all conditions, circumstances, and influences surrounding and affecting the development and behavior of individuals and groups." Environment is also a community of beings that includes complex set of interactions and rhythm. (Roy, 1984, p. 39; Roy and Corliss, 1993; Roy and Andrews, 1999; Senesac and Roy, 2015, p. 158; Swimme and Berry, 1992).
Focus	On persons, groups, families, communities, or societies with ineffective behavior, and on manipulation of stimuli so that they would fall within the patient's zone of positive coping. Increase, modify, decrease internal or external stimuli. Traditional interventions such as providing comfort or health teaching, or new undiscovered interventions (Roy, 1984, p. 28).

having been the advisee and student of Dorothy Johnson. Roy's first manuscript, conceptualizing man as an adaptive system, was based on Helson's (1964) theory of adaptation level and was written for Johnson's graduate class on conceptual models in nursing (Roy, 1970). Later influenced by Ralph Turner, a professor of sociology and a prominent scholar in collective behavior and role theory, Roy derived her explication of self-concept and role function.

Forces in the development of her model have been her administrative position at Mount St. Mary's College (Los Angeles, Calif.), which allowed her to further develop her theory through operationalizing it as a framework for the school's curriculum and allowed her the use of the expertise and support of faculty members who taught at that institution. Sister Callista Roy is an eloquent speaker and prolific writer, with a great deal of energy that has helped spread her ideas nationally and internationally. After completing a postdoctoral fellowship at the University of California, San Francisco School of Nursing (where she was trained as a clinical scholar on a Robert Wood Johnson fellowship in 1985), she embarked on a new phase in her research/practice theory career. As a clinical scholar and while in the program, she used her theory in a clinical neurology setting. During the 1990s, she also directed the doctoral program at Boston College, where she continues to be a faculty member. Roy continues to work on the further development of her theory, as well as on extensions through research (Whittemore, Chase, Mandle, et al., 2002) and proposals of middle-range theory (Whittemore and Roy, 2002). The formation of the Roy Adaptation Association (RAA, 2007), which followed the formation of the Boston Based Adaptation Research in Nursing Society (BBARNS, 1999), supported the continuity of scholarship and dissemination of publications and presentations based on RAM.

Paradigmatic Origins

Roy's theory is a synthesis of concepts developed outside the domain of nursing and redefined within the context of nursing. Although Helson's adaptation-level theory appears to be the impetus for the central concept in this theory—adaptation as a process—Roy clearly and admittedly was also influenced by her mentor and teacher, Dorothy Johnson. Johnson conceptualized a person as a behavioral system with seven subsystems, and Roy conceptualized a person as a system with two subsystems, as coping mechanisms, and four modes of coping. The similarities continue to encompass goals of nursing (homeostasis), focus (external regulatory mechanisms), the patients (maladaptive or potentially maladaptive people), and later, a person with ineffective behavior.

Roy's doctoral education in sociology and her work with Ralph Turner, a prominent role theorist, influenced her development of the role, interdependence, and self-concept (an interactionist approach) as effector modes. In the interactionist school of thought, one's self-concept is defined by interaction with others and, therefore, roles enacted by a person and significant others are predicated on their interdependence. These roles and their interdependence shape the concept of self. One-to-one interactions between individuals are characterized by the use of verbal and nonverbal symbolic communication, and it is through these symbolic interactions that roles are shaped. Adjusting this interactionist paradigm shaped a major component of Roy's theory, which she integrated with Helson's adaptation theory to form her conceptualization.

To be specific, Roy's theory evolved from a synthesis of concepts from the adaptation, systems, and interactional paradigms. Parallels exist between the list of concepts and the physiologic modes, Johnson's subsystems of behaviors, Henderson's activities of daily living, and unmet needs (e.g., rest, elimination, and circulation). Elements of systems theory influenced the development of the subsystems (Bertalanffy, 1968). Roy (1970) and Roy and Corliss (1993), acknowledged the influences of Levine (1966), Henderson (1960), Nightingale (1859), and Chardin (1965), among other theorists and philosophers. Further development of Roy's ideas incorporated philosophic principles that are informed by religious beliefs, humanistic ethos, cosmic unity, and integral relationships (Senesac and Roy, 2015).

The development of Roy's theory progressed rather rapidly to meet the curricular needs of Mount St. Mary's College. Therefore, some sense of urgency, as well as the backgrounds of existing faculty, may have contributed to some of the seemingly fragmented and overlapping concepts in its early development. This expediency may have created content to be used in a curriculum, rather than content that would enhance the development of nursing knowledge through questioning and refinement (Roy, 1989). All these influences and forces have been acknowledged in later writings (Andrews and Roy, 1986). The shift to more clinical and research focus is apparent in the later writings of Roy (Roy and Andrews, 1991; Roy and Corliss, 1993; Roy, 2009) and is credited to her postdoctoral education. At the turn of the century, a new phase in Roy's theory has been well established to advance, refine, and extend it. This is clearly the research phase of Roy's theory. Many utilizers of her theory operationalized concepts, developed research projects based on her theory, and ventured into developing middle-range theories.

Internal Dimensions

Roy's theory is a moderately abstract, logically deductive microtheory of the nursing client developed around descriptions of concepts; therefore, it is a concatenated theory developed around adaptation and its modes. Roy uses a field approach, connecting human beings with environment through interactions, although her approach started as monadic. The theory has a broad scope. It provides a framework with the potential of addressing a broad range of problem areas related to the client who has demonstrated ineffective responses to internal and external stimuli. The theory's goal is to conceptualize the nursing client (in Roy's early writings) as four coping modes, and (in later writing) as a system with two subsystems—the regulator and the cognator—and

even later as input, two subsystems, four effector modes, and output (Roy, 1984; Roy and Andrews, 1999). Roy and Roberts (1981) proposed the Roy theory as "a nursing practice theory . . . which is the knowledge of disorder" (p. 24); however, it provides a framework to organize knowledge that addresses modes and mechanisms of adaptation of effective as well as ineffective behavior.

Theory Critique

Roy's theory evolved from mental imagery of what nursing is, who the nursing client is, and what the goal of nursing care is. It was deductively derived from other theoretical formulations but was not based on research findings, nor did it generate many published research findings historically (Roy, 1976, p. 691; Roy and McLeod, 1981). This changed in the 1990s, when a decisive shift occurred from a focus on curriculum development to generating research and findings to lend support to theoretical propositions that evolved from theory. Establishing a focused program of research led Roy to develop two middle-range theories of cognitive processing and coping and adaptation processing (Roy, 2011b). During years of theory development, Roy has clarified her own philosophical assumptions and discussed them (Roy, 1988a; Roy and Corliss, 1993). Some of her assumptions could be propositions and therefore could be tested. One example is the conceptualization of human beings as having four coping modes. Furthermore, which behaviors are components of what mode of coping also needs to be subjected to evaluation. Roy acknowledges such directions in formulating propositions (Roy, 1980; Roy and Andrews, 1999) (Box 13-15).

Roy systematically developed theoretical propositions to promote research projects. Initially, the propositions were based more on neurologic and

BOX 13-15	PROPOSITIONS—ROY

- Nursing actions promote a person's adaptive responses.
- Nursing actions can decrease a person's ineffective adaptive responses.
- People interact with changing environment in an attempt to achieve adaptation and health.
- Nursing actions enhance the interaction of persons with environment.
- Enhanced interactions of persons with environment promote adaptation.

biologic sciences. Some of these propositions tended to reduce the person to responding to chemical or neural stimuli through neural inputs (Roy and Roberts, 1981, pp. 62–66). However, as she continued to develop her theory, the nursing perspective was demonstrated, with more attention paid to propositions that are more congruent with the nature of nursing, and that thereby incorporated a more wholistic aspect of human beings. On the basis of the assumptions of wholism, spirituality, and lived experiences, she promoted qualitative studies to uncover how clients tend to manifest models and mechanisms of adaptation (e.g., Gagliardi, Frederickson, and Shanley, 2002). Concept clarity could be enhanced by defining the theoretical distinctiveness of such related concepts as role, interdependence, and self-concept, as well as by providing valid empirical referents and reliable data related to each. The clarity of a theory in nursing could be enhanced by explicit relatedness between its central concepts. Roy's physiologic mode requires more clarity to better relate it to the other three modes of adaptation.

Many studies were conducted using Roy's theory, and a number of integrative analyses have contributed to advancing knowledge related to adaptation (Dobratz, 2008; Frederickson, 2000); some were directed to exploring and further developing concepts that are not as central to the theory, such as perceptions of the nursing clients. However, the patient's perceptions of her own situations were not central to the conceptualization of a person. Nevertheless, the earliest research projects focused on perceived adaptation levels of the elderly client (Idle, 1978) and perceptions of decision-making (Roy, 1977), rather than on empirically describing systems, effectors, or ineffective responses. When she later developed her theory, "perception" emerged as a central concept linking the regulator and cognator mechanisms (Bunting, 1988). Others, such as Randall, Poush-Tedrow, and Van Landingham (1982), provided support for the centrality of perceptions in understanding the experience and manifestations of adaptation. Although Roy acknowledged and supported the notion of client involvement in care, as alluded to in the following early quote, "According to this nursing model, the person is to be respected as an active participant in his care . . . The goal arrived at is one of mutual agreement between the nurse and patient. Intervention[s] are the options that the nurse provides for the patient" (Roy and Roberts, 1981, p. 47), the lack of integration of the concept perception in theory continued to be an issue. Several major recommendations for

revising the theory were subsequently provided by the BBARNS in 1999; among them is the need to give special attention to the roles of the concepts of perception and time in the theory. Perrett and Biley (2013) argued that perceptual processing, which Roy (2009) has identified as equal and one of four cognitive channels along with learning, judgment and emotion, is primary and vital to be engaged in, prior to any other cognitive process. In an integrative review of the qualitative research based on Roy's theory, Perrett (2007) concluded that the studies reviewed provided support for the propositions that time and perception influence adaptation. However, further thought should be given to how these concepts are interwoven into the theory's fabric. Theoretical propositions driven by the tenets of the theory and inclusive of these vital concepts to adaptation may enhance the potential of intervention-based research.

Many authors consider Roy's theory useful in integrating findings related to a particular patient's condition or set of problems. By providing a coherent framework to review findings, new meanings emerge and gaps in knowledge are identified. An example is Nayback (2009), who examined the posttraumatic stress disorders among military veterans and concluded that using Roy's theory is a more effective way to identify gaps in knowledge.

Roy's theory was used to develop research instruments, to describe responses to different health/illness concepts, and to evaluate interventions. Tools were developed early in the theory's history to measure perceptions of adaptation levels (Idle, 1978), perceptions of powerlessness in decision-making (Roy, 1979), health care outcomes for cancer patients (Lewis, Firsich, and Parsell, 1978, 1979), regaining functional abilities after delivery (Tulman and Fawcett, 1988). In total, and as of this writing, according to a very thorough review and critique of instruments developed and driven by the theory, 123 instruments were used in 231 studies over 30 years (Barone, Roy, and Frederickson, 2008). These instruments were developed to study the four adaptive modes and the cognator processing mechanism; other instruments were used with multiple adaptive modes. Of all these instruments, 21 met criteria for analysis by Barone et al. (2008). The authors identified 14 of them that are highly useful and should be used in the future to advance theory-based knowledge. Since the analysis by Barone and colleagues, Roy's theory has also been used as the basis for developing and using an instrument to assess antenatal behaviors in the four adaptive modes, an instrument that may be valuable for midwifery practice (Lee, Tsang, Wong, et al., 2011).

Roy's theory was used as a framework in multiple descriptive and exploratory research studies. In each of these studies, the use of the adaptation modes and the processes provided a framework to organize the questions and the categories in which responses could be housed. This framework helped facilitate data gathering, interpretation, and reporting, but perhaps not proposition confirmation. The theory was used as a framework to study the experiences and responses of clients to parental touch of preterm infants (Harrison, Leeper, and Yoon, 1990), of spinal cord–injured women during pregnancy (Craig, 1990), and of adult survivors of multiple traumas (Strohmyer, Noroian, Patterson, et al., 1993). It has been used to study spousal adaptation to mates' coronary artery bypass surgery (Artinian, 1991, 1992), the concerns and adaptation of new mothers after cesarean birth (Weiss, Fawcett, and Aber, 2009), and coping and adaptation of mothers during puerperium (Ospina, Munoz, and Ruiz, 2012). Its use helped to uncover the information needs of support in each one of the adaptation modes for patients who have undergone liver transplantation (Ordin, Karayurt, and Wellard, 2013); to describe how nausea and vomiting during pregnancy are manifested, influenced by, and affect each of the four adaptation modes (Isbir and Mete, 2013); and to determine the spiritual needs of cancer patients facing a terminal diagnosis (Granero-Molina, Cortes, Membrive, et al., 2014). It has also been used to explain factors that enhance healing after coronary bypass grafting (DiMattio and Tulman, 2003) as well as the complex relationship between social support and anxiety in pregnant and postpartum women and how they impact role function (Aktan, 2012). In the 21st century, Roy's theory continues to enjoy unusual research activity in describing relations between concepts as a framework for nursing intervention and for interpretation of results.

An example of another type of intervention that is well explained by Roy's theoretical framework is that of "touch." Certain types of touch (a focal stimulus in Roy's theory) were found to enhance the effectiveness of both the regulator and cognator adaptive systems in preterm infants. These then infer the preterm infant's ability to cope, as manifested in the physiologic and interdependence modes. Infants' responses included heart rate and oxygen saturation stability; decreased motor ability, which preserves energy; decreased behavioral stress cues;

and quiet sleep (Modrcin-Talbott, Harrison, Groer, et al., 2003).

Wendler (2003) used Roy's theory for another type of touch intervention for healthy adults receiving venipuncture (a noxious focal stimulus). "Tellington Touch" (redefined as a contextual stimulus) is a type of touch that was adapted from an approach used to calm horses. Wendler (2003) concluded that the touch intervention enhanced the regulator system and thus enhanced adaptation.

Different theories provide frameworks to study nursing needs and outcomes in different settings, as well as for clients at different times in the life span. Roy's theory has been used to study children (Waweru, Reynolds, and Buckner, 2008), adolescents (Ramini, Brown, and Buckner, 2008), and elders (Chen, 2005; Chen, Chang, Chyun, et al., 2005). It was used for acute and chronic conditions, and for adaptation to hospital and community settings.

In another group of studies, the researchers used Roy's theory as a framework to interpret data and connect findings with other similar findings (e.g., Gagliardi, 2003). Dobratz (2003) found that using a theoretical framework to teach undergraduate students about research helped the students integrate their research experience. Similarly, the theory was used as a foundation from which the dynamics of quality of life was researched and interpreted from the intersection of relationships between patients who had lung transplants and their caregivers (Lefaiver, Keough, Letizia, et al., 2007). Another way Roy's theory was used was to develop nursing interventions to help men who suffered childhood traumas to cope and adapt (Willis, DeSanto-Madeya, Ross, et al., 2015).

In addition to research utilization, it was used in practice, education, and for administration of health care systems. It was integrated with the process of clinical judgment, and it offered an excellent checklist for the assessment of variables responsible for problematic behavior resulting from environmental stimuli (i.e., focal, contextual, and residual stimuli) and the setting of priorities for action; for example, for understanding the lack of motivation to quit smoking (Villareal, 2003). The theory was also used in assessing and planning care for patients in surgical settings (Roy, 1971), in community settings (Cunningham, 2002; Hanchett, 1990; Schmitz, 1980), and in obstetric and pediatric settings—in short, in distributive and episodic settings (Wagner, 1976). The setting that created the most difficulty was the intensive care setting (Wagner, 1976). The theory has demonstrated its usefulness in assessing gerontology patients (Farkas, 1981; Janelli, 1980), young children (Galligan, 1979), cardiac patients (Gordon, 1974), patients with organic brain damage (Hamer, 1991), postpartum patients (Kehoe, 1981), and fathers whose mates undergo cesarean delivery (Fawcett, 1981a). It has been useful in neonatal care (Downey, 1974), in demonstrating depression and life satisfaction among a group of retired people (Hoch, 1987), and for acute psychiatric patients (Kurek-Ovshinsky, 1991). Although the theory discussed human development, human aging processes are not clarified (Wadensten and Carlsson, 2003). Despite these clinical examples of effective theory utilization in practice, there are indications of a lack of boundary clarity between role function, interdependence, and self-concept (Wagner, 1976).

In all these studies, the utility of a checklist to identify normal behavior and deviations from normal behavior was demonstrated, and the theory's potential for identifying outcomes criteria to be used for quality assurance was also demonstrated (Laros, 1977). At the same time, however, these studies demonstrated a lack of concept boundaries, which is a limitation of the theory's framework for understanding the nature of person–environment interactions, other than providing descriptive accounts of correlations between stimuli and individuals' responses (Young-McCaughan, Mays, Arzola, et al., 2003). There are some thoughtful and useful directions for developing nursing therapeutics based on theory.

The theory's circle of contagiousness in education is wide and extensive compared with other theories. Conferences were planned in the 1970s through 2010 for educators interested in using the theory as a framework for their curriculum. The annual conference planned by Mount St. Mary's College is another indication of the wide interest that continues for the theory (Wallace, 1993). For educational settings faced with the need to develop a conceptual framework for curricula, the availability of a theory that has been operationalized at Mount St. Mary's College School of Nursing, including the textbooks and literature to use, made for enthusiastic adoption of the theory. Roy's theory has been used in 11 states (27 schools) and also in Canada and Switzerland (Fawcett, 1984). The theory has also been used in specialty curricula (Brower and Baker, 1976). The challenges inherent in operationalizing and implementing Roy's theory drive faculty to develop some innovative approaches to promote a more adaptive implementation (Morales-Mann and Logan, 1990), ideas that have been extended internationally (Fawcett, 2003).

Clinical setting administrators have also attempted a further operationalization of the theory in several settings. In each instance, it provided a framework for assessment of patient needs in each of the modes and a ready-made, usable classification system for the stimuli. Recording of patient care needs was rendered more organized and simple, and there were indications of increased patient satisfaction and expanded professional practice (Laros, 1977; Mastal, Hammond, and Roberts, 1982). In a case study analysis, Gless (1995) demonstrated the clinical utility of Roy's theory in supporting and promoting a quadriplegic patient's ability to cope with living in a long-term care facility.

All concepts related to the physiologic mode, or effectors, are concrete and are most directly related to observable data; data related to this mode tend to predominate in the findings. Perhaps this is partially because concepts from the other three modes are generally abstract, less operationalized, and beset with unclear boundaries. The concepts are theoretically defined but lack both boundary validity and operational definition. Adaptation, the consequence of nursing care—a process and an end result—lacks both theoretical and operational definition and validity. Exemplars of adapted patients and patients with ineffective behavior (process and product) could help in advancing the theoretical development of concept definitions.

Concepts tend to be somewhat tautological, such as focal stimuli, which are also identified behaviors in each of the modes. The view of a person as an open interacting system and the view of input and output appear to be inconsistent, even though Roy, in her later writings, incorporated both input and output within her conceptualization of a person.

External Components of Theory

Society and other health care professionals would agree that nursing deals with the physiologic needs of the patient and the goal of adaptation in that mode, but there may be less agreement on the role of nursing in relation to other modes. Perhaps this is because of the decreasing time that nurses spend with patients in hospitals and the still-limited development of theory for utilization in home and community care. It is also because of the focus of the health care system on biologic and physiologic aspects of care. The systematic assessment potential that Roy's theory offers is congruent with the prevailing view of a need for an organized system in assessment and intervention, and utility of the nursing process in patient care.

The theory's simplicity and the available operationalized teaching-oriented literature enhanced its wide geographical spread but limited its more thoughtful and inquisitive use; coping mechanisms of cognator and regulator continue to require clarification. The complexity of the propositions has initially slowed the theory's operationalization for research projects. Educators and clinicians, however, in search of a coherent way to readily present and discuss their care or teaching, found the theory useful and provided more face validity to the theory's concepts. Conversely, researchers initially ignored the theory, found the complexity of the propositions and their physiologic perspective cumbersome or unrepresentative of the nursing perspective, or tended to use the theory as a framework without connecting its concepts to the whole research process from conceptualization to interpretation; these researchers, therefore, turned to other perspectives. For whatever reasons, creative projects proceeded from face validity studies to construct criterion validity, and, at the beginning of the 21st century, to relational research. This progression represents a strength of this theory.

Another major strength of Roy's theory lies in its exemplary nature of theory development. The theory evolved from a belief that nursing makes a unique contribution to patient care and that the recipient of care is an open adaptive system. After structurally identifying major components of theory, assumptions, and concepts, Roy and many others who have used the theory, provided evidence for its utility as a framework for the different missions in the discipline of nursing.

Theory Testing

Studies were conducted by Roy during her postdoctoral Robert Wood Johnson fellowship at the University of California, San Francisco, to determine the cognitive processes in patients with head injury and to test different propositions of the theory (Roy and Andrews, 1991). The results provided detailed descriptions of patterns of information processing of patients over the course of their illness due to head injury. Results also supported the proposition that nursing interventions using Roy's theory tended to improve cognitive processing of these patients (Roy and Andrews, 1991). Others have used the theory to describe responses to chronic illness (Pollock, 1986), perceptions of stressors of children in an intensive care unit (Munn and Tichy, 1987), the needs of spouses of surgical patients (Silva, 1987), and the differences between recovery rates in the

functional abilities of postpartum vaginal and cesarean delivery patients (Tulman and Fawcett, 1988).

Studies were conducted to test the relationships among several of the theory's concepts. Findings indicate that the four response modes (physiologic, self-concepts, interdependence, and roles) are not interrelated (Nuamah, Cooley, Fawcett, et al., 1999). Other findings provide support that focal, contextual, and one of the components of coping mechanisms, the passive–avoidance coping strategies, were related to psychological stress, which is one of the indicators for adaptation in the self-concept mode (Levesque, Ricard, Ducharme, et al., 1998).

Roy's propositions related to spirituality also received some attention (Malinski, 2002). Putting trust in God and speaking of religion during illness and recovery was found to be an important coping strategy for black patients on hemodialysis (Burns, 2004). Conceptualizing spirituality as a residual stimulus was associated with adjustment to end-stage renal diseases for women (Tanyi and Werner, 2003). Using role function mode as a framework, Dobratz (1984, 2004) conceptualized and discussed death as life-closing spirituality; she subsequently defined life closure as "behavior indicative of a reintegrated self-concept that reflects mastery, growth and transformation through life's meanings, values and purposeful existence," a definition that reflects a more inclusive view of spirituality (Dobratz, 2014, p. 55).

The effects of interventions designed within an adaptation framework were evaluated in several studies. Examples are evaluation of the effects of using a birth chair on mothers and infants (Cottrell and Shannahan, 1986, 1987) and of prenatal education on unplanned cesarean birthing (Fawcett and Henklein, 1987). Fawcett's (1981b) research in identifying the needs of parents facing cesarean section is an example of significant research offering support to Roy's modes of adaptation as a primary assessment framework. An example of particular significance is a study to identify the adaptation modes and needs of postpartum women after a cesarean birth, considering how common cesarean surgeries have become globally (Weiss et al., 2009). Levels of adaptation have been an elusive consequence but a most significant aid in understanding the nursing care process and its intended goals. The study of Lewis et al. (1979), geared toward developing an instrument to measure the adaptation level of chemotherapy patients, is a step in the right direction in the empirical definition of adaptation. Studies using experimental design to test the effectiveness of Roy-driven intervention by school nurses to empower adolescents with attention deficit hyperactivity disorder (Frame, 2003) and human touch to enhance the well-being of preterm infants (decreased motor activity, decreased behavior stress cues, increased quiet sleep, and stabilized heart rate and oxygen saturation) supported the proposition that by intervening in the regulator and cognator subsystem, coping response modes are enhanced (Modrcin-Talbott et al., 2003).

Roy's studies, reported in Roy and Andrews (1999) and Roy (2011b), also support the effectiveness of interventions driven by her theory in improving cognitive functioning in patients with head injury. Bakan and Akyol (2008) used the theory as a framework to develop and test Roy-based interventions to improve the quality of life and functional capacity of heart failure patients and found the intervention effective. Contributions of research findings synthesized by Pollock, Frederickson, Carson, et al. (1994) provided guidelines for further testing of the theory and the rationale for collaboration of researchers who are using the same theory. Akyil and Erguney (2013) used the theory to test the effects of an education program driven by each of the adaptation modes on patients with chronic obstructive pulmonary disease; the study's findings indicated that theory-guided interventions increased adaptation in only three modes (physiologic, self-concept, and role function). A care plan based on Roy's theory significantly increased adaptation of stroke patients in physiologic mode (Alimohammadi, Maleki, Shahriari, et al., 2015). When a formal orientation period was designed for new nurses, it facilitated their adaptation (Ashton, 2015). Relationships between study variables and theory concepts need further analysis (see Table 13-6 and Box 13-15). The BBARNS renamed the Roy Adaptation Association in 2001, enhanced the systematic testing and further development of Roy's theory (Fawcett, 2002; Fawcell and DeSanto-Madeya, 2013). Roy's theory was used to test the relationship between constant interaction with changing environment through an exercise program and its effect on sleep and quality of life (Young-McCaughan et al., 2003), and to test family adaptation to spinal cord injury (DeSanto-Madeya, 2006, 2009).

There was also support for the use of Roy's intervention-based theory that empowered preadolescents with attention deficit hyperactivity disorder and enhanced their perception of self-worth (Frame, 2003; Frame, Kelly, and Bayley, 2003). Likewise, it was used with adolescents in an asthma camp to change adaptive outcomes related to taking responsibility for one's own care. The results indicated that adolescents demonstrated responsibility in management in the interdependence mode (Buckner, Simmons, Brakefield, et al., 2007).

Roy provides a useful framework for testing environmental stimuli barriers and mobility. Shyu et al. (2004) found evidence in their study on the mobility of Taiwanese patients who had undergone hip surgery to support the proposed theoretical relationship that links environment and individual adaptive modes. On the other hand, Samarel, Tulman, and Fawcett's (2002) study on testing different types of support and education on adaptation to early-stage breast cancer did not yield significant differences between the different groups of women receiving different Roy-based interventions.

Roy's theory has been dynamic and actively pursued for the development of middle-range theories by many utilizers in two areas: (1) caregivers' effectiveness and well-being and (2) coping with pain and chronicity. Five middle-range theories were developed based on Roy's theory. Tsai (2003) developed a theory to describe stress of caregivers who are relatives of chronically ill individuals. A similar middle-range theory was developed by Smith and her colleagues to describe and predict family caregiving effectiveness and patient and caregivers' well-being (Smith, Pace, Kochinda, et al., 2002).

Roy's theory has been also used as a framework to develop and test a middle-range theory about chronic pain in older people with arthritis (Tsai, Tak, Moore, et al., 2003). A similar middle-range theory was modified to describe adaptation to chronic pain (Dunn, 2004), and to help women better manage their chronic illness (Weinert, Cudney, and Spring, 2008). Roy herself, in collaboration with Whittemore, developed a middle-range theory that extends her adaptation framework to explain coping with diabetes mellitus through theory, concept synthesis, and the use of empirical evidence (Whittemore and Roy, 2002). A review of Roy adaptation model demonstrates a cumulative pattern in conducting research and integrating the results toward developing two middle-range theories; cognitive recovery from mild head injury and coping and adaption processing (Roy, 2011b).

Roy's theory has been used as a framework to further develop concepts such as social isolation in older adults, in which five attributes were identified: number of contacts, feeling of belonging, fulfilling relationships, engagement wishes, and quality of network. The author concludes that, as conceptualized, social isolation may be a productive variable in research if incorporated with the Roy Adaptation Model (Nicholson, 2009). Another example is its use in developing the concept of quality of life as perceived by lung transplant candidates and their caregivers (Lefaiver, Keough, Letizia, et al., 2007).

Although time and cultural constraints may place some limits on international use of the theory, it enjoys a global presence and is considered a vehicle to promote better patient care, improve communication, and facilitate studies (Shah, Abdullah, and Khan, 2013). It has been used to describe the perceptions of children suffering from HIV/AIDS in Kenya (Waweru et al., 2008). It was adapted as a framework for a nursing curriculum in Colombia (Moreno, Durán, and Hernandez, 2009), and it was used to develop interventions to enhance the adaptation of patients with heart failure in Turkey (Bakan and Akyol, 2008). Yeh (2002, 2003) used Roy's theory to test the relationship between environmental stimuli and biopsychosocial responses of children with cancer in Taiwan. She found the theory translatable and the proposition that links environments with responses well supported. Others provided mixed reviews of translating the concepts of self-concept, interdependence, and role function into other cultures (Chung, 2004). However, a general review of the theory's international utilization reveals that it is effective for use in different cultures (Roy Adaptation Association, 2007), and that eastern and Latin American countries have used the theory extensively. Roy Adaptation Associations have been formed in Japan, Columbia, and Mexico (Roy, Whetsell, and Frederickson, 2009).

Roy believes her theory can be a framework for global health. She applies the four adaptive modes and that contributes to health and quality of life and end-of-life that focused on individuals and groups functioning, coordination, identity formation, integrated and collaborative processes, and interdependence. By doing that she planted the seeds of using the theory to meet changing global needs and advancing knowledge related to global functioning and adaptation (Roy, 2011a).

CONCLUSION

There is a growing contemporary dialogue in health care fields on patient-centered care and outcomes of care. This dialogue makes the client the focus of health care and health care outcomes the ultimate goal and test for quality care. The emphasis in nursing practice has always been on the client, in historical as well as contemporary times. Whether the client is an individual, a family, or a community, the nurse's work begins with a careful assessment of the client and plans for the appropriate intervention by focusing on the needs, resources, the problems, or the responses experienced and/or observed in the client. In this chapter, five nursing theorists spanning the decades of the 1950s, 1960s, and 1970s demonstrate an emphasis on client-centered care in their theories. There is also a focus on outcomes of care. Johnson defines a client as a behavioral system with seven subsystems, and a nurse's role and goal is to regulate and preserve the organization and integration of the patients' behaviors, particularly when the subsystems are threatened. Levine focuses on conserving and mobilizing energy. To Roy, the client is a person, a family, a group, or a community, and is a biopsychosocial adaptive system with two processor subsystems. The client is capable of adapting through the regulator and cognator processes. The goal of nursing is to enhance adaptation through four modes—the physiologic–physical mode, the self-concept mode, the role function mode, and the interdependent mode. To Neuman, nurses are concerned about keeping clients' systems stable. They do that through first addressing the concentric lines of resistance, then penetrating lines of defense, all to keep the client's central structure intact. The nurse's role is to prevent stressors from penetrating flexible lines of defense, preserve lines of resistance, and support a client's resources.

Although these theorists did not ignore the environment (environment is the focus for Rogers), it is clear that the core of their theories was to provide a framework to understand who the client is. The questions that these theories generated addressed stability and instability, adaptation, coping, and the consequences of nurses' interventions that facilitate and promote these processes.

In addition to Florence Nightingale, who introduced nursing to the notion of the centrality of environment in nurses' domain of practice, Martha Rogers is the person–environment relationship guru. Furthermore, her theory supports the essentiality of patterns and patterning in understanding the experiences of health and illness. She also reinforced the idea that nursing is based on science. She pioneered the connection between physics and nursing, and she provided the optimistic view of health that empowers the individual as well as the professional nurse. She was a visionary thinker, an

REFLECTIVE QUESTIONS

1. Why were these theorists grouped together in this chapter?

2. Compare and contrast how "client" was conceptualized by each of the five theorists presented in this chapter. What are some common propositions, and in what ways do they differ drastically?

3. Which, if any, of these definitions and views of client persist in contemporary nursing practice?

4. Compare and contrast the outcomes in each theory.

5. What are some paradigmatic origins shared by the five theorists discussed in this chapter and which appear to be contradictory?

6. Critics differ on how Martha Rogers' theory has influenced progress in the discipline of nursing. A group of critics considers her theory to completely miss the substance and goals of nursing. Others believe that she was a theorist who was ahead of her time. Where do you stand on your views of her theory? Be specific, support your analysis, and indicate why.

7. How does Rogers define the concepts of energy and interaction? Develop research questions that could advance knowledge about these two concepts.

8. Identify one research instrument that needs development to test one vital proposition in each theory.

9. Make a case for a different approach to categorizing the five theorists discussed in this chapter. Provide the rationale for the proposed categorization.

10. Select one of the theorists and develop a research project to test two or three propositions that could extend knowledge in your field of practice. In what ways would the results of the selected research questions extend the theory?

11. Identify three ways by which any of the theories may extend nursing knowledge in your field.

12. Rogers rejected reductionism, causality, the separation of person and environment, and what else? What scientific value did she embrace and in what ways did these values inform her theory? Compare and contrast her approach with Johnson's.

13. How would Rogers' theory explain hyperactivity, type A behavior, attention deficit hyperactivity, and sleep disorders? What research propositions may help support or refute her possible explanation?

14. Describe a program of research within your field of interest that is informed by any one of the theories.

15. Identify two middle-range theories that evolved from Rogers' and Roy's theories. Critically assess their congruence with explicit and implicit assumptions in Rogers' theory.

inspiring leader, and a theorist who was ahead of her time. She saw the world of nursing very differently, and provided a framework for others to experience this perspective. Despite many critics, many of her concepts and propositions continue to stimulate innovative nursing research.

These theories continue to generate fundamental as well as translational questions that could enhance nursing science, as well as enrich nursing practice.

REFERENCES

Johnson

Ainsworth, M. (1972). Attachment and dependency: A comparison. In J. Gewirtz (Ed.), *Attachment and dependency*. Englewood Cliffs, NJ: Prentice-Hall.

Alligood, M.R. (2014). Philosophies, models, theories: Critical thinking structures. In M.R. Alligood (Ed.), *Nursing theory: Utilization and applications* (5th ed., pp. 40–62). St. Louis, MO: Mosby.

Auger, J.A. (1976). *Behavioral systems and nursing*. Englewood Cliffs, NJ: Prentice-Hall.

Auger, J.A. and Dee, U. (1983). A patient classification system based on the behavioral system model of nursing: Part 1. *The Journal of Nursing Administration*, 13(4), 38–43.

Bluhm, R.L. (2014). The (dis)unity of nursing science. *Nursing Philosophy*, 15(4), 250–260.

Bruce, G.L., Hinds, P., Hudak, J., Mucha, A., Taylor, M.C., and Thompson, C.R. (1980). Implementation of ANA's quality assurance program for clients with end-stage renal disease. *Advances in Nursing Science*, 2(2), 79–95.

Buckley, W. (1968). *Modern systems research for the behavioral scientist*. Chicago, IL: Aldine.

Chen, C.J., Chen, Y.C., Sung, H.C., Kuo, P.C, and Wang, C.H. (2011). Perinatal attachment in naturally pregnant and infertility-treated pregnant women in Taiwan. *Journal of Advanced Nursing*, 67(10), 2200–2208.

Chin, R. (1961). The utility of system models and developmental models for practitioners. In W.G. Bennis, K.D. Beene, and R. Chin (Eds.), *The planning of change* (pp. 201–215). New York: Holt, Rinehart and Winston.

Colling, J., Owen, T.R., McCreedy, M., and Newman, D. (2003). The effects of a continence program on frail community-dwelling elderly persons. *Urologic Nursing*, 23(2), 117–127, 127–131.

Coward, D.D. and Wilkie, D.J. (2000). Metastatic bone pain: Meanings associated with self-report and self-management decision making. *Cancer Nursing*, 23(2), 101–108.

Damus, K. (1980). An application of the Johnson behavioral system model for nursing practice. In J.P. Riehl and C. Roy (Eds.), *Conceptual models for nursing practice* (2nd ed.). New York: Appleton-Century-Crofts.

Dee, V. (1986). *Validation of a patient classification instrument for psychiatric patients based on the Johnson model for nursing.* Unpublished doctoral dissertation. San Francisco, CA: University of California.

Dee, V. (1990). Implementation of the Johnson model: One hospital's experience. In M.E. Parker (Ed.), *Nursing theories in practice* (pp. 33–44). New York: National League for Nursing.

Dee, V. and Auger, J.A. (1983). A patient classification system based on the behavioral system model of nursing: Part 2. *The Journal of Nursing Administration*, 13(5), 18–23.

Dee. V. and Poster, E.C. (1995). Applying Kanter's theory of innovative change: The transition from a primary to attending model of nursing care delivery. *Journal of American Psychiatric Nurses Association*, 1(4), 112–119.

Dee, V. and van Servellen, G. (1998). Managed behavioral health care patients and their nursing care problems, level of functioning, and impairment at discharge. *Journal of American Psychiatric Nurses Association*, 4(2), 57–66.

Derdiarian, A. (1983). An instrument for theory and research development using the behavioral systems model for nursing: The cancer patient, Part I. *Nursing Research*, 32(4), 196–201.

Derdiarian, A. (1984). *An investigation of the variables and boundaries of cancer nursing: A pioneering approach using Johnson's behavioral systems model for nursing.* In Proceedings of the 3rd International Conference on Cancer Nursing. Melbourne, Australia: The Cancer Institute/Peter MacCallum Hospital and the Royal Melbourne Hospital.

Derdiarian, A.K. (1990a). Effects of using systematic assessment instruments on patient and nurse satisfaction with nursing care. *Oncology Nursing Forum*, 17, 95–101.

Derdiarian, A.K. (1990b). The relationships among the subsystems of Johnson's behavioral system model. *Image: Journal of Nursing Scholarship*, 22, 219–225.

Derdiarian, A.K. (1991). Effects of using a nursing model-based assessment instrument on quality of nursing care. *Nursing Administration Quarterly*, 15(3), 1–16.

Derdiarian, A.K. (1993a). Application of the Johnson behavioral system model in nursing practice. In M.E. Parker (Ed.), *Patterns of nursing theories in practice* (pp. 285–298). New York: National League for Nursing.

Derdiarian, A.K. (1993b). The Johnson behavioral system model: Perspectives for nursing practice. In M.E. Parker (Ed.), *Patterns of nursing theories in practice* (pp. 267–284). New York: National League for Nursing.

Derdiarian, A. and Forsythe, A.B. (1983). An instrument for theory and research development using the behavioral systems model for nursing: The cancer patient, Part II. *Nursing Research*, 32(4), 260–267.

Dickerson, S.S., Alqaissi, N., Underhill, M. and Lally, R.M. (2011). Surviving the wait: Defining support while awaiting breast cancer surgery. *Journal of Advanced Medicine*, 67(7), 1468–1479.

Dickoff, J., James, P., and Wiedenbach, E. (1968). Theory in a practice discipline, Part 1. Practice oriented theory. *Nursing Research*, 17(5), 415–435.

Draucker, C.B., Martsolf, D., and Stephenson, P.S. (2012). Ambiguity and violence in adolescent dating relationships. *Journal of Child and Adolescent Psychiatric Nursing*, 25(3), 149–157.

Feshback, S. (1970). Aggression. In P. Mussen (Ed.), *Carmichael's manual of child psychology* (3rd ed.). New York: John Wiley & Sons.

Grubbs, J. (1980). An interpretation of the Johnson behavioral system model. In J.P. Riehl and C. Roy (Eds.), *Conceptual models for nursing practice* (2nd ed., pp. 217–254). New York: Appleton-Century-Crofts.

Hadley, B.J. (1970, March). *The utility of theoretical frameworks for curriculum development in nursing: The happening at Colorado.* Paper presented at WICHEN General Session, Honolulu, Hawaii.

Harris, R.B. (1986). Introduction of a conceptual model into a fundamental baccalaureate course. *Journal of Nursing Education*, 25, 66–69.

Holaday, B. (1974). Achievement behavior in chronically ill children. *Nursing Research*, 23(1), 25–30.

Holaday, B. (1980). Implementing the Johnson model for nursing practice. In J.P. Riehl and C. Roy (Eds.), *Conceptual models for nursing practice* (2nd ed.). New York: Appleton-Century-Crofts.

Holaday, B. (1981). Maternal response to their chronically ill infants' attachment behavior of crying. *Nursing Research*, 30(6), 343–347.

Holaday, B. (1982). Maternal conceptual set development: Identifying patterns of maternal response to chronically ill infant crying. *Maternal Child Nursing Journal*, 11(1), 47–58.

Holaday, B. (1987). Patterns of interaction between mothers and their chronically ill infants. *Maternal Child Nursing Journal*, 16(1), 29–45.

Holaday, B. (2002). Johnson's behavioral system model in nursing practice. In M.R. Alligood and A. Marriner-Tomey (Eds.), *Nursing theory: Utilization and application* (2nd ed., pp. 149–171). St. Louis, MO: Mosby.

Holaday, B. (2014). Dorothy E. Johnson's behavioral system model. In M.R. Alligood (Ed.), *Nursing theorists and their work* (8th ed., pp. 332–355). St Louis, MO: Mosby

Holaday, B. (2015). Dorothy Johnson's behavioral system model and its application. In M.C. Smith and M.E. Parker (Eds.), *Nursing theories and nursing practice* (4th ed., pp. 89–104). Philadelphia, PA: F.A. Davis

Holaday, B. and Turner-Henson A. (1987). Chronically ill school-age children's use of time. *Pediatric Nursing*, 13, 410–414.

Holaday, B., Turner-Henson, A., and Swan, J. (1996). The Johnson behavioral system model: Explaining activities of chronically ill children. In P. Hinton Walker and B. Neuman (Eds.), *Blueprint for use of nursing models* (pp. 33–63). New York: NLN Press.

Johnson, D.E. (1959a). A philosophy of nursing. *Nursing Outlook*, 7(4), 198–200.

Johnson, D.E. (1959b). The nature of a science of nursing. *Nursing Outlook*, 7(5), 291–294.

Johnson, D.E. (1961). The significance of nursing care. *American Journal of Nursing*, 61(11), 63–66.

Johnson, D.E. (1964, June). *Is there an identifiable body of knowledge essential to the development of a generic professional nursing program?* Paper presented at First Interuniversity Faculty Work Conference Nursing Council, NEBHE, Stowe, VT.

Johnson, D.E. (1968a). Theory in nursing: Borrowed or unique. *Nursing Research*, 17(3), 206–209.

Johnson, D.E. (1968b, April). *One conceptual model of nursing.* Paper presented at Vanderbilt University, Nashville, TN.

Johnson, D.E. (1974). Development of theory: A requisite for nursing as a primary health profession. *Nursing Research*, 23(5), 372–377.

Johnson, D.E. (1978). State of the art of theory development in nursing. In *Theory development: What, why, how?* New York: National League for Nursing.

Johnson, D.E. (1980). The behavioral system model for nursing. In J.P. Riehl and C. Roy (Eds.), *Conceptual models for nursing practice* (2nd ed.). New York: Appleton-Century-Crofts.

Johnson, D.E. (1987). Evaluating conceptual models for use in critical care nursing practice. *Dimensions of Critical Care Nursing*, 6(4), 195–197.

Johnson, D.E. (1989). Some thoughts on nursing. *Clinical Nurse Specialist*, 3(1), 1–4.

Johnson, D.E. (1990). The behavioral system model for nursing. In M.E. Parker (Ed.), *Nursing theories in practice* (pp. 23–32). New York: National League for Nursing.

Johnson, D.E. (1992). The origins of the behavioral system model. In F.N. Nightingale (Ed.), *Notes on nursing: What it is, and what it is not* (Commemorative edition, pp. 23–27). Philadelphia, PA: Lippincott.

Johnson, D.E. (1996). Introduction to the Johnson behavioral system model: Explaining activities of chronically ill children. In P. Hinton Walker and B. Neuman (Eds.), *Blueprint for use of nursing models* (pp. 33–34). New York: NLN Press.

Kaya, N. (2012). Effect of attachment styles of individuals discharged from an intensive care unit on intensive care experience. *Journal of Critical Care*, 27(1), 103e7–103e14.

Lachicotte, J.L. and Alexander, J.W. (1990). Management attitudes and nurse impairment. *Nursing Management*, 21, 102–104, 106, 108, 110.

Lobo, M.L. (2002). Behavioral system model: Dorothy E. Johnson. In J.B. George (Ed.), *Nursing theories: The base for professional nursing practice* (5th ed., pp. 155–169). Upper Saddle River, NJ: Prentice Hall.

Lovejoy, N. (1983). The leukemic child's perceptions of family behaviors. *Oncology Nursing Forum*, 10(4): 20–25.

Lovejoy, N. (1985). *Needs of vigil and nonvigil visitors in cancer research units.* In Fourth Cancer Nursing Research Conference Proceedings. Honolulu, HI: American Cancer Society.

Majesky, S.J., Brester, M.H., and Nishio, K.T. (1978). Development of a research tool: Patient indicators of nursing care. *Nursing Research*, 27(6), 365–371.

Naguib, H.H. (1988). *Physicians', nurses', and patients' perceptions of the surgical patients' educational rights.* Unpublished doctoral dissertation. University of Alexandria, United Republic of Egypt.

Oyedele, O.A., Wright, S.C.D., and Maja, T.M.M. (2013). Prevention of teenage pregnancies in Soshanguve, South Africa: Using the Johnson behavioral system model. *Journal of Nursing and Midwifery*, 15(1), 95–108.

Parsons, T. (1951). *The social system.* New York: Free Press.

Porter, L. (1972). The impact of physical-physiological activity on infants' growth and development. *Nursing Research*, 21(3), 210–219.

Poster, E.C. and Beliz, L. (1988). Behavioral category ratings of adolescents in an inpatient psychiatric unit. *International Journal of Adolescence and Youth*, 1, 293–303.

Poster, E.C. and Beliz, L. (1992). The use of the Johnson behavioral system model to measure changes during adolescent hospitalization. *International Journal of Adolescence and Youth*, 4, 73–84.

Poster, E.C., Dee, V., and Randell, B.P. (1997). The Johnson behavioral system model as framework for patient outcome evaluation. *Journal of the American Psychiatric Nurses Association*, 3, 73–80.

Randell, B.P. (1991). NANDA versus the Johnson behavioral systems model: Is there a diagnostic difference? In R.M. Carroll-Johnson (Ed.), *Classification of nursing diagnoses: Proceedings of the ninth conference. North American Nursing Diagnosis Association* (pp. 154–160). Philadelphia, PA: Lippincott.

Rapaport, A. (1968). Forward. In W. Buckley (Ed.), *Modern systems research for the behavioral scientist* (pp. xiii–xxii). Chicago, IL: Aldine.

Rawls, A.G. (1980). Evaluation of the Johnson behavioral model in clinical practice. *Image*, 12, 13–16.

Reynolds, W. and Cormack, D.F. (1991). An evaluation of the Johnson Behavioral System Model of Nursing. *Journal of Advanced Nursing*, 16(9), 1122–1130.

Sears, R.R., Maccoby, E.E., and Levin, H. (1957). *Patterns of child rearing.* Evanston, IL: Row & Peterson.

Small, B. (1980). Nursing visually impaired children with Johnson's model as a conceptual framework. In J.P. Riehl and C. Roy (Eds.), *Conceptual models for nursing practice* (2nd ed., pp. 264–273). New York: Appleton-Century-Crofts.

Stamler, C. and Palmer, J.O. (1971). Dependency and repetitive visits to the nurse's office in elementary school children. *Nursing Research*, 20(3), 254–255.

von Bertalanffy, L. (1968). *General systems theory: Foundations, development, application.* New York: George Braziller.

Wilkie, D. (1990). Cancer pain management: State-of-the-art care. *Nursing Clinics of North America*, 25, 331–343.

Wu, R. (1973). *Behavior and illness.* Englewood Cliffs, NJ: Prentice-Hall.

Zetterberg, H.L. (1963). *On theory verification in sociology* (Rev. ed.). Totowa, NJ: Bedminster Press.

Levine

Abdellah, F.G. and Levine, E. (1986). *Better patient care through nursing research* (3rd ed.). New York: Macmillan.

Abumaria, I.M., Hastings-Tolsma, M. and Sakraida, T.J. (2015). Levine's conservation model: A framework for advanced gerontology nursing practice. *Nursing Forum*, 50(3), 179–188.

Allvin, R., Berg, K., Idvall, E., and Nilsson, U. (2007). Postoperative recovery: A concept analysis. *Journal of Advanced Nursing*, 57(5), 552–558.

Artigue, G.S., Foli, K.J., Johnson, T., Marriner-Tomey, A., Poat, M.C., Poppa, L.D., Woeste, R., and Zoretich, S.T. (1994). Myra Levine: Four conservation principles. In A. Marriner-Tomey (Ed.), *Nursing theorists and their work* (4th ed., pp. 199–210). St. Louis, MO: C.V. Mosby.

Bao, Y., Vedina, R., Moodie, S. and Dolan, S. (2013). The relationship between value incongruence and individual and organizational well-being outcomes: an exploratory study among Catalan nurses. *Journal of Advanced Nursing*, 69(3), 631–641.

Barnum, B.J.S. (1994). *Nursing theory: Analysis, application, and evaluation* (4th ed.). Philadelphia, PA: Lippincott.

Bates, M. (1967). A naturalist at large. *Natural History*, 76(6), 8–16.

Bernard, C. (1957). *An introduction to the study of experimental medicine*. New York: Dover.

Bertalanffy, L. (1968). *General system theory*. New York: George Braziller.

Buber, M. (1967). *Between man and man*. New York: Macmillan.

Burd, C., Langemo, D.K., Olson, B., Hanson, D., Hunter, S., and Sauvage, T. (1992). Skin problems: Epidemiology of pressure ulcers in a skilled care facility. *Journal of Gerontological Nursing*, 18(9), 29–39.

Burd, C., Olson, B., Langemo, D., Hunter, S., Hanson, D., Osowski, K.F., and Sauvage, T. (1994). Skin care strategies in a skilled nursing home. *Journal of Gerontological Nursing*, 20(1), 28–34.

Cannon, W.B. (1939). *The wisdom of the body*. New York: W.W. Norton.

Cox, R.A., Sr. (1991). A tradition of caring: Use of Levine's model in long-term care. In K.M. Schaefer and J.B. Pond (Eds.), *Levine's conservation model: A framework for nursing practice* (pp. 179–197). Philadelphia, PA: F.A. Davis.

Delmore, B.A. (2006). Levine's framework in long-term ventilated patients during the weaning course. *Nursing Science Quarterly*, 19(3), 247–258.

Donaldson, S.K. and Crowley, D.M. (1978). The discipline of nursing. *Nursing Outlook*, 26(2), 113–120.

Dubos, R. (1966). *Man adapting*. New Haven, CT: Yale University Press.

Erikson, E. (1968). *Identity, youth and crisis*. New York: W.W. Norton.

Esposito, C.H. and Leonard, M.K. (1980). Myra Estrin Levine: In The Nursing Conference Group (Ed.), *Nursing theories: The base for professional practice*. Englewood Cliffs, NJ: Prentice-Hall.

Fawcett, J. (1989). *Analysis and evaluation of conceptual models of nursing* (2nd ed.). Philadelphia, PA: F.A. Davis.

Fawcett, J. (2014). Thoughts about conceptual models, theories, and quality improvement projects. *Nursing Science Quarterly*, 17(4), 336–339.

Fawcett, J. and DeSanto-Madeya (2013). *Contemporary nursing knowledge: Analysis and evaluation of nursing models and theories* (3rd ed.). Philadelphia, PA: F.A. Davis.

Feynman, R. (1965). *The character of physical law*. Cambridge, MA: MIT Press.

Flaskerud, J.H. and Halloran, E.J. (1980). Areas of agreement in nursing theory development. *Advances in Nursing Science*, 3(1), 1–7.

Gagner-Tjellesen, D., Yurkovich, E.E., and Gragert, M. (2001). Use of music therapy and other ITNIs in acute care. *Journal of Psychosocial Nursing and Mental Health Services*, 39(10), 26–37, 52–53.

Grindley, J. and Paradowski M. (1991). Developing an undergraduate program using Levine's model. In K.M. Schaefer and J.B. Pond (Eds.), *Levine's conservation model: A framework for nursing practice* (pp. 199–208). Philadelphia, PA: F.A. Davis.

Hall, K.V. (1979). Current trends in the use of conceptual frameworks in nursing education. *Journal of Nursing Education*, 18(4), 26–29.

Hirschfeld, M.J. (1976). The cognitively impaired older adult. *American Journal of Nursing*, 76(12), 1981–1984.

Irvin, S.M. (2007). Sensorineural hearing changes after myelogram. *Journal of PeriAnesthesia Nursing*, 22(1), 27–39.

Levine, M.E. (1966a). Trophicognosis: An alternative to nursing diagnosis. In *Exploring progress in medical-surgical nursing practice* (Vol. 2, pp. 55–70). New York: American Nurses Association Regional clinical conference.

Levine, M.E. (1966b). Adaptation and assessment: A rationale for nursing intervention. *American Journal of Nursing*, 66(11), 2450–2453.

Levine, M.E. (1967). The four conservation principles of nursing. *Nursing Forum*, 6(1), 45–59.

Levine, M.E. (1969). The pursuit of wholeness. *American Journal of Nursing*, 69(1), 93–98.

Levine, M.E. (1971a). Holistic nursing. *Nursing Clinics of North America*, 6(2), 253–264.

Levine, M.E. (1971b, June). Time has come to speak of health care. *AORN Journal*, 13, 37–43.

Levine, M.E. (1973). *Introduction to clinical nursing* (2nd ed.). Philadelphia, PA: F.A. Davis.

Levine, M.E. (1979). The science is spurious [letter to the editor]. *American Journal of Nursing*, 79(8), 1379–1383.

Levine, M.E. (1989a). The ethics of nursing rhetoric. *Image: Journal of Nursing Scholarship*, 21(1), 4–6.

Levine, M.E. (1989b). The four conservation principles: Twenty years later. In J.P. Riehl (Ed.), *Conceptional models for nursing practice* (3rd ed.). East Norwalk, CT: Appleton & Lange.

Levine, M.E. (1989c). Ethical issues in cancer care: Beyond dilemma. *Seminars in Oncology Nursing*, 5(2), 124–128.

Levine, M.E. (1990). Conservation and integrity. In M.E. Parker (Ed.), *Nursing theories in practice* (pp. 189–202). New York: National League for Nursing.

Levine, M.E. (1991). The conservation principles: A model for health. In K.M. Schaefer and J.B. Pond (Eds.), *Levine's conservation model: A framework for nursing practice* (pp. 1–11). Philadelphia, PA: F.A. Davis.

Levine, M.E. (1995). The rhetoric of nursing theory. *Image: The Journal of Nursing Scholarship*, 27(1), 11–14.

Levine, M.E. (1996). The conservation principles: A retrospective. *Nursing Science Quarterly*, 9(1), 38–41.

Levine, M.E. (1999). On the humanities in nursing . . . originally published as a discourse in *Canadian Journal of Nursing Research*, 1995, 27(2), 19–23. *Canadian Journal of Nursing Research*, 30(4), 213–217.

Mantle, F. (2001). Complementary therapies and nursing models . . . originally published In D. Rankin-Box (Ed.). 2001 Nurse's handbook of complementary therapies. *Complementary Therapies in Nursing and Midwifery*, 7(3), 142–145.

Mefford, L.C. and Alligood, M.R. (2011). Evaluating nurse staffing patterns and neonatal intensive care unit outcomes using Levine's conservation model of nursing. *Journal of Nursing Management*, 19(8), 998–1011.

Mock, V., Pickett, M., Ropka, M.E., Lin, E.M., Steward, K.J., Rhodes, V.A., et al. (2001). Fatigue and quality of life outcomes of exercise during cancer treatment. *Cancer Practice*, 9(3), 119–127. ·

Mock, V., Ropka, M.E., Rhodes, V.A., Pickett, M., Grimm, P.M., McDaniel, R., et al. (1998). Establishing mechanisms to conduct multi-institutional research—fatigue in patients with cancer: An exercise intervention. *Oncology Nursing Forum*, 25(8), 1391–1397.

Mock, V., St. Ours, C., Hall, S., Bositis, A., Tillery, M. et al. (2007). Using a conceptual model in nursing research—mitigating fatigue in cancer patients. *Journal of Advanced Nursing*, 58(5), 503–512.

Netto, L., Moura, M.A., Queiroz, A.B., Tyrrell, M.A. and Bravo, M. (2014). Violence against women and its consequences. *Acta Paulista de Enfermagem*, 27(5), 458–464.

Newport, M.A. (1984). Conserving thermal energy and social integrity in the newborn. *Western Journal of Nursing Research*, 6, 176–197.

Nightingale, F. (1969). *Notes on nursing. What it is and what it is not*. New York: Dover Publications.

Piccoli, M. and Galvao, C.M. (2001). Perioperative nursing: Identification of the nursing diagnosis infection risk based on Levine's conceptual model [Portuguese]. *Revista Latino-Americana de Enfermagem*, 9(4), 37–43.

Pond, J.B. (1990). Application of Levine's conservation model to nursing the homeless community. In M.E. Parker (Ed.), *Nursing theories in practice* (pp. 203–216). New York: National League for Nursing.

Pond, J.B. (1991). Ambulatory care of the homeless. In K.M. Schaefer and J.B. Pond (Eds.). *Levine's conservation model: A framework for nursing practice* (pp. 167–178). Philadelphia, PA: F.A. Davis.

Pond, J.B. and Taney, S.G. (1991). Emergency care in a large university emergency department. In K.M. Schaefer and J.B. Pond (Eds.), *Levine's conservation model: A framework for nursing practice* (pp. 151–166). Philadelphia, PA: F.A. Davis.

Riehl, J.P. (1980). Nursing models in current use. In J.P. Riehl and C. Roy (Eds.), *Conceptual models for nursing practice* (2nd ed.). New York: Appleton-Century-Crofts.

Rogers, C.R. (1961). *On becoming a person*. Boston, MA: Houghton-Mifflin.

Rogers, M.E. (1964). *Reveille in nursing*. Philadelphia, PA: F.A. Davis.

Rogers, M.E. (1970). *An introduction to the theoretical basis of nursing*. Philadelphia, PA: F.A. Davis.

Selye, H. (1956). *The stress of life*. New York: McGraw-Hill.

Taylor, J.W. (1974). Measuring the outcomes of nursing care. *Nursing Clinics of North America*, 9(2), 337–348.

Taylor, J.W. (1989). Levine's conservation principles: Using the model for nursing diagnosis in a neurological setting. In J. Riehl-Sisca (Ed.), *Conceptual models for nursing practice* (3rd ed.). East Norwalk, CT: Appleton & Lange.

Teeri, S., Välimäki, M., Katajisto, J., and Leino-Kilpi, H. (2007). Nurses perceptions of older patients integrity in long-term institutions. *Scandinavian Journal of Caring Science*, 21(4), 490–499.

Tillich, P. (1961). The meaning of health. *Perspectives in Biology and Medicine*, 5, 92–100.

Tompkins, E.S. (1980). Effect of restricted mobility and dominance on perceived duration. *Nursing Research*, 29(6), 333–338.

Webster's Third New International Dictionary. (1986). Springfield, MA: Merriam-Webster.

Neuman

Angosta, A.D., Ceria-Ulep, C.D., and Tse, A.M. (2014). Care delivery for Filipino Americans using the Neuman systems model. *Nursing Science* Quarterly, 27(2), 142–148.

Barnum, B.J.S. (1998). *Nursing theory: Analysis, application, evaluation* (5th ed.). Philadelphia, PA: Lippincott Williams & Wilkins.

Baumann, S.L. (2012). What's wrong with the concept of self-management? *Nursing Science Quarterly*, 25(4), 362–363.

Beckman, S.J., Boxley-Harges, S.L. and Kaskel, B.L. (2012). Experience informs: Spanning three decades with the Neuman systems model. *Nursing Science Quarterly*, 25(4), 341–346.

Beddome, G. (1989). Application of the Neuman systems model to the assessment of community-as-client. In B. Neuman (Ed.), *The Neuman systems model* (2nd ed.). East Norwalk, CT: Appleton & Lange.

Benedict, M.B. and Sproles, J.B. (1982). Application of the Neuman model to public health nursing practice. In B. Neuman (Ed.), *The Neuman systems model: Application to nursing education and practice*. Norwalk, CT: Appleton-Century-Crofts.

Bergstrom, D. (1992). Hypermetabolism in multisystem organ failure: A Neuman systems perspective. *Critical Care Nursing Quarterly*, 15(3), 63–70.

Bertalanffy, L. (1968). *General system theory*. New York: George Braziller.

Bourbonnais, F.F. and Ross, M.M. (1985). The Neuman systems model in nursing education: Course development and implementation. *Journal of Advanced Nursing*, 10(2), 117–123.

Bourdeanu, L. and Dee, V. (2013). Assessment of chemotherapy-induced nausea and vomiting in women with breast cancer: A Neuman systems model framework. *Research and Theory for Nursing Practice: An International Journal*, 27(4), 296–304.

Breckenridge, D.M. (1989). Primary prevention as an intervention modality for the renal client. In B. Neuman (Ed.), *The Neuman systems model* (2nd ed.). East Norwalk, CT: Appleton & Lange.

Breckenridge, D.M. (2002). Using the Neuman systems model to guide nursing research in the United States. In B. Neuman and J. Fawcett (Eds.), *The Neuman systems model* (4th ed., pp. 176–182). Upper Saddle River, NJ: Prentice Hall.

Breckenridge, D. (2011). The Neuman systems model and evidence-based nursing practice. In B. Neuman and J. Fawcett (Eds.). *The Neuman systems model* (5th ed., pp. 245–252). Upper Saddle River, NJ: Pearson Education Press.

Brink, L.W., Neuman, B., and Wynn, J. (1992). Transport of the critically ill patient with upper airway obstruction. *Critical Care Clinics*, 8(3), 633–647.

Buchanan, B.F. (1987). Human environment interaction: A modification of the Neuman systems model for aggregates, families, and the community. *Public Health Nursing*, 4(1), 52–64.

Burke, Sr., M.E., Capers, C.F., O'Connell, R.K., Quinn, R.M., and Sinnott, M. (1989). Neuman-based nursing practice in a hospital setting. In B. Neuman (Ed.), *The*

Neuman systems model (2nd ed.). East Norwalk, CT: Appleton & Lange.

Cammuso, B.S. and Wallen, A.J. (2002). Using the Neuman systems model to guide nursing education in the United States. In B. Neuman and J. Fawcett (Eds.), *The Neuman systems model* (4th ed., pp. 244–253). Upper Saddle River, NJ: Prentice Hall.

Campbell, V. and Keller, K.B. (1989). The Betty Neuman health care systems model: An analysis. In J.P. Riehl-Sisca (Ed.), *Conceptual models for nursing practice* (2nd ed.). East Norwalk, CT: Appleton & Lange.

Capers, C.F. and Kelly, R. (1987). Neuman nursing process: A model of holistic care. *Holistic Nursing Practice*, 1(3), 19–26.

Capers, C.F., O'Brien, C., Quinn, R., Kelly, R., and Fenerty, A. (1985). The Neuman systems model in practice: Planning phase. *Journal of Nursing Administration*, 15(5), 29–39.

Caplan, G. (1964). *Principles of preventive psychiatry*. New York: Basic Books.

Casalenuovo, G.A. (2002). Fatigue in diabetes mellitus: Testing a middle-range theory of well-being derived from the Neuman theory of optimal client system stability and the Neuman systems model. *Dissertation Abstracts International*, 63, 2301B.

Chardin, P.T. (1955). *The phenomenon of man*. London: Collins.

Clarke, P.N. and Lowry, L. (2012). Dialogue with Lois Lowry: Development of the Neuman systems model. *Nursing Science Quarterly*, 25(4), 332–335.

Cobb, R.K. (2012). How well does spirituality predict health status in adults living with HIV-disease: A Neuman systems model study. *Nursing Science Quarterly*, 25(4), 347–355.

Cornu, A. (1957). *The origins of Marxian thought*. Springfield, IL: Charles C. Thomas.

Current Nursing. (2010). *Nursing theories*. Retrieved from http://currentnursing.com/nursing_theory/application_Betty_Neuman's_model.html

Dale, M.L. and Savala, S.M. (1990). A new approach to the senior practicum. *Nursing Connections*, 3(1), 45–51.

Delunas, L.R. (1990). Prevention of elder abuse: Betty Neuman health care systems approach. *Clinical Nurse Specialist*, 4(1), 54–58.

de Munck, R. and Murk, A. (2002). Using the Neuman systems model to guide administration of nursing services in Holland: The case of Emergis, Institute for Mental Health Care. In B. Neuman and J. Fawcett (Eds.), *The Neuman systems model* (4th ed., pp. 300–316). Upper Saddle River, NJ: Prentice Hall.

Drew, L.L., Craig, D.M., and Beynon, C.E. (1989). The Neuman systems model for community health administration and practice: Provinces of Manitoba and Ontario, Canada. In B. Neuman (Ed.), *The Neuman systems model* (2nd ed.). East Norwalk, CT: Appleton & Lange.

Dunn, S.I. and Trepanier, M. (1989). Applications of the Neuman systems model to perinatal nursing. In B. Neuman (Ed.), *The Neuman systems model* (2nd ed.). East Norwalk, CT: Appleton & Lange.

Edelson, M. (1970). *Sociotherapy and psychotherapy*. Chicago, IL: University of Chicago Press.

Fawcett, J. (2004). Conceptual models of nursing: International in scope and substance? The case of the Neuman systems model. *Nursing Science Quarterly*, 17(1), 50–54.

Fawcett, J. and DeSanto-Madeya (2013). *Contemporary nursing knowledge: Analysis and evaluation of nursing models and theories* (3rd ed.). Philadelphia, PA: F.A. Davis.

Fawcett, J. and Giangrande, S.K. (2001). Neuman systems model-based research: An integrative review project. *Nursing Science Quarterly*, 14(3), 231–238.

Fawcett, J. and Giangrande, S.K. (2002). The Neuman systems model and research: An integrative review. In B. Neuman and J. Fawcett (Eds.), *The Neuman systems model* (4th ed., pp. 120–149). Upper Saddle River, NJ: Prentice Hall.

Florczak, K., Poradzisz, M. and Hampson, S. (2012). Nursing in a complex world: A case for grand theory. *Nursing Science Quarterly*, 25(4), 307–312.

Foote, A.W., Piazza, D., and Schultz, M. (1990). The Neuman systems model: Application to a patient with a cervical spinal cord injury. *Journal of Neuroscience Nursing*, 22, 302–306.

Gehrling, K.R. and Memmott, R.J. (2008). Adversity in the context of the Neuman systems model. *Nursing Science Quarterly*, 21(2), 135–137.

Gigliotti, E. (2001). Empirical tests of the Neuman systems model: Relational statement analysis. *Nursing Science Quarterly*, 14(2), 149–157.

Gigliotti, E. (2003). The Neuman systems model institute: Testing middle-range theories. *Nursing Science Quarterly*, 16(3), 201–206.

Gigliotti, E. (2007). Improving external and internal validity of a model of midlife women's maternal-student role stress. *Nursing Science Quarterly*, 20(2), 161–170.

Gigliotti, E. (2011). Deriving middle range theories from the Neuman systems model. In B. Neuman and J. Fawcett (eds.). *The Neuman systems model* (5th ed., pp. 283–298). Upper Saddle River, NJ: Prentice-Hall Publications.

Gigliotti, E. and Fawcett, J. (2002). The Newman systems model and research instruments. In B. Neuman and J. Fawcett (Eds.), *The Neuman systems model* (4th ed., pp. 150–175). Upper Saddle River, NJ: Prentice Hall.

Gomez-Tovar, L.O., Diaz-Suarez, L. and Cortes-Munoz, F. (2016). Evidence and Betty Neuman's model-based nursing care to prevent delirium in the intensive care unit. *Enfermeria Global*, 41, 64–77.

Haggart, M. (1993). A critical analysis of Neuman's systems model in relation to public health nursing. *Journal of Advanced Nursing*, 18, 1917–1922.

Harris, S.M., Hermiz, M.E., Meininger, M., and Steinkeler, S.E. (1989). Betty Neuman: Systems model. In A. Marriner-Tomey (Ed.), *Nursing theorists and their work*. St. Louis, MO: C.V. Mosby.

Heffline, M.S. (1991). A comparative study of pharmacological versus nursing interventions in the treatment of postanesthesia shivering. *Journal of Post Anesthesia Nursing*, 6(5), 311–320.

Herrick, C.A. and Goodykoontz, L. (1989). Neuman's systems model for nursing practice as a conceptual framework for a family assessment. *Journal of Child and Adolescent Psychiatric and Mental Health Nursing*, 2(2), 61–67.

Hinton-Walker, P. and Raborn, M. (1989). Application of the Neuman model in nursing administration and practice. In B. Henry, C. Arndt, M. Di Vicenti, and A. Marriner-Tomey (Eds.), *Dimensions of nursing administration: Theory, research, education, practice*. Boston, MA: Blackwell Scientific Publications.

Hoeman, S., and Winters, D.M. (1990). Theory based case management: High cervical spinal cord injury. *Home Health Care Nurse*, 8, 25–33.

Johnson, S.E. (1989). A picture is worth a thousand words: Helping students visualize a conceptual model. *Nurse Educator*, 14(3), 21–24.

Jones-Cannon, S. and Davis, B. (2005). Coping among African-American daughters caring for aging parents. *The ABNF Journal*, 16(6), 118–123.

Kelley, J.A., Sanders, N.F., and Pierce, J.D. (1989). A systems approach to the role of the nurse administrator in education and practice. In B. Neuman (Ed.), *The Neuman systems model* (2nd ed.). East Norwalk, CT: Appleton & Lange.

Kottwitz, D. and Bowling, S. (2003). A pilot study of the elder abuse questionnaire. *Kansas Nurse*, 78(7), 4–6.

Kubsch, S., Linton, S.M., Hankerson, C., and Wichowski, H. (2008). Holistic interventions protocol for interstitial cystitis symptom control. *Holistic Nursing Practice*, 22(4), 183–190; quiz 191–192.

Lamb, K.A. (1999). Baccalaureate nursing students' perception of empathy and stress in their interactions with clinical instructors testing a theory of optimum student system stability according to the Neuman systems model. *Dissertation Abstracts International*, 60, 1028B.

Lancaster, D.R. and Whall, A.L. (1989). The Neuman systems model. In J.J. Fitzpatrick and A.L. Whall (Eds.), *Conceptual models of nursing: Analysis and application* (2nd ed.). East Norwalk, CT: Appleton & Lange.

Lillis, P.P. and Cora, V.L. (1989). A case study analysis using the Neuman nursing process format: An abstract. In B. Neuman (Ed.), *The Neuman systems model* (2nd ed.). East Norwalk, CT: Appleton & Lange.

Louis, M. (1995). The Neuman model in nursing research: An update. In Betty Neuman (Ed.), *The Neuman systems model* (pp. 473–495). East Norwalk, CT: Appleton & Lange.

Louis, M. and Koertvelyessy, A. (1989). The Neuman model in nursing research. In B. Neuman (Ed.), *The Neuman systems model* (2nd ed.). East Norwalk, CT: Appleton & Lange.

Lowry, L.W. (2002). The Neuman systems model and education: An integrative review. In B. Neuman and J. Fawcett (Eds.), *The Neuman systems model* (4th ed., pp. 216–237). Upper Saddle River, NJ: Prentice Hall.

Lowry, L.W. (2009, May). *A fresh look at the Neuman Systems Model*. Powerpoint presented at the 12th International Biennial Neuman Systems Model Symposium, Las Vegas, NV.

Lowry, L.W. (2012). A qualitative descriptive study of spirituality guided by the Neuman systems model. *Nursing Science Quarterly*, 25(4), 356–361.

Lowry, L.W. and Anderson, B. (1993). Neuman's framework and ventilator dependency: A pilot study. *Nursing Science Quarterly*, 6(4), 195–200.

Lowry, L.W., Beckman, S., Gehrling, K.R., and Fawcett, J. (2007). Imagining nursing practice: The Neuman systems model in 2050. *Nursing Science Quarterly*, 20(3), 226–231.

Lowry, L.W. and Jopp, M.C. (1989). An evaluation instrument for assessing an associate degree nursing curriculum based on the Neuman systems model. In J.P. Riehl-Sisca (Ed.), *Conceptual models for nursing practice* (3rd ed., pp. 73–85). Norwalk, CT: Appleton & Lange.

Martins, C.L., Echevarria-Guanilo, M.E., Silveira, D.T., Gonzales, R.I.C. and Pai, D.D. (2015). Risk perception of work-related burn injuries from the workers perspective. *Texto Contexto Enferm, Florianopolis*, 24(4), 1148–1156.

McClure, M. and Gigliotti, E. (2012). A medieval metaphor to aid use of the Neuman systems model in simulation debriefing. *Nursing Science Quarterly*, 25(4), 318–324.

McDowell, B.M., Chang, N.J., and Choi, S.S. (2003). Children's health retention in South Korea and the United States: A cross-cultural comparison. *Journal of Pediatric Nursing*, 18(6), 409–415.

Merks, A., Verberk, F., de Kuiper, M. and Lowry, L.W. (2012). Neuman systems model in Holland: An update. *Nursing Science Quarterly*, 25(4), 364–368.

Meyer, T. and Xu, Y. (2005). Academic and clinical dissonance in nursing education: Are we guilty of failure to rescue? *Nurse Educator*, 30(2), 76–79.

Mirenda, R.M. (1986). The Neuman systems model: Description and application. In P. Winstead-Fry, P. (Ed.), *Case studies in nursing theory*. New York: National League for Nursing.

Moore, D. (2009, May). *Expanding the least restrictive continuum in mental health practice*. Powerpoint presented at the 12th International Biennial Neuman Systems Model Symposium, Las Vegas, NV.

Moscaritolo, L.M. (2009). Interventional strategies to decrease nursing student anxiety in the clinical learning environment. *Journal of Nursing Education*, 48(1), 17–23.

Mrkonich, D.E., Hessian, M., and Miller M.W. (1989). A cooperative process in curriculum development using the Neuman health care systems model. In J.P. Riehl-Sisca (Ed.), *Conceptual models for nursing practice* (3rd ed.). East Norwalk, CT: Appleton & Lange.

Mrkonich, D.E., Miller, M., and Hessian, M. (1989). Cooperative baccalaureate education: The Minnesota intercollegiate nursing consortium. In B. Neuman (Ed.), *The Neuman systems model* (2nd ed.). East Norwalk, CT: Appleton & Lange.

Nelson, L.F., Hansen, M., and McCullagh, M. (1989). A new baccalaureate North Dakota-Minnesota nursing education consortium. In B. Neuman (Ed.), *The Neuman systems model* (2nd ed.). East Norwalk, CT: Appleton & Lange.

Neuman, B. (1982). *The Neuman systems model: Application to nursing education and practice*. Norwalk, CT: Appleton-Century-Crofts.

Neuman, B. (1989a). The Neuman systems model. In B. Neuman (Ed.), *The Neuman systems model* (2nd ed.). East Norwalk, CT: Appleton & Lange.

Neuman, B. (1989b). The Neuman nursing process format: Family case study. In J.P. Riehl-Sisca (Ed.), *Conceptual models for nursing practice* (3rd ed.). East Norwalk, CT: Appleton & Lange.

Neuman, B. (1989c). In conclusion–In transition. In B. Neuman (Ed.), *The Neuman systems model* (2nd ed.). East Norwalk, CT: Appleton & Lange.

Neuman, B. (1995). *The Neuman systems model* (3rd ed.). East Norwalk, CT: Appleton & Lange.

Neuman, B. (2002a). Betty's Neuman's autobiography and chronology of the development and utilization of the Neuman systems model. In B. Neuman and J. Fawcett (Eds.), *The Neuman systems model* (4th ed., pp. 325–346). Upper Saddle River, NJ: Prentice Hall.

Neuman, B. (2002b). The Neuman systems model. In B. Neuman and J. Fawcett (Eds.), *The Neuman systems model* (4th ed., pp. 3–33). Upper Saddle River, NJ: Prentice Hall.

Neuman, B. (2002c). Assessment and intervention based on the Neuman systems model. In B. Neuman and J. Fawcett (Eds.), *The Neuman systems model* (4th ed., pp. 347–359). Upper Saddle River, NJ: Prentice Hall.

Neuman, B. (2011a). Betty Neuman's autobiography and chronology of the development and utilization of the Neuman systems model. In B. Neuman and J. Fawcett (Eds.), *The Neuman systems model* (5th ed., pp. 330–337). Upper Saddle River, NJ: Pearson.

Neuman, B. (2011b). The Neuman systems model. In B. Neuman and J. Fawcett (Eds.), *The Neuman systems model* (5th ed., pp. 3–34). Upper Saddle River, NJ: Pearson.

Neuman, B. and Fawcett, J. (Eds.). (2002). *The Neuman systems model* (4th ed.). Upper Saddle River, NJ: Prentice Hall.

Neuman, B. and Fawcett, J. (Eds.) (2011). *The Neuman systems model* (5th ed). Upper Saddle River, NJ: Pearson.

Neuman, B. and Fawcett, J. (2012). Thoughts about the Neuman systems model: A Dialogue. *Nursing Science Quarterly*, 25(4), 374–376.

Neuman, B., Newman, D.M.L., and Holder, P. (2000). Leadership-scholarship integration: Using the Neuman systems model for 21st century professional nursing practice. *Nursing Science Quarterly*, 13(1), 60–63.

Neuman, B. and Reed, K.S. (2007). A Neuman systems model perspective on nursing in 2050. *Nursing Science Quarterly*, 20(2), 111–113.

Neuman, B. and Young, R.J. (1972). A model for teaching total person approach to patient problems. *Nursing Research*, 21(3), 264–269.

Newman, D.M. (2005). A community nursing center for the health promotion of senior citizens: Based on the Neuman Systems Model. *Nursing Education Perspective*, 26(4), 221–223.

Newman, D.M.L., Neuman, B., and Fawcett, J. (2002). Guidelines for Neuman systems model-based education for the health professions. In B. Neuman and J. Fawcett (Eds.), *The Neuman systems model* (4th ed., pp. 193–215). Upper Saddle River, NJ: Prentice Hall.

Newman, M.A. (2003). A world of no boundaries. *Advances in Nursing Science*, 26(4), 240–245.

Pierce, J.D., and Hutton, E. (1992). Applying the new concepts of the Neuman systems model. *Nursing Forum*, 27(1), 15–18.

Pothiban, L. (2002). Using the Neuman systems model to guide nursing research in Thailand. In B. Neuman and J. Fawcett (Eds.), *The Neuman systems model* (4th ed., pp. 183–190). Upper Saddle River, NJ: Prentice Hall.

Potter, M.L. and Zauszniewski, J.A. (2000). Spirituality, resourcefulness, and arthritis impact on health perception of elders with rheumatoid arthritis. *Journal of Holistic Nursing*, 18(4), 311–336.

Putt, A. (1972). Entropy, evolution and equifinality in nursing. In J. Smith (Ed.), *Five years of cooperation to improve curricula in western schools of nursing*. Boulder, CO: Western Interstate Commission for Higher Education.

Reed, K.S. (1989). Family theory related to the Neuman systems model. In B. Neuman (Ed.), *The Neuman systems model* (2nd ed.). East Norwalk, CT: Appleton & Lange.

Reed, K.S. (2002). The Neuman systems model and educational tools. In B. Neuman and J. Fawcett (Eds.), *The Neuman systems model* (4th ed., pp. 238–243). Upper Saddle River, NJ: Prentice Hall.

Reed, K.S. (2003). Grief is more than tears. *Nursing Science Quarterly*, 16(1), 77–81.

Ross, M.M. and Bourbonnais, F.F. (1985). The Betty Neuman systems model in nursing practice: A case study approach. *Journal of Advanced Nursing*, 10(3), 199–207.

Ross, M.M., Bourbonnais, F.F., and Carroll, G. (1987). Curricular design and the Betty Neuman systems model: A new approach to learning. *International Nursing Review*, 34(3), 75–79.

Sanders, N.F. and Kelley, J.A. (2002). The Neuman systems model and administration of nursing services: An integrative review. In B. Neuman and J. Fawcett (Eds.), *The Neuman systems model* (4th ed., pp. 271–187). Upper Saddle River, NJ: Prentice Hall.

Selye, H. (1950). *The physiology and pathology of exposure to stress*. Montreal: ACTA.

Sipple, J.A. and Freese, B.T. (1989). Transition from technical to professional-level nursing education. In B. Neuman (Ed.), *The Neuman systems model* (2nd ed.). East Norwalk, CT: Appleton & Lange.

Skalski, C.A., DiGerolamo, L., and Gigliotti, E. (2006). Stressors in five client populations: Neuman systems model-based literature review. *Journal of Advanced Nursing*, 56(1), 69–78.

Smith, M.C. (1989). Neuman's model in practice. *Nursing Science Quarterly*, 2(3), 116–117.

Sohier, R. (1989). Nursing care for the people of a small planet: Culture and the Neuman systems model. In B. Neuman (Ed.), *The Neuman systems model* (2nd ed.). East Norwalk, CT: Appleton & Lange.

Stepans, M.B. and Knight, J.R. (2002). Application of Neuman's framework: Infant exposure to environmental tobacco smoke. *Nursing Science Quarterly*, 15(4), 327–334.

Story, E.L. and Ross, M.M. (1986). Family centered community health nursing and the Betty Neuman systems model. *Nursing Paper*, 18(2), 77–88.

Sullivan, J. (1986). Using Neuman's model in the acute phase of spinal cord injury. *Focus Critical Care*, 13(5), 34–41.

Timmermans, O., van Linge, R., van Petergem, P., van Rompaey, B. and Denekens, J. (2013). A contingency perspective on team learning and innovation in nursing. *Journal of Advanced Nursing*, 69(2), 363–373.

Turner, S.B. and Kaylor, S.D. (2015). Neuman systems model as a conceptual framework for nurse resilience. *Nursing Science Quarterly*, 28(3), 213–217.

Wilson, L.C. (2000). Implementation and evaluation of church-based health fairs. *Journal of Community Health Nursing*, 17(1), 39–48.

Ziemer, M.M. (1983). Effects of information on postsurgical coping. *Nursing Research*, 32(5), 282–287.

Rogers

Barnum, B.J.S. (1994). *Nursing theory: Analysis, application, and evaluation* (4th ed.). Philadelphia, PA: Lippincott.

Barrett, E.A. (1986). Investigation of the principle of helicy: The relationship of human field motion and power. In V.M. Malinski (Ed.), *Explorations on Martha Rogers' science of unitary human beings* (pp. 173–187). Norwalk, CT: Appleton-Century-Crofts.

Barrett, E.A. (1990a). Visions of Rogers' science-based nursing. In E.A. Barrett (Ed.), *Visions of Rogers' science-based nursing* (pp. 31–44). New York: National League for Nursing.

Barrett, E.A. (1990b). A measure of power as knowing participation in change. In O.L. Strickland and C.F. Waltz (Eds.), *Measurement in nursing outcomes* (pp. 159–175). New York: Springer.

Barrett, E.A. (1990c). The continuing revolution of Rogers' science-based nursing education. In E.A. Barrett (Ed.), *Visions of Rogers' science-based nursing* (pp. 303–317). New York: National League for Nursing.

Barrett, E.A. (2002). What is nursing science? *Nursing Science Quarterly*, 15(1), 51–60.

Barrett, E.A. (2003). A measure of power as knowing participation in change. In O.L. Strickland and C.Diloria (Eds.), *Measurement in nursing outcomes* (2nd ed., Vol. 3), New York: Springer.

Barrett. E.A. (2010). Power as knowing participation in change: What's new and what is next. *Nursing Science Quarterly*, 23(1), 47–54.

Barrett, E.A. and Caroselli, C. (1998). Methodological ponderings related to the power as knowing participation in change tool. *Nursing Science Quarterly*, 11(1), 17–22.

Baumann, S.L., Wright, S.G. and Settecase-Wu, C. (2014). A science of unitary human beings perspective of global health nursing. *Nursing Science Quarterly*, 27(4), 324–328.

Benonis, B.C. (1989). The lived experience of recovering from addiction: A phenomenological study. *Nursing Science Quarterly*, 2(1), 37–43.

Biley, F.C. (1992). The perception of time as a factor in Rogers' science of unitary human beings: A literature review. *Journal of Advanced Nursing*, 17(9), 1141–1145.

Blair, C. (1979). Hyperactivity in children: Viewed within the framework of synergistic man. *Nursing Forum*, 18, 293–303.

Bultemeier, K. (1997). Rogers' science of unitary human beings in nursing practice. In M.R. Alligood and A. Marriner-Tomey (Eds.), *Nursing theory: Utilization and application* (pp. 153–174). St. Louis, MO: Mosby.

Bultemeier, K. (2002). Rogers' science of unitary human beings in nursing practice. In M.R. Alligood and A. Marriner-Tomey (Eds.), *Nursing theory: Utilization and application* (2nd ed., pp. 267–288). St. Louis, MO: Mosby.

Burr, H.S. and Northrop, F.S.C. (1935). The electrodynamic theory of life. *The Quarterly Review of Biology*, 10, 322–333.

Butcher, H.K. (1993). Kaleidoscoping in life's turbulence: From Seurat's art to Rogers' nursing science. In M.E. Parker (Ed.), *Patterns of nursing theories in practice* (pp. 183–198). New York: National League for Nursing.

Butcher, H.K. (2002). Living in the heart of helicy: An inquiry into the meaning of compassion and unpredictability within Rogers' nursing science. *Visions: The Journal of Rogerian Nursing Science*, 10(1), 6–22.

Butcher, H.K. and Malinski, V.M. (2010). Martha Rogers' science of unitary human beings. In M.E. Parker and M.C. Smith (Eds.), *Nursing theories and nursing practice* (3rd ed., pp. 253–276). Philadelphia, PA: F.A. Davis.

Caratao-Mojica, R. (2015). The science of unitary human beings in a creative perspective. *Nursing Science Quarterly*, 28(4), 297–299.

Carboni, J.T. (1995a). Enfolding health-as-wholeness-and-harmony: A theory of Rogerian nursing practice. *Nursing Science Quarterly*, 8(2), 71–78.

Carboni, J.T. (1995b). The Rogerian process of inquiry. *Nursing Science Quarterly*, 8(1), 22–37.

Caroselli, C. (1995). Power and feminism: A nursing perspective. *Nursing Science Quarterly*, 8(3), 115–119.

Caroselli, C. and Barrett, E.A.M. (1998). A review of the power as knowing participation in change literature. *Nursing Science Quarterly*, 11(1), 9–16.

Chardin, T. (1961). *The phenomenon of man*. New York: Harper Torchbooks.

Clarke, P.N. (1986). Theoretical and measurement issues in the study of field phenomena. *Advances in Nursing Science*, 9(1), 29–39.

Covington, H. (2001). Therapeutic music for patients with psychiatric disorders. *Holistic Nursing Practice*, 15(2), 59–69.

Cowling, W.R. (1986). The science of unitary human beings: Theoretical issues, methodological challenges, and research realities. In V. Malinski (Ed.), *Explorations on Martha Rogers' science of unitary human beings*. Norwalk, CT: Appleton-Century-Crofts.

Cox, T. (2003). Theory and exemplars of advanced practice spiritual intervention. *Complementary Therapies in Nursing and Midwifery*, 9(1), 30–34.

Farren, A.T. (2009). An oncology case study demonstrating the use of Rogers' science of unitary human beings and standardized nursing languages. *International Journal of Nursing Terminologies and Classifications*, 20(1), 34–39.

Fawcett, J. (2003a). The science of unitary human beings: Analysis of qualitative research approaches. *Visions: The Journal of Rogerian Nursing Science*, 11(1), 7–20.

Fawcett, J. (2003b). The nurse theorists: 21st century updates—Martha E. Rogers. *Nursing Science Quarterly*, 16(1), 44–51.

Fawcett, J. and DeSanto-Madeya (2013). Rogers' science of unitary human beings. In J. Fawcett and S. DeSanto-Madeya (Eds.), *Contemporary nursing knowledge: Analysis and evaluation of nursing models and theories* (3rd ed.). Philadelphia, PA: F.A. Davis.

Ference, H. (1986). The relationship of time experience, creativity traits, differentiation, and human field motion. In V. Malinski (Ed.), *Explorations on Martha Rogers' science of unitary human beings*. Norwalk, CT: Appleton-Century-Crofts.

Fitzpatrick, J. (1988). Theory based on Rogers' conceptual model. *Journal of Gerontological Nursing*, 14(9), 14–16.

Floyd, J.A. (1983). Research using Rogers' conceptual system: Development of a testable theorem. *Advances in Nursing Science*, 5(2), 37–48.

Garon, M. (1992). Contributions of Martha Rogers to the development of nursing knowledge. *Nursing Outlook*, 40(2), 67–72.

Gill, B.P. and Atwood, J.R. (1981). Reciprocity and helicy use related to EFT and wound healing. *Nursing Research*, 30(2), 68–72.

Goldberg, W.G. and Fitzpatrick, J.J. (1980). Movement therapy with the aged. *Nursing Research*, 29(6), 339–346.

Hardin, S.R. (2003). Spirituality a integrality among chronic heart failure patients: A pilot study. *Visions: The Journal of Rogerian Nursing Science*, 11(1), 43–53.

Hanchett, E.S. (1992). Concepts from eastern philosophy and Rogers' science of unitary human beings. *Nursing Science Quarterly*, 5(4), 164–170.

Heidt, P. (1981). Effect of therapeutic touch on anxiety level of hospitalized patients. *Nursing Research*, 30(1), 32–37.

Hektor, L.M. (1989). Martha E. Rogers: A life history. *Nursing Science Quarterly*, 2(2), 63–73.

Herdtner, S. (2000). Using therapeutic touch in nursing practice. *Orthopaedic Nursing*, 19(5), 77–82.

Hills, R.G.S. and Hanchett, E. (2001). Human change and individuation in pivotal life situations: Development and testing the theory of enlightenment. *Visions: The Journal of Rogerian Nursing Science*, 9(1), 6–19.

Jacono, J. and Jacono, B. (2008). The use of puppetry for health promotion and suicide prevention among Mi'Kmaq youth. *Journal of Holistic Nursing*, 26(1), 50–55.

Johnston, R.L., Fitzpatrick, J.J., and Donovan, M.J. (1982). Developmental stage: Relationship to temporal dimensions [Abstract]. *Nursing Research*, 31(2), 120.

Karnick, P.M. (2014). The science of unitary human beings continues to flourish. *Nursing Science Quarterly*, 27(1), 29.

Katz, V. (1971). Auditory stimulation and developmental behavior of the premature infant. *Nursing Research*, 20(3), 196–201.

Kelly, A.E., Sullivan, P., Fawcett, J., and Samarel, N. (2004). Therapeutic touch, quiet time, and dialogue: Perceptions of women with breast cancer. *Oncology Nursing Forum*, 31(3), 625–631.

Kim, H.S. (1983). Use of Rogers' conceptual system in research: Comments. *Nursing Research*, 32(2), 89–91.

Kim, M.J. and Moritz, D.A. (Eds.). (1982). *Classification of nursing diagnosis: Proceedings of the third and fourth national conference*. New York: McGraw-Hill.

Kim, T.S. (2001). Relation of magnetic field therapy to pain and power over time in persons with chronic primary headache: A pilot study. *Visions: The Journal of Rogerian Nursing Science*, 9(1), 27–42.

Kim, T.S. (2008). Science of unitary human beings: An update on research. *Nursing Science Quarterly*, 21(4), 294–299.

Kim, T.S., Kim, C., Park, K.M., et al. (2008). The relation of power and well-being in Korean adults. *Nursing Science Quarterly*, 21(3), 247–254.

Kim, T.S., Park, J.S., and Kim, M.A. (2008). The relation of meditation to power and well-being. *Nursing Science Quarterly*, 21(1), 49–58.

Krieger, D. (1976). Healing by the laying on of hands as a facilitator of bioenergetic change: The response of in vivo human hemoglobin. *International Journal of Psychoenergetic Systems*, 1, 121–129.

Leddy, S.K. (1995). Measuring mutual process: Development and psychometric testing of the Person-Environment Participation Scale. *Visions: The Journal of Rogerian Nursing Science*, 3(1), 20–31.

Leddy, S.K. (2003). A unitary energy-based nursing practice theory: Theory and application. *Visions: The Journal of Rogerian Nursing Science*, 11(1), 21–28.

Lewandowski, W.A. (2002). Patterning of pain and power with guided imagery: An experimental study with persons experiencing chronic pain. *Case Western Reserve University*, March 8.

Lewin, K. (1964). *Field theory in the social sciences*. New York: Harper Torchbooks.

Lowry, R.C. (2002). The effect of an educational intervention on willingness to receive therapeutic touch. *Journal of Holistic Nursing*, 20(1), 48–60.

Madrid, M. and Winstead-Fry, P. (1986). Rogers' conceptual model. In P. Winstead-Fry (Ed.), *Case studies in nursing theory*. New York: National League for Nursing.

Malinski, V.M. (1986). *Explorations on Martha Rogers' science of unitary human beings*. Norwalk, CT: Appleton-Century-Crofts.

Malinski, V.M. (2012). Meditations on the unitary rhythm of dying-grieving. *Nursing Science Quarterly*, 25(3), 239–244.

Mason, T. and Patterson, R. (1990). A critical review of the use of Rogers' model within a special hospital: A single case study. *Journal of Advanced Nursing*, 15(2), 130–141.

Maville, J.A., Bowen, J.E., and Benham, G. (2008). Effect of healing touch on stress perception and biological correlates. *Holistic Nursing Practice*, 22(2), 103–110.

Meleis, A.I. (1988). Book reviews (Malinski, V.M. [1986] *Explorations on Martha Rogers' science of unitary human beings*). *Research in Nursing and Health*, 11, 59–63.

Moccia, P. (1985). A further investigation of dialectical thinking as a means of understanding systems-in-development: Relevance to Rogers' principles [Commentary]. *Advances in Nursing Science*, 7(4), 33–38.

Newman, M.A. (1976). Movement, tempo, and the experience of time. *Nursing Research*, 25(4), 273–279.

Newman, M.A. (1979). *Theory development in nursing*. Philadelphia, PA: F.A. Davis.

Newman, M.A. (1989). The spirit of nursing. *Holistic Nursing Practice*, 3(3), 1–6.

Newman, M.A. (1994). *Health as expanding consciousness*. New York: National League for Nursing.

Newman, M.A. (2003). A world of no boundaries. *Advances in Nursing Science*, 26(4), 240–245.

O'Mathuna, D.P., Pryjmachuk, S., Spencer, W., Stanwick, M., and Matthiesen, S. (2002). A critical evaluation of the theory and practice of therapeutic touch. *Nursing Philosophy*, 3(2), 163–176.

Onieva-Zafra, M. D., Garcia, L.H. and del Valle, M.G. (2015). Effectiveness of guided imagery relaxation on levels of pain and depression in patients diagnosed with fibromyalgia. *Holistic Nursing Practice*, 29(1), 13–21.

Phillips, J.R. (1989). Science of unitary human being: Changing research perspective. *Nursing Science Quarterly*, 2(2), 57–60.

Phillips, J.R. (2000). Rogerian nursing science and research: A healing process for nursing. *Nursing Science Quarterly*, 13(3), 196–201.

Phillips, J.R. (2013). Creating an epiphany with Martha E. Rogers. *Nursing Science Quarterly*, 26(3), 241–246.

Phillips, J.R. (2015). Martha E. Rogers: Heretic and heroine. *Nursing Science Quarterly*, 28(1), 42–48.

Plummer, M. and Molzahn, A.E. (2009). Quality of life in contemporary nursing theory: A concept analysis. *Nursing Science Quarterly*, 22(2), 134–140.

Polanyi, M. (1958). *Personal knowledge*. Chicago, IL: University of Chicago Press.

Porter, L.S. (1972). The impact of physical-physiological activity on infant growth and development. *Nursing Research*, 21(3), 210–219.

Powers, C.P., Hart, V.A., Shattell, M. and MacCulloch, T. (2012). The concept of "the will to thrive" in mental health. *Issues in Mental Health Nursing*, 33(11), 805–807.

Quinn, J.F. (1989). Therapeutic touch as energy exchange: Replication and extension. *Nursing Science Quarterly*, 2(2), 74–78.

Reis, P.J. and Alligood, M.R. (2014). Prenatal yoga in late pregnancy and optimism, power, and well-being. *Nursing Science Quarterly*, 27(1), 30–36.

Ring, M.E. (2009a). Reiki and changes in pattern manifestations. *Nursing Science Quarterly*, 22(3), 250–258.

Ring, M.E. (2009b). An exploration of the perception of time from the perspective of the science of unitary human beings. *Nursing Science Quarterly*, 22(1), 8–12.

Rogers, M.E. (1970). *An introduction to the theoretical basis of nursing*. Philadelphia, PA: F.A. Davis.

Rogers, M.E. (1980a). Nursing: A science of unitary man. In J.P. Riehl and C. Roy (Eds.), *Conceptual models for nursing practice* (2nd ed.). New York: Appleton-Century-Crofts.

Rogers, M.E. (1980b). *The science of unitary man* [Audiotapes]. New York: Media for Nursing.

Rogers, M.E. (1980c, December). *Science of unitary man: A paradigm for nursing*. Paper presented at the International Congress on Applied Systems Research and Cybernetics, Acapulco, Mexico.

Rogers, M.E. (1983a). Science of unitary human being: A paradigm for nursing. In I.W. Clements and F.B. Roberts (Eds.), *Family health: A theoretical approach to nursing care*. New York: John Wiley & Sons.

Rogers, M.E. (1983b, June). *Nursing science: A science of unitary human beings*. Paper presented at the First National Rogerian Conference, New York University.

Rogers, M.E. (1985). A paradigm for nursing. In R. Wood and J. Kekahbah (Eds.), *Examining the cultural implications of Martha E. Rogers' science of unitary human beings*. Lecampton, KS: Wood-Kekahbah Associates.

Rogers, M.E. (1986). Science of unitary human beings. In V. Malinski (Ed.), *Explorations on Martha Rogers' science of unitary human beings*. Norwalk, CT: Appleton-Century-Crofts.

Rogers, M.E. (1987). Rogers' science of unitary human beings. In R.R. Parse (Ed.), *Nursing science: Major paradigms, theories, and critiques*. Philadelphia, PA: W.B. Saunders.

Rogers, M.E. (1988). Nursing science and art: A perspective. *Nursing Science Quarterly*, 1(3), 99–102.

Rogers, M.E. (1989). Nursing: A science of unitary human beings. In J.P. Riehl-Sisca (Ed.), *Conceptual models for nursing practice* (3rd ed., pp. 181–188). Norwalk, CT: Appleton and Lange.

Rogers, M.E. (1990). Space age paradigm for new frontiers in nursing. In M.E. Parker (Ed.), *Nursing theories in practice* (pp. 105–113). New York: NLN.

Rogers, M.E. (1992). Nursing science and the space age. *Nursing Science Quarterly*, 5(1), 27–34.

Rossi, L. and Krekeler, K. (1982). Small-group reactions to the theoretical framework "unitary man" (1980). In M.J. Kim and D.A. Moritz (Eds.), *Classification of nursing diagnosis: Proceedings of the third and fourth national conference*. New York: McGraw-Hill.

Schneider, P.E. (1995). Focusing awareness: The process of extraordinary healing from a Rogerian perspective. *Visions: The Journal of Rogerian Nursing Science*, 3(1), 32–43.

Schodt, C.M. (1989). Parental-fetal attachment and couvade: A study of patterns of human-environment integrality. *Nursing Science Quarterly*, 2(2), 88–97.

Shearer, N.B.C. (2009). Health empowerment theory as a guide for practice. *Geriatric Nursing*, 30(2), 4–10.

Shearer, N.B.C., Cisar, N., and Greenberg, E.A. (2007). A telephone-delivered empowerment intervention with patients diagnosed with heart failure. *Heart and Lung*, 36(3), 159–169.

Smith, D.W. (1995). Power and spirituality in polio survivors: A study based on Rogers' science. *Nursing Science Quarterly*, 8(3), 133–139.

Smith, M.C. and Kyle, L. (2008). Holistic foundations of aromatherapy for nursing. *Holistic Nursing Practice*, 22(1), 3–9.

Smith, M.C., Kemp, J., Hemphill, L., and Vojir, C.P. (2002). Outcomes of therapeutic massage for hospitalized cancer patients. *Journal of Nursing Scholarship*, 34(3), 257–262.

Smith, M.J. (1986). Human-environment process: A test of Rogers' principle of integrality. *Advances in Nursing Science*, 9(1), 21–28.

Smith, M.J. (1988). Testing propositions derived from Rogers' conceptual system. *Nursing Science Quarterly*, 1(2), 60–67.

Tettero, I., Jackson, S., and Wilson, S. (1993). Theory to practice: Developing a Rogerian-based assessment tool. *Journal of Advanced Nursing*, 18(5), 776–782.

Todaro-Franceschi, V. (2001). Energy: A bridging concept for nursing science. *Nursing Science Quarterly*, 14(2), 132–140.

Todaro-Franceschi, V. (2008). Clarifying the enigma of energy, philosophically speaking. *Nursing Science Quarterly*, 21(4), 285–290.

Ugarriza, D.N. (2002). Intentionality: Applications within selected theories of nursing. *Holistic Nursing Practice*, 16(4), 41–50.

von Bertalanffy, L. (1968). *General systems theory: Foundations, development, application*. New York: George Braziller.

Wall, L.M. (2000). Changes in hope and power in lung cancer patients who exercise. *Nursing Science Quarterly*, 13(3), 234–242.

Watson, J. and Smith, M.C. (2002). Caring science and the science of unitary human beings: A trans-theoretical discourse for nursing knowledge development. *Journal of Advanced Nursing*, 37(5), 452–461.

Whelton, B.J. (1979). An operationalization of M. Rogers' theory throughout the nursing process. *International Journal of Nursing Studies*, 16, 7–20.

Winstead-Fry, P. (1984). Personal Communication.

Winstead-Fry, P. (2000). Rogers' conceptual system and family nursing. *Nursing Science Quarterly*, 13(4), 278–280.

Wright, B.W. (2004). Trust and power in adults: An investigation using Rogers' science of unitary human beings. *Nursing Science Quarterly*, 17(2), 139–146.

Wright, B.W. (2007). The evolution of Rogers' science of unitary human beings: 21st century reflections. *Nursing Science Quarterly*, 20(1), 64–67.

Yarcheski, A. and Mahon, N.E. (1991). An empirical test of Rogers' original and revised theory of correlates in adolescents. *Research in Nursing and Health*, 14(6), 447–455.

Yarcheski, A. and Mahon, N.E. (1995). Rogers' pattern manifestations and health in adolescents. *Western Journal of Nursing Research*, 17(4), 383–397.

Yarcheski, A., Mahon, N.E., and Yarcheski, T.J. (2002). Humor and health in early adolescents: Perceived field motion as a mediating variable. *Nursing Science Quarterly*, 15(2), 150–155.

Roy

Aktan, N.M. (2012). Social support and anxiety in pregnant and postpartum women: A secondary analysis. *Clinical Nursing Research*, 21(2), 183–194.

Akyil, R.C. and Erguney, S. (2013). Roy's adaptation model-guided education for adaptation to chronic obstructive pulmonary disease. *Journal of Advanced Nursing*, 69(5), 1063–1075.

Alimohammadi, N., Maleksi, B., Shahriari, M. and Chitsaz, A. (2015). Effect of a care plan based on Roy adaptation model biological dimension on stroke patients' physiologic adaptation level. *Iranian Journal of Nursing and Midwifery Research*, 20(2), 275–281.

Andrews, H.A. (1991). Overview of the self-concept mode. In C. Roy and H.A. Andrews (Eds.), *The Roy adaptation model: The definitive statement* (pp. 269–279). East Norwalk, CT: Appleton & Lange.

Andrews, H.A. and Roy, C. (1986). *Essentials of the Roy adaptation model*. Norwalk, CT: Appleton-Century-Crofts.

Artinian, N.T. (1991). Stress experience of spouses of patients having coronary artery bypass during hospitalization and 6 weeks after discharge. *Heart and Lung*, 20, 52–59.

Artinian, N.T. (1992). Spouse adaptation to mate's CABG surgery: 1 year follow-up. *American Journal of Critical Care*, 1(2), 36–42.

Ashton, K.S. (2015). The orientation period: Essential for new registered nurses' adaptation. *Nursing Science Quarterly*, 28(2), 142–150.

Bakan, G. and Akyol, A.D. (2008). Theory-guided interventions for adaptation to heart failure. *Journal of Advanced Nursing*, 61(6), 596–608.

Barone, S.H., Roy, C.L., and Frederickson, K.C. (2008). Instruments used in Roy adaptation model-based research: Review, critique, and future directions. *Nursing Science Quarterly*, 21(4), 353–362.

Bertalanffy, L. (1968). *General system theory*. New York: George Braziller.

Boston-Based Adaptation Research in Nursing Society. (1999). *Roy Adaptation Model-Based Research: 25 Years of Contributions to Nursing Science*. Indianapolis, IN: Center Nursing Press.

Brower, H.T. and Baker, D.J. (1976). Using the adaptation model in a practitioner curriculum. *Nursing Outlook*, 24(11), 686–689.

Buckner, E.B., Simmons, S., Brakefield, J.A., Hawkins, A.K., et al. (2007). Maturing responsibility in young teens participating in an asthma camp: Adaptive mechanisms and outcomes. *Journal for Specialists in Pediatric Nursing*, 12(1), 24–36.

Bunting, S.M. (1988). The concept of perception in selected nursing theories. *Nursing Science Quarterly*, 1(4), 168–174.

Burns, D. (2004). Physical and psychosocial adaptation of blacks on hemodialysis. *Applied Nursing Research*, 17(2), 116–124.

Chardin, P.T. (1965). *Hymn of the universe* (S. Bartholomew, Trans.). New York: Harper & Row.

Chen, C.C.H. (2005). A framework for studying the nutritional health of community-dwelling elders. *Nursing Research*, 54(1), 13–21.

Chen, C. C.H., Chang, C.K., Chyun, D.A., and McCorkle, R. (2005). Dynamics of nutritional health in a community sample of American elders: A multidimensional approach using Roy adaptation model. *Advances in Nursing Science*, 28(4), 376–389.

Chung, S.C. (2004). Conceptual models of nursing: International in scope and substance? The case of the Roy adaptation model. *Nursing Science Quarterly*, 17(3), 281–282.

Cottrell, B. and Shannahan, M. (1986). Effect of the birth chair on duration of second stage labor and maternal outcome. *Nursing Research*, 35(6), 364–367.

Cottrell, B. and Shannahan, M. (1987). A comparison of fetal outcome in birth chair and delivery table births. *Research in Nursing and Health*, 10, 239–243.

Craig, D.I. (1990). The adaptation to pregnancy of spinal cord injured women. *Rehabilitation Nursing*, 15(1), 6–9.

Cunningham, D.A. (2002). Application of Roy's adaptation model when caring for a group of women coping with menopause. *Journal of Community Health Nursing*, 19(1), 49–60.

DeSanto-Madeya, S.A. (2006). A secondary analysis of the meaning of living with spinal cord injury using Roy's adaptation model. *Nursing Science Quarterly*, 19(3), 240–246.

DeSanto-Madeya, S.A. (2009). Adaptation to spinal cord injury for families post-injury. *Nursing Science Quarterly*, 22(1), 57–66.

DiMattio, M.J. and Tulman, L. (2003). A longitudinal study of functional status and correlates following coronary artery bypass graft surgery in women. *Nursing Research*, 52(2), 98–107.

Dobratz, M.C. (1984). Life closure. In S.C. Roy (Ed.), *Introduction to nursing: An adaptation model* (2nd ed.). Englewood Cliffs, NJ: Prentice-Hall.

Dobratz, M.C. (2003). Putting the pieces together: Teaching undergraduate research from a theoretical perspective. *Journal of Advanced Nursing*, 41(4), 383–392.

Dobratz, M.C. (2004). Life-closing spirituality and the philosophic assumptions of the Roy adaptation model. *Nursing Science Quarterly*, 17(4), 335–338.

Dobratz, M.C. (2008). Moving nursing science forward within the framework of the Roy adaptation model. *Nursing Science Quarterly*, 21(3), 255–259.

Dobratz, M.C. (2014). Life closure with the Roy adaptation model. *Nursing Science Quarterly*, 27(1), 51–56.

Downey, C. (1974). Adaptation nursing applied to an obstetric patient. In J.P. Riehl and C. Roy (Eds.), *Conceptual models for nursing practice*. New York: Appleton-Century-Crofts.

Dunn, K.S. (2004). Toward a middle-range theory of adaptation to chronic pain. *Nursing Science Quarterly*, 17(1), 78–84.

Farkas, L. (1981). Adaptation problems with nursing home application for elderly persons: An application of the Roy adaptation nursing model. *Journal of Advanced Nursing*, 6, 363–368.

Fawcett, J. (1981a). Assessing and understanding the cesarean father. In C.F. Kehoe (Ed.), *The cesarean experience: Theoretical and clinical perspectives for nurses*. New York: Appleton-Century-Crofts.

Fawcett, J. (1981b). Needs of cesarean birth parents. *Journal of Obstetric, Gynecologic, and Neonatal Nursing*, 10, 371–376.

Fawcett, J. (1984). *Analysis and evaluation of conceptual models of nursing*. Philadelphia, PA: F.A. Davis.

Fawcett, J. (2002). The nurse theorists: 21st century updates—Callista Roy. *Nursing Science Quarterly*, 15(4), 308–310.

Fawcett, J. (2003). Conceptual models of nursing: International in scope and substance? The case of the Roy adaptation model. *Nursing Science Quarterly*, 16(4), 315–318.

Fawcett, J. (2005). *Contemporary nursing knowledge: Analysis and evaluation of nursing models and theories*. (2nd ed.). FA Davis Company. Philadelphia, PA.

Fawcett, J. and DeSanto-Madeya, S. (2013). *Contemporary nursing knowledge: Analysis and evaluation of nursing models and theories* (3rd ed.). Philadelphia, PA: F.A. Davis.

Fawcett, J. and Henklein, J. (1987). Antenatal education for cesarean birth: Extension of a field test. *Journal of Obstetric, Gynecologic, and Neonatal Nursing*, 16, 61–65.

Frame, K. (2003). Empowering preadolescents with ADHD: Demons or delights. *Advances in Nursing Science*, 26(2), 131–139.

Frame, K., Kelly, L., and Bayley, E. (2003). Increasing perceptions of self-worth in preadolescents diagnosed with ADHD. *Journal of Nursing Scholarship*, 35(3), 225–229.

Frederickson, K. (2000). Nursing knowledge development through research: Using the Roy adaptation model. *Nursing Science Quarterly*, 13(1), 12–17.

Gagliardi, B.A. (2003). The experience of sexuality for individuals living with multiple sclerosis. *Journal of Clinical Nursing*, 12, 571–578.

Gagliardi, B.A., Frederickson, K., and Shanley, D.A. (2002). Living with multiple sclerosis: A Roy adaptation model-based study. *Nursing Science Quarterly*, 15(3), 230–236.

Galligan, A.C. (1979). Using Roy's concept of adaptation to care for young children. *American Journal of Maternal Child Nursing*, 4(1), 24–28.

Gless, P.A. (1995). Applying the Roy adaptation model to the care of clients with quadriplegia. *Rehabilitation Nursing*, 20(1), 11–16.

Gordon, J. (1974). Nursing assessment and care plan for a cardiac patient. In J.P. Riehl and C. Roy (Eds.), *Conceptual models for nursing practice*. New York: Appleton-Century-Crofts.

Granero-Molina, J., Cortes, M.D., Membrive, J.M., Castro-Sanchez, A.M., Entrambasaguas, O.M.L. and Fernandez-Sola, C. (2014). Religious faith in coping with terminal cancer: What is the nursing experience? *European Journal of Cancer Care*, 23(3), 300–309.

Hamer, B.A. (1991). Music therapy: Harmony for change. *Journal of Psychosocial Nursing and Mental Health Services*, 29(12), 5–7.

Hanchett, E.S. (1990). Nursing models and community as client. *Nursing Science Quarterly*, 3, 67–72.

Hanna, D.R. and Roy, C. (2001). Roy adaptation model and perspectives on the family. *Nursing Science Quarterly*, 14(1), 9–13.

Hannon-Engel, S.L. (2008). Knowledge development: The Roy adaptation model and bulimia nervosa. *Nursing Science Quarterly*, 21(2), 126–132.

Harrison, L.L., Leeper, J.D., and Yoon, M. (1990). Effects of early parent touch on preterm infants' heart rates and arterial oxygen saturation levels. *Journal of Advanced Nursing*, 15, 877–885.

Helson, H. (1964). *Adaptation-level theory: An experimental and systematic approach to behavior*. New York: Harper & Row.

Henderson, V. (1960). *Basic principles of nursing care*. London: International Council of Nurses.

Hoch, C. (1987). Assessing delivery of nursing care. *Journal of Gerontological Nursing*, 13(1), 10–17.

Idle, B.A. (1978). SPAL: A tool for measuring self-perceived adaptation level appropriate for an elderly population. In E.E. Bauwens (Ed.), *Clinical nursing research: Its strategies and findings* (Monograph series No. 2). Indianapolis, IN: Sigma Theta Tau.

Isbir, G.G. and Mete, S. (2013). Experiences with nausea and vomiting during pregnancy in Turkish women based on Roy adaptation model: A content analysis. *Asian Nursing Research*, 7(4), 175–181.

Janelli, L.M. (1980). Utilizing Roy's adaptation model from a gerontological perspective. *Journal of Gerontological Nursing*, 6(3), 140–150.

Kehoe, C.F. (1981). Identifying the nursing needs of the postpartum cesarean mother. In C.F. Kehoe (Ed.), *The cesarean experience: Theoretical and clinical perspectives for nurses*. New York: Appleton-Century-Crofts.

Kurek-Ovshinsky, C. (1991). Group psychotherapy in an acute inpatient setting: Techniques that nourish self-esteem. *Issues in Mental Health Nursing*, 12, 81–88.

Laros, J. (1977). Deriving outcome criteria from a conceptual model. *Nursing Outlook*, 25, 333–336.

Lee, L.Y.K., Tsang, A.Y.K., Wong, K.F., and Lee, J.K.L. (2011). Using the Roy adaptation model to develop an antenatal assessment instrument. *Nursing Science Quarterly*, 24(4), 363–369.

Lefaiver, C.A., Keough, V., Letizia, M., and Lanuza, D.M. (2007). Using the Roy adaptation model to explore the dynamics of quality of life and the relationship between lung transplant candidates and their caregivers. *Advances in Nursing Science*, 30(3), 266–274.

Levesque, L., Ricard, N., Ducharme, F., Duquette, A., and Bonin, J.P. (1998). Empirical verification of a theoretical model derived from the Roy adaptation model: Findings from five studies. *Nursing Science Quarterly*, 11(1), 31–39.

Levine, M.E. (1966). Adaptation and assessment: A rationale for nursing intervention. *American Journal of Nursing*, 66, 2450–2453.

Lewis, F., Firsich, S.C., and Parsell, S. (1978). Development of reliable measures of patient health outcomes related to quality nursing care for chemotherapy patients. In J.C. Krueger, A.H. Nelson, and M.O. Wolanin (Eds.), *Nursing research: Development, collaboration, utilization*. Germantown, MD: Aspen.

Lewis, F.M., Firsich, S.C., and Parsell, S. (1979). Clinical tool development for adult chemotherapy patients: Process and content. *Cancer Nursing*, 2(2), 99–108.

Malinski, V.M. (2002). Developing a nursing perspective on spirituality and healing. *Nursing Science Quarterly*, 15(4), 281–287.

Mastal, M.F. and Hammond, H. (1980). Analysis and expansion of the Roy adaptation model: A contribution to holistic nursing. *Advances in Nursing Science*, 2(4), 71–81.

Mastal, M.F., Hammond, H., and Roberts, M.P. (1982). Theory into hospital practice: A pilot implementation. *Journal of Nursing Administration*, 12(6), 9–15.

Modrcin-Talbott, M.A., Harrison, L.L., Groer, M.W., and Younger, M.S. (2003). The biobehavioral effects of gentle human touch on preterm infants. *Nursing Science Quarterly*, 16(1), 60–67.

Morales-Mann, E.T. and Logan, M. (1990). Implementing the Roy model: Challenges for nurse educators. *Journal of Advanced Nursing*, 15, 142–147.

Moreno, M.E., Durán, M.M., and Hernandez, A. (2009). Nursing care for adaptation. *Nursing Science Quarterly*, 22(1), 67–73.

Munn, V.A. and Tichy, A.M. (1987). Nurses' perceptions of stressors in pediatric intensive care. *Journal of Pediatric Nursing*, 2, 405–411.

Nayback, A.M. (2009). PTSD in the combat veteran: Using Roy's adaptation model to examine the combat veteran as a human adaptive system. *Issues in Mental Health Nursing*, 30(5), 304–310.

Nicholson Jr., N.R. (2009). Social isolation in older adults: An evolutionary concept analysis. *Journal of Advanced Nursing*, 65(6), 1342–1352.

Nightingale, F. (1859). *Notes on nursing: What it is and what it is not*. London: Harrison. Reprinted 1995. Philadelphia, PA: Lippincott.

Nuamah, I.F., Cooley, M.E., Fawcett, J., and McCorkle, R. (1999). Testing a theory for health-related quality of life in cancer patients: A structural equation approach. *Research in Nursing and Health*, 22(3), 231–242.

Ordin, Y., Karayurt, O. and Wellard, S. (2013). Investigation of adaptation after liver transplantation using Roy's adaptation model. *Nursing and Health Sciences*, 15(1), 31–38.

Ospina, A.M., Munoz, L., and Ruiz, C.H. (2012). Coping and adaptation process during puerperium. *Colombia Medica* 43(2), 167–174.

Perrett, S.E. (2007). Review of Roy adaptation model-based qualitative research. *Nursing Science Quarterly*, 20(4), 349–356.

Perrett, S.E. and Biley, F.C. (2013). A Roy model study of adapting to being HIV positive. *Nursing Science Quarterly*, 26(4), 337–343.

Pollock, S.E. (1986). Human responses to chronic illness: Physiologic and psychological adaptation. *Nursing Research*, 35(2), 90–95.

Pollock, S.E., Frederickson, K., Carson, M.A., Massey, V.H., and Roy, C. (1994). Contributions to nursing science: Synthesis of findings from adaptation model research. *Scholarly Inquiry for Nursing Practice*, 8(4), 361–372.

Ramini, S.K., Brown, R., and Buckner, E.B. (2008). Embracing changes: Adaptation by adolescents with Cancer. *Pediatric Nursing*, 34(1), 72–79.

Randall, B., Poush-Tedrow, M., and Van Landingham, U.J. (1982). *Adaptation nursing: The Roy conceptual model applied*. St. Louis, MO: C.V. Mosby.

Roy Adaptation Association. (2007). Cultural issues of the Roy adaptation model examined. *RAA Review*, 9(2), 2.

Roy, C. (1970). Adaptation: A conceptual framework for nursing. *Nursing Outlook*, 18(3), 42–45.

Roy, C. (1971). Adaptation: A basis for nursing practice. *Nursing Outlook*, 19(4), 254–257.

Roy, C. (1976). *Introduction to nursing: An adaptation model*. Englewood Cliffs, NJ: Prentice-Hall.

Roy, C. (1977). *Decision-making by the physically ill and adaptation during illness*. Unpublished doctoral dissertation, University of California, Los Angeles.

Roy, C. (1979). Relating nursing theory to education: A new era. *Nurse Educator*, 4(2), 16–21.

Roy, C. (1980). The Roy adaptation model. In J.P. Riehl and C. Roy (Eds.), *Conceptual models for nursing practice* (2nd ed.). New York: Appleton-Century-Crofts.

Roy, C. (1984). *Introduction to nursing: An adaptation model* (2nd ed.). Englewood Cliffs, NJ: Prentice-Hall.

Roy, C. (1987). Roy's adaptation model. In R.R. Parse (Ed.), *Nursing science: Major paradigms, theories, and critiques* (pp. 35–45). Philadelphia, PA: W.B. Saunders.

Roy, C. (1988a). An explication of the philosophical assumptions of the Roy adaptation model. *Nursing Science Quarterly*, 1(1), 26–34.

Roy, C. (1988b). Altered cognition: An information processing approach. In P.H. Mitchell, L.C. Hodges, M. Muwaswes, and C.A. Walleck (Eds.), *AANN's neuroscience nursing: Phenomenon and practice: Human responses to neurological health problems* (pp. 185–211). East Norwalk, CT: Appleton & Lange.

Roy, C. (1989). The Roy adaptation model. In J.P. Riehl-Sisca (Ed.), *Conceptual models for nursing practice* (3rd ed., pp. 105–114). East Norwalk, CT: Appleton & Lange.

Roy, C. (1991). The Roy adaptation model in nursing research. In C. Roy and H.A. Andrews (Eds.), *The Roy adaptation model: The definitive statement* (pp. 445–458). East Norwalk, CT: Appleton & Lange.

Roy, C. (2000a). A theorist envisions the future and speaks to nursing administrators. *Nursing Administration Quarterly*, 24(2), 1–12.

Roy, C. (2000b). The visible and invisible fields that shape the future of the nursing care system. *Nursing Administration Quarterly*, 25(1), 119–131.

Roy, C. (2008). Adversity and theory: The broad picture. *Nursing Science Quarterly*, 21(2), 138.

Roy, C. (2009). *The Roy adaptation model* (3rd ed.). Upper Saddle River, NJ: Prentice Hall Health.

Roy, C. (2011a). Extending the Roy adaptation model to meet changing global needs. *Nursing Science Quarterly*, 24(4), 345–351.

Roy, C. (2011b). Research based on the Roy adaptation model: Last 25 years. *Nursing Science Quarterly*, 24(4), 312–320.

Roy, C. and Andrews, H.A. (1991). *The Roy adaptation model: The definitive statement*. East Norwalk, CT: Appleton & Lange.

Roy, C. and Andrews, H.A. (1999). *The Roy adaptation model* (2nd ed.). Norwalk, CT: Appleton & Lange.

Roy, C. and Corliss, C.P. (1993). *The Roy adaptation model: Theoretical update and knowledge for practice* (pp. 215–229). New York: National League for Nursing.

Roy, C. and McLeod, D. (1981). Theory of the person as an adaptive system. In C. Roy and S.L. Roberts (Eds.), *Theory construction in nursing: An adaptation model*. Englewood Cliffs, NJ: Prentice-Hall.

Roy, C. and Roberts, S.L. (1981). *Theory construction in nursing: An adaptation model*. Englewood Cliffs, NJ: Prentice-Hall.

Roy, C., Whetsell, M.V., and Frederickson, K. (2009). The Roy adaptation model and research. *Nursing Science Quarterly*, 22(3), 209–211.

Samarel, N., Tulman, L., and Fawcett, J. (2002). Effects of two types of social support and education on adaptation to early-stage breast cancer. *Research in Nursing and Health*, 25, 459–470.

Schmitz, M. (1980). The Roy adaptation model: Application in a community setting. In J.P. Riehl and C. Roy (Eds.), *Conceptual models for nursing practice* (2nd ed.). New York: Appleton-Century-Crofts.

Senesac, P. and Roy, C. (2015). Sister Callista Roy's adaptation model. In M.C. Smith and M.E. Parker (Eds.), *Nursing theories and nursing practice* (4th ed.). Philadelphia, PA: F.A. Davis.

Shah, M., Abdullah, A., and Khan, H. (2013). Compare and contrast of grand theories: Orem's self care deficit theory and Roy's adaptation model. *International Journal of Science and Research*, 4(1), 1834–1837.

Shyu, Y., Liang, J., Lu, J.R., and Wu, C. (2004). Environmental barriers and mobility in Taiwan: Is the Roy adaptation model applicable? *Nursing Science Quarterly*, 17(2), 165–170.

Silva, M.C. (1987). Needs of spouses of surgical patients: A conceptualization within the Roy adaptation model. *Scholarly Inquiry for Nursing Practice: An International Journal*, 1, 29–44.

Smith, C.E., Pace, K., Kochinda, C., Kleinbeck, S.V.M., Koehler, J., and Popkess-Vawter, S. (2002). Caregiving effectiveness model evolution to a midrange theory of home care: A process for critique and replication. *Advances in Nursing Science*, 25(1), 50–64.

Strohmyer, L.L., Noroian, E.L., Patterson, L.M., and Carlin, B.P. (1993). Adaptation six months after multiple trauma: A pilot study. *Journal of Neuroscience Nursing*, 25, 30–37.

Swimme, B. and Berry, T. (1992). *The universe story*. San Francisco, CA: Harper Collins.

Tanyi, R.A. and Werner, J.S. (2003). Adjustment, spirituality, and health in women on hemodialysis. *Clinical Nursing Research*, 12(3), 229–245.

Tiedeman, M.E. (1983). The Roy adaptation model. In J.J. Fitzpatrick and A.L. Whall (Eds.), *Conceptual models of nursing: Analysis and application* (pp. 146–176). Bowie, MD: Robert J. Brady Company.

Tsai, P. (2003). A middle-range theory of caregiver stress. *Nursing Science Quarterly*, 16(2), 137–145.

Tsai, P.F., Tak, S., Moore, C., and Palencia, I. (2003). Testing a theory of chronic pain. *Journal of Advanced Nursing*, 43(2), 158–169.

Tulman, L. and Fawcett, J. (1988). Return of functional ability after childbirth. *Nursing Research*, 37(2), 77–81.

Villareal, E. (2003). Using Roy's adaptation model when caring for a group of young women contemplating quitting smoking. *Public Health Nursing*, 20(5), 377–384.

Wadensten, B. and Carlsson, M. (2003). Nursing theory views on how to support the process of ageing. *Journal of Advanced Nursing*, 42(2), 118–124.

Wagner, P. (1976). Testing the adaptation model in practice. *Nursing Outlook*, 24(11), 682–685.

Wallace, C.L. (1993). Resources for nursing theories in practice. In M.E. Parker (Ed.), *Patterns of nursing theories in practice* (pp. 301–311). New York: National League for Nursing.

Waweru, S.M., Reynolds, A., and Buckner, E.B. (2008). Perceptions of children with HIV/AIDS from the USA and Kenya: Self-concept and emotional indicators. *Pediatric Nursing*, 34(2), 117–124.

Weinert, C., Cudney, S., and Spring, A. (2008). Evolution of a conceptual model for adaptation to chronic illness. *Journal of Nursing Scholarship*, 40(4), 364–372.

Weiss, M., Fawcett, J., and Aber, C. (2009). Adaptation, postpartum concerns, and learning needs in the first two weeks after caesarean birth. *Journal of Clinical Nursing*, 18(21), 2938–2948.

Wendler, M.C. (2003). Effects of Tellington touch in healthy adults awaiting venipuncture. *Research in Nursing and Health*, 26(1), 40–52.

Whittemore, R. and Roy, C. (2002). Adapting to diabetes mellitus: A theory synthesis. *Nursing Science Quarterly*, 15(4), 311–317.

Whittemore, T., Chase, S.K., Mandle, C.L., and Roy, C. (2002). Lifestyle change in type 2 diabetes: A process model. *Nursing Research*, 51(1), 18–25.

Willis, D.G., DeSanto-Madeya, S., Ross, R., Sheehan, D.L. and Fawcett, J. (2015). Spiritual healing in the aftermath of childhood maltreatment: Translating men's lived experiences utilizing nursing conceptual models and theory. *Advances in Nursing Science*, 38(3), 162–174.

Yeh, C. (2002). Health-related quality of life in pediatric patients with cancer: A structural equation approach with the Roy adaptation model. *Cancer Nursing*, 25(1), 74–80.

Yeh, C. (2003). Psychosocial distress: Testing hypotheses based on Roy's adaptation model. *Nursing Science Quarterly*, 16(3), 255–263.

Young-McCaughan, S., Mays, M.Z., Arzola, S.M., Yoder, L.H., Dramiga, S.A., Leclerc, K.M., et al. (2003). Change in exercise tolerance, activity and sleep patterns, and quality of life in patients with cancer participating in a structured exercise program. *Oncology Nursing Forum*, 30(3), 441–454.

Part Five

ON DEVELOPING THEORIES OF DIFFERENT LEVELS

Part Four of this book discussed the pioneering theorists of the nursing discipline, the grand theorists who paved the way for subsequent generations. Part Five is intended to expand the historical examination of theoretical development into the present as well as to explore a framework by which future generations of theorists might continue to build on the work of those who preceded them.

Following the work of the grand theorists (first and second generation of theorists), the third-generation theorists (metatheorists), and the fourth-generation middle-range theorists (see discussion of theorists in Chapter 19), there was an increased focus on the need for development of nursing-specific concepts, the building blocks of nursing theory. Chapter 14, therefore, discusses various strategies used in concept development and provides contemporary examples of their application. Chapter 15 discusses the interrelationship among practice, research, and theory and explains how research and practice have influenced theory development in recent decades.

Chapter 16 discusses the development of middle-range theories, which are the focus of the current (fourth) generation of theorists. Since there is ample coverage of middle-range theory in other texts, this chapter is not presented as a comprehensive treatment of the topic; rather, it is intended to provide some operational examples of the processes involved in developing middle-range theories.

The next generation of theorists will be expected to enrich our discipline by effectively bridging the gaps that currently exist among practice, research, and theory. They will expand on the work of their forebears by developing theories that are less abstract, limited in scope, population-based, and readily operational. To explore ways in which this next generation might achieve these goals, I join Dr. Eun-Ok Im in Chapter 17 to provide a descriptive, analytical, and prescriptive framework for developing situation-specific theories.

14

Developing Concepts

Advancing knowledge in a discipline is predicated on the clarity of its concepts and their effective use in research programs, as well as on translation into practice. In continuing to build the scientific base of the discipline of nursing, developing the evidence for quality care, and translating the evidence into practice models, it is essential to clarify and sharpen the meaning attached to concepts. Defining, clarifying, evaluating, operationalizing, and subjecting concepts to theoretical and empirical testing are all essential and vital processes in advancing knowledge. Many lessons in our theoretical and research histories could inform the future of concept development.

The theoretical development of the discipline of nursing began historically with the compelling question of "How should nursing be defined?" Answers to this question resulted in numerous inclusive theories that attempted to identify the mission and goals of nursing, some of the actions involved in nursing care, and the scope of practice. This was followed by the attempts of a number of metatheorists to define the structure of the discipline, the strategies, and the tools for the further development of knowledge. One important stage that followed is concept development. The identification and development of concepts are vital stages in a discipline's progress. Concept development has evolved to take a central position in knowledge development in nursing. Weaver and Mitcham (2008) identified several forces that have been an impetus for the concept development movement in nursing. The first is the quest to define and delineate the boundaries of the discipline of nursing. The second impetus is the availability of funding that supports doctoral education. In identifying this force, they implicitly assure that the preponderance of writing about concepts is due to advanced degree preparation. The third factor is the organizational requirement that curricula be guided by conceptual frameworks, and the fourth is the numerous theory conferences that may have stimulated the theoretical

development of concepts. In addition to these forces, the articulation of frameworks and strategies for developing concepts and theories provided specific and easy-to-follow guidelines. In addition, as nurse scientists turned to developing the evidence for care, it became apparent that a need exists to clarify assumptions, properties, and referent parts for concepts and variables (Machado and Silva, 2007). Processes used in the development of concepts in nursing have received even more attention from nurse scholars, particularly in the last 20 years. The use of these strategies made major contributions to advancing the development of concepts that reflect the nature of the nursing discipline (Rodgers and Knafl, 2000; Walker and Avant, 2010). A present-day citation search for concept development yields an impressive body of literature.

One important premise to consider is that concepts, once formulated and labeled, tend to shape and guide what we see, and they provide order to observations and experiences that enhance understanding of situations and events. Before we had a concept labeled "burnout," we did not see burnout, even though the syndrome may have existed in one form or another. Because we did not have a label to give to that constellation of behaviors, we did not have a reservoir in which we could connect and deposit those seemingly discrete feelings and responses of apathy, irritability, impatience, and the urge to flee and change one's life. Therefore, describing the varied behaviors and actions related to them may have been limited and somewhat ineffective. For example, no burnout is described by people living in the Middle East; that is, no such concept exists, even though the experiences and the responses may exist and may have always been there, although not described as concisely or dealt with as effectively.

Labeling a concept should not be considered permanent or static. It should be a dynamic process that is responsive to new knowledge, experiences, perceptions, and data. In a human science discipline, participants should be able to articulate and label new concepts or redefine existing concepts. Consider the concept of "reflection," which has frequently been interpreted in practice and teaching as a way to "think" or "do." Bulman, Lathlean, and Gobbi (2012) conducted a qualitative study involving nursing students and faculty that revealed that reflection may instead be thought of as a "way of being."

Concepts evolve from experiences; their definitions and meanings reflect the theorists' educational background, perspectives, and the theoretical frameworks that guide their work. For example, interactionist theorists review a nurse–patient situation and may focus on interaction, role taking, symbols, and roles. Another theorist who has a psychoanalytical lens may explain and interpret the same situation through another set of concepts such as denial, repression, latent hostility, and maternal or paternal conflict.

In spite of the increase in the number of concepts identified, confusion has surrounded concept development. The term *concept development* has been used interchangeably with concept analysis and concept clarification. In addition, the philosophical foundations of concepts tended to be ignored in most of the strategies utilized in defining concepts (Duncan, Cloutier, and Bailey, 2007). There are many different processes for developing concepts, and all of them are vital for advancing knowledge development. The beginnings of concept analysis in nursing can be traced to Wilson (1963/1969), whose processes were used as the only guidelines for nurses' attempts at identifying and describing concepts. Walker and Avant's (1988, 1995, 2005, 2010) thoughtful strategies for concept and theory development, derivation, and integration further clarified the process and demonstrated its multidimensionality. There are many examples of the use of their strategies in the literature, for example, Dennis (2003). These pioneering efforts were followed by the introduction of other options that made the processes of concept development more congruent with the nature of the discipline of nursing as a human and caring science (Rodgers and Knafl, 2000). Each new strategy was developed to reflect the perspective of nursing as holistic and interactive, and with the natural domain of nursing and its dynamic concepts (Rodgers, 1989; Schwartz-Barcott and Kim, 2000; Wuest, 1994). The introduction of options in the development of concepts allowed for more congruency with the style and format of agents of knowledge development, as well as with the goals and levels of existing knowledge in the nursing discipline.

One of the most comprehensive discussions about concept development was provided by Beth L. Rodgers and Kathleen A. Knafl, first in 1992 and then in 2000. Their seminal text included chapters by many authors who discussed either the syntax or the substance of concepts or a combination of both. Several strategies were provided with exemplars of how the strategies were used. The strategies discussed are the Wilson method of concept analysis, the evolutionary method of concept analysis, the Hybrid model of concept development, concept clarification, simultaneous concept analysis, multiphase approach to concept analysis and development, and concept development within a critical paradigm (Rodgers and Knafl, 2000). Within all these different strategies are some fundamental processes that could be used as the bases for all types of concept development.

In this chapter, I have provided a framework for the most fundamental strategies that lead to advancing the progress of concept development. I have also discussed the different components of concept development, and have described those strategies that I believe are essential for advancing nursing science and for making a difference in the quality of nursing care. The reader will notice that those strategies described pay specific tribute to the centrality of clinical practice in developing concepts, no matter which strategy is used.

There are four major fundamental strategies for concept development. These are concept exploration, concept clarification, concept analysis, and integrated concept development. These strategies are used at various levels of nursing concept development. Each strategy has different processes to advance the concept to the next level of development.

CONCEPT EXPLORATION

Concept exploration is a strategy for concept development used when new concepts are identified and before they become an accepted component of the nursing lexicon. Similarly, a concept may have been accepted in the daily experience of nurses, yet because it is embedded in the nursing experience, its existence and properties are normalized, thereby camouflaging and limiting the concept's growth and meanings. *Sacrifice* is such a concept; this term was used to describe nurses' or patients' responses to work situations, plans of care, or changes in life styles. However, the how's, what's, when's, and why's were not described, and nurses have taken for granted that we knew its meaning (Florczak, 2004). Views of sacrifice from other fields, as well as from the humanities, helped provide an initial definition of sacrifice, so that the author could then begin to imbed this definition in nursing practice situations to further clarify it (Florczak, 2004). Therefore, concept exploration is a strategy used when a concept has only recently been introduced in the literature and it is too early to articulate its definite properties and potential explanatory power. Exploration of a concept presupposes that it is unknown to the readers of nursing literature, or that it is so familiar that it has been taken for granted, to the extent that members of the discipline are not aware of its significance to the development of knowledge. Concept exploration is also appropriate for concepts that have been uncritically adopted by nursing from other disciplines without consideration for the values, assumptions, and missions of the discipline (e.g., see the concept of empathy in (Morse, Anderson, Bottorff, et al. [1992]). Other examples are branding (Dominiak, 2004) and improvisation (Hanley and Fenton, 2007). Concept exploration is the process by which a phenomenon is identified and introduced to colleagues to raise their consciousness about the phenomenon, to claim its importance and significance for nursing, and to stimulate the members of the discipline to consider it further in their research. Another goal for concept exploration is to nurture curiosity about a particular concept. When a concept is introduced into the literature through concept exploration, the author should be raising and answering questions about its relevance to nursing and its meaning to nursing clients. Concept exploration is used when concepts are still ambiguous and their relationships to the discipline of nursing are still at the preliminary stages of consideration.

Concept exploration includes identifying the major components and dimensions of the concept through appropriate questions raised about each component. Then, triggers are proposed to continue the exploration process. Advantages to the discipline or nursing practice are identified and defined. The ultimate goal in concept exploration is to demonstrate whether or not there is the potential for further development of this concept. It is also to build a case for reasons to continue with or discontinue such explorations. Concept explorations are essential in a dynamic and changing discipline that is responsive to global, societal, and individual changes. It maintains the dynamism and responsiveness of the discipline.

Two examples of concept exploration are Norris' (1985) classic proposal of the concept of "primitive pleasure" as the basic human need and as a possible goal for nursing to nurture, preserve, and attend to in human beings. In proposing to give attention to primitive pleasure, she questioned physiologic homeostasis as a goal for nursing practice. She explored primitive pleasure as sensual, sensory, and carnal, as compared to cognitive and aesthetic. She defined pleasure as bodily pleasure at the basic and reflexive level and less at the intellectual level. Although it may call on some cognitive processes to perceive these pleasures, it reflects a certain level of awareness and consciousness, and does not require any cognitive processes to experience it or to modify it. Norris explored the meaning of this concept and its relationship to nursing, indicating that nurses' work has always included a focus on enhancing patients' pleasure by helping them to feel comfortable through touch and through other sensory stimuli. By offering a clinical exemplar to demonstrate the potential of better understanding patients' needs through the concept of primitive pleasure, she further supported her claim for the need to explore the development of this concept. However, because her goal was to raise nurses' consciousness to the competing goal of heightened pleasure, as compared with maintaining homeostasis, the major questions that she answered were: What is pleasure? And, what potential has it for nursing? She proposed that a range of patterned experiences to demonstrate it must be identified and examined. She also looked at other writings in nursing to document and support her arguments for developing the constellation of subconcepts related to primitive pleasures. She further explored the concept by examining others' seminal writing, such as Nightingale, who almost a century earlier proposed promoting the pleasure of her Crimean War patients. The ultimate goal for concept exploration is for a reader or a listener to say "this is worth considering and developing further."

Another example of exploration is provided by Laborde (1989), who proposed to consider the concept of torture as a nursing concern. She described the nature of the concept and situated the concept within the domain of nursing and within health care. In reviewing this exploration, a reader realizes that nurses can have different experiences of torture; they can be the subjects of torture; they may participate in torture, either willingly or unwillingly; and they may care for patients who have been tortured. Therefore, there is a need for further development of knowledge related to this concept, its implications in the health care of tortured individuals, and the roles that nurses play. With the world events of terrorism and torture in detention camps during the first decade of the 21st century, this beginning concept exploration points to nurses' potential roles in uncovering, understanding, researching, and preventing torture, and caring for patients who have been exposed to torture.

These two examples demonstrate what I mean by concept exploration. In neither example was the concept ready for a full-fledged concept analysis or for the development of any propositions. Both raised consciousness, both made the reader curious about their meanings and implications, both connected the concepts of nursing to the proposition, both challenged some levels of the status quo about what nurses need to know, and both provided support for why the concept is worth further development. These processes are essential for concept exploration, and concept exploration is a strategy for concept development.

In a dynamic and evolving science such as nursing, it is essential to promote communication and dialogue about concepts during the exploration phase of development. Concept exploration may be used more vigorously by different constituents, for example, by clinicians who are developing concepts based on their clinical practice, but equally by researchers who are discovering new concepts through their research programs. Concept exploration should be encouraged to enhance uncovering of new ideas.

CONCEPT CLARIFICATION

Concept clarification may be used to refine concepts that have been used in nursing without a clear, shared, and conscious agreement on the properties or the meanings attributed to them. The goal of concept clarification is to refine existing definitions, sharpen theoretical definitions, consider interrelationships between the different elements of the concept, discover new relationships, and discuss these relationships to resolve existing conflicts about meanings and definitions. Concept clarification may also help reveal previously unrecognized ambiguities in concepts. For example, the concept of "competence in nursing practice" has long been part of the nursing lexicon and has been applied internationally to professional practice; however, its definition has been elusive. Through a process that involved revisiting the different meanings provided in the literature, Garside and Nhemachena (2013) concluded that there is no universally accepted definition. Clarification enables nurse scholars, educators, and clinicians to agree upon a single definition to effectively guide their dialogues.

Concept clarification was proposed by Norris (1982) "to foster the development of increasingly meaningful descriptions of nursing phenomena" (p. xv). It was also defined by Kramer (1993) as "a highly creative, rigorous, and intuitive process that can generate multiple useful meanings for a single concept" (p. 407). This strategy includes processes of inclusion and exclusion, in which attempts are made to define what could be included and what could be excluded in the foundation, meaning, and attributes of the concept. One useful process is to clarify boundaries, to define contexts, and to define other subconcepts surrounding those concepts that are being clarified. Concept clarification reduces ambiguity; yet clarification includes a critical review of the properties of a concept, illuminating new dimensions to it that had not been considered beforehand, widening the sphere of the concept beyond previous views, while narrowing its boundaries for better definition to support its further development. Processes in concept clarification include comparing, contrasting, delineating and differentiating, providing exemplars, identifying assumptions and philosophical bases, identifying what events trigger the phenomena, and proposing questions from a nursing perspective. Answers to these questions help in the further development of a concept. In concept clarification, the implications for nursing research, theory, and practice are carefully discussed.

According to Norris' (1982) classical and pioneering article, which endures and transcends time, concept clarification has five steps:

1. After identification of the concept from within the discipline, as well as consideration of how it could be considered through the lens of other disciplines, repeatedly describe the phenomenon inherent in the concept.
2. Systemize the observations and the descriptions of the phenomenon. Establish categories and hierarchy; continue to observe, discover, communicate, and think about the concept; develop insights. Look for patterns and sequences of events. Ask and answer such questions as: What events trigger the phenomenon? What happened before to inspire the phenomenon? What happened as a result of the phenomenon?

3. Develop operational definitions, and ask yourself and others: How will I know the concept when I see it?

4. Construct a model. Models provide a better tool for communication, and help to depict the relationship between the responses, events, situations being clarified, and other related concepts.

5. Develop hunches and hypotheses to move to an experimental mode.

All strategies and processes for concept development are based on the ability of the developer to use critical thinking skills. Kramer (1993) and Chinn and Kramer (1999) made a compelling argument for the connection between critical thinking and concept clarification and for the rationale that concept clarification is a strategy that could enhance critical thinking. They identified several steps toward clarifying concepts, each with several processes; these are: formulating the purposes of clarification, selecting and synthesizing data sources, and developing a conceptualization. In clarifying concepts, the theorist identifies and examines assumptions, identifies and analyzes contexts, provides multiple interpretations, and engages in reflective analysis of the results.

Concept clarification does not require the development of contrary cases, propositions, hypotheses, antecedents, or consequences, which are essential processes in concept analysis. A clarified concept stimulates thinking and explains an aspect of nursing (Mairis, 1994). Concept clarification in nursing must be connected to health and to the goals of nursing. Concept clarification includes literature reviews and analysis of the literature to identify values and attributes and to compare and contrast the properties that may have been defined (Lackey, 2000).

I believe that the processes of concept clarification described in the preceding text may have contributed to the identification of the different meanings and conceptualizations of caring. Morse, Solberg, Neander et al. (1990) explored caring and described the different ways in which it appeared in the literature. They clarified caring by its epistemological perspectives, which resulted in five conceptualizations: caring as a human trait, as an emotion, as a moral imperative, as a mutual endeavor, or as a therapeutic intervention. Lewis (2003) further clarified four pathways for thinking about caring as "being." The properties identified are spirituality, moving beyond the self, creating healing environments, and being artistic. This is accomplished through a process of clarification that involves transforming the caregiver and the one being cared for.

Hall, Stevens, and Meleis (1994) and Hall (1999) introduced a concept to the nursing literature that had been taken for granted, and was accepted and used, yet its conscious use was limited. They defined marginalization as "the process through which persons are peripheralized on the basis of their identities, associations, experiences, and environments" (p. 25). Marginalization is defined as being away from the center, being at the borders or the periphery, being a part of the periphery of social networks. They defined its properties as intermediacy, differentiation, power, secrecy, voice, and liminality (perceptions of time, world, and self-image and its relationship to experiences). Each of these properties is defined, discussed, and related to the concept as a whole. They clarified the central components (peripheralization), some salient properties (associations), and some conditions (it is a process). They differentiated marginalization from alienation (focused on subjective experience), from stigmatization (one aspect), and from segregation (more physically oriented). Furthermore, marginalization is differentiated from vulnerability and from oppression.

Absent from this analysis were those processes used in developing exemplars and contrary cases. However, the authors made a case for the significance of the concept for nursing research, nursing practice, and the theoretical development of the discipline. The concept is studied in the discipline of nursing, and a case was made for its relevance to further knowledge development (Hall, 1999). One significant aspect of this concept is its origin and the process by which it is clarified. It is not a new concept. It has been used interchangeably with a number of other concepts, including vulnerability; therefore, the authors set out to clarify the concept and to propose its centrality in nursing. It evolved from individual research programs dealing with low-income women or women without incomes and their access to health care, patterns of self-care, lesbians' patterns of responses and relationships in the health care system, lesbians living with or dealing with substance abuse, low-income women with HIV, and lesbians dealing with sexual abuse. The common thread in all of these programs of research was the intense marginalizing experiences of women, which prompted the authors to take a closer look at the concept and its meanings, and its potential for further development. The other important aspect of this example of concept clarification is the collaborative effort of the authors/researchers and its influence on clarifying a concept transcending time, geography, and setting.

Another example of concept clarification is provided by Beeber and Schmitt (1986) in their clarification of the concept of group cohesiveness. Although this is a concept that has been previously described, discussed, and studied, the authors developed a case for its relevance to nursing, and for reexamining and redefining the potential contribution of nurses to the development of theory related to this concept. In clarifying the concept, they added a new perspective that allowed the questioning of the positive values that were automatically granted to this concept. Their critical examination of a broader view of the meaning of the concept, allowing the exploration of both the negative and positive, made the process more of clarification and less of analysis. The authors provided a history of the definition, identified the diffusion of the concept and the ambiguities inherent in the existing definitions, defined its properties, reviewed relevant literature in other disciplines, critically analyzed the use of group cohesiveness in the nursing literature, and provided alternative uses for the concept in nursing research and theory building for introducing students to group work, for further developing precise measures, and for the development of clinical indicators, among other uses. Similarly, by clarifying the concept of professionalism in Iranian nursing, Dehghani, Salsali, and Cherghi (2015) demonstrated that professional behaviors taught to students in an academic setting are different from the professional behaviors expected and observed in a practice setting; this enabled the authors to identify barriers and facilitators related to professionalism.

Some more mature concepts may be better explored by using more than one method. The concept of *hope* is an example. With the many definitions in the literature, analyzing existing definitions (Wilson) and exploring views from other disciplines (Norris) yielded a more comprehensive definition for one author (Sachse, 2007). Building on these definitions, others continued to clarify the nature of hope and its relationship to other concepts in nursing (Tutton, Seers, and Langstaff, 2009). Another form of clarification may require a research study, as was used to clarify the concept of "patient participation," a concept very often used to describe patients' involvement in the care process. It is a concept described as well in several nursing theories. By studying it through a grounded theory design, a group of Swedish authors clarified an important core category of mutuality in negotiation to explain how nurses understood participation. A clarification process added an important dimension to the concept's many other dimensions (Sahlsten, Larsson, Sjöstrom, et al., 2007).

CONCEPT ANALYSIS

Concept analysis is a strategy for further developing concepts. In using concept analysis processes to develop concepts, the assumption is made that the concepts have been introduced in the literature, that they have been defined and clarified, but that they are in need of further analysis to advance them to the next level of development. Concepts are analyzed when their significance is established and their relationship to the discipline of nursing has been clarified. Analysis implies a breaking down to well-defined components; it reflects building and rebuilding, and presumes the essential components are identified and defined. The goal of analysis is to bring the concept closer to being used for research or for clinical practice, as was done with the concept of wellness to render it more appropriately used with older adults (McMahon and Fleury, 2012). Concept analysis contributes also to instrument development and theory testing (Davis, 1992). Processes inherent in concept analysis include answering some significant questions and raising some new, pertinent questions.

Several strategies have been used in the nursing literature to analyze concepts: the Wilson method, the simultaneous concept analysis strategy, and the hybrid method. Each is described briefly.

Wilson's Method of Concept Analysis

One of the most cited references for concept analysis is Wilson's (1963/1969) method. The variations on this method have been described by Chinn and Kramer (1991) and Walker and Avant (2010), among other scholars in nursing. Examples of the use of the Wilson method in nursing are given by Avant (2000) and Avant and Abbott (2000). Wilson identified 11 steps to use in concept analysis.

1. Identify and isolate the questions of the concept. Three different sets of questions are described. The first set of questions is related to facts. He proposes that these questions should be answered by existing knowledge about the concept. The second

set of questions involves those related to values about the concept. These need to be answered based on moral principles of the "shoulds" and "should nots," as determined by society or other important bodies that influence moral judgment in a discipline. The third set of questions is related to meanings; these are best considered in terms of concepts; they do not concern facts or values. Although questions may appear to belong purely to only one category, in the broader sense they are not truly pure and may reflect more than one category.

2. Consider the possible answers to the questions and identify the essential elements of these questions. The goal here is clarity of communication in an attempt to find answers that are "right." Right answers are given within a context. Avant (2000) demonstrated how the "right" answer to a question differs in different contexts by using the concept "science," which is defined differently in different disciplines: a process, truth establishment, or a social activity. The "right" answers also change according to the context of the particular era. For example, titles of "Hispanic," "Latina," and "Mexican American" evolved new meanings over the years.

3. Identify and describe exemplars to reflect the different critical and essential characteristics of the concept. Identify the typical features, as well as those that may not be so typical. The question he proposes answering here is: "If that is not an example of it, then nothing is." These exemplars are considered model cases.

4. Identify "contrary cases," that is, those exemplars that do not include any of the properties of the concept. Just as with exemplary cases, contrary cases may be the extreme opposites of the exemplars, in that the concept is not readily visible or apparent. These are cases in which the concept and its properties are absent.

5. Identify, describe, and use some related cases in which the concept may be connected or similar in some way, or as it occurs in similar texts. Analyze which features are essential and which are not. For example, "change" is a concept related to the concept of "transitions."

6. Provide borderline cases as exemplars. Select exemplars that may have some features or attributes of the concept and in which ambiguity exists about whether the case belongs to the concept or not. Particularly consider cases that are difficult to classify because they help in the further development of the concept.

7. Develop and present invented cases. Wilson promoted the idea of developing an invented situation to exemplify the typical features and properties for the concept. The context for the invented case may be different, the exemplar may be totally out of the ordinary, and the method of recounting the case should be innovative. These invented cases are developed to highlight or enhance the major features of the concept. Examples may be found in poetry and in fables.

8. Identify and define the social contexts, and analyze concepts with an eye to who may use it, why it may be used, and how it could be used. Concepts occur within a social context that includes the past as well as the future. Meanings are derived from a social context, and interpretations differ across disciplines, time spans, regions, and cultures.

9. Beware of underlying anxiety related to concepts or generated by the concepts. Wilson encourages identifying, describing, and analyzing the feelings attached to the concept. This means identifying any controversy related to the concept, whether it has any stigma attached to it, and what debates exist related to it. These are the sentiments generated by the concept due to history, meanings, and unresolved issues.

10. Define and explain the potential practical results related to the concept. The practical uses of the concept need to be defined and identified, and a breakdown of its essential elements and their relationship to practice should be defined.

11. Carefully choose the language used to describe the results and label the concept. Finally, Wilson recommends making a decision on the best words to use to reflect the concept and its meaning. Because words often have different meanings, as well as ambiguous interpretations, it is essential to choose one meaning and label to reflect it. He suggests selecting a label with an eye on usefulness.

There are many variations to Wilson's method (Avant, 2000) in nursing. An example is analysis of pain management. Pain management is accepted in nursing as an integral component of the nurses' mission in providing nursing care to clients. The meaning of this concept is varied, and its goals are numerous. It could be based on a value system of reciprocity, patriarchy, or collaboration. Davis (1992) used a concept analysis strategy to identify the role of patient involvement in managing their own pain. On the basis of Walker and Avant's (1995) strategies, she examined patients' perceptions of pain management, explored the different definitions offered in the literature, defined the concept's attributes, developed an exemplary case, identified border and related cases, and identified ways by which pain management could be empirically referenced in clinical situations. The analysis provided the basis for patient involvement in the caring processes.

Walker and Avant's (2010) strategies, which are used extensively in developing nursing concepts, are based on Wilson's strategies. However, theirs differ in that the guidelines and the specific steps in their strategies are more user-friendly and better suited for nurses' needs for well-operationalized steps. By using one of the strategies that they outlined for developing concepts based on the phenomenon of *interruption*, the authors were able to identify several properties, including: interruptions could be planned or unplanned human experiences, internally or externally created, and they create discontinuity. As a process that nurses experience frequently, understanding the properties and outcomes of interruption could lead to an effective program of research related to its outcomes on nurses and patients (Brixey, Robinson, Johnson, et al., 2007). Similarly, Hawks' (1991) analysis of power resulted in identifying the properties of power as "power to" versus "power over" and in the development of a conceptual map that contains the different components inherent in power (sources, skills, and orientation) and the role of self-confidence in attaining the goals. The systematic analyses of these two concepts may lead to further development of the concepts and create the potential for more systematic research, with the ultimate result of developing client-sensitive and client-responsive theories. Many other examples in the literature utilize Walker and Avant's strategies in concept analysis, including analysis of concepts for multidisciplinary use (McNeill, 2014). It is of note that these strategies have been utilized in Sweden (Allvin, Berg, Idvall, et al., 2007), Canada (Campbell-Yeo, Laatimer, and Johnston, 2008), Egypt, Netherlands, Austria, Germany (Boggatz, Dijkstra, Lohrmann, et al., 2007), Australia (Levett-Jones, Lathlean, Maguire, et al., 2007), Ireland (Fogarty and Cronin, 2008), and Korea (Shin, Park, Ryu, et al., 2008).

Simultaneous Concept Analysis

Many concepts in nursing are interrelated and overlapping, such as interaction, communication, relating, and reciprocity, among others. The concepts of change, transition, coping, and adapting also have many common and uncommon attributes. One innovative and discipline-congruent strategy for analyzing concepts is the simultaneous analysis strategy used by Haase, Leidy, Coward et al. (2000) in analyzing spiritual perspective, hope, acceptance, and self-transcendence. This strategy is based on collaboration, critical thinking, expertise of participants, complementarity, mutual trust building, and mutual consensus building. These attributes are congruent with the nature of nursing as a human science and a caring discipline.

Colleagues interested in similar or different concepts may join efforts to clarify their concepts in relation to a larger whole, and in the process, clarify others' concepts and increase the clarity of the concept based on the common root of the related concepts. Although most other strategies used a more individual approach to concept development, the simultaneous concept analysis is based on a value system of connectedness and collaboration (Haase et al., 2000). Individual analysis, thinking, and conceptualizing form the first building blocks for this strategy. Antecedents, critical attributes, and outcomes for each concept are first identified and defined. Similarities and differences in attributes, antecedents, and consequences are then identified to create what the authors call a validity matrix.

The group reviews, compares, and contrasts the results of their development of similar components with each original concept and engages in critical assessment, paying particular attention to language, semantics, meanings, and goals. This process continues until some shared agreement is achieved and a visual diagram or table is constructed to reflect this agreement. This strategy supports the potential of refining concepts and developing them further. It is a strategy that is congruent with the nature of human science as dialogue and with the nature of scientific discovery as collaborative. Several examples illustrate the multiuse of this strategy. One example is considering a concept through the lens of different philosophical paradigms. This enriches our ability to uncover the multitude of dimensions of a concept, as well as deepening our understanding of clients' different perspectives. A second example is considering *spirituality* from empiricism, interpretivism, and poststructuralism (Tinley and Kinney, 2007), and a third is comparing and contrasting *presence* and *caring* (Finfgeld-Connett, 2008). Finally, another outcome of this strategy may be the ability to develop a middle-range theory, as demonstrated by a group of Swedish clinicians who used it to refine and develop a theoretical model of coping for families of patients in intensive care units (Johansson, Hildingh, Wenneberg, et al., 2006).

The Hybrid Strategy

This strategy synthesizes empirical with theoretical approaches. Schwartz-Barcott and Kim (1986, 2000) developed this method. This is another strategy more congruent with the evolving nature of methodology in nursing research, in that it combines quantitative and qualitative methods. The hybrid strategy is also based on the concept Wilson's analysis strategy (1963/1969) and the grounded theory approaches of Schatzman and Strauss (1973).

Schwartz-Barcott and Kim (2000) identified three major phases. The first is the theoretical phase, the second is field work, and the third is the analytical phase. These phases are not sequential or linear; work can be ongoing in each and all simultaneously. In the theoretical phase, the theorist defines a concept, searches the literature, identifies meaning and measurement issues, and selects a working definition. In the fieldwork phase, the theorist sets the stage for the proposed work, negotiates, selects participants, and collects and analyzes data. Comparing, contrasting, and weighing the results, and allowing time to revisit the theoretical and fieldwork phases, constitute the final analytical phase. Some similarities exist between the simultaneous and hybrid strategies. Both could deal with clusters of related concepts, and both are multidimensional.

Madden (1990) used this strategy to develop the concept of therapeutic alliance, and the author supports its utility in distinguishing the properties of one concept from other similar and related concepts. Similarly, DeNuccio and Schwartz-Barcott (2000) used the hybrid model to analyze the concept of withdrawal. They began with a review of the pervasiveness of the concept in nursing and discovered that it is relatively underdeveloped. They then defined the concept as a flight response used as a defense to an actual or anticipated threat. They described it in terms of biologic adaptation

and an instinctive physical response. Then, they discussed how it is measured in research through a literature review. Subsequently, they observed it clinically, developed a set of key questions related to observations, developed case studies to reflect the different responses, and validated earlier notions about withdrawal. It is through these processes that common factors were identified to describe and refine withdrawal.

Other effective examples of how the three phases of a hybrid strategy—theoretical, empirical, and analytical—were used is in developing the concepts of *health literacy* (Sykes, Wills, Rowlands, et al., 2013), *being sensitive* (Sayers and de Vries, 2008), *dance in mental health nursing* (Ravelin, Kylmä, and Korhonen, 2006), and *mindfulness* (White, 2014). In all cases, the hybrid method for developing the concepts provided step-by-step guidelines, helped increase the depth of the analysis, and produced rich definitions. In all situations, the authors concluded that using multisources to develop the concepts illustrated the significance of the concept, although a need remained for further support and development of the concepts.

Concept analysis of international nurse migration, that was completed utilizing extensive literature review, led to identifying its uses and describing its attributes, but it proved to be a challenging process requiring research, critical analysis, and synthesis of results. It is noteworthy that this extensive analysis resulted in considering the importance of focusing on the rights and freedom of choice for immigrants (Freeman, Baumann, Blythe, et al., 2012). The extensive multidimensional concept analysis demonstrated the complexities involved in nurse migration and added new dimension to understanding it.

AN INTEGRATIVE STRATEGY TO CONCEPT DEVELOPMENT

All of the previously mentioned strategies, in addition to the foresight of metatheorists who pioneered the movement toward developing knowledge in nursing (e.g., Chinn and Kramer [1999] and Walker and Avant [2010]), have made major contributions to elucidating the most appropriate strategies to use in a human science discipline. Strategies continued to evolve, most often based on Wilson's approach to concept development (Rodgers, 1989). The critics of these strategies point out the lack of contextualization of the process (Paley, 1996), as well as the tendency to view the concepts as static (Rodgers, 2000). Over the years, I have worked with colleagues and students to develop concepts, narratives, and theoretical propositions by using an integrative strategy to concept development.

This strategy evolved over years of teaching, mentoring, researching, and theorizing. Since the late 1960s and early 1970s, I have presented students in graduate theory classes with the request/requirement to participate in developing concepts from phenomena that have captured their interest and attention.

In reflecting on some of my rationale for not using existing strategies (none of the strategies was articulated at the time, except for Wilson's), three reasons become apparent. The first is well analyzed by Wuest (1994). Existing strategies appear limited in capturing context and are less direct about biases (sexism, politicism, and racism) that exist in the social structure in which health care is embedded. The strategies provide limited framework to uncover oppression, to analyze the status quo and its effect, or to reflect on the different realities and ways by which to change these situations that perpetrate inequities.

The second reason is their limited guidelines for approaching concept development from the perspective of clinical practice or from the experiences of clinicians. The strategies are also limited in their acknowledgment and affirmation of the experiences that students, clinicians, researchers, and theoreticians bring with them. These experiences affect the way they view and choose to focus on any particular situation and, therefore, should be part of the analysis and the development of the concept.

The third rationale is inherent in the "recipe" approach to concept development, which reduces the process of concept development to a series of ingredients, steps, and phases—rather than focusing on critical thinking, consciousness raising, and value clarification—which are components of knowledge development. The question that remained to nag me is how to build into any strategy opportunities for raising consciousness about what is, as well as what ought to be, in understanding, shaping, and developing concepts (Henderson, 1995). Reed and Leonard (1989) admonished nurses to "move beyond conceptual ruts" (p. 51) by ethically questioning the frameworks used in analyzing problems, and by allowing the process of concept analysis and development to raise more questions than it may answer (Rodwell, 1996). The selection of the phenomena

from which concepts are developed is a process of consciousness raising. These are some of the reasons that have prompted the development and refinement of an integrative strategy over the years. The starting point for concept development using the integrative strategy could be from any source, research, practice, or literature review.

With the level of maturity that the discipline of nursing has achieved, developing concepts could begin from different sources, as well as from a combination of sources. The impetus may be clinical observations, undefined phenomena from other theories (Peck, 2008), an existing concept (Takase, 2010), a synthesis from the literature (Bonis, 2009; Cypress, 2010; Weaver, Morse, and Mitcham, 2008), or from research (Izumi, Baggs, and Knafl, 2010; Wiseman, 2007). While one of the strategies described in this chapter may be the primary framework, increasingly, a combination of sources is essential for advancing knowledge about concepts. As we think about a future for knowledge development that is more informed and based on a solid foundation of evidence, using a combination of strategies will become the norm. A similar approach to using a combination of strategies is reflected in the use of the evolutionary strategy to concept development that was developed by Rodgers (2000) and well utilized in developing such concepts as community health (Baisch, 2009), social isolation (Nicholson, 2009), and cancer survivorship (Doyle, 2008). Just as there are more indications that we are moving toward more interdisciplinarity, interprofessional education and collaboration, more interconnection between disciplines and fewer silos, I propose that there should be fewer silos between the different strategies. An example of other authors who considered new strategies for developing theories that are more integrative and less siloed is known as ID-EA, which incorporates inductive and deductive inquiry, synthesis, and evaluation. An example of its use was to describe the concept of liminality in cultural transitions and advance it to theory-based practice (Baird and Reed, 2015).

In this section, I propose a strategy for developing concepts from different starting points, and I demonstrate the process from phenomenon to concept. There is no one way or approach for identifying phenomena. There is no one way of doing it, and there is no way by which the richness and haphazardness of the process can be fully captured. Conceptualizing is never reducible to a linear set of components or to a neat and tidy set of processes. A conceptualization could happen all at once, or it could take years and never quite evolve into a useful integrated view of reality. There are, however, six stages and several processes that are useful in engaging in the whole activity of theorization, whether theorization is used as a framework for research, for data interpretation, for concept development, for statistical model building, or for the development of a theory. The stages are: (1) sensing and taking in a phenomenon, (2) describing a phenomenon, (3) labeling, (4) concept development, (5) statement development, (6) explicating assumptions, and (7) sharing and communicating. Although these stages and processes are presented here linearly and sequentially, they could occur simultaneously, out of sequence, or in conjunction with other, yet undelineated, stages. It is useful for students of theory to deliberately and consciously experience each of these stages, even when such experiences are based on only a rehearsal of what they would use in the development of theory.

Sensing and Taking in a Phenomenon

Sensing, pausing, and taking in are processes of sizing up a situation that has attracted our attention for whatever reason, whether that reason is cognitive, affective, objective, or subjective, or whether it is a hunch or just an uneasy feeling. A phenomenon may attract and hold the attention of the observer, making her pause to think about it and reflect on its nature. This *attention grabbing* may happen when the phenomenon is occurring, or it may evolve retrospectively. A clinician may air the room whenever she changes a dressing without pausing to think about the relationship of increased fresh air in the room and healing. A clinician may want a family to be present during a painful procedure for a patient, or might change a patient's position, believing that either or both may decrease suffering and/or enhance well-being. These actions or their consequences may have been the reasons a clinician continues to practice them, but, because they have not grabbed her attention, she has not been able to develop them further. Attention grabbing includes observations, mental labor, and personal involvement, all so closely intertwined that it makes it hard to reduce them to linearity: What happens first? What happens next?

Observation is a complex process, more of a sensory experience than merely seeing. Accurate observation is difficult because of the tendency for selective observations and selective inattention. To know when one is observing with the eyes and when one is observing through mental activity helps to clarify and distinguish the dimensions of observation (Zderad and Belcher, 1968). Both activities are part of attention grabbing and are essential in developing theories, but they need to be deconstructed into components and distinguished from one another. We cannot totally separate what we observe from what we want to see or what we observe from our experiences; nor do we want to. However, we can allow ourselves to observe what we do not know, what we, at this time, do not understand, and what is out of the realm of our experience. Observation occurs both with the "naked eye" and within a "matrix of theory." Beveridge (1957) reminds us that:

> Accurate observation of complex situations is extremely difficult, and observers usually make many errors of which they are not conscious. Effective observation involves noticing something and giving it significance by relating it to something else noticed or already known; thus it contains both an element of sense-perception and a mental element. It is impossible to observe everything, and so the observer has to give most of his attention to a selected field, but he should at the same time try to watch out for other things, especially for anything odd. . . . Powers of observation can be developed by cultivating the habit of watching things with an active, inquiring mind. (pp. 104–105)

A deliberate attempt must be made to experience and practice naked-eye observations, as well as observations within the matrix of theory or those guided by a paradigm. Observation is not a new skill to nurses; it has been the cornerstone of practice. As King (1975) put it:

> Direct observation has been a primary function of nurses for centuries. Nurses collect voluminous data in their daily activities to gain immediate factual information to plan and give nursing care. They have been trained to make observations and to measure selected physiological and behavioral parameters of human beings to answer immediate questions. (p. 26)

After the initial serendipitous identification of a phenomenon, whether from a clinical setting or from careful review of research studies, attention grabbing is followed by *attention giving*. Attention giving is a more deliberate process. It is a process that includes a careful delineation of those situations or events that have the potential of demonstrating the phenomenon under consideration. Situations or incidents selected for observation should vary to consider different aspects of phenomena. An example may illustrate this process. A primary health care worker in Cali, Colombia, noticed over the years that per diem maids tended to ignore all attempts to bring them to the clinic early in their pregnancy for prenatal care. She also noticed that they tended to bring their sick children to the emergency room with the very first sign of any mild illness. The discrepancy between getting prenatal care and getting pediatric care caught her attention. The health care worker may then choose to give this matter her attention and deliberately look into the differences between the two clinics, the meanings attached to pregnancies and offspring, and to preventive and curative care, or she may choose to consider the environments of both clinics or a number of alternatives, depending on her interest, goals, and previous experiences as a theorist.

Sometimes a question—a patient's, a colleague's, one's own—may call attention to some phenomenon and provoke thinking. The beginning may be the absence of an expected response experienced by the nurse with surprise, anger, disappointment, or relief. These subjective responses may be used as clues to the nature of the phenomenon itself. (Zderad, 1978, p. 40)

It is looking at the experience with wide-open eyes, with knowledge, facts, theories held at bay; looking at the experience with astonishment. Concentrating on the experience is absolutely necessary. Becoming absorbed in the phenomenon without being possessed by it is equally important. (Oiler, 1982, p. 180)

During the taking-in and attention-getting processes, a dialogue with oneself, with one's theoretical journal, with others, or with all these may be helpful in delineating the phenomenon to further pursuit. The dialogue may include the following questions:

What is it that is attracting the attention of the observer?

Where does it happen?

Is it similar to or different from happenings under different sets of circumstances?

Under what conditions does the observer sense it, see it, hear it, observe it, read it, or touch it?

Can the observer describe it? What is the description?

Can the observer document it with model cases and prototype situations?

The objective of completing the taking-in stage with the two processes of attention grabbing and attention giving is to delineate a phenomenon for further theoretical development.

Describing a Phenomenon

The interest in some problem, question, situation, or event—theoretical or clinical—gnaws at the observer for some time. Our early theorists began their theoretical formulations with a nagging problem based on experience, observation, and thinking related to the organization of nursing curricula and the nature of the substantive knowledge that should be included in nursing courses. Some specific questions that baffled them were: What is nursing? And, what is nursing's mission? The combination of their questions and their clinical backgrounds resulted in several theories that have helped us distinguish the boundaries of our discipline. These theories have attempted, and succeeded in some ways, to provide some abstract concepts and propositions that can be generalized to different areas of specialization in nursing.

Nursing has gone beyond the beginnings of being concerned only with the disciplinary boundary questions that preoccupied our colleagues in theory. Members of the discipline are now capable of focusing inquiry with the goal of developing theories on phenomena surrounding health, transitions, interactions, nursing clients, and nursing therapeutics.

The observer should attempt to respond to the following questions in defining the phenomenon:

What is the phenomenon?

When does it occur?

What are the boundaries of the phenomenon?

What does it share with a larger class of phenomena?

Does the phenomenon vary? Under what circumstances?

Is the phenomenon isolated in reality?

Does it have a function? Are there multiple factors associated with it? Does it serve an explanatory purpose?

Does it refer to a long-term behavior, to characteristic or habitual modes of behaving, or to patterns of behavior detectable in repeated or similar acts?

Is the phenomenon related to time and place?

Is the phenomenon related to some theoretical framework, to one's basic philosophy of nursing or manner of being? In what way?

This sums up what the phenomenon is and where and when it occurs. Answers to each of these questions will help describe a phenomenon.

The description of a phenomenon may be first articulated in question form. An interest in sleeplessness in intensive care units may prompt one of the following questions (Landis, 1983):

Why do patients experience periods of lack of sleep in intensive care units?

What are the properties of sleeplessness or wakefulness in intensive care units?

Is sleeplessness an adaptive coping style or a maladaptive one?

Others' interests or clinical focuses may prompt other types of questions, such as:

What processes do nurses go through to decide whether or not to provide pain medication for patients experiencing pain?

What are the properties of effective transition into the sick or well role?

What are effective and ineffective transitions?

What are the predictors of occurrence of premenstrual stress?

What is a stressful menopausal experience?

Why do certain immigrant groups seem to be more consistently "satisfied" with health care than others?

What types of social support do different subcultural groups need during illness?

Once the general problem area is identified, questions are then asked to determine whether the problem of interest falls within the domain of nursing. They include:

In what way is the phenomenon related to nursing's substantive knowledge process?

In what way would understanding the phenomenon help in explaining some aspect of nursing care?

Can you think of some questions around that phenomenon, the answer to which would be significant to nursing?

How is the phenomenon related to the social policy statement of what nursing is?

Are there some biases that you could identify: background of the researcher, presence of the researcher?

Did the investigator provide contrasting observations, thereby demonstrating contexts in which phenomena are observed or not observed?

Are there repetitive patterns?

A phenomenon is not a thing in itself; it is not what exists, but rather is organized around perceptions. When experience, and sensory and intuitive data become coherent as a whole, and prior to attachment of any meaning, we have a phenomenon. A phenomenon, then, is an aspect of reality colored by the perception of the viewer of that reality. A phenomenon remains merely a phenomenon as long as we attach to it no cognitive, intuitive, or inferential interpretation. For example, separate and repetitive observations of the appearance of newly immigrated groups occurring more often in emergency rooms than in the regularly scheduled outpatient clinics is a beginning observation that may evolve into a phenomenon. When one observes that individuals belonging to the immigrant group tend to miss scheduled appointments and appear more often at unscheduled times, a vague pattern begins to emerge. When the observer further hears an individual from the same or another immigrant group rejecting the pace of life in the United States and complaining about having to plan activities and events so far in advance, then the vague pattern begins to form into a shape. The form could be concerns about planning, disenchantment with structured existence, or various abilities to deal with emergencies in preference to maintenance. The observer can then ask questions, observe, read, and structure situations in which planning is considered a norm (e.g., birthing preparation, rehabilitation, and discharge), and can therefore ascertain whether indeed a pattern is still apparent.

Delineation of phenomena is achieved through the analysis of models, situations, or exemplars. Model situations are vivid examples of the phenomenon and help to describe it. A model situation depicts reality in its prototype, its ideal form, and it allows demonstration of what the phenomenon is and where it exists (Chinn and Jacobs, 1987).

Labeling

Labeling is a stage that comes somewhere during the process of theorizing, and a label may change several times in the process. The function of labeling is to communicate succinctly, to relate to the written literature, to help to delineate what further observations to obtain, and to reduce a phenomenon that is usually described in a paragraph to a concept or statement. Labeling is more than selecting a Label X to describe Phenomenon Y. Labeling allows for semantic analysis (Scheffler, 1958). Semantic analysis permits the theorist to consider the normative use of the term, as well as other more esoteric uses. Labeling is associated with a kind of defining that ranges from a dictionary definition to a more complex definition that takes the perspective of the theorist into consideration. The label, "preference for spontaneity," emerged from further consideration of Middle Eastern immigrants' health and illness behaviors to denote their lack of enthusiasm about planning, preference for dropping in over making appointments, preference for missing appointments, and preference for showing up in the delivery room with no prenatal care (Olesen and Meleis, 1990). A label of "positioning" allows exploration of a patient's position in bed, ability to breathe, outcome of decrease in edema, and/or ability to feel empowered when communicating with others. A label and semantic analysis bring the theorist closer to concept development.

Some criteria must be considered when labeling concepts. Lundberg (1942) suggests Eubank's (1932) criteria, which insists on the use of precise labels that contain only one idea and that are consistent in their meaning whenever they are employed.

Labeling a concept is a highly individualized experience involving interpretations of the phenomenon. It includes hunches, opinions, and speculations. A labeled phenomenon is a concept or a statement, but it is predefined theoretically and operationally.

Concept Development

Somewhere in this process of theorizing, and not in linear progression, a concept begins to emerge. Concepts evolve out of a complex constellation of impressions, perceptions, and experiences. Conception in Kantian terms is an organized perception. Phenomena are perceived, and only when they are organized and labeled do they become concepts. Concepts are a mental image of reality, tinted with the theorist's perception, experience, and philosophical bent. They function as a reservoir and an organizational entity, and they bring order to observation and perceptions. They help to flag related ideas and perceptions without going into detailed descriptions.

Several processes are useful in concept development: defining, differentiating, delineating antecedents and consequences, modeling, analogizing, and synthesizing. *Defining* depends on the label given to the phenomenon. Therefore, the labeling stage should be carefully considered; premature labeling may prompt the theorist to review unrelated literature. Defining a concept helps to delineate subconcepts and dimensions of the concept. During the process of defining concepts theoretically and operationally, the theorist is smoothing rough edges, clarifying ambiguities, enhancing precision, and relating concepts to some empirical referents. Lundberg (1942) also suggests that:

Operational definitions, then, are merely definitions which consist as far as possible of words clearly designating observations of events and performable and observable operations subject to corroboration. Thus, they may consist of (1) "physical manipulations," such as reading the weight on a weight scale, (2) "objective verbal designations of these manipulations," or (3) "verbal designations of symbolical or mental operations," such as the definition of "preference for spontaneity."

Operational definitions of concepts in nursing have to be referenced in practice and put into context in reality. Otherwise, they would not be useful for nurses (Jacobs and Huether, 1978). A human response, a unit of analysis for nursing theorists, may not always lend itself to the same corroboration expected in the physical sciences and strived for by social scientists, nor should it.

Defining concepts could also be based on an extensive review of literature to further delineate a concept. Covington (2003) reviewed literature related to "caring presence" and articulated a definition that could be used to further develop a concept. A systematic review of analyses of the concept of quality of life in nursing resulted in the need for continuous investigation to differentiate it from other concepts (Fulton, Miller, and Otte, 2012).

Differentiating is a process of sorting in and sorting out similarities in and differences between the concept being developed and other like concepts. In developing the concept of transition as a central concept in nursing, Chick and Meleis (1986) discussed the similarities and differences between the priorities of the concepts of transition and change. Similarly, Reed and Leonard (1989) described how they saw the differences between self-neglect, the concept under development, and suicide and noncompliance. The importance in using the process of differentiation is in accessing related bodies of literature and in further refining the attributes of the concept under development.

In *delineating antecedents*, the theorist is attempting to define the contextual conditions under which the concept is perceived and is expected to occur. Antecedents to transitions that are of interest to the domain of nursing have been defined as events such as recovery, death, immigration, amputation, diagnoses of chronic illnesses, pregnancy, and admission to hospital (Chick and Meleis, 1986). The theorist may ask, "So what?" in attempting to identify the consequences of the concept. Consequences are those events, situations, or conditions that are related to and preceded by the concept under development.

To *delineate consequences*, a theorist can practice by listing every concept or statement that, in her opinion or as manifested in research findings, may result from the concept. It is important to deliberately attempt to delineate positive as well as negative consequences. Consequences of transition may be disorientation, confusion, growth, changes in body image, changes in self-concept, and role sufficiency (Meleis, 1975).

Modeling is the process of defining and identifying exemplars to illustrate some aspect of the concept. Exemplars could be clinical referents or research referents. Several types of models are used, each to illustrate different aspects of a concept. A like model is one that illustrates the concept in its entirety. A contrary model is a situation, a group, or an incident in which a contrasting aspect of the concept is absent or is present under a different set of contextual conditions. A population that is not in some major transition may be compared with one that is undergoing a significant transition, which may provide the contrary model. A like model and a contrary model help the theorist in articulating, demonstrating, and highlighting the differences between situations, events, and clients in which the phenomena related to the concept are demonstrated and not demonstrated, thus increasing the potential for clarifying it further. Paterson and Zderad (1988) described a technique of explanation through negation to help in describing the phenomena. Presenting another related phenomenon that does not describe the phenomenon under development helps sharpen the clarity of that phenomenon.

> *A phenomenon cannot be described completely by negation but it may be clarified to some extent by saying what it is not. For instance, empathy is not sympathy; it is not projection; it is not identification. (p. 90)*

Analogizing is a process by which a deliberate choice is made to describe the concept under development through another concept or phenomenon that is sufficiently like the one under study, but that has been studied more extensively, explored more systematically, and therefore is better understood than the concept under study. If the phenomenon and the concept are alike, but represent different domains, and we understand one more than the other, then perhaps the better-understood phenomenon will help shed some light, raise better questions, and offer greater insight into the lesser-understood phenomenon. An example of analogizing is the use of fables or fictional stories to illustrate a concept. One example of analogizing that I used is of aliens from other times and planets to illustrate the need for international collaboration in knowledge development (Meleis, 1987).

Synthesizing is a process of bringing together findings, meanings, and properties that have been amplified by each of the processes described previously. Synthesizing includes, but is not limited to, describing future steps in theorizing.

Statement Development

The development of a concept may be an end result for some theorists and an interim stage for others, one leading to further development of a concept through statement development or research implementation. However, concept development may not be possible because the situation requires statement development. The questions that we may be facing in nursing as a human science are: Is concept development the only avenue to the development of theory? Is it possible that the building blocks for nursing theories are statements, descriptions of situations without zeroing in on specific concepts?

Statement development is a stage during which explanations related to the phenomenon are provided. The explanations link the concepts, antecedents, consequences, and assumptions. Statements are developed to describe, explain, prescribe, or predict. They are developed as an end result or to synthesize other statements for research purposes.

To develop statements, several questions may be helpful. Examples are:

In what ways can we further explicate the concept being considered?

In what ways are nursing clients' health and environment affected by the concept?

What are some potential consequences of the concept?

What are some corollaries of the concept?

Propositions are tentative statements about reality and its nature. They describe relationships between events, situations, or actions. Propositions could be developed to describe the properties of the concepts; these descriptive propositions are called *existence propositions* (Zetterberg, 1963). They are factor-isolating propositions (Dickoff, James, and Wiedenbach, 1968), and the end result is therefore descriptive theory, as essential to science as any other theory. Consider, for example, descriptive theory of the atom and its significance to our knowledge of the atom.

Propositions may also be relational, describing the association between concepts or causal relationships between concepts (Reynolds, 1971). The process of developing propositions is also a process of identifying the central questions related to the concept. Propositions provide the central answers that help to explain, describe, or predict nursing reality. The more refined, developed, and advanced the relationship statements are, the more they are able to describe and predict the nature of the relationship, the direction of the relationship, and the strength of the relationship (Chinn and Jacobs, 1987).

Organizing propositions is one of the processes in the propositional stages. Proposition organization could be accomplished through different channels. Propositions may be arranged to represent the process of concept discovery and the process of proposition formation. In this case, a chronologic organization is achieved. A second way is to organize propositions around the central concepts in the theory. A third method is to organize propositions in terms of significance for testing, beginning with those whose test represents the central questions of the theory. Other ways are to organize around independent or dependent variables. Ordering propositions enhances their usefulness and their aestheticism (Zetterberg, 1963).

Explicating Assumptions

During every stage of the process, the observer pauses, reflects, and questions both implicit and explicit assumptions. To regard periods of wakefulness as sleeplessness, the observer has made an assumption that certain periods of wakefulness are disruptive and that disturbed behavior may result in sleeplessness. Imagine that the observer is beginning from an opposite point of view (i.e., that wakefulness promotes healing); observation will be more open to positive consequences, and to what promotes wakefulness. Therefore, reflection on and analysis of one's views, beliefs, and theoretical underpinnings will help delineate assumptions of the developing theory.

Sharing and Communicating

None of these stages and processes are entirely new to nurses, whether they are clinicians, theorists, or researchers. What may have made it appear new in the 1980s was the growing acceptance of conceptualization as a significant aspect of knowledge development in nursing. This acceptance is demonstrated in the journals devoted to conceptual development of the discipline and in the increasing productivity in metatheory and theory writing. No theorization process is complete without opportunities to share and communicate it with colleagues. Theorizing may happen in isolation, but it does not grow in isolation. Sharing and communicating goes beyond writing and publication. It should be defined as a daily happening in the lives of clinicians, theorists, and researchers.

Instead of staging opportunities for sharing and communicating conceptualizations, redefining existing opportunities and resources may enhance this process. Clinical conferences may be redefined to include a theoretical journal sharing hour. Faculty meeting time may be reorganized to permit discussion for evolving concepts or statements; students may use part of their class time for a juice or sherry hour to freely discuss phenomena of interest.

CONCLUSION

Concepts are the building blocks of theories and the cornerstones of every discipline. The rate of progress in the discipline of nursing can be measured by the extent to which members of the discipline are able to uncover and develop concepts that reflect the phenomena related to nursing care. These phenomena, neglected in the past because of the focus on more biomedical phenomena, are being identified, defined, and developed by nursing scholars. Strategies used in developing concepts that reflect these phenomena were initially borrowed from other disciplines. In the process of using these strategies, nursing scholars refined and further developed them. This chapter has described major strategies for the development of concepts, providing examples to ground each strategy in the experience of concept development. The strategies discussed in this chapter could also have use in nursing education; not only could they provide frameworks for educators to use in teaching concepts, they could also provide students with the tools for concept mapping, a visual approach that some educators use to represent students' knowledge levels and to determine gaps. By creating and studying these maps it harnesses students' critical thinking abilities and their clinical judgments as well (Atay and Karabacak, 2012; Gerdeman, Lux, and Jacko, 2013; Revell, 2012).

As you select one of these strategies to use in developing a concept of your choice, remember to

REFLECTIVE QUESTIONS

1. Select a phenomenon that interests you. Use the steps outlined by Wilson to define and develop it.

2. Compare and contrast the results in developing the phenomenon using the Wilson method to those you could achieve using the simultaneous strategy.

3. There was an attempt in this chapter to *not* present recipes for concept development, but rather to present guidelines. What do you consider are the strengths and weaknesses of each of the strategies presented in this chapter?

4. Select one published paper related to your phenomenon or concept of interest, and identify and critically analyze the processes in the development of the concept.

5. In what ways did the strategies used to define concepts support or stagnate the progress in developing knowledge in your field of interest?

6. In the integrative strategy, clinical practice, research, and conceptualizing are proposed to be used for concept development. Provide an example from literature in your field of interest for which you think this strategy is used. Critically describe how it was or was not utilized. Then, redevelop the concept using the integrative strategy.

7. Compare and contrast all strategies, identifying areas of agreement and those of disagreement.

8. Under the description of phenomena, the author identified a number of questions to define the phenomena of interest. Identify five critical/essential questions for this phase of integrative strategy for concept development.

use it as a guideline and not as a blueprint that must be implemented as is. The nature of the phenomena, the creativity of the user, the experience of the clinician, and the findings of the research should shape the nature of the concept. Do not sacrifice substance for method. The substance of nursing should continue to shape and drive the methods used. You, the reader, should also remember that you have a vital role in further developing and refining any and all strategies used in developing concepts.

REFERENCES

Allvin, R., Berg, K., Idvall, E., and Nilsson, U. (2007). Post-operative recovery: A concept analysis. *Journal of Advanced Nursing*, 57(5), 552–558.

Atay, S. and Karabacak, U. (2012). Care plans using concept maps and their effects on the critical thinking dispositions of nursing students. *International Journal of Nursing Practice*, 18(3), 233–239.

Avant, K.C. (2000). The Wilson method of concept analysis. In B.L. Rodgers and K.A. Knafl (Eds.), *Concept development in nursing* (pp. 55–64). Philadelphia, PA: W.B. Saunders.

Avant, K.C. and Abbott, C.A. (2000). Wilsonian concept analysis: Applying the technique. In B.L. Rodgers and K.A. Knafl (Eds.), *Concept development in nursing* (pp. 65–76). Philadelphia, PA: W.B. Saunders.

Baird, M.B. and Reed, P.G. (2015). Liminality in cultural transition: Applying ID-EA to advance a concept into theory-based practice. *Research and Theory for Nursing Practice: An International Journal*, 29(1), 25–37.

Baisch, M.J. (2009). Community health: An evolutionary concept analysis. *Journal of Advanced Nursing*, 65(11), 2464–2476.

Beeber, L.S. and Schmitt, M.H. (1986). Cohesiveness in groups: A concept in search of a definition. *Advances in Nursing Science*, 8(2), 1–11.

Beveridge, W.I.B. (1957). *The art of scientific investigation*. New York: W.W. Norton.

Boggatz, T., Dijkstra, A., Lohrmann, C., and Dassen, T. (2007). The meaning of care dependency as shared by care givers and care recipients: A concept analysis. *Journal of Advanced Nursing*, 60(5), 561–569.

Bonis, S.A. (2009). Knowing in nursing: A concept analysis. *Journal of Advanced Nursing*, 65(6), 1328–1341.

Brixey, J.J., Robinson, D.J., Johnson, C.W., Johnson, T.R., Turley, J.P., and Zhang, J. (2007). A concept analysis of the phenomenon interruption. *Advances in Nursing Science*, 30(1), E26–E42.

Bulman, C., Lathlean, J., and Gobbi, M. (2012). The concept of reflection in nursing: Qualitative findings on student and teacher perspectives. *Nurse Education Today*, 32(5), E8–E13.

Campbell-Yeo, M., Latimer, M., and Johnston, C. (2008). The empathetic response in nurses who treat pain: Concept analysis. *Journal of Advanced Nursing*, 61(6), 711–719.

Chick, N. and Meleis, A.I. (1986). Transitions: A nursing concern. In P.L. Chinn (Ed.), *Nursing research methodology*. Boulder, CO: Aspen.

Chinn, P.L. and Jacobs, M.K. (1987). *Theory and nursing: A systematic approach* (2nd ed.). St. Louis, MO: C.V. Mosby.

Chinn, P.L. and Kramer, M.K. (1991). *Theory and nursing: A systematic approach*. St. Louis, MO: Mosby–Year Book.

Chinn, P.L. and Kramer, M.K. (1999). *Theory and nursing: Integrated knowledge development* (5th ed.). St. Louis, MO: Mosby.

Covington, H. (2003). Caring presence: Delineation of a concept for holistic nursing. *Journal of Holistic Nursing*, 21(3), 301–317.

Cypress, B.S. (2010). Who is the emergency room patient? An evolutionary concept analysis. *Dimensions of Critical Care Nursing*, 29(4), 182–191.

Davis, G.C. (1992). The meaning of pain management: A concept analysis. *Advances in Nursing Science*, 15(1), 77–86.

Dehghani, A., Salsali, M., and Cheraghi, M.A. (2015, March). Professionalism in Iranian nursing: Concept analysis. *International Journal of Nursing Knowledge*, 27(2), 111–118.

Dennis, C.L. (2003). Peer support within a health care context: A concept analysis. *International Journal of Nursing Studies*, 40(3), 321–332.

DeNuccio, G. and Schwartz-Barcott D. (2000). A concept analysis of withdrawal: Application of the Hybrid Model. In B.L. Rodgers and K.A. Knafl (Eds.), *Concept development in nursing* (pp. 161–192). Philadelphia, PA: W.B. Saunders.

Dickoff, J., James, P., and Wiedenbach, E. (1968). Theory in practice discipline: Part 1. Practice oriented theory. *Nursing Research*, 17(5), 415–435.

Dominiak, M.C. (2004). The concept of branding: Is it relevant to nursing? *Nursing Science Quarterly*, 17(4), 295–300.

Doyle, N. (2008). Cancer survivorship: Evolutionary concept analysis. *Journal of Advanced Nursing*, 62(4), 499–509.

Duncan, C., Cloutier, J.D., and Bailey, P.H. (2007). Concept analysis: The importance of differentiating the ontological focus. *Journal of Advanced Nursing*, 58(3), 293–300.

Eubank, E.E. (1932). *The concepts of sociology*. Lexington, MA: D.C. Heath.

Finfgeld-Connett, D. (2008). Qualitative comparison and synthesis of nursing presence and caring. *International Journal of Nursing Terminologies and Classifications*, 19(3), 111–119.

Florczak, K.L. (2004). An exploration of the concept of sacrifice. *Nursing Science Quarterly*, 17(3), 195–200.

Fogarty, C. and Cronin, P. (2008). Waiting for healthcare: A concept analysis. *Journal of Advanced Nursing*, 61(4), 463–471.

Freeman, M., Baumann, A., Blythe, J., Fisher, A., and Akhtar-Danesh, N. (2012). Migration: A concept analysis from a nursing perspective. *Journal of Advanced Nursing*, 68(5), 1176–1186.

Fulton, J.S., Miller, W.R., and Otte, J.L. (2012). A systematic review of analyses of the concept of quality of life in nursing. *Advances in Nursing Science*, 35(2), E1–E12.

Garside, J.R. and Nhemachena, J.Z.Z. (2013). A concept analysis of competence and its transition in nursing. *Nurse Education Today*, 33(5), 541–545.

Gerdeman, J.L., Lux, K., and Jacko, J. (2013). Using concept mapping to build clinical judgment skills. *Nurse Education in Practice*, 13(1), 11–17.

Haase, J.E., N.K Leidy, Coward, D.D., Britt, T., and Penn, P.E. (2000). Simultaneous concept analysis: A strategy for developing multiple interrelated concepts. In B.L. Rodgers and K.A. Knafl (Eds.), *Concept development in nursing* (pp. 209–230). Philadelphia, PA: W.B. Saunders.

Hall, J.M. (1999). Marginalization revisited: Critical, postmodern, and liberation perspectives. *Advances in Nursing Science*, 22(2), 88–102.

Hall, J.M., Stevens, P.E., and Meleis, A.I. (1994). Marginalization: A guiding concept for valuing diversity in nursing knowledge development. *Advances in Nursing Science*, 16(4), 23–41.

Hanley, M.A. and Fenton, M.V. (2007). Exploring improvisation in nursing. *Journal of Holistic Nursing*, 25(2), 126–133.

Hawks, J.H. (1991). Power: A concept analysis. *Journal of Advanced Nursing*, 16, 754–762.

Henderson, D.J. (1995). Consciousness raising in participatory research: Method and methodology for emancipatory nursing inquiry. *Advances in Nursing Science*, 17(3), 58–69.

Izumi, S., Baggs, J.G., and Knafl, K.A. (2010). Quality nursing care for hospitalized patients with advanced illness: Concept development. *Research in Nursing and Health*, 33(4), 299–315.

Jacobs, M.K. and Huether, S.E. (1978). Nursing science: The theory-practice linkage. *Advances in Nursing Science*, 1(1), 63–74.

Johansson, I., Hildingh, C., Wenneberg, S., Fridlund, B., and Ahlström, G. (2006). Theoretical model of coping among relatives of patients in intensive care units: A simultaneous concept analysis. *Journal of Advanced Nursing*, 56(5), 463–471.

King, I.M. (1975). A process for developing concepts for nursing through research. In P.J. Verhonick (Ed.), *Nursing research* (Vol. 1). Boston, MA: Little, Brown.

Kramer, M.K. (1993). Concept clarification and critical thinking: Integrated processes. *Journal of Nursing Education*, 32(9), 406–414.

Laborde, J.M. (1989). Torture: A nursing concern. Image: *Journal of Nursing Scholarship*, 21(1), 31–33.

Lackey, N.R. (2000). Concept clarification: using the Norris method in clinical research. In B.L. Rodgers and K.A. Knafl (Eds.), *Concept development in nursing* (pp. 192–208). Philadelphia, PA: W.B. Saunders.

Landis, C. (1983). *Sleeplessness in intensive care unit: A developing concept*. Paper presented in the course Theory Development in Nursing at the University of California, San Francisco.

Levett-Jones, T., Lathlean, J., Maguire, J., and McMillan, M. (2007). Belongingness: A critique of the concept and implications for nursing education. *Nurse Education Today*, 27(3), 210–218.

Lewis, S.M. (2003). Caring as being in nursing: Unique or ubiquitous. *Nursing Science Quarterly*, 16(1), 37–43.

Lundberg, G.A. (1942). *Social research*. New York: Longman's Green.

Machado, A. and Silva, F.J. (2007). Toward a richer view of the scientific method: The role of conceptual analysis. *American Psychologist*, 62(7), 671–681.

Madden, B.P. (1990). The hybrid model for concept development: Its value for the study of therapeutic alliance. *Advances in Nursing Science*, 12(3), 75–87.

Mairis, E. (1994). Concept clarification in professional practice—dignity. *Journal of Advanced Nursing*, 19, 947–953.

McMahon, S. and Fleury, J. (2012). Wellness in older adults: A concept analysis. *Nursing Forum*, 47(1), 39–51.

McNeill, C. (2014). Risk: A multidisciplinary concept analysis. *Nursing Forum*, 49(1), 11–17.

Meleis, A.I. (1975). Role insufficiency and role supplementation: A conceptual framework. *Nursing Research*, 24(4), 264–271.

Meleis, A.I. (1987). *Pandemic images: Knowledge development for empowerment*. San Francisco, CA: Sigma Theta Tau.

Morse, J.M., Anderson, G., Bottorff, J.L., Yonge, O., O'Brien, B., Solberg, S.M., and McIlveen, K.H. (1992). Exploring empathy: Fit for nursing practice? *Image: Journal of Nursing Scholarship*, 24(4), 273–280.

Morse, J.M., Solberg, S.M., Neander, W.L., Bottorff, J.L., and Johnson, J.L. (1990). Concepts of caring and caring as concept. *Advances in Nursing Science*, 13(1), 1–14.

Nicholson, N.R., Jr. (2009). Social isolation in older adults: An evolutionary concept analysis. *Journal of Advanced Nursing*, 65(6), 1342–1352.

Norris, C.M. (1982). *Concept clarification in nursing*. Rockville, MD: Aspen Systems.

Norris, C.M. (1985). Primitive pleasure as the basic human state. *Advances in Nursing Science*, 8, 25–43.

Oiler, C. (1982). The phenomenological approach in nursing research. *Nursing Research*, 31(3), 178–181.

Olesen, V. and Meleis, A. (1990). *Spontaneity: A social phenomenon observed in Middle-Eastern immigrants*. Unpublished manuscript.

Paley, J. (1996). How not to clarify concepts in nursing. *Journal of Advanced Nursing*, 24(3), 572–578.

Paterson, J.G. and Zderad, L.T. (1988). *Humanistic nursing* (2nd ed.). New York: National League of Nursing.

Peck, S. (2008). Survivorship: A concept analysis. *Nursing Forum*, 43(2), 91–102.

Ravelin, T., Kylmä, J., and Korhonen, T. (2006). Dance in mental health nursing: A hybrid concept analysis. *Issues in Mental Health Nursing*, 27(3), 307–317.

Reed, P.G. and Leonard, V.E. (1989). An analysis of the concept of self-neglect. *Advanced Nursing Science*, 12(1), 39–53.

Revell, S.M.H. (2012). Concept maps and nursing theory: A pedagogical approach. *Nurse Educator*, 37(3), 131–135.

Reynolds, P.D. (1971). *Primer in theory construction*. Indianapolis, IN: Bobbs-Merrill.

Rodgers, B.L. (1989). Concepts, analysis and the development of nursing knowledge: The evolutionary cycle. *Journal of Advanced Nursing*, 14, 330–335.

Rodgers, B.L. (2000). Concept analysis: An evolutionary view. In B.L. Rodgers and K.A. Knafl (Eds.), *Concept Development in Nursing: Foundations, Techniques, and Applications* (pp. 77–102). Philadelphia, PA: W.B. Saunders

Rodgers, B.L. and Knafl, K.A. (2000). *Concept development in nursing*. Philadelphia, PA: W.B. Saunders.

Rodwell, C.M. (1996). An analysis of the concept of empowerment. *Journal of Advanced Nursing*, 23, 305–313.

Sachse, D. (2007). Hope: More than a refuge in a storm: A concept analysis using the Wilson method and the Norris method. *The International Journal of Psychiatric Nursing Research*, 13(1), 1546–1553.

Sahlsten, M.J.M., Larsson, I.E., Sjöstrom, B., Lindencrona, C.S.C., and Plos, K.A.E. (2007). Patient participation in nursing care: Towards a concept clarification from a nurse perspective. *Journal of Clinical Nursing*, 16(4), 630–637.

Sayers, K.L. and de Vries, K. (2008). A concept development of "being sensitive" in nursing. *Nursing Ethics*, 15(3), 289–303.

Schatzman, L. and Strauss, A.L. (1973). *Field research: Strategies for a natural sociology*. Englewood Cliffs, NJ: Prentice-Hall.

Scheffler, I. (1958). *Philosophy and education*. Boston, MA: Allyn and Bacon.

Schwartz-Barcott, D., and Kim, H.S. (1986). A hybrid model for concept development. In P.L. Chinn (Ed.), *Nursing research methodology: Issues and implementations* (pp. 91–101). Rockville, MD: Aspen Systems.

Schwartz-Barcott, D. and Kim, H.S. (2000). An expansion and elaboration of the hybrid model of concept development. In B.L. Rodgers and K.A. Knafl (Eds.), *Concept development in nursing* (pp. 129–160). Philadelphia, PA: W.B. Saunders.

Shin, H., Park, Y.J., Ryu, H., and Seomun, G.A. (2008). Maternal sensitivity: A concept analysis. *Journal of Advanced Nursing*, 64(3), 304–314.

Sykes, S., Wills, J., Rowlands, G., and Popple, K. (2013). Understanding critical health literacy: A concept analysis. *BMC Public Health*, 13(1), 150.

Takase, M. (2010). A concept analysis of turnover intention: Implications for nursing management. *Collegian*, 17(1), 3–12.

Tinley, S.T. and Kinney, A.Y. (2007). Three philosophical approaches to the study of spirituality. *Advances in Nursing Science*, 30(1), 71–80.

Tutton, E., Seers, K., and Langstaff, D. (2009). An exploration of hope as a concept for nursing. *Journal of Orthopaedic Nursing*, 13(3), 119–127.

Walker, L.O. and Avant, K.C. (1988). *Strategies for theory construction in nursing* (2nd ed.). New York: Appleton-Century-Crofts.

Walker, L.O. and Avant, K.C. (1995). *Strategies for theory construction in nursing* (3rd ed.). East Norwalk, CT: Appleton-Lange.

Walker, L.O. and Avant, K.C. (2005). *Strategies for theory construction in nursing* (4th ed.). Upper Saddle River, NJ: Pearson/Prentice Hall.

Walker, L.O. and Avant, K.C. (2010). *Strategies for theory construction in nursing* (5th ed). Upper Saddle River, NJ: Pearson/Prentice Hall.

Weaver, K. and Mitcham, C. (2008). Nursing concept analysis in North America: State of the art. *Nursing Philosophy*, 9(3), 180–194.

Weaver, K., Morse, J., and Mitcham, C. (2008). Ethical sensitivity in professional practice: Concept analysis. *Journal of Advanced Nursing*, 62(5), 607–618.

White, L. (2014). Mindfulness in nursing: An evolutionary concept analysis. *Journal of Advanced Nursing*, 70(2), 282–294.

Wilson, J. (1963/1969). *Thinking with concepts*. New York: Press Syndicate of the University of Cambridge.

Wiseman, T. (2007). Toward a holistic conceptualization of empathy for nursing practice. *Advances in Nursing Science*, 30(3), E61–E72.

Wuest, J. (1994). A feminist approach to concept analysis. *Western Journal of Nursing Research*, 16(5), 577–586.

Zderad, L.T. (1978). From here-and-now to theory: Reflections on how. In J.G. Patterson (Ed.), *Theory development: What, why, how?* New York: National League for Nursing.

Zderad, L.T. and Belcher, H.C. (1968). *Developing behavioral concepts in nursing*. Atlanta, GA: Southern Regional Education Board.

Zetterberg, H.L. (1963). *On theory and verification in sociology* (Rev. ed.). Totowa, NJ: Bedminster Press.

15

Developing Theories

The aim of nursing science is to develop theories to describe, explain, and understand the nature of phenomena, and anticipate the occurrence of phenomena, events, and situations related directly or indirectly to nursing care. Theories are also developed to provide nurses with the rationale and the guidelines for models of care to change unwanted aspects of phenomena, as well as to support other aspects of phenomena. Theories provide frameworks for nursing prescriptions as well. These emerging explanatory and prescriptive theories reflect abstract representations of response patterns of human beings to health and illness, to environments, to treatments, and to health care professionals. They also represent patterns of how and under what conditions and within what contexts healthy and therapeutic and unhealthy and nontherapeutic relationships are formed in the health care system. In nursing, a human science, such descriptions and explanations are developed within a context of time, history, environment (social sanctions and obligations), and human conditions (including human rights). These aims for the development of theories in human science are congruent with the aims of other human sciences that are focused on human beings and their lives (Schensul, 1985).

The nature of nursing science and the potential in its growth require a close relationship between theory, practice, and research. Theoreticians, clinicians, and researchers in nursing share one ultimate goal—understanding the health care needs of clients and communities for the purpose of enhancing their sense of well-being, promoting their health status, facilitating their transitions, and increasing their access and options for health care that is most appropriate for their situation.

Despite this shared goal, few would deny that, in the history of the discipline, some tension has existed among theorists, clinicians, and researchers. This tension has been caused by myths and confusion about each other's intentions, methods, and goals. Some nurses, who may hold any one of

these roles, may believe some myths about other unfamiliar roles. For example, some clinicians may believe that theorists are only "ivory tower" philosophers who dream up ideas unconnected with practice or research. Without delving into these ideas and studying them, they may tend to dismiss them. Researchers, the theorists counter, focus on small research projects using empirical approaches to the development of nursing knowledge. These research projects may confirm or refute propositions that are disconnected and may not reflect a coherent approach to illuminating phenomena within a coherent context. Some clinicians believe that researchers and theorists are too far removed from clinical practice to be able to develop models of care useful for implementation, so how could they possibly develop theories that could be helpful in understanding clinical phenomena? Some clinicians even go so far as to ask how theoreticians and researchers could presume to describe, explain, or predict outcomes of clinical practice when they have not been regularly involved in providing nursing care to patients, families, or communities? Educators also using similar arguments may contribute to the gaps between theory, research, and practice by not introducing philosophical discourses or by not engaging in dialogues about nursing theories in their teaching (McIntyre and McDonald, 2013).

Truth is multidimensional and tends to be dynamic and contextual; therefore, there are some truths in all these positions, but none represents all truths for any one position. The theorists have provided the discipline—and continue to do so—with a coherent vision of the core of its domain: the focus on patients as human beings; the interactional nature of clients, nurses, environment; and the primacy of health and well-being as the crux of the discipline's mission. The goals of self-care, adaptation, homeostasis, expanded consciousness, balance, and harmony with environments were articulated by theorists as the major goals of nursing care. They proposed concepts that have become the cornerstones of the discipline and about which there has been more agreement than was anticipated in the 1970s. Researchers, on the other hand, have developed instruments for some central concepts, such as wound healing, levels of confusion, social support, pain intensity, and symptom distress. Researchers also have tested some theoretical propositions related to clinical practice, such as the determinants of maternal role development, or the determinants of recovery in cardiovascular patients. Clinicians have used theory as the bases for their actions, even when they were not able to articulate which theories they use and under which circumstances.

In the 1980s, attempts were made to complete the practice–theory–research cycle. Mercer, for example, systematically worked on identifying responses to mothering in adult women, in adolescent women, and in women undergoing cesarean and vaginal deliveries (Mercer, 1984; Mercer, Ferketich, May, et al., 1987a, 1987b). Mercer identified clinical issues related to mothering, such as ways in which new mothers establish mothering role cues, as well as the timing in which these cues appear. Mercer continued to develop and refine her theoretical ideas. She relabeled and redefined mother role attainment theory to "becoming a mother," which is more congruent with nursing as a human science (Mercer, 2004). Benoliel's critical analyses on psychosocial responses of patients to cancer are another example. Benoliel is a researcher who was engaged in studying clinically relevant questions that are embedded in a theoretical tradition, and she has developed theoretical propositions from her clinical and investigative work. She also provided guidelines to using her findings and theoretical guidelines in holistic care for clients who have life-threatening diseases or who are grieving from losses related to terminal illness (Benoliel, 1977; Benoliel and De Valde, 1975; Benoliel, Tornberg, and McGrath, 1984). She bridged the gaps between education, research, and practice by providing guidelines for educators for curricular development related to transitions and life-threatening diseases (Benoliel, 1982, 1983). These are only two powerful examples that illustrate the notion that progress in the discipline of nursing is predicated on actualizing the relationship between the research, theoretical, clinical, and educational bases.

More recently, McCrae's (2012) concern about the absence of nursing theory in education, practice, and research led her to review the major debates in the literature about nursing theory. She identified several barrier themes: the lack of definition of the nursing discipline; the belief that theories do not provide prescriptions for practice; the belief that theories are incompatible with evidence-based practice; a de facto medical leadership that impedes utilization of nursing models; the lack of nurse autonomy; and the lack of relevance of theories with contemporary health care systems. In spite of these barriers, there is agreement among many that by engaging in nursing-focused theoretical dialogues, nurses may be more effective in bridging the gap between theory and practice (Hatlevik, 2012) and, more importantly, may enhance their abilities to develop theory.

One assumption that appears to receive approving nods from members of the discipline is that disciplines develop through scientific discoveries, and scientific discoveries are useful when they are organized into some coherent wholes. These wholes could be theories or theoretical statements. Theories provide the frameworks that help in describing, explaining, predicting, and prescribing. Therefore, theory construction and development are activities that are essential in all disciplines. In fact, the progress of any discipline is measured by the scope and quality of its theories and the extent to which its community of scholars is engaged in theory development. Completing isolated research projects that are not cumulative or that do not lead to the development or corroboration of theories has limited usefulness. Kuhn (1970) contends that disciplines that are in the preparadigmatic stage demonstrate a pattern of research equated with haphazard problem solving; the central questions of the field are not well identified. The results of the individual research projects do not lead to theoretical formulations that may explain phenomena; may predict events, situations, or responses; and may help in prescribing interventions. It is for all these reasons that we offer strategies for developing theories.

Activities of theory development are not new to nurses, despite another myth that persisted for many years, that nurses began their theoretical journey only in the mid-1970s and early 1980s. Whether they were aware of it or not, clinical nurses have actively participated in conceptualizing many aspects of the domain of nursing. These conceptualizations demonstrate different approaches to theory development. For example, the earliest attempts at capturing nursing practice conceptually are well illustrated by Florence Nightingale, who, through the wisdom she gained from her work in the Crimean War, linked health with environmental factors, linked care with systematic data collection, and linked hygiene with well-being. Her efforts resulted in conceptual views of patients as physical, spiritual, and intellectual beings needing warmth, nutrition, and quiet environments (Nightingale, 1992). She conceptualized the environment as external to the patient, comprised of air, water, drainage, light, and cleanliness. Her writings about data collection, graphics and statistics, and health and illness demonstrate many theoretical propositions, some of which have been tested by epidemiologists. Other aspects of her conceptualization, such as the relationship between health and clean environments, have been used in the development of other theories, such as Rogers' theory of unitary human beings (Rogers, 1970).

Many more attempts at theory development followed Nightingale's. Some are reported in the literature, and many more may have gone unreported. Any time that concepts are delineated, hunches are developed by linking concepts together to help describe, explain, predict, or prescribe, and those hunches are communicated and used in a number of situations (the genesis of generalization), the beginnings of a theory are formulated. The developer of those hunches has been engaged in a process of theory development. In most instances, the process and product go unreported; therefore, the process is not complete, and a theory does not formally develop. A theory is the articulation and communication of a mental image of a certain order that exists in the world, of the important components of that order, and of the way in which those components are connected. The mental image is an abstract representation of order that exists in reality as perceived by the theorist. It includes abstract concepts that then provide the potential of being generalized to a number of categorical events or situations. Some efforts in theory development go unrecognized, most probably because of a lack of communication and a limited potential for generalization beyond the one experienced situation. But perhaps it is also because nurses lack an awareness of their potential to articulate aspects of the discipline theoretically or are reluctant to accept the potential for theorizing in a practice discipline.

The 1980s were characterized by a multiplicity of strategies for theory development. For example, Walker and Avant (1988, 1995, 2005, 2010) proposed different beginning points for theorizing concepts, statements, or theories and different approaches for derivation, synthesis, or development. The 1980s also were characterized by a multiplicity of research approaches that would inevitably lead to different types of theories (Allen, Benner, and Diekelmann, 1986). The development of concepts important to nursing and central to its domain was another significant feature of the decade. Examples of these concepts are self-neglect (Reed and Leonard, 1989), environment (Stevens, 1989), dyspnea (Carrieri, Janson-Bjerklie, and Jacobs, 1984), cachexia (Lindsey, Piper, and Stotts, 1982), and comfort (Neves-Arruda, Larson, and Meleis, 1992).

Subsequent to the momentum that focused on the mechanics and processes of theory development, some rich dialogues in the literature are based on viewing nursing phenomena through the critical lens of theoretical assumptions and philosophical principles, with a continuation adherence to the confines of the syntaxes of concept development (Andershed and Ternestedt, 2001), derivations, development of taxonomies, and levels of theories as seen, for example, in such titles as "Implications of Taxonomy on Middle Range Theories" (Blegen and Tripp-Reimer, 1997, see Chapter 21). A new trend emerged toward the end of the 20th century in advancing the theoretical discourse in the literature by using tools of analysis to develop new less-developed phenomenon, such as the concept of "intentional action by clients" (Burks, 2001; Kulig, 2000).

In addition, the theoretical discourse of the new century was free from the boundaries imposed by the early, more structured theories and approaches to theory construction. This allowed a new breed of theory developer to use innovative and more contemporary approaches to developing theoretical nursing approaches to viewing phenomena (Cutcliffe and McKenna, 2005). I am using "approaches" here intentionally to contrast it with structures or theories. For example, Harden (2000) advances the argument that language analysis can be used as a framework to better understand patients' narratives and that understanding is enhanced by tapping into the narratives of both the patients (as recipients of care) and the providers of care.

In reviewing the theoretical dialogues during the first decade of the 21st century, it is apparent that there are many areas of agreements. Those who discussed theory development have a shared view of the proper domain for theoretical formulations. One such shared view is to include in theories the evidence accumulated from research that depicts situations or events related to responses or anticipated responses to health and illness (Smith and Liehr, 2003). Current and future theoretical work will focus on the further development of concepts emanating from the nursing domain and its mission and from the practice and actions of nurses. Central concepts in the nursing domain that continue to capture the attention of nurses are relationships with environments, well-being, interaction, coping with transitions, positioning, living with illness, presence of family, safety, quality of life, and nursing therapeutics, among others. Theory development may also occur in the functional areas of administration, teaching, and learning (Meleis, 1992).

THEORY DEVELOPMENT: EXISTING STRATEGIES

A review and analysis of the literature of theory in nursing yields four major strategies of theory development. These are differentiated primarily by their origin of theory, practice, or research, and by whether, in addition to their original source, other sources were used in developing the theory. These four major strategies are: (1) theory to practice to theory; (2) practice to theory; (3) research to theory; and (4) theory to research to theory. Each of the strategies is presented and discussed in this chapter. Another strategy, an integrative approach to theory development, is presented in Chapter 16 for the development of middle-range theories. Further refinement of this strategy is presented in Chapter 17 for the development of situation-specific theories. This ought-to-be strategy is the most congruent with the discipline of nursing and could be used by itself or in combination with any of the following approaches to theory development.

Theory-to-Practice-to-Theory Strategy

The theorist who uses this strategy begins the process of theorizing by selecting a theory to use in practice and then uses practice to refine the theory further. This strategy is based on several premises:
- An existing theory can help in describing and explaining nursing phenomena; however, the theory's assumptions are not completely congruent with the assumptions that guide nursing.
- The theory is not entirely useful in helping nurses meet their goals in nursing practice. The theory does not define phenomena in ways that are useful for the integrity of the nurse practice act definitions.

- The theory does not directly help in defining actions for nurses. The focus of the theory is different from the focus needed for nursing practice.
- The theory does not provide adequate definitions of the central concepts of nursing.

A theorist using this strategy attempts to explain and describe a clinical situation through the selected theory and discovers the need for a modification of concepts, redevelopment of others, and possible reconsideration of other definitions that better reflect the practice situation. She may also consider relationships between concepts that were not proposed in the original theory or ones that interpret these relationships from a nursing perspective. This strategy for theory development speaks only to circumstances in which we see the world through an established theory with delineated concepts. It is a particular theory then that guides actions and dictates how we see nursing and how we act in the world.

Many examples in the nursing literature demonstrate the use of this strategy in theory development (Table 15-1). Peplau's (1952) theory of interpersonal relations in nursing was based on psychoanalytical theory that she used as a framework to describe psychiatric nursing practice. Her theory of nursing reflects psychoanalytical concepts and her psychiatric nursing clinical expertise. Johnson's (1980) view of the client as consisting of subsystems of behavior and her theory about assessments and diagnoses of nursing problems as occurring due to imbalance, overload, or deprivation are based on biomedical and systems paradigms. Her background in pediatric care, her continuous interest in clinical nursing, and the paradigms guiding her nursing world resulted in her theory of nursing. Johnson's view of a client with subsystems of behavior is analogous, but not equal to, the biomedical system. Her notion of homeostasis as a goal of nursing is parallel to Parsons' (1951) idea of homeostasis of social systems. The structure and function of Johnson's subsystems are modeled after the structure and function of Parson's social systems. The result is a theory of nursing that describes a nursing client, explains some of the actions of the client and the nurse, and, perhaps, could in the future predict further action. Another example of this strategy is Benner's theory of novice and expert practice (1984) based on her clinical observations through the Dreyfus and Dreyfus model of skill acquisition in aircraft pilots (1986).

Some may say these are borrowed theories. Barnum (1990) disagreed. She stated that "borrowed

TABLE 15-1	Examples of Theory to Practice to Theory: Clinical and Paradigmatic Origins of Selected Nursing Theories	
Theory →	Practice →	Theory →
Psychoanalytic theory	Psychiatry	Peplau
Systems theory	Pediatrics	Johnson
Adaptation theory	Pediatrics	Roy
Existentialist	Psychiatry	Travelbee
	Adult/Med Surg	Paterson and Zderad
Biomedical systems	Med Surg	Orem
		Henderson
		Abdellah

theories remain borrowed as long as they are not adapted to the nursing milieu and the nursing image of human beings. Once such theories have been adapted to the nursing milieu, it is logical to refer to these boundary overlaps as shared knowledge rather than as borrowed theories" (p. 95). The strategy discussed here is based on deriving nursing theories from theories developed in other disciplines. These derived theories reflect unique nursing knowledge and its practice field. Dickoff and James (1968) contended that theories from biology, psychology, and sociology are "building blocks . . . in the mansion of nursing theory" (p. 202). A new meaning is given to the guiding theory or paradigm, a new meaning that is pertinent to nursing. Norbeck (1981), Mercer (1981), Millor (1981), and Meleis (1975) used a theory or viewed nursing through another paradigm to develop a conceptualization of social support, maternal role attainment, child battering, and role supplementation, respectively, describing and explaining behaviors related to nursing care.

Other modifications of this strategy are exemplified by Roy and Roberts (1981) and Paterson and Zderad (1988). Roy viewed nursing from systems, adaptation, and interactionist paradigms. Her theory combines those paradigms with nursing practice, and the result is the person as an adaptive system or with two internal control systems, the regulator and the cognator subsystems. The activities of these subsystems are demonstrated through four adaptive modes (effectors): the physiologic mode, the self-concept mode, the role-function mode, and the interdependence mode. The development of the modes, particularly the self-concept, the role-function, and the interdependence modes, is derived from an interactionist sociologic paradigm as exemplified by self-concept, role, and symbolic interactionist theories. Paterson and Zderad's (1988) uniqueness evolved from using existentialist philosophy as

the paradigm for the development of their nursing theory. There are several common processes in the development of theories through this strategy:

- Knowledge of non-nursing theories and of a practice field
- Analysis of theory and practice area (analysis is a process by which the object of analysis is reduced into components and each component is defined and evaluated; theories are reduced to assumptions, concepts, and propositions; and practice is described through exemplars and case models)
- Use of assumptions, concepts, and propositions of theory to describe the clinical area
- Redefinition of assumptions, concepts, and propositions to reflect the domain of nursing (redefining may also include modifications of some aspects of theory)
- Construction of theories involving the development and explanation of exemplars representing the redefined assumptions, concepts, and propositions (assumptions, concepts, and propositions reflect the original theory)

An example of these processes is provided by considering Johnson's theory of behavioral subsystem. Johnson (1980) used Parson's (1951) concept of behavioral system, redefining it from a nursing perspective as "all patterned, repetitive and purposeful ways of behaving that characterize each man's life, are considered to comprise his behavioral system" (Johnson, 1980, p. 209). She then identified seven subsystems, labeled each, and discussed the relationship between each subsystem and the whole system. Several characteristics of a theory evolve from this strategy. The parent theory is well described and parallels the new practice-based theory. Concepts, attributes, properties, and descriptions are similar both theories. The context for the evolving theory differentiated from the context of the parent the

Additional examples are provided by Dalton (2003) as well as Bender and Feldman (2015). Dalton used Kim's theory of collaborative decision-making in a dyad in practice and added concepts about caregiver coalition formation and outcomes to develop a theory that could be used in research for family decision-making. Bender and Feldman, aware that a healthy environment is necessary to promote healing (Nightingale, 1992) but cognizant of the fact that maintenance of that environment may no longer be central to current nursing practice (Kleffel, 2005), used existing conceptualization of environment to develop a practice theory lens to reorient the relationship of environment to nursing practice.

Finally, it might be helpful to differentiate between the *clinical theorist* and the *clinician who uses theory*. The clinical theorist is one whose goals include the refinement and development of theory. The clinician who uses theory has a goal of theory application. The clinical theorist is engaged in practice and in the development or refinement of theory. She uses such processes as analyses, syntheses, comparisons, refinements, extensions, and reflections, as well as other mental processes. She uses the process of theory development to understand, know, or further develop some coherent generalizations that go beyond the present situation. The clinician who uses theory uses mainly clinical strategies to apply theories for the purpose of understanding and knowing. The differences and similarities are presented in Table 15-2.

Practice-to-Theory Strategy

Some theories are driven by clinical practice situations and are inductively developed. They reflect experiences that evolve from practice and are based on clinical situations and on the experiences of theorists in practice. This strategy is built on several premises:

1. Whatever theories that exist are not useful in describing the phenomenon of interest to the person. Existing theories are not helpful in understanding problems a clinician is confronting. We may not know, for example, what is providing comfort to nursing clients, how comfort is defined, how it is achieved, who is expected to participate in providing it, what are the different ways in which it is manifested, and what is feasible and what is not feasible in comforting patients in various stages of health–illness. Answers to these questions could be articulated conceptually by clinical experts through descriptions of models of comforting acts derived from their practice, then by defining it and continuing to develop it (Kolcaba, 2004).

2. The person is able to develop theories; there are resources to support the process of developing theories. Each theory, whether developed from practice or from research, was developed over a long span of time.

3. The phenomenon is significant enough to pursue, as developing knowledge about a phenomenon is a long process. The significance of the phenomenon is established historically, and supported by present imperatives or through reflection about breaking new future grounds.

4. There may be clinical understanding and wisdom about the phenomenon, but that

TABLE 15-2	The Clinical Theorist (Theory to Practice to Theory) and the Clinician Who Uses Theory (Theory to Practice)	
Theory to Practice to Theory		*Theory to Practice*
Goal		
Development; strategies for development		Application; strategies for application
Strategies		
Analyses, synthesis, comparison, refinement, extension, mental processes, reflection, creation		Analyses, description, interpretation, application
Uses		
Understand, know, develop		Understand, know
Evaluation		
Authenticity, congruency, context for discovery, context for justification, other criteria for evaluation of theory		Authenticity, congruency, context for justification
Person		
Clinical theorist		Clinician

understanding has not been articulated into a meaningful whole. Nurses may be viewing the phenomena individually and independently.

The clinician begins the process of theory development with a nagging question that evolves from a practice situation (Henderson, 1995; Kolcaba, 2004; Orlando, 1961). The insight is grounded in the practice situation, and the result has the potential for understanding other similar situations through the development of a set of propositions. This strategy depends on observing new phenomena in a practice situation; developing sensitizing concepts; and labeling, describing, and articulating the properties of these concepts. The properties are the subconcepts included in them, the boundaries, the definitions, the examples, the meaning, and so forth.

The development of theory using this strategy is based heavily on the work of Glaser and Strauss (1967). While collecting data, the researcher keeps diaries, observes, analyzes similarities and differences, compares and contrasts responses, and develops concepts and then linkages (Clarke, 2005). The grounded theory approach is credited to sociologists Schatzman and Strauss (1973) and Glaser and Strauss (1968), who have done a great deal to articulate the process and share its nuances, providing us with a multitude of examples to demonstrate its utility. It is a strategy not entirely foreign to nursing; the Yale school of thought in nursing produced many examples of theoretical development that are parallel to the work done by Glaser and Strauss (1968). Theories evolving from the Yale approach are those related to interpersonal relations and interactions in nursing, as viewed by Orlando, Travelbee, and Wiedenbach (see Chapter 12). These theorists developed their ideas by being totally immersed in clinical work, either giving care themselves or observing care being given. They used a variety of methods to collect their clinical data, such as case studies, interviews, and observations. It appears that they then isolated the central phenomenon of nursing related to the client's interaction with the nurse and those phenomena related to the development of nurse–patient relationships. Categories emerged, concepts were labeled, and beginning propositions were developed.

These were theories based on and evolving from clinical practice, with the intention of describing and explaining extant nursing practice. One may presume that the theorists did not use any existing paradigm or theories. This may or may not be true. An equal presumption may be that these theorists had an interactionist background, prompting them to see nursing practice in one particular way. This strategy is most useful for clinicians, particularly when they deliberately begin to use the process to develop theories, then articulate and communicate them. (Backscheider [1971] offers a useful example of this process.)

One of the most significant processes used by the pre-1980s theorists who demonstrated this strategy is their knowledge of their clinical areas. They had the resources to identify exemplars and to compare and contrast different exemplars. They may have used the same components defined and discussed in this chapter under the heading "Theory-to-Practice-to-Theory Strategy." However, without more information published about their strategies, it is not possible to use their work as an example of the modified practice–theory method.

Theorists using this strategy (such as [Olshansky, 1962] on chronic sorrow) tended to describe the clinical situation and processes that supported and/or inspired the evolving theories. An example of the use of this strategy is that provided by theorists who were interested in describing noncompliant behaviors. Clients who do not follow and "comply" with prescribed regimens have been labeled noncompliant or difficult. Some nursing scholars provided analyses demonstrating that neither concept adequately described the roles of intention and environment in not adhering to a regimen. Therefore, Reed and Leonard (1989) proposed instead the concept of *self-neglect*, which is defined as intentional neglect despite available resources. The authors described a clinical situation that prompted their conceptualization, reviewed existing theories, compared and contrasted self-neglect with other like concepts, such as suicide and noncompliance, then provided more clinical exemplars to refine the properties and attributes of the concept. This strategy is also exemplified by Maeve's (1994) "carrier bag theory of nursing practice." Her theory of nursing practice was modeled after Fisher's (1979) carrier bag theory of human evolution, positing that human beings evolved not through developing weapons, tools, and hunting, but through collecting, gathering, and accumulating. Instead of viewing human evolution as based on "man the hunter," she proposed "women as the carriers," and suggested that instead of viewing evolution through the innovation of hunting, that we consider the spectacular development of containers by women, the heroines, as the impetus for evolution and development. Maeve (1994) used this theory to reflect the everyday practices of nurses that evolve from storytelling of lived experiences in practice situations. She proposes that theories should be the result of capturing practice through articulating those ideas that represent nursing phenomena. The theory components are bedside nurses sharing their experiences, and the process of sharing and articulating these experiences, with practice-driven theories as the outcome of the narrative. Eakes (1995, 2004) integrated different published clinical observations on chronic sorrow into a middle-range theory, supported by research. Kahn-John (2016) used the practice-to-theory strategy to develop a resilience model that highlighted harmony, respect, and spirituality as cornerstones for wellness among the Navajo Indians. Although the impetus was practice, she integrated review of other theories as well as preliminary research results.

The processes used in developing practice-driven theoretical formulation are dynamic, changing to reflect the participants in theory development. Keeping journals, writing notes, reflecting in diaries, writing stories about clinical practice, talking with others, exposing our ideas for discussion, uncovering meaning, challenging assumptions, and most importantly, using critical thinking throughout these processes are methods to develop theories (Benner, 1984; Gadow, 1988; Habermas, 1984).

Research-to-Theory Strategy

The research-to-theory strategy is the most acknowledged and accepted strategy for theory development, both by scientists in other fields as well as by many within the discipline of nursing. This strategy is used to develop theories that are based on research. In fact, for empiricists, postempiricists, and postpositivists, theory development is considered exclusively a product of research. Therefore, according to this perspective, the strategy *par excellence* is research to theory. Theorists who adhere to this strategy believe that theories evolve from replicated and confirmed research findings and a series of falsifications (Allmark, 2003). From this perspective, theories are referred to as *scientific theories*, and the purpose for developing such theories as described by Jacox (1974) is because:

[I]solated facts are of little interest to scientists, they try to put the knowledge of their respective fields together in such a way that the various events or phenomena with which they are concerned are systematically related to one another. A biologist, for example, wants to know not only about cells,

species, and adaptation, but also how all of these are related to each other and to other biological phenomena. Scientific knowledge is systematically organized into "theories." The purpose of a scientific theory is to describe, explain, and predict a part of the empirical world. (p. 4)

Reynolds (1971) refers to this strategy in the construction of theories as the "Baconian approach." It is also most commonly known as the inductive method. Reynolds proposed four steps to this strategy.

1. Select a phenomenon that occurs frequently and list all the characteristics of the phenomenon.
2. Measure all the characteristics of the phenomenon in a variety of situations (as many as possible).
3. Analyze the resulting data carefully to determine if there are any systematic patterns among the data worthy of further attention.
4. Once significant patterns have been found in the data, formalization of these patterns as theoretical statements constitutes the laws of nature (axioms, in Bacon's terminology). (p. 140)

The strategy presupposes two significant conditions: (1) that there is agreement in the field on the major concepts that should concern its community of researchers and (2) that each research concerns itself with a manageable number of variables with easily detectable patterns. Social science research could not guarantee these conditions (Reynolds, 1971); nursing is similar in some ways. Until the 1980s, there was very little agreement on the central questions in the field. Therefore, isolated research projects were launched to explore questions that were either tangentially related to the mission of nursing or the answers that were central to other disciplines.

As nurse scholars began to agree that nursing deals with human beings who are constantly influencing and being influenced by their environment, there was more appreciation of the complexities inherent in the phenomena central to the care processes. Therefore, although some theories may evolve from research findings, others may continue to capture nursing practice and still others may be derived from other theories. In a dynamic science, all strategies for theory development will continue to inform the discipline.

The development of theory from research will be enhanced by completing research projects that answer questions that are central to the discipline and that are driven by common and shared conceptualizations.

Often, we find that research findings were designed to answer questions that are either not central to nursing or are not translatable to connect with other findings to form a coherent conceptualization. This limitation in potential coherence results from lack of articulated theory to drive the questions; the consequences may be research findings, but not theory development.

This strategy is built on the assumption that there is truth out there in real life that can be captured through the senses and that this truth can be verified or falsified. Repeated verification is an indication of the existence of this truth, and repeated support of a hypothesis leads to the development of scientific theories. There are numerous examples in the literature of nurse researchers who have used this strategy in developing theories; among them are Johnson (1972), Barnard (1973), Lindeman and Van Aernam (1973), and Johnson and Rice (1974).

Not all proponents of this method advocate sensory data as the basis of truth, and not all of them speak of validation and falsification. The grounded theorists have proposed another approach within this strategy, one based on the discovery of concepts and on the identification of patterns, processes, and explanations. The research design proposed by Glaser and Strauss (1968), and further developed by Strauss and Corbin (1994), is that of field study, in which not only theories evolve from research but the research question also evolves from the data gathered. The sole purpose of research, as proposed by this group of field researchers, is the development of theory. Numerous theories have been developed using this second approach, the grounded theorists' approach (Fagerhaugh, 1974; Stern, 1981). A similar approach was used by Smith (1981) in conceptualizing health. She identified four modalities to describe how her research participants tended to view health. These were clinical, role–performance, adaptation, and eudaemonistic modes of viewing and conceptualizing health. Hopkinson, Hallett, and Luker (2005) used phenomenological philosophy to frame a qualitative study, the results of which were articulated in a theory of how new graduates in nursing tend to cope with caring for dying patients.

Two examples will be offered here of the steps to use in the research-to-theory strategy. The first is by Lindeman (1980), who advocated the development of theory from research in her keynote address to the Western Society for Research in 1980. Lindeman used her own research to illustrate the research to theory process and to identify the steps to use in developing theory from research. The second example is Dluhy's proposal (1995) which is discussed on page 369.

The Research-to-Theory Method: Exemplar by a Researcher, Carole A. Lindeman (1980)

The first study, designed to determine the value of preoperative teaching, led to the conclusion that structured preoperative teaching significantly improved the adult surgical patient's ability to cough and deep breathe postoperatively and also significantly reduced the mean length of hospital stay.

A second study was conducted to determine the most efficient way to implement a structured preoperative teaching program. That study, "The Effects of Group and Individual Preoperative Teaching," led me to conclude that group teaching was as effective and more efficient than individual teaching. These findings and those from the first study were consistent with educational research and theory. However, other results from that second study could not be explained by existing theory and continued to trouble me. Those results were:

1. Site of incision does interact in a significant way with teaching method. Subjects receiving group instruction and having "other" incisions had a shorter length of hospital stay than the same group receiving individual instruction. Ventilatory function scores were not different for the two groups. Interpretation required consideration of psychosocial factors in contrast to the physiologic factors associated with the stir-up regime.

2. Age, per se, does not alter postoperative ventilatory function when preoperative teaching and practice are provided. Mean postoperative values on ventilatory function tests were not significantly different for subjects in the various age ranges. In fact, older subjects having major procedures did significantly better than their younger counterparts.

3. Smoking history, per se, does not affect postoperative ventilatory function, length of hospital stay, or number of analgesics administered when preoperative teaching and practice are provided. There were no significant differences between smokers and nonsmokers.

According to the medical literature, these were factors associated with high-risk groups. However, when these so-called "high-risk" patients received structured preoperative teaching, their postoperative ventilatory function measures were comparable to those of other patients. The conceptual/theoretical framework for the research did not explain these results. I was left with a big unanswered "Why?"

Before pursuing those unanswered questions, I conducted a third study dealing with the effects of preoperative visits by operating room nurses. Although a large array of dependent variables was included, the data led to the conclusions that the preoperative visit was useful to the operating room nursing personnel for creating a safe, effective, and efficient intraoperative experience, but it did not produce measurable health status benefits for the patient. Coming from an educational psychology framework, I focused on the content of the teaching encounter as a way to explain why the one intervention, structured preoperative teaching, produced measurable benefits and the second intervention, preoperative interview, did not. I concluded that patients could learn and recall psychomotor behaviors taught in the preoperative period, but material that only served a cognitive structuring process, if learned, would not be retained.

However, I was then involved in a fourth study that refuted my interpretation and led me to propose a different set of theoretical statements. The fourth study was a descriptive study of significant nursing interventions in the preoperative and intraoperative periods and postoperative welfare. The study used Donabedian's structure, process, and outcome framework; however, due to observations made in our pilot study, we added patient baseline data to the overall framework. Much to my surprise, the data showed that patient baseline and organizational data were more strongly correlated with patient welfare than were specific nursing interventions.

I continued to mull over the conclusions from these various studies in an attempt to bring order to the data. Although each study by itself had been useful in making decisions about nursing practice, it seemed that they would be more useful if the results—the expected and the unexpected—could be tied together in some meaningful way in the form of nursing practice theory.

It is difficult, if not impossible, to describe one's thought processes as data and concepts are analyzed. Let it suffice to say that I continued to focus on three concerns:

1. A nursing intervention relating to skill development had a significant impact; a nursing intervention involving cognitive structuring did not.
2. Interactions between the patient and the intervention were not totally predictable and, in fact, were quite surprising.
3. Interactions between the institution and the intervention were not totally predictable.

Emerging from these data, from observations made during the research, and from my further analysis was the conclusion that patient welfare is [affected] by three major sets of variables: organizational, content of care, and patient characteristics. It also seemed clear to me that the critical variable is the patient, with nursing care only effective to the extent that it facilitates the patients' management of their own care.

Having identified the major concepts, the next step in this inductive process involves formulation and validation of relational statements.

The following statements have validity in terms of the research cited earlier:

1. The recipient of health care is the single most important variable in determining actual health status.
2. Those organizations having a potential for enhancing self–health care management are most likely to have a positive influence on actual health status.
3. Those interventions having a potential for enhancing self–health care management are most likely to have a positive influence on actual health status.
4. Characteristics of the caregiver as a person are not significant in determining actual health status.
5. The presurgical nursing interventions designed to enhance the self–health care management abilities of the patient will influence postoperative health status.

Within this inductive process, I am now at the point of theory construction. To complete this step of the process I have had to reconsider the nature or definition of nursing. Without this broader perspective, any theory would exist in limbo. Its ability to predict and its test in reality would remain unknown. Again, for my own efforts, I have conceptualized nursing as a profession that exists because society has needs for health care. These needs generate from three factors: environmental and social factors, disease factors, and health factors. Those health issues or needs that arise because of the interaction of these three factors are the primary focus of nursing. Included are such issues as child abuse, maternal attachment, teenage suicide, the chronically ill, and so forth. Nursing may also assist other professionals by coordinating or implementing components of their plan of care. The social workers, nutritionists, physicians, psychologists, and others all have a role in dealing with issues generating from one or more of these three factors. I personally believe that nursing does have a unique and independent practice role, and it is defined in terms of the point of interplay of these factors.

Now, back to theory development. My next step is to analyze already completed research in terms of the five relational statements presented earlier. I need to consider patients other than presurgical. I need to explore settings other than acute care. I need to explore further interventions—those that relate to health maintenance more than disease prevention. I need to reexamine my major construct, "self–health care management," in terms of the label—does it truly and clearly communicate the nature of the variable? Is it really the variable producing the observable effects? Only when a review of this nature is completed will I be ready to construct a formal theory that can then be tested, modified, and expanded by other researchers and scholars.*

The Research-to-Theory Method: Dluhy's Proposal

Dluhy's (1995) proposal for a method to map pluralistic knowledge for the purpose of generating theory is another example of the research-to-theory strategy. She proposes to identify the core elements, the implicit and explicit assumptions, and the relationship between variables from studies that have been done in nursing and other disciplines. The purposes of knowledge mapping are to answer the questions of what are the best explanations of a central question in the discipline and what are the optimal ways by which these explanations tend to complement each other. Mapping findings is a strategy to integrate massive amounts of knowledge by linking multiple variables and considering these variables from within multiple contexts. Developing theory from research, particularly theory that could inform the discipline of nursing, requires knowledge of the nursing discipline, knowledge

of its mission and its perspective, knowledge of philosophical views of science, and knowledge of the various theoretical perspectives that drive the kind of questions explored.

Several steps support the processes needed for integrating research knowledge into theoretical wholes. These steps are used to develop a coherent map of findings (Blalock, 1979; Dluhy, 1995):

1. Know well the substantive area for which mapping is proposed by identifying all relevant literature, findings, and dialogues.
2. Identify the different ontological beliefs and epistemological approaches used in this area of research.
3. Identify major philosophical and theoretical issues that can clearly divide the findings related to the question under review.
4. Develop a grid reflecting the ontology on one axis and epistemology on another axis.
5. Identify major concepts that evolve as core in the literature. This process may entail counting the number of times that a concept may have been the focus of an investigation, or it may require a qualitative analysis of the centrality of the concept. The context of the particular question may dictate the ways by which a concept is declared central. Identify and analyze similarities and differences between the evolving central concepts.
6. Analyze the core concepts and the findings to reflect patterns and themes by placing them at different points on the four quarters of the grid.
7. Engage in scholarly dialogues to identify assumptions, conceptual areas, and epistemological approaches.
8. Validate axes of grid and placement of conceptual themes and areas through some established methods of validation, such as constant comparisons, Q-sort, or use of different validation teams.

Dluhy (1995) mapped knowledge related to chronic illness by identifying two ontological vertical axes representing the ability to control and be controlled (determinism to free will), and the nature of person (reductionism to idealism). She then identified the horizontal axis as the epistemological axis ranging from positivism to subjectivism. She placed conceptual areas in each quadrant that resulted from a review of more than 300 research and theoretical references. Placement in a particular quadrant was based on the conceptual area within the context of

*Quoted by permission from the author and publisher. Lindeman, C.A. (1980). The challenge of nursing research in the 1980s. In *Communicating nursing research: Direction for the 1980s*. Boulder, CO: Western Interstate Commission for Higher Education.

the related ontology and epistemology. Examples of conceptual areas are fatigue, dyspnea, pain, defense mechanisms, and support. A large cluster of conceptual areas in any quadrant is an indication of their predominance within the context of a certain set of ontological assumptions and epistemological approaches.

Determining agreements on concepts, on findings related to these concepts, and on translating findings that reflect diverse contexts are steps toward developing coherent conceptualizations that may lead to developing theory from research.

Synthesizing and integrating findings and theoretical discourses has proved to be an effective strategy in developing new theoretical frameworks and models. Lenz, Suppe, Gift, et al. (1995) pooled their individual work and collaborated in developing a middle-range theory to describe "unpleasant symptoms." The processes they used are similar to the processes used in mapping, with the difference that this group primarily worked on mapping their own findings. The original work on this theory was done by Pugh and Gift when they combined efforts to write a chapter on dyspnea and fatigue and subsequently combined efforts with others to develop a theory for unpleasant symptoms. Gift (2004) provides a clear trajectory on how the theory was developed from research related to fatigue, dyspnea, and pain. Similarly, Slatyer, Conventry, Twigg, et al. (2015) critically integrated a plethora of professional models developed by others to recognize and delineate the critical components of effective models. These components are leadership; independent and collaborative practice; and a structure and environment that promote professional development, that focus on patient outcomes, and that nurture innovation and research (Slatyer et al., 2015).

Theory-to-Research-to-Theory Strategy

In this strategy, theory drives the research questions, and the results that answer these research questions inform and modify the theory. The difference between this strategy and the research-to-theory strategy lies in the use or nonuse of theory as a guiding framework for the research questions. Theorists who begin the research by defining a theory and determining propositions for testing, and then go further to modify and develop the original theories, are considered users of this strategy. Theories also may be modified and or extended through research.

An original theory of genetic vulnerability due to family experience (BRCA mutation for breast cancer) was modified and extended through inductive analysis of qualitative research to include the effect of living with the risk that they may have the genetic tendency though relieved not to have the BRCA mutation (Hamilton and Kopin, 2013). Researchers may begin from review of a number of theories from which they develop a theoretical model and with the interpretation of new results to develop another more effective theory that better describes, explains, and predicts outcomes. Examples of this strategy are offered by Berg and Sarvimaki (2003). Berg and Sarvimaki (2003) used three theories to study health promotion and developed a framework of health promotion. And while many have developed theoretical models meant to predict the inclination of a nurse to leave a clinical position, Cowden's and Cummings' (2012) research based on those earlier theories lead them to develop their own original theory.

Although many researchers use processes similar to the ones that theorists may use, some significant differences are apparent between researchers and theorists using this strategy. The researcher using theories aims at testing, confirming, refuting, or replicating theories. She uses theory as a framework for the operational definitions for variables and statements, and she uses mental processes, problem solving, and interpretive processes to describe findings. The theorist who uses research as a means for the development of theory ends investigation with a refined, modified, or further-developed coherent theoretical explanation of theory. The impact on the discipline is different, and is needed for different purposes such as translation, refinement, or development. The theorist researcher's findings are specific to selected phenomena and selected findings, whereas the theorist's impact may be through integrated theoretical statements that explain and predict a wider range of phenomena (Table 15-3).

The processes used for the theory-to-research-to-theory method are:

1. A theory that is compatible with the domain of nursing is selected to explain the phenomenon of interest.
2. Concepts of the theory are redefined and operationalized for the research.
3. Findings are synthesized and used to modify, refine, or develop the original theory.
4. In some instances, the result may be a new theory.

TABLE 15-3	Differences Between Theory-to-Research-to-Theory Strategy and Theory-to-Research Strategy	
Theory to Research to Theory	**Theory to Research**	
Goal		
Test, refine, develop theory; openness to options for further developments	Test, accept, refute, replicate; aim to conclude	
Uses		
A framework for research and for modification of theory; define concepts for future use; generate new propositions; explain, define questions	A framework for research; define variables and questions; prove/disprove	
Strategies		
Mental processes; creative, abstract, reflective thoughts; interpretation; synthesis; intuitive leaps	Mental processes; problem solving; interpretation	
Evaluation		
Theoretical thinking, conceptual definitions, other theory analyses criteria	Variable definitions, validity, reliability, other research criteria	
Impact on Discipline		
Through integrated theoretical statements that explain and predict with a wider scope	Through selected scientific findings that explain and predict specifics	
Future		
Generates more propositions; inspires	Provides support for existing propositions and for clinical actions	

CONCLUSION

Knowing and experimenting with strategies for theory development enhance members of the discipline's capacity to advance knowledge and subsequently translate it into models of care. Another probable result of such knowledge is the integration of philosophical processes with empirical processes, resulting in a more integrated knowledge. The rift between scientists and philosophers that marked the era of empirical positivism is decreasing. Our early philosophers believed that science is based totally on philosophical processes; our scientists believed that it is based on the intellectual labor inherent in philosophical processes. This chapter demonstrated this latter process as essential for embarking on research and for interpreting research. Both processes are processes of theorizing. The end result may or may not be a theory; the end result may be clarification of a concept or the articulation of a number of propositions that may be an extension of another theory. Systematic research is an essential step in the process of completing the practice-to-theory-to-research loop. Eventually, a theory will have to respond to the analytical and critical evaluative criteria presented in Chapter 10.

REFLECTIVE QUESTIONS

1. What assumptions must be made to engage in theory development in nursing? Identify and discuss the implicit and explicit assumptions in this chapter.

2. Identify one theory in your field of interest; indicate the rationale for which it is considered a theory and why it is or it is not a nursing theory.

3. Describe how the author developed this theory and what strategies you may use to develop it further.

4. Select a phenomenon for which a theory may be developed. Develop a theory using one of the strategies discussed in this chapter. Why did you select this strategy? How might you refine it?

5. Prepare a manuscript for publication using one of the strategies in developing a theory reflecting your field of interest.

REFERENCES

Allen, D., Benner, P., and Diekelmann, N.L. (1986). Three paradigms for nursing research: Methodological implications. In P.L. Chinn (Ed.), *Nursing research methodology: Issues and implications*. Rockville, MD: Aspen Systems.

Allmark, P. (2003). Popper and nursing theory. *Nursing Philosophy*, 4(1), 4–16.

Andershed, B. and Ternestedt, B.M. (2001). Development of a theoretical framework describing relatives' involvement in palliative care. *Journal of Advanced Nursing*, 34(4), 554–562.

Backscheider, J. (1971). The use of self as the essence of clinical supervision in ambulatory patient care. *Nursing Clinics of North America*, 6(4), 785–794.

Barnard, K. (1973). The effect of stimulation on the sleep behavior of the premature infant. In M.V. Batey (Ed.), *Communicating nursing research, collaboration and competition*. Boulder, CO: Western Interstate Commission of Higher Education.

Barnum, B.J. (1990). *Nursing theory: Analysis, application, and evaluation* (2nd ed.). Boston, MA: Little, Brown.

Bender, M. and Feldman, M.S. (2015). A practice theory approach to understanding the interdependency of nursing practice and the environment. *Advances in Nursing Science*, 38(2), 96–109.

Benner, P. (1984). *From novice to expert: Excellence and power in clinical nursing practice*. Menlo Park, CA: Addison-Wesley.

Benoliel, J.Q. (1977). Social characteristics of death as a recorded hospital event. *Communicating Nursing Research*, 8, 245–265.

Benoliel, J.Q. (1982). Educating nurses for community-based care of advanced cancer patients. AACE Abstracts. *Medical and Pediatric Oncology*, 10(1982), 30A–31A.

Benoliel, J.Q. (1983). The historical development of cancer nursing research in the United States. *Cancer Nursing*, 6(4), 261–268.

Benoliel, J.Q. and De Valde, S. (1975). As the patient views the intensive care unit and the coronary care unit. *Heart and Lung*, 4(2), 260–264.

Benoliel, J.Q., Tornberg, M.J., and McGrath, B.B. (1984). Oncology transition services: Partnerships of nurses and families. *Cancer Nursing*, 7(2), 131–137.

Berg, G.V. and Sarvimaki, A. (2003). A holistic approach to health promotion. *Scandinavian Journal of Caring Sciences*, 17(4), 384–391.

Blalock, H.M., Jr. (1979). Measurement and conceptualization problems: The major obstacle to integrating theory and research. *American Sociological Review*, 44, 881–894.

Blegen, M.A. and Tripp-Reimer T. (1997). Implications of nursing taxonomies for middle-range theory development. *Advances in Nursing Science*, 19(3), 37–49.

Burks, K.J. (2001). Intentional action. *Journal of Advanced Nursing*, 34(5), 668–675.

Carrieri, V.K., Janson-Bjerklie, S., and Jacobs, S. (1984). The sensation of dyspnea: A review. *Heart and Lung*, 13(4), 436–447.

Clarke, A.E. (2005). *Situational analysis: Grounded theory after the postmodern turn*. Thousand Oaks, CA: Sage Publications.

Cowden, T.L. and Cummings, G.G. (2012). Nursing theory and concept development: A theoretical model of clinical nurses' intentions to stay in their current positions. *Journal of Advanced Nursing*, 68(7), 1646–1657.

Cutcliffe, J.R. and McKenna, H.P. (2005). *The essential concepts of nursing*. London, UK: Elsevier, Churchill Livingstone.

Dalton, J.M. (2003). Development and testing of the theory of collaborative decision making in nursing practice for dyads. *Journal of Advanced Nursing*, 41(1), 22–33.

Dickoff, J. and James, P. (1968). A theory of theories: A position paper. *Nursing Research*, 17(3), 197–203.

Dluhy, N.M. (1995). Mapping knowledge in chronic illness. *Journal of Advanced Nursing*, 21, 1051–1058.

Dreyfus, H. and Dreyfus, S. (1986). *Mind over machine: The power of human intuition and expertise in the era of the computer*. New York: Free Press.

Eakes, G.G. (1995). Chronic sorrow: The lived experience of parents of chronically mentally ill individuals. *Archives of Psychiatric Nursing*, 9(2), 77–84.

Eakes, G.G. (2004). Chronic sorrow. In S.J. Peterson and T.S. Bredow (Eds.), *Middle range theories: Application to nursing research* (pp. 165–175). Philadelphia, PA: Lippincott Williams & Wilkins.

Fagerhaugh, S.Y. (1974). Pain expression and control on a burn care unit. *Nursing Outlook*, 22, 645–650.

Fisher, E. (1979). *Women's creation: Sexual evolution and the shaping of society*. Garden City, NJ: Anchor Press/Doubleday.

Gadow, S. (1988). Covenant without cure: Letting go and holding on in chronic illness. In J. Watson and M. Ray (Eds.), *The ethics of care and the ethics of cure. Synthesis in chronicity* (pp. 5–14). New York: National League for Nursing.

Gift, A. (2004). Unpleasant symptoms. In S.J. Peterson and T.S. Bredow (Eds.), *Middle range theories: Application to nursing research* (pp. 78–94). Philadelphia, PA: Lippincott Williams & Wilkins.

Glaser, B.G. and Strauss, A.L. (1967). *The discovery of grounded theory: Strategies for qualitative research*. Chicago, IL: Aldine.

Glaser, B.G. and Strauss, A.L. (1968). *Time for dying*. Chicago, IL: Aldine.

Habermas, J. (1984). *The theory of communicative action: Vol. 1. Reason and the rationalization of society*. London, UK: Heinmann.

Hamilton, R. and Kopin, S. (2013). Theory development from studies with young women with breast cancer who are BRCA mutation negative. *Advances in Nursing Science*, 36(2), E41–E53.

Harden, J. (2000). Language, discourse and the chronotope: Applying literary theory to the narratives in health care. *Journal of Advanced Nursing*, 31(3), 506–512.

Hatlevik, I.K.R. (2012). The theory-practice relationship: Reflective skills and theoretical knowledge as key factors in bridging the gap between theory and practice in initial nursing education. *Journal of Advanced Nursing*, 68(4), 868–877.

Henderson, D.J. (1995). Consciousness-raising in participatory research: Method and methodology for emancipatory nursing inquiry. *Advances in Nursing Science*, 17(3), 58–69.

Hopkinson, J.B., Hallett, C.E., and Luker, K.A. (2005). Everyday death: How do nurses cope with caring for dying people in hospital? *International Journal of Nursing Studies*, 42(2), 125–133.

Jacox, A. (1974). Theory construction in nursing: An overview. *Nursing Research*, 23(1), 4–13.

Johnson, D.E. (1980). The behavioral system model for nursing. In J.P. Riehl and C. Roy (Eds.), *Conceptual models for nursing practice* (2nd ed.). New York: Appleton-Century-Crofts.

Johnson, J.E. (1972). Effects of structuring patients expectations on their reactions to threatening events. *Nursing Research*, 21(6), 499–504.

Johnson, J.E. and Rice, V.H. (1974, May/June). Sensory and distress components of pain. *Nursing Research*, 23, 203–209.

Kahn-John, M. (2016). The path to development of the Hozho Resilience Model for nursing research and practice. *Applied Nursing Research*, 29, 144–147.

Kleffel, D. (2005). The evolution of the environmental metaparadigm of nursing. In L.C. Andrist, P.K. Nicholas and K.A. Wolf (Eds.), *A history of nursing ideas* (pp. 97–108). Sudbury, MA: Jones and Bartlett.

Kolcaba, K. (2004). Comfort. In S.J. Peterson and T.S. Bredow (Eds.), *Middle range theories, application to nursing research* (pp. 255–273). Philadelphia, PA: Lippincott Williams & Wilkins.

Kuhn, T.S. (1970). The structure of scientific revolutions. In O. Neurath (Ed.), *International encyclopedia of unified science* (2nd ed., Vol. 2). Chicago, IL: University of Chicago Press.

Kulig, J.C. (2000). Community resiliency: The potential for community health nursing theory development. *Public Health Nursing*, 17(5), 374–385.

Lenz, E.R., Suppe, F., Gift, A.G., Pugh, L.C., and Milligan, R.A. (1995). Collaborative development of middle-range nursing theories: Toward a theory of unpleasant symptoms. *Advances in Nursing Science*, 17(3), 1–13.

Lindeman, C.A. (1980). The challenge of nursing research in the 1980s. In *Communicating nursing research: Direction for the 1980s*. Boulder, CO: Western Interstate Commission for Higher Education.

Lindeman, C.A. and Van Aernam, B. (1973). Nursing intervention with the presurgical patient: The effects of structured and unstructured preoperative teaching. In F. Downs and M. Newman (Eds.), *A source book in nursing research*. Philadelphia, PA: F.A. Davis.

Lindsey, A., Piper, B., and Stotts, N. (1982). The phenomenon of cancer cachexia, review. *Oncology Nursing Forum*, 9(2), 38–42.

Maeve, M.K. (1994). The carrier bag theory of nursing practice. *Advances in Nursing Science*, 16, 9–22.

McCrae, N. (2012). Whither nursing models? The value of nursing theory in the context of evidence-based practice and multidisciplinary health care. *Journal of Advanced Nursing*, 68(1), 222–229.

McIntyre, M. and McDonald, C. (2013). Contemplating the fit and utility of nursing theory and nursing scholarship informed by the social sciences and humanities. *Advances in Nursing Science*, 36(1), 10–17.

Meleis, A.I. (1975). Role insufficiency and role supplementation: A conceptual framework. *Nursing Research*, 24(4), 264–271.

Meleis, A.I. (1992). Directions for nursing theory development in the 21st century. *Nursing Science Quarterly*, 5, 112–117.

Mercer, R. (1981). A theoretical framework for studying factors that impact on the maternal role. *Nursing Research*, 30(2), 73–77.

Mercer, R. (1984). Predictors of maternal role attainment at one year post birth. *Western Journal of Nursing Research*, 6(3), 62.

Mercer, R. (2004). Becoming a mother versus maternal role attainment. *Journal of Nursing Scholarship*, 36(3), 226–232.

Mercer, R., Ferketich, S., May, K., and de Joseph, J. (1987a). *A comparison of maternal and paternal responses during pregnancy*. Proceedings—Council of Nurse Researchers Conference, Arlington, VA, October 13–16. Silver Spring, MD: American Nurses Association.

Mercer, R., Ferketich, S., May, K., de Joseph, J., and Sollid, D. (1987b). *Maternal and paternal responses in high- and low-risk pregnancies*. Symposium. Proceedings Sigma Theta Tau International Biennial Conference, San Francisco, November 10. Indianapolis, IN: Sigma Theta Tau International.

Millor, G.K. (1981). A theoretical framework for nursing research in child abuse and neglect. *Nursing Research*, 30(2), 78–83.

Neves-Arruda, E.N., Larson, P.J., and Meleis, A.I. (1992). Comfort. Immigrant hispanic cancer patients' views. *Cancer Nursing*, 15(6), 387–394.

Nightingale, F. (1992). *Notes on nursing: What it is, and what it is not*. Philadelphia, PA: J.B. Lippincott.

Norbeck, J. (1981). Social support: A model for clinical research and application. *Advances in Nursing Science*, 3, 43–59.

Olshansky, S. (1962). Chronic sorrow: A response to having a mentally defective child. *Social Casework*, 43, 190–193.

Orlando, I. (1961). *The dynamic nurse–patient relationship*. New York: G.P. Putnam's Sons.

Parsons, T. (1951). *The social system*. New York: Free Press.

Paterson, J.G. and Zderad, L.T. (1988). *Humanistic nursing* (2nd ed.). New York: National League for Nursing.

Peplau, H.E. (1952). *Interpersonal relations in nursing*. New York: G.P. Putnam's Sons.

Reed, P.G. and Leonard, V.E. (1989). An analysis of the concept of self-neglect. *Advanced Nursing Science*, 12(1), 39–53.

Reynolds, P.D. (1971). *Primer in theory construction*. Indianapolis, IN: Bobbs-Merrill.

Rogers, M.E. (1970). *An introduction to the theoretical basis of nursing*. Philadelphia, PA: F.A. Davis.

Roy, C. and Roberts, S. (1981). *Theory construction in nursing: An adaptation model*. Englewood Cliffs, NJ: Prentice-Hall.

Schatzman, L. and Strauss, A.L. (1973). *Field research: Strategies for a natural sociology*. Englewood Cliffs, NJ: Prentice-Hall.

Schensul, S.L. (1985). Science theory and application in anthropology. *American Behavioral Scientist*, 29(2), 164–185.

Slatyer, S., Coventry, L.L., Twigg, D., and Davis, S. (2015). Professional practice models for nursing: A review of the literature and synthesis of key components. *Journal of Nursing Management*, 24(2), 139–150.

Smith, J. (1981). The idea of health: A philosophical inquiry. *Advances in Nursing Science*, 3(3), 43–50.

Smith, M.J. and Liehr, P.R. (2003). *Middle range theory for nursing*. New York: Springer.

Stern, P.N. (1981). Solving problems of cross-cultural health teaching: The Filipino child-bearing family. *Image*, 13, 47–50.

Stevens, P.E. (1989). A critical social reconceptualization of environment in nursing: Implications for methodology. *Advances in Nursing Science*, 11(4), 56–68.

Strauss, A. and Corbin, J. (1994). Grounded theory methodology: An overview. In N.K. Denzin and Y.S. Lincoln (Eds.), *Handbook of qualitative research*. Thousand Oaks, CA: Sage.

Walker, L.O. and Avant, K.C. (1988). *Strategies for theory construction in nursing* (2nd ed.). Norwalk, CT: Appleton-Century-Crofts.

Walker, L.O. and Avant, K.C. (1995). *Strategies for theory construction in nursing* (3rd ed.). East Norwalk, CT: Appleton-Lange.

Walker, L.O. and Avant, K.C. (2005). *Strategies for theory construction in nursing* (4th ed.). Upper Saddle River, NJ: Pearson/Prentice Hall.

Walker, L.O. and Avant, K.C. (2010). *Strategies for theory construction in nursing* (5th ed.). Upper Saddle River, NJ: Pearson/Prentice Hall.

16

Developing Middle-Range Theories

To advance nursing knowledge, we must continue to build a robust scientific base and develop coherent frameworks that drive the science, as well as become a reservoir for the accumulating evidence that results from research. Middle-range and situation-specific theories are at those levels of conceptualization that could inform nursing practice and research and thus continue the cycle of advancing foundational knowledge and enhancing quality care. The theories discussed in this book have had a transformational effect on the entire discipline of nursing. They were conceptualized to answer questions about the overall mission, goals, and nature of the discipline of nursing and to differentiate the substance of the discipline from other disciplines. The theories of Martha Rogers, Dorothy Johnson, and other theorists of their era in nursing helped provide the framework for the discipline, and their theories set the boundaries for the nature of questions to be explored and investigated in the process of building and advancing the discipline. Without these fundamental theories to build on, we would not have been able to progress to the next level: the middle-range and situation-specific theories. Both of these types of theories are defined in this and the next chapter, and exemplars will be provided for each one. The goal for this chapter, then, is to discuss and propose strategies and processes that could be used to develop middle-range theories. The strategies described in Chapter 15 will undoubtedly continue to inform the discipline; that is, scientists will use theories to develop research projects, which in turn will modify other theories, and clinicians will propose theories based on their clinical observations. However, patterns of scientific discovery and the progress of certain disciplines, particularly nursing, tend to demonstrate a more integrative strategy to theory development. Similarly, the tendency is to progressively develop middle-range and situation-specific theories, rather than grand theories. The differences among the three types of theories—grand, middle-range, and situation-specific—are illustrated in Table 16-1.

DEFINITION OF MIDDLE-RANGE THEORY

Middle-range theory is defined as the coherent articulation of a set of concepts that describe and explain relationships that are related to a particular phenomenon. Middle-range theories are less abstract than grand theories, are more accessible to researchers and clinicians, but reside at a higher level of abstraction than do empirical findings, and they contain propositions that reflect generalizations that go beyond specific clinical case studies. Middle-range theories were defined by their inventor, the sociologist Robert Merton, in 1968, as lying in the middle—between the hunches developed in a practice situation and the highly abstract, all-encompassing theory. Middle-range theories deal with more specific phenomena (Meleis, 1997); they usually have a limited number of concepts and propositions (Fawcett and DeSanto-Madeya, 2013), they are more operational and amenable to testing (Walker and Avant, 2010), they avail themselves more to empirical work (Meleis, 1997), and they provide a limited view of reality (Smith and Liehr, 2003) (Table 16-1). They are closer than grand theories to nursing practice issues, challenges, opportunities, and responses.

There is a clear indication that our discipline has undergone a turning point toward producing more accessible and functional theories that guide productive research programs, as well as providing theory- and research-based evidence to nursing practice. Middle-range theories also support the notion that the discipline of nursing's mission, goals, and focus have been defined and that we are ready for more specific questions about nursing care. The majority of middle-range theories describe and provide frameworks to deal with clients' experiences of symptoms, and they provide the means to understand responses to health and illness situations. The language of these middle-range theories is that

TABLE 16-1	Properties and Examples of Grand, Middle-Range, and Situation-Specific Theories		
Properties	**Grand Theories**	**Middle-Range Theories**	**Situation-Specific Theories**
Level of abstraction	High	Medium	Low
Scope	The nature, mission, and goals of nursing	Specific phenomena or concepts transcending and crossing different nursing fields	Specific nursing phenomena limited to specific populations or to a particular field
Level of context	Low	Medium	High
Connection to nursing research and practice	Too broad to connect	Limited	Relationship readily apparent (may prescribe for clinical practice)
Diversities, generalizations, and/or universalization	Ensuring universalization and generalization, but negating diversities	Crossing different nursing fields and reflecting a wide variety of nursing care situations, but rarely respecting diversities in them	Respecting diversities in nursing phenomena, but negating universalization and limiting generalization
Examples	Theories by Peplau, Henderson, Hall, Johnson, Abdellah, King, Wiedenbach, and Rogers (See Chapters 9, 11–13)	Theories by Hagerty, et al. (Also see Fawcett and DeSanto-Madeya [2013]; Peterson and Bredow [2013]; and Smith and Liehr [2003])	Theories by Braden, Im and Meleis, and Hall, et al. (See Chapter 17)

Reprinted with permission from Im, E. and Meleis, A.I. (1999). Situation-specific theories: Philosophical roots, properties, and approach. *Advances in Nursing Science*, 22(2), 11–24.

used in nursing practice to deal with patient care phenomena such as pain, unpleasant symptoms, empathy, uncertainty, comfort, change, lifestyle, health promotion, relationships, and deliberative planning for care. This language reflects the early theorists' attempts to move the discipline away from adopting biomedical language that focuses on disease, pathology, and malfunctioning and to focus on individuals' responses and experiences within the context of health, illness, and encounters with the health care system.

Indications of this turning point are edited books developed with compilations of the middle-range theories. Among these analyses are those edited by Smith and Liehr (2003) and Peterson and Bredow (2013). The book by Smith and Liehr presents and discusses the middle-range theories of uncertainty in illness, self-efficacy, unpleasant symptoms, family stress and adaptation, community empowerment, meaning, and self-transcendence. Peterson's and Bredow's goals for their book are to present and discuss a number of middle-range theories and to apply them to nursing research. They categorize the middle-range theories they selected for discussion in terms of their origin and emphasis. Therefore, they use the broad categories of physiological, psychological, social, and integrative practices to discuss the most widely used middle-range theories.

Under the physiologic framework, they present and analyze two theories of pain: unpleasant symptoms and a balance between analgesia and side effects. Under the psychological framework they focus on self-efficacy and chronic sorrow. Under the social framework, they discuss social support, caring, interpersonal relations, and attachment. And they create an integrative category under which they include modeling and role modeling, comfort, health-related quality of life, health promotion, deliberative nursing process, and resilience. They also created a category for models that did not fit well in any other category and called it the practice models category. Examples are the Shuler Nurse Practitioner Practice Model and the American Association of Critical Care Nurses' Synergy Model. These examples demonstrate that the potential exists for different classifications that could prompt different approaches to advancing knowledge and, therefore, yield different outcomes.

SOURCES FOR MIDDLE-RANGE THEORIES

The different approaches to developing theories and to understanding the sources of theories that are presented in Chapter 15 should be viewed as broad categories for the origin of all types of theories. The following discussion explicates these approaches with examples that are specific to developing middle-range theories.

There are many sources for developing middle-range theories; however, it is important to note research findings must inform them. These research findings could be an integration of several projects conducted either by the same group of researchers or an integration of findings of research conducted by different researchers who focused on a similar set of phenomena. Forsberg, Lennerling, Fridh et al. (2015), after years of studying the threats that face organ transplant recipients and through identifying the risks they face that culminate into rejection, developed a middle-range theory about the perceived threat of the risk of graft rejections. This theory enabled the theorists, and undoubtedly subsequent utilizers of the theory, to develop clinical actions to mitigate these risks. A similar strategy was used by Perry (2015) to develop the theory of transcendent pluralism, which helps nurses to identify and advance actions against devaluation and to enhance human dignity, particularly for those who are disadvantaged. Perry developed the theory by synthesizing the findings of four empirical quantitative and qualitative studies that explored how individuals make decisions related to devaluation and dignity and then identifying related concepts and propositions; she went further by using an evaluation framework to develop credibility for the theory. Carr (2014) provides yet another example of research-based middle-range theory with the theory of family vigilance. On the basis of the results of three qualitative studies, this theory helps identify the meaning and the commitment to caring for a hospitalized family member from the family's perspective and how understanding this perspective informs the care provided and ways to engage family members.

Another familiar source for middle-range theory is the use of an inductive process utilizing grounded theory research (Strauss, 1987; Strauss and Corbin, 1994, 1998). In this approach, data is systematically collected and analyzed with the purpose of developing a theory. In one example of this approach, researchers who explored the holistic provision of health care in faith communities uncovered several components that contribute to sustaining health: entering into the private world of others, connecting faith with health, and experiencing mutual transformation of the nurse and

the patient (Dyess and Chase, 2012). The result of defining and connecting these components was a middle-range theory that describes the uniqueness of faith community nursing.

Theorists can develop middle-range theories by combining findings from their own research projects with other findings gleaned from reviewing the literature. One example is the middle-range theory of flight nursing expertise, which combines quantitative literature from cognitive sciences and qualitative literature from nursing to develop a framework to understand the relationship among experience, training, knowledge, expanded decision-making, and actions of flight nurses (Reimer, Clochesy, and Moore, 2013). When integrated, the concepts from the two sets of studies reflecting different disciplines provide a broader scope of explanation than either discipline on its own.

Many middle-range theories have been developed from research or clinical care models that were themselves inspired by the work of existing grand theorists such as those of Roy, King, Neuman, and Roger. From these theories, clinical care models or research evolved and were implemented, eventually leading to the development of middle-range theories. One effective and productive example is the middle-range theory of self-care of chronic illness (Riegel, Jaarsma, and Stromberg, 2012). The authors identified factors that affect self-care for individuals faced with the challenges of chronic illness. These factors included experience and skills, motivation, cultural beliefs and values, confidence, habits, functional and cognitive abilities, support from others, and access to care. To succeed in self-care management, the individuals with chronic illness must engage in monitoring health-promoting practices. Orem's self-care was also the spring board for a theory of weight management developed by Pickett, Peters, and Jarosz (2014). The authors developed their middle-range theory from Orem's assumptions and the concepts of self-care as well as from the synthesis of published empirical literature.

Another well-utilized and effective source for developing middle-range theory is the use of expert panels for integrative reviews of literature and the development and support of a consensus for emerging categories. An example based on this strategy is a new theoretical model developed to explain and understand different types of dependence-related lesions (e.g., moisture lesions, friction lesions) that had previously been misidentified as pressure ulcers (Garcia-Fernandez, Agreda, Verdu, et al., 2014). On the basis of an expert panel review of the results of extensive searches of international health sciences databases, the authors developed a model that nurses could use in practice to diagnose specific lesion types and provide appropriate interventions. The theory is likely to generate many research questions as well.

A final source for the development of middle-range theory is integration of different theories. The question that Fearon-Lynch and Stover (2015) started from was "why do some people with diabetes mellitus gain mastery over the illness-related stress and emerge with positive attitudes and fortitude and some do not?" After exploring the theory of mastery, which addresses responses to stress from illness, and the organismic integration theory, which focuses on motivational forces, Fearon-Lynch and Stover integrated the concepts related to human responses and behavior change outcomes to generate their own theory. Geary and Schumacher (2012) used a similar approach to create a theoretical framework to describe the care needs and responses of patients who are experiencing health care transitions. Although researchers had previously utilized multiple theories and considered a variety of contexts in attempting to address issues surrounding hospital discharge, readmission, and the transition between caregivers, Geary and Schumacher concluded that none adequately addressed the increasing complexity of the care situations and the systems involved. To address this, they integrated transition theory and complex science concepts to develop a framework that takes into account the multiple relationships, the multifaceted situations, and the dynamic, constantly changing realities of the informal and formal caregivers and the discharged patients. Their formulation provides a more powerful tool that could guide research and practice to uncover and respond to the many more specific and dynamic issues patients and caregivers encounter in more modern times.

TOOLS FOR DEVELOPING MIDDLE-RANGE THEORIES

Theory development includes mental processes that incorporate analysis, discovery, formulation, and validation of uniformities. These may come as a result of sensory observation or as a consequence of a logical or rational analysis of the problem or the phenomenon. They may also result from intuitive reasoning, from an insight that occurs over an extended period of time, or from a "click" that comes as quick as lightning. The thought processes can be spontaneous or premeditated—the timing is never predictable (Sorokin, 1974)—but a conscious effort to look at the phenomenon or the question is infinitely more helpful in bringing the process to closure. It does not guarantee the "click," but it increases its chances.

Just as the process of researching is enhanced by a knowledge of substantive content, a knowledge of research methodology, experience, and the ability to critique research, all processes of theory development are also supported and enhanced by the knowledge of what constitutes theory, knowledge of what major issues confront theorizing, ability to critique theory, knowledge of existing theories, and knowledge of major pitfalls in the development of theory. Knowledge of theory's context, such as the clinical area, is essential. Theorizing is a process that is refined through a deliberate experience. The processes of reflecting, analyzing, questioning, relating, thinking, writing, changing, and communicating are integral parts of philosophical analysis, essential to theory development, and a prelude to and a consequence of research. Keeping a theory diary or journal in which observations, reflections, and relationships are systematically logged helps the theorist to sort out thoughts, develop documentation, and synthesize empirical reasoning with intuitive reasoning (Zderad, 1978).

Norms used to enhance science also are useful in enhancing theory development and they drive the utilization of other tools. Merton (1968, 1979) identified a number of these norms, two of which are pertinent here: the norms of *communality* and *organized skepticism*. Communality encourages nurses to share developing ideas and expose beginning theories for review by peers, to help sharpen the theory and to allow the norm of organized skepticism to prevail. This latter norm "requires detached scrutiny of work according to empirical and logical criteria" (Meleis and May, 1981, p. 38). Dialogues with colleagues in practice, in theory, and in research promote other ways of looking at concepts—other angles and other perspectives.

Collaboration is another significant tool for theory development. In a human science such as nursing, theory development is increasingly a collaborative effort. Collaboration allows the constant comparison and evaluation of competing ideas, provides the medium for a scholarly dialogue to refine concepts, and enhances the integration of seemingly diverse findings, all of which are important processes in developing coherent theories. Theorists of the future are not individual workers; they are team participants (Meleis, 1992). There is support for this current generation of collaborative theorists: for example, the team that proposed the use of simultaneous concept analysis in the development of concepts started from the assumption of collaboration (Haase, Britt, Coward, et al., 1992). (See Chapter 14) Other examples of collaborative theories are the theory of unpleasant symptoms (Lenz, Suppe, Gift, et al., 1995) and the conceptualization of symptom management (University of California, San Francisco, School of Nursing Symptom Management Faculty Group, 1994).

Intuition is another essential tool that has been discussed in the nursing literature. Intuition is defined as reaching some decision or conclusion without the conscious or apparent availability of information (Rew, 1986; Westcott, 1968). Rew (1986) defines the attributes of intuition as: "Knowledge of a fact or truth, as a whole; immediate possession of knowledge; and knowledge independent of the linear reasoning process" (p. 23). Whether this tool is intuition or the expert speaking, several authors have encouraged allowing that inner voice to surface, believing in it, and trusting it (Agan, 1987; Benner, 1984; Rew, 1986; Rew and Barrow, 1987); others argue that intuition is grounded in cognitive science and psychology and could be tested through a combination of soft and hard methods (Gobet and Chassy, 2008). While all agree that intuition is the result of subjective experiences and responses, Green (2012) argued that it is a valid form of knowledge and that it is correlated with objective reality. Therefore, it is essential and a credible tool for developing theoretical connections that could lead to theory development.

Closely related to intuition are *introspection* and *reflection*. Silva (1977) reminded us "to value truths arrived at by intuition and introspection as much as those arrived at by scientific experimentation" (p. 62). Reflection is a process of thinking that may or may not be bound by the need for problem solving.

DEVELOPING MIDDLE-RANGE THEORIES: THE INTEGRATIVE STRATEGY

Although there are strategies and tools that are common to the development of all levels of theory (see Chapter 15), and though in the future all strategies may be integrated at this juncture in the development of theories and in advancing nursing knowledge, I choose to separate the processes involved in developing each level of theory and to progressively develop them in each subsequent chapter with specific examples related to the level of abstraction of each theory category. I urge the reader to mix and match strategies (those presented in Chapters 15–17), to critically consider which are more effective, and to be aware of other strategies that may evolve through their attempts to develop theories. And, future scholars, be warned! There are no specific recipes for developing theories; there are only guidelines, patterns, and guideposts. Ultimately, the processes may be different in each episode of theory development.

It is apparent from the review of the sources for developing middle-range theories that there is a level of sophistication in our discipline that prompts contemporary scholars to use more integrative strategies to developing theories. I call this the integrative strategy for developing middle-range theory. This ought-to-be strategy is intended to be used by itself or in combination with other strategies. Also see Chapter 17 for further development of this strategy.

Developing all levels of theories is a dynamic process, not based on static steps or strategies. It is driven by different sources, and although it starts at many different points, it always ends with a middle-range theory. While it must start by selecting a particular area of knowledge, either from a specific clinical question or from a research finding, the selection process may be a deliberate one or it may be the result of serendipity. In any case, a critical assessment of the rationale for selection is an essential component of the development process. *However, I must emphasize again to the reader that the process for developing theories is not a linear one, nor does it ever follow any one specific path.* The components should be viewed as parts of a segmented puzzle; the full picture becomes manifest when all the pieces of the puzzle are put together. The different pieces of the puzzle may fit together at a different pace and not in any systematic fashion. The theory emerges slowly, just as a very complex puzzle takes shape in slow motion, with different shapes manifesting themselves as several pieces come together to form a recognizable whole. At a certain point when putting a puzzle together, several pieces fit together and a shape begins to emerge faster than expected, then a slow period ensues. Building a theory is also a very dynamic

BOX 16-1 THE INTEGRATIVE STRATEGY: DEVELOPING A MIDDLE-RANGE THEORY

- Clinical observations of different groups to whom nurses were providing care, and facilitation of developing new roles for patients and significant others.
- Identifying similarities and differences in groups and in nursing care provided.
- Developing a conceptually based nursing intervention.
- Testing the intervention clinically and through a series of research studies.
- Integrating the research findings, and finding commonalities and themes.
- Asking the next set of questions to reveal any lack of knowledge about the concept.
- A thorough review of research and clinical publications in nursing about the concept.
- An analysis of commonalities and differences in the literature, and an identification of concepts depicting the nature of questions about theory.
- Communicating and reporting theory at different stages.

process. Just as shapes and images in a puzzle may project one image midway, the end image may be completely different. The process for developing a middle-range theory is depicted in Box 16-1.

Theories that tend to be rich in explaining responses, illuminating situations, enhancing wisdom about events, and providing directions for actions have evolved through this integrative strategy. Such theories may have emerged primarily from any one source; however, the complexity of situations that give rise to these theories usually compels theorists to gather clinical evidence, identify exemplars, collect solutions, and garner support from other sources. In using an integrative strategy, theorists add in any combination experience that is based on clinical practice, evidence from research, and knowledge that is based on theoretical formulations. This knowledge depends on the type of evidence and support that is needed, based on the phenomenon for which they are developing a theory.

Clinical practice has been one of the most significant sources for theory development. Subsequent to the group of nurse theorists discussed in this volume, some more contemporary theories may be deemphasizing the role of practice in theory development and are favoring more the role of research evidence in formulating theories. Theorists who use the integrative strategy, however, recognize the significance of the relationship among practice, theory, and research and understand that each plays a role in the development of nursing theory. In addition, when using an integrative strategy, the person, theorist, clinician, or researcher also becomes an integral part of the theoretical formulation. Even when a deliberate attempt is made to distance the agent (the theorist or researcher) from the subject matter, and even when such attempts are carefully guarded and implemented, the

infiltration of previous experiences in shaping the clinical situation and subsequently the theoretical formulation is inevitable. These experiences are part of a nursing perspective that is then reflected in the evolving conceptualization. All these factors become the context that shapes what we see, how we see it, and how we analyze it. They are part of an integrative strategy.

Phenomena seen from a nursing perspective are not seen in exactly the same way as phenomena seen from a sociologic perspective. A nursing perspective is focused on considering the phenomena holistically and dynamically and within a context. Nurses are concerned with phenomena related to the experience of, and response to, health and illness, such as transitions, comfort, care, the nursing process, supporting, coping, grieving, mourning, suffering, and monitoring; in other words, phenomena that will eventually make a difference in some aspect of health care. Phenomena are described or explained through the interaction of health–illness events, person–environment relationships, and the human-responses perspective. Different perspectives provide different lenses through which phenomena are viewed. Each perspective identifies the limits within which inquiries are made (Donaldson and Crowley, 1978). (See Chapter 6 for a discussion on nursing perspective.) Another assumption for this strategy is that some kind of reality exists out there, and that there is a pattern and order in the universe around us, as well as, paradoxically, a certain degree of uniqueness. Because we live in an orderly, nonrandom world, this order is comprehensible to a certain extent and within a certain context. The concept of uniqueness, however, deserves a closer look.

If each event or process of a phenomenon was absolutely unique or occurred randomly, without order or pattern, then no generalizations could be made. Without some degree of generalization, there is no science because all sciences attempt to generalize about recurrent phenomena. Scientists, unlike philosophers, must also assume some logical connection between perceivable events, as well as a certain degree of predictability. In practice, nurses focus on the uniqueness of individuals for the purpose of individualizing care. However, we must consider seriously Ellis' (1982) everlasting admonition against using the uniqueness of man as a crutch to avoid patterning and order, which remain the essential components of theory and science. Uniqueness reminds us to consider patterns of diversity and individuality, which, when examined, could add to the complexity and richness of theory. Therefore, uniqueness and patterning are also significant premises on which the integrative strategy of theory development is based.

With this caveat, and with the necessity of considering a rich contextual background, it may seem difficult to isolate a beginning point for the integrative strategy in theory development. However, like the strategies discussed in the previous chapter, some essential stages and processes may facilitate theorizing.

An integrative strategy must be grounded in clinical practice at many different stages in theory development. An integrative strategy requires collaboration and dialogue. The beginning hunches and conceptual schemes are shared and communicated with others to allow for critique and further development. An integrative strategy requires the development of a framework and a theoretical vision, as well as opportunities to test these hunches or evolving conceptualizations with colleagues and other participants. Other components of this integrative strategy are research (of different designs) and different methods to clarify, support, or test some of the evolving hunches. Research documentation may be supplemented by reflective clinical diaries, descriptive journals, and dialogues about analyses, among other sources and approaches. An example of a theory in which the theorists used an integrative strategy is the *Theory of Human Relatedness* (Hagerty, Lynch-Sauer, Patusky, et al., 1993). The authors of this theory experienced situations in clinical practice that prompted them to think of various states of connectedness and disconnectedness. They dialogued, observed, kept notes, conducted research in the library, and identified the social processes inherent in relating, as well as the different states of relatedness, including connectedness, disconnectedness, parallelism, and enmeshment.

The evolving theory explains, describes, and has the potential for clarifying situations in which nurses relate to others (which is most of the time). The potential power of this theory in enhancing the understanding of such situations is directly related to its integrative strategy of development.

DEVELOPING TRANSITION THEORY: AN EXEMPLAR OF INTEGRATIVE STRATEGY

As an example of the integrative strategy, consider the development of the concept of transition into a middle-range theory (Meleis, 2010, 2015). In the same way that an emerging shape takes form in a puzzle, different team members develop different parts of the theory at different times in its development. Although the journey, as presented here, may make the process of development appear linear and systematic, it is not. Questions that I asked in the 1960s led to the development of a conceptual framework–based intervention that I called *Role Supplementation*. After testing the intervention empirically, I questioned whether we knew which patient responses may have necessitated such an intervention, and with my colleagues, I began a more systematic approach to developing the experience and outcomes of transitions. We then moved on to a full circle of theory-based intervention.

In the following sections, I reconstruct the components of the theoretical journey that led to developing the middle-range theory of transitions (Meleis, 2010).

Clinical Observations

First, the theorist (who may or may not perceive him- or herself as a theorist) asks questions about a particular client or a situation. For the theory of transitions, the impetus was triggered by clinical observations. It was the experience of people and their responses to changes in their lives—specifically, becoming new mothers—that attracted my intellectual curiosity. My interest was triggered by how nurses facilitate individuals' acquisition of new roles to support healthy lifestyles and diminish the potential for becoming ill in patients facing changes in their lives. In addition, in a world where people are in constant movement and change, and one in which individuals are constantly learning to cope with short- and long-term changes, the human experiences and responses during transition become central to nursing interests. Assisting individuals and communities in dealing with transitions that affect their health emerged as a challenge for nurses, both before a change occurs, as well as during and after the change.

Developing theories is a long, laborious process. My interest in transitions dates back to the mid-1960s, when many support groups evolved to help people deal with a variety of problems. Support groups were initiated by nurses or lay people to help clients deal with the demands of new parenting responsibilities, with loss of family members, or with understanding a devastating diagnosis of mastectomy, as well as with anything in a person's life that was deemed out of the ordinary. As Ph.D. students and new graduates, we found ourselves practicing what was preached, and we asked questions, such as: "What are some common threads among all these groups?" We became aware of the need to consider the presence of some universal features in creating and conducting these groups and in their outcomes. I guess this awareness and the need to find some order in seemingly unrelated events was also driven by a growing interest in theory, and in theorizing about nursing.

This awareness was also nurtured by an interest in the phenomena that surrounded planning pregnancies, in the processes involved in caring for spouses with long-term illness, and in the experiences of becoming a new parent and mastering parenting roles, which were the subjects of my master's and Ph.D. dissertation researches. I studied the process of decision-making in family planning and discovered the significance of spousal communication and interaction in effective or ineffective planning of the number of children in families (Meleis, 1971). Although there were minimal data and interest at the time in the processes of and responses to changes, my colleague and I assumed that the knowledge needed was not about transitions, but rather about how nurses can make a difference in helping people achieve healthy outcomes after their transitions (Meleis and Swendsen, 1978). We focused on nurses' actions, on developing interventions, and on defining outcomes. In doing so, we were influenced by the context of justifying nursing actions to demonstrate that these actions make a difference in patients' outcomes.

Preliminary Research

Therefore, my next research questions were about what happens to people who do not make healthy transitions, and what nursing interventions nurses use to facilitate their clients' healthy transitions. The theoretical background of symbolic interactionism led to a focus on the symbolic world that shapes those interactions and responses that get organized into coherent sets of roles. We began observing people in transition with lenses that could organize and order these observations in terms of the roles enacted by both the actors and reactors. When people are not able to understand and enact particular new roles, they experience deficiencies. Roles, from a symbolic interactionist perspective, are defined in terms of behaviors, sentiments, and goals (Turner, 1962). That is where our clinical observations of health-oriented groups came in. So, first, we defined unhealthy or ineffective transitions as leading to role insufficiency, and we defined role insufficiency as any difficulty in the cognizance and/or performance of a role or of the sentiments and goals associated with the role behavior as perceived by the self or by significant others. Role insufficiency is characterized by behaviors and sentiments affiliated with the perception of disparity in fulfilling role obligations or expectations (Meleis, 1975).

Defining Concepts

In developing the middle-range theory of nursing intellectual capital, so that we could understand the relationship between organizational members' (in one case, nurses) knowledge, skills, and experiences on organizational outcomes, it was necessary to define and differentiate between the key concepts of human, social, structural, and relational capital and potential patient outcomes (Covell, 2008). Similarly, in our work on developing transitions, we defined the goal of healthy transitions as a mastery of the behaviors, sentiments, cues, and symbols associated with new roles and identities and nonproblematic transitions. Although the nature of transitions and the nature of responses to different transitions were still a mystery, this was not a mystery we felt compelled to uncover. We believed that knowledge development in nursing should be geared toward the development of nursing therapeutics and not toward understanding the phenomena related to responses to health and illness situations. In retrospect, we think that it is this belief in the need for developing nursing therapeutics and in finding out what difference nursing makes that may have been the driving force toward our development of role supplementation as a nursing therapeutic and for the research that occupied us during all of the 1970s

(Meleis, 1975; Meleis and Swendsen, 1978). The reader should note how a particular philosophy on theory shapes how a phenomenon is defined and the nature of questions asked.

Research Program

Subsequently, role supplementation as a nursing therapeutic was used in a number of research projects. The major questions in each research project sought to further define the components, processes, and strategies related to role supplementation, and to answer the question of whether it made a difference in helping patients complete a healthy transition. At that time, I defined health as *mastery*, and in different research projects mastery was tested through such proxy outcome variables as "fewer symptoms," "perceived well-being," and/or "ability to assume new roles." Role supplementation was used to help couples assume the new role of parenting (Meleis and Swendsen, 1978) and to help postmyocardial infarction patients develop an at-risk identity, which led to better compliance with a rehabilitation regimen (Dracup, Meleis, Baker, et al., 1984). It was also used to describe how the elderly maintained their sexuality (Kass and Rousseau, 1983) and how parental caregiving roles are acquired effectively (Brackley, 1992). Similarly, it was used to ease the caregivers' roles for Alzheimer's patients (Kelly and Lakin, 1988). The framework was also used to better describe women who were not successful in becoming mothers and who manifested role insufficiency (Gaffney, 1992). Having a coherent framework helped articulate new research questions and provided a reservoir for accumulating the answers and refining the framework. The results demonstrated that nurses' actions tended to anticipate, facilitate, and enhance transitions and healthy outcomes. Having research programs that continue the development of middle-range theories may require the development of new or the refinement of existing research instruments (Räsänen, Backman, and Kyngäs, 2007). By articulating a coherent theory, researchers can continue to refine it through research conducted in other countries.

Clinical Observations Post Research Findings

Once again, it was time to go back for clinical observations. The growing interest in the discipline to uncover the lived experiences of people in health and illness prompted the need for more clinical immersion. Dr. Norma Chick of Massey University, Palmerston North, New Zealand, came to work with me during her sabbatical and agreed to collaborate with me in further developing the phenomena of how people respond to change. We both observed people undergoing changes due to immigration, and due to critical and intensive care. In 1985, we completed and published the results of our findings in an article that we entitled, "Transitions: A Nursing Concern" (Chick and Meleis, 1986). During this phase, "transition" was defined conceptually and was connected to the discipline of nursing. I believe that the result of our analysis positioned transition as a central concept in nursing thought. After developing a conceptualization of a phenomenon, a periodic determination of research and theory gaps may require revisiting care situations. In fact, clinical observations and periodic immersion in clinical situations are vital to the process of developing theories in human science. This periodic revisiting of caring episodes is one of the hallmarks of an integrative strategy to developing middle-range theories. Theories identify gaps in the science of self-management of chronic health problems through knowledge gained from concrete experiences (Reed, 2006). Ryan and Sawin (2009) developed an individual and family self-management theory to describe and predict quality of life, perceived well-being, and cost. They point out that interventions that are both person- and family-centered must address the context of care by fostering structural conditions or the self-management process itself by enhancing knowledge, beliefs, and self-regulatory behaviors. The need to focus on families is driven by actually working in clinical situations and recognizing that the management of chronic health conditions is both influenced by families and acts to affect families. The authors identified gaps in research and previous conceptualizations that led to a new, more comprehensive middle-range theory.

Integrative Literature Review

Flight nurses have existed since flying became a mode of transportation. The properties of the experiences and actions of those nurses who are involved in the safe care of people in flight are similar in some ways and different in others from those of nurses who care for patients in hospitals or communities. To develop a coherent understanding of these properties, actions, and responses, Reimer and Moore (2010) conducted an extensive review of the literature spanning about five decades. They then developed nine concepts and five propositions that formed the middle-range theory of flight nurses' expertise, skills, knowledge, and subsequent actions.

A vital component in the process of developing a middle-range theory is extensive, comprehensive, and integrative literature review to define concepts or identify the existing evidence. Extensive literature searches should be conducted at different critical points in developing a middle-range theory. In continuing the dynamic and integrative strategies to develop transitions, 10 years marked a critical point to revisit the literature in a more systematic way, and to integrate and analyze it. With Dr. Karen Schumacher, then a doctoral student at the University of California at San Francisco, I wondered about the extent to which transitions were used as a concept or a framework in nursing literature. A search of the literature yielded 310 articles that focused on transitions. We then analyzed these articles and identified more support for transitions as a central concept in nursing (Schumacher and Meleis, 1994).

During this part of theory development, clinical observations and findings from the literature are integrated. Literature reviews are also used to refine, support, or refute previous formulations. The review and analysis of the literature on transitions (Schumacher and Meleis, 1994) reaffirmed what we previously conceptualized; however, it also provided evidence to refine earlier conceptualizations. Instead of only three types of transitions: developmental, situational, and health–illness (Chick and Meleis, 1986), a fourth type of transition emerged. This new type of transition received much attention in the literature—we called it "organizational transition." Organizational transition was another type of transition explored by nurses, and it also represented an environmental transition. All the results of the literature analysis and interpretation indicated that transition is an area that requires more systematic, scholarly attention in the discipline of nursing.

Reviewing literature should not be confined to nursing literature. In developing and explicating transition, certain authors emerged as important to our continuous development of the theory of transitions. Bridges (1980, 1991), the guru of transitions and author of two significant books (*Making Sense of Life's Changes: Transitions,* and *Managing Transitions: Making the Most of Changes*), described three phases of going through transitions. These are an ending phase, characterized by disenchantment; a neutral phase, characterized by disintegration and disequilibrium; and a beginning phase, characterized by anticipations and taking on new roles. Each one of these phases requires different coping strategies and congruent nursing therapeutics. His work affirmed the significance and universality of transitional experiences and responses, and provided the impetus to continue in our journey to further clarify and develop transition, conceptually as well as empirically.

We then asked the question, "What happens to people during transitions?" We began answering this question through clinical observations, literature reviews, and research findings. Coping with transitions is a dynamic process that includes different processes, some of which are creatively constructed, such as those attached to caregivers' role acquisitions (Schumacher, 1995). Further, the complexity of transitions is manifested in the different team members and organizations that are involved in discharge planning and management of patients and families (Geary and Schumacher, 2012).

Critical Reviews Through Dialogues

Having established the significance of transitions to nursing, and having demonstrated the extent to which nurses participate in patients' transitions, we were led to extensive dialogues with many colleagues. This is another important component in the process of developing theories. The question presented in these dialogues was: "What nursing therapeutics could be used to enhance healthy outcomes in individuals who are experiencing a transition?" Most of the care that nurses provide happens during individuals' transitions, and the goal of nursing care is to enhance healthy outcomes. Therefore, we defined the mission of nursing within a framework of transition. Developing the concept of transition and supporting its significance through review and analysis of literature related to transition led us to define nursing as the art and science of facilitating the transition of a population's health and well-being. Nursing is also defined as "being concerned with the processes and the experiences of human beings undergoing transitions where health and perceived well-being is the outcome" (Meleis and Trangenstein, 1994, p. 257). Within this definition, areas for knowledge development that have some universality and that could support a more systematic effort in knowledge development were identified. Examples are knowledge related to the processes and experiences of human beings undergoing transitions, the nature of emerging life patterns that result from transitions, the nature of environments that support or constrain healthy transitions, and the nature of nursing therapeutics that could be used to prevent unhealthy transitions, to augment healthy transitions, or to promote wellness during transitions (Meleis, 1993).

The cycle of theory development continues to be informed by practice, the literature, and research, and it subsequently leads to further identification of more integrated and coherent areas of investigation. Strategies used during the cycle for theory development, as indicated previously, are clinical observations, literature reviews, critical thinking, analytical dialogue, questioning, empirical testing, describing, searching for and articulating exemplars, and communicating the results. In the following section, I demonstrate that utilizing transitions in research projects leads to further development of transitions as a middle-range theory.

Researching Again

Once again, it is time to ask specific research questions. The transitions framework, as conceptualized in the analyses I have provided thus far, was then used as a conceptual framework in a number of studies. It has been used as a framework for transition in the elderly (Schumacher, Jones, and Meleis, 2010), and to describe immigrants' transitions (Meleis, Dallafar, and Lipson, 1998), the experience of women living with rheumatoid arthritis (RA; Shaul, 1995), the process of recovery from cardiac surgery (Shih, 1995), the process of developing family caregiving roles for patients in chemotherapy (Schumacher, 1995), the experience of early memory loss for patients in Sweden (Robinson, Ekman, Meleis, et al., 1997), and the experience of African American women's transitions to motherhood (Sawyer, 1999).

I asked some of the authors of these studies to describe in their own words how they used transitions as a framework. Here is how Karen Schumacher described her interest in transitions and how transitions shaped her work:

As a doctoral student, I conceptualized the process of taking on the caregiving role as a transition, specifically as a transition that involved the acquisition of a new role. Using the nursing and social psychology literature on transitions, I developed a model of caregiver role acquisition. In this model, caregiver role acquisition is conceptualized as a role transition that involves creative role-making through interaction with the role partner (the care receiver) within a particular social structural context. The model emphasizes the interactional

processes that occur in taking on the family caregiving role. The model was published in Scholarly Inquiry for Nursing Practice in an article entitled "Family Caregiver Role Acquisition: Role-Making Through Situated Interaction."

In the dissertation, I also identified critical periods in the cancer experience in which caregivers and patients had difficulty in managing cancer-related care. These critical periods were times of disruption and disconnectedness, in which both emotional stress and uncertainty about what to do occurred. Four critical periods were identified: the diagnostic period, the side-effect intensive period in the chemotherapy cycle, the junctures between treatment modalities, and the end of treatment. An interesting finding was that access to nurses was limited or nonexistent during these critical periods. The support and continuity of care that are nursing ideals do not appear to be made available to patients and caregivers at critical periods in the cancer experience. The findings raise questions about what nursing care organized from a transitions perspective, rather than in relation to medical treatment, might be like.

During my postdoctoral fellowship at Oregon Health Sciences University, I turned to skill development as one aspect of the transition into the caregiving role. Family caregiving skill has not been systematically conceptualized, although assisting caregivers to develop skill in taking care of an ill person is a routine part of home care nursing. Nine caregiving processes were identified (monitoring, interpreting, making decisions, taking action, making adjustments, providing hands-on care, accessing resources, working together with the ill and family members, and working with health care providers). For each of these processes, indicators of the caregiver's level of skill were identified. These indicators will be used as the basis for an instrument that nurses will be able to use for assessment with family caregivers. The instrument will enable nurses to develop a profile of caregiving skill with their clients, which then could be used to target interventions. A long-term goal is to develop an instrument with which to measure family caregiving skill in research. Such an instrument would make it possible to measure changes in family caregiving skills during transitions in the caregiving experience. It could also be used to measure the effect of nursing interventions. (Schumacher, personal communication, 1996)

Schumacher continued her work in developing transitions by integrating it with complexity science to provide a new lens through a framework to improve the potential of patients' and families' transition outcomes by carefully attending to a complex array of variables that also reflect the more current structures of health care systems (Geary and Schumacher, 2012).

Petra Robinson is another graduate student who worked with me on the analysis of data from patients with early memory loss. It became apparent to us that realizing and coming to grips with memory loss is a long process that includes stages, in-between stages, and periods of spillover and overlap. The major experience could be captured in the category of "suffering in silence." While they suffer in silence, people losing their memory go through stages for which they develop different strategies. These we called "forgetfulness," "something is wrong," and "in search of meaning." These stages occur before patients receive care congruent with their needs. During the stage of forgetfulness, individuals try their best to normalize their experience, gloss over it, and not take it seriously, but they suffer from it nevertheless. They watch and analyze as soon as they become aware that something is wrong. Finally, they use the strategy of avoidance and vigilance as they search for a meaning. Their experience is characterized by solitary suffering, and we believed that, by uncovering that suffering, we could support the strategies they use, share in their suffering, and enhance their resources until a definite diagnosis is made (Robinson et al., 1997).

The process of developing mothering in African American women was described by Sawyer as getting diagnosed with pregnancy, getting ready, dealing with reality, settling in, dreaming, and ending up becoming an engaged mother (Sawyer, 1996b). She defined *engaged mothering* as "an active, involved, and mutual process in which a woman is preparing to be a mother, caring for herself and her infant, and dreaming about and planning for the future" (Sawyer, 1996b, p. 73). Sawyer found that the identity women develop of being a mother was reflected by being engaged on many levels:

[E]ngaged with baby, partner, parent, family, friends, coworkers, and the general community; engaged with their care during pregnancy; engaged in sorting through information and advice and choosing a role model; engaged in dealing with the daily hassles they faced in society; engaged in handling problems during the pregnancy and after the baby was born; engaged in figuring out the baby and adapting to changes in their lives; and engaged in planning for and dreaming about a 'good life' for their child and family. Motherhood is incorporated into the women's sense of self and is a synthesis of motherhood into the woman's

identity rather than merely the attainment or addition of a role. Engaged mothering is dynamic and interactive and embedded within the context of the woman's family, history, life experiences and dreams. (Sawyer, 1996b, pp. 73–74)

Understanding women's roles and how they mother their babies, which is part of nursing's mission, cannot be understood without understanding the process that women go through to develop this mothering identity. Nursing actions to support the process are more effective when they are matched to the different stages and critical points in the process.

Here, Linda Sawyer (personal communication, 1996a) describes how she used transition to guide her study and interpretations:

In this study on African American women, transitions theory provided a framework which allowed motherhood to be studied as a complex, longitudinal, and multidimensional process, focused on patterns of response over time. Common themes in the definition of transitions are disruption, disconnectedness, and emotional upheaval—certainly themes common to expectant and new mothers. Compared to all transitions, which are of interest to nursing, the transition to motherhood has received the most attention in the nursing literature. Maternal role attainment (MRA) is the construct used in nursing to describe the transition to motherhood. MRA has focused on the dyad of mother and child, on motherhood as a role, has not described the meaning of motherhood, has been studied through quantitative methods using multiple tools, and has not been tested cross culturally. Since the construct of MRA has not been studied cross culturally, this theory cannot be generalized to all mothers, and the cultural equivalence of this construct needs testing.

This grounded theory study described the transition to motherhood for a group of African American women as a longitudinal process which spanned the time period between the woman's decision to get pregnant or to continue a pregnancy and the time when mothering was incorporated into her identity. For some women, the transition was planned and hoped for, and for others it occurred earlier than planned but was still welcome. In this study, women exhibited success in the transition through their active involvement in preparing, caring, and dreaming. Women developed a sense of comfort in caring for their child, sought out sources of support and connection within their families and the community, and planned for and actively pursued their dreams and vision for a good future for themselves and their child.

Conditions for transitions usually include meanings, expectations, level of knowledge and skill, the environment, level of planning, and emotional and physical well-being. Women described their meaning of becoming a mother, which evolved out of their experiences and dreams. Expectations were formed from hearing other women talk about their experiences and observing other mothers, reading or watching videos, and by fantasy. The level of knowledge was high among this group of women because of their active involvement in preparing during pregnancy through classes, written materials, role models, questioning, obtaining advice, and seeking formal prenatal care. Mothering skills were developed through figuring out the baby, "maternal instinct," and for some women, through previous experience in caring for children. The environment for this group of women increased their stress during pregnancy. Women were faced with and dealt with incidents of racism, stereotyping, and negativity frequently in their daily lives. The environment mediated the transition through both providing support and increasing stress. The level of planning, illustrated by the condition of intentionality of the pregnancy, affected the transition, since women who were actively trying to get pregnant proceed through the transition easier. A second condition of prior miscarriage or history of health problems of the mother diminished the woman's sense of both emotional and physical well-being and was an inhibitor of the transition.

Several critical points in this transition may require nursing intervention. Early in the prenatal period, an assessment needs to occur regarding the woman's history of prior miscarriage or health problems and the intentionality of the pregnancy. Worries will need to be solicited and appropriate reassurance and support provided. Nursing interventions may not be successful if offered before the woman has passed the critical point—i.e., after the time the previous miscarriage occurred. Additional options to prepare for motherhood may need to be utilized for women with a history of previous problems, since this group of women was less likely to attend traditional classes. Special care or additional support may also need to be provided for the women with prior problems. Nurses need to ensure that care is provided in a culturally congruent manner and be sure that African American women receive information about the progress of the pregnancy and the size and condition of the baby at each visit. Labor and delivery is a particularly stressful time, and nurses need to intervene to ensure that mothers receive support and that their birth plans are respected as much as possible. After the baby was born, women had many questions and a need for reassurance. This is a time when nursing interventions are welcome and heeded. Nursing support from a consistent person with whom the

woman is comfortable is important to assist new mothers in settling-in until they gain confidence in making decisions regarding the care of the baby, usually at four months postpartum.

Shaul (1995) found in her doctoral dissertation research that women with RA went through three stages before settling into the business of caring for themselves. The first stage is becoming aware, when the symptoms are nagging but are still ignored. The second stage is learning to live with RA. During this stage, women felt alienated from their environment while trying to cope with the many symptoms they experience, such as fatigue, stiffness, depression, and swelling. During stage three, they master the new knowledge and know that the condition has its ups and downs, but they have a sense of control that comes from knowing about the disease and knowing how to manage their own daily care.

Integrative Findings

The next step in our journey toward developing a middle-range theory for transition was to analyze the research findings related to transition experiences and responses. Similarities and differences in utilizing transitions as a framework and in the findings were then compared, contrasted, and integrated. Extensive reading, reviewing, and dialoguing about each research study and finding led to the final stage of developing transition as a middle-range theory, complete with components, conditions, responses, outcomes, and nursing therapeutics. One of the nursing therapeutics thus identified is role supplementation, which was the very early impetus for finding a coherent way to facilitate clients' transitions and enhance their mastery of their roles and health in a new situation. The middle-range theory was then articulated and published (Meleis, Sawyer, Im, et al., 2000). By communicating the theory in literature and exposing it for critique and utilization, other researchers and clinicians can complete the cycle of theory development.

Summary of Process

The process we used to develop transition as a middle-range theory is depicted in Box 16-1. The impetus for this process was triggered by clinical observations. Generalizations about these observations were articulated in a more coherent whole within a conceptual framework. The conceptual framework evolved from a "lens" that was colored by symbolic interactionism as a philosophy and role theory as a theoretical framework. Empirical research, as well as clinical observations, drove the development of a more modified conceptual framework. Extensive review of the literature helped build on previous conceptualizations by refining, extending, modifying, and developing a more nuanced framework. Clinical exemplars illustrated the rationale for the changes. Several empirical research studies used the most recent conceptualizations. Critical analyses of the findings, dialogues about the researchers' experiences with the framework, and reframing of the findings in comparison to other findings led to a more refined middle-range theory. Concepts then were defined using the most recent findings, with exemplars provided from the completed research. Box 16-1 summarizes this process, which ends with communication and reporting of the middle-range theory.

CONCLUSION

The integrative strategy for middle-range theory development and the tools used are described and discussed in this chapter. The future for advancing nursing knowledge depends on the extent to which we are willing to commit to developing coherent frameworks to drive future research programs and practice models. The future theoretical development in nursing is in presenting our science in middle-range and situation-specific theories. I strongly believe that the nature of nursing as a human science focused on the experiences and responses to health and illness lends itself to the development and use of middle-range and situation-specific theories (American Nurses Association, 2010). To continue developing and refining middle-range theories, concepts and propositions must be subjected to evaluation and testing. Testing could be performed using quantitative, qualitative, or mixed methods, regardless of whether the theory is inductively or deductively developed (Elo, Kaariainen, Isola, et al., 2013). Another way of evaluating a theory (see Chapter 10 for theory evaluation) is assessing the extent to which it is used and utilized by educators, scientists, clinicians, or theoreticians. And if it is not used, the question should be "why not?" Marsh (2013) poses such a question about the well-developed middle-range theory of teetering on the edge, a substantive theory of postpartum depression that was developed and researched over many years by Beck (1993). March, who has been a woman's health nurse for 12 years, questioned why she had not been provided the opportunity to learn about the theory in her education or clinical programs since, after she discovered it, she found the theory to be very effective in her practice. The question then that I leave with readers, whether educators, clinicians, or researchers, is: "Are middle-range theories well-utilized in the discipline and profession of nursing?" In this chapter, I provide the process used to develop middle-range theories and give examples of each component of the process. In particular, the integrative strategy to theory development was used to describe the journey toward the development of a middle-range theory of transition, as well as in developing other theories.

REFLECTIVE QUESTIONS

1. What are the relationships between grand theories, middle-range theories, and situation-specific theories?

2. Select two middle-range theories that reflect your field of study, and critically discuss ways by which they stimulate, or fail to stimulate, a program of research.

3. Compare and contrast the sources, tools, and strategies that the theorists used in developing these two theories.

4. Review the middle-range theories that may be effective in advancing knowledge in your field of specialization. Discuss why and in what ways they are or are not effective.

5. Select one theory that you wish to study and develop two propositions that reflect the assumptions and the concepts of the theory. If you were to prove or refute these propositions, what research questions would you ask?

REFERENCES

Agan, R.D. (1987). Intuitive knowing as a dimension of nursing. *Advances in Nursing Science*, 10(1), 63–70.

American Nurses Association. (2010). *Nursing is a social policy statement* (2nd ed.). Washington, DC: Author.

Beck, C.T. (1993). Teetering on the edge: A substantive theory of postpartum depression. *Nursing Research*, 42(1), 42–48.

Benner, P. (1984). *From novice to expert: Excellence and power in clinical nursing practice*. Menlo Park, CA: Addison-Wesley.

Brackley, M.H. (1992). A role supplementation group pilot study: A nursing therapy for potential parental care givers. *Clinical Nurse Specialist*, 6(1), 14–19.

Bridges, W. (1980). *Making sense of life's changes: Transitions*. Menlo Park, CA: Addison-Wesley.

Bridges, W. (1991). *Managing transitions: Making the most of changes*. Menlo Park, CA: Addison-Wesley.

Carr, J.M. (2014). A middle-range theory of family vigilance. *MEDSURG Nursing*, 23(4), 251–255.

Chick, N. and Meleis, A.I. (1986). A nursing concern. In P.L. Chinn (Ed.), *Nursing research methodology: Issues and implementation* (pp. 237–257). Rockville, MD: Aspen.

Covell, C.L. (2008). The middle-range theory of nursing intellectual capital. *Journal of Advanced Nursing*, 63(1), 94–103.

Donaldson, S.K. and Crowley, D. (1978). The discipline of nursing. *Nursing Outlook*, 26(2), 113–120.

Dracup, K., Meleis, A.I., Baker, K., and Edlefsen, P. (1984). Family-focused cardiac rehabilitation: A role supplementation program for cardiac patients and spouses. *Nursing Clinics of North America*, 19(1), 113–124.

Dyess, S.M. and Chase, S.K. (2012). Sustaining health in faith community nursing practice: Emerging processes that support the development of a middle-range theory. *Holistic Nursing Practice*, 26(4), 221–227.

Ellis, R. (1982). Conceptual issues in nursing. *Nursing Outlook*, 30, 406–410.

Elo, S., Kaariainen, M., Isola, A., and Kyngas, H. (2013). Developing and testing a middle-range theory of the well-being supportive physical environment of home-dwelling elderly. *The Scientific World Journal*, 2013, Article ID 945635.

Fawcett, J. and DeSanto-Madeya (2013). *Contemporary nursing knowledge: Analysis and evaluation of nursing models and theories* (3rd ed.). Philadelphia, PA: F.A. Davis.

Fearon-Lynch, J.A. and Stover, C.M. (2015). A middle-range theory for diabetes self-management mastery. *Advances in Nursing Science*, 38(4), 330–346.

Forsberg, A., Lennerling, A., Fridh, I., Karlsson, V., and Nilsson, M. (2015, January–December). Understanding the perceived threat of the risk of graft rejections: A middle-range theory. *Global Qualitative Nursing Research*, 2, 1–9.

Gaffney, K.F. (1992). Nursing practice model for maternal role sufficiency. *Advances in Nursing Science*, 15(2), 76–84.

Garcia-Fernandez, F.P., Agreda, J.J., Verdu, J., and Pancorbo-Hidalgo, P.L. (2014). A new theoretical model for the development of pressure ulcers and other dependence-related lesions. *Journal of Nursing Scholarship*, 46(1), 28–38.

Geary, C.R. and Schumacher, K.L. (2012). Care transitions: Integrating transition theory and complexity science concepts. *Advances in Nursing Science*, 35(3), 236–248.

Gobet, F. and Chassy, P. (2008). Towards an alternative to Benner's theory of expert intuition in nursing: A discussion paper. *International Journal of Nursing Studies*, 45(1), 129–139.

Green, C. (2012). Nursing intuition: A valid form of knowledge. *Nursing Philosophy*, 13(2), 98–111.

Haase, J.E., Britt, T., Coward, D.D., Leidy, N.K., and Penn, P.E. (1992). Simultaneous concept analysis of spiritual perspective, hope, acceptance, and self-transcendence. *Image: Journal of Nursing Scholarship*, 24(2), 141–147.

Hagerty, B.M., Lynch-Sauer, J., Patusky, K.L., and Bouwsema, M. (1993). An emerging theory of human relatedness. *Image: Journal of Nursing Scholarship*, 25(4), 291–296.

Kass, M.J. and Rousseau, G.K. (1983). Geriatric sexual conformity: Assessment and intervention. *Clinical Gerontologist*, 2(1), 31–44.

Kelly, L.S. and Lakin, J.A. (1988). Role supplementation as a nursing intervention for Alzheimer's disease: A case study. *Public Health Nursing*, 5(3), 146–152.

Lenz, E.R., Suppe, F., Gift, A.G., Pugh, L.C., and Milligan, R.A. (1995). Collaborative development of middle-range nursing theories: Toward a theory of unpleasant symptoms. *Advances in Nursing Science*, 17(3), 1–13.

Marsh, J.R. (2013). A middle-range theory of postpartum depression: Analysis and application. *International Journal of Childbirth Education*, 28(4), 50–54.

Meleis, A.I. (1971). Self-concept and family planning. *Nursing Research*, 20(3), 29–36.

Meleis, A.I. (1975). Role insufficiency and role supplementation: A conceptual framework. *Nursing Research*, 24(4), 264–271.

Meleis, A.I. (1992). Directions for nursing theory development in the 21st century. *Nursing Science Quarterly*, 5, 112–117.

Meleis, A.I. (1993). *A passion for substance revisited: Global transitions and international commitments*. Published keynote speech given at the 1993 National Doctoral Forum, St. Paul, MN, June 1993.

Meleis, A.I. (1997). *Theoretical nursing: Development and progress* (3rd ed.). Philadelphia, PA: Lippincott-Raven.

Meleis, A.I. (2010). *Transitions theory: Middle-range and situation-specific theories in nursing research and practice*. New York: Springer Publishing Company.

Meleis, A.I. (2015). Transitions theory. In M.C. Smith and M.E. Parker (Eds.) *Nursing theories and nursing practice* (4th ed., pp. 361–380). Philadelphia, PA: FA Davis Co.

Meleis, A.I., Dallafar, A., and Lipson, J.G. (1998). The reluctant immigrant: Immigration experiences among Middle Eastern immigrant groups in California. In Baxter, D. and Krulfeld, R. (Eds.), *Selected papers on refugees and immigrants* (Vol. V, pp. 214–230). Arlington, VA: American Anthropological Association.

Meleis, A.I. and May, K.M. (1981). Nursing theory and scholarliness in the doctoral program. *Advances in Nursing Science*, 4(1), 31–41.

Meleis, A.I., Sawyer, L.M., Im, E.O., Schumacher, K., and Messias, D.K. (2000). Experiencing transitions: An emerging middle-range theory. *Advances in Nursing Science*, 23(1), 12–28.

Meleis, A.I. and Swendsen, L. (1978). Role supplementation: An empirical test of a nursing intervention. *Nursing Research*, 27(1), 11–18.

Meleis, A.I. and Trangenstein, P.A. (1994). Facilitating transitions: Redefinition of a nursing mission. *Nursing Outlook*, 42(6), 255–259.

Merton, R. (1968). *Social theory and social structure* (3rd ed.). New York: Free Press.

Merton, R.K. (1979). *The sociology of science: An episodic memoir*. Carbondale and Edwardsville, IL: Southern Illinois University Press.

Perry, D.J. (2015). Transcendent pluralism: A middle-range theory of nonviolent social transformation through human and ecological dignity. *Advances in Nursing Science*, 38(4), 317–329.

Peterson, S.J. and Bredow, T.S. (2013). *Middle-range theories: Application to nursing research* (3rd ed.). Philadelphia, PA: Wolters/Kluwer-Lippincott Williams & Wilkins.

Pickett, S., Peters, R.M., and Jarosz, P.A. (2014). Toward a middle-range theory of weight management. *Nursing Science Quarterly*, 27(3), 242–247.

Räsänen, P., Backman, K., and Kyngäs, H. (2007). Development of an instrument to test the middle-range theory for the self-care of home-dwelling elderly. *Scandinavian Journal of Caring Sciences*, 21(3), 397–405.

Reed, P. (2006). Commentary on neomoderinism and evidence-based nursing: Implications for the production of nursing knowledge. *Nursing Outlook*, 54(1), 36–38.

Reimer, A.P., Clochesy, J.M., and Moore, S.M. (2013). Early examination of the middle-range theory of flight nursing expertise. *Applied Nursing Research*, 26(4), 276–279.

Reimer, A.P. and Moore, S.M. (2010). Flight nursing expertise: Towards a middle-range theory. *Journal of Advanced Nursing*, 66(5), 1183–1192.

Rew, L. (1986). Intuition: Concept analysis of a group phenomenon. *Advances in Nursing Science*, 8(2), 21–28.

Rew, L. and Barrow, E.M. (1987). Intuition: A neglected hallmark of nursing knowledge. *Advances in Nursing Science*, 10(1), 49–62.

Riegel, B., Jaarsma, T., and Stromberg, A. (2012). A middle-range theory of self-care of chronic illness. *Advances in Nursing Science*, 35(3), 194–204.

Robinson, P.R., Ekman, S.L., Meleis, A.I., Wahlund, L.O., and Winbald, L.O. (1997). The experience of early memory loss. *Health Care in Later Life*, 2(2), 107–120.

Ryan, P. and Sawin, K.J. (2009). The individual and family self-management theory: Background and perspectives on context, process, and outcomes. *Nursing Outlook*, 57(4), 217–225.

Sawyer, L.M. (1996a). Personal Communication.

Sawyer, L.M. (1996b). *Engaged mothering within a racist environment: The transition to motherhood for a group of African American women*. San Francisco, CA: UCSF, doctoral dissertation.

Sawyer, L.M. (1999). Engaged mothering: The transition to motherhood for a group of African American women. *Journal of Transcultural Nursing*, 10(1), 14–21.

Schumacher, K.L. (1995). Family caregiver role acquisition: Role-making through situated interaction. *Scholarly Inquiry for Nursing Practice*, 9(3), 211–226.

Schumacher, K.L. (1996). Personal Communication.

Schumacher, K.L., Jones, P., and Meleis, A.I. (2010). Helping elderly persons in transition: A framework for research and practice. In A.I. Meleis (Ed.), *Transitions theory: Middle-range and situation-specific theories in nursing research and practice* (pp. 129–144). New York: Springer Publishing Company.

Schumacher, K.L. and Meleis, A.I. (1994). Transitions: A central concept in nursing. *Image: Journal of Nursing Scholarship*, 26(2), 119–127.

Shaul, M.P. (1995). From early twinges to mastery: The process of adjustment in living with rheumatoid arthritis. *Arthritis Care and Research*, 8(4), 290–297.

Shih, F.J. (1995). *The experience of Taiwanese patients during recovery transition from cardiac surgery*. Doctoral dissertation, University of California at San Francisco, U.M.I., Ann Arbor, MI: University Microfilms, no. 9502643, 1995.

Silva, M.C. (1977). Philosophy, science, theory: Interrelationships and implications for nursing research. *Image*, 9(3), 59–63.

Smith, M.J. and Liehr, P.R. (2003). *Middle-range theory for nursing*. New York: Springer Publishing.

Sorokin, P. (1974). How are sociological theories conceived, developed and validated. In R.S. Denisoff, O. Callahan, and M.H. Levine (Eds.), *Theories and paradigms in contemporary sociology*. Itasca, IL: F.E. Peacock.

Strauss, A. (1987). *Qualitative analysis for social scientists*. Cambridge, UK: Cambridge University Press.

Strauss, A. and Corbin, J. (1994). Grounded theory methodology – An overview. In N.K. Denzin and Y.S. Lincoln (Eds.), *Handbook of qualitative research* (pp. 273–285). Thousand Oaks, CA: Sage Publications.

Strauss, A. and Corbin, J. (1998). *Basics of qualitative research – technologies and procedures for developing grounded theory* (2nd ed.). Thousand Oaks, CA: Sage Publications.

Turner, R. (1962). Role taking: Process vs. conformity. In A. Rose (Ed.), *Human behavior and social processes*. Boston, MA: Houghton-Mifflin.

University of California, San Francisco School of Nursing Symptom Management Faculty Group. (1994). A model for symptom management. *Image: Journal of Nursing Scholarship*, 26(4), 272–276.

Walker, L.O. and Avant, K.C. (2010). *Strategies for theory construction in nursing* (5th ed.). Upper Saddle River, NJ: Pearson/Prentice Hall.

Westcott, M.R. (1968). *Antecedents and consequences of intuitive thinking*. Final report to U.S. Department of Health, Education, and Welfare. Poughkeepsie, NY: Vassar College.

Zderad, L.T. (1978). From here-and-now to theory: Reflections on how. In J.G. Patterson (Ed.), *Theory development: What, why, how?* New York: National League for Nursing.

Developing Situation-Specific Theories

EUN-OK IM • AFAF MELEIS

INTRODUCTION

The discipline of nursing is at a level of maturity that allows theorists to develop theories that are more congruent with the nature of nursing, the diversity of nursing clients, the complexity of experiences, the responses of human beings in the face of illness situations or calamities, and the dynamic nature of environments. These theories answer more specific questions and provide frameworks that are more accessible to researchers and clinicians. We believe that the future of advancing knowledge in the discipline could best be supported by developing these situation-specific theories, which are closer to operationalization and implementation, closer to the clinical realities of caring for clients, and more reflective of variations in the contexts and situations of populations than middle-range theories.

Situation-specific theories are differentiated from grand and middle-range theories by level of abstraction, degree of specificity, scope of context, level of accessibility to clinical practice and research findings, extent of reflection of population diversity, and by the extent to which they limit or claim generalizability. (See Table 16-1 in the previous chapter for a comparison of the three levels of theory.) Im and Meleis (1999a) provided a useful comparison between the grand theories of Peplau, Henderson, Hall, Johnson, Abdellah, King, and Wiedenbach, the middle-range theories of Hagerty et al., and situation-specific theories of Braden, Im, and Meleis, and Hall, et al. (Im and Meleis, 1999b; Meleis and Im, 2000).

Development of situation-specific theory is at an early state of maturity. The majority of these theories were created early in the 21st century, and the scholars' works tend to be limited to the reports of their own situation-specific theories rather than actual usages and/or evaluation of the theories (Im, 2014a). Many nursing scholars have developed theories that fit the definition and description of situation-specific theories without having labeled them as such (Im, 2014a).

Within this chapter, we define situation-specific theories, discuss their philosophical roots, identify their major properties, and propose an integrative strategy for developing them. We also discuss the current status of the situation-specific theory by examining several contemporary examples as they are depicted in published nursing literature.

DEFINITION OF SITUATION-SPECIFIC THEORIES

Situation-specific theories are coherent representations and descriptions of a set of concepts, an explanation of the relations between those concepts, and a prediction of outcomes related to these relationships. The representation is grounded in clinical, teaching, policy, or administrative situations. It is focused on a specific set of phenomena, more subscribed situations, and has a limited set of conditions.

More specifically, Im and Meleis (1999b) defined situation-specific theories as "theories that focus on specific nursing phenomena that reflect clinical practice and that are limited to specific populations or to particular fields of practice." They asserted that situation-specific theories would be necessary because grand theories and middle-range theories rarely reflect the diversities in nursing phenomenon, and have inherent limitations in describing, explaining, and understanding of increasingly diverse and complex nursing phenomenon (Im and Meleis, 1999b). Moreover, the lack of sociopolitical, cultural, and/or historic contextual considerations in grand theories and middle-range theories also necessitates situation-specific theories because situation-specific theories are placed in social and historical context and they are limited to a socially constraining structure, or a politically limiting situation (Meleis, 1997).

Situation-specific theories are less abstract than middle-range theories and are limited in the number of concepts described, in the range of explanations offered, in the scope of research propositions they drive, and in the outcomes claimed. These limitations are not a reflection of the significance of the potential contributions to the science that may be generated, but rather are a reflection of the depth of explanation that such theories offer the user for a particular, specific area or field of concern. Depth and richness also emanate from the consideration of such significant contextual conditions that are thought to be vital for the explanatory power of a situation-specific theory but that may otherwise be perceived as noise and deviation in a more abstract middle-range theory. For example, in the development of a situation-specific theory on any health experience or responses (e.g., pain experience or management), the theorist should consider marginalization of clients due to racism, ageism, nationalism, or other –isms; consideration of these factors would be less vital in middle-range theories. Situation-specific theories are more tolerant of multiple truths and more congruent of an increasingly integrative theory of truth, as presented in Chapter 8, pages 146–150.

In some ways situation-specific theories are similar to the *single-domain* or *microtheories* defined by Merton (1968) and the *practice theories* defined by Jacox (1974). All are at a lower level of abstraction than middle-range theories (Merton, 1968). Practice theories are single-domain or microtheories that are specific to nursing; as the name implies, they start from practice, and their goal is to influence practice. Still, there are unique aspects of situation-specific theories—their philosophical bases, their properties, the approach to development—that certainly distinguish them from single-domain/micro theories and practice theories.

PHILOSOPHICAL ROOTS OF SITUATION-SPECIFIC THEORIES

Situation-specific theories are based on an assumption of philosophical, theoretical, and methodological plurality. There are four major philosophical roots that could drive the development of situation-specific theories: (1) post-empiricism, (2) critical social theory and feminism, (3) hermeneutics, and (4) neo-pragmatism.

Post-empiricism is somewhat different from positivism, especially logical positivism and the Vienna Circle. Although post-empiricism still has belief in observables and is based on careful scientific strategies, it does not view common patterns or universal laws governing all of health as rigidly as logical positivism. Rather, it assumes that reasonable predictions are possible and that these predictions can estimate expected human responses under certain health/illness conditions and provide directions for nursing care.

Critical social theory and feminism provide the rationale for respecting diversities of framework as well as providing the framework to consider the sociopolitical and historical contexts in situation-specific theories (Im and Meleis, 1999b). Feminists and critical theorists could also highlight the subjective and social construction of nursing phenomenon, sociopolitical and economic influences, and the influences of racism, classism, and sexism. However, because critical theory disagrees with classical social and economic theories, Im and Meleis (1999b) were cautious in connecting critical theory with situation-specific theories. Since feminism focuses on the world of women in male-dominated societies, feminist theories provide a framework that highlights the lived experience and the historical context as the basis for knowing, generating, documenting, and analyzing.

Hermeneutics was also proposed to be a philosophical root of situation-specific theories because they assume historical consciousness and humanistic and historical knowledge (Im and Meleis, 1999b). Hermeneutics considers the human state or essence as supreme, and it highlights the interactive circle—"hermeneutic circle"—between patient and nurse or subject and scientist. Hermeneutics emphasizes awareness of meaning (including embedded meaning) and self-reflection, and considers "understanding" as the basis of knowing. However, because hermeneutics (except the objective, validation hermeneutics) negates objectifying the human state or the modeling of the human state, we should be careful in developing situation-specific theories based on the assumptions of hermeneutic philosophies (Im and Meleis, 1999b).

Finally, neo-pragmatism could be another philosophical root for development of situation-specific theories. The properties of situation-specific theories (discussed in the next section) agree with the stance of neo-pragmatism represented by Rorty (1999) that emphasizes multiple realities. According to neo-pragmatism, the truth is what is approved by the scholars who agreed on the truth. Subsequently, the truth is time-dependent and situation-dependent. This stance of neo-pragmatism agrees more with the tenants and properties of situation-specific theories; situation-specific theories do not transcend time, place, a socially constraining structure, or politically limiting situations. All these conditions shape and define situation-specific theories; if any condition changes, then the theory no longer applies.

PROPERTIES OF SITUATION-SPECIFIC THEORIES

Situation-specific theories have unique properties that distinguish them from grand theories and middle-range theories. The first such property is their *low level of abstraction*. Since the increasing diversity and complexity of nursing phenomena negates the application of broad, overarching theory, there is a need for theories that focus on specific phenomena. Situation-specific theories fit this need by answering a set of coherent questions about situations with a limited scope and focus. Situation-specific theories are much less abstract than grand theories or middle-range theories, but they are more abstract than individuals' frameworks or stories about practice (Im and Meleis, 1999b).

The second property of situation-specific theories is the *specificity* of the particular nursing phenomenon that the theories aim at explicating. Grand theories and middle-range theories are broader in scope and the phenomena addressed within them tend to transcend fields of practice. Phenomena defined within situation-specific theories are confined to a particular field of practice or single specialty. Therefore, situation-specific theories are more likely to provide guidelines for practice model generation that drive the development of nursing therapeutics. An example of such specific phenomena is: patterns of living with rheumatoid arthritis or with irritable bowels.

A third property of situation-specific theory that must be fulfilled is the *specific context*. Since situation-specific theories are placed in social, cultural, and historic contexts, their scope could be limited to specific situations or specific populations. For instance, the situation-specific theory of menopausal symptom experience of low-income Korean immigrant women developed by Im and Meleis (1999b) specifically reflects the context that the women are living within the United States.

Thus, the theory cannot be used to describe and explain Korean immigrant women in other countries or Korean women in their country of origin. Similarly, in the last example, the theorist would be considering patterns of living with rheumatoid arthritis or irritable bowels for women in Tromsø, Norway (specific gender properties, certain weather patterns, and specific policies).

A fourth property of situation-specific theories is their *strong connection to a limited set of research questions*. Both situation-specific theories and middle-range theories can provide the framework from which to generate research questions. However, situation-specific theories provide closer linkages to research because, unlike middle-range theories, they are confined to phenomena and questions within the context of a single specialty or field.

In addition, because situation-specific theories are usually developed by synthesizing and integrating a limited set of research findings, as well as clinical exemplars, they could be more easily linked to research projects and clinical practice situations.

The final properties of situation-specific theories are their *incorporation of diversities* in nursing phenomena and the resulting *limitations in generalization* (Im and Meleis, 1999a). Grand theories aim to extract and universalize the essence of observations, data, or themes. Middle-range theories aim to reflect the diversities in the sense that they provide a framework for specific nursing phenomenon and reflect a wide range of nursing situations, but they are based on the assumption that theories are universal; they therefore cannot fully describe, explain, interpret, and understand diversities within participants. Situation-specific theories, however, inherently consider diversities in culture, gender, educational background, religion, sexual orientation, and political preference. This consideration of diversities inherently limits making generalizations.

SOURCES FOR SITUATION-SPECIFIC THEORIES

The sources of situation-specific theories are multiple. Whether the impetus is research, practice, or theory, the integration of all sources is the hallmark of these theories. The context and the population tend to be the criteria for the development of such theories; generalizations tend to be limited, and a specific time in history may be integral to developing situation-specific theories. Im (2005) goes even further in suggesting that the integrated strategy of practice, theory, and research as proposed by Meleis (1997) is the strategy of choice when developing situation-specific theory. The integrative strategy described in Chapters 14, 15, and 16—and elaborated on later in this chapter—is actually the strategy of choice for both middle-range and situation-specific situations. It is imperative in situation-specific theories to include the history of the clinical situation, the involvement and engagement of the theorist, a clear nursing perspective, a holistic dynamic, the changing framework, and the phenomenon (described and explained through the interaction of health–illness events, personal environment, relationships, and human response), as well as other defining aspects of the context. The integrative strategy also includes research findings and other data from clinical experiences or other theories. This integrated strategy contrasts with practice-to-theory strategy, research-to-theory strategy, and theory-to-theory strategy. It combines the best of all in an integrative way. Im (2005) is explicit in including the criteria of "multiple truths" as an essential assumption for using the integrated strategy to developing situation-specific theories.

Any nursing and non-nursing conceptual models, grand theories, and middle-range theories could provide the foundation for situation-specific theories. On the basis of an existing theory, theory derivation could be conducted by using analogy for explanations, understandings, or predictions of a particular situation of a specific population of interest as well. For example, Riegel and her colleagues (Riegel and Dickson, 2008; Riegel, Dickson, and Faulkner, 2015) developed a scale to measure self-care, applied the scale in a practice setting, and then used both the results and the original self-care theory to develop their own situation-specific theory to uniquely describe and explain self-care for patients with heart failure. Willis, DeSanto-Madeya, and Fawcett (2015) used Rogers' theory of unitary human beings as the framework used to guide the development of a situation-specific theory to describe and explain the process of healing from childhood maltreatment for men.

Im and Meleis, recognizing that the middle-range theory of transitions (discussed in Chapter 16) lacked specificity, used it to develop several situation-specific theories to describe and explain how certain populations experience transition (e.g., Korean American women experiencing menopause, Asian American cancer patients in their health/illness transition)

within the context of their daily lives (Im, 2008; Im and Meleis, 1999a). And the same theory was used by a number of other scholars who developed nine more situation-specific theories that were analyzed and discussed by Im (2014b). In developing these theories, though based and driven by a middle-range theory of transitions, the theories they developed described patient's responses to health–illness experiences more accurately and fully. Similarly, Clingerman (2007) used transition theory to develop her theory about migrants' transitions. Theory triangulation and theory derivation were used as a source and a strategy to develop a theory to explain complex adaptive systems for patients in transition. Geary and Schumacher (2012) used major concepts on complex adaptive systems from complex science and from middle-range transition theory.

Finally, multiple theories can be combined with the published literature and findings from research studies to form the integrated sources for situation-specific theory. Two examples are the situation-specific theories on immigrant women's physical activity experience (Im, Chang, Nguyen, et al., 2015) and quality of life among older South Korean adults with type 2 diabetes (Chang and Im, 2014). Below we describe the integrative approach to developing situation-specific theories.

THE INTEGRATIVE STRATEGY FOR DEVELOPING SITUATION-SPECIFIC THEORIES

The integrative strategy for the development of situation-specific theories was originally proposed by Meleis (1997) and further developed and operationalized by Im (2005). While there are some similarities to the integrative strategy proposed and used in developing concepts (see Chapter 14) and in developing middle-range theories (see Chapter 16), there are some subtle and not-so-subtle differences. The reader is encouraged to critically identify differences and similarities as well as to identify and develop new strategies. We provide these processes only as guidelines to be modified and updated. Furthermore, while we provide these processes in what appears to be a linear progression, we are cognizant that in developing theories, processes are neither linear nor do they ever go in the same order (Box 17-1). It is important to note that research and practice reviews and exemplars are incorporated into each component below.

BOX 17-1	THE INTEGRATIVE STRATEGY FOR DEVELOPING SITUATION-SPECIFIC THEORIES

- Grounding in nursing domain and perspective
- Selection of a theory
- Specify population characteristics and context
- Review of literature (practice, education and research)
- Collaborate (reflect, analyze, critique through dialogue)
- Check assumptions
- Document process
- Report and share

[Also based on Im, E.O. and Meleis, A.I. (1999a). Situation-specific theory of Korean immigrant women's menopausal transition. *Image: Journal of Nursing Scholarship*, 31(4), 333–338.]

Grounding in Nursing Domain and Perspectives

First and foremost, in developing a situation-specific theory that could enhance nursing science, the theorist must be grounded in the discipline of nursing, scope of practice, and the discipline's domain and perspective, as discussed in Chapter 6. Identifying the phenomenon and the problematics that need to be explicated, as well as the population for which the theory will be developed, are important aspects to be considered in theory development. Being cognizant of and driven by the goals and the mission of nursing will require immersion and understanding of the clinical situation and the conditions for which the theory is developed. In developing a situation-specific theory on breast-feeding, Nelson (2006) was inspired by clinical observations of the maternal effort to breast-feed and the limited support these mothers received from their providers. She became aware that existing theories did not help in achieving the desired outcomes.

Another example is elderly transitions. Although the starting point for this situation-specific theory was the transition theory (Schumacher and Meleis, 1994), the clinical experiences of the authors and their research findings in the literature helped them develop a more specific model in which healthy and unhealthy processes in elderly transitions were articulated, reflecting the aging situation and the experiences of gains and losses that occur through the biological, social, and psychological aging processes. The literature reviews, combined with

clinical experiences of working with the elderly experiencing transitions, were integrated to produce seven healthy processes that could be the triggers for healthy outcomes.

This situation-specific theory proposes that those elderly who are aware of the transition, experiences, and responses, and who positively and realistically redefine the meaning of their transition, modify their expectations of themselves and others, and engage and modify the daily routines of their lives to become more congruent with new demands in their lives. Similarly, those who are not only willing, but who actually develop new skills and competencies that are based on knowledge of the situation, and who maintain some continuity in their lives, go on to also create new choices, find opportunities for growth, and tend to have a healthier transition outcome. It does not matter whether the transitions they are experiencing are developmental, situational, or one of health and illness. The outcome of a healthy transition is the experience of minimal symptoms; these people tend to have optimal functional status, and they tend to feel connected and to experience a sense of empowerment and integrity. These outcomes are mediated by the patterns of transition and are a function of whether the events that triggered the transition are single or multiple occurrences, and whether the transitional events are sequential, simultaneously related, or simultaneously unrelated. Unhealthy transition processes, in their extremes, are opposite from the healthy processes, and the process indicators will include compromised functional status and feelings of disempowerment, in addition to a tendency to experience a variety of symptoms. A coherent approach to elderly care and scholarship was suggested by utilizing the transitions framework and through immersion in clinical observations, both of which shaped this situation-specific theory (Schumacher, Jones, and Meleis, 2010).

Selection of a Theory

As indicated in the previous example, review, study, and analysis of middle-range theory is the more common starting point than grand theories for developing a situation-specific theory. Dialogue, analysis, critique, identifying exemplars, affirming and/or modifying assumptions, defining and redefining concepts, and explaining relationships are processes used in developing situation-specific theories when based on middle-range theories. During such review, it may be determined that the theory does not quite allow a comprehensive and inclusive explanation of clinical situations for scientists or clinicians. Riegel and Dickson (2008, 2010) found that no integrated and coherent set of explanations of self-care existed for patients with heart failure. They identified several concepts that specifically reflect this population of patients and several propositions that were tested offering preliminary support for the theory. Their starting point was self-care theory; they pointed out the existing confusion between the various self-care concepts, and they opted to further clarify self-care from a number of other concepts. Several related situation-specific theory examples that emerged from other theories exist in the literature: Im (2005) describes Falk-Rafael's (2001) empowered caring, LaCoursiere's (2001) online social support, and Poss' (2001) synthesis of health belief model and theory of reasoned action as examples of situation-specific theories based on other theories.

Specifying Populations Within a Context

Narrowing a theory's scope can increase its power explanation, but it limits the theory application and utility to certain populations and repertoire of conditions. Therefore, developing a coherent situation-specific theory that drives science and practice requires detailed specificity about the populations for which the theory is developed. An example is pain experiences of Caucasian patients diagnosed with cancer (Im, 2006). Furthermore, it requires attention to, and incorporation of, the sociocultural and historical context to explain the clinical situation, as well as the conditions that affect care. Additionally, it requires attention to a particular set of genetic markers that may characterize this population. Many examples illustrate this population focus.

A situation-specific theory of breast-feeding included a broad contextual history surrounding breast-feeding and the sociocultural norms that influenced whether women breast-feed or bottle-feed. Few would deny the influence of the media, society, and the bottle-feeding industry in influencing the decisions of women and their families. Therefore, a review of these conditions, as well as other factors, is vital in developing a theory about women's choices, options, decisions, and actions (Nelson, 2006). Another example is the menopausal transition of Korean immigrant women (Im and Meleis, 2010, p. 121). Unlike women who are not recent immigrants, Korean immigrant women tended to pay less attention to menopause and tended not to

attribute changes in their lives to menopause, but rather more to work and the immigration transition. Menopause was a silent experience for them, either normalized or ignored. In a research study exploring how new Korean immigrants tended to experience and respond to menopause, the findings indicated a need for developing a more contextual and specific conceptualization of the menopausal transition. The research findings by Im (1997) then led to developing a more specific conceptualization of transition, one that embraced menopause as a transition, the immigration experience, and the centrality of gender, context, and socioeconomic status, as well as the ability to manage symptoms (Im and Meleis, 1999b). These concepts then helped to modify the middle-range theory of transitions and made it more specific for the purpose of illuminating the situation and experience of immigrant women. Such specificity leads to more focused future research questions, as well as to a different level of understanding (e.g., Korean immigrant women's experiences in the health care system as they manifest resistance and reluctance to discuss what the symptoms of menopause may be). A diagram depicting the situation-specific theory is presented in Figure 17-1, with asterisks indicating how specificity to the Korean immigrant women uncovered by research led to modifications or extensions of the Schumacher and Meleis (1994) model. Within the immigration transition framework, Clingerman (2007) further modified the transition middle-range theory by adding the context for migrant farm workers. She sharpened the propositions by considering immigration documentation, citizenship status, and personal U.S. identity; this led her to consider a sense of peace as a more congruent outcome for this population.

Using population characteristics as a starting point for the development of situation-specific theories is another productive approach. Im used her cumulative wisdom from research evidence about vulnerable women and their health to develop several situation-specific theories to explain different phenomena and generate propositions for further research. Among them are situation-specific theories about the cancer pain experience (Im, 2008) and women's attitudes toward physical activity (Im, Stuifbergen, and Walker, 2010).

Review of Literature

An integrative review of interdisciplinary and interprofessional literature that encompasses the theory,

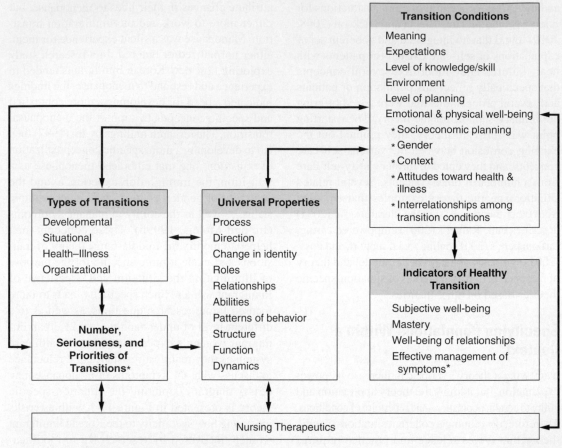

*Additions to the model of Schumacher and Meleis (1994).

Figure 17-1   Model of a situation-specific theory: The menopausal transition experience of Korean immigrant women. Reprinted with permission from Im, E.O. and Meleis, A.I. (1999a). Situation-specific theory of Korean immigrant women's menopausal transition. *Image: Journal of Nursing Scholarship*, 31(4), 333–338.

research, and practice will illuminate the emerging situation-specific theory throughout the process of development. Although Sakraida (2005) did not call her conceptualization of the divorce transition of midlife women a situation-specific theory, the results of her research program could eventually lead to a coherent situation-specific theory. She offers an example of an extensive review of divorce transition literature, the transition for midlife women, and the determinants of outcomes based on initiators and noninitiators of the divorce.

An integrated systematic review of literature could also be used to perform a comprehensive analysis of currently existing knowledge about a nursing phenomenon. While theorists may start their theorization from a literature review that may be the impetus for their theoretical thinking about a specific nursing phenomenon, they may also be inspired by their clinical, research, or educational experiences that trigger a theoretical journey. In any of these situations it is essential that a thorough review includes reviewing existing theories, interdisciplinary and interprofessional literature, as well as research, education, and practice literature.

Collaboration

International and interdisciplinary collaborative efforts could be a source for theory development in the situation-specific theories. Collaborative works provide diverse views and different sets of findings, allow for comparison of ideas, enhance scholarly dialogues, and promote integration of visions. Furthermore, collaborative efforts could also provide a source for theory development that strongly links theory to practice. International collaborative efforts could provide different cultural perspectives on a single nursing phenomenon.

Theorizing could be done by a single person or a group of colleagues, and by incorporating experiences and reflexivity of the theorists, clinicians, and researchers through diverse sources of theorizing.

Checking Assumptions

At different points during the development of a theory, the theorist pauses to check assumptions upon which the theory is built. For situation-specific theories, the assumptions checked include those related to connection to nursing practice values, perspective, domain, and mission, as well as those that emanate from the sociopolitical and historical context, particularly to diversity of populations and principles of equity in the provision and access to care. Situation-specific theories do not transcend time or existing policies that constrain the care provided.

Documenting the Process

Documentation of all the processes involved in the theorization is essential to confirm the theoretical and analytic decision trails created by the theorist. Questions on conceptualization and theorization, critiques of each step of the development process, and reflection on possible impact of the theories within the social and political environment need to be systematically documented through theoretical diaries and/or memos. This documentation on the rationale, outcome, and evaluation of all actions related to conceptualization and theorization is an important component in the integrative strategy, and this will allow well grounded, cogent, justifiable, relevant, and meaningful theory development processes and outcomes.

Reporting and Sharing

The final step of the integrative strategy is to report and share the documented theorization as a manuscript, a model, or a research report with nursing communities. By reporting and sharing, theorists may receive critiques by peers, and these reviews can be used to continue to develop the theory. Also, the documented and disseminated theory could be further developed through validation processes that ideally should include nursing clients. If the theory is perceived by nursing clients as a representative of their real experience, the theory could be more easily used to describe and explain the nursing phenomenon, and result in better nursing outcomes.

THE STATUS OF SITUATION-SPECIFIC THEORIES

The identification and use of situation-specific theories and the support for their use has been increasing (Lee, Hann, Yang, et al., 2011; Lee, Fawcett, Yang, et al., 2012). Several themes that reflect the status of situation-specific theories emerged from an extensive literature review by Im (2014a). She categorized the results of the review of the literature from 1999 to 2013, which yielded 19 articles, into four nonexclusive publication patterns: (1) publications in which the authors explicitly identified their work as a situation-specific theory, (2) publications in which the work met the defining characteristics of situation-specific theory even though the authors didn't explicitly identify the work as such, (3) publications in which the authors proposed that their conceptualization may evolve into a situation-specific theory, and we add here another category, and (4) publications describing situation-specific theories that drove the development of practice models but that were not the impetus for research projects. In addition, Im identified several strategies that were used to develop situation-specific theories. In her review of published situation-specific theories, Im (2014a) reports that 12 (63%) were explicitly labeled as situation-specific theories.

It is of historical note that the first publication to identify a situation-specific theory was by Im and Meleis (1999a), in which they described the development of their theory to explain the menopausal transition of Korean immigrant women in the United States. (See *Specifying Populations Within a Context* on page 395 for a more extensive discussion.) Other examples of those explicitly defined as situation-specific theories include works by Riegel and Dickson (2008), Riegel, Dickson, and Faulkner (2015), Nelson (2006), Clingerman (2007), and Willis et al. (2015). Riegel, Dickson, and Faulkner identified their work as "a situation-specific theory of health failure self-care," and it is a clear example of a theory that embodies the properties and sources discussed previously in this chapter. Nelson's theory was titled as "a situation-specific theory of breastfeeding," and it was also clear on differences and uniqueness of the theory from other existing theories on breast-feeding. Clingerman's theory was explicitly called "the situation-specific theory of migration transition for migrant farmworker women," and the limitation of the situation-specific theory to the particular context described was well acknowledged. "Moving beyond dwelling in suffering" is presented as a situation-specific theory and it, also, models the property to be included in situation-specific theories (Willis et al., 2015).

Works that meet our definition of situation-specific theories but that weren't explicitly identified as such include Ohlén, Andershed, Berg, et al.'s (2007) theory and Alizadeh, Hylander, Kocturk, et al.'s (2010) theory. Ohlen and colleagues aimed to explain the nursing phenomenon around safety for relatives of an adult or older patient who was close to end of life. Although they never claimed that their theory was a situation-specific theory, the article clearly identifies the necessary properties of that theory type (e.g., context, specific nursing phenomenon). Additionally, they used an integrative strategy for theorization that incorporated an existing theory (Ricoeur's [1992] ethical intention theory), their clinical experience with relatives, and a literature review on existing studies on relatives' experiences during end-of-life situations. While the use of integrative strategy in itself is not a property of situation-specific theories, its use for specific phenomena, population setting, and context adds another dimension supporting situation-specific theories. Alizadeh and colleagues developed their theory specifically to explain the perception and management of "family honor" by youth clinic personnel in Swedish primary care; again, the specificity clearly identifies this as a situation-specific theory, even if the authors did not label it as such.

Examples of those theories that the authors proposed may evolve into situation-specific theory include those of Bennett, Sauvé, and Shaw (2005) and Polivka, Chaudry, Crawford, et al. (2013). Polivka and colleagues did not identify their theory as situation-specific, but they acknowledged that they used Im's (2005) integrative strategy to develop their theory and that they derived their theory from an existing situation-specific theory.

Im observed that all the situation-specific theories since 1999 provided clear directions for nursing interventions. This includes both theories explicitly labeled situation-specific by their creators as well as those subsequently identified as situation-specific by Im during her review. For example, Nelson's situation-specific theory (2006) could provide directions for future practice for breast-feeding planning among mothers and significant others. Similarly, Ohlén et al.'s theory (2007) could provide directions for future nursing practice for end-of-life care to enable safety for relatives.

Methods and sources informed the development of situation-specific theories. Multiple methodologies were used to develop seven of the reviewed (Im, 2014a) situation-specific theories. It is important to note that while methods may specifically be related to research projects or programs of research, methodologies are also mostly driven by implicit or explicit philosophical principles. For example, grounded theory methodology is a systematic qualitative research methodology in general (Glaser and Strauss, 2012); it is based on theoretical assumptions about induction (rather than deduction) and based on the goal of developing grounded theory. Therefore, it was considered a theorizing method by Suh (2008), Bull and McShane (2008), and Alizadeh et al. (2010). Other methodologies used were feminist research methods (Clingerman, 2007), interpretive ethnography (Baird, 2012), and qualitative focus groups (Polivka et al., 2013) that were used to develop their theories. Each of these methods evolved from particular philosophical bases that also inform the particular situation-specific theory.

Only two theories (Artinian, Magnan, Sloan, et al., 2002; Riegel and Dickson, 2008; Riegel et al., 2015) were developed and tested through the use of quantitative methods based on post-empiricism; Riegel and colleagues used a literature review of research findings on self-care along with utilizing and integrating findings from their previous studies as sources for the development of their theory (mostly quantitative studies), while Artinian and colleagues used a descriptive correlational study design in their work.

Mixed methods were used in the development of the other situation-specific strategies. Several theories employed both feminism and ethnography: Im (2008) used the findings from a mixed-method study on cancer pain of Asian Americans; Im and Meleis (1999a) used the findings from a *mixed-method* study on low-income Korean immigrant women's menopausal transition experience; and Lee et al. (2012) used their multiple studies (both quantitative and/or qualitative) on hepatitis B virus health-related behaviors of Korean Americans. *Critical thinking/ reasoning processes* are also other methods used in developing situation-specific theories. These processes include analysis, discovery, formulation, and validation, using several different methods (e.g., deductive, inductive, abductive, dialectical). The contexts for the reasoning process include norms and standards, knowledge and skills, conceptual scheme, and reflexivity. A theorist could start theorization by initially developing and refining conceptual schemes through *reasoning dialogues* with others, as well as with self. *Writing memos and* journals as methods could help start and retain the theorist's internal and external dialogue. *Discussions* with other colleagues and research participants and participation in seminars, conferences, and/or panel discussions could also help initiate and maintain the theorist's external dialogue. Finally, *reflexivity* helps in considering social, cultural, and historical contexts by uncovering deep-seated, but rarely identified perspectives on the specific situations and/or the specific populations, and through the use of a full account of the theorists' perspectives, thoughts, and conduct. In the reasoning process, reflexivity on the theorists' own values helps determine the meanings attached to the specific situations and/or the specific populations.

As mentioned previously, literature reviews were major sources that have been frequently used in the development of situation-specific theories. (See also discussion of *Sources for Situation-Specific theories* section on page 392.) Examples are Nelson's theory (2006) that was developed based on a literature review and existing theories of breast-feeding. Using Ricoeur's ethical intention theory as a starting point, and Ohlén et al.'s theory (2007) was developed mainly through a literature review and theoretical reasoning based on clinical experiences from end-of-life care.

Finally, national or international collaborative efforts were also a source of theorizing in some situation-specific theories. Several theories were developed by multiple theorists working within a single country, including Sweden (Alizadeh et al., 2010; Ohlén et al., 2007) and South Korea (Suh, 2008). Others were developed through international collaboration between theorists from the United States and other countries (Davidson, Dracup, Phillips, et al., 2007; Lee et al., 2012).

EVALUATING SITUATION-SPECIFIC THEORIES IN THE LITERATURE

Despite the increasing number of situation-specific theories that have been developed during the past decade, theory evaluation of situation-specific theories tends to be limited (Im, 2015), and virtually no specific criteria to evaluate situation-specific theories have been developed. In spite of that, we found the beginning of a trend for evaluating these types of theories. For example, Vellone, Riegel, D'Agostino et al.'s theory (2013) was evaluated in 417 patients with heart failure by testing several propositions from the theory. Reynolds and O'Connell's theory (2012) was evaluated among 428 parents of 9- to 18-year-old girls using factor analysis and logistic regression analyses; the findings supported the major propositions of the theory. In addition, situation-specific theories have been evaluated by focusing on specific populations. Because a situation-specific theory targets a specific population, it is expected that this type of theory should be evaluated by testing it on that specific population. For instance, Ezer, Ricard, Bouchard, et al. (2006) evaluated their situation-specific theory through a prospective correlational study among 70 women following their partners' diagnosis of prostate cancer, the population for which the theory was developed.

It is important to note that specific examples of future research projects were provided in almost all situation-specific theories. One example of the connection between research and theory that focused on a particular population was offered by a group of international collaborators (Vellone et al., 2013) who connected the development of instrument, middle-range theory, and situation-specific theory. Therefore, we consider that an explicit indication of potential research connection as an important criteria in evaluating theories.

CONCLUSION

The future for advancing nursing knowledge depends on the extent to which we are willing to commit to developing coherent theoretical background that could drive future research programs and practice models. The nature of nursing as a human science that is rooted in the experiences and responses to health and illness lends itself far better to the development and use of situation-specific theories than middle-range or grand theories. In this chapter, an overview of situation-specific theories was provided. The current status and examples of situation-specific theories from the literature were discussed, and suggestions were proposed for future development and use of situation-specific theories in nursing research and practice.

REFLECTIVE QUESTIONS

1. Compare and contrast a middle-range and a situation-specific theory. What are the similarities and differences in the processes of development, the sources, and the testing?

2. Select a middle-range theory in your field and use it to develop a situation-specific theory using the guidelines outlined in this chapter. How would you refine these guidelines?

3. Identify, discuss, and critique the role of research in developing situation-specific theories.

4. There are situation-specific theories that evolved from practice, those that were articulated from research, and yet others that evolved from other theories. Select one of each from your field of practice or research and critically discuss the potential power of each in advancing knowledge.

5. Select a situation-specific theory, a middle-range theory, and a grand theory, and develop a research question from each. Compare and contrast the nature and specificity of the questions and the potential population of the study.

6. Develop a defensible argument for and the rationale against the development of situation-specific theories.

REFERENCES

Alizadeh, V., Hylander, I., Kocturk, T., and Törnkvist, L. (2010). Counselling young immigrant women worried about problems related to the protection of "family honour"--from the perspective of midwives and counsellors at youth health clinics. *Scandinavian Journal of Caring Sciences*, 24(1), 32–40.

Artinian, N.T., Magnan, M., Sloan, M., and Lange, M.P. (2002). Self-care behaviors among patients with heart failure. *Heart & Lung*, 31(3), 161–172.

Baird, M.B. (2012). Well-being in refugee women experiencing cultural transition. *Advances in Nursing Science*, 35(3), 249–263.

Bennett, S.J., Sauvé, M.J., and Shaw, R.M. (2005). A conceptual model of cognitive deficits in chronic heart failure. *Journal of Nursing Scholarship*, 37(3), 222–228.

Bull, M.J. and McShane, R.E. (2008). Seeking what's best during the transition to adult day health services. *Qualitative Health Research*, 18(5), 597–605.

Chang, S.J. and Im, E.O. (2014). Development of a situation-specific theory for explaining health-related quality of life among older South Korean Adults with type 2 diabetes. *Research and Theory for Nursing Practice: An International Journal*, 28(2), 113–126.

Clingerman, E. (2007). A situation-specific theory of migration transition for migrant farmworker women. *Research and Theory for Nursing Practice*, 21(4), 220–235.

Davidson, P.M., Dracup, K., Phillips, J., Padilla, G., and Daly, J. (2007). Maintaining hope in transition: a theoretical framework to guide interventions for people with heart failure. *The Journal of Cardiovascular Nursing*, 22(1), 58–64.

Ezer, H., Ricard, N., Bouchard, L., Souhami, L., Saad, F., Aprikian, A., and Taguchi, Y. (2006). Adaptation of wives to prostate cancer following diagnosis and 3 months after treatment: a test of family adaptation theory. *International Journal of Nursing Studies*, 43(7), 827–838.

Falk-Rafael, A.R. (2001). Empowerment as a process of evolving consciousness: A model of empowered caring. *Advances in Nursing Studies*, 24(1), 1–16.

Geary, C.R. and Schumacher, K.L. (2012). Care transitions: integrating transition theory and complexity science concepts. *Advances in Nursing Science*, 35(3), 236–248.

Glaser, B.G. and Strauss, A.L. (2012). *The discovery of grounded theory: strategies for qualitative research*. New Brunswick, NJ: Aldine Transaction.

Im, E.O. (1997). *Neglecting and ignoring menopause within a gendered multiple transitional context: Low income Korean immigrant women*. San Francisco, CA: UCSF, doctoral dissertation.

Im, E.O. (2005). Development of situation-specific theories: An integrative approach. *Advances in Nursing Science*, 28(2), 137–151.

Im, E.O. (2006). A situation-specific theory of Caucasian cancer patients' pain experience. *Advances in Nursing Science*, 29(3), 232–244.

Im, E.O. (2008). The situation-specific theory of pain experience for Asian American cancer patients. *Advances in Nursing Science*, 31(4), 319–331.

Im, E.O. (2014a). The status quo of situation-specific theories. *Research and Theory for Nursing Practice*, 28(4), 278–298.

Im, E.O. (2014b). Situation-specific theories from the middle-range transitions theory. *Advances in Nursing Science*, 37(1), 19–31.

Im, E.O. (2015). The current status of theory evaluation in nursing. *Journal of Advanced Nursing*, 71(10), 2268–2278.

Im, E.O., Chang, S.J., Nguyen, G., Stringer, L., Chee, W., and Chee, E. (2015). Korean immigrant women's physical activity experience: A situation-specific theory. *Research and Theory for Nursing Practice: An International Journal*, 29(1), 10–24.

Im, E.O. and Meleis, A.I. (1999a). A situation-specific theory of Korean immigrant women's menopausal transition. *Image: Journal of Nursing Scholarship*, 31(4), 333–338.

Im, E.O. and Meleis, A.I. (1999b). Situation-specific theories: philosophical roots, properties, and approach. *Advances in Nursing Science*, 22(2), 11–24.

Im, E.O. and Meleis, A.I. (2010). A situation-specific theory of Korean immigrant women's menopausal transition. In A.I. Meleis (Ed.), *Transitions theory: Middle-range and situation-specific theories in nursing research and practice* (pp. 121–129). New York: Springer Publishing Company.

Im, E.O., Stuifbergen, A.K., and Walker, L. (2010). A situation-specific theory of midlife women's attitudes toward physical activity. *Nursing Outlook*, 58(1), 52–58.

Jacox, A. (1974). Theory struction in nursing: An overview. *Nursing Research*, 23(1), 4–13.

LaCoursiere, S.P. (2001). A theory of online social support. *Advances in Nursing Science*, 24(1), 60–77.

Lee, H., Fawcett, J., Yang, J.H., and Hann, H-W. (2012). Correlates of hepatitis B virus health-related behaviors of Korean Americans: A situation-specific nursing theory. *Journal of Nursing Scholarship*, 44(4), 315–322.

Lee, H., Hann, H.W., Yang, J.H., and Fawcett, J. (2011). Recognition and management of HBV infection in a social context. *Journal of Cancer Education*, 26(3), 516–521.

Meleis, A.I. (1997). *Theoretical nursing: Development and progress*. Philadelphia, PA: Lippincott Williams & Wilkins.

Meleis, A.I. and Im, E.O. (2000). From fragmentation to integration: Situation-specific theories. In N.L. Chaska (Ed.), *The nursing profession: Tomorrow's vision* (pp. 881–891). Thousand Oaks, CA: Sage Publications.

Merton, R. (1968). *Social theory and social structure* (3rd ed.). New York: Free Press.

Nelson, A.M. (2006). Toward a situation-specific theory of breast-feeding. *Research and Theory for Nursing Practice*, 20(1), 9–27.

Ohlén, J., Andershed, B., Berg, C., Frid, I., Palm, C.-A., Ternestedt, B.-M., and Segesten, K. (2007). Relatives in end-of-life care--part 2: A theory for enabling safety. *Journal of Clinical Nursing*, 16(2), 382–390.

Polivka, B.J., Chaudry, R., Crawford, J.M., Wilson, R., and Galos, D. (2013). Application and modification of the integrative model for environmental health. *Public Health Nursing*, 30(2), 167–176.

Poss, J.E. (2001). A new model for cross cultural research: Synthesizing the health belief model and the theory of reasoned action. *Advances in Nursing Science*, 23(4), 1–15.

Reynolds, D. and O'Connell, K.A. (2012). Testing a model for parental acceptance of human papillomavirus vaccine in 9- to 18-year-old girls: A theory-guided study. *Journal of Pediatric Nursing*, 27(6), 614–625.

Ricoeur, P. (1992). *Oneself as another*. Chicago, IL: The University of Chicago Press.

Riegel, B. and Dickson, V.V. (2008). A situation-specific theory of heart failure self-care. *The Journal of Cardiovascular Nursing*, 23(3), 190–196.

Riegel, B. and Dickson, V.V. (2010). Self-care of heart failure: A situation-specific theory of health transition. In A.I. Meleis (Ed.), *Transitions theory: Middle-range and situation-specific theories in nursing research and practice* (pp. 320–326). New York: Springer Publishing Company.

Riegel, B., Dickson, V.V., and Faulkner, K.M. (2015). The situation-specific theory of heart failure self-care: Revised and updated. *The Journal of Cardiovascular Nursing*, 31(3):226–235.

Rorty, R. (1999). *Philosophy and social hope by Richard Rorty*. London, UK: Penguin Books. Retrieved from http://www.penguin.co.uk/nf/Book/BookDisplay/0,,9780140262889,00.html

Sakraida, T.J. (2005). Divorce transition differences of midlife women. *Issues in Mental Health Nursing*, 26(2), 225–249.

Schumacher, K. and Meleis, A.I. (1994). Transitions: A central concept in nursing. *Image: Journal of Nursing Scholarship*, 26(2), 119–127.

Schumacher, K.L., Jones, P., and Meleis, A.I. (2010). Helping elderly persons in transition: A framework for research and practice. In A.I. Meleis (Ed.), *Transitions theory: Middle-range and situation-specific theories in nursing research and practice* (pp. 129–144). New York: Springer Publishing Company.

Suh, E.E. (2008). The sociocultural context of breast cancer screening among Korean immigrant women. *Cancer Nursing*, 31(4), E1–E10.

Vellone, E., Riegel, B., D'Agostino, F., Fida, R., Rocco, G., Cocchieri, A., and Alvaro, R. (2013). Structural equation model testing the situation-specific theory of heart failure self-care. *Journal of Advanced Nursing*, 69(11), 2481–2492.

Willis, D.G., DeSanto-Madeya, S., and Fawcett, J. (2015). Moving beyond dwelling in suffering: A situation-specific theory of men's healing from childhood maltreatment. *Nursing Science Quarterly*, 28(1), 57–63.

Part Six

OUR THEORETICAL FUTURE

After reviewing the rich theoretical past that helped in capturing and articulating the essence, the goals, the meaning, and the outcomes of nursing care, the question that we should be addressing is, "How do we use this significant progress in the development of the discipline as a launch pad toward an even richer theoretical future?"

In Chapter 18, I propose an answer to an important question: "How do we measure progress in a discipline?" What patterns do we look for? Alternatively, what are the markers for a stagnating discipline? Different theories are proposed to analyze the levels of the progress and development of nursing. The meaning of each of these theories and the contribution they make to the discipline and its scientific base are discussed.

In Chapter 19, I look at the future of advancing theory. I examine some of the imperatives that we must nurture and in which we must invest intellectual and human resources to continue on a path that ensures progress of theory and benefits the health and well-being of populations. I discuss several imperatives, such as having a clear disciplinary identity, promoting theoretical thinking, and facilitating the development of fifth generation theories. These are also guided by philosophical assumptions that embrace social justice and equity in providing health care to achieve equitable distribution of resources and health care. I also present some of the major threats and opportunities that could be a context for advancing the discipline.

18

Measuring Progress in a Discipline

As scholars continue to advance nursing science, develop knowledge, refine models of care, answer critical disciplinary questions, and articulate theories, the question becomes: **What are the best ways to measure progress in the discipline?** What are the quantitative and qualitative indicators and metrics to allow members of the discipline to argue that progress has been made? How do we determine trends or outcomes of growth and advancement in a discipline? How do we recognize that a knowledge base is growing and that a discipline is progressing? These questions become more complex as epistemic diversity grows in the discipline, and with the increasing acceptance of multiple theories of truth and interdisciplinarity. How does this diversity translate into ways by which to determine progress in a discipline?

Within the halls of academia in the western and northern hemispheres, progress in research is currently measured by a handful of gold standards. Chief among these standards is the level of funding (governmental or otherwise) awarded to a research program or project deemed by peer reviewers as significant in answering pressing questions. A second gold standard in many parts of the world, whether developed or developing, is the number of accepted publications a particular researcher has amassed in leading journals (Hofmeyer, Newton, and Scott, 2007). Publications in leading journals denote the ability to disseminate knowledge and competitively communicate advancement in knowledge in the literature, though they may not provide as clear an indication of the translation and implementation of findings. Finally, there has been a growing practice to measure progress through the number of citations of a particular publication and the level of impact of the journals in which the results are published.

In most of these gold standards for determining progress, theoretical progress has been somewhat ignored or minimized (Chinn, 2014). The quest for evidence-based practice also presumed the dominance of empirics and positivism over many other philosophies and patterns of knowing, even though the meaning of evidence in human science has been questioned and a consensus on defining it has not been reached (Thorne and Sawatzky, 2014). Among those patterns of knowing that may be eclipsed by a focus on evidence and by using only these gold standards are the person (knowing through the individual self), aesthetic (the art of nursing), and ethics (moral knowledge), which are essential for understanding and providing quality, comprehensive, person-based contextual care (Porter, 2010). Others have also argued that another way of knowing is through reciprocal interdependence, which incorporates different worldviews into a more coherent and comprehensive whole (Pitre and Myrick, 2007). These different ways of knowing call for different approaches to measuring progress.

More importantly, and equally problematic for a human science discipline, knowledge has been deconstructed to reflect mostly research findings, rather than knowledge in all its complexity, which is based on accepting epistemic diversity and which includes interpretation, understanding, and critical questioning of the status quo in quality of care. How is a discipline's progress measured within a context that reflects theoretical development and attention to the inclusion of constituents' views of such progress and epistemic diversity? Several philosophers and scientists have studied scientific growth and have advanced many theories to describe patterns of scientific progress based on retrospective analysis of physical and social science progress. The question of how sciences develop, which has occupied philosophers of science, has also become one of nursing's significant questions; it should drive many intellectual dialogues in our discipline, beginning with, "What processes did nursing go through to achieve its current stage of development?" To answer these questions, nurses have resorted to patterns that have been previously identified by other disciplines. However, describing growth using patterns that are more congruent with scientific progress in the physical sciences may not be congruent with patterns that manifest in a human discipline such as nursing (Lazenby, 2013). Using such patterns, then, may become a constraint in making progress, and may impede further theoretical growth.

Tentative answers to these questions are proposed in this chapter. Three theories are used to describe growth in the discipline. Each is presented with exemplars, and each could be used to analyze progress in areas of practice. The strengths and weaknesses of each theory are presented. I have used these theories to discuss progress as achieved through the turn of the 21st century. As we go forward, these same theories could be used to determine progress in real-time. Let me say at the outset that questions about advancement, growth, and progress in a discipline beg many thoughtful and critical dialogues that transcend contemporary and more mainstream views about knowledge development, acquisition of new knowledge, and cutting-edge discoveries. Dialogues

about progress must be made within the context of patterns of knowing and theories of truth, as discussed in Chapter 8. To help in this discussion, I tentatively offer thoughts about how to review progress through these three theories (see Table 18-1).

A THEORY OF REVOLUTION

Thomas S. Kuhn (1970, 1971), a prolific American writer and speaker and a physicist by training, gave credence to the philosophy of science as a field worthy of exploration and investigation. He is credited with developing the revolutionary theory of scientific development. *Revolution* is defined in *Webster's Third New International Dictionary* as "a sudden, radical or complete change" characterized by "overthrowing" fundamental changes. Kuhn's theory is congruent with these sentiments. Sciences, to Kuhn, develop by leaps and bounds only through periods of crisis. During these crises, theories

TABLE 18-1	Comparison Among Three Processes of Progress on the Discipline: Revolution, Evolution, and Integration		
Analytical Unit	**Revolution**	**Evolution**	**Integration**
Sentiment	Aggression: crises	Adaptation	Change
Interaction	Competition	Cumulation	Collaboration
Goals	Conquering	Building	Progressing
	Overthrowing	Developing	Understanding
Process	Substitution	Lower to higher	Openness
	Elimination	Selection	Flexibility
	Discontinuity	Simple to complex	Contemporary and traditional
		Continuity	Innovation
Pattern of development	Convergence	Mutation	Diversion
		Slow, long range	
Reasoning	Adversarial	Logical	Dialectical
Mode	Rejection	Acceptance	Understanding
Evaluation	Criticize to destroy	Analyze to construct	Dialogue to develop
Environment	Critical	Restrictive	Supportive
	Challenge		
Options	No option during normal science	Limited options	Open/unlimited options
Units of analysis	Paradigms	Merits	History
	Changes	Competitions	Pattern
		Demands	Development of members
		Successes	Number of unique phenomena identified
			Quality of questions answered
			Actualizing relationships between research, theory, and practice
Nursing	Preparadigmatic	Would-be discipline	Discipline

compete, anomalies are identified, and inadequacies are highlighted. This period of scientific unrest is followed by a tranquil period that Kuhn calls "normal science," in which members of the field unify and accept one theory as a common paradigm.

Kuhn's central ideas regarding paradigms are as follows:

1. A *paradigm* is defined as an entire repertoire of beliefs, values, laws, principles, theory methodologies, ways of application, and instrumentation.
2. A paradigm encompasses substantive theoretical assumptions about the subject matter of the discipline and methodological strategies, as well as a degree of consensus about theory methods and techniques.
3. A paradigm includes the questionable areas in the field and some puzzle solutions that could act as examples to help members of that scientific community solve remaining *normal science* problems in the discipline.
4. A discipline matures when it has such a paradigm. Before its paradigmatic stage, however, fact-finding is haphazard and variable in the processes the discipline uses to answer questions. This period is characterized as the preparadigmatic stage of the discipline.

The transition from crisis to normal science marks a scientific revolution. Kuhn asserts that scientific revolutions are inevitable for the development of a science, and these revolutions occur when earlier paradigms no longer work. This revolutionary process is characterized by sudden changes, and its cornerstone is competition. Development is not possible without competition, the result of which is the predominance of one paradigm and the rejection of all others. Members of a discipline may discard one paradigm and replace it with another competing paradigm because they find the model of the new paradigm more successful or agree more strongly with it.

Kuhn also believes that scientific development is *noncumulative*, meaning that a useful aspect of one theory is not added to another competing theory to render it more useful. Thus, competition between paradigms does not evolve into collaborative paradigms; rather, only one paradigm prevails. In other words, old paradigms, regardless of their usefulness, are incompatible with newly conceived paradigms (Kuhn, 1970).

Once a paradigm dominates and a discipline enters "normal science," competition is halted.

Collaboration, then, replaces competition, and the scientific community prevents any alternative paradigms from emerging during this period. Even when theoretical or methodological issues evolve, the scientific community avoids and ignores them, permitting the continuing dominance of the prevailing paradigm.

Kuhn's ideas led to a belief that disciplines develop by convergence. Converging on one paradigm is then accepted as the goal of disciplines leading to progress. A *convergent process* is a closed process rather than an *open process*. One may question the notion of a closed converging process to define science, a process antithetical to the nature of science, which is characterized as being open to new developments and tolerant of competition.

In his later writing, Kuhn replaced the term *paradigm* with *disciplinary matrix*, denoting the same definition of paradigm but with the addition of *shared exemplars* (Kuhn, 1970, pp. 181–210). Because the content boundaries of paradigms are not entirely explicit, but rather implicit, exemplars are provided to identify problems and solutions in the discipline. They are models for problems and solutions that scientists accept during the period of normal science (Table 18-1).

Challenges to Using Kuhn's Theory to Define Progress

Kuhn's ideas have been both revered and criticized. Many writers have taken issue with his admonitions and questioned the capability of his theory to describe and predict the developmental process in the progress of science. More specifically, Kuhn's notion of the development of scientific disciplines through crises and scientific revolutions has fostered numerous debates in the field of philosophy of science. Some have pointed to historical inconsistencies between Kuhn's analysis of several of the established scientific disciplines and his generalization about such developments; these inconsistencies point to the harmonious coexistence between numerous competing paradigms in disciplines that have progressed despite the multiplicity and competitiveness of paradigms. This existing truth negates his theory of revolution.

In view of those who have pointed out such inconsistencies, coexistence between competing paradigms leads to appropriate debates within a given field. Critics point out disciplines that were established despite having no single guiding framework. Why, Dudley Shapere (1981, p. 58) asks, should we only have the extremes, the absolute differences in competing paradigms (thus a crisis), or the absolute identity within one paradigm (thus a revolution) followed by normal science? Is it not possible to have, at any one point in time, both similarities and differences, both competition and collaboration?

Larry Laudan also challenged Kuhn's assertion, proposing that competition is continuous and that scientific disciplines include a variety of coexisting research traditions (Laudan, 1981, p. 153). Laudan identified five major flaws in Kuhn's philosophical view of the development of scientific discipline (Kuhn, 1977, pp. 74–76). These have implications for nursing.

1. "Kuhn's failure to see the role of conceptual problems in scientific debates and in paradigmatic evaluation." Kuhn appears to be using only a positivistic view of science by comparing the number of facts a theory can address and the congruence between these facts in theory and in real life. An empirical view addresses elements in verification and falsification of theories, but not conceptual coherence, logic, social congruence, or other significant components of usefulness.

2. "Kuhn never really resolves the crucial question of the relationship between a paradigm and its constituent theories." Does a paradigm encompass all theories? Do theories explain and describe the paradigm, or vice versa? Which gives evidence to the other?

3. The notion of a prevailing paradigm does not allow for the changes and discoveries that characterize our present science, in which misconceptions are corrected, parts of theories are justified, and other parts are changed. Scientific discovery is a continuous process; present tools allow for a fast pace. Kuhn's theory of scientific development appears to provide a rigid structure that limits the continuous development of theories and the continuous correction of the paradigm's weaknesses, which may become apparent only with time.

4. Kuhn does not advocate the explicit articulation of paradigms or disciplinary matrices. Therefore, such implicitness does not account for nursing's attempt to make the boundaries of the discipline explicit or its assumptions debatable. Nor does such implicitness promote the many controversies that Kuhn considers essential to the development of science.

Scientists can debate explicit matrices but can avoid implicit ones.

5. "Because paradigms are so implicit and can be identified only by pointing to their *exemplars* (basically an archetypal application of a mathematical formulation to an experimental problem), it follows that whenever two scientists use the same exemplars they are, for Kuhn, *ipso facto* committed to the same paradigm" (Laudan, 1981, p. 85). If more scientists work in this way, we come closer to a revolution. In nursing, some nurses have used the same exemplars even though they held divergent views about the most basic conceptual and methodological questions. Helping people cope with transitions is an area providing exemplars in health–illness transitions, developmental transitions, or situational transitions. These exemplars have been treated effectively by those who adhere to psychoanalytical views, and just as effectively by those adhering to sociocultural views in nursing. Therefore, the exemplars themselves would not mean commitment to some paradigm. Commitment to one paradigm over another is apparent only by making paradigms explicit and not by maintaining implicitness.Finally, Toulmin (1972) identified a sixth flaw apparent in Kuhn's philosophy:

6. How the transitions from competing paradigms to revolution to normal science occur is not clear in Kuhn's writing. Does a community of scholars hold a mass meeting to denounce one competing paradigm and adopt another? Considering that, according to Kuhn, followers of each paradigm are supposedly entrenched in the paradigm they use and do not always seem to communicate, nor do they always share a common language or worldview, how could they agree on one rather than another paradigm? Contrary to Kuhn's ideas regarding the lack of communication during the crisis period, Toulmin offers many historical examples of careful communication, debate, discussion, or proposed modification in physics before any minute change was made or any modification was incorporated into the established body of the discipline (Toulmin, 1972, p. 10).

Many nurse scholars have hoped for a revolution that would result in a single relevant and dominant paradigm that unites nursing knowledge and denotes progress. However, the outcome of paradigmatic shifts that have occurred in nursing may better be described in terms of a revolution toward accepting the simultaneous existence of multiple paradigms. This paradigmatic pluralism is discussed later in this chapter.

Revolutionary Theory of Progress and the Discipline of Nursing

Some nursing scholars seem to have accepted Kuhn's theory of progress and have adhered to the position that nursing is following the same patterns of revolutionary development as the other physical sciences analyzed by Kuhn. Nursing progress has thus been measured against the canons proposed by him (Hardy, 1978). The result has been a negatively critical assessment of nursing progress and anticipation of a scientific revolution in nursing, in which one paradigm prevails and is accepted by the nursing community. According to these scholars, nursing is in its preparadigmatic stage. It is possible that the scientific revolution in nursing may never come, not because nursing is not progressing, but because there may never be periods of normal science. Other natural and behavioral science disciplines continue to progress and have competing paradigms to describe and predict the phenomena of their disciplines.

Some nurses have presented a view of nursing as something that has arrived at the beginnings of a paradigm (Fawcett and DeSanto-Madeya, 2013; Munhall, 1982; Newman, 1983), or is undergoing a paradigm shift. The processes depicted, however, do not demonstrate competition, rejection, and dominance as much as an evolutionary process, and the focus on a single dominant paradigm suggests that revolutionary theory, by itself, is inadequate to measure the progress of nursing, a discipline in which there is growing support for the coexistence of multiple paradigms. Indeed, the notion of having only one paradigm is unacceptable to nursing and other sciences that deal with human beings and complex health–illness situations. There is growing support for pluralistic paradigms for knowledge development that value empiricism, theoretical knowledge, and practice-based knowledge (Reed and Lawrence, 2008). In fact, emerging paradigms in nursing, such as molecular and systems biology and genetic biomarkers that define human beings, as well as robotic care, while competing in defining the nature of caring, are not substitutable nor is there only one that dominates. Each is driving sets

of new questions to be examined and answers to be integrated to advance nursing knowledge (Founds, 2009; Grady and Gough, 2015; Monteiro, 2016). Theories in nursing have been integrated with practice, and all types and categories of theoretical formulations are coexisting (Im and Chang, 2012).

Even when revolution does occur within nursing, it may be that it is a revolution of addition, rather than the revolution of replacement that is central to Kuhn's theory. Consider, for example, how maternity-care nurses in Brazil promoted the substitution of a hospital-based, biomedically driven, physician-led framework with one that is personalized, community-based, women-driven, feminist, humanistic, and subject to minimal medical intervention (Quitete, Mouta, Progianti, et al., 2013). Both paradigms of care coexist, and there is no indication that total substitution will occur anytime soon. This is an example of coexistence of very different paradigms in nursing simultaneously; hence, an example of paradigmatic pluralism. However, I suggest that the appropriateness of using the revolutionary theory to describe progress and the development of nursing knowledge should continue to be debated, other theories should be discussed, and analyses of consequences should be carefully considered (Table 18-1).

A THEORY OF EVOLUTION

A second approach to critically assessing progress in knowledge development is by using an evolutionary lens. Evolution denotes change in a certain direction, unfolding from lower to higher, from simpler to more complex, and in the direction of greater coherence. It gives the impressions of continuity and long-term cumulative changes. An evolutionary view of a scientific discipline combines instances of intellectual innovation complemented by a continuing process of critical assessment and selection. It acknowledges competition but accepts the inevitability of cumulation in knowledge development. An evolutionary stance also acknowledges the significance of the genealogy of ideas in the progress of knowledge.

Toulmin (1972) used Darwin's evolutionary theory as the basis for a framework to explain the process of knowledge development. He identified four basic principles for Darwinian theory, each of which has a counterpart in the evolution of scientific disciplines.

1. Each discipline contains its own body of concepts, areas of concern, methodologies,

and goals, all of which can change drastically but slowly through a mutable process. Nevertheless, a definite continuity can be detected in the major ideas of the discipline. Conceptual thoughts in each of the disciplines, while having coherence and continuity, also manifest slow, long-term changes, with each new conceptual thought based on previous ideas, and with the more developed concepts superseding older ones.

2. All ideas, concepts, and methodologies are given a chance to compete, to be discussed, and to be weeded out. Only those discoveries and innovations that fit will flourish and survive from one generation to the next. This process of the retention of some conceptual thoughts, mutation of others, and rejection of still others explains the stability of intellectual thoughts in disciplines and accounts for transformations into new theories.

3. Marked substantive changes in the field are possible when several conditions exist. One important condition is qualified people in the discipline who are capable of inventing new ideas, exploring new problems, and developing new theories. An evolutionary position presupposes an arena for debate, critique, and competition. Another necessary condition is sufficient openness in the discipline to allow for new ideas to develop and survive long enough to prove their suitability or to be refuted.

4. The selection of the more useful ideas, concepts, and theories is based on how well they meet the demands of the local intellectual environment within the discipline. The selection process is also based on congruence of the demands, issues, current problem areas, and innovative ideas that are being offered (Toulmin, 1972, pp. 139–143). Other competing ideas continue to be adhered to, refined, and further developed.

An evolutionary process of knowledge development contains such units of analysis as merits, competitions, demands, and successes. When contrasting Darwinian biological evolutionary process with the Toulmin intellectual evolutionary process, one finds a pattern of development based on survival of the fittest, innovation, comparison of ideas, and systematic patterns of selection of the best among competing paradigms. One theory, one set of ideas that may have more explanatory power to resolve some significant conceptual problem, is generally

selected over another theory, however well-established it may have been. The newly adopted theory may incorporate parts of the previous theory and reject other parts. Therefore, progress in the physical sciences is not revolutionary, according to Toulmin, but evolutionary. It has taken on a cumulative pattern.

The evolutionary theory of knowledge presupposes agreement within a discipline about the problem areas of the field and the criteria for truth and explanation. In addition, certain conditions should exist as indicators that a discipline has developed cumulatively. Freese (1972) identified the first four conditions, and I have added an additional one:

1. *Modification of truth value*: Generalizations are cumulative when one generalization modifies a previous generalization; that is, one generalization causes change to occur to or from truth, falsity, or indetermination. An empirical confirmation of the second generalization modifies the truth inherent in the first.

2. *Modification of antecedent value*: Generalizations are cumulative if the empirical verification or falsification of a second subsequent generalization modifies the antecedent in the first generalization. Change of one to the other of the following would fulfill this condition: necessary but not sufficient, sufficient but not necessary, necessary and sufficient, sufficient with necessity indeterminate, and necessary with sufficiency indeterminate.

3. *Premise or derivation in a deductive chain*: This applies to cases in which a confirmed proposition in one theory becomes a premise preceding another proposition in another theory. Theory is cumulative when the propositions of one theory are based on or help modify the premises of another theory.

4. *Space–time independence*: Theories are cumulative when their propositions transcend geography and time.

5. *Practice–research–practice–dependent link*: This link presupposes modification of practice based on theory or research, or vice versa. Accumulation stems from a direct ripple effect between practice and research.

If we accept these premises for cumulative knowledge, then the physical sciences, using both the revolutionary criteria and the evolutionary process, are established disciplines. The social and behavioral sciences, on the other hand, are classified as being in a preparadigmatic stage or are, in Toulmin's terms, "would-be disciplines." One can readily detect conditions of cumulation in the physical sciences, very little of which exists in the social and behavioral sciences or, indeed, in nursing (Table 18-1).

Propositions emanating from theoretical nursing do not fit in a deductively tight, logically interrelated cumulative model. Systematic cumulative development that begins from a common point and expands upward to become another canon cannot be detected in nursing knowledge. If cumulation is the unit of analysis for the evolution of disciplines, then nursing scientific development is not closely congruent with either a revolutionary or an evolutionary concept. Rather, if we impose on it the two theories that we have just discussed, the discipline of nursing theoretical development has followed a course that may be considered unsystematic, haphazard, and lacking direction.

A THEORY OF INTEGRATION

As a discipline and a profession, nursing does not lend itself to assessment through theories that are solely revolutionary or solely evolutionary. Any attempt to measure progress must consider the uniqueness of the discipline, the level and nature of integration, its different components (practice, theory, research, and policy), the different sources of its theories, the quality of questions that drive programs of research, the practice models that evolved from translating research, and the level and quality of a scientific preparation and engagement of the human nursing capital. The extent to which a society values and acknowledges a discipline is also an indicator of progress. To fully account for all these factors—to account for the discipline's uniqueness—requires recognizing that nursing progress has involved aspects of both revolution and evolution. For this reason, a theory of integration is proposed here. The rationale is also provided to support the congruency of this integrative theory with the nature and mission of nursing.

One unique feature of nursing is its *theory development*. The development of nursing theory was not based on the research of the discipline, nor did every research project contribute to the development of theory (Batey, 1977; Fawcett, 1978). Another unique feature of the discipline is that its competing ideas exist simultaneously and have existed for decades (different research methodologies; conceptual approaches to care, comfort, and pain). In fact, competing theories are used even within the same research programs and institutions. To be sure, areas of agreement do exist; for instance, there is acknowledgment of the significance of environment in assessing health of individuals and in planning and implementing intervention, and there is agreement that the discipline of nursing is focused on health and coping, health and illness transitions, and human responses to health and illness. Although each of these concepts may be viewed from a different theoretical background, agreement is growing that these concepts are central to the discipline.

One may argue that the discipline has been in continuous crisis over the origins of its knowledge base for many years (practice, teaching, or administration) and that the agreement now is that advancing its knowledge base is predicated, for the most part, on connection with clinical practice. Is this a paradigm shift, an evolution, or integration? There is growing consensus that it is probably the latter. The discipline of nursing incorporates knowledge for and from practice, research, education, and teaching. While there were also areas of philosophical disagreement about the methods of inquiry that are most congruent with the subject matter of dynamic nursing practice and its philosophical stand, normalization and integration processes may have occurred to increase consensus. But, this integration of philosophies and methods (more congruent with either practice, research, or education) may have led to avoiding the exploration of new risky subjects that would have required using very different methods. Creativity may have been undermined and may have been replaced with well-established and more fundable areas (Heinrich, 2010).

In a discipline that deals with human beings, it is perhaps not feasible for only one theory to explain, describe, predict, and provide practice guidelines for all the discipline's phenomena. For example, medicine, which has long depended on the biomedical model and its basis in the structure and function of biologic systems, has expanded with new discoveries to use genetics and neurosciences to better explain systems and signs and to drive the development of more congruent interventions. It also incorporates various means for auscultation, palpation, and laboratory tests, all of which are accompanied by different competing but coexisting theories (Frank, 1957, pp. 356–358).

A case for paradigmatic pluralism has been made in nursing because there is a need for theories about people, interactions, illness, health, and nursing interventions. In fact, many different current theories, although seen by some as competing with each other, address different relationships and focus on different phenomena, thereby actually complementing each other. These theories evolved from many paradigms (adaptation, system, and interactionist, among others). Nursing deals with human behavior, and human behavior in all its complexity could not be explained through a single general and comprehensive theory. In fact, the desire for a single, all-embracing "scientific psychology" may itself prove to be a "will-o'-the-wisp." Certainly, a similar will-o'-the-wisp had to be disregarded before modern physics could become the discipline it now is; the reasons why this was so throw some light on the contemporary state of behavioral science (Toulmin, 1972, p. 386).

Another feature of nursing that supports its uniqueness is that, as a profession, it exists in an open system, and it must be influenced by and be responsive to society's needs at all times, and through collaboration with many constituents (Andrew and Wilkie, 2007). Therefore, nurse scientists and clinicians could not afford to converge on any one paradigm to the exclusion of others. Nurses' and clients' actions continue to be shaped by each other and by their social environments. This is where the analogy between nursing and sociology appears (Urry, 1973); both disciplines are dynamic and changing, and both develop through integration, rather than revolutions or evolutions. Nursing has many communities, fields, organizations, and constituents. No one of these can be exclusive in promoting and supporting one competing theory over another.

Another pattern of knowledge development in nursing is the changing nature of what constitutes units of analyses that incorporated and reflected different schools of thought. Researchers in nursing have long focused on the community, family, and on individuals as whole; more recently, though, researchers have also focused on patients at the cellular, molecular, and genetic levels. They use quantitative and qualitative techniques and explore administrative and clinical questions. In instances in which changes occur, old paradigms are redefined rather than being totally rejected. For example, even as Nightingale's concept of environment is revived, new definitions, such as Rogers' definition of environment as an energy field, are redefining her ideas.

There has been an evolution in nursing theoretical approaches that has been defined as coexisting paradigmatic perspectives (Doucet and Merlin, 2014; Newman, Sime, and Corcoran-Perry, 1991) or evolving commonalities of nurse-designed models of health care (Mason, Jones, Roy, et al., 2015). Evolutionary approach to nursing knowledge may better explain progress based on these coexisting ideas that are built on, and evolve from, integrating existing theories or existing practice models. Evolution may provide a framework to describe the emerging coexistence of paradigms that are built on nursing theories. Several paradigms coexist that could be considered evolutionary as they evolved cumulatively by building on early conceptual ideas. One example is *the interactive*—an integrative paradigm that focuses on defining human beings as adaptive biopsychosocial and spiritual beings in constant interaction with an environment, and capable of self-care. Another is *the simultaneity* paradigm, in which a human being is defined as an irreducible whole forming an integral energy field with the environment. Another yet is *the transformative* paradigm, which considers human beings as changing and unpredictive and as cocreative with their human becoming (Doucet and Merlin, 2014; Newman et al., 1991).

Evolutionary progress may also be measured by examining innovative redesign of care modalities and identifying their commonalities. The American Academy of Nursing recently identified "Edge Runners," individuals who are associated with innovative care delivery systems that are impacting health care. The Academy identified several commonalities in the care models led by Edge Runners, including a holistic definition of health and care that is community-based, relationship-based, and continuous (Mason et al., 2015).

It is the presence of competing theories, competing schools of thought, and debatable ideas that makes a discipline scholarly. The right to question, critique, and challenge has characterized all advanced disciplines (Toulmin, 1972, p. 110). If nursing were to adopt a revolutionary philosophy for its growth, it could put an end to this significant property of scholarliness (Laudan, 1977, pp. 73–76). Competition, creativity, and innovation are the hallmarks of scientific growth.

The discussion thus far has attempted to address the unique features of nursing that may make a solely revolutionary or solely evolutionary theory of development incongruent with the nature of the discipline. Using either theory may even interrupt further advancement of the discipline (Table 18-1). The thesis of this discussion is that nursing progress seems to have charted its own path; ideas that were rejected in one stage of development have been accepted at a different stage. Examples of this are the early rejection of nursing theories, the revived acknowledgment of spirituality (Macrae, 1995) and of Nightingale's focus on health and environment, the preoccupation with quantitative research methodology in the 1960s, the more recent revival of meaning of experience, the greater acceptance of alternate designs for research such as phenomenology, and the arguments for reclaiming our traditions (Bradshaw, 1995). Ideas have been cumulative at times and unrelated to previous stages at others. Toulmin (1972), despite his interest in cumulation, observed that:

[T]he leading ideas current at any stage in the development of the 20th century social science have tended to resemble those current two or three generations before, more than they have resembled those of the immediately previous generation (p. 385).

The discipline of nursing, with its perspective, domain, theories, and research, is increasingly used as the organizing framework and as substantive content for education, clinical practice, and research. There is less need for advocacy of nursing as a serious profession with a major impact on the health of populations. There is less focus on justifying nursing theory. Nursing programs discuss and use nursing theories in addition to theories from other disciplines. Graduates of programs that use nursing theories are aware of the strengths and limitations in utility of nursing theory, and the strengths and limitations of theories that were developed to answer questions that are more central and more relevant to other disciplines.

The syntactical debates (theory versus conceptual framework, nursing theory versus borrowed theory, and qualitative versus quantitative methods) are fading, giving way to substantive debates (determinants of health, the impact of environment on lifestyle, and the impact of lifestyle on self-management of care). Indications of theory refinement and extension began in the early 1980s, and gained momentum at the turn of the 21st century. Relationships between domain concepts were being explored using existing nursing theories and other pertinent theories, such as interpersonal relations and the delivery of nursing care (nursing therapeutics), resulting in theoretical exemplars that could guide nursing research (Kasch, 1984).

Theory and science exist because they are created by *human beings*. Therefore, progress in theoretical

development should also be measured by progress in the *human capital* of a discipline. If human capital in nursing is examined as a criterion for progress, then there is no doubt that the discipline of nursing has progressed by leaps and bounds. Nurses globally are better educated with bachelor, master, and doctorate degrees, and they have achieved many prominent leadership positions as ministers of health, presidents of foundations, board chairpersons, and executives in major international organizations.

The development and engagement of nurses in different communities is also an indication of progress (Burrage, Shattell, and Habermann, 2005; Duke and Moss, 2009). Because our scholarly work centers around and emanates from a *nursing domain*, special-interest groups emerged as (what Merton calls) a *"community of scholars"* who, in turn, helped in the refinement and extension process (Merton, 1973). These communities of scholars are organized and active locally and globally, focused on different theories, and/or organized around substantive nursing areas such as sleep, self-management and symptom management, women's health, nursing diagnosis, interventions, and outcomes. An example of engagement in a defined community of scholars is manifested in the development of research centers in some of the leading schools of nursing. Members of these centers ask coherent sets of questions leading to integrated projects that shed light on fundamental health problems. For example, at the University of Pennsylvania, faculty belong to research centers as they focus on different sets of phenomena and concepts such as transitions, history, and outcomes. These communities of scholars, organized around phenomenon and particular areas of investigation, drive organized and coherent scientific productivity that goes beyond a single study or one person's program of research. Progress is demonstrated in the nature of questions asked in as much as the answers produced.

Another criterion to determine progress is the degree to which societies value the contribution of a discipline. Therefore, it is also progress when leading organizations and foundations choose to focus on studying the issues and the opportunities that the discipline of nursing offers societies and their health care. The National Academy of Medicine (NAM, formerly called the Institute of Medicine [IOM]), in collaboration with the Robert Wood Johnson Foundation, produced an elaborate study (IOM, 2010) about the future of nursing. The very existence of that study, along with its recommendations, the subsequent formation of action coalitions for implementation of the recommendations, and a subsequent 5-year review of results (NAM, 2016), are indications of how the discipline is acknowledged and valued. They are indications that assessing nursing's issues, opportunities, and progress are worthy of leading institutions' serious attention. This valuation is a result of the knowledge and the evidence provided that links nursing actions with population outcomes. Similar commissions were appointed in other countries to study progress in the discipline of nursing and to make recommendations that improve health care (Campbell, Fauveau, ten Hoope-Bender, et al., 2011; Dussault, Buchan, Sermeus, et al., 2010).

We have achieved, as members of the discipline, an incredible level of wisdom about our discipline. What Johnson referred to as "practical wisdom" (1959, p. 294) characterizes nursing well into the second decade of the 21st century. Practical wisdom is manifested in the strategic plan that was developed by and for the National Institute of Nursing Research, defining future areas of nursing research as symptom science, wellness, self-management to improve quality of life for people with chronic illness, and end-of-life and palliative care (Grady and Gough, 2015). All of these areas reflect societal needs and pressing health care issues, thus declaring that nurses have a major knowledge development role in these areas of health care. Practical wisdom is also manifested in the discipline's mission of translating and implementing actions that are theoretically sound and are designed to make a difference in the lives of people. It includes deliberate actions that are subjected to evaluation, reflection, and analysis. Lauder (1994) differentiated between theoretical knowledge and practical wisdom, with the former ending up with an intellectual conclusion and the latter with action that is morally good for human beings. The age of wisdom encompasses all the properties of the stages that the discipline of nursing has experienced, not in a cumulative way but rather synergistically and developmentally, with experience and practice as the hallmarks. Wisdom is reflected in the mounting acceptance of the complexity and the fluidity of nursing concepts and the significance of the temporal dimensions in our research and theory development. Natural turns and detours are made with more ease and comfort, just as Newton made a natural turn to astronomy because, at that time, finding one's way at sea had been a preoccupation of the time, or just as Kepler turned to astrology and used it during the Thirty Years' War.

Using theories and developing new theories has benefited from temporal experiences. From such use and further development came wisdom. Although we must not forget Bacon's reasoning for empirical testing or Kant's insistence on *a priori* conceptual schemata independent of experience, a practice discipline such as nursing cannot exist if it forgets Kaplan's advice that the pursuit of wisdom expresses a deep concern with the good that can be achieved in human life. Those benefits resulting from nursing practice have to be conveyed to the public, to whom nursing is ultimately accountable. Public awareness and accountability are the main pillars on which the discipline of nursing will rest.

Popular theories of knowledge development call for a pattern of progress that is not manifested in its entirety in nursing. Therefore, nursing progress may have been underestimated and its scientific impact not duly acknowledged. An integrative process of development allows for an explanation of competitions and collaborations, acceptances and rejections, cumulations and innovations, peaks and valleys, reconsideration and development, evolution and convolution (complex, twisting, winding form, or design) (*Webster's Third New International Dictionary,* 1986).

Integration is neither a nonpattern nor a negative pattern; rather, it allows for pendulum swings and is explained as a *pattern in progress*. It is not a pattern that follows the conventional idea of progress, toward a paradigm. Rather, it is a pattern of progress that depicts nursing's accomplishments and its solid theoretical present through accommodation, refinement, and collaboration among thoughts, ideas, and individuals, and through its impact on health care (Gottlieb, 2007). This pattern of progress does not underestimate the further need for progress that is inherent in all scientific disciplines. It allows for careful critique of what has been and what is yet to be accomplished.

Table 18-1 illustrates the differences and similarities among the three processes of knowledge progress discussed in this chapter. When the progress of nursing is analyzed through each of these three philosophical views, different conclusions can be drawn. To a revolutionist, nursing is in a preparadigmatic stage; to an evolutionist, nursing is a would-be discipline; to an integrationist, nursing has achieved a disciplinary status. A careful assessment of patterns of growth and development, milestones, stages, and phenomena identified in nursing demonstrate the quality and significance of questions asked and answers provided. These

REFLECTIVE QUESTIONS

1. Articulate an area or field of interest using two of the theories of progress to describe advancement in that field. Compare and contrast your conclusions about progress in that field. Why did you arrive at this conclusion?

2. Discuss the wisdom, or lack of it, in using integration theory as a theory to determine the level of progress and development in the discipline.

3. Extrapolating from theories of progress discussed in this chapter, discuss what indicators of progress you would use in evaluating the developmental stages of the scholars/scientists in the field of nursing. Use similar analysis to develop criteria and benchmarks for academicians and clinicians.

4. What are the major conclusions that you would draw from reviewing this chapter? Compare and contrast these conclusions with the author's conclusions. Provide the rationale for your conclusions and support from contemporary literature in nursing theory.

units of analyses represent a synthesis of research, theory, and practice. When nursing is analyzed in these terms, it has achieved a disciplinary status.

At any particular time, a recognized domain will include many phenomena that are not entirely clear or apparently consequential, and these might create genuine and inquisitive stances. This does not reflect lack of maturity in a discipline, but rather indicates its continuing growth (Chinn, 2008). The bond between scientific endeavors and reflection is becoming stronger; adaptation and demand are becoming key forces of progress, instead of structure and inflexibility. It is accepted that limitations in the nursing discipline stem from limitations of time, not from some perceived shortcoming. To paraphrase McBride (1986), the future should not be viewed with apologies nor should we highlight and focus on our inadequacies; rather, we should develop and nurture a sense that theoretical nursing has contributed a great deal to the present maturity of the discipline and, even more importantly, to the health and well-being of populations.

CONCLUSION

Reviewing progress in the discipline demonstrates that a considerable level of wisdom has been achieved. Wisdom is the "capacity to take account of all important factors in a problem and to attach to each its due weight" and to know which ends to pursue (Russell, 1957, p. 29). It combines knowledge, feelings, morals, and practice. Wisdom is a sense of proportion. Knowledge can give us nursing therapeutics to enhance self-care, increase mother–infant attachment, increase social support or networks, ease

the effects of transition, or maintain the integrity of the individual. Only wisdom and understanding can ensure their appropriate use for our clients without imposing our own values. Wisdom is a total perspective, seeing an object, event, or idea in all its pertinent relationships. Spinoza defined wisdom as seeing things "*sub specie aeternitatis*," in view of eternity (Copleston, 1963, p. 253); Durant (1957) suggested defining wisdom as seeing things "*sub specie totius*," in view of the whole. Considering the stages of knowledge development in nursing and considering nursing as a whole leads to the proposition that nursing is currently encountering a scholarly evolution, characterized by some revolutions as well as by integration of pluralistic approaches to developing and advancing nursing knowledge base.

Emerson once said, "To the philosopher, all things are friendly and sacred, all events profitable, all days whole, all men [or women] divine." To nursing, all stages were essential to bring us to the stage of scholarliness, and from all stages will emerge the age of wisdom. "Knowledge is power, but only wisdom is liberty" (Durant, 1957, p. 9). *Once there was a there.* Now "there" is here. Let us acknowledge and enjoy our accomplishments, but also remember that there is no end to what lies ahead because it is the process that is the future. The future presents many challenges and opportunities to be discussed in the next chapter.

REFERENCES

Andrew, N. and Wilkie, G. (2007). Integrated scholarship in nursing: An individual responsibility or collective undertaking. *Nurse Education Today*, 27(1), 1–4.

Batey, M.V. (1977). Conceptualization: Knowledge and logic guiding empirical research. *Nursing Research*, 26(5), 324–329.

Bradshaw, A. (1995). What are nurses doing to patients? A review of theories of nursing past and present. *Journal of Clinical Nursing*, 4(2), 81–92.

Burrage, J., Shattell, M., and Habermann, B. (2005). The scholarship of engagement in nursing. *Nursing Outlook*, 53(5), 220–223.

Campbell, J., Fauveau, V., ten Hoope-Bender, P., Matthews, Z., and McManus, J. (2011). *The state of the world's midwifery 2011. Delivering health saving lives*. New York: United Nations Population Fund. Retrieved from https://www.unfpa.org/sites/default/files/pub-pdf/en_SOWMR_Full.pdf

Chinn, P.L. (2008). The discipline of nursing-letter from the editor. *Advances in Nursing Science*, 31(1), 1.

Chinn, P.L. (2014). Nursing theories for the 21st century-letter from the editor. *Advances in Nursing Science*, 37(1), 1.

Copleston, S.J. (1963). *A history of philosophy. Volume 4, Modern philosophy: Descartes to Leibniz* (Baruch Spinoza, pp. 211–269). Garden City, NY: Image Books.

Doucet, T.J. and Merlin, M.D. (2014). Conceptualizations of health in nursing practice. *Nursing Science Quarterly*, 27(2), 118–125.

Duke, J. and Moss, C. (2009). Re-visiting scholarly community engagement in the contemporary research assessment environments of Australasian universities. *Contemporary Nurse*, 32(1–2), 30–41.

Durant, W. (1957). What is wisdom? *Wisdom: The Magazine for Knowledge for All America*, 20(8), 25.

Dussault, G., Buchan, J., Sermeus, W., and Padaiga, Z. (2010). *Investing in Europe's health workforce of tomorrow: Scope for innovation and collaboration*. Summary report of the three Policy Dialogues. European Observatory on Health Systems and Policies. Retrieved from http://www.euro.who.int/en/about-us/partners/observatory

Fawcett, J. (1978). The relationship between theory and research: A double helix. *Advances in Nursing Science*, 1(1), 49–62.

Fawcett, J. and DeSanto-Madeya, S. (2013). *Contemporary nursing knowledge: Analysis and evaluation of nursing models and theories* (3rd ed.). Philadelphia, PA: F.A. Davis.

Founds, S.A. (2009). Introducing systems biology for nursing science. *Biological Research for Nursing*, 11(1), 73–80.

Frank, P. (1957). *Philosophy of science*. Englewood Cliffs, NJ: Prentice-Hall.

Freese, L. (1972). Cumulative sociological knowledge. *American Sociological Review*, 37(4), 472–482.

Gottlieb, L.N. (2007). Canadian nursing scholarship: A time to celebrate, a time to stand guard. *Canadian Journal of Nursing Research*, 39(1), 5–10.

Grady, P.A. and Gough, L.L. (2015). Nursing science: Claiming the future. *Journal of Nursing Scholarship*, 47(6), 512–521.

Hardy, M.E. (1978). Practice oriented theory: Part 1. Perspectives on nursing theory. *Advances in Nursing Science*, 1(1), 37–48.

Heinrich, K.T. (2010). Passionate scholarship 2001-2010: A vision for making academe safer for joyous risk-takers. *Advances in Nursing Science*, 33(1), E50–E64.

Hofmeyer, A., Newton, M., and Scott, C. (2007). Valuing the scholarship of integration and the scholarship of application in the academy for health sciences scholars: Recommended methods. *Health Research Policy and Systems*, 5(5), 1–8.

Im, E.O. and Chang, S.J. (2012). Current trends in nursing theories. *Journal of Nursing Scholarship*, 44(2), 156–164.

Institute of Medicine (IOM). (2010). *The future of nursing: Leading change, advancing health*. Washington, DC: The National Academies Press.

Johnson, D.E. (1959). The nature of a science of nursing. *Nursing Outlook*, 7(5), 291–294.

Kasch, C. (1984). Interpersonal competence and communication in the delivery of nursing care. *Advances in Nursing Science*, 6(2), 71–88.

Kuhn, T.S. (1970). The structure of scientific revolutions. In Neurath, O. (Ed.), *International encyclopedia of unified science* (2nd ed., Vol. 2). Chicago, IL: University of Chicago Press.

Kuhn, T.S. (1971). The relations between history and history of science. *Daedalus*, 100, 271–304.

Kuhn, T.S. (1977). *The essential tension: Selected studies in scientific tradition and change*. Chicago, IL: University of Chicago Press.

Laudan, L. (1977). *Progress and its problems: Toward a theory of scientific growth*. Berkeley, CA: University of California Press.

Laudan, L. (1981). A problem solving approach to scientific growth. In I. Hacking (Ed.), *Scientific revolutions*. Oxford, UK: Oxford University Press.

Lauder, W. (1994). Beyond reflection: Practical wisdom and the practical syllogism. *Nurse Education Today*, 14(2), 91–98.

Lazenby, M. (2013). On humanities of nursing. *Nursing Outlook*, 61(1), E9–E14.

Macrae, J. (1995). Nightingale's spiritual philosophy and its significance for modern nursing. *Image: Journal of Nursing Scholarship*, 27(1), 8–10.

Mason, D.J., Jones, D.A., Roy, C., Sullivan, C.G., and Wood, L.J. (2015). Commonalities of nurse-designed models of health care. *Nursing Outlook*, 63(5), 540–553.

McBride, A.B. (1986). Theory and research. *Journal of Psychosocial Nursing*, 24(9), 27–32.

Merton, R.K. (1973). *The sociology of science: Theoretical and empirical investigations*. Chicago, IL: University of Chicago Press.

Monteiro, A.P. (2016). Cyborgs, biotechnologies, and informatics in health care – new paradigms in nursing sciences. *Nursing Philosophy*, 17(1), 19–27.

Munhall, P.L. (1982). Nursing philosophy and nursing research: In apposition or opposition. *Nursing Research*, 31(3), 176–177, 181.

National Academy of Medicine (NAM). (2016). *Assessing progress on the Institute of Medicine report the future of nursing*. Washington, DC: The National Academies Press.

Newman, M.A. (1983). The continuing revolution: A history of nursing science. In N.L. Chaska (Ed.), *The nursing profession: A time to speak*. New York: McGraw-Hill.

Newman, M.A., Sime, A.M., and Corcoran-Perry, S.A. (1991). The focus of the discipline of nursing. *Advances in Nursing Science*, 14(1), 1–16.

Pitre, N.Y. and Myrick, F. (2007). A view of nursing epistemology through reciprocal interdependence: Towards a reflexive way of knowing. *Nursing Philosophy*, 8(2), 73–84.

Porter, S. (2010). Fundamental patterns of knowing in nursing: The challenge of evidence-based practice. *Advances in Nursing Science*, 33(1), 3–14.

Quitete, J.B., Mouta, R.J.O., Progianti, J.M., and da Costa Vargens, O.M. (2013). Applying the theory of scientific revolutions in the construction of a new field of obstetric nursing. *Journal of Nursing UFPE On-Line*, 7(12), 3–20.

Reed, P.G. and Lawrence, L.A. (2008). A paradigm for the production of practice-based knowledge. *Journal of Nursing Management*, 16(4), 422–432.

Russell, B. (1957). The world's need for wisdom. *Wisdom: The Magazine for Knowledge for all America*, 14, 29.

Shapere, D. (1981). Meaning and scientific change. In I. Hacking (Ed.), *Scientific revolutions*. New York: Oxford University Press.

Thorne, S. and Sawatzky, R. (2014). Particularizing the general: Sustaining theoretical integrity in the context of an evidence-based practice agenda. *Advances in Nursing Science*, 37(1), 5–18.

Toulmin, S. (1972). *Human understanding: The collective use and evolution of concepts*. Princeton, NJ: Princeton University Press.

Urry, J. (1973). Thomas S. Kuhn as sociologist of knowledge. *British Journal of Sociology*, 24(4), 462–473.

Webster's Third New International Dictionary. (1986). Springfield, MA: Merriam-Webster.

19

Fifth-Generation Theorists: Passion for Advancing Theory

Theory development and utilization have matured in the discipline of nursing. However, according to Grace, Willis, Roy et al. (2016), our profession is at a crossroads because of a tilt toward the empirical and away from the philosophical and theoretical inquiry. Whereas the discipline has moved through four earlier dimensions—absence of theory, debate about theory, development of grand visions of the discipline, and development of theories at different levels of abstraction, scope, utility, and contagiousness—members of the discipline are ready to move to the *fifth dimension*. This *fifth dimension* is characterized by integrating theory in all aspects of the discipline, and by unapologetic ease in developing theories from practice, from other theories, and from research. It is also characterized by integrating knowledge driven by theories and using it to refine, identify, update, refute, or support existing theories. Similarly, the *fifth-dimension* era for theory development is characterized by integrating research findings to develop new theories. This era in theoretical nursing signals going beyond concept development and ensuring that when new concepts are developed the focus is on asking and answering questions that are fundamental to the discipline of nursing and that they are translatable toward making a difference in the quality care provided for populations.

To continue advancing theoretical nursing, members of the discipline—whether engaged in clinical practice, in educating students, in conducting research projects, or in developing policies—must be able to demonstrate embodied knowledge of the discipline's domain and perspective, theoretical thinking, and a propensity toward developing *fifth-generation theories*. Educators and mentors must instill these same competencies in future graduates. In addition, it is imperative to consider several threats and opportunities for theorizing, for advancing interprofessional knowledge while taking advantage

of revolutions that have occurred and continue to occur in health sciences and in health technologies. The three components for theorizing—disciplinary identity, theoretical thinking, and fifth-generation theories—as well as potential threats and opportunities are presented and discussed in this chapter. These discussions are intended to stimulate thinking about the future of theory in nursing, to promote dialogue, and to foster debate.

DISCIPLINARY IDENTITY

To be a member of a particular discipline means being able to articulate a view of the discipline, its values, its mission, and its boundaries, however flexible, dynamic, and expandable they are. In addition, an important component of this identity is to engage in advancing its knowledge base that is predicated on the extent to which its members recognize its foci, define its significant questions, and continuously work on providing relevant answers to its practice. Articulating a vision about a discipline requires knowing, understanding, and continuing to provide health care for the populations; it also requires being able to articulate coherent frameworks that drive the relevant questions while also using the frameworks as reservoirs to integrate the answers related to the social mission of a discipline. For our discipline of nursing, the vision is providing quality care; it is ultimately our "moral imperative" (Grace et al., 2016). To engage in a relevant and significant dialogue in a discipline requires a strong sense of identity, pride in its history, and a passion to fulfill its mission. This is manifested through articulating a perspective, utilizing disciplinary knowledge, and taking responsibility for continuing to advance this knowledge (Fawcett, 2006; Willis, Grace, and Roy, 2008).

The task of developing theoretical frameworks that reflect clinical practice and that could better inform practice and drive the research agenda in the discipline of nursing is not complete yet, nor will it ever be finished in dynamic and responsive disciplines. Theory as the link between research findings and practice utilization is dynamic, changing, and constantly evolving. Clinicians need and use theory to inform their practice. What helps clinicians is not only that a patient's uncertainty about a particular diagnosis and prognosis is related to slow progress in wound healing; it is also knowing that patients who have lifestyles based on the ability to plan and to be certain, or who function better with a sense of control over their environments, tend to have different recovery patterns than others who have already experienced lives of more uncertainty. The first is a research hypothesis; the second is a theoretical proposition that reflects a discipline's established assumptions about the importance of the environment and patterns of behavior, as well as how responses to a current illness situation must be understood within the context of the person's total life patterns.

Theory is also the link between fragmented research projects and a coherent research program, and it provides the language that reflects an identity in a field. How patients experience symptoms and interpret them, and the strategies they use to care for their symptoms in particular and their health in general, is a theoretical question that may drive a number of research studies with populations who have experiences with different symptoms. The results of these studies add knowledge to self-care theories, provide support to develop new theories, and may refine existing theories on managing a number of illness experiences, such as pain and shortness of breath.

Theory also provides the contextual interpretation of research findings and the framework to connect the different experiences nurses encounter, again providing the means for a disciplinary identity. A theory on transition and health may alert nurses to use knowledge that illuminates the experiences and responses of patients and provide them with strategies to enhance the health and well-being of patients undergoing this transition. Being aware of what to anticipate, what to observe, and what to assess may also provide the nurse with the opportunity to modify the theoretical interpretations that emanate from the theory. Theories allow the more complex interrelationships to be considered and, therefore, responses could be viewed more within a context of antecedents and consequences, as well as patterns, rather than isolated relationships, events, or responses.

The production of nursing theories and the strategies and analyses provided by metatheorists have been the impetus for promoting many theoretical and philosophical dialogues in the discipline as well for the development of strategic definitions of areas of research to guide our research enterprise. Among these are the study of self-care, self-management of chronic illness, and the relationships between compassion and meaning of life for end-of-life patients (Grady, 2014, 2015). These theoretical dialogues also produced many theory-based research projects that continue to support or refute theories or to drive the development of middle-range and situation-specific theories as evidenced in the reviews presented in this book in Chapters 11 to 13. In spite of the increasing number of research and clinical publications based on the different theories (see Chapter 21), there is an alarming tendency in U.S. graduate programs (particularly those focused on educating nurse practitioners) to omit nursing theory from their curricula (Chinn, 2014). This tendency may eventually produce graduates who lack the language and the knowledge base that may undermine their ability to develop or nurture a strong disciplinary identity, and graduates who may be ill-equipped to utilize and develop theories. This pattern may interrupt the theoretical growth of the discipline, which may in turn be a barrier to forming a well-defined disciplinary identity that incorporates nursing values, mission, and goals. Therefore, advancing nursing knowledge requires a cyclical process of being able to access and use the theoretical heritage to develop a strong disciplinary identity, and theoretical thinking is vital for insuring the continuity in this cycle.

THEORETICAL THINKING

At the turn of the 21st century, there was a movement to minimize the role of theory, and theoretical development of the discipline was also manifested in educational institutions in the United States, while, interestingly, they became more prominent in curricula in European (especially in the Scandinavian and eastern European countries), South American, and southeast Asian countries. In the United States, evidence-based practice discourse tended to substitute for theoretical dialogues (Chinn, 2008), but without careful attention to ontological analyses of the evidence, clinical practice may not fully reap the benefit of the integration of theoretical and research evidence (Sharts-Hopko, 2013;

Whall, Sinclair, and Parahoo, 2006). Theoretical and philosophical dialogues enrich the potential of engaging with significant phenomena in the discipline and encourage not only application of theory but the development of theory as well (McIntyre and McDonald, 2013).

Theoretical thinking in the discipline of nursing—which deals with the study of human health, caring, healing, recovery, and living with illness, as embedded in relationships with environment and within a historical, political, and social context—must be informed by social justice and equity theories. For how could individuals be defined in human science without understanding the influence of the political, economic, social, and cultural context? Therefore, an overall guiding ontological framework for any theoretical discourse in nursing must incorporate principles of health equity, the meaning of power differential, the goals of a just environment, and the opportunities to review frameworks that uncover inequalities in health care and in the work environments, structure, and organization. Promoting theoretical thinking in our discipline while embracing our rich theoretical history requires incorporation of the fundamental tenets of inclusiveness, advocacy, equity, and justice (Thorne, 2014, pp. 79–92) and their relationship to the delivery of quality health care.

Theoretical nursing includes a discourse about the structure of nursing knowledge, the sociopolitical structures in which nursing is embedded, the philosophical bases of nursing science, theory development, the history of nursing knowledge, and nursing theories. For many years, aspects of these components have been included in doctoral nursing programs in the United States (Jacobs-Kramer and Huether, 1988) and internationally. A more limited version has been included in master's programs, with more emphasis placed on presentations and critique of existing nursing theories (Jacobson, 1987). Although nursing theories were used as frameworks for nursing curricula in undergraduate programs during the 1970s and 1980s, only a limited number have included opportunities to discuss theoretical nursing and approaches to theory development (Jacobs-Kramer and Huether, 1988; Meleis and Price, 1988), and increasingly, there is a paucity of these discussions (Fawcett and Alligood, 2005; Fawcett, 2012).

Although theory has been instrumental in the general progress of the discipline of nursing, the most cogent and significant contribution that the nursing theorists have made is the promotion of theoretical thinking in the discipline among faculty and students. Theoretical thinking is about identifying and using assumptions and concepts and recognizing patterns. It is characterized by the ability to use frameworks to promote understanding, as well as the ability to be skeptical about frameworks and their utility in exploring any, all, or part of health–illness situations. It is the ability to connect seemingly discrete, unconnected thoughts, observations, or facts, and to see a coherent whole. It is abstract thinking grounded in exemplars from practice. A theoretical thinker is a reflective thinker who suspends "fragmentedness" to allow for the exploring, explaining, and reinterpreting of wholes. A critical thinker is someone who is able to explore and describe patterns, not only discrete facts, and who engages in individual ontological dialogues, as well as similar dialogues with others. A theoretical thinker is a critical thinker with a goal of discerning patterns, connecting ideas, and developing explanatory models; to ask and answer the "whats," "why nots," and "what ifs." A critical thinker is one who is inquisitive, truth seeking, systematic, and analytical (Dewey, 1982; Facione, Facione, and Sanchez, 1994). A theoretical thinker does not allow procedures and rules alone to drive his or her focus or explorations; rather, he or she uses them only as tools that must be considered, revisited, and revised. Theoretical thinking includes critical consideration of the discipline's central phenomena and questions. Theories are dynamic and always changing, and, as Levine (1995) admonished, they "are not written in stone."

A theoretical thinker questions the prevailing models that have governed his or her nursing care. An example of a model that has been critically analyzed is the biomedical model. The biomedical model, as a framework for health care, has been challenged because of its limited effectiveness (Engel, 1977), and has been challenged by nurses as inappropriate for the mission of nursing (Allan and Hall, 1988; Shaver, 1985). Others have described the differences in perspectives between nursing and other health fields and the uniqueness of the nursing perspective, despite its dependent and interdependent functions (Visintainer, 1986).

Nursing theorists have demonstrated theoretical thinking and are among those nurses who not only challenged the biomedical model, but who also proactively conceptualized different aspects of the territory of nursing. Their conceptualizations provided the bases for identifying nursing perspectives and for defining our nursing domain. It is because of their pioneering work that members of the discipline continue to discuss the theoretical bases of practice and pose and answer theoretically driven questions. This theoretical thinking must continue to be promoted in nursing education, administration, and research.

Theoretical thinking, the pride that discipline's member has in the theoretical threads of her discipline, a belief in the self as a proactive developer of knowledge, and an identity that incorporates the ability to structure nursing knowledge are values essential for quality care and for the continuous development of the discipline (Meleis, 1992). If nurses expect to have a significant impact on health care through development and use of theory, content related to the purpose, generation, and use of theory must be integrated into the curricula much earlier than it currently is (Jacobs-Kramer and Huether, 1988, p. 376). In fact, the seeds for such values could and should be planted in students as early as possible in nursing education. It is not enough to promote these values in doctoral or master's programs; they should be incorporated all through nursing education beginning in the very first year (Batra, 1987; Rafferty, Allcock, and Lathlean, 1996).

Having the time and the space to reflect on the discipline's progress and future is essential not only to learn how to engage in dialogues on these topics, but also for building on and for advancing the substance of these discourses (Holt, 2014). However, when theory and its development are introduced as separate components of a nursing curriculum, students and faculty may find it difficult to relate them to practice, to research, and to policy. These artificial content silos may have been necessary during the decades when the primacy of theoretical nursing was still debated, but the progress that has occurred in our discipline should allow us to now integrate theory in all the clinical and research components of the curriculum. To capture students' attention, to sensitize them to the significance of theory in their practice or research, and to demystify theory, teaching of theory must come out of its closet, and it must be innovatively integrated in curricula (Karmels, 1993). When faculty are skeptical about theoretical nursing, they cannot persuade students of its importance (Levine, 1995), and when theory is sequestered into separate courses, its meaning and its role in practice and in research are questioned and minimized.

Theoretical nursing provides *nursing curricula* with a perspective that is uniquely nursing's, it provides nursing students with frameworks that help them define their values and the concepts used in their practice, the significant problems in their fields, and approaches to structuring and developing knowledge. More importantly, a theoretical nursing perspective promotes the primacy of discovering, developing, and structuring nursing knowledge.

The relationship between theory and nursing curricula is similar to the relationship between research and nursing curricula. In the past, educators asked whether research courses should be included in the curriculum, at what level they should be introduced, and what should be included (Wilson, 1985). The questions related to theory, theoretical nursing, and philosophy are no longer whether theory should be a component of nursing programs, or at what level it should be introduced; rather, the questions educators will grapple with during the next decade are what aspects of theory should be introduced at every educational level, and what are the most effective and meaningful ways by which they should be included.

Similar dialogues must continue to consider the role of theoretical nursing in *nursing administration*. What role should nursing administrators play in advancing theoretical nursing? Nursing administrators are critical constituencies who, through their vision and leadership role, have tremendous influence on nurses in the practice arena. They can act as role models in promoting theoretical thinking, in creating and nurturing a scholarly environment, in providing the incentives and the rewards, and in investing time, money, and effort in advancing nursing knowledge. This sentiment of the close connection between nursing administration and nursing knowledge, and of the potential of nursing theory construction by or as promoted by nursing administrators, was expressed repeatedly in the late 1980s (examples are the volume edited by Henry, Arndt, DiVincenti, et al., 1989; also DeGroot, Ferketich, and Larson, 1987, p. 38). Until the late 1980s, there was a limited dialogue about the relationship of nursing theory and nursing administration (Christmyer, Catanzariti, Langford, et al., 1988). Some addressed the shortcomings of that limited dialogue, indicating that specialty nursing, such as nursing leadership or administration, should not be claiming that nursing theories do not represent them (Dashiff, 1988), as this may distance them from the core of the domain of nursing. These dialogues continue to be important during the third decade of the 21st century, suggesting that administrative, organizational, and clinical decision-making needed for patient care require theory and outcome measurements (Jeffs, Sidani, Rose, et al., 2013).

Nursing administrators and nursing practice are a source and resource for these theories.

Viewing nursing administration from a domain perspective and investigating theoretical and clinical questions from that perspective could lead to a more coherent approach to structuring knowledge that is as useful to clinicians as it may be to administrators. Theories for the future must address the innovative relationship between practice, information, computer usage, skills acquisition, and clinical judgments (Anderson, Dobal, and Blessing, 1992), as well as the use and outcomes of health-enabling technologies that are particularly used for monitoring chronic illness and empowering patients for effective self-care (Knight and Shea, 2014). Theoretical aspects of the nursing domain may provide clinicians and administrators with a unifying framework that could further contribute to the development of coherent theories to guide nursing care (Jennings and Meleis, 1988; Meleis and Jennings, 1989), particularly in light of the dramatic changes and advances in health care technology, as well as the increasing numbers of populations that are aging and living with chronic illnesses, all of which require the use of new tools by nursing administrators (an example is the use of mobile health technology in Moore, Holaday, Meehan et al., 2015).

The question remains: What are the best approaches to incorporating theoretical thinking in nursing in educational and administrative organizations? I propose several approaches for the integration of theoretical knowledge to promote theoretical thinking in educational and clinical institutions.

- A deliberate plan to engage in *theoretical dialogues* should be developed and implemented in educational and clinical institutions. The extent to which the discipline of nursing will continue to evolve with a theoretical base depends on the ability of its members to engage in theoretical discussion and debates at all levels of education and practice (such as Allen, 1987). Opportunities for theoretical thinking could be found in the daily routines of students' lives (classroom teaching as well as clinical mentorship), and in clinicians' lives (shift reports as well as supervisory education).
- Analytical and critical consideration of nursing theories should be a cornerstone of curricula in nursing, from community college to doctoral programs, with different goals at each educational level. For example, the choice of a discussion of human beings as nursing clients may be organized around nursing theories that

discuss human beings and the different goals of the different perspectives.
- Consideration of research and clinical exemplars that are related to different domain concepts and questions and beginning attempts at a thorough review may help in creating some coherence and may delineate further avenues of investigation.
- In preparing for "Magnet review designation," members of an organization may engage in a theoretical and philosophical dialogue to uncover values and define shared mission and framework.
- The advanced clinicians and clinical specialists can be coached to develop and share wisdom gleaned from their clinical practice in the form of exemplars. Exemplars identify, model, and direct problems of concern to nursing and ways of solving these problems.
- Finally, just as theoretical discourses are provided to compare and contrast models of care delivery such as total patient care, functional care, team nursing care, and primary care, similar discourses should be provided on nursing theories that drive patient care interventions (Tiedeman and Lookinland, 2004).

As much as philosophical discussions and theoretical exchanges are vital and useful, their utility is limited without considering related research as an integral part of these discussions (Whall et al., 2006), a view that is congruent with how science is viewed (Laudan, 1981). Theorists, researchers, clinicians, and educators should explicitly state the theoretical underpinnings of their work and engage in dialogues with self and others to help in identifying relationships or the lack of them with other components of the domain of nursing. Such discussions will help the continuity in refining both the domain and the work being done to advance its knowledge base.

FIFTH-GENERATION THEORISTS

Nursing theories of the past, present, or the future do not answer all the questions that nurses may ask; neither do sociological, psychological, physiologic, or engineering theories. Different theories in each of these disciplines answer different questions, and yet some questions still have not been answered because of the complexity of the environment within which each discipline functions. Other questions that appeared to have been answered have later been challenged by new data and new competing explanations; for example, Margaret Mead's cultural determinism and Sigmund Freud's seduction theories have been debated and questioned because of new evidence developed years after they developed their theories. Therefore, theories are dynamic and should not be expected to receive total support for all their propositions at any one time.

Because of the scientific maturity of our discipline that has been informed by the results of many theory-based research programs, our discipline is ready to inspire and support the development of fifth-generation theorists. *First-generation theorists* are the original thinkers in the discipline who developed enduring coherent visions of the discipline. They are the group of theorists that Dorothy Johnson chose to build around in the first theory course for master's students in the United States at the University of California, Los Angeles. I had the privilege of teaching this course in 1969 to 1970 and became very acquainted with the wealth and depth of these theorists' offerings. These giants— Virginia Henderson, Dorothy Johnson, Myra Levine, Florence Nightingale, Dorothea Orem, Ida Orlando, Hildegard Peplau, Martha Rogers, and Ernestine Wiedenbach—inspired, in my opinion, the *second-generation theorists,* who include Imogene King, Betty Neuman, Margaret Newman, Rosemarie Parse, Josephine Paterson, Callista Roy, Jean Watson, and Loretta Zderad. These thinkers, as well as the *third-generation metatheorists,* such as Kay Avant, Jacqueline Fawcett, Margaret Harding, Hesook Kim, Afaf Meleis, and Lorraine Walker (Kim, 2010), may have contributed to the development of *fourth-generation theorists* and the explosion of

middle-range theories pioneered by such theorists who based their theories on research, including Katharine Kolcaba (comfort) and Merle Michele (uncertainty), among many others (Alligood, 2014; Smith and Liehr, 2013).

The *fifth generation of theorists* will benefit from this rich theoretical history, the current progress in research, and the increasing sophistication in the delivery of nursing care. These next-generation theorists are those who will be developing theories at all levels of abstraction and scopes (Table 19-1). Among them are those who develop situation-specific theories to describe, explain, or predict phenomena within a specific explanatory context. These are also theories that focus on uncovering voices, identifying patterns, and interpreting themes (Chapter 17). These theories are contextualized and represent many truths about similar situations with different populations. They help illuminate the experiences of populations, as well as the situation for nurses. Situation-specific theories respect mind–body wholeness and environment–person connections; they allow for a multiplicity of truth, for tentativeness of interpretation, and for complexity of contexts. Situation-specific theories are generally used to formulate questions and answer questions within a context. They help in explaining situations that are limited in scope and in focus. An example of such theories is symptom-specific theory versus a theory of symptom management or a theory of unpleasant symptoms. Another example is a theory of identity and health versus African American identity and the psychotherapeutic environment (Brown, 1996; Lenz, Suppe, Gift, et al., 1995; Meleis, Isenberg, Koerner, et al., 1995; University of California, San

TABLE 19-1	Patterns of Theorizing		
Component	**Clinical**	**Conceptual**	**Empirical**
Phenomena	Discovered	Discovered	Created
Concepts	Emerge from phenomenon	Used as per theory or redefined	Used as is redefined
			Modified due to research
Propositions	Linkages evolve from experience	Theoretical properties evolve from theory	Deduced from theory
Theory	Descriptive/explanatory	Descriptive	Descriptive
	Prescriptive	Explanatory	Predictive
Purpose	Explain	Explain	Explain
	Prescribe	Development of theory	Development of theory
	Development of theory		Researcher
	Clinical practice		
Approach	Clinical experience	Conceptualization	Measurement testing
Evaluation	Guided by practice situation	Guided by theory	Guided by research

Francisco, School of Nursing Symptom Management Faculty Group, 1994).

Fifth-generation theorists, however, may not be confined to only developing situation-specific theories, because they are among those who would have benefited from the full scope of the discipline's theoretical and research progress. What characterizes this group of theorists is not only the type of theory they develop but it is also their use of integrative strategies for developing theories that reflect significant and fundamental problems and solutions related to care supported by clinical, theoretical, or research evidence. Thus theorizing, for them, evolves from extending other theories, abstracting from practice, or synthesizing research findings, or any combination of these types. An example is Glenister (2011), who integrated theories to develop a general systems theory in nursing.

Theories for fifth-generation theorists may be driven by clinical knowledge that results from engaging in the gestalt of doing and caring. Florence Nightingale, a definite first generation theorist, developed her ideas based and grounded by her work with wounded soldiers in the Crimean War, and her theory of the significance of attending to the environment evolved from clinical work. Clinical knowledge could be the result of personal and subjective knowing, and there are numerous examples of theoretical propositions in the literature, particularly in the clinical literature, that evolved from the sum total of the wisdom of clinicians. The question is: How can we advance these clinical-based theoretical propositions that reflect the wisdom of the experiences of clinicians and establish the credibility of that knowledge and, thus, the acceptability of utilizing it to make a difference in patient care? In the past, this credibility may have been based on the fact that a given practice or procedure worked as used by a single nurse. However, because we are trying to establish a case for the significance of this knowledge, guidelines need to be developed for what makes this type of knowledge credible and acceptable beyond the single use for the purpose of providing guidance for an entire practice area.

Theories evolving from clinical practice use what feminist psychologists call "connected knowing," developing theories collaboratively through interpersonal relations with clients and through being connected with what individuals may be experiencing. These theories have been described in different ways by different authors. They have been defined as narrative, naturalistic, or clinical concepts. Theories that evolve from a clinical setting have richer clinical context and a longer life span and may have been used without being publicly championed and acknowledged as theories. However, while clinical practice may inform the beginning development of these theories, fifth-generation theorists will and must address and integrate research findings and evidence to render them more credible, and hence more acceptable.

Fifth-generation theorists may also develop theories from existing conceptualization or theories. Even then, there is a need to integrate research findings and evidence related to the phenomena for the purpose of refining, revising, or extending the scope of the new conceptualization as well as developing other related theories. Also, integrating existing theories to develop more effective frameworks that are more congruent, for example, with mobile technology and use of electronic health records, while at its embryonic stages, could become the impetus for fifth-generation theories (examples are Moore et al., 2015; Strudwick, Booth, and Mistry, 2016).

Fifth-generation theorists could influence knowledge advancement, quality of nursing care, and policies if they have been educated as critical and theoretical thinkers and if they have developed the capacity and skills in utilizing the integrative strategy in theory development or similar other strategies. It goes without saying that fifth-generation theorists will be grounded in a disciplinary identity, have a strong scholarly passion in an area and a field of study, and give special intellectual attention to oppressive social structures, disempowering practices, and strategies to promote healing, health, and well-being, while empowering clients, families, and communities.

THREATS AND OPPORTUNITIES IN THEORIZING

Threats to a sustainable theoretical development in the discipline exist in four areas—in establishing an interprofessional identity, in utilizing scientific revolutions in health care, in incorporating innovations and entrepreneurship, and in attempting to reflect national and international diversity and inclusiveness—each of which are briefly discussed here. I ask the reader to contemplate ways by which these threats could be changed to opportunities for the purpose of developing more relevant and responsive theories that could be used by health care teams that are interprofessional and interdisciplinary.

These threats and opportunities are connected and are not mutually exclusive.

Interprofessional Identity and Voice

There is a body of evidence pointing to the importance of creating effective health care teams in achieving positive outcomes in patient care, in enhancing health and well-being, and in decreasing errors, unsafe practices, and infections (NAM, 2010). There have also been ongoing dialogues about the need to revolutionize education in the health professions to avoid the educational silos and to promote integrative, interdisciplinary, and interprofessional education without which effective and functioning health care teams are not guaranteed (Bhutta, Chen, Cohen, et al., 2010; Josiah Macy Jr. Foundation, 2013). These publications have spurred important conversations about how to develop interprofessional educators, curricula, and future graduates who benefit from innovative and integrated strategies (NAM, 2013). These dialogues point to threats and opportunities that are driven by a fundamental challenge of the existing power differential among members of the different professions and the entitled supremacy of medical science and physician leadership (Meleis, 2015).

The first of two specific threats related to interprofessional identity and voice is the intentional or unintentional trivialization of nursing knowledge or nurses' roles and their contributions by other professions. Knowledge and perspectives of members of the discipline of nursing have not been consistently recognized and valued, even though they focus on contributing to theories that address the daily lived experiences and needs of populations, on ways to promote their comfort, and on providing care that is based on compassion and which address responses and experiences to illness by using qualitative methodologies that are more congruent with human sciences. Yet as an example, findings from an ethnographic study demonstrated that when a team includes health care assistants, there is both a perceived and real marginalization of members of teams who bring in different expertise (Lloyd, Schneider, Scales, et al., 2011). The lack of focus on discipline-driven questions as a product of bias and trivialization can result in the loss of a nursing voice in advocacy and in developing relevant health policies. (As discussed in the next section, it can also result in the loss of relevant theories). To transform this threat to opportunity and provide nurses with the platform for a more effective voice, members

of the discipline must recognize the historical oppression of nurses' roles, voices and actions—by physicians, by administrators, and sometimes by societies at large—and using their awareness of that second-class status to understand other marginalized populations. And since 90% of nurses are women, it is also essential to uncover how women's status and position are viewed globally. These views are created and strengthened by the presence of privilege that historically has been given to men and physicians. Awareness of such injustices for themselves helps uncover injustices experienced by the population they care for (Van Herk, Smith, and Andrew, 2011). Changing the narrative to the power of nurses associated with their focus on the whole person and their environment, on the research findings that have made a difference in health care, and on the developed theories that led to more effective models of care will influence a more positive identity and empower nurses to have a voice (Peter and Liaschenko, 2013).

The second threat stems from the still undefined and less developed and evaluated frameworks for interprofessional functioning, shared decision-making and clinical care outcome goals. While the relationship between team functioning and health outcomes have been well established, prompting ongoing dialogues about insuring the establishment of functioning teams, theories that guide the forming of collaborations have not been given the attention needed.

There have been many theories in the interprofessional field and growing syntheses that resulted in a 2013 issue of the *Journal of Interprofessional Care*, which is entirely devoted to dialogues about theories for interprofessional practice (Reeves and Hean, 2013). Yet there has not been careful examination and analysis of whether these evolving interprofessional theories respect and reflect nursing interest and phenomena in health care. And no models have been developed to describe how roles of the team members are singularly different and collectively similar, or how partnerships are enacted to achieve equitable interprofessional decision-making (Lewis, Stacey, Squires, et al., 2016). The threat in forming teams in which each member may provide and participate equally and up to their full capacity requires an ability of each member of the different professions to yield their territoriality and to find common grounds, combine perspectives, and develop shared perceptions of clinical situations (Barr, 2013; Meleis, 2015). An imperative common ground to allow collaboration and partnership to evolve and mature may be through interprofessional education and developing the capacity for critical thinking (Papp, Huang, Clabo, et al., 2014).

There are ways to change this threat to an opportunity as the interest is growing in interprofessional education, teamwork, interdependence, and collaboration. *Fifth-generation theorists* will need to engage in developing theories that incorporate the domain concepts, values, mission, and outcomes in ways that could be used by other members of the health care team and could lead to shared decision-making. As evidenced below, revolutions and advances in science also add to the challenge of ensuring the sustainability of a nursing perspective and voice.

Revolutions in Sciences

The threats that may occur due to the many scientific revolutions are the unintentional marginalization of nursing knowledge by disciplines in which these revolutions are claimed, the loss of nursing perspective, and less utilization of the rich theory development strategies that have been unique to nursing in favor of those used in other disciplines. Advancements in neurosciences and genetic science require a shift of focus of determinants of health, disease, and behavior. Consider, for example, how the discovery of telomeres is revolutionizing fundamental knowledge about health and illness. These new discoveries make it very apparent that the work to be done to continue to advance knowledge for the health and health care of populations, more than ever before, must become interdisciplinary.

The 21st century will be known as the century in which the hybridization of disciplines evolved and became the norm. It is the century when realization about pressing questions in health, illness, interventions, and recovery could not be addressed within the perspective and skill sets of one discipline or one science. It will be known as the century of partnership, collaboration, and interdisciplinarity. Members of disciplines who have existed in silos and who created boundaries, real or imaginary, will no longer compete in advancing the knowledge base of their discipline. The National Institutes of Health have already developed road maps for the future based on interdisciplinary science and teams. The Institute of Medicine has deliberated and advocated for quality care through partnerships (Grey and Mitchell, 2008). Nursing and medical organizations have developed competitive projects to promote the formulation of interdisciplinary teams. Universities have helped advance the hybridization

of disciplines by creating collaborative programs that draw on the expertise of relevant professions and disciplines. The University of Pennsylvania, for instance, developed an institute that brings together urban developers, epidemiologists, nurses, and social scientists to address the effects of the increasing global urbanization on the social fabric of communities, as well as on the health and illness of populations. None of the disciplines above can singularly address the cumulative and integrative outcomes or ways to ameliorate the ill-effects of urbanization while promoting opportunities for healthy and effective economic and community growth. Forward-looking foundations as well have captured the imperativeness of interdisciplinarity as exemplified by the Macy Foundation, which invited scientists and scholars to dialogue about integrating the disciplines of neuroscience, psychology, nursing, and behavioral science to better understand human responses (Macy Foundation, personal communication, 2004) and also assembled a group representing many health professions to discuss best practices in providing primary care and in deciding who should provide it (Cronenwett and Dzau, 2010). The collective wisdom of the invited members representing the different disciplines and professionals results in integrated frameworks and recommendations that reflected their different perspectives and different goals. These are examples of how members of different disciplines may work together, equally, to glean the most benefit from each other's perspectives and advance knowledge that is utilized by all for understanding phenomena and for decision-making.

Interdisciplinarity connotes researchers from different fields working together and utilizing integrated theoretical frameworks. A consequence may be the development of a new discipline—*transdisciplinarity* (Grey and Connolly, 2008), which is considered the future of science. Interdisciplinarity requires "permeable boundaries" (Frickel, 2004). However, for disciplines to develop permeable boundaries they must first have strong boundaries. Disciplines that have achieved a certain level of maturity in their science base and knowledge development, as well as a strong disciplinary identity in their scientists, will develop those strong boundaries and thus its members become more secure for making those boundaries more permeable. The threat is if members of a discipline embark on a journey of interdisciplinarity before such maturity is achieved, the central phenomena and the significant questions of that discipline and the approach to investigating these questions may be totally overshadowed by other, more mature disciplines. This may also lead to funding and support that follows the dominant discipline's questions and methodologies, thus impeding the potential of synthesis and integration of knowledge that true and equal interdisciplinarity promises. How such integration of theories is achieved and what can be gained and lost will depend on the level of each discipline's scientific maturity. Another potential tension is between the promise of interdisciplinarity and the more familiar and accepted norms in developing productive careers that are more discipline-specific (Rhoten and Parker, 2004). Similarly, the tension exists in the paradox of the need for disciplinary specialization and subspecialization while creating interdisciplinarity (Strober, 2006).

I fear that the phenomena of nursing discipline, the pressing questions of our profession, will be minimized, ignored, or replaced by the pressing questions of other disciplines (Chinn, 2007; Fawcett, 2008). This fear is also echoed by others who have dialogued about interdisciplinarity (Grey and Connelly, 2008). So, the questions to consider are: What does it mean to have a disciplinary domain and perspective? And, how do we preserve that core of the discipline as we become more interdisciplinary? What should members of the discipline guard as they become interdisciplinary? Advantages to interdisciplinarity are obvious. It provides more comprehensive answers to questions about quality care. Answers to pressing questions related to health care involve biobehavioral as well as sociocultural bases and hence require interdisciplinary teams to address their complexity. Interdisciplinarity can work without undermining one discipline or another through the principles of equality, partnership, reciprocity, synthesis, and integration to achieve a whole that is better than the distinct parts that each discipline represents. To what

extent will nurses, who are emerging from a history of inequity and oppression, be able to honor and value the core values and mission of our discipline as interdisciplinarity becomes the norm?

As we nurture and support interdisciplinarity, we must also continue to invest in our achieved disciplinary identity, we need to support more coherent approaches to knowledge development—ones that encompass, and do not neglect, knowing, understanding, and caring; ones that support models of knowledge development that are congruent with our mission. Support of such identities includes tangible support from granting agencies, as well as publishing support from editors of nursing journals.

There are possibly two complementary models for developing theories, offered here only to stimulate dialogues about the consideration of other models as well (Table 19-2). Should both models be supported? Should one prevail? These are questions to consider for a clearer future for advancing theory. By being clear about our mission, our values, and the models we choose to use for knowledge development, we are empowering ourselves to empower our consumers. To become clear and to consolidate efforts, we are challenged to further develop and structure knowledge using either one or both of the models. I believe both models will continue to exist side by side in the 21st century and perhaps beyond. What are your thoughts on these models? What other models exist? How will these models influence the progress and development of theoretical nursing?

There are many challenges facing interdisciplinary research that could be shifted to opportunities for more integrated theories. The challenge is to avoid intellectual centrism and to truly develop strategies to transcend discipline theories and to advance interdisciplinary knowledge (Kneipp, Gilleskie, Sheely, et al., 2014).

TABLE 19-2	Models for Theory Development	
Unit of Analysis	*Model 1*	*Model 2*
Unit of observation	Defined, concise, operational Predefined A particular aspect	Behaviors, events, or situations embedded in a context Human being and environment
Assumptions	Axioms Value free	Context Value laden, beliefs, action
Concepts	Defined, operationalized *a priori*	Emerge from clinical, research, or theory
Propositions	Operationalized	Descriptive, explanatory statements
Theory development	Relationship between concepts Theory evolves from a research tradition	Theory evolves from theory, practice, research

TABLE 19-2	Models for Theory Development (*continued*)	
Unit of Analysis	*Model 1*	*Model 2*
Conditions	Conciseness, source, facts	Perceptions, meanings, patterns, context
Tools for development	Observation Research designs Research findings	Collaboration Dialogue Intuition Experiences Diaries Self
Reasoning		Connective
Context	Logical development	Documentation of discovery
Theorist	Documentation of justification Distanced, objectified, not active participant	Engaged, attached, acting, developing
Purpose		Describe, explain, understand
Theory use	Explain, predict	Congruency with human values
Focus	Congruency with evidence Knowing	Understanding Caring
Criteria for evaluation of phenomena	Centrality and closeness to cutting edge in discipline	Significance to discipline, to theorist, to humanity
Evaluation	Validity, reliability Critique Testing	Description Analysis Testing
Criteria for analysis	Validity and reliability of concepts Operationalizability	Theorist experiences Social structure
Criteria for testing	Research Empirical evidence Statistical methods Corroboration	Values Understanding Usefulness Intuition Coherence Comprehensiveness Support from experience Diversity of exemplars
Validity	Universality Replicability	
Norms	Stands the test of time Universal Observation Ordered	Contextual Reflection
Time	Defined time period Transcends time	Time and historically embedded
Approach	Analysis of findings Not contextual	Reflection Analysis Forward leaps Historical and structural context
Language	Evidence Generalizability Replicability	Understanding Intersubjectivity Consistency Consensus
Goals	Probability Prescription	Pattern Identification Liberation Change Consciousness-raising
Dissemination	Professional audience	Subjects Policy makers

Innovations and Entrepreneurship

Major changes have occurred in technology and in computerization, digitalization, and information systems, all of which affected the discipline of nursing (Davidson, 2016). Theories of the past have focused on individuals and on establishing face-to-face relationships in contiguous space, usually a hospital setting. Assessment was focused on the professional worker, and information-giving was more didactic, profession-centric, and reliant on the use of handouts and brochures. With the increasing emphasis and focus on recycling, energy, and environmental sustainability, and with proliferation of information sources, paperless environments and transparent and accessible information make it all the more feasible to utilize new innovative resources such as telehealth for communication between and among clients and health care professionals. The challenge is how to maintain what characterizes nursing as a human science whose members use interaction as a vital and essential tool for assessment, diagnosis, and caring. And the question is how to continue to reap the full benefits of interactions, which include being able to read another human being's body and facial language and expressions and to interpret these symbols toward a more wholistic understanding of experiences and responses. All this may be challenged with communication through technology.

With the increasing emphasis on precision medicine (or precision nursing!), there is also an imperative to understand advances in technologies that make this precision feasible to implement. Precision medicine is about ensuring that people's unique differences in lifestyles, in genes, and in environments are taken into consideration in assessing, diagnosing, treating, and preventing diseases (Gillman and Hammond, 2016). There are also the many diagnostic technologies that have become the gold standards for precision medicine diagnosis and intervention. Among these new technologies are sequencing of genes, imaging, and electronic health records (Jameson and Longo, 2015).

Future fifth-generation theorists will be profoundly influenced and challenged by the nature of technological development and by how technology is used in practice, research, teaching, and administration. We have moved steadfastly into an era of client-centered information systems and organized data sets, one of an increasing availability of health care information that is disseminated to the public through network systems, mobile technology, social media, and telehealth for self-monitoring of health care and remote assessment by clinicians. In addition, these technologies allow the sharing of information among members of the different professions promoting (or hindering) collaborative care of patients. These innovative technologies also allow sharing of aggregate information among researchers and policy makers. Our challenge is to address ways by which theoretical frameworks and technology will interface, especially while nurses continue to adopt pluralistic philosophies in defining, connecting, and using data for nursing practice, research, and policy development. Although there is equal concern in prematurely selecting a system to guide these processes, the risks may be higher in not settling on one shared framework. The challenge is to resolve these conflicts and to settle on a framework or frameworks that will facilitate exchanges and drive a more common and congruent set of outcomes. The challenge to face in the future continues to be in the development of processes and theories to integrate the development of informatics, computerization and other technologies, and theoretical nursing, and to guide the development of innovative technologies that inform the mission, the goals, and the theories that reflect the goals of health care in general, as well as those that embrace the holistic caring of individuals and their families, which are the hallmarks of nursing (Hays, Norris, Martin, et al., 1994; Nagel, Pomerleau, and Penner, 2013).

Because of the increased use of technology, insurance-driven policies related to hospitalization and discharge, and increased costs of hospitalization worldwide, patients tend to leave hospitals earlier and continue their complex and long-term recovery and rehabilitation transition at home. Therefore, the transition to recovery is somewhat more protracted, and patients need expert and competent care at home. These trends will drive the development of theories to reflect a new set of emerging care needs for patients. However, many of the medical information systems continue to depend more on biomedical knowledge and less on what is essential for nursing care processes. In what ways will the nursing perspective and domain inform informatics, health care records, telehealth, and computer-driven instruction for self-care?

The challenges inherent in this technological and information revolution also present unique new opportunities for nurse scholars to develop innovative practices that facilitate and drive quality care. There are many examples of new devices to ensure proper feeding of babies whose sucking is challenged by congenital anomalies (Penn Nursing, 2016a). Other examples are apps to monitor management of diabetes (Penn Nursing, 2016b). With the challenge of technology coupled with economic constraints in resources and limited or deprived organizations, there are more opportunities for nurses to develop and evaluate innovative inventions for assessment, diagnosis, and caring of populations (Adams, 2014).

There are also golden opportunities for entrepreneurship. Developing a theoretical identity is congruent with an entrepreneurial identity; both are based on a strong sense of what is best for populations' care, what to advocate for, what are fundamental foci of the discipline, how best to use resources to enhance well-being of people, and how best to use innovations to achieve valued disciplinary defined outcomes. Entrepreneurship is about using a business-driven model for the common good (Kovalainen and Osterberg-Hogstedt, 2013). It is about harnessing the capacity of the discipline of nursing and its members to deliver quality care that positions people to be able to achieve their maximum well-being and supports their abilities to function up to their full capacities in spite of illness, chronicity, and poorly functioning systems. An example of effective entrepreneurship is the company established by Dr. Kathryn Bowles, RightCare Solutions, which is based on extensive research that reflects nursing's mission of providing theory-based care through the continuum of care. On the basis of extensive research and influenced by nursing knowledge, the 'Discharge Decision Support System (D2S2)' was developed and marketed to allow clinicians and administrators to identify rehabilitation and recovery needs of patients and match them with the best strategies to facilitate meeting their health care needs and enhance their well-being (Bowles, Dykes, and Demiris, 2015; Bowles, Hanlon, Holland, et al., 2014).

Considering the use of innovative technology and the potential for entrepreneurship provides a context, as well as the means, to advance theoretical nursing. However, as scholars utilize these new and innovative approaches to assess and deliver care based on communication and interaction models of care, the focus must continue to be articulated through the lens that defines our discipline, which is the well-being of people and their environments (Nilsson, Hofflander, Eriksen, et al., 2012). Clinical research, educational innovation, and entrepreneurship are predicated on the belief that nurses have an innovative, entrepreneurial identity, the wisdom of knowing their discipline domain, and the experiences they accumulated in practice (Cioffi, 2015).

Diversity and Inclusiveness

There is a threat to develop theories and knowledge that reflects only the majority of populations, as well as the developed region of the world, and less of the developing countries. Developing theories that reflect the diversity of our country as well as global diversity, and theories that promote inclusiveness and prevent disparities, require recognition of inequality, mindfulness, and deliberate and systematic strategies. Starting from a framework of equity and justice to drive theory development of the future will naturally and inevitably guide theoretical thinkers and fifth-generation theorists to consider our diverse world. Diversity includes diversity in ethnicity, culture, religion, socioeconomic status, gender, sexual orientation, roles of nurses, sites of care; and advancing nursing knowledge requires accounting for each of them.

Let's first discuss country and cultural diversity. To enhance the power of theories, they must be inclusive. One of the principles that could empower nurses and enrich future theories is to participate in the development of cross-national knowledge building that benefits from participation by colleagues from different parts of the world. Although certain aspects of nursing interventions are culturally contexted, the phenomena themselves transcend cultures and societies (Falk-Rafael, 2006). Comforting patients, helping wounds heal, feeding the elderly, increasing mobility and activity, rehydrating populations, preserving the integrity of clients, promoting health, developing healthy environments, promoting rest, supporting sleep, intubating, monitoring, managing symptoms, and decreasing pain are examples of phenomena that nurses deal with around the globe.

Long ago, Dr. Hiroshi Nakajima, the Director General of the World Health Organization (WHO), warned us of what continues to be true—that history will judge the 20th century as the "era when human development faltered and gave rise to a wave of poverty" (Nakajima, 1995, p. 25). The same could be said about the 21st century. Growing inequality between and within countries is, in his words, "a matter of life and death." There is an urgent need to develop knowledge about marginalization and about responses to that marginalization on the quality of health care delivered to marginalized people. Several components of marginalization are pertinent to nursing. At the core is a quest to eliminate social and economic disparities (Crigger, 2008). The definition of marginalization highlights the effects of being in stigmatized jobs, being from another culture, having a sexual preference different from the prevailing norms, lacking those mainstream characteristics that represent those who are at the center of communities, and being at the peripheries of communities. The elderly who live alone, or who have memory loss, are marginalized. These are the people who "fall between the cracks"; for example, in earthquakes, rescue workers and bystanders may not be direct victims, but they nevertheless experience traumas that have profound impact on their well-being (Taylor and Frazer, 1982). Those whose gender is in question, or those who are transgender, continue to be singled out and marginalized, whether in their needs of their daily lives or in their quest to assert their identities. When people are marginalized, they are stripped of their voices, stripped of their power, and stripped of their rights to resources.

Marginalized people tend to be reflective about their own situations and develop their own symbols and language, and these marginalize them even further. Having unique symbols, languages, dress codes, and places to meet further marginalizes them. Having delayed reactions may marginalize people. Although they may not represent another culture, their language, responses, and reactions reflect their own lexicon and their own symbols. This lexicon and the symbolism in it may not be well understood by others, and this marginalized group is pushed to the periphery even further and becomes even less powerful. Marginalized people tend to be more sensitive to the needs of others, know more about nonmarginalized people, and be less demanding of other people (Hall, Stevens, and Meleis, 1994). Future theories must address the situation of marginalized clients in the health care system and reflect health and illness responses within a context of marginalization.

However, nurses care for members of the population that also hold privileged statuses as well. With growing theoretical discussions in nursing on women's health, the elderly population, the poor, the underrepresented minorities, and the homeless population, are we marginalizing those who hold privileged societal positions and who reflect more the majority than the minority? Sellman (2005) argues that all individuals who are patients are "more than ordinarily vulnerable." In what ways are we developing knowledge that reflects and addresses the experiences of minorities—vulnerable, underserved, and marginalized—and the privileged? What arguments do we hold for either or for both? A social justice framework and engagement in diverse dialogues may promote the development of concepts and theories that reflect global health and illness responses and experiences of populations regardless of their positions in societies (Anderson, Rodney, Reimer-Kirkham, et al., 2009).

Covering the various dimensions about the nature of phenomena through international work creates knowledge that is more culturally sensitive and empowers nurses to influence policy changes related to health care. Committing to globally relevant topics, particularly ones with relevance to social problems, produces passionate scholars and may increase scholarly productivity (Heinrich, 2010). Sharing and reciprocating findings about phenomena increases nurses' repertoires of therapeutics that would, in turn, enhance their effectiveness in caring for diverse populations. The principle of a global view could ensure that nurses' efforts in knowledge development become more cumulative, more culturally sensitive, more attuned to oppressive power relations, and more responsive to the concerns of the world (Georges, 2008). Culturally sensitive theories help nurses become more culturally competent in a world that is constantly in transition, one in which patients tend to reflect diversity. This principle mandates thinking internationally in every aspect of our work and in the theories that we attempt to develop, with attention to the common good. A framework of social and economic justice geared toward addressing disparities is more congruent with global concerns (Crigger, 2008). Yet relativism in developing knowledge, limited resources, and constraints in creating global teams may act as barriers to developing global theories. Our international colleagues continue to remain skeptical about the ability of nurses to collaborate on an equal basis to develop theories that address nursing phenomena from a global perspective. They remind us that theories developed in the United Kingdom, Sweden, Finland, Brazil, and France are barely recognizable in the United States. (And this U.S.-centric book is an example; page limitation is an excuse, but not a totally convincing one!). Our knowledge is U.S.-based, but since the empowerment of nurses and the enhancement of quality care require a global application, such application should be informed by global theories. How will we be able to reconcile these differences in the future? What will it be—local or global theories? Robust dialogues between East and West and North and South must be the norm in the future (Salas, 2005).

The nature of nursing practice is profoundly influenced by the sociocultural and political events in any society, as well as its technological advancements. Major changes occurred in the health care system during the 1990s that will continue to influence the types of theories that nurses may develop, as well as the utility of these theories. The movements to primary health care and managed care increase the potential of educating more primary caregivers, because the scarcity of primary care providers decreases the length of time that nurses spend with patients. Theories of the late 1990s—which provided guidelines for developing trust and strong interpersonal ties with patients, the role of the self in the healing processes, and the extensive assessment and monitoring that nurses were able to perform during long hospitalizations or repeated visits—will be limited. Models to promote patient–nurse relationships within the constraints dictated by time, technology, and more economically driven health care encounters will be developed. Therefore, the nature of relationships that incorporates technology needs to be redefined, and ways by which such relationships may be established must be reconsidered (Betts, 2005).

Diversity is also about the different sites where nurse–patient encounters occur. Most of the theories that have been developed have started from the premise that the nursing client is a hospitalized person. Over the years, patients have moved out of the hospitals earlier, and, whenever possible, are cared for on an outpatient basis. Although public health nurses have always given care to patients in communities and in their homes, the practice of public health nursing is undergoing drastic changes simultaneously, and patients are also going home with more acute conditions and with a need for monitoring of their critical needs, within the limitations of time and budgetary constraints.

The nature of practice is also changing in another major way. Old international mandates (WHO, 1978) for better health care have advocated community-based primary health care as the practice of choice to ensure better health care for people and better access to health care have become more urgent in the 21st century. Community-based health care requires the development of models for care that are more complex and contextual and that are created with clients' involvement.

There is also a growing diversity in the roles that nurses and other caregivers perform. More specifically, the nature of practice is influenced by the changing roles of advanced nursing practice clinicians, which may require rethinking theories needed for their practice (Davies and Hughes, 1995). Another example is the increasing number of generalists and primary health care providers in medicine and the changes in their educational preparation and training. Another is the increasing number of care assistants and physician's assistants. Similarly, the interface between technology, genomic technology, and nursing practice is changing, and this requires careful development of theories that incorporate this progress (Loescher and Merkle, 2005).

There is also diversity in nurses' knowledge, roles, and actions that must inform theory development. It has been advocated that the development of theories in the future must avoid what Bradshaw (1995) warned against in the past; that is, ignoring the nursing tradition of practical tasks and the techniques of physical care and focusing only on a psychosocial approach to patient care and knowledge development. She proposes that nurses engaged in the development of knowledge must consider rediscovering theories that hold together the personal, the relational, the scientific, and the technological aspects of patient care. Similarly, a focus only on what nurses do rather than on what nurses know and on the context in which they practice contributes to disempower and silence nurses (Canam, 2008). Development of the discipline and members of the discipline must include the pragmatics of what nurses do and the expansive scope of knowledge that incorporates past, present, and future (Litchfield and Jónsdóttir, 2008). Diversity and inclusiveness are challenges in all aspects of nursing education, practice, research, and policy development. But, it is through an inclusive framework that fifth-generation theories will provide the frameworks for providing quality care that makes a difference in the lives of populations.

CONCLUSION

This chapter discusses the urgency of creating the future of theoretical nursing and the challenges and opportunities that could hinder or facilitate development, refinement, and progress in nursing theory. To jump-start again our theoretical future, discipline members must continue investing in and nurturing a strong disciplinary identity, promoting theoretical and philosophical discourses, and facilitating the education and the development of fifth-generation theorists. They also must address threats that may slow progress and use these threats as futuristic opportunities. Among them are the threat to losing a nursing identity and voice through interprofessionalism, developing theories that are guided by revolutions in science but are not reflective of the goals and mission of nursing, and utilizing dynamic and innovative technology to become entrepreneurs, which may lead to a reductionist approach to caring. There is also the threat of developing and advancing knowledge that does not reflect the increasing diversity of the U.S. population, as well as providing a global perspective. The significance of futuristic theories is in answering the pressing global questions in nursing and in developing

REFLECTIVE QUESTIONS

1. Identify two paradoxes that may promote or impede advancing nursing knowledge.

2. Take one side of each paradox, and develop compelling arguments toward promoting it.

3. In what ways is the support for evidence-based practice an indication of progress in the discipline? Discuss the pros and cons of using it as a framework for education and practice.

4. What might be some best practices for incorporating theoretical discourses in nursing education and nursing practice? What might be some least effective practices? Identify and critique one of these practices.

5. Select one of the challenges presented in this chapter and discuss ways by which you may choose to integrate it as an opportunity in your field of interest.

6. In your opinion, what is the most pressing challenge currently facing the further advancement of nursing knowledge?

7. Will we be able to develop theories that honor the technical aspects of nursing and continue to inform equally the psychosocial and biobehavioral aspects of nursing? Can a theory comprehensively address these different components of human beings? Reflect on these questions and develop a defensible argument.

fifth-generation theories that reflect the history and practice of nursing. While each threat may lead to a different outcome, together they may lead to the loss of nursing identity, voice, and influence in what matters the most, which is the well-being of populations. Recognizing these threats could lead to many opportunities for innovations in health care.

REFERENCES

Adams, J.M. (2014). How do we know if we're innovating? Setting the strategy for innovation evaluation – Guest editorial. *Journal of Nursing Administration*, 44(2), 63–64.

Allan, J. and Hall, B. (1988). Challenging the focus on technology: A critique of the medical model in a changing health care system. *Advances in Nursing Science*, 10(3), 22–34.

Allen, D.G. (1987). The social policy statement: A reappraisal. *Advances in Nursing Science*, 10(1), 39–48.

Alligood, M.R. (2014). *Nursing theorists and their work* (8th ed.). St Louis, MO: Mosby

Anderson, J.A., Rodney, P., Reimer-Kirkham, S., Browne, A.J., Khan, K.B., and Lynam, M.J. (2009). Inequities in health and health care viewed through the ethical lens of critical social justice: Contextual knowledge for the global priorities ahead. *Advances in Nursing Science*, 32(4), 282–294.

Anderson, R.A., Dobal, M.T., and Blessing, B. (1992). Theory-based approach to computer skill development in nursing administration. *Computers in Nursing*, 10(4), 152–157.

Barr, H. (2013). Toward a theoretical framework for interprofessional education. *Journal of Interprofessional Care*, 27(1), 4–9.

Batra, C. (1987). Nursing theory for undergraduates. *Nursing Outlook*, 35(4), 189–192.

Betts, C.E. (2005). Progress, epistemology and human health and welfare: What nurses need to know and why. *Nursing Philosophy*, 6(3), 174–188.

Bhutta, Z.A., Chen, L., Cohen, J., Crisp, N., et al. (2010). Education of health professionals for the 21st century: A global independent commission. *Lancet*, 375(9721), 1137–1138.

Bowles, K.H., Dykes, P. and Demiris, G. (2015). The use of health information technology to improve care and outcomes for older adults. *Research in Gerontological Nursing*, 8(1), 5–10.

Bowles, K.H., Hanlon, A.L., Holland, D.E., Potashnik, S., and Topaz, M. (2014). Impact of discharge planning decision support on time to readmission among older adult medical patients. *Professional Case Management*, 19(1), 29–38.

Bradshaw, A. (1995). What are nurses doing to patients? A review of theories of nursing past and present. *Journal of Clinical Nursing*, 4(2), 81–92.

Brown, S.J. (1996). [Letter to the editor]. *Advances in Nursing Science*, 18(4), vi–vii.

Canam, C.J. (2008). The link between nursing discourses and nurses' silence: Implications for a knowledge-based discourse for nursing practice. *Advances in Nursing Science*, 31(4), 296–307.

Chinn, P.L. (2007). Challenge to action. In C. Roy and D.A. Jones (Eds.), *Nursing knowledge development and clinical practice*. New York: Springer

Chinn, P.L. (2008). A postmodern view of evidence – letter to the editor. *Advances in Nursing Science*, 31(4), 281.

Chinn, P.L. (2014). Nursing theories for the 21st century – letter from the editor. *Advances in Nursing Science*, 37(1), 1.

Christmyer, C.S., Catanzariti, P.M., Langford, A.M., and Reiz, J.A. (1988). Bridging the gap: Theory to practice–Part I, clinical applications. *Nursing Management*, 19(9), 42–50.

Cioffi, J.M. (2015). Insight and discovery in clinical nursing practice. *Collegian*. doi:10.1016/j.colegn.2015.10.004

Crigger, N.J. (2008). Towards a viable and just global nursing ethics. *Nursing Ethics*, 15(1), 17–27.

Cronenwett, L. and Dzau, V. (2010). Who will provide primary care and how will they be trained? In B.J. Culliton and S. Russell (Eds.), *Proceedings of a conference sponsored by the Josiah Macy, Jr. Foundation*. Durham, NC: Josiah Macy, Jr. Foundation

Dashiff, C. (1988). Theory development in psychiatric mental health nursing: An analysis of Orem's theory. *Archives of Psychiatric Nursing*, 2(6), 366–372.

Davidson, P.M. (2016). Rockefeller Foundation-Lancet Commission report: A call for action for human health. *International Journal of Nursing Studies*, 53, 1–2.

Davies, B. and Hughes, A.M. (1995). Clarification of advanced nursing practice: Characteristics and competencies. *Clinical Nurse Specialist*, 9(3), 156–160.

DeGroot, H.A., Ferketich, S.L., and Larson, P.J. (1987). Theory development in a non-university service setting. *Journal of Nursing Administration*, 17(4), 38–44.

Dewey, J. (1982). *How we think*. Lexington, MA: Heath (originally published in 1910).

Engel, G.L. (1977). The need for a new medical model: A challenge for biomedicine. *Science*, 196, 129–137.

Facione, N.C., Facione, P.A., and Sanchez, C.A. (1994). Critical thinking disposition as a measure of competent clinical judgment. The development of the "California Critical Thinking Disposition Inventory." *Journal of Nursing Education*, 33(8), 345–350.

Falk-Rafael, A. (2006). Globalization and global health: Toward nursing praxis in the global community. *Advances in Nursing Science*, 29(1), 2–14.

Fawcett, J. (2006). Commentary: Finding patterns of knowing in the work of Florence Nightingale. *Nursing Outlook*, 54(5), 275–277.

Fawcett, J. (2008). On 'evidence-based practice': Purpose of research is to develop theory. *Nursing Science Quarterly*, 21(1), 89.

Fawcett, J. (2012). Thoughts on concept analysis: Multiple approaches, one result. *Nursing Science Quarterly*, 25(3), 285–287.

Fawcett, J. and Alligood, M.R. (2005). Influences on advancement of nursing knowledge. *Nursing Science Quarterly*, 18(3), 227–232.

Frickel, S. (2004). Building an interdiscipline: Collective action framing and the rise of genetic toxicology. *Social Problems*, 51(2), 269–287.

Georges, J.M. (2008). Bio-power, Agamben, and emerging nursing knowledge. *Advances in Nursing Science*, 31(1), 4–12.

Gillman M.W. and Hammond, R.A. (2016). Precision treatment and precision prevention: Integrating 'below and above the skin.' *Journal of the American Medical Association Pediatrics*, 170(1), 9–10.

Glenister, D. (2011). *Towards a general systems theory of nursing: A literature review*. In Proceedings of the 55th annual meeting of the ISSS. Hull, UK.

Grace, P.J., Willis, D.G., Roy, C., and Jones, D.A. (2016). Profession at the crossroads: A dialog concerning the preparation of nursing scholars and leaders. *Nursing Outlook*, 64(1), 61–70.

Grady, P.A. (2014). Charting future directions in nursing research: NINR's innovative questions initiative – guest editorial. *Journal of Nursing Scholarship*, 46(3), 143.

Grady, P.A. (2015). A pathway for the future: An update on NINR's innovative questions initiative – guest editorial. *Journal of Nursing Scholarship*, 47(2), 105.

Grey, M. and Connolly, C.A. (2008). Coming together, keeping together, working together: Interdisciplinary to transdisciplinary research and nursing. *Nursing Outlook*, 56(3), 102–107.

Grey, M. and Mitchell, P.H. (2008). Guest editorial: Nursing and interdisciplinary research. *Nursing Outlook*, 56(3), 95–96.

Hall, J.M., Stevens, P.E., and Meleis, A.I. (1994). Marginalization: A guiding concept for valuing diversity in nursing knowledge development. *Advances in Nursing Science*, 16(4), 23–41.

Hays, B.J., Norris, J., Martin, K.S., and Androwich, I. (1994). Informatics issues for nursing's future. *Advances in Nursing Science*, 16(4), 71–81.

Heinrich, K.T. (2010). Passionate scholarship 2001–2010: A vision for making academe safer for joyous risk-takers. *Advances in Nursing Science*, 33(1), E50–E64.

Henry, B., Arndt, C., DiVincenti, M., and Marriner-Tomey, A. (Eds.). (1989). *Dimensions of nursing administration: Theory, research, education, practice*. Boston, MA: Blackwell Scientific Publications.

Holt, J. (2014). Nursing in the 21st century: Is there a place for nursing philosophy? *Nursing Philosophy*, 15(1), 1–3.

Jacobs-Kramer, M. and Huether, S.E. (1988). Curricular considerations for teaching nursing theory. *Journal of Professional Nursing*, 4(5), 373–380.

Jacobson, S. (1987). Studying and using conceptual models of nursing. *Image: Journal of Nursing Scholarship*, 19(2), 78–82.

Jameson, J.L. and Longo, D.L. (2015). Precision medicine – personalized, problematic, and promising. *New England Journal of Medicine*, 372(23), 2229–2234.

Jeffs, L., Sidani, S., Rose, D., Espin, S., Smith, O., et al. (2013). Using theory and evidence to drive measurement of patient, nurse and organizational outcomes of professional nursing practice. *International Journal of Nursing Practice*, 19(2), 141–148.

Jennings, B.M. and Meleis, A.I. (1988). Nursing theory and administration practice: Agenda for the 1990s. *Advances in Nursing Science*, 10(3), 56–69.

Josiah Macy Jr. Foundation. (2013). *Interprofessional care coordination: Looking to the future. Issue brief* (Vol. 1, Issue 2). New York, NY: The Josiah Macy Jr. Foundation.

Karmels, P. (1993). Conundrum game for nursing theorists Neuman, King, and Johnson. *Nurse Educator*, 18(6), 8–9.

Kim, H.S. (2010). *The nature of theoretical nursing in nursing* (3rd ed.). New York: Springer.

Kneipp, S.M., Gilleskie, D., Sheely, A., Schwartz, T., Gilmore, R.M., and Atkinson, D. (2014). Nurse scientists overcoming challenges to lead transdisciplinary research teams. *Nursing Outlook*, 62(5), 352–361.

Knight, E.P. and Shea, K. (2014). A patient-focused framework integrating self-management and informatics. *Journal of Nursing Scholarship*, 46(2), 91–97.

Kovalainen, A. and Osterberg-Hogstedt, J. (2013). Entrepreneurship within social and health care: A question of identity, gender and professionalism. *International Journal of Gender and Entrepreneurship*, 5(1), 17–35.

Laudan, L. (1981). A problem solving approach to scientific growth. In I. Hacking (Ed.), *Scientific revolutions*. Oxford, UK: Oxford University Press.

Lenz, E.R., Suppe, F., Gift, A.G., Pugh, L.C., and Milligan, R.A. (1995). Collaborative development of middle-range nursing theories: Toward a theory of unpleasant symptoms. *Advances in Nursing Science*, 17(3), 1–13.

Levine, M.E. (1995). The rhetoric of nursing theory. *Image: Journal of Nursing Scholarship*, 27(1), 11–14.

Lewis, K.B., Stacey, D., Squires, J.E., and Carroll, S. (2016). Shared decision-making models acknowledging an interprofessional approach: A theory analysis to inform nursing practice. *Research and Theory for Nursing Practice: An International Journal*, 30(1), 26–43.

Litchfield, M.C. and Jónsdóttir, H. (2008). A practice discipline that's here and now. *Advances in Nursing Science*, 31(1), 79–91.

Lloyd, J.V., Schneider, J., Scales, K., Bailey, S., and Jones, R. (2011). Ingroup identity as an obstacle to effective multiprofessional and interprofessional teamwork: Findings from an ethnographic study of healthcare assistants in dementia care. *Journal of Interprofessional Care*, 25(5), 345–351.

Loescher, L.J. and Merkle, C.J. (2005). The interface of genomic technologies and nursing. *Journal of Nursing Scholarship*, 37(2), 111–119.

Macy Foundation. (2004). Personal Communication.

McIntyre, M. and McDonald, C. (2013). Contemplating the fit and utility of nursing theory and nursing scholarship informed by the social sciences and humanities. *Advances in Nursing Science*, 36(1), 10–17.

Meleis, A.I. (1992). Theoretical thinking progress in the discipline of nursing. In K. Kraus and P. Astedt-Kurki (Eds.), *International perspectives on nursing* (pp. 1–12). Tampere, Finland: University of Tampere Department of Nursing.

Meleis, A.I. (2015). Interprofessional education: A summary of reports and barriers to recommendations. *Journal of Nursing Scholarship*, 48(1), 106–112.

Meleis, A.I., Isenberg, M., Koerner, J.E., Lacey, B., and Stern, P. (1995). *Diversity, marginalization, and culturally competent health care issues in knowledge development*. Washington, DC: American Academy of Nursing.

Meleis, A.I. and Jennings, B.M. (1989). Theoretical nursing administration: Today's challenges, tomorrow's bridges. In B. Henry, C. Arndt, M. DiVincenti, and A. Marriner-Tomey (Eds.), *Dimensions of nursing administration: Theory, research, education, practice*. Boston, MA: Blackwell Scientific Publications.

Meleis, A.I. and Price, M.J. (1988). Strategies and conditions for teaching theoretical nursing: An international perspective. *Journal of Advanced Nursing*, 13, 592–604.

Moore, S.E., Holaday, B., Meehan, N., and Watt, P.J. (2015). Exploring mHealth as a new route to bridging the nursing theory-practice gap. *Research and Theory for Nursing Practice: An International Journal*, 29(1), 38–52.

Nagel, D.A., Pomerleau, S.G., and Penner, J.L. (2013). Knowing, caring, and telehealth technology: Going the distance in nursing practice. *Journal of Holistic Nursing*, 31(2), 104–112.

Nakajima, H. (1995, May 20). Growing inequity is a matter of life and death [editorial]. Michigan State University IIH, Newsletter, p. 25.

National Academy of Medicine-formerly Institute of Medicine (NAM). (2010). *The future of nursing: Leading change, advancing health*. Washington, DC: The National Academies Press.

NAM. (2013). *Establishing transdisciplinary professionalism for improving health outcomes: Workshop summary*. Washington, DC: The National Academies Press.

Nilsson, L., Hofflander, M., Eriksen, S., and Borg, C. (2012). The importance of interaction in the implementation of information technology in health care: A symbolic interactionism study on the meaning of accessibility. *Informatics for Health and Social Care*, 37(4), 277–290.

Papp, K.K., Huang, G.C., Clabo, L.M.L., Delva, D., Fischer, M., Konopasek, L., Schwartzstein, R.M., and Gusic, M. (2014). Milestones of critical thinking: A developmental model for medicine and nursing. *Academic Medicine*, 89(5), 715–720.

Penn Nursing. (2016a). University of Pennsylvania School of Nursing Health Technology Innovation Incubator featuring Dr. Barbara Medoff-Cooper: Neonur – Big breakthrough for the tiniest hearts. Retrieved from http://www.nursing.upenn.edu/innovation/health-technology-lab/Pages/Our-Projects.aspx?itemID=4

Penn Nursing. (2016b). University of Pennsylvania School of Nursing Health Technology Innovation Incubator featuring Dr. Terri Lipman: MyDiaText – Healthy motivations for kids with Type 1 diabetes. Retrieved from http://www.nursing.upenn.edu/innovation/health-technology-lab/Pages/Our-Projects.aspx?itemCategory=mHealth

Peter, E. and Liaschenko, J. (2013). Moral distress reexamined: A feminist interpretation of nurses' identities, relationships, and responsibilities. *Journal of Bioethical Inquiry*, 10(3), 337–345.

Rafferty, A.M., Allcock, N., and Lathlean, J. (1996). The theory/practice 'gap': Taking issue with the issue. *Journal of Advanced Nursing*, 23, 685–691.

Reeves, S. and Hean, S. (2013). Why we need theory to help us better understand the nature of interprofessional education, practice and care. *Journal of Interprofessional Care*, 27(1), 1–3.

Rhoten, D. and Parker, A. (2004). Risks and rewards of an interdisciplinary research path. *Science*, 306(5704), 2046.

Salas, A.S. (2005). Toward a north-south dialogue: Revisiting nursing theory (from the south). *Advances in Nursing Science*, 28(1), 17–24.

Sellman, D. (2005). Towards an understanding of nursing as a response to human vulnerability. *Nursing Philosophy*, 6(1), 2–10.

Sharts-Hopko, N.C. (2013). Tackling complex problems, building evidence for practice, and educating doctoral nursing students to manage the tension. *Nursing Outlook*, 61(2), 102–108.

Shaver, J. (1985). A biopsychosocial view of human health. *Nursing Outlook*, 33(4), 186–1101.

Smith, M.J. and Liehr, P.R. (2013). *Middle-range theory for nursing* (3rd ed.). New York: Springer.

Strober, M.H. (2006). Habits of the mind: Challenges for multidisciplinary engagement. *Social Epistemology*, 20(3/4), 315–331.

Strudwick, G., Booth, R., and Mistry, K. (2016). Can social cognitive theories help us understand nurses' use of electronic health records? *CIN: Computers, Information, Nursing*, 34(4), 169–174.

Taylor, A.J.W. and Frazer, A.G. (1982). The stress of post-disaster body handling and victim identification work. *Journal of Human Stress*, 8, 4–12.

Thorne, S. (2014). Nursing as social justice: A case for emancipatory disciplinary theorizing. In P.N. Kagan, M.C. Smith and P.L. Chinn (Eds.), *Philosophies and practices of emancipatory nursing: Social justice as praxis*. New York: Routledge.

Tiedeman, M.E. and Lookinland, S. (2004). Traditional models of care delivery. *Journal of Nursing Administration*, 34(6), 291–297.

University of California, San Francisco, School of Nursing Symptom Management Faculty Group. (1994). A model for symptom management. *Image: Journal of Nursing Scholarship*, 26(4), 272–276.

Van Herk, K.A., Smith, D., and Andrew, C. (2011). Examining our privileges and oppressions: Incorporating an intersectionality paradigm into nursing. *Nursing Inquiry*, 18(1), 29–39.

Visintainer, M. (1986). The nature of knowledge and theory in nursing. *Image: Journal of Nursing Scholarship*, 18(2), 32–38.

Whall, A.L., Sinclair, M., and Parahoo, K. (2006). A philosophic analysis of evidence-based nursing: Recurrent themes, metanarratives, and exemplar cases. *Nursing Outlook*, 54(1), 30–35.

Willis, D.G., Grace, P.J., and Roy, C. (2008). A central unifying focus for the discipline: Facilitating humanization, meaning, choice, quality of life, and healing in living and dying. *Advances in Nursing Science*, 31(1), E28–E40.

Wilson, H.S. (1985). *Research in nursing*. Menlo Park, CA: Addison-Wesley.

World Health Organization. (1978). *Primary health care. Report on primary health care*. Geneva, Switzerland: Alma Ata, USSR.

Part Seven

OUR HISTORICAL AND CURRENT LITERATURE

Literature in nursing is rich with writings in theory, of theory, and on theory. Some of the writings provided significant milestones in the shaping of the theoretical progress in nursing. Chapters 20 and 21 of this book are organized around these writings. They provide an **analytical review of the central and classical literature** in metatheory and theory up to the beginning of the 1980s. Chapter 21 provides a **categorized listing of literature related to theory** through 2016.

These chapters are offered for students, faculty, clinicians, and researchers. The serious theory student needs analytical familiarity with the significant writing that shaped progress in the discipline of nursing. The cursory theory student can find these chapters helpful as an overview of writing related to nursing theory. All concerned with the discipline of nursing will find that the literature relates, in some way, to their specific area of expertise. This literature is a significant component of our heritage, without which our practice, teaching, and research are limited.

20

Historical Writings in Theory

To develop, analyze, or critique theories, a theory student, user, or developer needs a background that includes all the significant writings related to theoretical nursing. This chapter provides the reader with a critical assessment of the central writing contained in the nursing literature of the 1980s. With the publication of *Advances in Nursing Science*, as well as of other theoretically oriented journals and books, theory literature has developed and proliferated exponentially, and it is therefore no longer possible to include a comprehensive critical assessment of writings in theory. As many as possible of those writings on theory up to the early 1980s that are considered classic are included in this chapter.

The chapter is divided into two sections. Section I includes analysis and critique of the metatheory literature. Section II includes analysis and critique of the literature on nursing theory, written by nurse theorists or by others who have used nursing theory in research, practice, education, and administration. All analytical abstracts are listed alphabetically within the sections.

A reader can use this chapter in many ways: *first*, the reader can use it in conjunction with the contents of various chapters in the book; *second*, when studying a particular theorist's work, the reader can identify citations related to the theorist and can pull out those that have been abstracted for review; *third*, Section I could be read in its entirety as a way to prepare for a general overview of nursing theory; *fourth*, the reader can divide the writings in Section II into those relating to a particular theory or read the abstracts related to each theorist separately; and *fifth*, readers interested in the development of theoretical nursing may wish to have a temporal perspective by reading abstracts according to year of citation.

The intent of the abstracts is to challenge readers to different interpretations, not to critique the writing. *Readers are encouraged to read original writings and to use these analytical abstracts only to provide them with one perspective of the writings.* Finally, the reader should remember that the analyses here include the interpretation of the authors who abstracted them, which may or may not agree with others' interpretations.

SECTION I

Abstracts of Writings in Metatheory, 1960–1984
ELLEN MAHONEY • AFAF MELEIS

Abdellah, F. (1969). The nature of nursing science. Nursing Research, 18(5), 390–393.

This article seeks to move toward the "identification of nursing science." History is reviewed, and nursing scientists are exhorted to build on the work of nurse pioneers who were mainly theorists. Nursing science is defined as a body of cumulative scientific knowledge (drawn from the physical, biologic, and behavioral sciences) that is uniquely nursing. Emphasis is on

an evolving science. The more that nursing research is directed by scientific theory, the more likely its results will contribute to the development of a nursing science. There are too few nursing scientists (should be 1%), but the numbers are growing. "It is the inescapable role of the nurse–scientist to point the way for change in nursing."

This is a short overview article, but it contains details of nursing history and random observations of interest.

Andreoli, K.G. and Thompson, C.E. (1977).
The nature of science in nursing. **Image, 9(2),**
32–37.

The theoretical basis of practice is the science of
nursing, and it defines nursing's uniqueness. Science is defined as a system of knowledge based on
scientific principles. Its ultimate goal is the discovery of new knowledge, the expansion of existing
knowledge, and the reaffirmation of previously held
knowledge. Nursing is defined by abstracting the
major elements from the conceptions of several
nursing theorists. Science in nursing (the body of
verified knowledge found within the discipline of
nursing) is distinguished from the science of nursing (that body of verifiable knowledge that will be
derived from nursing practice, the unique way in
which nursing uses borrowed knowledge). Nursing
will attain the status of a science once it has clearly
identified a verifiable knowledge base that can be
contested and corroborated. This knowledge base
will come from practice. Specific attention is given
to the scientific methodologies of nursing research,
conceptual models in nursing, the nursing process,
and nursing diagnosis as a means of developing a
knowledge base.

The fact that the article offers more than the
others in the category is an interesting argument
for the integration of basic and applied science and
the sections on scientific methodologies in nursing
that stress the theory–practice–research link. One
might argue that the "unique" elements of nursing
presented are really not so unique. The definition of
"science" comes from the dictionary; the conceptions of nursing science presented (especially by
Johnson and Rogers) should be read in the original.

Batey, M.V. (1972). Values relative to research
and to science in nursing as influenced by a
sociological perspective. **Nursing Research,**
21(6), 504–508.

Central to the development of the science of nursing
is the continuing issue of the function of values in
research and in science. This article is a response
to the question: How does preparation in one of the
disciplines related to nursing bear on the identification
and conceptualization of nursing research problems
and approaches used to design and carry through
an investigation? Batey's response is organized
in three topics: (1) an overview of her conceptual
and methodological orientation in sociology; (2)

illustrations of the research in her work; and (3)
contrasting perspectives of science with thought
geared toward nursing science. It is to the third
topic that the abstract is addressed.

Research is a tool of science; the goal of science
is the continuing advancement of an objective body
of knowledge. Batey contrasts two perspectives
of science: (1) as a social system with values (expressed) as the desired goal toward which science
strives (i.e., an advancing and objectively verified
body of knowledge), *norms* (expected standards of
behavior, including disinterest, organized skepticism, and communality), and *pertained relations*
(the expectation of a competent response to one's
creative effort) versus (2) as a means (knowledge
for use). An investigator's perspective will influence types of research problems identified, as well
as the selection of knowledge brought to bear for
their conceptualization and research methodologies.
In nursing, where knowledge is valued for its use
(perspective 2), it is hypothesized that a greater
emphasis is placed on descriptive studies than on the
subsequent stages of the discovery process toward
an objectively verified body of knowledge. Until
we alter our normative system in nursing relative
to science, we can expect little movement toward
nursing science.

Whereas a major thrust of the article focuses on
the dilemma of conflicting values for nurses educated
in other fields, the section "Perspectives of Science"
(pp. 507–508) is provocative and well worth reading, particularly after exposure to explications of
nursing science and arguments for practice theory.
Does the reader agree with Batey's hypothesis that
a discipline emphasizing knowledge for use will
emphasize descriptive research?

Batey, M.V. (1977). Conceptualization:
Knowledge and logic guiding empirical
research. **Nursing Research, 26(5), 324–329.**

This is an excellent article analyzing functions and
processes of research conceptualization. Analyzing
a systematic sample of articles published in *Nurs-*
ing Research, Batey identified "limiting features"
representing problems of: (1) the *conceptual phase*
("fallacies of reasoning, specification of meaning,
and use of knowledge in conveying the problem,
conceptual framework, and/or purpose"); (2) the
empirical phase ("technical processes related to
the methods and procedures of data production
and reduction"); and (3) the *interpretative phase*

("analytical processes related to deriving meanings of findings"). Batey judged that the vast majority of problems are due to limitations of the conceptual phase, particularly the lack of clear definition and inadequate development or utilization of a conceptual framework. Factors contributing to conceptual limitations are identified, as are their consequences.

The remainder of the paper is an explication of the conceptual phase of research to achieve a reduction of the limitations noted. Components of the conceptual phase are: (1) The *problem* determines the context of the study by setting the major parameters of the phenomenon of concern; it includes what, how, why, or under what conditions phenomena occur, and a normative statement; (2) the *conceptual framework* involves background knowledge that delineates the present knowledge state about the problem and that yields the theoretical statement through which the investigator attempts to construct an accurate image of the phenomenon of study; it includes background (review of literature) and rationale (theoretical framework); and (3) the *purpose* is derived from the rationale; the research purpose is the hypothesis to be tested.

The article also includes brief but helpful sections on purposes and methods for literature review, scientific versus commonsense meanings of concepts, tips on critical reading, and guidelines for the interpretative phase and its dynamic relation to conceptualization.

There is some overlap and lack of clarity in defining the three components of the conceptual phase, and it would have been appropriate to explicate more on the theoretical background of a study. This article should be read in the context of other articles that address conceptualization and conceptual frameworks. Besides tying these phases together, this article provides useful criteria for the design and evaluation of research.

Becker, C.H. (1983). A conceptualization of concept. Nursing Papers: Perspectives in Nursing, *15(2), 51–58.*

The first part of this article is a series of lists. The first list has to do with characteristics of concepts: ambiguity, conventional meaning, dependent on context, neither false nor true, and either significant or nonsignificant. The author inserts an observation: "Concepts arise in the mind of an individual as a result of attempts to make order out of what is observed."

The next list describes modes of concept analysis (from Edel, 1979): Socratic (general and essential), element analysis, genetic (how evolved), functional, systems, pragmatic, logical, operational, and phenomenological. A summary list gives the requirements for an appropriate use of concepts in theory development: "(1) concepts have intention; (2) concepts are seen as models of some aspect of reality; (3) the concepts selected are significant; (4) the mode of concept analysis dictates the method of investigation of the concept; (5) the value bias and semantic overtones are inherently present in the concepts selected for study; and (6) concepts are subject to continual analysis and refinement."

Then, micro-concepts are endorsed: "micro-concepts rather than general macro-concepts may have the potential to contribute more to the structuring of nursing knowledge." An example is given: self-esteem (micro) versus personality (macro). The author presents the following reasoning: "Macro-concepts, because of their generalness, have a loose flexibility of meaning. Micro-concepts would not allow this looseness." There are also lesser variables in micro-level concepts: (1) the intention of the author is easily understood; (2) meaning is not so easily distorted; (3) the most appropriate mode of analysis is easily identified; and (4) there is no polarity.

Beckstrand, J. (1978). The notion of a practice theory and the relationship of scientific and ethical knowledge to practice. Research in Nursing and Health, *1(3), 131–136.*

Beckstrand critiques several authors who have supported a "practice theory" (Dickoff and James, Jacox, etc.). For such notions to be meaningful, practice knowledge must be shown to be different from scientific knowledge or ethical knowledge, or else "no need for a separate practice theory would exist." Two primary aspects of practice knowledge, the knowledge of how to make changes, and the knowledge of what is "good" are examined. First *science*, "the knowledge of lawlike empirical relationships," is studied to determine if it includes the knowledge used to control phenomena in practice. Beckstrand provides an extended summary discussion of the nature of scientific knowledge, relating it to the notion of "control." "The potential for controlling a phenomenon is synonymous with lawlike relationships and the potential for prediction that they provide. . . . Science seeks to establish the knowledge that allows for this kind of control." To make changes one must have some control. Although practice often seeks this control through invalid argument, "functional argument," and empirical generalization, these are "based on the knowledge of scientific laws and lawlike relationships." The controls possible in scientific experimentation are impossible in the practice situation, but despite uncertainty of outcome, practice methodology nonetheless proceeds by valid deduction from scientific laws.

Next is a review of the field of ethics. Ethics is concerned with the knowledge of what is right, good, or obligatory. Both normative ethics and metaethics have relevance to practice. But theories of the moral obligations of practitioners "are identical in form" to other theories of moral obligation; theories of moral value in practice do not represent unique forms of theory. The goals defined in practice are not moral values that may be determined by the methods of ethical philosophy and no others. In short, "it would appear that there is no need for a practice theory distinct from a scientific or ethical theory."

The bulk of the article is Beckstrand's reading in the philosophy of science and ethical theory. Her more abbreviated attempts to apply these readings to Dickoff and colleagues are dependent on crucial unargued and unevidenced assertions. For example, (1) the relation of "practice knowledge," (Beckstrand's term) to "practice theory," which is the focus of the authors she surveys, after all, to have a theory of teaching is not to have the knowledge to teach a course in Russian history; (2) the assertion that practice knowledge can be broken down into two generalizations—"how to make changes" and "what is good"—without oversimplification or distortion; and (3) the assertion that unscientific reasoning and procedures are "based" on scientific reasoning and procedures. Although Beckstrand argues that the knowledge on which practice is based is science knowledge, she admits outright that the reasoning process in practice is often unscientific, and she ignores experience, tradition, or even nonscientific logic as bases.

Beckstrand emphasizes what might be called "content" with regard to science and practice theory (i.e., concern only for the knowledge in science and practice and not the reasoning processes, and concern only for just what information, basically, is used in it and not for the descriptive shape of the activity, its form, nor its outline definition). Beckstrand reverses herself when discussing ethics, saying that although there may be specific ethical obligations or directives especially and uniquely

applicable to a practice, the form of the theory is that of an ethical theory. Might one not ask her then, why a theory of practice (although the information used in it may well be the same as ethics and science) cannot remain unique because its shape and its form is that of a practice theory?

Beckstrand, J. (1978). The need for a practice theory as indicated by the knowledge used in conduct of practice. Research in Nursing and Health, 1(4), 175–179.

Beckstrand's aim is to extend her previous argument. Her first article said that "much of the knowledge required for practice is the knowledge of science and ethics." Here, she "examines" practice to see if "the theoretical knowledge used in practice is completely defined by science, ethics, and logic." To determine this, she turns to the definition of the purpose of practice: "Practice attempts to *change* an entity or phenomenon in such a way that a greater good is realized." Accomplishing change in practice necessitates the knowledge of both change and action. This knowledge can be reduced to limited categorization, but Beckstrand broadens the base of necessary knowledge here to include "the domain of logic in general."

Following this is the logical analysis of the conduct of practice. First, she discusses conditions. She asserts that "[t]o say that an interaction is meaningful is to say that the interaction has logical implications in relation to existing scientific or ethical knowledge." She argues that although the combination of conditions in each situation can draw on infinite numbers for infinite variance, and that because the "human potential" to perceive or the "personal knowledge" of the practitioner are limited, only a finite number of conditions are attended to or identified, and they are identified in a way "most dependent on the practitioner's scientific and ethical knowledge."

Next, under the rubric of "description" of the conduct of practice, Beckstrand discusses values and goals. She restates that the goal of practice is change toward the greater good. Determination of this greater good depends on the values of the practice discipline, values that "reflect normative ethical theories." A practitioner sometimes accepts a hierarchy of values "implicitly and uncritically, but these hierarchies and their implementation represent ethical decisions." She concludes that the knowledge of practice "depends not on some special aspects of practice, but on science and ethics alone."

Immediately in her introduction, Beckstrand, without calling attention to it, puts forward two new factors missing from her first article: "theoretical knowledge" presumably now will bridge her pass from "theory" to "knowledge" (whereas this formulation does not appear at all in her first essay, it is seen three times in this introduction to her second), and "logic" is added (again, without comment) to science and ethics, to subsume practice theory. One might hypothesize that these additions reflect a reaction to criticism (her own or that of others) of the first piece, and therefore that these problems are to be addressed. The body of the article never again mentions "theoretical knowledge" but instead substitutes "knowledge" alone, as in the first essay. What is more, because she freely interchanges "theoretical knowledge used in practice" with "knowledge used in practice," one may deduce a confusion in the use of the concept "theoretical." What of the goal to maintain health *against* changes?

In addition, it would have been helpful if Beckstrand had considered, even as an error to be refuted, that a theory of nursing might be as relevant to "nursing ethics" as a theory of ethics. Finally, her conclusion forgets her introduction and its specificities of "theoretical" and "logic." "Thus, the knowledge of practice depends not on some special aspects of practice, but on science and ethics alone." Both articles are thought-provoking and central readings in metatheory.

Beckstrand, J. (1980). A critique of several conceptions of practice theory in nursing. Research in Nursing and Health, 3, 69–79.

Although the title and summary suggest a survey of ideas about "practice theory," half of this article (roughly five pages) is devoted to what Beckstrand characterizes as the "set-of-rules" conception of practice theory, which she attributes to Ada Jacox. Other writers, most notably Dickoff, James, and Wiedenbach, who provide the opening focus of the essay, are given remarkably short shrift. The initial section, "The notion of Dickoff et al.," attempts to explain their notion, mixing restatement of their formulations with a series of asserted exemplifications of what they mean: "the articulation of the conceptual frameworks . . . practitioners actually use"; "in changing a flat tire a practice theory is being employed"; an identity between their notions and "technology" (i.e., "the totality of a plan of action used to bring about a goal that is presumed desirable").

The big interest for Beckstrand is Jacox (1974). Jacox's is presented as an incorrect interpretation of Dickoff and colleagues—incorrect because Beckstrand appears to interpret Dickoff and James' position in terms of each practitioner having her own practice theory formula. Jacox, according to Beckstrand, suggests a rigid, compulsion-carrying deck of directives, which one shuffles on each occasion to find the right rules of procedure. Nurses are "compelled to conform . . . to a set of rules imposed by an external authority." Under this conception, "prescriptive practice theory becomes a set of universally prescribed rules for practice."

Following this is the longest section of the essay (by far)—an attack on the Jacox position so characterized. Beckstrand produces a discussion of ethics intended to demonstrate that one cannot prescribe a goal without making an unjustifiable value judgment. Then she makes a series of "practical arguments." Prescriptions cannot take into account all the variables in a given situation. Sometimes, two prescriptions will conflict. The practitioner will be forced to make an "arbitrary" decision between them. She takes time to "demonstrate" that you could not have a prescription specific to every situation. She responds to objections by saying that, even under such a theory, scientific and ethical judgment would still be required. Granted this, Beckstrand asserts that the change would be nil. She argues that such a theory will not be valuable in the education of practitioners because she has already shown it is not valuable in practice. Nursing education does not involve prescriptions of this kind because those in education "are not imperatives carrying sanctions for their adoption or violation." Sets of rules for practice are no aid in research because "as prescriptions, they imply no deductively derivable empirically true or false consequences (predictions)."

Other notions of practice theory are briefly examined. Conceptual frameworks of nursing, such as Roy's or Jones' "are not scientific theories but ideologies" because they are "legitimately alterable on the sole basis of personal or public discretion." Beckstrand also differs with those (like Peterson) who wish to try to delineate the bounds of nursing inquiry. In theory development and in research, one does not know *a priori* what is relevant, rather, one lets the characterizations and categorizations emerge and evolve from the situation.

In this article, Beckstrand provides a unique interpretation of Dickoff and colleagues and of Jacox. Although the problem with Dickoff and colleagues inevitably represents some difficulties with their exposition, most attempts like this at reduction can be problematic (as they dismiss and refute such approaches in their 1975 article) simply because they fail to include all the elements Dickoff, James, and Wiedenbach insist on (i.e., a conceptual framework with built-in goal orientation, prescriptions, and a survey list). The set-of-rules theory attributed to Jacox also has some flaws. We would assume that Jacox would argue that her proposed system is not intended to be a straightjacket and that provisions for "breaking" rules are made. Beckstrand's arguments against Jacox would seem to apply to any attempts to teach practice, or to any potential contributions from research. She sees the possibility of this objection: "one might argue that if a prescriptive practice theory of the set-of-rules type cannot be justified, then no decision can be made about what to do in practice."

As to her paragraph on metatheory, first, under Carnap's definition, all theories of nursing are metatheories. Second, after all these attempts to discredit practice theory, she says that, if one will call it metatheory, it is okay, and Dickoff and colleagues' may be considered a beginning (and worthy) metatheory of nursing practice. Beckstrand notes that because Dickoff and colleagues "did not fully explicate or formalize their theory," they have only offered "undeveloped ideas." Dickoff and colleagues, of course, do not have a theory. (That is to say, they do not have a "practice theory.") These appear to be unfortunate mix-ups. Despite our analytical arguments, we consider Beckstrand's writing stimulating, challenging, and an absolute must for a theory student.

Benoliel, J.Q. (1977). The interaction between theory and research. Nursing Outlook, 25(2), 108–113.

This essay explores relationships between theory and research as reciprocal elements in an ongoing process through which scientific knowledge relevant to nursing is created, expanded, tested, and refined. Practice can serve as a stimulus to research and can therefore form part of the cyclical process. There is also a brief section on sources of knowledge in nursing.

This is a simple account of the "constantly flowing interchange between the realities of practice, theory development, and scientific investigation." The inductive/deductive cycle is demonstrated, as is an example of building a body of knowledge by the

"application of different philosophical approaches to the study of a particular human phenomenon." Better "sources of knowledge" include Rogers, Carper, and Beckstrand.

Berthold, J.S. (1968). Prologue: Symposium on theory development in nursing. Nursing Research, 17(3), 196–197.

According to the author, no substantive definition of "theory" can be applied with any generality due to the ambiguity and complexity of the concept "theory." Differential use of terms necessitates clear understanding of their use to avoid semantic confusion and to allow for attention to the substance of various positions.

In this introduction to the symposium, Berthold states: "The questions . . . involve a discussion of various positions about and approaches to developing a conceptual structure of knowledge useful and necessary to attain the goals established by nurses." In elaborating on this statement, the author stresses thought processes that result in theoretical constructs, ordered in a systematic way; knowledge that is verified; theory that is useful in stimulating new observations and insights and in generating propositions concerning relevant events; and goals that are established and controlled by nurses for nursing.

This is a brief overview that succinctly captures the major issues, questions, and debates about nursing theory development addressed in the symposium. (See articles by Schrag, Crowley, Folta, and Brown, as well as Panel Discussion.)

Brown, M.I. (1964). Research on the development of nursing theory: The importance of a theoretical framework in nursing research. Nursing Research, 13(2), 109–112.

Two major questions are addressed: (1) How far have we progressed through research toward the development of an integrated body of nursing theory? And (2), how can we determine if a research project has a theoretical framework that will make possible a contribution to scientific knowledge? Sections of the paper include the need for nursing theory, concept validation through research, and assessment of the theoretical framework of a research project. A research project that contributes to nursing theory can be identified by certain characteristics, such as an aim to pursue knowledge for its own sake, the statement of the relationship of the problem to research and nursing literature, the use of established meaningful terms, the association of findings to the work of others, and the logical but creative exposition of implications and further hypotheses for testing.

This early, easy-to-read article is a brief reminder of the theory–research symbiosis. The article emphasizes rationale rather than criteria for selecting theoretical frameworks. Would Brown's conclusions be different if this article were written in the 1980s?

Brown, M.I. (1968). Theory development in nursing: Social theory in geriatric nursing research. Nursing Research, 17(3), 213–217.

This is an exemplification of Brown's theme—the nature of nursing research and its relation to theory formation. The article is a descriptive account of the use of the concept of socialization in a gerontologic research project.

Although Brown asks how theories of the basic and other applied sciences relate to nursing research, her response stresses problems intrinsic to the theories. Other authors (see especially Klein, Crawford, and Johnson et al.) emphasize the implications of "borrowing" theories formulated in other disciplines. The article is part of the 1968 Symposium on Theory Development in Nursing.

Brown, M.L. (1983). Research questions and answers: The use of theory and conceptual frameworks in nursing research and practice. Oncology Nursing Forum, 10(2), 111–112.

The author presents an initial distinction: "A theory explains the nature of phenomena and a conceptual framework identifies what variables are important." Both are important to "identify, categorize, and expand nursing knowledge in an organized and thoughtful way." A catalog of notions of theory is then offered. The author summarizes: "Theory, then, helps identify the research problem, defines . . . appropriate evidence . . . and determines methods to obtain, organize, and integrate information."

In dealing with conceptual frameworks, on the other hand, the author simply presents a definition: "A conceptual framework is an organized grouping of ideas or concepts that assists in providing overall structure to the research project and the nursing process."

The author follows Derdiarian's delineation of the need for order and systematization in nursing research, education, and practice. Finally, she cites Marino's conceptual framework for cancer nursing.

This article is actually a columnist's response to a question by readers about the terms "theory" and "conceptual framework." More elaborate and somewhat different presentations are available elsewhere in the literature.

Burgess, G. (1978). The personal development of the nursing student as a conceptual framework. Nursing Forum, 17(1), 96–102.

Burgess proposes "personal development" of the student nurse as a conceptual framework in professional nursing education. Rationales are presented (enhanced potential for professional effectiveness, improved quality of care, criteria for retention of students), as well as means of operationalizing personal development (ability to articulate goals and philosophy and to evaluate accomplishments and needs, change in attitudes, increased sensitivity to others).

A conceptual framework is defined, by analogy, as a unifying central theme that provides the mechanism for articulating and relating all parts of the curriculum. Course objectives are the means of providing attachment to the central theme, and the courses themselves (content plus learning experiences) are "free to respond to currents of movement and creative expression," while maintaining their attachment to the central theme.

The proposed conceptual framework provides a provocative, if controversial, alternative to more common subject- or process-oriented curricula. The major value of this article, however, is its simple, yet creative and helpful explanation of the characteristics and purposes of the conceptual framework and its emphasis on the need to operationalize concepts.

Bush, H.A. (1979). Models for nursing. Advances in Nursing Science, 1(2), 13–21.

This article examines types of models, the relationship between models and theories, and the use of models in nursing research, education, and practice.

Models provide a means for ordering, clarifying, and analyzing concepts and their relationships; they provide analogs to reality and stimulate the scientific process by identifying new possibilities. A model primarily expresses structure, whereas a theory provides substance. Models used in nursing must represent the ordered reality of focus on human beings, their environment, their health, and nursing itself (i.e., isomorphic). Models are used: (1) in research, to conceptualize the research process itself and to facilitate thinking about concepts and their relationships; (2) in education, to guide curricula planning; and (3) in practice, to guide assessment, intervention, and evaluation.

This article provides a good summary of types of models and their purposes in nursing. More pragmatic information on the development of models may be found in Jacox and McKay.

Carper, B.A. (1978). Fundamental patterns of knowing in nursing. Advances in Nursing Science, 1(1), 13–23.

A classification of the patterns of knowledge in nursing is presented here. The article addresses the question: "What kinds of knowledge are most valuable to the discipline of nursing?" Answers are meant to provide (1) perspective and significance to the discipline, (2) awareness of the complexity and diversity of nursing knowledge, and (3) an operational definition of nursing.

Four patterns of knowing are identified:

1. *Empirical* (the science of nursing). The science of nursing is in a healthy but embryonic stage; theoretical models are presenting new perspectives.
2. *Aesthetics* (the art of nursing). Aesthetics is achieved by empathy, "dynamic integration" of parts into the whole, and the recognition of particulars versus universals.
3. *Personal knowledge.* Personal knowledge is concerned with the quality of interpersonal contacts, promoting therapeutic relationships, and individualized care.
4. *Ethics* (the moral component) "what ought to be done." Each individual pattern of knowing is necessary, but not sufficient, for achieving the goals of nursing. It is their interrelationship that defines the whole. These patterns provide structure and boundaries, dictate subject matter for nursing education, and, together, represent a complete approach to the problems and questions of the discipline of nursing.

The reader of this article should consider several points. The "Aesthetics of Nursing" section appears to confuse knowledge with action ("a science teaches us to know, and an art to do") and blurs distinctions between intuition, perception, instinct, and what we more ordinarily call knowledge. Perhaps most important, the identification of aesthetic with *empathy* loses any sense of clear distinction between this and her third category, described as "acceptance."

In this case, Carper is rejecting an approach to the client as an "object," and is rejecting establishing "authentic personal relationships."

In addition, the "Ethics of Nursing" obscures a major oversight of this paper (something emphasized by Donaldson and Crowley)—that nursing involves history and philosophy, as well as science and art. The delineation of goals, principles, and values and of the hierarchies among these that are specific to nursing are the continuing products of nursing experience and of thought in nursing that is broadly theoretical. The value of this article lies in its provision of a broader perspective of nursing knowledge than has been previously presented in the literature.

Chapman, C.M. (1976). The use of sociological theories and models in nursing. Journal of Advanced Nursing, 1, 111–127.

Theory development has not kept pace with expanding roles in nursing and does not support nursing actions. Nursing and sociology are similarly defined as interactive processes between individuals, and the author therefore suggests the potential contribution of sociological theories and models to the development of nursing theory.

Social exchange theory is proposed to explain how patients and nurses satisfy their own needs and goals, and organizational theories are considered in the context of their effect on goal achievement, communication, and compliance. Concluding remarks stress that (1) borrowed theories must be validated in the new situation, and (2) theories in the behavioral sciences can describe and explain more accurately than they can predict due to the variability in human behavior.

The bulk of this article focuses on the effects of organizational structure on nurse roles and behaviors in the United Kingdom. The reader might question comparisons between nursing and sociology and assumptions about nurses and patients. The article emphasizes theories related to the delivery of care and the development of nursing theory that would support clinical practice. Whereas the ideas presented in the conclusions are important, their development is somewhat limited.

Chinn, P.L. and Jacobs, M.K. (1978). A model of theory development in nursing. Advances in Nursing Science, 1(1), 1–11.

The process of theory development is a means of facilitating the evolution of nursing science and is the most critical task facing the nursing profession. Theory is defined as "an internally consistent body of relational statements about phenomena which is useful for prediction and control." Conceptual frameworks are presented as less developed theoretical statements allowing description and explanation.

The model of theory development contains four separate but interrelated components: (1) examination and analysis of concepts, (2) formulation and testing of relational statements, (3) theory construction, and (4) practical application of theory. These components may be differentiated by the nature of the operations involved: cognitive (1 and 3); empirical (2 and 4); and by their functions: description and explanation (1 and 2); prediction and control (3 and 4). As a whole, the model demonstrates, "how different types of research yield varying types of products, each contributing to the total development of the science." Also included in the model are boundaries that delimit areas of nursing concern, while allowing free exchange of content and processes among sciences, and a central core denoting the influence of history on theory development in nursing. The importance of the theory–practice linkage and the dynamic and contextual nature of the process of theory development are emphasized.

Two major arguments are developed: (1) "The process of theory development has greater value for nursing than the product," and (2) the emphasis in theory development should be prediction and control. These positions should be contrasted with authors who emphasize the preliminary importance of descriptive and explanatory theories, the importance of the "product" for building a science of nursing, and the guiding influence of a clear conception of nursing.

Clark, J. (1982). Development of models and theories on the concept of nursing. Journal of Advanced Nursing, 7(2), 129–134.

This article aims to show that models and theories in nursing have "practical value for the ordinary clinical nurse." One must relate theoretical work to what nurses actually do, built around concepts that can be operationalized. The failure to do this explains "the relative lack of impact on nursing practice . . . of the work in theory development undertaken in recent years."

Clark presents a "simple model of nursing." The model is a "gross simplification," but deliberately so, as more elaborate models are less universal. Often, models do not easily fit all fields of nursing.

How can such a model help the ordinary practicing nurse? (1) It purports explicitly that there is something called "nursing" that has an identity of its own ("versus those who still see nursing merely as a collection of tasks undertaken on the initiative of . . . doctors"); (2) it stresses the reciprocity of the nurse–patient relationship and the significance of environment; and (3) it stresses cause and effect relationships; "considerably more attention must be paid than in the past to outcomes of nursing care."

The remainder of the article is an application to her own situation. Clark demonstrates by considering her own nursing care in light of the model.

More popularizing than theory or scholarship, the article provides a role model of informal, thoughtful, and conscious practice, and does a good job of presenting serious ideas in attractive and readily understandable ways. It is a well-written example of what it argues—relating scholarship in nursing to practice, making it available to "consumers." It is a soft-sell for theory-based practice and is effective.

Cleland, V.S. (1967). The use of existing theories. Nursing Research, 16(2), 118–121.

Theory serves two major functions: as a tool, it gives direction to empirical investigation; as a goal, it tends to abstract, summarize, and order research findings. The goal function of theory, which is the basis for progression of science, has been less adequately used in nursing. The functional method of research, which begins with a significant problem or question and then searches for relevant theoretical formulations, enables the nurse researcher to take advantage of advances made in other disciplines, while ensuring nursing relevance. It permits the researcher to work inductively from existing empirical data and deductively from other theoretical formulations. An example of this is given to illustrate the inherent limitation of research that has no theoretical framework (and, of course, the superiority of one that does).

This rationale for conceptual frameworks is similar to others on the subject, and may be contrasted with the "grounded" approach (see Quint). Although the authors in this group of articles agree on the values of a framework, consider the integral relationship of this section and the one on theory critique.

Colaizzi, J. (1975). The proper object of nursing science. International Journal of Nursing Studies, 12(4), 197–200.

The beginning of a science should be a philosophical inquiry into its appropriate domain. In initiating a science of nursing, considerable theoretical ambiguity has resulted from the assumption that nursing science is synthetic. Although we have amassed a body of scientific findings (that can be properly called health technology), what we have failed to do is circumscribe that which is uniquely nursing. Although nursing takes place within both technical and existential dimensions, the proper object of nursing science is the human experience of health and illness. Therefore, the research methods of human science, rather than those of natural science, must be used to investigate the questions that arise within this (existential) dimension.

This article offers an intelligent support of prevalent and influential conceptions of nursing science that emerged in the 1980s.

Collins, R.J. and Fielder, J.H. (1981).
Beckstrand's concept of practice theory:
A critique. **Research in Nursing and Health,**
4(3), 317–321.

The authors find two major flaws in Beckstrand's analysis. First, they attack her claim that "the knowledge nurses need to effect changes is scientific knowledge." Specifically, they follow Toulmin's suggestion that there is a "plurality of different types of medical knowledge," and they quickly collapse it into two "modes." Beckstrand has overlooked or ignored the subjective, the knowledge of the particular, "knowing the client as a particular human being." Several of the authors' statements on this issue are memorable: "The role of the nurse and the biographer are similar; both must turn their attention to knowing individuals in all of the uniqueness and particularity. . . . The nurse's role is perhaps closer to that of the priest, intimate friend, or therapist—seeking not only knowledge of the individual but also the person's well-being. Understanding is not the primary goal, but a way of becoming an effective adviser and advocate for the person's interest."

Second, there are moral issues in nursing that will not be resolved by appeal to ethics but are specific to nursing. The authors point to activities or goals that are not obligatory but that are praiseworthy; these are characterized as, "[M]oral ideal. . . . The questions of which, if any, moral ideals an individual pursues is not answered by an ethical theory. The theory may be used to justify an ideal as a moral ideal, but the choice of which ones to pursue must flow from an individual's concept of what kind of life the person wishes to lead. . . . The profession

of nursing has only recently emerged from the role of being the physician's handmaiden and is now in the process of defining itself as a profession in its own right, embodying certain moral ideals. Just what those ideals should be is one of the major elements of a practice theory."

This is an interesting, analytical article. It nicely adjusts and fills out Beckstrand's work, without any excessive negativity. It is a good example of the sense of a shared enterprise: Beckstrand is a colleague whose work is to be built on.

Crawford, G., Dufault, S.K., and Rudy, E.
(1979). Evolving issues in theory development.
Nursing Outlook, *27(5), 346–351.*

This review of nursing theory literature addresses issues in historical perspective: Is nursing theory borrowed or unique? Is nursing a basic or applied science? Should there be theories *of* nursing or *for* practice? What are the approaches to theory development? The purpose of the article is to redefine these issues in light of Donaldson and Crowley's article.

A strong bias for unique, practice-oriented, "situation-producing" theories is presented. Problems of borrowing are presented (e.g., lack of isomorphism). Authors agree with Johnson that the nature of knowledge required for nursing will foster theory development that is unique to nursing.

As defined in the 1968 nursing science conference, basic science supports knowledge for its own sake, whereas applied science demonstrates knowledge with practical aims and applications. Donaldson and Crowley present the need to increase understanding of phenomena (basic), demonstrate applicability of basic knowledge in real situations (applied), and explain how to use knowledge to achieve goals in practice (prescriptive theory). Together, these comprise nursing science.

Regarding the issue of theory *of nursing* (delineation of definition and scope of or about nursing and the nursing process) versus *for practice* (conceptualizations guiding nursing action to achieve desired goals), these authors address the question of unified versus diverse theories, supporting Jacox's "middle-range theories." It is possible that they confuse "unified theory" with the values of a theoretical framework. The complexities of the arguments for and against unified and diverse theories are not addressed.

This approach to theory development lends support to inductive, deductive, historical, and philosophical methods. Theories should be developed to generate new knowledge and to organize knowledge about the discipline of nursing (supporting Donaldson and Crowley). The author states McKay's questions about which methods are most appropriate and what are the criteria for acceptance of findings. She also supports Stevens' advice to ask the significant questions and only then to seek appropriate research methodologies.

This article provides a good overview of critical issues in nursing theory development from a historical perspective. Although one is attempting to resolve these issues, the complexities of the arguments and contrasting positions are not always fully addressed, precluding comprehensive, definitive resolution. Nevertheless, this article is a good synthesis of supporting positions and contains an excellent bibliography on theory development in nursing.

Dickoff, J. and James, P. (1968). Researching research's role in theory development.* Nursing Research, *17(3), 204–205.

Research is for the sake of theory and theory is for practice. However, research alone will not produce theory, and theory produced without research has little hope of viability. Research is a tool to be used in conjunction with adequate conceptualization and with a level of precision that, although scientifically sound, does not preclude practical usefulness. The purpose of research (creating or testing theory) should determine the methodology used.

This excellent, humorous, and atypically brief article by Dickoff and James is one of the best articles on the research–theory–practice link available in the literature.

Dickoff, J. and James, P. (1968). A theory of theories: A position paper.* Nursing Research, *17(3), 197–203.

Dickoff and James begin by defining theory as a conceptual system or framework invented for some purpose. (There are other kinds of theory besides "predictive theory.") Because a profession shapes reality, nursing theory must provide conceptualizations to guide the shaping of reality to nursing's professional purpose. Therefore, nursing theory is at the fourth or highest level—situation-producing theory—because the nursing aim is practice. Nursing has an advantage to offsetting the difficulty of producing so complex a theory, namely, "the privileged and habitual intercourse with empirical reality carried on in a practice discipline," together with

the practical wisdom passed on in apprenticeship. (There follows a summary of "Theory in a Practice Discipline"—see abstract of that article for this information.) Natural and social science theories will be offered by contributors, but one should realize that conceptualization at a sophisticated level constitutes the integration of these into nursing theory. The authors' summary indicates that definition and types of theory delineated are the crucial points made. They suggest that valuation of their theory or theories rests on "whether or not the proposed position constitutes a fruitful view of theory."

This is a stimulating introduction to the ideas of Dickoff and James and contains some knowing asides (e.g., the authors encourage nurses to persist in theory building despite "the smoother sailing and quicker payoff in status and funds to be found in repetition or imitation of inquiry" in other disciplines). Nevertheless, the article is simply an overview and depends on more elaborate articulations ("Theory in a Practice Discipline," etc.) for substantive support.

Dickoff, J., James, P., and Wiedenbach, E. (1968a). Theory in practice discipline: Part 1. Practice oriented theory.* Nursing Research, *17(5), 415–435.

This is the first of two articles on the nature and development of theory in a practice discipline. A major thesis is made explicit at the outset: theory is relevant to practice, practice to theory, and both are relevant to research. The movement is delineated from felt discomfort/criticism to articulation of a problem, and then to speculative and eventual practical resolution. This "epitomizes that theory is born in practice and must return to practice." What is theory? Theory is a "conceptual framework to some purpose." There is some discussion of the nature of theory and misconceptions about theory.

The four levels of theory are: (1) factor-isolating theories; (2) factor-relating theories (descriptive); (3) situation-relating theories (predictive, etc.); and (4) situation-producing theories (prescriptive). Each of these is then described: (1) involves naming, classifying; (2) is depicting or "natural-history-stage" theory; (3) extends from predictive theory into "promoting and inhibiting" theories; (4) is the primary subject of the article, situation-producing theory. The three essential ingredients of a situation-producing theory are: (1) goal content specified as an aim for activity; (2) prescriptions for activity; and (3) a survey list to serve as a supplement.

Each of these ingredients is discussed, the first two briefly, the survey list at some length. As to the first, "No more feeling of reverence to some shadowy high ideal can substitute in theory for the conception of goal as goal." As to prescriptions, they are commands giving a directive, aimed at a specified end, and directed toward some specified agent. The survey list accounts for the agent's judgment, experience, and practical insight. It bridges the gap between particular activity and the goal content and prescriptions. Such activity has six salient aspects: agency, patiency, framework, terminus, procedure, and dynamics.

What is nursing theory? It must be a theory at the most sophisticated level, a situation-producing theory. This article suggests what might be expected in a nursing theory. Again, the discussion is structured on the tripartite division—goal, prescription, and survey-list ingredients. The discussion of goal content identifies the goals as "beforehand specifications of situations the theorist deems worthy to produce," as well as "explicit conceptualizations subject to revision." The treatment of the prescription ingredient merely expands on the original statement, using examples of what has been said already. Furthermore, "appropriate specificity of goal content and prescription is an important consideration in any practice theory."

The survey list ingredients are explained and illustrated at some length. Under *agency*, the question is asked, "Who might be agents of activity that realizes the nursing goal?" The conclusion is that there is no theoretical reason that all nursing agents must be nurses or even persons. *Patiency*, similarly, is mainly the extension of that term to cover "[a]ny person or thing that receives the activity of a registered nurse." *Framework* asks: What in the context of activity, practically speaking, is relevant? *Terminus* is activity in terms of outcomes. This and *procedure* are fairly obvious discussions of viewing activity in terms of means and ends. *Dynamics* introduces interesting questions about the motivations of nurses and how these may be influenced. The question is of the "power sources" for successful nursing activity.

The article closes with a brief look at existing nursing theory. Actually, this is mainly a look at nursing literature. Beginning with the observation that there is no existing nursing theory to meet their paradigm, the authors argue nonetheless that extant nursing literature constitutes a contribution to, or preparation for, such a theory. They discuss the difficulties of "would-be" nursing theorists, they observe that there may be more than one good nursing theory, and then they propose to consider types of nursing literature (other than research studies): the "inspirational" literature of nursing, treatises and textbooks, and procedure and policy books. These constitute "a rich mine, if we know how to exploit the veins." The existence of something concrete to be examined critically—written materials and existing practice—is a necessary stepping stone. "In other words, even now, practice is guided in some incipient way by embryonic theory."

Dickoff and colleagues have much to offer: "As Einstein's theory of relativity is . . . so is our theory of theories." In fact, it is this very insistence that they are introducing a *new kind* of theory, substantively different, that provides the major ground for doubt or dispute. Whereas some parts of this article are dense and full of ideas, whole sections seem diffuse, rambling, simplistic, and often unnecessary. There is no bibliography. However, their pretensions to metatheory are the main objectionable elements (except for an occasional condescension to nurses and "would-be" nurse theorists). This is the major substantive article by these authors, and it is a "must read" because of the contagion and impact of their ideas. Critical reading of this article should be followed by reading of the article by Jacox and the series by Beckstrand.

Dickoff, J., James, P., and Wiedenbach, E. (1968b). Theory in a practice discipline: Part II. Practice oriented research. Nursing Research, 17(6), 545–554.

To have a nursing theory, three sources must be tapped: awareness of practice theory, interest in developing it, and "openness to relevant empirical reality." The authors see the first two of these as covered in Part I of this article, which is briefly reviewed. Research and practice are the constituents of the required "openness." The essential aspect of practice, as opposed to "mere" research, lies in the accomplishment of something in the here and now. Research has as its goal "[i]nput to knowledge beyond the immediate particular." Possible research objectives are to stimulate conception and to validate a conception already formed. "We can say that research has two objectives or that research has theory as its immediate objective but in two different ways." Simply put, though, research tests theory or stimulates theory.

There are two ways to stimulate theory: the researcher "encounters again and again, and with as many variations as possible, empirical reality." This is called planned "staring." A second way is to test theory at the just-preceding level. As for testing, only fourth-level theory testing is considered; it is "fairly well-accepted" that the others can be tested. The purpose of situation-producing theory is threefold: (1) to achieve its goal; (2) that these results be desirable when achieved; and (3) that guiding action by the theory is feasible in terms of cost, etc. Testing means testing all three dimensions: the theory's *coherency* must be tested; its *palatability* must be assessed; and the *feasibility* claim must be evaluated. Research methodology is not absolute and can be expected to vary with the level of theory tested, and with its being strictly "test" *or* stimulation. The conditional nature of methodology is stressed to approach creatively the kind of research needed or to stimulate practice theory for nursing. Summary and conclusions follow. Noteworthy among these observations are: "Research is for theory, theory for practice, so that practice fittingly has first place and theory has the mediating role."

"There is a thorough-going, mutual interdependence as among the three activities of practice, theorizing, and research."

"In short, to supply nursing image is to venture a nursing theory."

The authors are mostly to be commended for certain emphases, certain stressed elements, especially concerning the place and importance of theory in nursing. As with their other productions, this article fails to provide any bibliography. This article is not so controversial and seems not so valuable as their other contributions.

Donaldson, S.K. and Crowley, D. (1978). The discipline of nursing. Nursing Outlook, 26(2), 113–120.

This article poses a series of significant questions. It begins by noting the question of the nature of nursing, but addresses this through a subquestion: What are the recurrent themes in nursing inquiry? These could suggest "boundaries" for a systematic study of the discipline of nursing. There follows a long discussion of the nature of classification of disciplines. Nursing is seen as a "professional" discipline. It is noted as a discipline different from nursing science (doctoral training for nursing historians, as well as for nursing scientists, is endorsed) and different from nursing practice (the discipline should be governing practice instead of

vice versa). Finally, the structure of the discipline of nursing is considered, a generalization is offered ("nursing studies the wholeness or health of humans"), and some "major conceptualizations in nursing" are presented.

The article is poorly organized. The opening ideas are not developed and are unrelated to what follows (except for the assertion, not discussed, that they provide "boundaries"). On the second page, the authors state that what is truly important is to define the discipline of nursing. Having discussed the nature and relations of disciplines, one expected the next section to be entitled "The Discipline of Nursing." Instead, the authors launch into a discussion of nursing-as-practice versus the discipline of nursing. The structure (as opposed to the nature or definition?) and nursing's "perspective" are not clearly delineated or related. Definition is never mentioned, and what is given is somewhat vague, broad, and unspecific to nursing, such as "Major conceptualizations in nursing: 1. Distinctions between human and nonhuman beings; 2. Distinctions between living and non-living. . . . 7. Human characteristics . . . such as consciousness, abstraction . . . aging, dying, reproducing."

Nevertheless, this seminal work is challenging, and it has had a wide and significant impact on the theory development literature because of the importance of the topic and its timeliness. It makes the point successfully that nursing is a discipline and gives support to its focus.

Ellis, R. (1968). Characteristics of significant theories. Nursing Research, 17(3), 217–222.

Significant theories for nursing are those that (1) improve practice by addressing the goal of nursing (represented by Henderson's definition) and (2) include the patient as a component. The purposes of theory development are (1) to distinguish fact from pseudofact, (2) to structure and synthesize facts from other fields, (3) to give direction to practice, and (4) to provide a framework for retrieval and use of generated and stored knowledge.

Seven characteristics of significant theories are enumerated: (1) *Scope* (the number of concepts related). Scope provides framework for ordering observations about a variety of phenomena, and it must include psychological and biologic variables; the broader the scope, the greater the significance. (2) *Complexity* (the notion that theory should treat multiple variables or relationships of a single variable in its full complexity). The strength of this argument is Ellis' admonition that "incomplete conceptualizations lead to hazards of illusory comprehension." (3) *Testability* (focuses chiefly on the importance of recognizing theories as hypothetical constructs, amenable to change). (4) *Usefulness* (the ultimate criterion is that theories help develop and guide clinical practice). (5) *Implicit value* must be recognized and made explicit. (6) *Capability* of generating new information, new ideas, and practices must be there. (7) *Terminology* can be used meaningfully with, or applied to, phenomena observed in nursing.

These "characteristics of significant theories" speak directly or indirectly to evaluative methodologies and criteria for internal and external validity presented elsewhere, providing a succinct presentation of major considerations. Ellis' positions on scope and complexity should be compared with those of Jacox, Hardy, Stevens, Duffey and Muhlenkamp, and Hage. The major area of disagreement between Ellis and other authors is related to the characteristic of testability, which, she states, can be sacrificed in favor of scope, complexity, and clinical usefulness. Ellis argues that "elegance and complexity of structure are to be preferred to precision in the meaning of concepts in the present state of knowledge." This view should be contrasted with the more prevalent argument for testability as the ultimate determinant of significance.

Fawcett, J. (1980). A framework for analysis and evaluation of conceptual models of nursing. Nurse Educator, 5(6), 10–14.

The purpose of this article is to provide a clear definition of conceptual models, to delineate the confused distinction between conceptual models and theories, and to develop a framework for analysis and evaluation of conceptual models.

A conceptual model is defined as a set of abstract concepts and the assumptions that integrate them into a meaningful configuration. By identifying relevant phenomena (person, environment, health, and nursing), a conceptual model provides a perspective for scientists; by describing these phenomena and their interrelationships in general and abstract terms, the model represents the first step in developing the theoretical formulations needed for scientific activities.

A theory is a set of interrelated concepts, definitions, and propositions that present a systematic view of phenomena by specifying relations among variables (Kerlinger). It postulates specific relations

among concepts and takes the form of a description, explanation, prediction, or prescription for action. Any theory presupposes a more general abstract conceptual system. The crucial distinction between a conceptual model and a theory is the level of abstraction; a theory is both more precise and more limited in scope than its parent conceptual scheme.

On the basis of this distinction between conceptual models and theories, different frameworks are required for analysis and evaluation. The remainder of the article is devoted to the presentation of a framework for analysis (philosophical base, context, scope) and evaluation (internal validity, etc.) of conceptual models of nursing.

This is an excellent, substantive article that is of value both in its articulation of differences between conceptual models and theories and its eclectic framework.

Gebbie, K. and Lavin, M.A. (1974). Classifying nursing diagnoses. American Journal of Nursing, 74(2), 250–253.

As the Report of the First National Conference on the Classification of Nursing Diagnoses, this article describes the process of developing a classification system and a list of tentative nursing diagnoses.

It is an example of what Dickoff and James call a factor-isolating theory. The relationship of nursing diagnoses to theory development, while observed in the article, is made explicit and developed in detail by Kritek (1978).

Gortner, S.R. (1983). The history and philosophy of nursing science and research. Advances in Nursing Science, 5(2), 1–8.

Only in the past few years have philosophy of science issues attracted serious attention in nursing research, as the research tradition moves into a new phase of development. Questions regarding method, discovery (as opposed to justification or proof), ethics, politics, and so forth are now prompting comment. This article presents an overview of this philosophical component of emerging nursing science and research and does so in part through a historical perspective.

In the early years, practice was the source of knowledge. Efforts to generate a knowledge base for nursing through research have been much more prominent in the past two decades. Early research approaches included development of critical resources, surveys, conferences, studies of procedure, case analyses, and alliance with other disciplines. More recent times have seen the enlargement of critical resources (especially in doctoral education) and public support and new development of colleagueship, communication, and research designs and methods.

On this last subject, Gortner addresses a major point of discussion: "To assume that the choice of research methods used in nursing was influenced by a particular philosophy of science (e.g., logical positivism) is to attribute too much deliberation or rationality to what was the result of social, political, and economic events." With doctoral training in fields other than nursing, nursing scientists brought with them methods that had served them well. They also had to face the pragmatics of funding. "Granting agencies prefer controlled studies in which variables are well-specified and instrumentation is precise." Finally, generalizability has become a critical element because "the capacity to affect practice depends heavily on this factor."

Consensus has emerged about the definition and subject matter of nursing and the research paradigms of its science. However, the philosophical orientation of the science remains chiefly empirical and naturalistic. Attempts to incorporate theoretical propositions are now being made, and the search is on to discover relationships. "Science (empirics), art (esthetics), morality (ethics), and intuition (personal or subjective) all represent sources of knowledge. . . . The profession surely can accommodate multiple paradigms (analytic, humanistic) and modes of inquiry (naturalistic, experimental, historical)." In the formation of research questions and the choice of areas of inquiry, it can be expected that inquiry will be of a more fundamental nature in the future than was true in the past. Examples of phenomena that have relevance for nursing include self-care, social support, family functioning, and stress. Two other important areas are clinical therapeutics and investigation of environments.

Gortner concludes that "nursing science will make a major contribution, as science, in the interface of the biological and social sciences concerned with illness and health."

This article is significant because of its comprehensiveness and currency; it points to the shape of nursing's future.

Green, J.A. (1979). Science, nursing and nursing science: A conceptual analysis. Advances in Nursing Science, 2(1), 57–64.

This article examines the term "science" historically, linguistically, and contextually. The scientific method is considered ("science includes both methodology and knowledge"), and the functions of science are indicated. Various definitions are cited (Conant, Nagel, Fischer), and a synthetic definition is offered. The usefulness of this definition of science for nursing is said to be its potential for evaluating the status of nursing science: "It provides a standard to determine whether or not a designated body of knowledge constitutes a science." A distinction is established between science and technology.

A series of definitions of nursing are considered, with attention given to chronologic development of the nurse's role (Henderson, Wiedenbach, Yura and Walsh, King, Travelbee). Following Travelbee, an analytical course is set. Nursing is seen as involving content and process. A comparison of nursing and medicine is made. Knowledge drawn from natural, behavioral, social, and medical sciences constitutes the science in nursing. This is then transformed through application in clinical practice. So, a definition of nursing becomes "a service discipline that provides care, concern, and comfort to recipients experiencing a broad range of health–illness phenomena through the synergetic combination of its art and science." This definition precludes the separate classification of technical and professional nursing.

The main value of this article is that it collects and presents good basic materials on the questions "What is science?" and "What is nursing?" Green's only argument for "nursing science" is a reference to Gortner and colleagues, who, she says, document its existence. Also, her synthetic definitions seem to be inferior to her citations from other sources.

Hall, B.A. (1981). The change paradigm in nursing: Growth versus persistence. Advances in Nursing Science, 3(4), 1–6.

Questions of emerging and competing paradigms in nursing theory development are addressed as they relate to shaping the values of the professional. The "change paradigm," which postulates continuous flux, has been pervasive in nursing theory (e.g., adaptation, development). It is argued that: (1) a paradigm based on change may not be the most productive departure for the study of humans and health; (2) a focus on change leads to the illusion that things are changing when they are actually staying the same; and (3) nursing's attention may have been drawn to the phenomena of change at the expense of increasing our understanding of the capacity for stability and persistence.

Hall's attention to the heuristic value of a paradigm is an interesting example of the sociology of science, and her admonitions about the acceptance of unverified assumptions underlying theory are provocative and important. Several interesting questions are raised, based on Kuhn's work, and have generalizability beyond the specific example: What is the process by which a paradigm is accepted? Why and when does a paradigm's shift occur? What is the relationship between theory and value? Can competing paradigms exist simultaneously, and with what implications?

The presentation of change and stability as competing theoretical notions may be somewhat oversimplified. Although Hall explicitly refrains from dropping models of change, her presentation is strongly biased in the direction of stability (albeit perhaps for the sake of balance). Perhaps change and stability are better viewed as which/when versus either/or phenomena. Kuhn's paradigm, espoused by Hall, would seem to preempt the possibility of dialectical theory development. This article should be read by the student with some background in theory development.

Hardy, M.E. (1978). Perspectives on nursing theory. Advances in Nursing Science, 1(1), 37–48.

Nursing theory development and evaluation are viewed within the context of stages of scientific development. Applying Kuhn's thesis on the development of scientific knowledge, Hardy argues that nursing is in a "preparadigmatic" stage of theory development, "characterized by divergent schools of thought which, although addressing the same range of phenomena, usually describe and interpret these phenomena in different ways." Nursing needs to struggle through and beyond the preparadigmatic stage of scientific development because confusion, wasted energy, and poorly focused, systematic research result from this lack of a well-defined perspective.

A "metaparadigm," or prevailing paradigm, on the other hand, presents a general orientation that holds the commitment and consensus of the scientists of a particular discipline. It determines the general parameters of the field, provides focus to scientific endeavor, and may subsume several "exemplar" paradigms, which are more concrete and specific in directing the activities of scientists. The existence of a prevailing paradigm facilitates the "normal work of science." Research is purposeful,

orderly, and raises few unanswerable questions. Whereas the adoption of a metaparadigm cannot be decreed but rather will be based on its scientific credence and its potential for advancing scientific knowledge, nursing scientists can facilitate this process by being well informed in a substantive area and participating actively in theory construction and research.

Subsequent sections of this article address the nature of theory, the relationship between theory and practice, criteria for "borrowing" theory from other disciplines, types (levels) of theory, and criteria for theory evaluation, including logical adequacy, empirical adequacy, usefulness, and significance. Each of these criteria is clearly elaborated.

Whereas Hardy's "perspectives" are not clearly interrelated, they are well worth reading. Before reflecting on the implications of nursing's "preparadigmatic" stage of theory development, consider: (1) the applicability of Kuhn's thesis to nursing and (2) evidence for other conclusions on the status of nursing science. The sections on development and evaluation of theory are excellent. Hardy's criteria should be compared with other taxonomies.

Jacobs, M.K. and Huether, S.E. (1978). Nursing science: The theory-practice linkage. Advances in Nursing Science, 1(1), 63–73.

Nursing science is defined as both process and product: "the process of nursing science requires that concepts be defined, operationalized, linked into relationships, and verified. From verified conceptual linkages accrue the product, which is theory; and the theory explains and predicts nursing phenomena." The goal of nursing science is to define goals and guide practice; it is prerequisite to professional autonomy and impact.

The complementary and mutually dependent interrelationship of theory and practice are emphasized and demonstrated. Concepts, the building blocks of theory, must be empirically derived and operationalized in a clear and useful manner. They are then linked in theoretical formulations that are subject to empirical verification. Theory without practice is vacuous; practice without theory is intuitive rather than scientific. The contributions of both researchers and practitioners are crucial.

These authors present nursing as an evolving science. The current status of nursing science is illuminated by historical perspective; education and "cohesiveness will facilitate the advancement of nursing science." The article includes brief sections on the nature of science, the structure and function of science, and the process of concept selection and definition. The theory–practice linkage is clearly articulated and appropriately emphasized.

Jacox, A. (1974). Theory construction in nursing: An overview. Nursing Research, 23(1), 4–13.

Three levels or stages of theory development are discussed: (1) a period of specifying, defining, and classifying the concepts used in describing the phenomena of the field; (2) developing statements or propositions that propose how two or more concepts are related; and (3) specifying how all the propositions are related to each other in a systematic way.

Concepts are abstract representations of reality that indicate the subject matter of a theory. They may vary both in complexity (concepts, "higher-level" concepts, constructs), and in the degree to which they are observable versus symbolic (empirical–theoretical continuum). Precise operational definitions are emphasized.

Propositions are statements of constant relationships between two or more concepts or facts. All scientific propositions are based on empirical generalizations that may be proved false in the future. Types of relational statements include laws, axioms, theorems, hypotheses, and principles—all differentiated on the basis of degree of tentativeness. Although nursing has made wide use of principles on which to base nursing action, Jacox observes little attempt to relate these principles to one another systematically.

Scientific theory is defined as "a systematically related set of statements, including some law-like generalizations, that is empirically testable." The purpose of theory "to describe, explain, and predict a selected aspect of empirical reality" requires the use of both inductive and deductive reasoning and a close relationship among theory, practice, and research.

Jacox espouses nursing practice theory as that which guides the nurse's actions in attaining nursing goals in patient care. While presupposing and building on theory that explains, describes, and predicts, nursing practice theory must allow the investigator to go beyond these levels to prescribe and control. She describes nursing as a discipline "in which the major concern is *use* of knowledge."

Other topics discussed in this article include: (1) definition and use of models to guide research, (2) arguments for "middle-range theories" in nursing

(versus "grand theory" or "abstracted empiricism"), and (3) a discussion of the nature and source of knowledge and theory in (of, for) nursing and the proper use of nursing resources in theory development.

This article is a good overview of theory construction, emphasizing the relationships between various elements of theories and emphasizing as well issues in the development of nursing theory. Jacox's nursing practice theory should be compared with Dickoff and James and the contrasting position of Beckstrand. Comparisons should also be made with Hardy, Donaldson and Crowley, and Green. Reflection on Jacox's description of the "state of the art" of theory construction in nursing is recommended.

Johnson, D.E. (1959). The nature of a science of nursing. Nursing Outlook, 7(5), 291–294.

The basis for the concepts set forth in this article is found in the earlier article by this author on the philosophy of nursing. Here, the focus is on exploring the nature of nursing as a science and as a discipline. Johnson identifies professional disciplines as representing applied sciences. One might be interested in comparing her thoughts on this with a more recent article by Donaldson and Crowley, noting that Johnson and Crowley were colleagues at the University of California, Los Angeles in the mid-1960s and that Crowley was influenced by Johnson (1978).

Johnson believes that the goals of nursing must be established in precise terms to give direction to the search for a body of knowledge. Although nursing shares the ultimate goal held by all health workers, its specific and unique goal is not as clearly understood or as widely accepted as that of medicine's. It is through a discussion of nursing's professional goal that Johnson elaborates on her conceptions as a way of illustrating how the development of science can be given direction. Her conception of nursing care is borrowed from general systems theory, and the primary purpose of nursing care is expressed in terms such as tension, equilibrium, and dynamic state.

For nursing to achieve its goals, it is hypothesized that two kinds of knowledge are needed: the knowledge of people, which is shared knowledge common to all health workers, and knowledge of the science of nursing. Furthermore, it is this author's thesis that "the science of nursing is developed through the reformulation of concepts drawn from the basic sciences to yield a body of knowledge fundamental to the development of theories of nursing diagnosis and nursing intervention."

Borrowing theory is a controversial approach to the development of nursing knowledge but is nonetheless a useful one, as demonstrated by a number of other nursing theorists, as well as Johnson. Here, Johnson develops a rationale for that approach. We will later see how she does this using systems theory as a prototype to develop her behavioral systems model.

This article makes an important contribution to the early thinking about a science of nursing, in addition to showing us Johnson's early thinking about the behavioral systems model. The writing is clear, and the presentation is logically developed and expressed. This article should be read by those who are interested in Johnson's model, especially by those who wish to see how the model unfolded, and by all who are interested in the development and organization of nursing knowledge. Responses and patterns, part of the lexicon in nursing in the 1980s, were introduced as early as 1959, as is evident in this publication.

Johnson, D.E. (1968). Theory in nursing: Borrowed and unique. Nursing Research, 17(3), 206–209.

Differentiation of "borrowed" and "unique" theory in nursing may help clarify nursing's appropriate place and focus in theory development. Borrowed theory is defined as that knowledge developed in the main by other disciplines and drawn on by nurses. Unique theory is defined as that knowledge derived from the observation of phenomena and the asking of questions unlike those that characterize other disciplines.

The question of borrowed and unique is analyzed first in respect to the nature of knowledge required for nursing practice and the availability of the knowledge. This knowledge may be divided into: (1) knowledge of order, that which describes and explains the "normal" state of people and the "normal" scheme of things (this kind of knowledge is the focus of the basic sciences); (2) knowledge of disorder, that which helps us understand events that pose a threat to the well-being or survival of the individual or society; and (3) knowledge of control, that which allows the prescription of a course of action that, when executed, changes the sequence of events in desired ways predicated on the knowledge of disorder and geared toward specified outcomes. Although all these types of knowledge are basic to

nursing practice, it is in the area of disorder that efforts at nursing theory development should be concentrated.

A second perspective for analysis of the borrowed/unique issue considers the problem of nursing's objects in scientific investigation. Nursing is ill-defined as a field of practice and as a field of inquiry. The lack of definition constitutes a serious obstacle to professional and scientific development. If there is an area for study and theory development unique to nursing, it will evolve only through the study of phenomena and through asking questions in a way that is uncharacteristic of any other discipline. Behavioral system disorders represent such a focus.

Part of the 1968 Symposium on Theory Development in Nursing. This article is a "must read" because: (1) it is a cogent and effective analysis of one of the major issues in theory development; (2) Johnson's framework of order, disorder, and control is one of the major typologies in the literature; and (3) it serves as an introduction and rationale for Johnson's Behavioral Systems Model.

Johnson, D.E. (1978). Development of theory: A requisite for nursing as a primary health profession. In N. Chaska (Ed.), The nursing profession: Views through the mist. New York: McGraw-Hill.

The development of a theoretical body of nursing knowledge is a means of acquiring professional status. Impediments to the development of nursing science are surveyed, and two questions are presented as means of providing direction: For what purpose is a theoretical body of knowledge intended? And, what phenomena must be studied and what kinds of questions must be asked to develop the needed knowledge?

In response to these questions, Johnson discusses the evaluation of scientific disciplines and the professions as sciences. Sciences become differentiated on the basis of the distinctive perspective for observation and interpretation of selected phenomena. The focus of any profession's scientific concern is interdependent with its service (social function). Johnson discusses the implication of different conceptual models and alternative routes to theory development and presents three social criteria for evaluating models: congruence (Do nursing decisions and actions that are based on the model fulfill social expectations?); significance (Do nursing decisions and actions based on the model lead to outcomes for patients that make an important difference in their lives or well-being?); and utility (Is the conceptual system on which the model is based sufficiently well-developed to provide clear direction for nursing practice, education, and research?).

This is a good theoretical treatise on problems in nursing theory development and the evaluation of solutions to these problems. Direct responses to Johnson's guiding questions, however, must be supplemented from other sources (see sections on philosophy, practice, research, guidelines). Johnson's theory evaluation criteria, based on factors extrinsic to the substance of the model, represent an often-neglected yet important dimension.

Kramer, S. (1969). Behavioral science and human biology in medicine. The New Physician, 18(11), 965–978.

The question is raised whether information in the biologic, behavioral, and medical sciences can be used to develop a comprehensive theory of the human organism. Kramer presents the thesis that "in human development, the social environment, through its influence on genetically determined patterns of behavior together with the normal process of growth, is capable of modifying the development of every individual in characteristic ways." Examples of the interrelated nature of bio-psychosocial variables are given, using growth and development as a frame of reference. One major concept—"character structure"—is developed to define the psychic, somatic, and social unity of the individual to explain the empirical finding that alterations of behavior in one realm are capable of influencing all other realms (as in stress reactions).

The proposed "medical–ecological model" of the human organism represents an attempt to develop an eclectic "grand theory." The rationale is presented intelligently, and recognition is given to some major obstacles; for example, the fact that individual disciplines use words in different ways and use different units of analysis, ranging from the molecular (physiology) to the molar (behavioral sciences). Implications for conceptualization or viable theory development are left to the reader.

Kritek, P.B. (1978). The generation and classification of nursing diagnosis: Toward a theory of nursing. Image, 10(2), 33–40.

In building nursing theory, we have skipped the first stage of specifying, defining, and classifying our concepts, and this has led to problems. To the degree that first-level theory (descriptive) is dissonant with or unclear when related to "what is" in nursing, the eventual level-four theory (prescriptive) will be dissonant or unclear. Returning to the level-one theory, building and doing first things first may be a worthwhile place to redirect our energies. This is being done through the generation and classification of nursing diagnoses (see Gebbie and Lavin, 1974). This level-one theory is evaluated in terms of Ellis' criteria of a significant theory.

Read this article after Dickoff, James, and Wiedenbach (1968a, 1968b), Ellis (1968), and Gebbie and Lavin (1974). It is most insightful in the application and implications of Dickoff, James, and Wiedenbach's framework. Would you call nursing diagnoses theory?

Leininger, M.M. (1969). Introduction: Nature of science in nursing. Nursing Research, 18(5), 388–389.

This is a statement of conference goals to explore approaches and methods that will support a scientific discipline and a body of nursing knowledge. A core of nurses is eager to develop both a scientific and a humanistic discipline of nursing within institutions of higher education. Although "a theory" of nursing is spoken of, it is healthy and desirable that there be multiple theories, models, and conceptual frameworks. An attitude of constructive skepticism and collegial critique is urged.

In addition to induction and deduction, an ethnoscientific approach is suggested: a systematic and descriptive documentary study of phenomena through the eyes of people in their situations. Nursing lacks systematic ethnologic studies of concrete nurse–patient–other situations.

We must be tolerant of one another's failures and frustrations. Finally, change must be accommodated. Students should be encouraged to explore problems and test ideas that seem "exotic, highly radical, or out of this world." This is a brief overview of concerns facing the conference.

McCarthy, R.T. (1972). A practice theory of nursing care. Nursing Research, 21(5), 406–410.

Can this format (of Dickoff, James, and Wiedenbach), applied to a real-life situation, produce useful theories of nursing (practice)?

The purpose of this article is to illustrate how a practice theory can be developed on four levels.

McCarthy presents data from her survey of postoperative patterns of voiding in patients with spinal anesthesia to demonstrate the four levels of theory as described by Dickoff and colleagues (1968a). Under first-level theory (factor-isolating), she categorizes patients according to type of surgery. Second-level theory (factor-relating) involves analyzing the relationships between need for catheterization, duration of surgery, fluid intake, and so on. So far, so good. When we get to the third level, we find that "a statement that 'patients who have not voided within 14 hours may have to be catheterized' could be said to constitute predictive theory." The highest level of theory—situation-producing or prescriptive—is a nursing care plan (e.g., "note time of last voiding," "note when patient expresses desire to void, offer assistance," etc.).

The article also includes an example of a survey list in operation. Is the reader's response to the opening question affirmative or negative? Does your response reflect comment on McCarthy or on Dickoff, James, and Wiedenbach?

McKay, R. (1969). Theories, models, and systems for nursing. **Nursing Research, 18(5), 393–400.**

Theory is the cornerstone of all scientific work because the understanding, which is the goal of science, is expressed in terms of theoretical formulations. The article gives much space to defining various senses of the term "theory." Nursing, at present, should use the word in a modest sense. "Models" are defined and analyzed. Models vary in two ways: level of abstraction and metaphor used. Two metaphors have been dominant—the machine and the organism. The organism is currently the dominant model in many fields, and, for both philosophic and practical reasons, it is dominant in nursing.

The concept of "systems" is the ultimate central focus of the article. Various definitions of systems are offered. Open and closed systems are discussed. Properties of open systems are articulated, and the suggestion is made that nursing could be represented by such a systems approach. Theorems or propositions based on general systems theory developed by James Miller are endorsed as particularly appropriate for nursing. Finally, a systems approach to the study of nursing education is proposed for the study of students and of curricula.

This is a valuable treatment of the subjects considered. Its value is due in great part to the many clear and careful definitions and to its detailed

application of systems theory to nursing. A crucial question is posed about models and metaphor: Is the model merely a restatement in other terms, or does it accomplish extension or clarification? The late Dr. McKay was a central figure in metatheory. This represents a fine example of her writing.

McKay, R.C. (1977). What is the relationship between the development and utilization of a taxonomy and nursing theory? **Nursing Research, 26(3), 222–224.**

This essay is a brief description of the purposes and principles of classification schemes. The definition and arrangement of concepts in a taxonomy, presuming it reflects the natural system, is a descriptive model of reality and can be considered a theoretical design (factor-isolating or naming). The value of taxonomies for clinicians and educators are briefly listed.

This is another example of first-level theory; how it relates to the second level is not discussed. This article is really McKay's response to a reader's question.

Menke, E.M. (1978). Theory development: A challenge for nursing. In N.L. Chaska (Ed.), **The nursing profession: Views through the mist.** *New York: McGraw-Hill.*

Menke considers three issues related to theory development in nursing: the importance of theory development, the present status of theory development, and strategies to facilitate theory development in nursing.

Theory development is important for any discipline because it prescribes the conceptual framework for describing, explaining, and predicting phenomena. It serves as a means to isolate and classify facts, and it points to gaps in the available knowledge. Definitions and components of theories are discussed, as well as levels (Dickoff and James) or stages (Jacox) of theory development. The importance of lower-level theory development as a sound basis is emphasized, and the consideration of theories *about* nursing rather than *of* nursing is proposed. Lack of theory development may have been caused by the lack of systematic direction and collaboration among theory developers. An eclectic approach to theory development is advocated.

This is an excellent, well-written, and substantive review of major issues in theory development.

Moore, M. (1968). Nursing: A scientific discipline? **Nursing Forum,** *7(4), 340–348.*

Moore argues that, in our eagerness to break away from the apprenticeship tradition, nurses are trying to develop a scientific discipline without setting the foundation that is characteristic of every well-structured discipline. The fallacies and shortcomings of such practices as searching for a theory of nursing; borrowing concepts, tools, methods, and even questions from other disciplines; and allowing values to interfere with science are discussed, along with their ramifications. The only sensible basis for the development of a content area to be labeled "nursing" involves empirical generalizations regarding the effects on the patient of the activities we carry out as nurses.

This short, easy-to-read article should be read early in a nursing theorist's career because it provides an excellent overview of major issues and pitfalls in the development of nursing theory and nursing science. Moore's emphasis on a clear, precise definition of terms is refreshing. Although you can, now or later, argue about "the only sensible basis . . .," Moore is obviously interested in the theory–practice–research linkage.

Murphy, S.A. and Hoeffer, B. (1983). Role of the specialties in nursing science. **Advances in Nursing Science,** *5(4), 31–39.*

There is some conceptual movement away from specialization in nursing. Three trends have impact in this regard: (1) defining nursing as a discipline separate from medicine, (2) educating entry-level generalists, and (3) developing conceptual frameworks.

As to the first, perspectives of the two professions— medicine and nursing—are now clearly different. Medicine has become more specialized in an attempt to keep abreast of technologic changes and increased knowledge, whereas nursing has become more generalized and holistic in its approach to health care.

Second, medical-surgical nursing was disease-based, psychiatric nursing was patient-based, and community health nursing was locus-based. Many schools determined that using specialty departments as organizing components of the curriculum was no longer efficient; many now offer a series of concepts basic to nursing, along with the nursing process, and they loosely refer to these as an integrated curriculum. One of the outcomes is that the specialties are no longer clearly distinguishable.

Also, movement from the hospital setting to the university, as well as changing patterns of illness, has reinforced this direction.

Third, the new conceptual system in nursing provides direction for practice and education. However, none have delineated the role of the specialties. The role of nursing specialties is supported, nonetheless. The authors bring to their aid the social policy statement on nursing by the American Nursing Association: "The effectiveness of the profession is increased when specialists are available to focus their efforts on a particular aspect of clinical nursing, to test application of newly available theory to conditions germane to that clinical aspect, and to translate those theory applications into nursing approaches considered more useful than prevailing ones."

It appears that nursing specialties can best contribute to nursing science by generating and testing middle-range or limited-size theories. This type of theory is more directly relevant for addressing practice concerns. As practice-relevant theory is developed and refined in each specialty from its particular vantage point, the specialty contributes to nursing science through both cumulative and didactic processes.

The article concludes with a brief discussion of the theory development process (inductive, deductive, adapted) and a sustained example drawn from mental health nursing, where a concept from nursing, "mutual withdrawal," is identified and traced through its history.

This article is especially important for its focus on a perhaps as yet unassimilated consequence of recent developments in nursing: the de-emphasis of the specialties.

Newman, M.A. (1972). Nursing's theoretical evolution. **Nursing Outlook,** *20(7), 449–453.*

Following a brief discussion of the evolution of nursing science, Newman elaborates on three main approaches to the discovery of nursing knowledge that emerged during the 1960s: (1) the borrowing of theory from other disciplines with an intent to integrate it into a science of nursing; (2) an analysis of nursing practice situations in search of the theoretical underpinnings; and (3) the creation of a conceptual system from which theories could be derived. While limitations and difficulties in the first two approaches are discussed, Rogers is credited with initiating the third phase. The clear-cut delineation of the individual as the focus of nursing gave direction to the development of theory that is basic to nursing.

Newman cites Hempel to evidence the value of the Rogerian approach and, by comparing Rogers with other nurse theorists, concludes that a conceptual system of nursing is evolving and does provide meaningful direction for research. Whether the theory evolves inductively from ideas conceived in clinical practice or deductively from broad generalizations within the theoretical framework does not seem particularly important. What is important is that the nursing investigator should determine the relationship of her study question to the overall conceptual system in nursing and should therefore expand and elaborate the system by the testing of theories that have derived from it. Nursing is coming of age.

Newman's article should be contrasted with that of Hardy, who sees nursing in a "preparadigmatic" stage (from Kuhn). She cites the problem of the past as a dearth of nursing knowledge, while "the problem of the future will be an acceleration of that knowledge." Has this prediction been realized in the 20 years since this article was written? How does your answer attest to the veracity of Newman's characterization?

Notter, L.E. (1975). The case for nursing research. Nursing Outlook, 23(12), 760–763.

Slow progress in nursing research is attributed to views of nursing and women, too little cumulative effort, and the relatively new idea of nursing as an intellectual profession. The following are areas for concentrated effort: the need for more research based on theories consonant with nursing's domain of responsibility; the need for replication; the need for postdoctoral research and for individual researchers who select a problem area and continue to study it over time; and the need for more service agencies to develop clinical research programs that encourage staff participation in research.

Payne, G. (1973). Comparative sociology: Some problems of theory and method. British Journal of Sociology, 24(1), 13–29.

Comparative sociology is a method of inquiry that allows "explicit testing of sociological theories with data from various sources" and that examines "the nature of society as revealed by . . . the operation and interrelation of key processes in different societies, or areas of societies (historical, geographical, social)" (p. 13). The interrelationship of theory and method in the generation of social theory is examined, with emphasis on methodological issues in comparative analysis.

Societies that are similar in regard to a specific variable (e.g., form, function, or structure) are studied to generate laws that explain that one type of society only. Problems inherent in this approach are categorization (defining categories and determining an acceptable level of similarity) and generalization (producing theories that have more than specific application). The purpose of comparing dissimilar societies is to yield universal laws. Defining and determining the appropriate scope of variables, as well as developing specific, meaningful hypotheses, are major difficulties. In both approaches, problems develop in selecting study variables and studying them outside of their cultural context. Nevertheless, the comparative method provides not only understanding and insight but also a means of verifying theory and developing a science of sociology.

This is an excellent, substantive article on a particular methodology for the development of theory and science. Issues and problems of comparative study are addressed, and insight is given on the relationship of theory and methodology. What is missing in clarity of expression in this article is more than counterbalanced by the salience of ideas and the potential for applicability to nursing science development.

Payne, L. (1983). Health: A basic concept in nursing theory. Journal of Advanced Nursing, 8(5), 393–395.

The article traces the historical evolution of the concept of health. For centuries, disease has been the central focus for the examination of the phenomenon of health. Only one major formulation (Sigerist's in 1941) preceded the critical turning point statements in the constitution of the World Health Organization (1958): "Health is a state of complete physical, mental, and social well-being and not merely the absence of disease and infirmity."

Various paradigms have subsequently been developed, among them the ecological model, based on the relationship of people to the total environment (Blum, 1974; Rogers, 1960), and the equilibrium model, based on the body's self-regulatory powers to maintain constancy of the internal milieu (Dubos, 1965). Psychosocial models came later: sociocultural, philosophical, or relating health to notions or normality. A new emphasis on quality of life and high-level wellness emerged (Dunn, 1959) due to people's dissatisfaction with life despite their affluence; the idea of holism, originating in Gestalt theory, grew to a multidimensional approach, emphasizing self-responsibility, the whole person, and the process of caregiving; and the "salutogenic" model of health (Antonovsky, 1979) originated, in which "the origin of health lies in a 'sense of coherence,' that is, the way in which one sees life as meaningful, manageable, and comprehensible."

Assumptions based on traditional paradigms have bound nursing curricula and practice to the negative view of health in terms of absence of disease. "The concept of health constitutes a basic building block for nursing theory. . . . If the goal of nursing is the promotion of health, making this concept operational is essential for nursing practice." Finally, a definition of health is offered (a nursing concept of health): "Health is the effective functioning of self-care resources that ensures the operation and adequacy of self-care actions."

The article combines some history, some popularization, some commonplace information, and perhaps some helpful reminders.

Peterson, C.J. (1977). Questions frequently asked about the development of a conceptual framework. Journal of Nursing Education, 16(4), 22–32.

The relationship between theory and conceptual frameworks in nursing is examined. A conceptual framework is defined as "a loosely organized set or complex of ideas . . . that provides the overall structure of a curriculum (p. 25)." A theory is defined as a group of systematically interrelated propositions that provides organization to a body of content and, by allowing explanation and prediction, provides a guide for practice. A conceptual framework is an earlier evolutionary step that may be developed into theory, thus generating testable hypotheses.

Essential elements of a conceptual framework include the nature of the service provided (nursing/nursing process), goal or outcome (health), rationale for services (nonhealth or illness), characteristics of the caregiver (nursing practitioner), characteristics of the recipient (patient/client), and context for service (care setting or environment). Explanations of the relationships of these concepts provide the framework.

The relationship of the conceptual framework to borrowed theories, program philosophy and objectives, and curricular threads, as well as its role in the development of a nursing curriculum, are also addressed.

This is an excellent article that demystifies the conceptual framework in a thorough, organized, and articulate manner. While emphasizing the use of conceptual frameworks in nursing curricula, the article provides much useful material on theory components (including simple but excellent definitions) and theory development. Excellent figures summarize major points. Peterson's selection of concepts may be compared with those of Dickoff and James, and her presentation of the conceptual framework should be contrasted with that of Torres and Yura.

Phillips, J.R. (1977). Nursing systems and nursing models. Image, 9(1), 4–7.

Because the primary goal of nursing theory is the generation of knowledge specific to nursing, the process of theory building must be couched in a nursing frame of reference. Otherwise, the obtained knowledge will not be nursing knowledge that can be used to build or expand nursing science, or that can be used for nursing education, practice, or research. Models that nursing has borrowed (medical, psychological, ecological, social) are criticized on the grounds that not one of them views the person as a totality in interaction with the environment. Models of Rogers and Johnson are proposed as frameworks for nursing theory construction.

There are many points of agreements between the arguments of this article and one by Newman (1972). Although some good points are made about shortcomings (e.g., of the medical model), many of the arguments could be further developed. Are there any legitimate prototypes outside of nursing?

Putnam, P. (1965). A conceptual approach to nursing theory. Nursing Science, 3, 430–442.

A theoretical framework is valuable as a stimulus in the development of nursing science. In the absence of adequate theory, nursing is limited by the concrete here and now; nursing then becomes restricted to immediate impressions and is unable to explain the past, evaluate the present, or predict the future. Despite the clear necessity of a generalized theory, development has been slow and piecemeal; contributing factors include complexity of the subject matter, the proximity (and therefore influence) of the scientist to the empirical data, and the necessity of delimiting a knowledge base that will encompass changing objects in changing environmental fields.

A key to the conceptual maze is the identification of the unique domain of nursing. The knowledge base of the nursing process, nursing science, is at least a four-dimensional synthesis of knowledge relating to biological function, psychological function, social function, and variations in organization of these factors. The operational identification of the intermixture of components in the synthesis, defined and tested through nursing research, would be a genuine contribution to science. Nurses make it possible for patients to accomplish their own energy exchanges with the external environment. The abstraction of the idea of how nursing makes these exchanges possible is an essential step in theory construction. The constant interplay among theory, practice, and research is stressed.

Although other articles provide more cogent arguments for the value of nursing theory, more enlightened definitions of nursing, or more pragmatic suggestions for theory development, Putnam is particularly eloquent on the problems of lack of adequate theory, the characteristics of conceptual difficulties in nursing theory, and the need to identify the unique domain of nursing.

Quint, J.C. (1967). The case for theories generated from empirical data. Nursing Research, 16(2), 109–114.

This work discusses a research approach in which a given problem area is studied for the purpose of developing a conceptual framework. Sections are devoted to the research problem and its overall design, the collection and analysis of data, and the reporting and interpretation of the findings.

This article is the precursor of an approach that has gained increased interest and credibility in the ensuing years.

Rogers, M.E. (1963). Some comments on the theoretical basis of nursing practice. Nursing Science, 63(1), 11–13, 60–61.

This substantive article contains many of the elements that would later be incorporated into Rogers' *Introduction to the Theoretical Basis of Nursing* (1970). It is recommended that this be read prior to reading the book, but it is not a requisite to understanding the theory.

There is a mix of philosophy, definitions, concepts, and goals—all about life, human beings, nursing, and nursing science. Elements of the prototype theory—systems theory—are also present. These are presented not as a theoretical basis of the nursing process but rather "to stimulate logical and creative thinking concerning its identification and development." Despite Rogers' intent, however, a rudimentary structure of the future theory appears to be taking shape here.

First, the philosophical statements and beliefs are presented, along with assumptions about human beings. Nursing is defined as a process, and the goal of nursing is also stated. The concept-building process is discussed, with one concept—the life process—presented. Principles rest on the definitions of the concepts, and principles are integral to nursing science. As an example of a basic principle in nursing science, the adaptive mechanism in human beings is identified. Rogers states, "The human organism has an amazing, innate capacity to adapt: physically, biologically, socially." (An assumption!) The purpose of a principle is not discussed in detail.

Finally, Rogers says that the theoretical basis of nursing practice must include a philosophy and a concept of death as well as life. However, she does not undertake that task. Furthermore, although the term "health" was used, it was not defined. Nor does Rogers discuss the role of nursing as it relates to or interfaces with other health care givers. These, then, are a few limitations of this article.

The purpose of this article is to stimulate thinking concerning the identification and development of nursing science—the theoretical basis of nursing practice. Nursing science is a body of scientific knowledge characterized by descriptive, explanatory, and predictive principles about the life process of human beings. These principles rest on the review of the person as a unified "biophysicalpsychosocial" phenomenon in constant interaction with all parts of the environment. The body of knowledge develops through synthesis and resynthesis of selected information from the humanities and the biologic, physical, and social sciences to form new concepts and understanding about the person and environment. It assumes its own "unique scientific mix" through selection and patterning of this information. The focus of nursing science is central to the formation and understanding of its theories. This focus is elaborated in the remainder of the article.

This is one of the original and the most influential articles by one of nursing's true sages. This article, along with that of Johnson (1959), ushered in the era of nursing theory and nursing science. Rogers' characterization of nursing science has been a source of challenge and inspiration, and sometimes conflict, to all subsequent nurse philosophers and theorists.

For its historical importance and strength of argument, this article should definitely be read. An introduction to Rogers' theory is an added bonus.

Rubin, R. (1968). A theory of clinical nursing. Nursing Research, 17(13), 210–212.

This article is part of the 1968 Symposium on Theory Development in Nursing. It is a brief and simple example of development of a model and its use in research.

Silva, M.C. (1977). Philosophy, science, theory: Interrelationships and implications for nursing research. Image, 9(3), 59–63.

This is an overview of the relationships among philosophy, science, and theory, with implications for the conduct of nursing research. Science developed into specializations; philosophy "unifies scientific findings so that man as a holistic being might emerge." Science aims to describe, understand, predict, control, or explain phenomena. Theory refers to a set of related statements that have been derived from scientific data and from which plausible hypotheses can be deduced, tested, and verified.

Implications for nursing research: (1) All nursing theory and research is derived from or leads to philosophy, (2) philosophical introspection and intuition are legitimate methods of scientific inquiry, and (3) nursing knowledge arrived at by the scientific method too often sacrifices meaningfulness for rigor.

The author argues that no real distinctions are made between different kinds of knowledge until the Industrial Revolution; Darwin and Freud set off a proliferation of knowledge. This appears to ignore much great work, including the obvious contributions of Francis Bacon. Silva's comparisons of the realms of philosophy, science, and theory are good beginnings in nursing. Her pleas for the recognition of nonscientific ways of knowing deserve attention.

Silva, M.C. and Rothbart, D. (1984). An analysis of changing trends in philosophies of science on nursing theory development and testing. Advances in Nursing Science, 6(2), 1–13.

The philosophy of science and nursing theory are in states of transition. Has nursing theory kept pace with new trends in the philosophy of science?

Two competing schools in the philosophy of science are traced and examined: logical empiricism (1940s–1960s) and historicism (1960s–present). The schools are compared in terms of their views of science: (1) its components, (2) its characterization, and (3) its outcomes.

Components: For logical empiricism—deductive system, theories linked to and tested through empirically observable properties; for historicism—research tradition that includes many theories, ontological commitments, and methodological commitments.

Characterization: For logical empiricism—product, scientific knowledge, theory validation; for historicism—the human activity of working scientists, theory discovery.

Outcome: For logical empiricism—verification leading to a body of truth; for historicism—problem-solving effectiveness.

There follows a review of the literature in nursing theory. Three time periods are examined: 1964–1969, 1970–1975, and 1976–present.

1964–1969: Logical empiricist position everywhere (e.g., Dickoff and James, Abdellah. The exception—Leininger offered an ethnoscience research methodology.

1970–1975: Culmination of logical empiricism in Jacox and Hardy; conceptual frameworks; "The irony is that . . . the logical empiricist viewpoints espoused were being strongly repudiated by a growing number of philosophers of science. . . . [N]ursing's theoretical link to philosophy of science was . . . about a decade behind the times."

1976–present: Continued commitment to logical empiricism; a beginning trend toward historicism (e.g., in Newman, Hardy); revisions of conceptual frameworks and introduction of new ones, moving more explicitly toward logical empiricism; questioning of strictly quantitative methods.

Implications: (1) There should not be a single conceptual framework for nursing; (2) there will never emerge a static set of eternal truths; (3) historicism strongly encourages a careful study of actual practices, belief systems, and external factors; (4) the assessment of progress will be more practical (i.e., problem solving).

Important recommendations: (1) Cooperation among nursing theorists, researchers, clinicians, and scholars; (2) exploration of innovative qualitative methods.

Because this article presents itself as expository rather than argumentative, the major questions are: Should one, after all, be trendy and in line with the latest fashion in the philosophy of science? In what ways do the ultimate recommendations differ from what Dickoff and James would suggest?

Stainton, M.C. (1982). The birth of nursing science. The Canadian Nurse, 78(10), 24–28.

"The birth of nursing science" celebrates the coming-to-terms of the new science by reviewing its history and describing the conditions necessary for its development. The history is detailed despite its brevity and is told in a lively style, with the added perspective of the author's Canadian nationality and focus.

The list of developmental requirements includes a perception of nursing as a developing science in the minds and hearts of all nurses; a sense of the significance of each nurse's contribution; a cadre of nursing scientists; the conceptualization of nursing as a science; nursing research teams; monies; the introduction of nursing science to science in general; research and facilities in major centers of nursing; collaboration and international networks; replication of studies; nursing education at all levels of career development; an individual goal of professionalism; and an expectation that 1 day a nurse will be the recipient of the Nobel Prize for excellence in contributing to science.

The significance of this article should be considered in terms of its effects on the intended readership.

Tinkle, M.B. and Beaton, J.L. (1983). Toward a new view of science: Implications for nursing research. Advances in Nursing Science, 5(2), 27–36.

This article begins by pointing to two oppositions: the "hard" versus the "soft" science debate, and the opposition between traditional historians of science and the "historicist" revisionists, such as Kuhn and Laudan. These oppositions are associated and identified in Sampson's formulation as Paradigm I versus Paradigm II. "Context-free generalizations" comprise the object of Paradigm I; research guided by the view of Paradigm II is "often conducted in naturalistic settings, using observational methods."

The authors further contend that the dominance of Paradigm I science is a result of "nourishment it has received from a male-dominant, Protestant-ethic oriented, middle-class, liberal, and capitalistic society." The implications for nursing are multiple. If scientific truth is acontextual, then little attention is likely to be paid to the values and biases underlying

research endeavors, so that methodological biases or determinations of proper research subjects may go unexamined.

Further, nursing is, at its most basic level, a relational profession. However, acontextual study is not likely to focus on interpersonal or person–situation interactions. Such studies are apt to lack "ecological validity" and to be removed from the "real world."

The overarching conceptualization of nursing that can be abstracted from nursing theory is centered around the view of a human being as a holistic being. Nursing involves each person's unique bio–psycho–social context. The impact of the environment is a recurrent theme. Sociocultural context is stressed. However, the experimental method is also held in the highest regard.

"What is proposed is a blending of both methodologies to produce a science that retains a critical concern for objectivity while ensuring that the research it produces has validity in the real world and the influence of contextual variables is acknowledged."

This article suffers from the very problems it indicts. It is too abstract and general (i.e., it rarely provides *examples* of the kinds of studies it talks about), and when, as in two references to women's studies in psychology, it moves toward some specificity, the work is simply alluded to. It is also too far from real life; the proposal for blending the two methodologies in a future state moves toward the mystical: "This new synthesis will not consist of the use of Paradigm II methods in the context of discovery and the use of Paradigm I in matters of verification. Rather, a convergence will involve the higher organization of the opposites in both paradigms."

Nevertheless, the point of the article—that we must have an explicit awareness of the assumptions and biases underlying our methods (particularly, in this case, sexist ones)—commands our assent.

Tucker, R.W. (1979). The value decisions we know as science. Advances in Nursing Science, 1(2), 1–12.

Tucker argues that the processes of science necessarily involve the making of value judgments (versus the ubiquitous image of science as "value-free"). After classifying value judgments along their dimensions: rationale (personal versus objective), subscribership (individual versus "market"), and explicitness (formal versus contextual), he discusses the "value decision-making contexts in research." Tucker's position is that each step of the research process—from selection of a problem, theoretical framework, and methodology to analyzing and reporting data—involves value judgments. The principal activity of science is to make well-supported value judgments.

Tucker encourages an explicit awareness of "the value decisions we know as science." There are some valuable insights in this article—if you can avoid getting hung up on the personal value judgments (PVJs), contextual value judgments (CVJs), and value decision-marking contexts in research (VDMCRs).

Wald, F.S. and Leonard, R.C. (1964). Towards development of nursing practice theory. **Nursing Research, *13(4), 309–313.***

Nursing practice theory—based on the empirical approach of building knowledge directly from systematic study of nursing—is proposed as an alternative to "making borrowed concepts fit." In developing its own theories, nursing would become an independent discipline in its own right. In freeing themselves from the burden of looking only for applications of the basic sciences in their practice, nurses would at the same time take on the responsibility of developing their own science. This calls for the development of nursing practice theory.

Major sections of this article deal with: (1) the fallacy of nursing as an applied science ("accepted" principles may be invalid or inappropriate to nursing, nursing problems are being rephrased as social science cues rather than cues of practice); (2) characteristics of research methods for practice versus descriptive science (the difference lies in the selection of variables and the kinds of hypotheses that are entertained); (3) characteristics of practice versus descriptive theory (practice must contain causal hypotheses); and (4) barriers to the development of research of practice theory in nursing (related to research attitudes, need to generalize, and skill in research methods).

This is the first article written on practice theory in nursing and should definitely be read. Those interested in nursing theory should certainly contrast "the fallacy of nursing as an applied science" with the more prevalent view of how nursing science is developed. In addition, consider the process of practice theory development presented by Wald and Leonard (p. 311) that is clearly a precursor to the influential work of Dickoff, James, and Wiedenbach.

Weatherston, L. (1979). Theory of nursing: Creating effective care. Journal of Advanced Nursing, *4(7), 365–375.*

Effective nursing care requires a *theory of nursing* —a phrase that connotes the interdependence between the two concepts. Conceptual analysis of "nursing," using Wilson's "model case" method is presented as a way to determine the "essence of nursing," and provides a basis for deciding what nursing theory is. The purpose of theory is to explain, predict, or control phenomena. In order to be a theory of nursing, "the theory must be created and used with reference to the unique functions and intentions of nursing and the nature of nursing activity." The relationship between "microtheory" and "paradigmatic theory" are described. A model is developed to demonstrate the relationship of theory, practice, and education.

This article addresses several key issues, including the "essence" of nursing; the relationships among theory, practice, and education; and the rationale for and process of theory building in nursing. However, more sophisticated treatments of each of these subjects are available elsewhere, and should be read first. Many of the article's shortcomings are related to the nonevaluative use of several frameworks and definitions: Wilson's Model Case method, Peter's criteria for education, and conceptions of nursing that do not stress its scientific aspects.

SECTION II

Abstracts of Writings in Nursing Theory, 1960–1984

AFAF MELEIS • SANDRA SCHEETZ

The citations abstracted in this section pertain to selected central writings related to only six of the nurse theorists presented in this text (Johnson, Levine, Orem, Rogers, Roy, and Travelbee). Only selected writings related to each of the theorists and

others' writings (based on theories) are described and analyzed below. The abstracts presented in this section are organized alphabetically, according to theorist and author. This section is best used in conjunction with Chapters 5 and 9 and with the corresponding chapters in the text that focus on the analysis of the particular theory (Chapters 11–13).

DOROTHY JOHNSON

Auger, J.A. and Dee, V. (1983). A patient classification system based on the behavioral system model of nursing: Part 1. **Journal of Nursing Administration,** *13, 38–43.*

This first article of a two-part series focused on the development of a patient classification system based on a nursing model, and it was presented from the combined perspectives of administration and clinical practice. Part 2 (Dee and Auger), to follow, focused on the implementation of the classification system in the clinical setting. The nursing model used was Johnson's behavioral system model and the clinical setting was psychiatric.

The specific intent of such a classification system was for use "as a clinical measure of patient progress in addition to the administrative determination of staffing levels" (p. 38). The importance of a framework common to both was stressed. The rationale for such a classification system versus the use of an existing classification system was discussed.

The rationale for using the Johnson behavioral systems model as the theoretical framework for the classification system in this psychiatric setting was threefold: (1) it could be used with the existing programs based on social learning theory; (2) it could be applied to all clinical settings because of the emphasis on bio-psychosociocultural factors; and (3) it identified universal patterns of behavior applicable to all individuals. The model addresses the eight subsystems outlined by Johnson: ingestive, eliminative, sexual, dependency, affiliative, achievement, aggressive–protective, and restorative. These subsystems of behavior are "assumed to be universal and of primary significance to all persons" (p. 39).

Integrated with the nursing process, the model provided a focus for the assessment phase and is intended to link specific patient behaviors with their corresponding nursing interventions. Furthermore, the model can be used in clinical settings other than psychiatry.

The development of the classification tool began with certain people addressing the nursing care requirements for patients admitted to either the adult or child psychiatric units of the agency where it was developed. Therefore, the tool had to be both comprehensive and flexible enough to describe behaviors reflective of a wide variety of diagnoses

and age groups. To meet this challenge, a group of expert clinicians and nursing administrators was organized to develop the tool.

The criteria for item inclusion reflected several dimensions. First, each of the eight subsystems of the Johnson behavioral system model was operationalized in terms of both adaptive and maladaptive behaviors. The behavioral statements had to meet four criteria: "measurable, relevant to the clinical setting, observable, and specific to the subsystem" (p. 39). A panel of experts then evaluated the statements to make certain that they met the four criteria. The behaviors were also ranked in one of three categories according to their level of adaptiveness, with one being the most adaptive and three being the least adaptive, or maladaptive. Nursing interventions were also ranked according to requirements for intensity and frequency of nursing contact. A fourth level was included to reflect the intensity of one-to-one nursing care required for extremely maladaptive behavior.

After the initial set of critical behaviors were formulated, they were tested by letting a sample of 28 registered nurses, in pairs, serve as observers on seven inpatient units. "Each pair of observers was asked to rate each subsystem of behavior for all patients present on the unit during the shift. In addition, the observers rated the overall level of behavior for each patient" (pp. 39–40). Several exhibits were included to illustrate some components of the process thus far: first, the eight subsystems, definitions of behaviors, and critical behavior characteristics; second, characteristic patient behaviors and the requisite nursing intervention; and third, samples of level-three (maladaptive) patient behaviors and nursing interventions for the eliminative and affiliative subsystems.

The implementation of the system was described briefly, with mention of the steps taken. The description does not provide adequate information for anyone trying to duplicate the process. However, more depth was included in Part 2.

Preliminary testing of the tool revealed several problem areas associated with patient assessment. There were disagreements among staff about ratings of patient behaviors, although it was recognized that these reflected difficulties inherent in defining and measuring behaviors. Observer bias was also an uncontrolled variable associated with measurement of patient behaviors. The two subsystems with the highest level of agreement were eliminative and sexual, probably because these required the least inference on the part of the observers. The subsystems of affiliative, dependency, and achievement—requiring a higher level of observer inference—were found to have lower levels of observer agreement in this preliminary testing.

The importance of minimizing the influence of observer interpretation was recognized, but only one suggestion about how to accomplish this was made, other than through the use of a model to structure the observed behaviors. The suggestion was for staff to "consistently identify and discuss their observations of patient behavior to develop a common frame of reference and achieve a higher degree of agreement (p. 43)." Instrument testing (specifically, measures of content validity), reliability, and improving interrater reliability would also be important contributions to theory validation. In the long run, these would do more to contribute to the overall theory development and concept measurement. This is the next important step to be taken with the work done this far on the classification tool.

A number of the classification tool's administrative benefits were listed. They all reflected factors influencing decisions that considered cost-effectiveness and quality-of-care issues.

Broncatello, K.F. (1980). Auger in action: Application of the model. Advances in Nursing Science, 2(2), 13–23.

It has long been proposed that continued development of conceptual models is an important part of the development of nursing as a science; it is also given that a part of the continued development of models is application of the models in a variety of practices. However, what has become increasingly apparent in the 1980s is that application of the model to practice is insufficient for theory refinement. This article is a good example; although it demonstrates application to practice, it does not offer extension or refinement, neither of which are possible in single-case application.

There are several other limitations. After giving a fairly extensive review (summary) of Auger's application of the Johnson behavioral system model to the chronically ill hemodialysis patient, the author attempts to apply the model using new concepts that are not central to either Johnson's model or the extension offered by Auger. The section about applying the model begins with a discussion of self-concept and body image. A reader could rightfully question the fit of these concepts with the behavioral systems model.

Stressors are identified that could be extrapolated from the model, including diet, which affects the eliminative subsystem, and dependence on a machine, which sounds as if it were related to the aggressive–protective subsystem, although logically, it is more directly a problem of the dependence subsystem. Careful analysis of relationships with Auger was better provided in the next section, on the model in practice. Here, the author proposes to examine the consequences of hemodialysis on the eight subsystems outlined by Auger. The reader may continue to remain at a loss as to where body image and self-concept fit in the analysis.

This article provides labeling of nursing problems experienced by the chronically ill hemodialysis patient. The author also discusses interventions within the Johnson–Auger subsystems.

Dee, V. and Auger, J.R. (1983, May). A patient classification system based on the behavioral system model of nursing: Part 2. Journal of Nursing Administration, 13, 18–23.

The patient categorization tool (see Auger and Dee, Part 1), a major component of the classification system outlined in Part 1, provided a basis for the clinical application in terms of the nursing process in a child psychiatry inpatient setting. It was designed to be both comprehensive and flexible enough to allow its use with clients with a variety of diagnoses, as well as a wide age range. (How this was implemented was the subject of Part 1.) What was required by way of inpatient unit revisions is the focus of this second part.

The plan for developing materials and teaching strategies required revision of nursing assessment forms, teaching materials, staff seminars, and orientation of new employees. First of all, inpatient unit nursing assessment forms had to be revised to reflect the model. What had previously been two six-page assessment forms were replaced by four-page forms designed to assess patient factors or behaviors based on the Johnson model. Whereas the earlier forms had been specific to the patient populations, the new assessment form was specific to the Johnson model and was therefore useful in all clinical settings. In view of the fact that nurses vary in levels of education, clinical experience, and abilities, an interview guide was constructed to assist the nurses in eliciting information from the patient and family. The questions included reflected content from the eight subsystems of the Johnson Behavior

System Model (JBSM) as they related to the specific psychiatric setting and patient population.

The clinical nurse specialists (CNS) and the nursing coordinators of each unit developed a package of the teaching materials to illustrate the clinical application of the model. "The materials consisted of samples of completed nursing assessment forms, nursing care plans, and a list of recommended readings pertinent to the behavioral systems model and each subsystem" (Dee and Auger, 1983, p. 19).

Two exhibits contribute to the overall presentation of the teaching materials developed; these stand alone, not needing additional narrative to describe them to the reader. Exhibit 1 illustrates two pages of the nursing assessment form (with sample data) developed for one of the specific inpatient units; Exhibit 2 shows portions of a sample nursing care plan based on the assessment.

Staff seminars conducted totaled 4 hours and were required for all nursing staff on each unit. These were followed up by actual application on the units. All newly admitted patients were assessed, and care plans were developed based on the model using the new materials. Integration and follow-up of the nursing process was provided by the CNS through weekly nursing care plan meetings or individual clinical supervision.

The orientation of new employees consisted of didactic presentations of purpose and theory, audiovisual materials of examples of different levels of patient behaviors and the corresponding nursing intervention, and unit orientation. Subsequently, the orientee was required to complete a nursing assessment and care plan with supervision from an experienced registered nurse.

While theoretical advantages of using the model were anticipated, the practical advantages were realized only with continued use. There were many practical advantages. Some of the clinical advantages included more systematic patient behavioral assessment, resulting in a comprehensive baseline of behavior at time of hospitalization; more specific and expedited nursing care plans; a focus on patient strengths versus pathology; and improved monitoring of patient behavior over the course of hospitalization. These factors consequently provided more objective means for evaluating the quality of nursing care.

Administrative advantages included improved ability to determine required levels of staffing based on more accurate assessment of patient behaviors, and also a more appropriate assignment of new admissions to a unit based on the level of patient need and level of staffing available, thus achieving a better match of patient needs with staff resources. The corollary would then be that, as the overall identified need rose and fell, staffing levels could be raised or lowered accordingly, affecting (conversely influencing) scheduling, budgeting, and nursing hours. Overall efficiency in the integration and balance of scheduling, budgeting, and nursing hours would be improved, resulting in more cost-effective management.

Although the work was written primarily for administrators and clinicians, this scholarly approach to applying theory to practice demonstrates the utility of the JBSM for practice in various inpatient psychiatric units and gives direction to research. It also provides a working model of the "how to" in implementing theory in a practice setting and provides a blueprint for those who might choose to implement this or another theoretical model. (See more recent publications by Dee under Johnson references in Chapter 21.)

Derdiarian, A.K. (1983). An instrument for theory and research development using the behavioral systems model for nursing: The cancer patient, Part I. Nursing Research, 32(4), 196–201.

Clearly stated by the author in the introduction are both the main purposes of the research carried out and the scope and content of each part of this two-part series. The purpose was to develop a valid and reliable research tool to describe the behavioral changes of cancer patients as perceived by them. The research was conceptualized from the behavioral system perspective, and therefore much of the content of Part I is a synopsis of the Johnson behavioral systems model for nursing. For a reader who is unfamiliar with the model, this is an excellent review. The author's concise writing style makes the theoretical overview quite understandable, and the author remains true to Johnson's original work. Each of the seven subsystems (achievement, affiliation, aggressive–protective, dependence, eliminative, ingestive, and sexual) and the eighth subsystem that was added later (restorative) are reviewed, terms are defined, and relationships among concepts are spelled out. The goal of nursing is also stated.

In the rest of the article, the author reviews the support from the literature for the existence of each subsystem, both from work by Johnson and Auger, as well as from others writing on the same topic. The author then identifies the major dimensions extrapolated for each of the subsystems. The impact of cancer on each subsystem is then described using previously reported research. The Johnson model provides a conceptual reservoir within which research findings find a coherent existence.

This is a fine example of how theory can be used to guide research findings. The author then presents a table containing each subsystem, the determinants of behavior, and behavioral manifestations. It is upon these that the variables of interest for measurement were based. These then comprised the items of the instrument developed by the author. The development of the items and the frequencies in the table are not clear to the reader, and are incongruent with the theoretical discussion. The table fits in with Part II of the article, published in the next issue, where it is discussed and described.

Derdiarian, A.K. and Forsythe, A.B. (1983). An instrument for theory and research development using the behavioral systems model for nursing: The cancer patient, Part II. Nursing Research, 32, 260–267.

The focus and scope of Part II of this two-part series is on the process of establishing validity and reliability for an instrument that will test perceived behavioral changes of cancer patients, based on Johnson's behavioral systems model. One hundred twenty-one change items, based on each subsystem, were delineated from previous research and were given to a homogeneous sample of 163 cancer patients. The criteria for subject inclusion and exclusion are listed. The authors' rationale for the "limitation of selection criteria was to maximize the homogeneity of the sample in terms of salient intervening variables such as visible, extensive body disfigurement, level of awareness, comprehension, absence of additional stress caused by a new treatment or procedure, and variables of adult life cycle (p. 261)." What is not clear is why there are such broad parameters for inclusion of subjects. The extreme age variation (20–70 years), various cancer diagnoses, and range of treatments do not logically suggest a homogeneous sample to achieve the desired results.

Patients were asked to identify changes they perceived happening due to or since they became ill and to add or subtract changes. They were also asked to indicate quantitatively and quantitatively the extent of the changes and, finally, their perceptions of the consequences of the changes. Figure 1 in Part I presents the frequency distribution of responses. The authors did not discuss what decisions they made based on these frequency distributions.

Several approaches were used to estimate the instrument's content validity and reliability. What appears to be the first step was to use an expert panel of six members, divided into two groups. "The first group evaluated the comprehensiveness of the theoretical framework and its consistency with known theories, and the consistency of the operational definitions with the theoretical framework. The second group evaluated the consistency of the operational definitions with the categories and the times. The panel judged independently" (p. 262). A supplemental assessment of empirical validity was done using the theta coefficient estimation, which was derived from a factor analysis.

Described later in the "method" section are two other methods of evaluation of comprehensiveness. Here, a panel of three clinical nurse specialists in oncology independently judged the "other" changes added by the patients (p. 262). Because of these various methods used to evaluate comprehensiveness, some confusion is generated about the sequential timing of these evaluations, as well as about when the pilot testing and the reliability testing were completed.

The Derdiarian behavioral system model instrument was pilot tested after construction and estimation of content validity, using three male and three female subjects. Test–retest reliability was assessed by administering the instrument to, apparently, all 163 subjects. The instrument did not have identifying information on it, and "a randomized permutation schedule always places a subsystem questionnaire designed for retesting for reliability in the third place in the sequence of the subsystem questionnaires" (p. 262). Time to complete the instrument as reported by subjects was approximately 1.75 hours. After a 15-minute respite, the patient was asked to complete the retest subsystem questionnaire.

Also evaluated in the overall process was the performance of each of the eight trained research assistants. Interviewer reliability was an ongoing concern, as manifested by regular review of the tapes and rating of the interviewer behavior by two independent raters who were not involved in the data-gathering process.

Grubbs, J. (1980). An interpretation of the Johnson behavioral system model for nursing practice. In J.P. Riehl and C. Roy (Eds.), Conceptual models for nursing practice. New York: Appleton-Century-Crofts.

The purpose of this article is an attempt to operationalize the model so that it could be used as a systematic guide to nursing practice. The author indicates that this is her own interpretation of the Johnson behavioral system model.

The most obvious difference between Grubbs' interpretation and the original model is the addition of the restorative subsystem, with its goal being "to relieve fatigue and/or achieve a state of equilibrium by reestablishing or replenishing the energy distribution among the other subsystems" (p. 228). The additional subsystem was articulated by faculty members at the University of California, Los Angeles, after long discussions and debates. Johnson continued to remind the faculty that restoration is a requirement for each subsystem, and its addition may therefore be teleological and tautological. Also described are the functional requirements, which are better defined in Auger (1976).

This article makes an important contribution to the use of this model in the prospective development of tools (e.g., sample flow sheet and work sheet, which illustrate use of the model to guide the nursing process). There is even an appendix describing items, by system, that should be included in the assessment. Furthermore, the language and terminology used in the examples are consistent both with systems theory in general and with the behavioral system model more specifically.

Overall, this article is a contribution to the understanding of the behavioral system theory and, if read with Johnson's own account of her theory in the same book, will help to clarify the theory components. The process demonstrated here shows thought and solid construction based on the model.

Holaday, B. (1980). Implementing the Johnson model for nursing practice. In J.P. Riehl and C. Roy (Eds.), **Conceptual models for nursing practice** *(2nd ed.). New York: Appleton-Century-Crofts.*

The focus of this article, which follows the Grubbs article, is the operationalization of the model and application of the nursing process to care of the individual patient, using Johnson's model. The author designed a new assessment tool and synthesized Piaget's definition of cognition with Johnson's view of a human being as a system of behavior.

This author devotes the entire article to cognition— not even one of the behavioral subsystems—and to the eliminative system, which was defined by Johnson to include the excretion of physiologic wastes and which was expanded by Grubbs (and the faculty of University of California, Los Angeles)

to include the expulsion of one's feelings, beliefs, and emotions.

Had the author developed a rationale for incorporating Piaget's theory and refined the integration of it within either a subsystem or a cultural or psychological variable, the argument would have been more defensible.

Overall, the article is limited because of its narrow focus on the redefined eliminative subsystem, even though the author does follow through with each phase of the nursing process in accord with the purpose of the article. The article offers some clarification of the use of the behavioral systems model in practice. Refinement and extension were not provided.

Johnson, D.E. (1959). A philosophy of nursing. **Nursing Outlook,** *7(4), 198–200.*

At the time this article was written, the author had identified factors impinging on nursing that resulted in a confusion of goals and the division of nursing into two camps. The camps were divided into those who believed the professional nurse of the future would have largely supervisory and managerial responsibilities and, on the other side, those who believed that nursing could and would take its place as a professional discipline in relation to direct service to people who are "in need of nursing care."

Johnson belonged to the latter camp: the science of nursing and the art of nursing. The first of these—the discussion of the science of nursing, centered around the patient, the recipient of care—is phenomenal in that it is as relevant today as it was in the late 1950s. In fact, the discussion might almost be considered prophetic because three decades later, the client was identified as one of the nursing phenomena. Nursing process, nursing diagnosis, and nursing science are no longer as esoteric as they seemed in 1959 when Johnson's article was published. Nursing art, to Johnson, represented ministration of the basic unmet needs of the patient. Also identified are those activities that are delegated and controlled by the physician.

A sociologic analysis of the nursing role is used as a vehicle for understanding the division of labor between nurses and physicians. We will also see, much later in time, just how much of an impact this sociologic analysis has had on Johnson's own theory.

Johnson, D.E. (1961). The significance of nursing care. **Nursing Outlook,** *61(11), 63–66.*

This is a very significant—indeed, classic—work in nursing knowledge. Here, Johnson introduces the notion of stability rather than change as the goal of nursing. Meeting the needs of the patient helps bring about that stability.

Because of pressures from the medical and hospital management on nursing to take on non-nursing tasks, Johnson believes that the view of nursing as a direct and individualized service has become less goal-oriented and more blurred. Three major components or types of nursing services were identified: (1) nursing care, (2) delegated medical care, and (3) health care. Of the three, only one—nursing care—has "no well-delineated theoretical framework or conceptual basis to give it meaning or direction (p. 64)."

The purpose of this article, then, is to delineate such a framework within the context of nursing's distinctive contribution to patient welfare and the specific purpose of nursing care.

Using concepts of physiologic homeostasis borrowed from Cannon and stability in patterns of social interaction from Parsons, Johnson synthesized them and related them to individuals who are ill. Instability causes tension; if tension is intense, an individual experiences discomfort and displeasure.

Speculating from these, Johnson attempted to evolve a basis for nursing care using concepts of equilibrium, stress, and tension. Each of these is defined in general terms, and then as it applies to an individual patient (or group) or how the nurse might identify or assess stress, tension, or equilibrium. The conceptualization of equilibrium, stress, and tension presents a way of viewing the nature of disturbances that a patient might have, as well as the purpose of nursing care, or what might be considered nursing's specific responsibility in nursing care.

Two nursing interventions within this framework are also suggested. First, reduction of the stressful stimuli through the management of the physical and psychological environment, and second, support of the patient's "natural defenses and adaptive processes" through "protective and sustaining measures." The focus of nursing is on immediate situations, universal needs, and patterns that belong to the patient and are gratifying to him. The seeds for Johnson's theory were planted in this writing.

Johnson, D.E. (1980). The behavioral system model for nursing. In J.P. Riehl and C. Roy (Eds.), **Conceptual models for nursing practice** *(2nd ed.). New York: Appleton-Century-Crofts.*

Dorothy Johnson, for the first time in writing, clearly presents the whole of her theory. Much of her unpublished work had been alluded to by her protégées and, although available in manuscript form, it suffered from limited distribution. This was the first time the original behavioral systems theory for nursing was published in its entirety.

According to its author, the behavioral systems model has its origins in a philosophical perspective and has been supported by an expanding empirical and theoretical base (i.e., systems theory). (It would be helpful to read three of the author's early publications, two in 1959 and one in 1961, in conjunction with this one.) It is Johnson's perspective that both nurses and physicians theoretically have viewed a human being as a system. However, nurses view the patient as a behavioral system, whereas physicians view him as a biologic system. It is the nursing view of the human being as a behavioral system that underlies this model. A review of this article shows that the underlying assumptions of the model are explicit. The concepts are embedded in the context and are not specifically defined. The system is identified as having seven subsystems, which are briefly defined. The four structural elements of each subsystem are listed and discussed.

The basic elements of the model, which are briefly touched upon and that are implicit rather than explicit, include values, goal of action, patiency, and source of difficulty. The latter is discussed only minimally; noticeably missing is a discussion of intervention.

In summarizing, the author indicated that the behavioral systems model "seems defensible and promising by three criteria." The criteria were named in the 1974 article and are social congruence, social significance, and social utility. She also said that the model has "proved its utility in providing clear direction for practice, education, and research." Although the present work does not provide any evidence to support this, some available documentation exists and is discussed in the section on Johnson in this book.

Despite these limitations of the model—that is, underdevelopment of some of the elements and lack of supportive evidence for the model's utility—this theoretical model for nursing is one of the major contributions to nursing theory development in the past two decades. Furthermore, Johnson's thinking has impacted on a great number of graduate students in nursing who have since gone on to develop other theoretical models. Johnson's stimulus for progress should not be underestimated; it has resulted in the advancement of nursing as a science.

Lovejoy, N.C. (1983). The leukemic child's perceptions of family behaviors. Oncology Nursing Forum, *10(4), 20–25.*

Contributing to theory development and testing through the development of instruments to measure concepts is of utmost importance to the advancement of nursing science.

The author states that the Johnson model was selected as the theoretical framework "because of its basic premise that human behavior in health and illness is the independent domain of nursing" (Lovejoy, 1983, p. 20). In table form, as part of the background materials, the author presented a comparison of the Johnson behavioral system model (JBSM) goals by subsystem and by theorist, showing differences between theorists. The theorists compared are Johnson, Grubbs, Auger, and Lovejoy, all of whom have elaborated upon and used the model. This provides a helpful summary and review of the subsystems for the reader familiar with the model. It is assumed, however, that the reader has some knowledge of the model. The author notes the disparity among the theorists regarding the scope of the goal-directed behaviors of the subsystems, but concludes that "the goals used in this research appeared to parsimoniously and discretely define special domains of behavior (Lovejoy, 1983, p. 21)." The reader is left wondering where the support for such a conclusion is. Little additional elaboration of or support for "discretely defined domains of behavior" was given.

The Family Relations (FR) test, the instrument upon which the family assessment instrument was modeled, was then described. The FR test situation was designed as a play situation in which a child was to decide what feelings fit which members of the family. The family assessment instrument (Lovejoy) consists of 47 items apparently designed to reflect the eight subsystems of the JBSM. The number of questions ranges from four to eight for each subsystem. No explanation is provided for having a variable number of items per subsystem. The items are shown in Table 2 and stand alone without additional explanation. Items for the assessment tool were generated and formulated based on a review of major growth and development theorists and a review of chronic illness research. Statements reflecting functional and dysfunctional family member behaviors were formulated from this review. The statements describing these behaviors were then placed on individual cards for later test administration. Noticeably missing was reference to how items were formulated to reflect the eight subsystems of the JBSM. This is an important omission, given that the author purported that the instrument was "based on the Johnson Model for nursing (1983, p. 20)."

There are several major limitations with this instrument. First, there is little or no evidence of content and face validity within the context of either growth and development theory or the Johnson model. No evidence is presented indicating that the items were subjected to a review by experts, either in growth and development or the Johnson model. This was also true of the review of the scoring guide, as discussed previously. Although it is a time-consuming and arduous task, some attempt to develop content validity is crucial, even for initial instrument development, and this was overlooked in the development of this instrument.

Second, the scoring guide and the method of scoring described suggest that the rating of 0 to 2 is a scale, with equal distances between each measure. In application, these appear to be discrete categories and therefore not conducive to the summation-scoring method used.

It may be more appropriate to standardize the instrument by developing norms for each age group.

Rawls, A.C. (1980). Evaluation of the Johnson behavioral model in clinical practice: Report of a test and evaluation of the Johnson theory. Image, *12, 13–16.*

In the introduction, the author clearly identifies the importance of model testing for the future of nursing in general and, specifically, her rationale for choosing to evaluate the application of the Johnson theory. The purpose and scope of the report are also identified. The title might suggest that the "test" was research when, actually, it was an exercise in whether or not the theory was clinically useful.

As background for the study, a brief history and an overview of other authors' contributions to the model is presented. Johnson's model is briefly reviewed to provide readers with an outline of how the model was used as a framework by the author. The subsystems and their components and the structure and function of the theory are all defined. For purposes of discussion only, the structure, function, and functional requirements of the subsystems are discussed in detail. After clarification of a few other components of the model, the use of the Johnson model (JM) as a guide for the nursing process is illustrated.

Each stage of the nursing process—assessment through evaluation—is described within the context of the JM subsystems using the Grubbs assessment tool and nursing process worksheet. These processes and description are similar to those described by Janelli (1980) with Roy's model. Prior to the beginning of the "study," variables that may have influenced the outcome were explored. The identified variables were: "limited knowledge of Johnson's theory," "lack of experience in utilizing Grubbs' assessment tool and nursing process worksheet," and patient's response to the researcher, to the assessment tool, and to the plan of care developed. Time available for the study and the size of the study group were also identified. The author chose to limit the sample size to one "due to the variables cited previously" (Rawls, 1980, p. 13).

The study focused on a case presentation of one subject, beginning with patient background, followed by first- and second-level assessments. The patient selected for the study was a white male who had been hospitalized for evaluation of an accidental injury, resulting in painful amputation of the left hand and distal phalanges approximately 6 months earlier. The first-level assessment appeared to be more in keeping with the medical model, in that information about past and present history of the problem, psychological assessment, family, and social, environmental, and development history were reviewed.

From the perspective of the JM, no examples of subsystem assessments were presented. An exception was a statement indicating that, because no problems were noted in the review to that point, a complete review of the behavior subsystems was conducted using Grubbs' assessment tool. Two problem areas in the achievement subsystem were identified. Because there were problem areas in only this one subsystem, the discussion was limited to it. Second-level assessment proceeded from there. One concept—the concept of body image—was explored in depth.

The assessment phase was followed by a plan for care, again focusing on intervention for the two problems in the achievement subsystem only. The plan focused on how the patient's loss of his left hand and its function prevented him from meeting the conceptual goal of the achievement subsystem (i.e., to achieve or master). Variables that might have influenced the patient's care were explored and identified. "The developmental, psychological, sociological, and level-of-wellness variables were all viewed as influencing variables that could be manipulated to benefit the patient" (Rawls, 1980, p. 16).

The next step was the identification of nursing problems. This step may be confusing in that problems were identified earlier in the assessment phases of the nursing process. Furthermore, the author did not clarify why this additional step of problem identification was necessary. Further reading led me to conclude that these additional problems were refinements of previously identified problems in the achievement subsystem. The nursing interventions for these problems were detailed, with numerous examples used for illustration. Both long- and short-term goals of nursing intervention were formulated. The plan of care was evaluated and found to be appropriate, as measured by changes consistent with the short-term goals. The plan of care, with minor revisions, was also found to be appropriate to the patient's postoperative course.

The author's "evaluation of the JM" was more of an evaluation of the usefulness of the model for clinical practice than a critical review of the model itself. The author recommended that the model be tested further in a variety of settings with clients who have a variety of complex problems in each of the subsystems. To have stated this limitation is to the author's credit. Disadvantages of the model, as perceived by the author, included complex and unique terminology and the requirement of knowledge of systems theory to use the model more effectively. The author concluded that the advantages of the model for practice, in essence, outweighed the disadvantages; she believed that the JM "offers the nurse a tool which will allow her to accurately predict the results of nursing interventions prior to care," and "formulate standards for care" (1980, p. 16).

The nursing educator who is interested in teaching the JM or in demonstrating the application of theory to practice (as well as the nursing theorist concerned about the utility of the model for practice) would find this article of some interest. The beginnings of the elaboration of the concept of body image as it relates to the achievement subsystem are present in this author's assessment phase.

Small, B. (1980). Nursing visually impaired children with Johnson's model as a conceptual framework. In J.P. Riehl and C. Roy (Eds.), Conceptual models for nursing practice (2nd ed., pp. 264–273). New York: Appleton-Century-Crofts.

Although nursing research that tests hypotheses of nursing theories is critical for the advancement of a particular theory, this study does not test hypotheses evolving from Johnson's theory, but it demonstrates that the theory could be utilized in working with visually impaired children.

The report of a research study forms the first of two parts of this chapter. The second includes implications for nursing. The major assumptions underlying the theoretical framework of the study were derived from Piaget and cognitive developmental psychology. Two null hypotheses were tested and rejected. The first stated that "there would be no significant difference between the perceived body image of visually impaired and normally sighted preschool children." The second stated that there would be no significant difference between the spatial awareness of visually impaired preschoolers and those who were normally sighted.

The author explains results of the study using Johnson's theory. Vision plays an important role in the development of object permanence and the relation of objects in space. These two concepts are necessary for the development of a child's body image and for his awareness of his body in space. Therefore, if a child is visually handicapped, the implications are that nurses can intervene to meet his needs and to facilitate the development of his self-concept.

Once this line of reasoning was developed, and once a brief description of Johnson's model was presented, the author tended to focus more on interventions with the parents than with the child, therefore supporting Johnson's recommendations for intervention: manipulation of the environment to reduce tension.

MYRA LEVINE

Esposito, C.H. and Leonard, M.K. (1980). Myra Estrin Levine: In The Nursing Theories Conference Group (Ed.), **Nursing theories: A base for professional practice** *(pp. 150–163). Englewood Cliffs, NJ: Prentice-Hall.*

The content of this article is organized to include a summary of the components of Levine's theory, its application to the nursing process, and the relationship of the theory to five major concepts (humanity, society, health, learning, and nursing). In addition, a brief case study is included to demonstrate application to practice (i.e., the utility of the theory for clinical practice).

One of the major contributions of this chapter is the identification of the explicit assumptions underlying Levine's theory. This is helpful because the assumptions are implicit in Levine's writing.

There is one important omission in this discussion of Levine's theory: the major theoretical underpinning—namely, systems theory—is not identified. Given that systems theory is not acknowledged, it becomes clearer why Levine's theory is identified as having a close kinship to Maslow's hierarchy of needs. One might agree that parallels could be drawn between the conservation principles and Maslow's levels of needs, but Maslow's theory must not be construed as the prototype for Levine's principles. Nowhere in Levine's writing is there any reference to Maslow's needs hierarchy.

Two potential problems in this chapter are the lack of identification between Levine's and Esposito's and Leonard's additions, and that the parallels between Maslow's hierarchy of needs and conservation principles (tenuous at best) may be accidental and therefore do not justify this as a prototype paradigm. More support could be given to system or adaptations as guiding paradigms.

Hirschfeld, M.J. (1976). The cognitively impaired older adult. **American Journal of Nursing,** *76(12), 1981–1984.*

In a very straightforward discussion of the possible cognitive impairments of older adults, and in the only published work on utilization of Levine's theory in practice, Hirschfeld demonstrates how Levine's four principles of conservation can be applied to give direction to nursing interventions when impairments are present. The goal of the interventions is specified as trying to keep remaining cognitive capacities intact and in use.

Each conservation principle, and examples demonstrating problems in the area it covered, is discussed separately. For example, a variety of problems are described wherein the balance of activity and rest were disturbed. Focusing on conservation of energy in this case gave the nurse direction for intervention.

Levine, M.E. (1966). Adaptation and assessment: A rationale for nursing intervention. **American Journal of Nursing,** *66(11), 2450–2453.*

Levine introduced "trophicognosis" as an alternative concept to replace "nursing diagnosis" (Levine, M.E. [1966]. Trophicognosis: An alternative to nursing diagnosis. In *Exploring progress in medical surgical nursing practice* [pp. 55–70]. New York: American Nurses Association. A series of papers presented at the 1965 Regional Clinical Conferences, November 3–5, 1965, Washington, D.C.). The latter conjures up medicine and disease orientation, whereas the former focuses attention on judgments related to nursing care utilizing the scientific method. In that earlier writing, it becomes apparent that Levine is interested in delineating nursing goals and differentiating them from medical goals.

In this second of four articles that precede the publication of her book, *Introduction to Clinical Nursing,* Levine further demonstrates her conceptualization of nursing as utilizing the scientific method and as a coherent theory in guiding nursing actions. She argues that nursing practice and education have long been influenced by the prevailing beliefs about health and disease. As a result of a carryover or a carrythrough of earlier theories, nursing care has become "an unsynthesized 'total,' a sum of many disparate parts" (p. 2451). Thus, there is an urgent need, as Levine sees it, for a restatement of the theoretical basis for nursing practice. This is what she attempted to do in this article.

Drawing from a variety of sources—philosophy, physiology, and sociology—a few basic ideas about human beings become implicit assumptions of the theory. Central ideas are: (1) a human being's life is multidimensional, (2) a human being is in constant interaction with the environment, (3) a human being's internal environment is integrated and is dynamically balanced, (4) a human being responds to forces in the environment in a unique but integrated manner, (5) health and disease are patterns of adaptive change, and (6) the nurse is part of every patient's environment. One sees here the influence of systems theory: wholeness of human being, dynamic equilibrium, human being–environment interactions, and adaptation.

The author revived Nightingale's ideas of multicausality of illness, disease as a "reparative process," and nursing's goal as establishing a health environment that would enhance healing and reparative processes. Levine refocused nursing's attention on the wholeness of human beings, the uniqueness of each human being, and on the fact that a broad knowledge base is required by the nurse to give nursing care.

Levine's discussion of adaptation raises some questions. Adaptation is introduced but not really defined per se. For example, "all the processes of living are processes of adaptation," "diseases represent patterned responses or adaptations," "health and disease are patterns of adaptive change" (p. 2452). But what is adaptation? Levine indicates that

a criterion of successful adaptation is the attainment of social well-being, which is neither defined nor related to the preceding physiologic discussion.

The major ideas expressed about nursing are that the nurse is an agent who intervenes between a patient and his environment to facilitate adaptation and that the interventions are based on coherent and systematic knowledge and a scientific process in collecting data about the patient.

Levine, M.E. (1967). The four conservation principles of nursing. Nursing Forum, 6(1), 45–59.

This article is the third that this author wrote in an attempt to lay down a framework for nursing intervention. It is helpful to read this after reading the first two, on trophicognosis and on adaptation and assessment, to fully understand the process that Levine used in theory development: redefining central concepts, reconceptualization of nursing goals, and then nursing actions. She identified central concepts, stated assumptions, and proposed four central propositions.

The concept of adaptation as developed by Levine in her earlier article remains undefined. In the introduction alone, adaptation may be conceived or interpreted in three different ways. First, one can infer that it "can be manifested in patterns" and "has a course." One could also infer that adaptation is an outcome because it can be measured by "renewed social well-being." Third, in another context, one can infer that adaptation can be a capability or a characteristic of a person.

Aside from adaptation, the major focus of this article and Levine's major contribution to theory is the introduction of four conservation principles that are central to the mission of nursing. Levine identifies nursing principles as "fundamental assumptions which provide a unifying structure for understanding a wide variety of nursing activities" (p. 45). Here, each principle (labeled assumptions, but they may be the theory's propositions) is listed separately, along with a statement about nursing intervention, and is then followed by a discussion that supports the principle and the rationale for it. Clinical examples are included as supportive evidence. The four principles are all conservation principles. Conservation is defined as "keeping together," but the author emphasizes that this "should not imply minimal activity," especially on the part of the nurse.

The four principles are: "(1) The Principle of the Conservation of Patient Energy, (2) The Principle of the Conservation of Structural Integrity, (3) The Principle of Conservation of Personal Integrity, (4) The Principle of Conservation of Social Integrity." For each of these, nursing intervention is based on the conservation of the particular patient's need in focus. The four principles evolved from an assumption of the unity and integrity of the individual; they are well-developed and supported with clinical examples; and they are, in part, consistent with some assumptions from the systems theory.

Three critical questions are raised: (1) How did the author come to the point of identifying four and only four principles? (2) In principle 2, given the complex interrelationships of human structure and function (which Levine does discuss), why is the principle not stated in terms of both structural and functional integrity, or why weren't two separate principles for these developed? What is the rationale for focusing on structural integrity versus both structure and function? (3) Why aren't personal integrity and social integrity specifically defined?

Considering the dearth of theoretical frameworks for nursing available in the late 1960s, this framework made a substantial contribution to the science of nursing. Levine proved herself to be an insightful, forward-looking theorist.

Levine, M.E. (1969). *The pursuit of wholeness.* American Journal of Nursing, *69(1), 93–98.*

Consistent with the first three articles and with systems theory, Levine views a human being as a system in constant interaction with the environment: "patients are complete persons, not groups of parts."

This article provides a view of the human being from a nursing perspective, as a system in a constant dynamic interchange with the environment and as part of a larger ecosystem. Information is exchanged between the human system and the larger ecosystem by way of the perceptual subsystem. Disturbances in the perceptual subsystem, as well as the levels of organismic response used to protect the organism as it responds to the environment, give direction to nursing.

When the environment changes, the human being must change. Levine makes a fairly succinct theoretical statement here about what adaptation is. This process of change "whereby the individual retains his integrity—his wholeness—within the realities of his environment" is labeled adaptation (p. 95). The goal of the individual is to defend his wholeness.

There are at least four levels of organismic response, each physiologically predetermined. (This is an implicit assumption on Levine's part.) The responses are used to protect the organism, so that it can make a viable adaptation to the environment. The four levels include: response to fear, inflammatory response, response to stress, and sensory response. These four levels are fairly well-documented.

Alone, this article does not contribute substantially to our understanding of Levine's theory; it must not be read in isolation. In the context of earlier articles and ones that come later, the perspective of this one becomes clearer.

Levine, M.E. (1971). *Holistic nursing.* Nursing Clinics of North America, *6(2), 253–264.*

No new material is presented here. Instead, this is a synthesis of previously published material that contributes to a better general understanding of the theory. The author brings together all the ideas, the separate parts, of the earlier four articles into a whole. The parts of Levine's theory—the assumptions, central concepts, definitions of person (who is the nursing client), goals of nursing, and nursing intervention—are put together, and the interrelationships between parts are then described.

Levine views holistic nursing as a challenge before nurses. This approach to nursing takes place at the interface between the organism (human being) and the environment. In other words, nursing is an interaction, and the nurse, in a sense, mediates between the organism and his environment, whether the environment in question is the organism's internal or external environment.

For the person desiring an overview of the theory, or some help in piecing together the earlier parts of the theory, this article could be most helpful and should then be read before the first four articles.

Levine, M.E. (1971). *Time has come to speak of . . . health care.* AORN Journal, *13, 37–43.*

In a speech to the annual congress of the Association of Operating Room Nurses, focusing on the viability concerns of that group, Levine indirectly presents arguments in support of her theoretical framework for nursing. Ostensibly, the focus of the speech is the threat of increased technologic change and innovation to the roles of nurses, especially with the concomitant requirement for technicians to manage the machinery. The health care field has responded to technologic advances by increasing the number of technicians. Although operating room nurses were the first to be threatened by this influx, they are not the only ones inundated by technicians. For example, ICUs, CCUs, trauma, dialysis, burn, coma, respiratory, and hyperbaric units each require its own complement of technicians.

Nevertheless, Levine argues that, in all these settings, both technical and professional roles remain to be filled. She further argues that, although new threats from increasing numbers of technician positions continue to appear, the real concern is for the quality of patient care. What will happen if physician assistants, for example, go into underserved areas to provide a second- class kind of medical care? If this becomes a trend, then nursing must make itself heard to prevent these inadequacies from occurring. Those in society who are already underserved, already suffering, would be most affected by these health care inadequacies.

Confusion in the roles of workers, both professional and technical, has been a result of the great changes in health care. However, there still remains one need that nurses can recognize and sustain: self-respect and humanity of the patient. The nurse traditionally has been and must remain the patient's advocate. Unless the effort is made to reach out and establish human contact, the patient will become just another part of the elaborate machinery of technology. The technical role in this situation is supportive and essential, but it is the professional nurse who must be the patient's advocate, the humanizing agent, the one who brings "compassion, protection, and commitment to the bedside."

Given the changes in health care, the education of nurses must change too. To be the professional nurse, as described previously, Levine believes that the achievement of the education of a patient's advocate requires knowledge and skills of a global kind. Furthermore, there needs to be a conceptualization of nursing. She presents her formulations as valid forms of nursing intervention. She also suggests that the concepts inherent in the generalizations can be readily applied to all kinds of nursing intervention. It is here that we see Levine's support for her theoretical framework for nursing as one way to counter the threat of technologic advances to nursing, patients, and health care.

DOROTHEA OREM

Allison, S.E. (1973). A framework for nursing action in a nurse-conducted diabetic management clinic. **Journal of Nursing Administration,** *3(4), 53–60.*

This article is based on and follows the 1974 Backscheider article, although this one was published first. The author provides a comprehensive picture of the health care system, using the self-care model as a basis for the nurse-conducted diabetic management clinic. The author synthesizes some of Orem's and Backscheider's concepts: universal self-care, health deviation self-care (Orem), and mental, physical, motivational, emotional, and orientational capacities to follow a therapeutic regimen (Backscheider). The article provides a highly useful example of the use of Orem's ideas in a nurse-run diabetic clinic. Three models— self-care, health status, and environment—are offered as a framework for assessment and intervention. The author provides a very useful discussion of areas of responsibility, and differentiates between traditional nursing roles (administrative) and practitioner roles (clinically oriented) as shared and as delineated for nursing, medicine, and other health services. Although this is an ideal setting for theory testing, the focus of the article is on application.

Anna, D.J., Christensen, D.G., Hohn, S.A., Ord, L., and Wells, S.R. (1978). Implementing Orem's conceptual framework. **Journal of Nursing Administration,** *8(11), 8–11.*

The authors present a descriptive account of the implementation of Orem's model by a group of graduate students in a nursing home setting for adult patients (geriatric setting). In doing so, the authors provide a short summary of the theory, the use of the nursing process according to Orem, the strategies the students used in implementing the theory in the setting, and the obstacles preventing implementation by students, patients, and nursing staff. Difficulties experienced by the students in shifting to Orem's conceptualization (terminology, concept definitions, mechanization) are those that could be universal and could apply to all initial attempts at implementing any nursing theory. The conceptualization of a patient's role as that of a significant decision maker and eventually a performer of self-care activities presented another obstacle. Patients felt more comfortable as recipients of care. As expected, the nursing staff was resistant to change initiated by a group of temporary students. Evaluation of the implementation process was done by review of students' personal diaries. Themes were an increase in patient participation, motivation, and cooperation.

Backscheider, J.E. (1974). Self-care requirements, self-care capabilities, and nursing systems in the diabetic nurse management clinic. **American Journal of Public Health,** *64(12), 1138–1146.*

This author provides a conceptualization of the diabetic-related component of therapeutic self-care, encompassing a set of patient responsibilities (related to the patient's own condition and therapy and to the effects of his condition and therapy) and a set of action capabilities (physical, mental, motivational, emotional, and orientational). Nursing care is needed when a patient has limited capability to meet therapeutic self-care goals (self-care deficit). Nursing is a mediating system and is divided into four types. Nursing care (nursing system) is focused on the patient as a recipient of one-time guidance or teaching, on long-term assistance that is oriented toward maintenance and support, on more permanent compensatory care oriented toward some changes in the patient, or on compensatory care using changes in the environment.

When a given health care deviation occurs, the capabilities essential to meet that portion of therapeutic self-care are determined first and foremost. Criteria can then be established. The nurse can assess the patient's capabilities against the established criteria to determine whether or not the patient can meet self-care demands. This is a more positive approach, a more scientific one to establishing nursing interventions than by estimating the patient's abilities or limitations.

This is an important article to read in relation to the theory of self-care. It demonstrates the interaction between practice and theory development and shows potential for researchable questions.

Bromley, B. (1980). Applying Orem's self-care theory in enterostomal therapy. **American Journal of Nursing,** *80(2), 245–249.*

The author, an enterostomal therapist, begins with a discussion of her own personal philosophy of nursing practice, with the most useful tool being the nurse. Her choice of Orem's theory was made because of the apparent congruency between her own and Orem's philosophies. The usefulness of this article lies in the author's synthesis of her perceptions of Orem's theory and the use of an exemplar to demonstrate the theory–practice fit, particularly around nursing interventions. The author writes clearly and does a particularly nice job of showing how the nursing systems of self-care are implemented in an inpatient (hospital) setting. Using an example, she shows how she has moved with a client from a wholly compensatory system, through the partly compensatory system, to the supportive–educative system.

For those interested in the appropriateness of Orem's model for inpatient practice in a surgical setting, this is a good example because the author followed the theory closely throughout.

Buckwalter, K.C. and Kerfoot, K.M. (1982). Teaching patients self-care: A critical aspect of psychiatric discharge planning. **Journal of Psychiatric Nursing and Mental Health Services,** *20(5), 15–20.*

While ostensibly presenting clinical applications under the umbrella of Orem's self-care framework, this article is about discharge planning and teaching; it appears that the notion of self-care has been added after the fact. The abstract clues us in to the fact that self-care is not an integral part of the conceptualization of discharge planning.

The content covers understanding the diagnosis, stressors, signs and symptoms, resocializing issues, community support, and medication compliance. Each topic is briefly described and illustrated with clinical examples. A sample standardized protocol for depressed patients and their families is included.

The only references to Orem are the use of her definition of self-care and two references to kinds of nursing assistance, namely, teaching and self-care guidance. Self-care concepts are not applied to the content. To be consistent with the theoretical framework, the content must also follow. For example, the summary of the five areas to be covered with patient and family in the discharge planning interview (p. 16) lend themselves to the six health deviation self-care requisites as elaborated by Orem (1980, pp. 48–51).

This article covers an important topic of present concern for all mental health practitioners—not just nurses—regarding maintaining the mentally ill in the community. Overall, the article is written in a straightforward and understandable style, and presents important clinical content. Of concern is that the authors state that they are using Orem's perspective; although they do include topics under the rubric of self-care, Orem's framework in fact does not guide the conceptualization of the teaching and guidance plan.

Caley, J.M., Dirksen, M., Engalla, M., and
Hennrich, M.L. (1980). The Orem self-care
nursing model. In J.P. Riehl and C. Roy
(Eds.), **Conceptual models for nursing**
practice *(2nd ed., pp. 302–314). New York:*
Appleton-Century-Crofts.

The intent of the chapter is to offer an example of
the use of Orem's theory in a psychiatric setting,
using a suicidal patient as the case study. The discussion of the model, brief and limited, is organized
around the goal of action, patiency, actor's role,
source of difficulty, intervention focus/mode, and
consequences, both intended and otherwise.

It would be helpful for a theory novice who
is focused on a theory–psychiatric practice link
to read this chapter in conjunction with Orem's
work, with the understanding that it is a limited
exposé and does not do complete justice to Orem's
theories. The authors freely used concepts from
Backscheider (1971, 1974) and the Nursing Development Conference Group (1973) in addition
to Orem (1971).

Chang, B.L. (1980). Evaluation of health care
professionals in facilitating self-care: Review
of the literature and a conceptual model. **Ad-**
vances in Nursing Science, *3(1), 43–58.*

The purpose of this article is stated in terms of needs.
"A need exists for the evaluation of health professionals in facilitating self-care. Such an evaluation must
take into account lay persons' judgments regarding
the health care received. A conceptual framework
is needed for the evaluation of the role of health
professionals in facilitating self-care" (p. 44). The
"why" of this, its importance, is not spelled out.

The author states that the derivation of her
framework for the evaluation of health professionals is in part from Orem's work and in part from
other literature related to the evaluation of quality
of care. The dimensions of the framework are
listed as "(1) patient or layperson characteristics,
(2) health care professional characteristics, and (3)
patient outcomes" (p. 44). A diagram illustrates
the relationship of these dimensions and serves
to introduce the components of these dimensions.
The diagram contains all the dimensions and their
components and the direction of the linkages. The
third and last dimension, influenced by the preceding
two, is the focus of the review of literature. Why
only the third dimension—evaluation of outcomes
of self-care—is reviewed in detail is not stated.

Although the author has presented a broad
definition of self-care, a strong statement about
the overall importance of the topic and why this
particular definition of self-care was chosen over
others commonly used in the literature has thus far
not been presented.

There are numerous opportunities to use
Orem's framework to guide the conceptualization
of the model proposed, and they are not taken
advantage of. In the review of literature on evaluation of outcomes of self-care—specifically the
three components—the author appears to have
neglected to use important articles relevant to the
framework presented. Examples of this include
writings by Allison (1973), who addresses nurses
and other health team members and their role in
assisting patients to perform self-care regarding diabetic management, and by Backscheider
(1974), who also addresses the role of nurses in
assisting with the self-care practices of diabetics and the self-care competencies required by
ambulatory diabetics.

Although the author may have accomplished
her overall goals of presenting a conceptual model
and reviewing some literature related to evaluation
of health care professionals, conceptual linkages
between the different dimensions are missing.

Coleman, L.J. (1980). Orem's self-care
concept of nursing. In J.P. Riehl and C. Roy
(Eds.), **Conceptual models for nursing**
practice *(2nd ed., pp. 315–328). New York:*
Appleton-Century-Crofts.

The primary purpose of this article is to describe
the implementation of Orem's theory in one nursing
service department of a large metropolitan hospital. Therefore, Orem's model is first summarized
by the author, with particular emphasis on those
concepts and ideas that would be most useful for
the nursing service department of a hospital (e.g.,
nursing assistance, nursing process). The language
of the chapter, to be sure, is the language of nursing
administration, such as classification of patients,
techniques essential for nursing practice, utilization
of nursing personnel, and operational documents.
The author then describes what is involved in revising operational documents of a nursing service,
including departmental philosophy and goals,
departmental policies, divisional philosophy and
objectives, position descriptions, nursing tools, and
nursing care evaluation instruments in the process
of operationalizing Orem's model. Also briefly

described is the preparation of the nursing personnel for understanding and using Orem's concepts.

This chapter offers a "how to" contribution to the nursing administrator who wishes to implement the theory in practice.

Dickson, G.L. and Lee-Villasenor, H. (1982). Nursing theory and practice: A self-care approach. **Advances in Nursing Science, 5, 29–40.**

The stated purpose of this article is "to bridge the gaps between theory and practice through the research of the application of an evolving theory" (p. 29). The authors also present a "new nursing model in which to 'think nursing'" (p. 30). The findings described were from a field study carried out by the authors in their own independent practice settings using their own clients.

The framework of self-care developed by Orem and modified by Kinlein was chosen as the theoretical model for practice and research because the beliefs underlying the model were in keeping with the authors' philosophy. The authors adequately describe and document these background materials sufficiently for those familiar with the model. For those unfamiliar with the model, the review is not adequate.

A nonexperimental, descriptive design was used. The source of data was the written recording of nurse–patient interactions from 35 time periods with four clients. Although the authors describe the four female subjects, they do not tell us why eight other prospective subjects were not included.

The research process proceeded as follows: during the clients' appointments and during the process of providing nursing care, the nursing researchers recorded their clients' words. At the time that a "need" was expressed, the nurse then identified self-care assets, the self-care demands, and the self-care measures with the client. The next step was a period of introspection for reflection on the nursing phenomena observed. Operational definitions were established, and four research questions were generated.

The data analysis yielded four categories of care: (1) the client's expression of need, (2) self-care asset, (3) self-care demand, and (4) self-care measures. These were analyzed using content analysis from the grounded field theory methodology. Further analysis, in keeping with the inductive method of research being used (Glaser and Strauss), focused on the integration of categories and their properties.

Specifically, data were analyzed to determine properties of expressions of need and self-care assets. The latter were found to be similar to the indicators of self-care agency as identified by Kearney and Fleischer (1979).

In summary, the authors reflect on the limitations of the research, namely, sample size and bias, implications for practice and research, and directions for future research. The authors demonstrate clarity in describing both the procedures and the process of their experiences in relating theory to practice and research. The complex helical relationship of the three is clearly illustrated, and the scholarliness of their approach and writing adds to the overall readability. The model was their guide for practice and research and, with the model in mind, it helped to maintain their focus on their goals. For these reasons, this study would be of interest to theorists, researchers, and clinicians alike who espouse the self-care framework. More important, the article provides an exemplar for theory development using the practice-theory strategy.

Karl, C.A. (1982). The effect of an exercise program on self-care activities for the institutionalized elderly. **Journal of Gerontological Nursing, 8, 282–285.**

Although the title of this short report of a research study includes the concept of self-care, and although Orem is mentioned in the section, "Program Background," the self-care framework does not seem to guide the conceptualization of the study. The review of the research literature focuses on general topics of feelings of well-being and physiologic benefits of exercise rather than on self-care. Furthermore, liberties are taken with Orem's framework when the author states that "the theoretical defense for a study of the positive effects an exercise program can have on the institutionalized elderly and their ability to care for themselves has been formulated by Orem in her theory of self-care" (p. 283). Also misstated were the "assumptions"; in fact, these are really the hypotheses tested by the study.

Miller, J.F. (1980). The dynamic focus of nursing: A challenge to nursing administration. **Journal of Nursing Administration, 10(1), 13–18.**

Although the title of this article suggests that the focus will be on nursing administration, and despite the introductory statement that "nursing administrators are challenged to establish a climate that facilitates the use of appropriate frameworks to guide nursing" (p. 13), this article is really about the application of a nursing framework—Orem's—to acute care. However, there is very little evidence of the self-care theory, which the author purports to use. What the author did, in fact, was to pull out the idea of changes in the health–illness continuum, suggesting that nurses focus on changes in the patient's health status as a model to guide intervention. The author presents three conceptual phases for acute care patients (acute illness, convalescence, and restored health), problems and nursing care strategies related to each, and a patient case study to demonstrate application. Only phases 2 and 3 are linked to patient development of self-care skills.

Although it takes into account where the person is on the health–illness continuum (which phase), the proposed "model for dynamic nursing practice" essentially ignores Orem's nursing systems, which give direction for nursing intervention based on the person's health self-care needs or self-care deficits regardless of where he is on the health–illness continuum. Therefore, this article offers a very limited application of Orem's theory.

Miller, J.F. (1982). Categories of self-care needs of ambulatory patients with diabetes. **Journal of Advanced Nursing,** *7, 25–31.*

The stated purpose of this paper is to report a study of the identification of need categories of ambulatory diabetic patients within the context of the self-care nursing framework. The title of the article reflects this purpose. The method used to discover the categories of self-care needs was that of participant observation. The need for the research was identified, but why the self-care framework is "especially appropriate" (p. 25) was not explained.

The sample of 65 men and women, ranging in age from 22 to 83 years, came from different socioeconomic classes and were from various cultural backgrounds. No rationale for sample selection was presented. The clinic where the subjects were treated used the self-care concept for nursing practice. Data collection initially involved an assessment of the patient's self-care agency using an instrument designed by the researcher and published elsewhere. Additional self-care evaluation was completed during later patient contacts, with all patients in the study having a minimum of three contacts. "The evaluation consisted of four parts: an interview, physical assessment, interpretation of findings,

and mutually determined goals" (p. 26). During this process, nursing care was provided during the contact. "Data gathered were recorded on a care plan and collection continued until no new categories were discovered and each category had been saturated with examples" (p. 27). Ten categories of needs were identified: "acquire skills for self-care management, receive feedback regarding self-care management, become aware of own resources, have feelings of self-esteem enhanced, grieve over losses, work towards acceptance of chronic disease, have new or continuing health concerns evaluated, obtain services from various support agencies, alleviate physical and mental discomforts, identify positive role of the health care agency and feel like a full participant in determining care goals, and maintain family solidarity and support or assist ill member" (p. 27).

These findings reveal an interesting contrast to the findings of Dickson and Lee-Villasenor (1982), who similarly used the method of participant observation. The latter also made observations in a clinical setting with a quite different sample and gleaned their need categories from statements of needs as expressed by their subjects.

In the discussion and conclusions, there is a certain eagerness to apply the findings to the practice setting as the next step. Here, that application is premature. More appropriate to the Orem's present stage of theory development is the phase of reanalysis and refinement of the self-care need categories for this subpopulation.

This study makes an important contribution to nursing science by using the theoretical formulations of Orem to guide the organization into need categories of the observations made of 65 ambulatory diabetic clients. These data and categories contribute important information for continued theory development, for the inductive approach, and, more specifically, for the development of the concept of self-care needs.

Murphy, P.P. (1981). A hospice model and self-care theory. **Oncology Nursing Forum,** *8(2), 19–21.*

This brief article describes how Orem's self-care framework was used as a guide for nursing practice in a hospice setting. The focus of the article is on the role of nursing in this setting, using the three basic systems of nursing care described by Orem: (1) supportive–educative, (2) partially compensatory, and (3) wholly compensatory. Examples of interaction level between the nurse and the patient for each system and a diagram illustrate how the hospice team operates using the self-care framework.

Although this article is not based on research but rather on clinical application, and although it does not provide any new insights or interpretations of Orem's work, it does demonstrate that the self-care framework is a useful guide for practitioners in a setting with terminally ill patients.

Petrlik, J.C. (1976). Diabetic peripheral neuropathy. American Journal of Nursing, 76, 1794–1797.

While this article does not mention Orem's theory as a basis for the discussion of self-care, it is based on the earlier article by Backscheider on self-care requirements and self-care abilities and should be read in conjunction with it. In this case, the author focused on assessment of the self-care abilities of patients who have peripheral neuropathy and the concomitant long-term problems. The theory–practice analysis is useful in helping the reader delineate some research propositions.

Porter, D. and Shamian, J. (1983). Self-care in theory and practice. Canadian Nurse, 79(8), 21–23.

Self-care as theory originated in the early 1950s. Orem was perceived as visionary, and the theory was labeled as revolutionary by the authors. Self-care was defined, and the assumptions of the theory and the goal of nursing were identified; the scope of practice—the role of nurse in relation to the client—was also discussed. How nurses might achieve the goal of nursing according to Orem was also explored in this article.

The basic needs of clients, which nurses assist in meeting, are classified by Orem as universal, developmental, and health deviational. While these are consistent with Orem's theory, only brief listings suggest what makes up each of these categories of needs. Citing Orem, the authors suggested that nursing interventions corresponding to the first two categories of needs could be considered primary prevention. Secondary and tertiary prevention would be those interventions related to health deviation self-care needs.

Within the context of Orem's theory, nursing care planning is facilitated by the development of nursing systems. Nursing system was defined, and the hierarchical components of the nursing system were outlined. These included wholly compensatory, partly compensatory, and supportive–educative, all of which were defined indirectly within the context of examples. Patients were to be categorized into one of these three systems through the nursing process when the nurse planned care.

The nursing process within the context of self-care theory included the identification of a number of factors influencing a person's ability to perform self-care. Some were listed. This concluded the brief description of the assessment phase. Likewise, the intervention phase was only briefly described.

Intervention is required when self-care abilities are inadequate to meet self-care demands. Nursing measures that help the client to achieve the goal of self-care as defined by Orem include: (1) acting or doing for; (2) guiding; (3) teaching; (4) supporting; and (5) providing a developmental environment. None of these was discussed by the authors. The meanings of major terms and concepts were illustrated within the context of a clinical situation and were offset for emphasis. This clinical example was titled "Self-care theory in practice at the JGH" (Jewish General Hospital).

Overall, the authors' description was in keeping with the theory, and the few omissions of concepts were not significant in terms of the model. The article provides a clear distillation or synopsis of the theory presented in an easy reading style, and although it is merely informative, it might be of interest to the newcomer to Orem's model. It might also be of interest to clinicians wishing a quick overview of the model and its potential utility in the practice setting.

Smith, M.C. (1979). Proposed metaparadigm for nursing research and theory development: An analysis of Orem's self-care theory. Image, 11(3), 75–79.

The purpose of this article is to "propose a classification scheme to structure the analysis of existing research and the design of future research in nursing." The author uses Orem's theory to illustrate the proposed scheme. The ultimate purpose is to "formulate a cohesive, organized body of knowledge for theory building and development in nursing" (p. 75), as well as to organize existing research and design future research studies from a nursing framework.

Having developed a scheme and labeled a metaparadigm, the author illustrated how the premises and propositions of this particular nursing theorist are or can be classified. The author acknowledges and makes explicit her personally biased assumptions regarding the *sine qua non* of professional nursing practice.

This article is relevant to discussions of central phenomena in nursing and to the relationships among nursing research, theory development, and nursing practice.

Sullivan, T.J. (1980). Self-care model for nursing. *In* New directions for nursing in the '80s. *Kansas City, MO: American Nurses' Association.*

The introduction to this article is very broad, discussing the issues for nursing and society for the 1980s. This leads the reader to the present focus of self-care and its appropriateness for clients and for the nursing profession, specifically because of the values it embraces and their similarity to those embedded in our American sociocultural value system. Nowhere in the introduction is the reader made aware that the author has taken what she perceived to be a broad, abstract, and otherwise static grand-level theory and operationalized the concept of self-care to make it more usable. She undertook to organize a body of knowledge for nursing the aged, which resulted in a self-care model for nursing the aged.

More than one-half of the article focuses on a review of Orem's self-care model. This review includes a fairly comprehensive picture of the model and a description of its components. The nature, philosophy (including four underlying assumptions), and conceptual framework of the self-care model are all presented. The conceptual framework includes definitions of the three major conceptual constructs: therapeutic self-care demand, self-care agency, and nursing agency. The relationships among these parts of the framework are also explicated. Nursing agency is defined, and the hierarchical systems and their hierarchical subsystems—technologic, interpersonal, and social—of nursing care are further described and linkages noted.

In the author's discussion of the philosophy of self-care—more specifically within the discussion of the nurse–patient relationship—the author has taken what she described as a "lawlike generalization" and restated it as a proposition. Another statement of a corollary could also have been restated as a propositional statement. These statements were almost incidental to the purpose of this paper, yet they are critically needed to move this theory to the point of being tested by research. Elaboration of

the concepts, development of propositional statements, and subsequent hypothesis generation are basic requirements for validation of the self-care model. This author's brief discussion provides an important step in this direction.

The development of the self-care model for the aged was accomplished following "analysis and review of nursing literature on the aged and self-care." The outcome was a self-care model for nursing the aged. The four levels of the self-care system that emerged were listed and discussed. Conclusions that were reached following identification of these four self-care systems were also listed. The author also addressed the reality that clients might be functioning partly on one level and partly on another, and that the four levels of the self-care system are therefore fluid; they represent a continuum. The model also allows for movement over time, indicating that clients may move vertically from one level of self-care to another as well, in several identifiable directions.

The technological and interpersonal subsystems of the nursing systems overlap in the process of accomplishing the goals of self-care. These were discussed, and approaches for applying methods of assistance to the aged emerged as a result of the study. These approaches were listed from the highest level to the lowest level of client capability for self-care. Also listed from the highest level of client capability to the lowest were four interpersonal subsystems. The social subsystem dimension of the nursing subsystem was also briefly discussed. Horizontal linkages with the model were also discussed. The author noted that, while it was not within the scope of the paper to present the concrete referents identified in the model, they had been identified.

Implications for use of the self-care theory in general, and the self-care model for nursing the aged more specifically, were succinctly summarized. Implications for model development for nursing groups other than the aged, for nursing practice with an emphasis on health versus illness, for hypothesis generation leading to research, for nursing leadership roles in health care, and for issues in nursing such as accountability, legal and ethical, were all presented.

This article would be of interest to practitioners, educators, and researchers who desire to use the self-care model for any of those areas, and it is recommended for reading. For the student of the self-care model, it would be helpful as a succinct summary of the model, with examples of statements of propositions. It would also be of interest to those working with the elderly and those who are interested in the self-care model. Furthermore, for students of epistemology, it illustrates the process of model development through the operationalization of a grand-level theory. The article is clearly written and logically developed; overall, it is a scholarly work that suggests that the model can be used as a curriculum model for gerontologic nursing.

MARTHA ROGERS

Egbert, E. (1980, January). Concept of wellness. **JPN and Mental Health Services,** *18(1), 9–12.*

On the basis of the opening sentence in this article, it appears that Rogers' use of the term *health* (not wellness) in a statement about what nursing is was the stimulus for developing the concept of wellness. At no other time is there any reference to Rogers' work, nor is the concept of wellness, as it is developed, related back to her theory.

The concept of wellness, as developed here, was, in essence, distilled from a variety of definitions as a result of a literature review. On the basis of the review, the author determined that wellness could not be clearly defined. Instead, she delineated a list of characteristics of wellness from the conceptions described by several authors and institutions that attempted to define health, such as Freud, Maslow, Jourard, Perls, Jahoda, Wu, and the World Health Organization. The author suggested that, although health and wellness could not be clearly defined, the list, a synthesis of many definitions, could provide guidelines for nursing intervention and prevention.

This article does not contribute to our understanding of Rogers' theory but provides us with a summary of some of the definitions of health.

Falco, S.M. and Lobo, M.L. (1980). Martha E. Rogers. In The Nursing Theories Conference Group (Ed.), **Nursing theories: The base for professional nursing practice.** *Englewood Cliffs, NJ: Prentice-Hall.*

Consistent with the other chapters in this edited volume, there is a brief history about the theoretician whose theory is presented. This summary of Rogers' *Theoretical Basis of Nursing* by Falco and Lobo is generally written clearly and concisely.

The authors present Rogers' definition of nursing and the five major assumptions about human beings that underlie the nursing science explicated by Rogers. Not listed are the more general, broader assumptions underlying the four principles of homeodynamics, which are explicitly stated by Rogers. The second set of assumptions, similar to those about human beings, is grounded in systems theory. The four principles of homeodynamics are identified and elaborated on by the authors.

In the remainder of the article, the authors compare Rogers' theory with others, present clinical examples, and demonstrate the principles of homeodynamics, and then show how the principles might be used in the nursing process. This illustration shows the potential application of the model to clinical practice. Examples include series of questions to be used in the assessment phase to reflect each of the principles of homeodynamics. Examples are also given of nursing diagnoses, planning, and implementation within the framework. Tables illustrate the relationship of the principles of homeodynamics to the nursing process. This use of Rogers' principles in the nursing process is only one of two known published uses (see also Whelton, 1979) and is an important contribution to the theory.

The authors also discuss limitations of Rogers' principles (i.e., that they are too abstract and that terms have not been sufficiently operationalized).

For the reader unfamiliar with Rogers' *Theoretical Basis of Nursing,* this article presents a brief overview and summary. The examples of application to practice using the nursing process show the utility of the theory for practice, and this makes it more useful for the practitioner. In this way, the article contributes to our understanding and use of this theory and therefore to the science of nursing.

Katz, V. (1971). Auditory stimulation and developmental behavior of the premature infant. **Nursing Research,** *20(3), 196–201.*

Although not explicitly stated by the author, she was a student in Martha Rogers' program, and because this research was based on other research carried out at the same institution, it is assumed that Katz's study was developed based on assumptions of Rogers' theory. If this is correct, not presenting the theoretical framework would be a limitation.

If one were to try to guess which of Rogers' assumptions underlie this study, the following might be included: (1) a human being and his environment are continuously exchanging matter and energy with one another, (2) the life process evolves irreversibly and unidirectionally along the space/time continuum, (3) pattern and organization identify a human being and reflect his innovative wholeness (Rogers, 1970).

"The focus of this study was to determine whether a variation in the environment of the low-birth-weight premature infant by the introduction of the maternal voice can influence behavior" (p. 196). The design of the study was quasi-experimental, using a control group; it had a sample size of 62. The major statistical analysis was an analysis of variance, comparing those premature infants who received a regimen of auditory stimulation with those who did not. The behavioral outcomes measured were motor, tactile-adaptive, auditory, visual, muscle-tension, and irritability responses. All tools used had reliability and validity data available.

The same two raters (not the investigator) who were used to test all infants were blind as to which groups the infants were in. Interscorer agreement between the raters and the investigator was obtained after the raters were trained. These and other measures are important safeguards that were used in this study to reduce the potential for bias in the data. In general, based on the write-up, it appears that the study was well-designed.

The study supported previous findings that had indicated that variations in behavioral development are evident after changes are made in sensory input in low-birth-weight premature infants. More important, and consistent with Rogers' belief that the purpose of nursing as an empirical science is to describe and explain the phenomena central to its concern (i.e., persons) and to predict about them, this study provides empirical data from which nursing intervention can then be planned. In Rogers' terms, "the identification of relationship between events provides for an ordering of knowledges and for the development of nursing's hypothetical generalizations and unifying principles" (1980, pp. 84–85).

For these reasons, this study supports Roger's theory and contributes both to empirical validation of it as well as to the science of nursing in general by the rigor of the research. An important omission in the write-up, however, is that the researcher did not indicate other potentially testable hypotheses generated by this research.

Porter, L.S. (1972). The impact of physical-physiological activity on infants' growth and development. Nursing Research, 21(3), 210–219.

This rigorous experimental study was explicitly based on two assumptions of Martha Rogers' theory: (1) the human organism is an open system

in constant interaction with the environment, and (2) growth and developmental processes are unitary and integrative. The study was developed with the conceptualization that the human organism is an energy field in continuous motion. The researcher postulated a direct relationship between environmentally imposed motion and a speeding up of infant growth and development.

The research was built on earlier studies that also used Rogers' theory as a conceptual framework, as well as the researcher's own earlier study of infants. Because the researcher believed that the results of her earlier study were not generalizable enough, this study was undertaken as a follow-up study to corroborate the earlier findings. (An earlier study by Luz Sobong tested Johnson's proposition of stimulation and growth.)

The study is methodically and systematically described, clearly enough so as to be reproducible. Background, hypotheses, methodology, data collection, and results are all described in detail. Tables showing the data are included, as well as a summary of the analyses performed on the six measures of growth and development used in the study. The six measures of growth and development were gains in weight, length, motor, adaptive, language, and personal–social behavior. The design of the study was experimental, with random assignment of subjects who were then matched with a control group. One limitation in the data collection was that the investigator collected the data and was not blind to whether subjects were in the experimental or control group (or so it appears from the write-up).

A question is raised here regarding the data analysis. For example, the subjects were pretested on the six measures. Results presented showed that the heaviest control subject initially weighed 325 ounces, while the corresponding experimental subject weighed 369 ounces. There is a difference between these two of 44 ounces. In the discussion, the author indicated that there was "no important initial difference" (p. 216) between the groups. The question is, Is this a significant difference between the two groups? A t-test would have provided this information and, although it may have been done by the investigator, the results were not reported here.

This research study has contributed to the science of nursing not only by contributing to knowledge about infants, with implications for nursing intervention, but also by providing support for the assumptions upon which it was based, namely those of Martha Rogers. This was a rigorous study and a scholarly report.

Rogers, M.E. (1970). **An introduction to the theoretical basis of nursing.** *Philadelphia, PA: F.A. Davis.*

In this book, Martha Rogers first formally presents her ideas about the theoretical basis of nursing. Some of the origins of her ideas, her earlier thinking, are seen in her 1963 article, which is helpful to read either prior to or in conjunction with this book. (Rogers uses "man" to refer to the nursing client in this early writing.)

Essentially, the book is divided into three main sections. In the first section, "Book of Modern Nursing," she presents background material related to man's beginnings, the evolution of man's thinking, and theories of this century about how man and life originated. "The Phenomenon of Man: Nursing's Concern" is the second section. Here, Rogers states what she sees as the central concern of nursing: man in his entirety. Man as a whole, man as a system, is the prototypic theory used to present the underlying assumptions Rogers makes about man. The assumptions are explicitly numbered and labeled as such. Five assumptions upon which nursing science builds are identified.

In the third section, "Nursing's Conceptual System," Rogers clearly points out the aims of nursing, nursing's conceptual model, the principle of nursing science, the principles of homeodynamics, evidence to support the concepts, ideas about formulating testable hypotheses, ways in which to translate the conception into practice and, finally, some ideas about the future. The essence of the theory is expressed in the first part of this section. The assumptions about man, the focus of nursing, were identified in the earlier section, but it is here that the concepts and principles are defined—the internal structure, aspects of the goals and consequences, and some dimensions of the theory are outlined.

An important chapter in this section relates to the potential of this theory for research. In fact, a whole body of research attempting to verify the principles of the real world (being carried out by doctoral students under Rogers' direction) is presented. The limitation in this chapter discussing the findings is that about 95% of it includes unpublished doctoral dissertations and is not generally available. Nevertheless, the important thing is that numerous studies, including cluster studies, have been and continue to be undertaken in attempts to accumulate evidence in support of the principles postulated by Rogers. This fact alone makes Rogers' formulations stand out from all of the other nursing theories and

models, even to this day. Furthermore, implications of many of the studies give direction for practice as well as provide direction for additional research.

The major limitations of Rogers' formulations are well known. These are that the principles of homeodynamics—reciprocity, synchrony, helicy, and resonance—are all quite abstract and have not been adequately operationalized. Some would say that because the principles are not easily understood, they are difficult to translate into practice. Also, because of the lack of operational definitions, the research carried out to verify the principles provides questionable results. The major counter argument, if one were to think along the lines of Rogers' theory and writing, is that research must focus on the range of human phenomena and that this will give substance to nursing's abstract system. There is, to a degree, an element of inductive reasoning, and an inductive approach is suggested; that is, the principles provide the framework, the direction for research, but the research results really provide the substance of the theory.

A chapter in the third section, in addition to discussing research, addresses the potential of the theory for practice. With the exception of citing four research studies suggesting direction for nursing practice, the discussion is more or less an abstract discussion of nursing interventions that purportedly are based on the different principles of homeodynamics. It does not indicate whether the theory is actually used in any practice settings.

In closing, we would recommend to anyone interested in Rogers' theory to read, at the minimum, the third section of the book; then for additional understanding of the assumptions about human beings, the second section, and for background in general, the first. The book is clearly and logically developed and very readable. In general, reading the whole book, elegant in its simplicity, sophisticated in its presentation, and as erudite as its author, is highly recommended. Rogers stands out among nursing theorists, and her work in theorizing, research, and education presents a major contribution to nursing as a science.

Rogers, M.E. (1975). **Euphemisms in nursing's future.** *Image, 7(2), 3–9.*

The focus of this paper is an argument against the many forms of nursing services parading under the guise of nice-sounding titles, when in fact they are cover-ups for physicians' assistants. This controversy was at its height in the early to mid-1970s, and

Rogers was strongly opposed to the development of new roles or any new title, such as family health practitioner, pediatric associate, and primary care nurse. She believed that these acted as cover-ups for physician's assistants, were "perpetrated to deny a future to nurses and nursing" (p. 3), and were coined to enhance the economic gains of the physicians.

This article bears little if any relevance to Rogers' theoretical basis of nursing per se. What comes through are her beliefs about the roles and levels of education needed to prepare nurses and what the scope of nursing is. Her theme that a baccalaureate preparation for nursing is important is repeated here.

For those unfamiliar with the more personal side of the professional Martha Rogers, this article provides a touch of that side. It gives one a feel for the spontaneous way in which she makes her arguments and for the strength of her convictions. Her wit, sense of humor, and a touch of cynicism are well demonstrated in this article. For this alone, this article is worth reading.

Rogers, M.E. (1980). Nursing: A science of unitary man. In J.P. Riehl and C. Roy (Eds.),* Conceptual models for nursing practice *(2nd ed.). New York: Appleton-Century-Crofts.

In this chapter, Rogers brings us up to date on her thinking about nursing and a conceptual system in nursing. She in fact presents a few changes in the underlying assumptions and in the principles of homeodynamics, compared with her earlier book (1970). No explanation is set forth as to why the ·changes were made. In essence, no specific assumptions about man are identified. Rather, Rogers states that four building blocks are essential in the conceptual system presented in this paper. They are: (1) energy fields, (2) universe of open systems, (3) pattern and organization, and (4) four-dimensionality. Each is briefly discussed.

The principles of homeodynamics have been reduced from four to three, and one of the three is different from the original. The original four were the principles of reciprocity, synchrony, helicy, and resonance. The new three are the principles of helicy, resonance, and complementarity. The first two remain essentially the same in definition. The principles of complementarity have elements of the original principle of reciprocity, with the added idea of interaction between man and environment.

Some elements of the theory appear to have been updated; for example, the title. Here, the underlying assumptions are broadened to include more than those five assumptions about the human being. And, they are also described as building blocks rather than assumptions. As already discussed, the principles of homeodynamics have changed somewhat.

Also updated are the theories deriving from the proposed conceptual system. Only a few of these are discussed. These include theory of accelerating evolution, explanations of paranormal events, and rhythmical correlates of change. Rogers also takes into account the implications that advances in technology have for change.

The last of these updates is in the discussion of implications for practice. Changes in nursing practice must result from changes in man, such as the evolutionary emergence of new behavior patterns (e.g., hypertension and hyperactivity), new knowledge, and changes in values. This is an interesting point that Rogers makes and, indeed, one not commonly mentioned by most theorists.

It is recommended that this chapter be read in conjunction with Rogers' 1970 book.

Whelton, B.J. (1979). An operationalization of Martha Rogers' theory throughout the nursing process.* International Journal of Nursing Studies, *16, 7–20.

This is the second of only two known articles referring to situations in which Rogers' theory is used throughout the nursing process. This whole article essentially focuses on that, whereas Falco and Lobo (1980) only present the nursing process in a section of their chapter.

The introduction clearly states the purpose of the paper and describes the content to be covered and then, clearly and precisely, the authors carry out their plan. This makes the paper very readable.

The version of Rogers' theory used here is the earlier (1970) version rather than the 1980 updates. In the presentation of the theory, the structural components are clearly spelled out; that is, basic assumptions about man, the five nursing concepts (stated more explicitly than Rogers really did), and the nursing principles of homeodynamics derived from the concepts. The five nursing concepts identified by this author are wholeness, openness, pattern and organization, unidirectionality, and sentience and thought.

The clinical population of interest identified as the focus of the operationalization of Rogers' theory are those patients with decreased cardiac output and impaired neurologic function. For example, the assessment of these patients would include data related to the five general concepts already mentioned. Tables are included that show what is assessed under each of these categories. For example, under wholeness, physical integrity and psychological integrity are listed. Then, in a later table for a patient with impaired neurologic functioning, the subitems are listed.

The general format is carried out in detail through each phase of the nursing process, here identified as assessment, nursing diagnosis, plan of care (including goal), and implementation and evaluation. Detailed tables present an actual nursing care plan showing diagnosis, plan, and goal. No examples are given for implementation and evaluation.

At least one example in this area would have complemented the other phases. In summarizing, Whelton indicates that assessment tools will vary with the patient population. However, it is not entirely reasonable to have an assessment tool for each and every different patient population. Therefore, the tool described here could be developed in more general terms and could thus be more generalizable to other patient populations.

This article has contributed significantly to the applicability of Rogers' theory to practice by making the somewhat abstract notions of the theory more concrete and by operationalizing the theory within the nursing process.

SISTER CALLISTA ROY

Brower, H.T. and Baker, D.J. (1976). Using the adaptation model in a practitioner curriculum. **Nursing Outlook, 24(11), 686–689.**

The practitioner curriculum described here is a geriatric nurse practitioner program that uses Roy's adaptation model. The authors forthrightly state that Roy's model meets the following criteria: it outlines the features of the discipline and provides direction for practice, research, and education; it considers the values and goals of nursing, the client, and practitioner interventions; and, in essence, it is a theory at the prescriptive or situation-producing level. Because these criteria were met, the model was incorporated into this curriculum.

Another important identified aspect of the model was that it was helpful in differentiating between those aspects of care unique to nursing versus medical practice within the context of Roy's four modes of adaptation. Furthermore, in describing the application of the model, it appeared that examples used are the authors' interpretation of Roy's model.

Although the potential of the model for practice is supported (e.g., another area of practice is covered), the application offers neither refinement nor extension. On the other hand, some insights in the form of interventions for nursing are suggested. For example, to promote client adaptation, nursing interventions might include facilitation of adaptive tasks of aging through counseling, effective communication techniques, health education, active manipulation, providing support, and identifying resources. However, here the points of entry for the nursing intervention are not clearly spelled out. It is stated: "If inadequate adaptation is occurring, the practitioner can attempt to modify or manipulate focal stimuli, thereby making a positive response possible" (p. 687). This example simply is not specific enough; it suggests where to intervene but not when.

The third focus in this article is curriculum application. In this section, an elaboration of the content taught provides information about what these authors draw on from other fields and other theoretical models for a knowledge base as it relates to this model. For example, crisis intervention theory, health anthropology, attitudes, life review, stage theory, and role theory are all included. This information may be interesting to those who want to plan a similar practitioner program.

Farkas, L. (1981). Adaptation problems with nursing home application for elderly persons: An application of the Roy adaptation nursing model. **Journal of Advanced Nursing, 6(5), 363–368.**

The author suggested at the outset that the elderly are often dependent on significant others to provide care supplementary to home care, so that they can remain at home. The importance of this study, then, was to "assess the life circumstances surrounding nursing home applications for elderly people" (p. 364), and the Roy adaptation model was chosen as the framework to organize data collected about adaptation problems of elderly people and their significant others.

Three research questions were identified:

1. In what way can a conceptual framework in nursing provide for the understanding of adaptation problems of elderly persons and significant others that contribute to nursing home applications?

2. If two groups of elderly persons are receiving at least one home care service, what

similarities and differences exist in adaptation problems that allow one group to remain at home while the other group must apply for admission to a nursing home?

3. To what extent do the adaptation problems on the part of the elderly person and of those persons closest to him contribute to the nursing home application for the elderly person? (p. 364)

The discussion of the conceptual framework that followed those research questions briefly presented the underlying beliefs of the Roy adaptation model and identified the four adaptive modes and what was considered an "adaptive response." The nurse's role within the model was identified as promoting adaptation that involved two factors in the nursing process: assessment and intervention. Other than this brief overview, the author assumed that the reader was familiar with the model. Only one study was cited that documented characteristics or problems of elderly applicants to long-term care facilities, and no research, related to adaptation or to use of the adaptation model, was cited.

In the purpose statement, the general purpose to assess factors associated with nursing home application was repeated. A general statement that five hypotheses were formulated and tested was made, as well as a statement that they related to overall adaptation problems, powerlessness, role reversal guilt, and knowledge and utilization of services, but the hypotheses were not explicitly stated. Furthermore, no theoretical connections between the hypotheses and the Roy model were explicated. It is not clear that all the hypotheses flowed from the research question. This led me to conclude that the conceptualization of this research within the Roy model was extremely limited; that is, it was conceptually inadequate.

The study group and the control group were described, but criteria for each subject group were not specific.

The method used in this study was described as an *ex post facto* design, appropriate to this population because admission to a nursing home is not a variable that can be controlled. Statistical analyses were completed using chi-square. Both the elderly subjects and their significant others were interviewed in their homes.

The limitations of this research outweigh the contributions it might have made to the testing of the Roy adaptation model. What is more, in the conclusion, neither the limitations of the research nor the implications for future research are discussed.

Galligan, A.C. (1979). Using Roy's concept of adaptation to care for young children. American Journal of Maternal Child Nursing, 4(1), 24–28.

Given the psychosocial as well as the physical needs of hospitalized children, this author has chosen Roy's concept of adaptation "as a means of guiding nurses in a more conscious effort to assist the child during hospitalization." Rationale for the choice of this model was not provided.

The author has divided the hospital stay into four different stages: prehospitalization, preoperative, postoperative, and discharge. The rationale for these divisions was that, because "man" (child?) is in constant interaction with a changing environment, the nursing assessment and appropriate interventions must be revised periodically during the patient's stay. Each stage is briefly discussed regarding the potential for assessment and intervention. Then, to illustrate how the Roy adaptation model might be used to assess and intervene with a young child, a hypothetical case was presented.

For three of the four stages of hospitalization, omitting discharge, each mode is discussed with examples of assessment—including focal, contextual, and residual stimuli—and intervention. In the second and third stages, the dimensions of diagnosis and evaluation were added. The discharge stage was discussed only very briefly, indicating that the child should be evaluated again in each of the four adaptive modes, and a discharge plan should be formulated.

For those interested in the applicability of the model for practice, especially with patients other than adults, this is an important contribution, demonstrating that the model is useful in the nursing care of children. On the whole, however, it does not increase our understanding of the Roy model itself.

Janelli, L.M. (1980). Utilizing Roy's adaptation model from a gerontological perspective. Journal of Gerontological Nursing, 6(3), 140–150.

The title of this article clearly indicates its focus, but more specifically, the author discusses two purposes. The first is general background about how the author came to use the theory and an overview of the model. Selye's stress theory was identified as the paradigmatic origin of the theory. The second purpose of the article is to present use of the model with specific clinical examples in gerontologic nursing.

As far as contributions to the theory, the author presents her conception, in diagrammatic form, of a human being as a biopsychosocial being interacting with the environment. Although the Roy adaptation model is basically a systems model, Roy does not use the word "tension" as it is used in this description. Other than the diagram, this article does not substantially add to our understanding of the model. It does, or at least did in this case, provide enough direction for practice with an elderly clientele.

This article is useful for those interested in gerontologic nursing. Tables of needs and the schematic presentation of the human being–environment interactions are also useful.

Jones, P.S. (1978). An adaptation model for nursing practice. American Journal of Nursing, 78(11), 1900–1906.

The adaptation model described here is not related to the Roy adaptation model and, in fact, uses a different prototype theory as a basis for its development. The author suggested that having this second framework based on the idea of adaptation (in this case modeled after Selye) might be confusing, but she thought her model might have more to offer than other theories. She suggested that there were difficulties with other existing theories; however, the difficulties were not identified.

In addition to using Selye's theory as a prototype, Maslow's hierarchy of needs was also used "to provide structure and guidance for assessing all needs." Based on the hierarchy, the author developed an elaborate assessment tool.

In terms of the structural components of the model, assumptions and concepts were explicit. Eight underlying assumptions were listed. The major concepts used included wholeness, needs, adaptability, illness, and wellness. The author did not specifically develop propositional statements that described the relationship of the concepts.

On the whole, this article does not contribute to our understanding of Roy's adaptation model, although it may have contributed another perspective to the concept of the health–illness continuum (in this case, illness–wellness continuum), which is not terribly clear in Roy's model. Jones illustrates her model using a triangle to demonstrate the interaction of the three variables in an average person. This conceptualization helps to determine wellness when the person is physically ill but "well" in other areas, a problem in Roy's model.

Mastal, M.F. and Hammond, H. (1980). Analysis and expansion of the Roy adaptation model: A contribution to holistic nursing. Advances in Nursing Science, 2(4), 71–81.

Although believing that the Roy adaptation model has much to offer nursing by way of providing a framework to organize its body of nursing knowledge, these authors are highly critical of the model in its present form. Specifically, the criticisms focus on a lack of explicit theoretical components of assumptions and concepts, simple propositions, and relational propositions (criticisms noted in earlier critiques also).

The purpose of this article, then, is to make up for some of these deficits. Assumptions underlying the mode, heretofore implicit, are explicitly stated. (Roy's 1980 edition of *Conceptual Models* was not yet published when this article was written because in that edition, the assumptions are outlined by Roy. Readers are encouraged to compare the two sets of assumptions.)

The five major concepts within the framework are identified, summarized, and discussed. These include: (1) person, (2) environment, (3) adaptation, (4) health–illness, and (5) nursing.

The authors focus on the lack of theoretical and operational definitions, as well as on the narrow scope of health–illness. In attempting to elucidate this concept and to answer some questions, a continuum is defined, a new idea of transition is introduced, and nursing assessment along the continuum is clarified. This addition is justified on the basis that it expands the model's scope. However, based on this brief discussion, this is a critical addition to the concept of health–illness.

Two other major additions to the theory are a diagram depicting the relationships between the major concepts of the model and a set of propositional statements. The latter is a particularly important contribution because it is what the model lacked at the time this article was published.

Overall, the article is clearly written and adds to our understanding of the theory. The contribution of propositional statements adds to the researchability of the theory, and ultimately to nursing as a science.

Mastal, M.F., Hammond, H., and Roberts, M.P. (1982). Theory into hospital practice: A pilot implementation. Journal of Nursing Administration, 12(6), 9–15.

This article describes both the process involved when the Roy adaptation model was implemented in one unit of a small community hospital, and how the process contributed to the validation of nursing theory. The description of the process is detailed enough to give guidance to clinicians or administrators who might choose to implement a theoretical model. Each step of the process is outlined and described.

Adequate review and understanding of any theoretical model to be used in a clinical setting is requisite. In this case, the review revealed that not all components (philosophical basis, assumptions, concepts, and propositions) had been specifically identified and defined. This led the authors to pursue this end directly with the theorist, Sister Callista Roy. From this, specific components were clarified, and what were perceived by the authors to be the model's components were depicted visually. This effort was later used to make the model understandable and usable for the hospital's nursing staff. (This process of clarification of the components of the model and the communications with Sister Roy would also make another significant contribution to the theory's validation.) Once components of the model had been clarified, the administrative processes were initiated.

Planning and organizing were the major steps required administratively to start the pilot. Approval was sought, starting with the top levels of hospital and nursing administration. Congruence with the hospital philosophy, standards of patient care, and cost-effectiveness were all explored. One unit was selected for the pilot, with justification for that choice outlined.

Organization was based on Di Vincenti's theoretical framework for change and required three major steps: (1) establishing the change structure, (2) developing appropriate procedures, and (3) determining requirements and allocating resources. Each of these steps was described and discussed in some detail. In the change structure, shared power was the category of "how" to change. Group problem-solving and group decision-making, as part of shared power, was emphasized. Open communication and a method for addressing problems in an ongoing way were also important to the success of the project.

The development of procedures included review of existing forms and required revision of nursing assessment, although not of the nursing care plan. Procedures affecting unit function required guidelines for the following: "(1) using the assessment and planning tools, (2) nursing reports and rounds, (3) patient care conferences, (4) nursing documentation, (5) orientation of new personnel, (6) standards of performance and job descriptions for nurses involved in the project, and (7) audit criteria" (p. 13). Costs for these services and required materials were assumed

by the hospital. The planning and organizational phase was reported to have taken 5 months.

Staff education required the next major block of time. One-hour sessions weekly for a period of 15 weeks were structured for all the staff—registered nurses and licensed vocational nurses—on the pilot unit. Cooperation of the head nurse and other departmental heads to cover staffing on the unit during this time period was critical to the success of the classes.

The authors believed that the overall components of success of the pilot implementation were authority, leadership, and communication. Clear lines of authority and administrative sanction for the implementation of the adaptation model were critical. Furthermore, open communication was fostered and facilitated through weekly group meetings, through frequent one-to-one talks between project directors and staff nurses, and through the use of an on-unit community logbook for staff to express feelings.

Outcomes were measured indirectly, both by improved patient care and by nurses' satisfaction with enhanced professional practice. Since then, patient satisfaction is being documented by conducting further research. There were more concrete measures of enhanced nursing practice. Namely, the development of a new tool to assess the biopsychosocial status of patients (illustrated by Exhibit 1), more complete nursing care plans phrased in terms consistent with the model, and greater collegial sharing and rapport were reported.

This report was written clearly in a conversational style, without sacrificing scholarliness and thoroughness. It would be of interest to theorists, researchers, and clinicians alike who are interested in the Roy model because it clearly illustrates the helical nature of theory, research, and practice. What is more, it makes an important contribution to the science of nursing by demonstrating application to practice and by stimulating research.

Roy, C. (1970). Adaptation: A conceptual framework for nursing. Nursing Outlook, 18(3), 42–45.

The purpose of this article is to describe the framework of a conceptual model for nursing that was in the early stages of development by a nursing faculty group. Implications of the model for nursing science, practice, and education are suggested.

Implicit in the section "Theoretical Model" are the functional components of assumptions and concepts. Examples of the underlying assumptions are: (1) man is a biopsychosocial being, (2) man is constantly interacting with a changing environment, and (3) man has both innate and acquired coping mechanisms. The major concepts of the model are adaptation and coping, health and illness, and man and the environment. However, Roy, in this first publication on her theory, does not yet explicitly identify either the assumptions or the concepts.

In the discussion of the concepts, the major concept of adaptation is described in terms of its origin in the physiologic theory of Harry Helson. The definition is technical and somewhat tautological and does not answer the questions raised by the author, which are: "How does this adaptation take place?" and "What is behind the process?" These are difficult questions, and it was too early to answer them. Furthermore, when the author tries to answer the question about how the concept of adaptation applies to nursing, the answer is in terms of the function of nursing, which is "to support and promote patient adaptation."

Although the term "elements," as applied to conceptual models, was not used at the time this article was published, except in a course taught by Dorothy Johnson at the University of California, Los Angeles, where Roy was studying for her master's degree, this analysis reveals that the following elements are present: *goal of action* —to support and promote patient adaptation; and *actor's role* —to assess and intervene and to promote adaptation. Less clear are the elements of *patiency*, which is when the nurse becomes involved with the patient on the health–illness continuum, and the *source of difficulty* (although it is similar to patiency). The recipient of nursing care is the human being. The *intervention focus* or *mode* is to promote adaptation by changing the person's response potential. Specific examples are given. Understanding man in health and illness is the essential focus of adaptation nursing.

That this developing theoretical model presents rudimentary outlines of a nursing science is an overstatement on the part of the author. However, considering that this is one of the earlier theoretical models developed in nursing, it is an important contribution to the growth of nursing as a science. This is a useful article to read for those interested in analyzing the development of theoretical thinking in nursing.

Roy, C. (1971). Adaptation: A basis for nursing practice. Nursing Outlook, 19(4), 254–257.

This article picks up where the earlier one (1970) left off; it is helpful to read both together. It offers a description of man as an adaptive system with four modes of coping. Assumptions underlying the model are offered; the four modes of adaptation and their components, as well as examples, are listed. The four modes—later called effector modes—are physiologic needs, self-concept, role mastery (later, role function), and interdependence. All four modes were identified based on samples of behavior collected by the author's nursing students, as well as on a synthesis of work done by other nurses. The other nursing sources included Abdellah and McCain. Ultimately, it appears that the categories are a synthesis of several sources, which may raise some questions about the validity of the categories. What data and what research supported these four choices? Are there other modes, such as the cognitive mode, which might be included?

A more rigorous approach that may have helped in the development of nursing knowledge would have been for the author to develop a research orientation and a scientific approach, rather than a curricular one. Hindsight aside, the leap was immediately made to clinical application. Within the context of clinical application, new concepts then came up that had had insufficient elaboration. Examples of these included health–illness continuum, "positive" responses versus "negative" needs, and a diagram/figure describing the nursing process and first-level assessment.

The nursing goal, clearly stated, is "to bring about an adapted state in the patient, which frees him to respond to other stimuli which may be present." This remains a nursing goal of the theory in 1984, and continues to raise questions about what the nature of the adapted state is and its intended consequences (being [in 1984] the quality of life and the integrity of the individual).

To demonstrate the applicability of the model of adaptation to nursing, two case studies were presented. In each, the nurse used the model as a basis for assessment and intervention. Because it is clearly stated that the nurse establishes a nursing care plan and later evaluates it, and because the nursing process as it was known at the time encompasses four stages—assessment, planning, intervention, and evaluation—one wonders why Roy chose instead to use a nursing process including only two of the four—assessment and intervention. That question aside, the steps grew to six in 1984.

Although there is a discussion about planning, the "how to" of choosing nursing approaches is left to the process of nursing judgment outlined by McDonald and Harms. Additionally, the unintended consequences of the nursing intervention are not discussed.

Overall, this article continues to contribute to our understanding of processes, strategies, and phases of theory development in nursing.

Roy, C. (1976). The Roy adaptation model:
Comment. **Nursing Outlook,** *24(11), 690–691.*

Sister Callista Roy, who developed the Roy adaptation theory, herein presents her reactions to two articles by Brower and Baker (1976) and by Wolfer (1976). She thinks that the authors did a fine job in implementing ideas from her writings, considering that they used only her published material as a basis.

After more general reactions to Brower and Baker's article regarding the importance of a nursing model as a basis for role identification, Roy goes on to clarify her views, to identify what could be considered limitations, and to acknowledge difficulties with the model. Among these are the fact that the model "has not yet been submitted to the rigors of clinical research that will be necessary to establish its validity," and that the model is a deductive one and has not been developed by formal theory construction methods.

This interaction and feedback is an important process for the growth of nursing knowledge, and the thinking of scholars was evident later on in the development of Roy's theory.

Roy, C. (1979). Relating nursing theory to
education: A new era. **Nurse Educator,** *4(2),*
16–21.

This article examines the relationship between nursing theory and nursing education, from the meaning of theory to mechanisms of theory utilization, within a department of nursing.

Roy, C. (1980). The Roy adaptation model.
In J.P. Riehl and C. Roy (Eds.), **Conceptual**
models for nursing practice *(2nd ed.).*
New York: Appleton-Century-Crofts.

Data from research are notably still missing in this updated version of the Roy model, published a decade after the first publication appeared in *Nursing Outlook.*

Presented here is the more formal theory construction work that was promised in the earlier "Comment" (1976). Clearly presented and labeled as such are the basic assumptions underlying the model and the elements of the model, namely, values, goal of action, patiency, source of difficulty, and intervention. What is still missing is an elaboration of the major concepts and the propositions, or those statements that show the relationship among the concepts. This important omission is not acknowledged by the author. More seriously

at issue here is that the model is now 10 years old, is widely used as a curricular framework and in nursing practice settings, and yet research is still not being carried out.

A new diagram depicting the "source of difficulty" is not clarified in the text. The source of difficulty is first "described as the originating point of deviations from the desired state or condition." However, the discussion continues in the vein of how the modes and coping mechanisms are called into play (i.e., like a feedback system), rather than truly defining the source of difficulty. The discussion closes with this summary explanation: "'The source of difficulty,' then, is coping activity that is inadequate to maintain integrity in the face of a need deficit or excess." This does not match the diagram, which shows that there can exist either adaptive or maladaptive behaviors. The question unanswered by either the diagram or the text description is: When does a source of difficulty really exist? And, particularly and more importantly, when does the nurse intervene: at the originating point of deviation, or at a later time, when the coping mechanisms called up are inadequate? The diagram is somewhat confusing in light of the discussion in the text.

In summarizing, the author points to areas in which "continuing development" is needed, such as validation of assumptions, explication of values, and clarification of elements.

Schmitz, M. (1980). The Roy adaptation model:
Application in a community setting. In J.P.
Riehl and C. Roy (Eds.), **Conceptual models**
for nursing practice *(2nd ed., pp. 193–206).*
New York: Appleton-Century-Crofts.

The Roy adaptation model was applied here in the home setting, which is different from the inpatient setting where it has heretofore exclusively been applied. This necessitated an expansion of the concept of client from individual with an identified need to include the "family of care." If this broadened definition of the client is accepted, and it seems appropriate to do so, this will be an important contribution to the model.

In the introduction, the author is careful to identify differences between the home and hospital, especially in terms of nursing goals and nursing interventions. Also identified in the home setting were variables influencing care. The introductory remarks laid the groundwork for a detailed case study, with a family requiring home nursing care, which was the major focus of the study.

The care presentation included six detailed tables describing the client behaviors with focal, contextual, and residual stimuli for each mode and an accompanying nursing care plan for each.

The author summarized how the Roy adaptation model was used to assess and intervene with a family. Application of the model was the focus of this article. A more theoretical discussion would also have been appropriate because an expansion of the concept of client resulted from the thinking and work of this author, which is an important theoretical contribution.

Starr, S.L. (1980). Adaptation applied to the dying client. In J.P. Riehl and C. Roy (Eds.), Conceptual models for nursing practice (2nd ed.). New York: Appleton-Century-Crofts.

In this brief descriptive article, the author has elaborated on "elements of adaptive death" within four modes (Roy's): (1) physiologic mode, (2) self-concept mode, (3) role mode, and (4) interdependence mode. Within each mode, adaptive behaviors of the dying client are identified, stimuli affecting the behaviors are listed, and the nursing goal and interventions appropriate to each mode are presented.

Although this article is included in a set of three articles about the Roy adaptation model, there is no direct reference to Roy's work by the author. If one assumes that this is an application of the Roy model to practice, it is clear that it is timely, that the model can be applied to this group of patients, and that it is appropriate to nursing practice in this area. However, the article does not extend the Roy adaptation model.

Wagner, P. (1976). The Roy adaptation model: Testing the adaptation model in practice. Nursing Outlook, 24(11), 682–685.

According to this author, the potential for practice in both episodic and distributive settings using the Roy adaptation model has been realized. Graduate students who tested the feasibility of the model for practice concluded that "the model provided a good framework for ordering a variety of observations," and using the model for nursing enhanced assessment and intervention as well as the overall nursing process.

Before field testing the model, the graduate students reviewed materials published about the model. They found discrepancies between sources and also, although not stated directly, they found limitations in the original assessment tools. They also identified limitations with a tool they subsequently developed, even though their tool met the criterion that it was both theoretical and practical.

These authors also expressed concern with overlap between the four modes as developed by Roy.

The author gives an indication that the model provides enough direction to affect practice in a variety of settings. Who is acted upon is not as clearly described as where or in what setting the person is acted upon. We are not any clearer as to the focus of the theory, nor are any definitions clarified such as health–illness, modes, positive and negative behavior, and adaptation.

Wagner added two dimensions—nursing diagnosis and evaluation—to Roy's nursing process of assessment and intervention. These later (1984) became an integral part of Roy's nursing process.

Overall, this article supports the notion that the conceptual model currently applies to practice and that it does have relevance for the way nursing is practiced today.

JOYCE TRAVELBEE

Travelbee, J. (1963). What do we mean by rapport? American Journal of Nursing, 63(2), 70–72.

This article provides an excellent example of an attempt to conceptualize a phenomenon. It could be used as an early exemplar in concept development. However, the lack of clinical referents limits its wide utility and curtails its research potential. The term "rapport" is commonly used in nursing but had previously been neither conceptualized, operationally defined, nor researched. Frequently, rapport is defined by what it is not rather than by what it is. The explicit assumption underlying this development is that a controlled type of emotional involvement with the patient is allowed to establish and maintain rapport. Implicit in this is the value judgment that rapport is good or positive and to be valued.

Rapport is described in a number of ways here. It is a process in the way people perceive and relate to each other. It is an entity with empathy, compassion, and sympathy as components. It is also an outcome, being the ability to communicate creatively and intelligently to others. To establish rapport, certain ingredients are essential. A patient has to feel a sense of trust in the nurse. The nurse's needs should have been met in the past to be able to give of herself, but a bit of previous "suffering" would help nurses in understanding others. Stages of rapport development begin with empathy, then sympathy (equated in 1964 with caring), and then rapport.

Travelbee's major concepts, which later evolved into her theory, were introduced in this article.

21

Historical and Current Theory Bibliography

The purpose of this chapter is to provide the reader with a comprehensive bibliography related to nursing theory and theorizing in nursing. The chapter is divided into 54 sections. Sections 1 through 12 include literature related to metatheory and theorizing in nursing. Sections 13 through 37 include nursing theories organized alphabetically by theorist. Sections 38 through 48 include major paradigms that have influenced nursing or have been used in nursing. Sections 49 through 54 include websites and media tapes on theory. More specifically, the sections are:

THEORY AND THEORIZING IN NURSING

NURSING THEORY AND THEORISTS

PARADIGMS THAT HAVE INFLUENCED NURSING

MIDDLE-RANGE THEORY (P. 615)

SITUATION-SPECIFIC THEORY (P. 616)

WEBSITES AND MEDIA ON THEORY

There are several points to remember when using the bibliography.

1. Citations preceded by *asterisks* refer to works that have been abstracted in Chapter 20, Section I. Citations

preceded by *daggers* refer to works that have been abstracted in Chapter 20, Section II.

2. Most of the abstracts in Chapter 20 are expansions of citations in Chapter 21, Sections 3, 6, 7, 8, 10, and 11. The emphasis was on providing a comprehensive view of literature cited in Sections 3 and 11.

3. There are many ways to use the bibliography, such as systematically reading within a section, reading within chronological themes, selecting readings according to years or decades of publication, and reading sections in conjunction with appropriate book chapters.

THEORY AND THEORIZING IN NURSING

1. Philosophy and Methods

Barber, B. and Hirsch, W. (Eds.). (1962). *The sociology of science*. New York: Free Press of Glencoe.

Beckstead, J.W. and Beckstead, L.G. (2006). A multidimentional analysis of the epistemic origins of nursing theories, models, and frameworks. *International Journal of Nursing Studies*, 43(1), 113–122.

Benner, P. (2000). Links between philosophy, theory, practice, and research. *Canadian Journal of Nursing Research*, 32(2), 7–13.

Bennis, W.G., Benne, K.D., and Chin, R. (1976). *The planning of change* (3rd ed.). New York: Holt, Rinehart & Winston.

Blake, R.M., Ducasse, C.J., and Madden, E.H. (1960). *Theories of scientific method: The Renaissance through the nineteenth century*. Seattle, WA: University of Washington Press.

Blalock, H.M. (1969). *Theory construction*. Englewood Cliffs, NJ: Prentice-Hall.

Blumer, H. (1954). What is wrong with social theory? *American Sociological Review*, 19(1), 3–10.

Boykin, A., Parker, M.E., and Schoenhofer, S.O. (1994). Aesthetic knowing grounded in an explicit conception of nursing. *Nursing Science Quarterly*, 7, 158–161.

Brodbeck, M. (1956). The philosophy of science and educational research. *Review of Educational Research*, 26(5), 427–441.

Brodbeck, M. (1959). Models, meanings, and theories. In L. Gross (Ed.), *Symposium on sociological theory* (pp. 373–403). Evanston, IL: Row, Peterson & Co.

Brody, J.K. (1988). Virtue ethics, caring, and nursing. *Scholarly Inquiry for Nursing Practice*, 2(2), 87–96.

Bruner, R.S. (1966). The social construction of social theory. In R.S. Rudner (Ed.), *Philosophy of social science*. Englewood Cliffs, NJ: Prentice-Hall.

*Burgess, G. (1978). The personal development of the nursing student as a conceptual framework. *Nursing Forum*, 17(1), 96–102.

Campbell, N. (1953). The structure of theories. In H. Feigl and M. Brodbeck (Eds.), *Readings in the philosophy of science* (pp. 288–308). New York: Appleton-Century-Crofts.

Carnap, R. (1966). *An introduction to the philosophy of science*. New York: Basic Books.

Chafetz, J.S. (1978). *A primer on the construction and testing of theories in sociology*. Itasca, IL: F.E. Peacock Publisher.

*Chapman, C.M. (1976). The use of sociological theories and models in nursing. *Journal of Advanced Nursing*, 1, 111–127.

Chinn, P.L. (2006). A universal and fundamental nursing philosophy. *Advances in Nursing Science*, 29(3), 193.

Clarke, D.J. and Holt, J. (2001). Philosophy: A key to open the door to critical thinking. *Nurse Education Today*, 21(1), 71–78.

Cohen, M.R. and Nagel, E. (1962). *An introduction to logic and the scientific method* (Rev. ed.). New York: Harcourt Brace Jovanovich.

Copi, I.M. (1972). *Introduction to logic* (4th ed.). New York: Macmillan. (Note especially: Chapter 3, "Informal Fallacies," and Chapter 6, "Categorical Syllogisms.")

Copleston, F. (1963). *A history of philosophy: Vol. 8. Modern philosophy: Bentham to Russel, Part II, Idealism in America. The Pragmatic movement, the revolt against idealism*. Garden City, NJ: Image Books.

Costner, H. (1969). Theory, deduction, and rules of correspondence. *American Journal of Sociology*, 75, 245–263.

Costner, H. and Leik, R.K. (1964). Deductions from axiomatic theory. *American Sociological Review*, 29, 819–835.

Darbyshire, P., Diekelmann, J., and Diekelmann. N. (1999). Reading Heidegger and interpretive phenomenology: A response to the work of Michael Crotty. *Nursing Inquiry*, 6(1), 17–25.

Davis, K. and Glass, N. (1999). Contemporary theories and contemporary nursing—advancing nursing care for those who are marginalized. *Contemporary Nurse*, 8(2), 32–38.

Denisoff, R.S., Callahan, O., and Levine, M.H. (1974). *Theories and paradigms in contemporary sociology*. Itasca, IL: F.E. Peacock Publisher.

deRaeve, L. and Wainwright, P. (2001). Conference report. Philosophy of nursing: Theory and evidence, Swansea, 18–20 September 2000. *Nursing Philosophy*, 21(1), 95–97.

Dewey, J. (1958). *Experience and nature* (Rev. ed.). New York: Dover Publications.

Dewey, J. (1964). *Reconstruction in philosophy* (Rev. ed.). Boston, MA: Beacon Press.

Dewey, J. (1980). *The quest for certainty* (Rev. ed.). New York: Perigee Books.

DiBartolo, M.C. (1998). Philosophy of science in doctoral nursing education revisited. *Journal of Professional Nursing*, 14(6), 350–360.

Dubin, R. (1978). *Theory building*. New York: Free Press.

Durbin, P.R. (1968). *Philosophy of science: An introduction*. New York: McGraw-Hill.

Edwards, S. (1997). Philosophy in nursing. *Nursing Times*, 93(51), 48–49.

*Ellis, R. (1968). Characteristics of significant theories. *Nursing Research*, 17(3), 217–222.

Emden, C. (1998). Conducting a narrative analysis. *Collegian*, 5(3), 34–39.

Fry, S.T. (1999). The philosophy of nursing. *Scholarly Inquiry in Nursing Practice*, 13(1), 5–15.

Gadow, S. (1988). Covenant without cure: Letting go and holding on in chronic illness. In J. Watson and M. Ray (Eds.), *The ethics of care and the ethics of cure. Synthesis in chronicity* (pp. 5–14). New York: National League for Nursing.

Gastaldo, D. and Holmes, D. (1999). Foucault and nursing: A history of the present. *Nursing Inquiry*, 6(4), 231–240.

Geanellos, R. (2000). Exploring Ricoeur's hermeneutic theory of interpretation as a method of analysing research texts. *Nursing Inquiry*, 7(2), 112–119.

Gibbs, J. (1972). *Sociological theory construction*. Hinsdale, IL: Dryden Press.

Gibson, Q. (1960). *The logic of social inquiry*. New York: Humanities Press.

Goode, W.J. and Hatt, P.K. (1952). *Methods in social research*. New York: McGraw-Hill. (Note especially: Chapter 5, pp. 41–55, "Basic Elements of the Scientific Method: Concepts.")

Gouldner, A.W. (1961). Theoretical requirements of the applied social sciences. In H.J. Bennis, K.D. Benne, and R. Chin (Eds.), *The planning of change* (2nd ed.). New York: Holt, Rinehart & Winston.

Grey, J. (2014). Spinoza on composition, causation, and the mind's eternity. *British Journal for the History of Philosophy*, 22(3), 446–467.

Grinker, R.R. (Ed.). (1967). *Toward a unified theory of human behavior: An introduction to general systems theory* (2nd ed.). New York: Basic Books.

Habermas, J. (1984). *The theory of communicative action: Vol. 1. Reason and the rationalization of society*. London, UK: Heinmann.

Hage, J. (1972). *Techniques and problem of theory construction in sociology*. New York: John Wiley & Sons.

Hall, J.M. (1990). Towards a psychology of caring. *British Journal of Clinical Psychology*, 29, 129–143.

Harden, J. (2000). Language, discourse and the chronotope: Applying literary theory to the narratives in health care. *Journal of Advanced Nursing*, 31(3), 506–512.

Hardy, M.E. (1974). Theories: Components, development, evaluation. *Nursing Research*, 23(2), 100–107.

Harris, S. (1977). *What's so funny about science?* (Rev. ed.). Los Altos, CA: William Kaufmann.

Hempel, C.G. (1952). *Fundamentals of concept formation in empirical science*. Chicago, IL: University of Chicago Press.

Hempel, C.G. (1965). *Aspects of scientific exploration and other essays in the philosophy of science*. New York: Free Press.

Heslop, L. (1997). The (im)possibilities of poststructuralist and critical social nursing inquiry. *Nursing Inquiry*, 4(1), 48–56.

Holmes, C.A. and Warelow, P.J. (2000). Some implications of postmodernism for nursing theory, research, and practice. *Canadian Journal of Nursing Research*, 32(2), 89–101.

Husserl, E. (1962). *Ideas: General introduction to pure phenomenology* (Rev. ed.). W.R. Boyce Gibson (Trans.). New York: Collier Books.

Inkeles, A. (1964). *What is sociology?* Englewood Cliffs, NJ: Prentice-Hall. (Note especially: "Models of Society in Sociological Analysis," pp. 28–67.)

Johnson, J.L. (1991). Nursing science: Basic, applied, or practical? Implications for the art of nursing. *Advances in Nursing Science*, 14(1), 7–16.

Johnson, J.L. (1994). A dialectical examination of nursing art. *Advances in Nursing Science*, 17(1), 1–14.

Kaplan, A. (1964). *The conduct of inquiry: Methodology for behavioral science*. San Francisco, CA: Chandler.

*Kramer, S. (1969). Behavioral science and human biology in medicine. *The New Physician*, 18(11), 965–978.

Kuhn, T.S. (1970). The structure of scientific revolutions. In O. Neurath (Ed.), *International encyclopedia of unified science* (2nd ed., Vol. 2). Chicago, IL: University of Chicago Press.

Kuhn, T.S. (1977). *The essential tension: Selected studies in scientific tradition and change*. Chicago, IL: University of Chicago Press.

Lachman, R. (1963). The model in theory construction. In M.H. Marx (Ed.), *Theories in contemporary psychology*. New York: Macmillan.

Laudan, L. (1977). *Progress and its problems: Toward a theory of scientific growth*. Berkeley, CA: University of California Press.

LeBlanc, R.G. (1997). Definitions of oppression. *Nursing Inquiry*, 4(4), 257–261.

Lemaire, G., Macleod, R., Mulkay, M., and Weingart, P. (Eds.). (1976). *Perspectives on the emergence of scientific disciplines*. Chicago, IL: Aldine.

Lister, P. (1997). The art of nursing in a "postmodern" context. *Journal of Advanced Nursing*, 25(1), 38–44.

Losee, J. (1980). *A historical introduction to the philosophy of science* (2nd ed.). Oxford, UK: Oxford University Press.

MacKinnon, C.A. (1982). Feminism, Marxism, method, and the state: An agenda for theory. *Signs: Journal of Women in Culture and Society*, 7, 515–544.

Maris, R. (1970). The logical adequacy of Homan's social theory. *American Sociological Review*, 35, 1069–1081.

Marx, M.H. (1963). *Theories in contemporary psychology*. New York: Macmillan. (Note especially "The General Nature of Theory Construction," pp. 4–46.)

McCall, R.J. (1963). *Basic logic: The fundamental principles of formal deductive reasoning* (2nd ed.). New York: Barnes & Noble.

McCance, T.V., McKenna, H.P., and Boore, J.R. (2001). Exploring caring using narrative methodology: An analysis of the approach. *Journal of Advanced Nursing*, 33(3), 350–356.

*McKay, R. (1969). Theories, models and systems for nursing. *Nursing Research*, 18(5), 393–399.

Merton, R.K. (1973). *The sociology of science: Theoretical and empirical investigations* (edited with an introduction by N.W. Storer). Chicago, IL: University of Chicago Press.

Merton, R.K. (1977). *The sociology of science: An episodic memoir*. Carbondale, IL: Southern Illinois University Press.

Miller, E.F. (1980). Epistemology and political inquiry: Comment on Kress' "Against epistemology." *Journal of Politics*, 42, 1160–1167.

Monti, E.J. and Tingen, M.S. (1999). Multiple paradigms of nursing science. *Advances in Nursing Science*, 21(4), 64–80.

Morgan, G. (1982). Cybernetics and organizational theory: Epistemology or technique? *Human Relations*, 35, 521–538.

Mulholland, J. (1997). Assimilating sociology: Critical reflections on the "sociology in nursing" debate. *Journal of Advanced Nursing*, 25(4), 844–852.

Murphy, J.F. (Ed.). (1971). *Theoretical issues in professional nursing*. New York: Appleton-Century-Crofts. (Note especially Chapters 1, 2, and 3.)

Nolan, P.W., Brown, B., and Crawford, P. (1998). Fruits without labour: The implications of Friedrich Nietzsche's ideas for the caring professions. *Journal of Advanced Nursing*, 28(2), 251–259.

Northrup, F.S.C. (1965). *The logic of the sciences and the humanities* (Rev. ed.). New York: The World Publishing Co.

Paley, J. (1998). Misinterpretive phenomenology: Heidegger, ontology and nursing research. *Journal of Advanced Nursing*, 27(4), 817–824.

Parsons, C. (1995). The impact of postmodernism on research methodology: Implications for nursing. *Nursing Inquiry*, 2(1), 22–28.

Paul, R.W. and Heaslip, P. (1995). Critical thinking involving nursing practice. *Journal of Advanced Nursing*, 22, 40–47.

*Payne, G. (1973). Comparative sociology: Some problems of theory and method. *British Journal of Sociology*, 24(1), 13–29.

*Peterson, C.J. (1977). Questions frequently asked about the development of a conceptual framework. *Journal of Nursing Education*, 16(4), 22–32.

Pierson, W. (1999). Considering the nature of intersubjectivity within professional nursing. *Journal of Advanced Nursing*, 30(2), 294–302.

Polanyi, M. (1962). *Personal knowledge*. New York: Harper & Row.

Popper, K. (1976). *Unended quest: An intellectual autobiography*. La Salle, IL: Open Court.

Popper, K.R. (1959). *The logic of scientific discovery*. New York: Basic Books.

Popper, K.R. (1971). *The open society and its enemies: The spell of Plato* (Rev. ed.). Princeton, NJ: Princeton University Press.

Reed, P.G. (1995). A treatise on nursing knowledge development for the 21st century: Beyond postmodernism. *Advances in Nursing Science*, 17(3), 70–84.

Reynolds, P.D. (1971). *A primer in theory construction*. New York: Bobbs-Merrill.

Rolfe, G. (1999). The pleasure of the bottomless: Postmodernism, chaos and paradigm shifts . . . Reconstructing nursing: Evidence, artistry and the curriculum. *Nurse Education Today*, 19(8), 668–672.

Rolfe, G. (2015). Foundations for a human science of nursing: Gadamer, Laing, and the hermeneutics of caring. *Nursing Philosophy*, 16, 141–152.

Rorty, R. (1999). *Philosophy and social hope by Richard Rorty*. London, UK: Penguin Books.

Roy, C.L. (1995). Developing nursing knowledge: Practice issues raised from four philosophical perspectives. *Nursing Science Quarterly*, 8(2), 79–85.

Rudner, R.S. (1966). *Philosophy of social science*. Englewood Cliffs, NJ: Prentice-Hall. (Note especially: "The Construction of Social Theory.")

Russell, B. (1965). *On the philosophy of science*. New York: Bobbs-Merrill.

Rutty, J.E. (1998). The nature of philosophy of science, theory and knowledge relating to nursing and professionalism. *Journal of Advanced Nursing*, 28(2), 243–250.

Sahakian, W.S. (1968). *History of philosophy from the earliest times to the present*. New York: Barnes & Noble.

Sarter, B. (1988). Philosophical sources of nursing theory. *Nursing Science Quarterly*, 1(2), 52–59.

Schoenhofer, S.O. (2002). Theoretical concerns. Philosophical underpinnings of an emergent methodology for nursing as caring inquiry. *Nursing Science Quarterly*, 15(4), 275–280.

Schultz, P.R. and Meleis, A.I. (1988). Nursing epistemology: Traditions, insights, questions. *Image: Journal of Nursing Scholarship*, 20(4), 217–221.

Sheridan, A. (1980). *Michel Foucault: The will to truth*. New York: Tavistock.

Shils, E. (Ed.). (1968). *Criteria for scientific development, public policy, and national goals*. Cambridge, MA: MIT Press.

Sidorsky, D. (Ed.). (1977). *John Dewey: The essential writings*. New York: Harper Torch-books.

Simon, H.A. and Newell, A. (1963). The uses and limitations of models. In M.H. Marx (Ed.), *Theories in contemporary psychology* (pp. 89–104). New York: Macmillan.

*Silva, M.C. (1977). Philosophy, science, theory: Interrelationships and implications for nursing research. *Image: Journal of Nursing Scholarship*, 9(3), 59–63.

Silva, M.C. and Rothbart, D. (1984). An analysis of changing trends in philosophies of science on nursing theory development and testing. *Advances in Nursing Science*, 6(2), 1–13.

Silva, M.C., Sorrell, J.M., and Sorrell, C.D. (1995). From Carper's patterns of knowing to ways of being: An ontological philosophical shift in nursing. *Advances in Nursing Science*, 18(1), 1–13.

Sorrell, J.M. (1994). Remembrance of things past through writing: Esthetic patterns of knowing in nursing. *Advances in Nursing Science*, 17(1), 60–70.

Stacy, J. and Thorne, B. (1985). The feminist revolution in sociology. *Social Problems*, 32(4), 301–315.

Stein, K.F., Corte, C., Colling, K.B., and Whall, A. (1998). A theoretical analysis of Carper's ways of knowing using a model of social cognition. *Scholarly Inquiry in Nursing Practice*, 12(1), 43–60.

Stevenson, J.S. and Woods, N.F. (1986). Nursing science and contemporary science: Emerging paradigms. In G.E. Sorensen (Ed.), *Setting the agenda for the year 2000: Knowledge development in nursing* (Publication No. G-a170, 3M, 5/86). Kansas City, MO: American Nurses Association.

Stinchcombe, A.L. (1968). *Constructing social theories*. New York: Harcourt Brace Jovanovich.

Suppe, F. and Jacox, A.K. (1989). Philosophy of science and the development of nursing theory. *Annual Review of Nursing Research*, 3, 241–267.

Thorne, S.E., Kirkham, S.R., and Henderson, A. (1999). Ideological implications of paradigm discourse. *Nursing Inquiry*, 6(2), 123–131.

Torres, G. and Yura, H. (1974). *Today's conceptual framework: Its relationship to the curriculum development process* (Publication No. 15–1529). New York: National League for Nursing.

Toulmin, S. (1977). *Human understanding: The collective use and evolution of concepts*. Princeton, NJ: Princeton University Press.

Toulmin, S. (1981). The tyranny of principles. *Hastings Center Report*, 11, 31–39.

Traynor, M. (1997). Postmodern research: No grounding or privilege, just free-floating trouble making. *Nursing Inquiry*, 4(2), 99–107.

Van Laer, P.H. (1956). *Philosophy of science: Part One—Science in general*. Pittsburgh, PA: Duquesne University Press.

Van Laer, P.H. (1962). *Philosophy of science: Part Two— A study of the division and nature of various groups of sciences*. Pittsburgh, PA: Duquesne -University Press.

Wainwright, S.P. (1997). A new paradigm for nursing: The potential of realism. *Journal of Advanced Nursing*, 26(6), 1262–1271.

Wallace, W. (1971). Theories: Logical deduction, hypothesis, interpretation, instrumentation, scaling, and sampling. In *The logic of science in sociology* (pp. 63–74). New York: Aldine Atherton.

Warms, CA. and Schroeder, C.A. (1999). Bridging the gulf between science and action: The "new fuzzies" of neopragmatism. *Advances in Nursing Science*, 22(2), 1–10.

Watson, J. (1995). Postmodernism and knowledge development in nursing. *Nursing Science Quarterly*, 8, 60–64.

Weaver, W. (1970). *Science of change: A lifetime in American science*. New York: Charles Scribner's Sons.

White, J. (1995). Patterns of knowing: Review, critique, and update. *Advances in Nursing Science*, 17(4), 73–86.

Wolfer, J. (1993). Aspects of "reality" and ways of knowing in nursing: In search of an integrating paradigm. *Image: Journal of Nursing Scholarship*, 25, 141–146.

Wolman, B.B. and Nagel, E. (Eds.). (1965). *Scientific psychology: Principles and approaches*. New York: Basic Books.

2. Nursing Theory: General

Algase, D.L. and Whall, A.F. (1993). Rosemary Ellis' views on the substantive structure of nursing. *Image: Journal of Nursing Scholarship*, 25, 69–72.

Alligood, M.R. (2005). Influences on advancement of nursing knowledge. Interview by Jacqueline Fawcett. *Nursing Science Quarterly*, 18(3), 227–232.

Alligood, M.R. (2013). Nursing theorists and their work (8th ed.). St. Louis, MO: Mosby

Anderson, R.M., Funnell, M.M., and Hernandez, C.A. (2005). Choosing and using theories in diabetes education research. *Diabetes Educator*, 31(4), 513, 515, 518–520.

Andrews, G.J. and Moon, G. (2005). Space, place, and the evidence base: Part II—rereading nursing environment through geographical research. *Worldviews on Evidence Based Nursing*, 2(3), 142–156.

Andrist, L.C., Nicholas, P.K., and Wolf, K. (2005). *A history of nursing ideas*. Sudbury, MA: Jones & Bartlett Publishers.

Aquino-Russell, C., Struby, F.V., and Reviczky, K. (2007). Living attentive presence and changing perspectives with a web-based nursing theory course. *Nursing Science Quarterly*, 20(2), 128–134.

Barnum, B.J.S. (1994). *Nursing theory: Analysis, application and evaluation* (4th ed.). Philadelphia, PA: J.B. Lippincott.

Beckerman, A. (1994). A personal journal of caring through esthetic knowing. *Advances in Nursing Science*, 17(1), 71–79.

Beeber, L.S. and Schmitt, M.H. (1986). Cohesiveness in groups: A concept in search of a definition. *Advances in Nursing Science*, 8, 1–11.

Benner, P. (1984). *From novice to expert: Excellence and power in clinical nursing practice*. Menlo Park, CA: Addison-Wesley.

Benner, P. (Ed.). (1994). *Interpretive phenomenology: Embodiment, caring, and ethics in health and illness*. Thousand Oaks, CA: Sage.

Benner, P. and Wrubel, J. (1989). *The primacy of caring*. Menlo Park, CA: Addison-Wesley.

Bennett, J.A. (1997). A case for theory triangulation. *Nursing Science Quarterly*, 10(2), 97–102.

Bjork, I.T. (1995). Neglected conflicts in the discipline of nursing: Perceptions of the importance and value of practical skill. *Journal of Advanced Nursing*, 22, 6–12.

Booth, K., Kenrick, M., and Woods, S. (1997). Nursing knowledge, theory and method revisited. *Journal of Advanced Nursing*, 26(4), 804–811.

Bottorff, J.L. (1991). Nursing: A practical science of caring. *Nursing Science*, 14(1), 26–39.

Bunkers, S.S. (2012). Presence: The eye of the needle. *Nursing Science Quarterly*, 25(1), 10–14.

Cash. K. (1997). Social epistemology, gender and nursing theory. *International Journal of Nursing Studies*, 34(2), 137–143.

Chinn, P.L. (1983). *Advances in nursing theory development*. Rockville, MD: Aspen Systems.

Chinn, P.L. (1994). *Developing substance: Mid-range theory in nursing* [Preface]. Gaithersburg, MD: Aspen Systems.

Chinn, P.L. (Ed.). (1986). *Nursing research methodology issues and implementation*. Rockville, MD: Aspen Systems.

Chinn, P.L. and Jacobs, M. (1987). *Theory and nursing: A systematic approach* (2nd ed.). St. Louis, MO: C.V. Mosby.

Chinn, P.L. and Kramer, M.K. (1991). *Theory and nursing: A systematic approach* (3rd ed.). St. Louis, MO: C.V. Mosby.

Chinn, P.L. and Kramer, M.K. (2011). Integrated theory and knowledge development in nursing. St. Louis, MO: Elsevier Health Sciences.

Clift, J. and Barrett, E. (1998). Testing nursing theory cross-culturally. *International Nursing Review*, 45(4), 123–126.

Cull-Wilby, B.L. and Pepin, J.I. (1987). Towards a coexistence of paradigms in nursing knowledge development. *Journal of Advanced Nursing*, 12(4), 515–521.

Dean, J.M. and Mountford, B. (1998). Innovation in the assessment of nursing theory and its evaluation: A team approach. *Journal of Advanced Nursing*, 28(2), 409–418.

Donohue-Porter, P., Forbes, M., and White, J. (2011). Nursing theory in curricula today: Challenges for faculty at all levels of education. *International Journal of Nursing Education Scholarship*, 8(1), 1–18, Article 14.

Dudley-Brown, S.L. (1997). The evaluation of nursing theory: A method for our madness. *International Journal of Nursing Studies*, 34(1), 76–83.

Edwards, S.D. (1998). The art of nursing. *Nursing Ethics*, 5(5), 393–400.

Engebretson, J. (1997). A multiparadigm approach to nursing. *Advanced Nursing Science*, 20(1), 21–33.

Fawcett, J. (1993). *Analysis and evaluation of nursing theories*. Philadelphia, PA: F.A. Davis.

Fawcett, J. (1995). *Analysis and evaluation of conceptual models of nursing* (3rd ed.). Philadelphia, PA: F.A. Davis.

Fawcett, J. (1995). Notes on book review of analysis and evaluation of nursing theories. *Nursing Science Quarterly*, 8, 58–59.

Fawcett, J. and Madeya, S.D. (2013). Contemporary nursing knowledge: Analysis and evaluation of nursing models and theories (3rd ed.). Philadelphia, PA: F.A. Davis.

Fawcett, J., Watson, J., Neuman, B., Walker, P.H., and Fitzpatrick, J.J. (2001). On nursing theories and evidence. *Image: Journal of Nursing Scholarship*, 33(2), 115–119.

Fitzpatrick, J. and Whall, A. (1989). *Conceptual models of nursing: Analysis and application* (2nd ed.). East Norwalk, CT: Appleton & Lange.

Fitzpatrick, J., Whall, A., Johnston, R., and Floyd, J. (1982). *Nursing models and their psychiatric mental health applications*. Bowie, MD: Robert J. Brady Co.

Funk, S.G., Tornquist, E.M., Champage, M.T., Copp, L.A., and Wiese, R.A. (Eds.). (1990). *Key aspects of recovery: Improving nutrition, rest, and mobility*. New York: Springer Publishing Company.

Gastaldo, D. and Holmes, D. (1999). Foucault and nursing: A history of the present. *Nursing Inquiry*, 6(4), 231–240.

Gebbie, K. (Ed.). (1976, March 4–7). *Summary of the second national conference: Classification of nursing diagnosis*. St. Louis, MO: C.V. Mosby.

Gioiella, E.C. (1996). The importance of theory guided research and practice in the changing health care science. *Nursing Science Quarterly*, 9(2), 47.

Hagerty, B.M., Lynch-Sauer, J., Patusky, K.L., and Bouwsema, M. (1993). An emerging theory of human relatedness. *Image: Journal of Nursing Scholarship*, 25(4), 291–296.

Harden, J. (2000). Language, discourse and the chronotope: Applying literary theory to the narratives in health care. *Journal of Advanced Nursing*, 31(3), 506–512.

Henly, S.J., Vermeersch, P.E., and Duckett, L.J. (1998). Model selection for covariance structures analysis in nursing research. *Western Journal of Nursing Research*, 20(3), 344–355.

Hilton, P.A. (1997). Theoretical perspectives of nursing: A review of the literature. *Journal of Advanced Nursing*, 26(6), 1211–1220.

Holmes, C.A. and Warelow, P.J. (1997). Culture, needs and nursing: A critical theory approach. *Journal of Advanced Nursing*, 25(3), 463–470.

Holmes, C.A. and Warelow, P.J. (2000). Some implications of postmodernism for nursing theory, research, and practice. *Canadian Journal of Nursing Research*, 32(2), 89–101.

Im, E.O. and Chang, S.J. (2012). Current trends in nursing theories. *Journal of Nursing Scholarship*, 44(2), 156–164.

Im, E.O. and Meleis, A.I. (1999). A situation-specific theory of Korean immigrant women's menopausal transition. *Image: Journal of Nursing Scholarship*, 31(4), 333–338.

Im, E.O. and Meleis, A.I. (1999). Situation-specific theories: Philosophical roots, properties, and approach. *Advances in Nursing Science*, 22(2), 11–24.

Johnson, J. (1994). A dialectical examination of nursing art. *Advances in Nursing Science*, 17(1), 1–14.

Kahn, S. and Fawcett, J. (1995). Continuing the dialogue: A response to Draper's critique of Fawcett's 'Conceptual models and nursing practice: The reciprocal relationship.' *Journal of Advanced Nursing*, 22, 188–192.

Ketefian, S. and Redman, R.W. (1997). Nursing science in the global community. *Image: Journal of Nursing Scholarship*, 29(1), 11–15.

Kim, H.S. (1983). *The nature of theoretical thinking in nursing*. Norwalk, CT: Appleton-Century-Crofts.

Kim, H.S. (1994). Practice theories in nursing and a science of nursing practice. *Scholarly Inquiry for Nursing Practice*, 8, 145–166.

Kim, H.S. and Kollak, I. (Eds.). (2006). *Nursing theories: Conceptual and philosophical foundations* (2nd ed.). New York: Springer Publishing Company.

Kleffel, D. (2005). The evolution of the environmental metaparadigm of nursing. In L.C. Andrist, P.K. Nicholas, and K.A. Wolf (Eds.), *A history of nursing ideas*. Sudbury, MA: Jones and Bartlett.

Kolcaba, K.Y. and Kolcaba, R. (1991). An analysis of the concept of comfort. *Journal of Advanced Nursing*, 16, 1301–1310.

Laurent, C.L. (2000). A nursing theory for nursing leadership. *Journal of Nursing Management*, 8(2), 83–87.

Laustsen, G. (2006). Environment, ecosystems, and ecological behavior: A dialogue toward developing nursing ecological theory. *Advances in Nursing Science*, 29(1), 43–54.

Lauver, D. (1992). A theory of care-seeking behavior. *Image: Journal of Nursing Scholarship*, 24, 281–287.

Lenz, E.R., Suppe, F., Gift, A.G., Pugh, L.C., and Milligan, R.A. (1995). Collaborative development of middle-range nursing theories: Toward a theory of unpleasant symptoms. *Advances in Nursing Science*, 17(3), 1–13.

Liaschenko, J. and Fisher, A. (1999). Theorizing the knowledge that nurses use in the conduct of their work. *Scholarly Inquiry for Nursing Practice*, 13(1), 29–41.

Liehr, P. and Smith, M.J. (1999). Middle range theory: Spinning research and practice to create knowledge for the new millennium. *Advances in Nursing Science*, 21(4), 81–91.

Lundh, U., Soder, M., and Waerness, K. (1988). Nursing theories: A critical view. *Image: Journal of Nursing Scholarship*, 20, 36–40.

Maeve, M.K. (1994). The carrier bag theory of nursing practice. *Advances in Nursing Science*, 16, 9–22.

Manias, E. and Street, A. (2000). Possibilities for critical social theory and Foucault's work: A toolbox approach. *Nursing Inquiry*, 7(1), 50–60.

Marck, P. (1990). Therapeutic reciprocity: A caring phenomenon. *Advances in Nursing Science*, 13(1), 49–59.

Marriner-Tomey, A. (1989). *Nursing theorists and their work* (2nd ed.). St. Louis, MO: C.V. Mosby.

McCance, T.V. (1999). Caring: Theoretical perspectives of relevance to nursing. *Journal of Advanced Nursing*, 30(6), 1388–1395.

McIntyre, M. and McDonald, C. (2013). Contemplating the fit and utility of nursing theory and nursing scholarship informed by the social sciences and humanities. *Advances in Nursing Science*, 36(1), 10–17.

Meleis, A.I. (1992). Directions for nursing theory development in the 21st century. *Nursing Science Quarterly*, 5(3), 112–117.

Meleis, A.I. (1996). Theory development: A blueprint for the 21st century. In P. Hinton Walker and B. Neuman (Eds.), *Blueprint for use of nursing models*. New York: National League for Nursing.

Mischel, M.H. (1990). Reconceptualizing of the uncertainty in illness theory. *Image: Journal of Nursing Scholarship*, 22, 256–262.

Monti, E.J. and Tingen, M.S. (1999). Multiple paradigms of nursing science. *Advances in Nursing Science*, 21(4), 64–80.

Morse, J.M., Anderson, G., Bottorff, J.L., Yonger, O., O'Brien, B., Solberg, S.M., and Hunter McIlveen, K. (1992). Exploring empathy: A conceptual fit for nursing practice? *Image: Journal of Nursing Scholarship*, 24, 273–280.

Morse, J.M., Bottorff, J., Neander, W., and Solberg, S. (1991). Comparative analysis of conceptualizations and theories of caring. *Image: Journal of Nursing Scholarship*, 23, 119–126.

Morse, J.M., Miles, M.W., Clark, D.A., and Doberneck, B.M. (1994). "Sensing" patient needs: Exploring concepts of nursing insight and receptivity used in nursing assessment. *Scholarly Inquiry for Nursing Practice*, 8, 233–254.

Morse, J.M., Solberg, S.M., Neander, W.L., Bottorff, J.L., Johnson, J.L. (1990). Concepts of caring and caring as a concept. *Advances in Nursing Science*, 13(1), 1–14.

Newman, M. (1979). *Theory development in nursing*. Philadelphia, PA: F.A. Davis.

Nicoll, L.H. (Ed.). (1992). *Perspectives on nursing theory* (2nd ed.). Philadelphia, PA: J.B. Lippincott.

Nolan, M., Lundh, U., and Tishelman, C. (1998). Nursing's knowledge base: Does it have to be unique? *British Journal of Nursing*, 7(5), 270–276.

Norris, C. (Ed.). (1969, October 9–10). *Proceedings: Second nursing theory conference*. Kansas city, MO: University of Kansas Medical Center, Department of Nursing Education.

Nursing Development Conference Group. (1977). *Concept formalization in nursing: Process and product*. Boston, MA: Little, Brown.

Oberst, M.T. (1995). To what end theory? *Research in Nursing & Health*, 18, 83–84.

Parse, R.R. (1987). *Nursing science: Major paradigms, theories, and critiques*. Philadelphia, PA: W.B. Saunders.

Parse, R.R. (1995). Nursing theories and frameworks: The essence of advanced practice nursing. *Nursing Science Quarterly*, 8, 1.

Pilkington, F.B. (2005). Myth and symbol in nursing theories. *Nursing Science Quarterly*, 18(3), 198–203.

Pilkington, F.B., Frederickson, K., and Velsasco-Whetsell, M. (2006). The glass menagerie as heuristic for explicating nursing theory. *Nursing Science Quarterly*, 19(3), 190–196.

Reed, P.G. (1997). Nursing: The ontology of the discipline. *Nursing Science Quarterly*, 10(2), 76–79.

Richer, M.C. and Ezer, H. (2000). Understanding beliefs and meanings in the experience of cancer: A concept analysis. *Journal of Advanced Nursing*, 32(5), 1108–1115.

Riehl-Sisca, J.P. (1989). *Conceptual models for nursing practice* (3rd ed.). East Norwalk, CT: Appleton & Lange.

Rutty, J.E. (1998). The nature of philosophy of science, theory and knowledge relating to nursing and professionalism. *Journal of Advanced Nursing*, 28(2), 243–250.

Santos Salas, A. (2005). Toward a North-South dialogue: revisiting nursing theory (from the South). *Advances in Nursing Science*, 28(1), 17–24.

Sarvimki A. and Stenbock-Hult, B. (1992). *Caring: An introduction to health care from a humanistic perspective*. Helsinki, Finland: Foundation for Nursing Education.

Severinsson, E.I. (1998). Bridging the gap between theory and practice: A supervision programme for nursing students. *Journal of Advanced Nursing*, 27(6), 1269–1277.

Silva, M.C. (1987). Conceptual models of nursing. *Annual Review of Nursing Research*, 5, 229–246.

Simpson. J. (1998). The perplexities of conceptual frameworks. *Canadian Nurse*, 94(10), 51.

Spear, H.J. (2007). Nursing theory and knowledge development: A descriptive review of doctoral dissertations, 2000–2004. *Advances in Nursing Science*, 30(1), E1–E14.

Stiles, K.A. (2011). Advancing nursing knowledge through complex holism. *Advances in Nursing Science*, 34(1), 39–50.

Taylor, J.S. (1997). Nursing ideology: Identification and legitimation. *Journal of Advanced Nursing*, 25(3), 442–446.

Thompson, C. (1999). A conceptual treadmill: The need for "middle ground" in clinical decision making theory in nursing. *Journal of Advanced Nursing*, 30(5), 1222–1229.

Thorne, S., Canam, C., Dahinten, S., Hall, W., Henderson, A., Kirkham, S.R. (1998). Nursing's metaparadigm concepts: Disimpacting the debates. *Journal of Advanced Nursing*, 27(6), 1257–1268.

Thorne, S.E., Kirkham, S.R., and Henderson, A. (1999). Ideological implications of paradigm discourse. *Nursing Inquiry*, 6(2), 123–131.

Thorne, S. and Sawatzky, R. (2014). Particularizing the general: Sustaining theoretical integrity in the context of an evidence-based practice agenda. *Advances in Nursing Science*, 37(1), 5–18.

Tierney, A.J. (1998). Nursing models: Extant or extinct? *Journal of Advanced Nursing*, 28(1), 77–85.

Timpson, J. (1996). Nursing theory: Everything the artist spits is art? *Journal of Advanced Nursing*, 23, 1030–1036.

Torres, G. (1986). *Theoretical foundations of nursing*. Norwalk, CT: Appleton-Century-Crofts.

University of California, San Francisco, School of Nursing Symptom Management Faculty Group. (1994). A model for symptom management. *Image: Journal of Nursing Scholarship*, 26, 272–276.

Vicenzi, A.E. (1994). Chaos theory and some nursing considerations. *Nursing Science Quarterly*, 7(1), 36–42.

Wainwright, P. (2000). Towards an aesthetics of nursing. *Journal of Advanced Nursing*, 32(3), 750–756.

Walker, L.O. and Avant, K.C. (1995). *Strategies for theory construction in nursing* (3rd ed.). East Norwalk, CT: Appleton & Lange.

Winstead-Fry, P. (1986). *Case studies in nursing theory*. New York: National League for Nursing.

Wolf, L.A. (2015). Research as problem solving: Theoretical frameworks as tools. *Journal of Emergency Nursing*, 41(1), 83–85.

Younger, J.B. (1991). A theory of mastery. *Advances in Nursing Science*, 14(1), 76–89.

Zbilut, J.P. and Staffileno, B. (1994). Chaos theory and nursing revisited. *Nursing Science Quarterly*, 7(4), 150–152.

3. Metatheory and Theory Development in Nursing

Ahern, N.R. (2006). Adolescent resilience: An evolutionary concept analysis. *Journal of Pediatric Nursing: Nursing Care of Children and Families*, 21(3), 175–185.

Algase, D.L. and Whall, A.F. (1993). Rosemary Ellis' views on the substantive structure of nursing. *Image: Journal of Nursing Scholarship*, 25, 69–72.

Allan, H. (1998). Issues in infertility nursing: Broadening the debate. *Nursing Standard*, 12(27), 39–41.

Allchin-Petardi, L. (1998). Weathering the storm: Persevering through a difficult time. *Nursing Science Quarterly*, 11(4), 172–177.

Allen, D.G. (1987). The social policy statement: A reappraisal. *Advances in Nursing Science*, 10(1), 39–48.

American Nurses Association. (1995). *Nursing's social policy statement* (Publication No. NP-107). Washington, DC: Author.

An, J.Y., Hayman, L.L., Panniers, T., and Carty, B. (2007). Theory development in nursing and healthcare informatics: A model explaining and predicting information and communication technology acceptance by healthcare consumers. *Advances in Nursing Science*, 30(3), E37–E49.

Andershed, B. and Ternestedt, B.M. (2001). Development of a theoretical framework describing relatives' involvement in palliative care. *Journal of Advanced Nursing*, 34(4), 554–562.

Anderson, R.A., Dobal, M.T., and Blessing, B. (1992). Theory-based approach to computer skill development in nursing administration. *Computers in Nursing*, 10(4), 152–157.

Atay, S. and Karabacak, U. (2012). Care plans using concept maps and their effects on the critical thinking dispositions of nursing students. *International Journal of Nursing Practice*, 18(3), 233–239.

Avant, K.C. (1993). The Wilson method of concept analysis. In B.L. Rodgers and K.A. Knafl (Eds.), *Concept development in nursing* (pp. 51–60). Philadelphia, PA: W.B. Saunders.

Baker, C. (1999). From chaos to order: A nursing-based psycho-education program for parents of children with attention-deficit hyperactivity disorder. *Canadian Journal of Nursing Research*, 31(2), 71–75.

Banks-Wallace, J. (2000). Womanist ways of knowing: Theoretical considerations for research with African American women. *Advances in Nursing Science*, 22(3), 33–45.

Barker, P. (1998). The future of the theory of interpersonal relations? A personal reflection on Peplau's legacy. *Journal of Psychiatric and Mental Health Nursing*, 5(3), 213–220.

Barker. P.J., Reynolds, W., and Stevenson, C. (1997). The human science basis of psychiatric nursing: Theory and practice. *Journal of Advanced Nursing*, 5(4), 660–667.

Barnett, K. (1972). A theoretical construct of the concepts of touch as they relate to nursing. *Nursing Research*, 21(2), 102–110.

Barrett, E.A. and Caroselli, C. (1998). Methodological ponderings related to the power as knowing participation in change tool. *Nursing Science Quarterly*, 11(1), 17–22.

*Batey, M.V. (1977). Conceptualization: Knowledge and logic guiding empirical research. *Nursing Research*, 26(5), 324–329.

Baumann, S.L. (1997). Contrasting two approaches in a community-based nursing practice with older adults: The medical model and Parse's nursing theory. *Nursing Science Quarterly*, 10(3), 124–130.

*Becker, C.H. (1983). A conceptualization of concept. *Nursing Papers: Perspectives in Nursing*, 15(2), 51–58.

Beckstead, J.W. and Beckstead, L.G. (2006). A multidimensional analysis of the epistemic origins of nursing theories, models, and frameworks. *International Journal of Nursing Studies*, 43(1), 113–122.

*Beckstrand, J. (1978). The notion of a practice theory and the relationship of scientific and ethical knowledge to practice. *Research in Nursing and Health*, 1(3), 131–136.

*Beckstrand, J. (1978). The need for a practice theory as indicated by the knowledge used in conduct of practice. *Research in Nursing and Health*, 1(4), 175–179.

*Beckstrand, J. (1980). A critique of several conceptions of practice theory in nursing. *Research in Nursing and Health*, 3(2), 69–80.

Bell, A., Horsfall, J., and Goodin, W. (1998). The Mental Health Nursing Clinical Confidence Scale: A tool for measuring undergraduate learning on mental health clinical placements. *Australian and New Zealand Journal of Mental Health Nursing*, 7(4), 184–190.

Bergenson, B.S. (1971). Adaptation as a unifying theory. In J.F. Murphy (Ed.), *Theoretical issues in professional nursing*. New York: Appleton-Century-Crofts.

*Berthold, J.S. (1968). Prologue: Symposium on theory development in nursing. *Nursing Research*, 17(3), 196–197.

Bibace, R. and Walsh, M.E. (1982). Conflict of roles: On the difficulties of being both scientist and practitioner in one life. *Professional Psychology*, 13, 389–395.

Blegen, M.A. and Tripp-Reimer, T. (1997). Implications of nursing taxonomies for middle-range theory development. *Advances in Nursing Science*, 19(3), 37–49.

Blix, A. (1999). Integrating occupational health protection and health promotion: Theory and program application. *Official Journal of the American Association of Occupational Health Nurses*, 47(4), 168–171.

Bohny, B.J. (1980). Theory development for a nursing science. *Nursing Forum*, 19(1), 50–67.

Botha, M.E. (1989). Theory development in perspective: The role of conceptual frameworks and models in theory development. *Journal of Advanced Nursing*, 14(1), 49–55.

Bournes, D.A. and DasGupta, T.L. (1997). Professional practice leader: A transformational role that addresses human diversity. *Nursing Administration Quarterly*, 21(4), 61–68.

Boutain. D.M. (1999). Critical nursing scholarship: Exploring critical social theory with African American studies. *Advances in Nursing Science*, 21(4), 37–47.

Bowers, R. and Moore, K.N. (1997). Bakhtin, nursing narratives, and dialogical consciousness. *Advances in Nursing Science*, 19(3), 70–77.

Boychuk Duchscher, J.E. (1999). Catching the wave: Understanding the concept of critical thinking. *Journal of Advanced Nursing*, 29(3), 577–583.

Brixey, J.J., Robinson, D.J., Johnson, C.W., Johnson, T.R., Turley, J.P., and Zhang, J. (2007). A concept analysis of phenomenon interruption. *Advances in Nursing Science*, 30(1), E26–E42.

*Brown, M.I. (1964). Research on the development of nursing theory: The importance of a theoretical framework in nursing research. *Nursing Research*, 13(2), 109–112.

*Brown, M.I. (1968). Theory development in nursing: Social theory in geriatric nursing research. *Nursing Research*, 17(3), 213–217.

*Brown, M.L. (1983). Research questions and answers: The use of theory and conceptual frameworks in nursing research and practice. *Oncology Nursing Forum*, 10(2), 111–112.

Bulman, C., Lathlean, J., and Gobbi, M. (2012). The concept of reflection in nursing: Qualitative findings on student and teacher perspectives. *Nurse Education Today*, 32(5), E8–E13.

Bunkers, S.S. (1998). Considering tomorrow: Parse's theory-guided research. *Nursing Science Quarterly*, 11(2), 56–63.

Burks, K.J. (2001). Intentional action. *Journal of Advanced Nursing*, 34(5), 668–675.

*Bush, H.A. (1979). Models for nursing. *Advances in Nursing Science*, 1(2), 13–21.

Butt, G. (2008). Stigma in the context of hepatitis C: Concept analysis. *Journal of Advanced Nursing*, 62(6), 712–724.

*Carper, B.A. (1978). Fundamental patterns of knowing in nursing. *Advances in Nursing Science*, 1(1), 13–23.

Carr, J.M. (1998). Vigilance as a caring expression and Leininger's theory of cultural care diversity and universality. *Nursing Science Quarterly*, 11(2), 74–78.

Carson, M.G. and Mitchell, G.J. (1998). The experience of living with persistent pain. *Journal of Advanced Nursing*, 28(6), 1242–1248.

Carter, P.A. (1998). Self-care agency: The concept and how it is measured. *Journal of Nursing Measurement*, 6(2), 195–207.

*Chapman, C.M. (1976). The use of sociological theories and models in nursing. *Journal of Advanced Nursing*, 1, 111–127.

*Chinn, P.L. and Jacobs, M.K. (1978). A model for theory development in nursing. *Advances in Nursing Science*, 1(1), 1–11.

*Clark, J. (1982). Development of models and theories on the concept of nursing. *Journal of Advanced Nursing*, 7(2), 129–134.

Cleary, F. (1971). A theoretical model: Its potential for adaptation to nursing. *Image: Journal of Nursing Scholarship*, 4(1), 14–20.

*Cleland, V.S. (1967). The use of existing theories. *Nursing Research*, 16(2), 118–121.

Clift, J. and Barrett, E. (1998). Testing nursing theory cross-culturally. *International Nursing Review*, 45(4), 123–126.

Cohen, S.S. and Milone-Nuzzo, P. (2001). Advancing health policy in nursing education through service learning. *Advances in Nursing Science*, 23(3), 28–40.

*Colaizzi, J. (1975). The proper object of nursing science. *International Journal of Nursing Studies*, 12(4), 197–200.

*Collins, R.J. and Fielder, J.H. (1981). Beckstrand's concept of practice theory: A critique. *Research in Nursing and Health*, 4(3), 317–321.

Conway, M.E. (1985). Toward greater specificity in defining nursing's metaparadigm. *Advances in Nursing Science*, 7(4), 73–81.

Cooley, M.E. (1999). Analysis and evaluation of the Trajectory Theory of Chronic Illness Management. *Scholarly Inquiry in Nursing Practice*, 13(2), 75–95.

Copnell, B. (1998). Synthesis in nursing knowledge: An analysis of two approaches. *Journal of Advanced Nursing*, 27(4), 870–874.

Cormack, D.F.S. and Reynolds, W. (1992). Criteria for evaluating the clinical and practical utility of models used by nurses. *Journal of Advanced Nursing*, 17, 1472–1478.

Cowley, S. and Billings, J.R. (1999). Resources revisited: Salutogenesis from a lay perspective. *Journal of Advanced Nursing*, 29(4), 994–1004.

Cowden, T.L. and Cummings, G.G. (2012). Nursing theory and concept development: A theoretical model of clinical nurses' intentions to stay in their current positions. *Journal of Advanced Nursing*, 68(7), 1646–1657.

Cowling, W.R., III. (2000). Healing as appreciating wholeness. *Advances in Nursing Science*, 22(3), 16–32.

*Crawford, G., Dufault, S.K., and Rudy, E. (1979). Evolving issues in theory development. *Nursing Outlook*, 27(5), 346–351.

Croom, S., Procter, S., and Couteur, A.L. (2000). Developing a concept analysis of control for use in child and adolescent mental health nursing. *Journal of Advanced Nursing*, 31(6), 1324–1332.

Crossan, F. and Robb, A. (1998). Role of the nurse: Introducing theories and concepts. *British Journal of Nursing*, 7(10), 608–612.

Crow, R. (1982). Frontiers of nursing in the 21st century: Development of models and theories on the concept of nursing. *Journal of Advanced Nursing*, 7, 111–116.

Cull-Wilby, B.L. and Pepin, J.I. (1987). Towards a coexistence of paradigms in nursing process. *Journal of Advanced Nursing*, 12, 515–521.

Deatrick, J.A., Knafl, K.A., and Murphy-Moore, C. (1999). Clarifying the concept of normalization. *Image: Journal of Nursing Scholarship*, 31(3), 209–214.

DeMong, N.C. and Assie-Lussier, L.L. (1999). Continuing education: An aspect of staff development relating to the nurse manager's role. *Journal of Nurses Staff Development*, 15(1), 19–22.

Derdiarian, A.K. (1979). Education: A way to theory construction in nursing. *Journal of Nursing Education*, 18(2), 36–47.

DeSantis, L. and Ugarriza, D.N. (2000). The concept of theme as used in qualitative nursing research. *Western Journal of Nursing Research*, 22(3), 351–372.

DiBartolo, M.C. (1998). Philosophy of science in doctoral nursing education revisited. *Journal of Professional Nursing*, 14(6), 350–360.

*Dickoff, J. and James, P. (1968). A theory of theories: A position paper. *Nursing Research*, 17(3), 197–203.

Dickoff, J. and James, P. (1971). Clarity to what end? *Nursing Research*, 20(6), 499–502.

*Dickoff, J., James, P., and Wiedenbach, E. (1968). Theory in practice discipline: Part I. Practice oriented theory. *Nursing Research*, 17(5), 415–435.

*Dickoff, J., James, P., and Wiedenbach, E. (1968). Theory in practice discipline: Part II. Practice oriented theory. *Nursing Research*, 17(6), 545–554.

Dierckx de Casterle, B., Roelens, A., and Gastmans, C. (1998). An adjusted version of Kohlberg's moral theory: Discussion of its validity for research in nursing ethics. *Journal of Advanced Nursing*, 27(4), 829–835.

Dluhy, N.M. (1995). Mapping knowledge in chronic illness. *Journal of Advanced Nursing*, 21, 1051–1058.

Dolan, K. (1997). Children in accident and emergency. *Accident and Emergency Nursing*, 5(2), 88–91.

*Donaldson, S.K. and Crowley, D. (1978). The discipline of nursing. *Nursing Outlook*, 26(2), 113–120.

Donnelly, G.F. (1986). Nursing theory: Evolution of a sacred cow. *Holistic Nursing Practice*, 1(1), 1–7.

Doyle, N. (2008). Cancer survivorship: Evolutionary concept analysis. *Journal of Advanced Nursing*, 62(4), 499–509.

Dubin, R. (1978). *Theory building*. New York: Free Press.

*Ellis, R. (1968). Characteristics of significant theories. *Nursing Research*, 17(3), 217–222. (See Section 2.)

Ellis, R. (1971). Commentary on Walker's "Toward a clearer understanding of the concept of nursing theory." *Nursing Research*, 20(6), 493–494.

Ellis, R. (1982). Conceptual issues in nursing. *Nursing Outlook*, 30(7), 406–410.

Emden, C. (1998). Conducting a narrative analysis. *Collegian*, 5(3), 34–39.

Engebretson, J. (1997). A multiparadigm approach to nursing. *Advances in Nursing Science*, 20(1), 21–33.

English, I. (1993). Intuition a function of the expert nurse: A critique of Benners' novice to expert model. *Journal of Advanced Nursing*, 18(3), 387–393.

Evangelista, L.S. (1999). Compliance: A concept analysis. *Nursing Forum*, 34(1), 5–11.

Fawcett, J. and Boubonniere, M. (2001). Utilization of nursing knowledge and the future of the discipline. In N.L. Chaska (Ed.), *The nursing profession—Tomorrow and beyond* (pp. 311–320). Thousand Oaks, CA: Sage.

Fealy, G.M. (1997). The theory-practice relationship in nursing: An exploration of contemporary discourse. *Journal of Advanced Nursing*, 25(5), 1061–1069.

Fernandez, E. (1997). Just "doing the observations": Reflective practice in nursing. *British Journal of Nursing*, 6(16), 939–943.

Fisher, M.A. and Mitchell, G.J. (1998). Patients' views of quality of life: Transforming the knowledge base of nursing. Comment in: *Clinical Nurse Specialist*, (1998) 12(3), 98. *Clinical Nurse Specialist*, 12(3), 99–105.

Flaskerud, J.H. and Halloran, E.J. (1980). Areas of agreement in nursing theory development. *Advances in Nursing Science*, 3(1), 1–7.

Flaskerud, J.H. and Halloran, E.J. (1981). Areas of agreement in nursing theory development. *Advances in Nursing Science*, 3(3), 31–42.

Fogarty, C. and Cronin, P. (2008). Waiting for healthcare: A concept analysis. *Journal of Advanced Nursing*, 61(4), 463–471.

Forbes, M.A. (1999). Hope in the older adult with chronic illness: A comparison of two research methods in theory building. *Advances in Nursing Science*, 22(2), 74–87.

Freshwater, D. (1998). From acorn to oak tree: A neoplatonic perspective of reflection and caring. *Australian Journal of Holistic Nursing*, 5(2), 14–19.

Fry, S.T. (1999). The philosophy of nursing. *Scholarly Inquiry in Nursing Practice*, 13(1), 5–15.

Fulton, J.S., Miller, W.R. and Otte, J.L. (2012). A systematic review of analyses of the concept of quality of life in nursing. *Advances in Nursing Science*, 35(2), E1–E12.

Gaberson, K.B. (1997). What's the answer? What's the question? *Journal of the Association of Perioperative Registered Nurses*, 66(1), 148–151.

Garrett, B.M. and Cutting, R.L. (2015). Ways of knowing: Realism, non-realism, nominalism and a typology revisited with a counter perspective for nursing science. *Nursing Inquiry*, 22(2), 95–105.

Garside, J.R. and Nhemachena, J.Z.Z. (2013). A concept analysis of competence and its transition in nursing. *Nurse Education Today*, 33(5), 541–545.

Gassner, L.A., Wotton, K., Clare, J., Hofmeyer, A., and Buckman, J. (1999). Evaluation of a model of collaboration: Academic and clinician partnership in the development and implementation of undergraduate teaching. *Collegian*, 6(3), 14–21.

Gastaldo, D. and Holmes. D. (1999). Foucault and nursing: A history of the present. *Nursing Inquiry*, 6(4), 231–240.

Geanellos, R. (1997). Nursing knowledge development: Where to from here? *Collegian*, 4(1), 13–21.

*Gebbie, K. and Lavin, M.A. (1974). Classifying nursing diagnoses. *American Journal of Nursing*, 74(2), 250–253.

Gerdeman, J.L., Lux, K. and Jacko, J. (2013). Using concept mapping to build clinical judgment skills. *Nurse Education in Practice*, 13(1), 11–17.

Goode, W.J. and Hatt, P.K. (1952). Science: Theory and fact. In W.J. Goode and P.K. Hatt (Eds.), *Methods in social research* (pp. 7–17). New York: McGraw-Hill.

Gordon, N.S. (1998). Influencing mental health nursing practice through the teaching of research and theory: A personal critical review. *Journal of Psychiatric and Mental Health Nursing*, 5(2), 119–128.

Gormley, K.J. (1997). Practice write-ups: An assessment instrument that contributes to bridging the differences between theory and practice for student nurses through the development of core skills. *Nurse Education Today*, 17(1), 53–57.

*Gortner, S.R. (1983). The history and philosophy of nursing science and research. *Advances in Nursing Science*, 5(2), 1–8.

Gottlieb, L.N. and Gottlieb B. (1998). Evolutionary principles can guide nursing's future development. *Journal of Advanced Nursing*, 28(5), 1099–1105.

Gramling, L.F. (2007). Women in young and mid-adulthood: Theory advancement and retroduction. *Advances in Nursing Science*, 30(2), 95–107.

Gramling, L.F., Lambert, V.A., and Pursley-Crotteau, S. (1998), Coping in young women: Theoretical retroduction. *Journal of Advanced Nursing*, 28(5), 1082–1091.

Green, C. (2012). Nursing intuition: A valid form of knowledge. *Nursing Philosophy*, 13(2), 98–111.

Greenwood, J. (1998). Establishing an international network on nurses' clinical reasoning. *Journal of Advanced Nursing*, 27(4), 843–847.

Greenwood, J. (2000). Critical thinking and nursing scripts: The case for the development of both. *Journal of Advanced Nursing*, 31(2), 428–436.

Gulzar, L. (1999). Access to health care. *Image: Journal of Nursing Scholarship*, 31(1), 13–19.

Haas, B.K. (1999). Clarification and integration of similar quality of life concepts. *Image: Journal of Nursing Scholarship*, 31(3), 215–220.

Haase, J.E., Britt, T., Coward, D.D., Leidy, N.K., and Penn, P.E. (1992). Simultaneous concept analysis of spiritual perspective, hope, acceptance and self-transcendence. *Image: Journal of Nursing Scholarship*, 24, 141–147.

Hadley, B.J. (1969). Evolution of a conception of nursing. *Nursing Research*, 18(5), 400–405.

*Hall, B.A. (1981). The change paradigm in nursing: Growth versus persistence. *Advances in Nursing Science*, 3(4), 1–6.

Hall, J.M., Stevens, P.E., and Meleis, A.I. (1994). Marginalization: A guiding concept for valuing diversity in nursing knowledge development. *Advances in Nursing Science*, 16(4), 23–41.

Hamilton, R. and Kopin, S. (2013). Theory development from studies with young women with breast cancer who are BRCA mutation negative. *Advances in Nursing Science*, 36(2), E-41–E53.

Hardy, L.K. (1986). Janforum: Identifying the place of theoretical frameworks in an evolving discipline, the nursing profession. *Journal of Advanced Nursing*, 11(1), 103–107.

Hardy, M.E. (1974). The nature of theories. In M.E. Hardy (Ed.), *Theoretical foundations for nursing* (pp. 10–22). New York: MSS Information Corp.

*Hardy, M.E. (1978). Perspectives on nursing theory. *Advances in Nursing Science*, 1(1), 37–48.

Harris, I.M. (1971). Theory building in nursing: A review of the literature. *Image: Journal of Nursing Scholarship*, 4(1), 6–10.

Hart, M.A and Foster, S.N. (1998). Self-care agency in two groups of pregnant women. *Nursing Science Quarterly*, 11(4), 167–171.

Hawley, P., Young, S., and Pasco, A.C. (2000). Reductionism in the pursuit of nursing science: (In)congruent with nursing's core values? *Canadian Journal of Nursing Research*, 32(2), 75–88.

Henderson, D. (1997). Intersecting race and gender in feminist theories of women's psychological development. *Issues in Mental Health Nursing*, 18(5), 377–393.

Herbert, C.L. (1997). "To be or not to be"—An ethical debate on the not-for-resuscitation (NFR) status of a stroke patient. *Journal of Clinical Nursing*, 6(2), 99–105.

Herth, K. (1998). Hope as seen through the eyes of homeless children. *Journal of Advanced Nursing*, 28(5), 1053–1062.

Hinshaw, A.S. (1987). Response to "Structuring the nursing knowledge system: A typology of four domains." *Scholarly Inquiry for Nursing Practice*, 1(2), 111–114.

Hisama, K.K. (1999). Towards an international theory of nursing. *Nursing and Health Sciences*, 1(2), 77–81.

Holmes, C.A. and Warelow, P.J. (1997). Culture, needs and nursing: A critical theory approach. *Journal of Advanced Nursing*, 25(3), 463–470.

Holmes, C.A. and Warelow, P.J. (2000). Some implications of postmodernism for nursing theory, research, and practice. *Canadian Journal of Nursing Research*, 32(2), 89–101.

Hopkinson, J.B. (1999). A study of the perceptions of hospice day care patients: My phenomenological methodology. *International Journal of Nursing Studies*, 36(3), 203–207.

Horsburgh, M.E. (1999). Self-care of well adult Canadians and adult Canadians with end stage renal disease. *International Journal of Nursing Studies*, 36(6), 443–453.

Hurley, B.A. (1979). Why a theoretical framework in nursing research? *Western Journal of Nursing Research*, 1(1), 28–41.

Im, E.O. (2005). Development of situation-specific theories: An integrative approach. *Advances in Nursing Science*, 28(2), 137–151.

Im, E.O. and Meleis, A.I. (1999). A situation-specific theory of Korean immigrant women's menopausal transition. *Image: The Journal of Nursing Scholarship*, 31(4), 333–338.

Jaarsma, T., Halfens, R., Senten, M., Abu Saad, H.H., and Dracup, K. (1998). Developing a supportive-educative program for patients with advanced heart failure within Orem's general theory of nursing. *Nursing Science Quarterly*, 11(2), 79–85.

Jacobs-Kramer, M.K. and Chinn, P.L. (1988). Perspectives on knowing: A model of nursing knowledge. *Scholarly Inquiry for Nursing Practice*, 2(2), 129–139.

Jacobson, M. (1971). Qualitative data: As a potential source of theory in nursing. *Image: Journal of Nursing Scholarship*, 4(1), 10–14.

*Jacox, A. (1974). Theory construction in nursing: An overview. *Nursing Research*, 23(1), 4–13.

Janes, N.M. and Wells, D.L. (1997). Elderly patients' experiences with nurses guided by Parse's theory of human becoming. *Clinical Nursing Research*, 6(3), 205–222.

Jennings, B.M. (1987). Nursing theory development: Successes and challenges. *Journal of Advanced Nursing*, 12(1), 63–69.

Johansson, I., Hildingh, C., Wenneberg, S., Fridlund, B., and Ahlstrom, G. (2006). Theoretical model of coping among relatives of patients in intensive care units: A simultaneous concept analysis. *Journal of Advanced Nursing*, 56(5), 463–471.

*Johnson, D.E. (1959). The nature of a science of nursing. *Nursing Outlook*, 7(5), 291–294.

*Johnson, D.E. (1968). Theory in nursing: Borrowed and unique. *Nursing Research*, 17(3), 206–209.

Johnson, D.E. (1974). Development of theory: A requisite for nursing as a primary health profession. *Nursing Research*, 23(5), 372–377.

*Johnson, D.E. (1978). Development of theory: A requisite for nursing as a primary health profession. In N. Chaska (Ed.), *The nursing profession: Views through the mist*. New York: McGraw-Hill.

Johnson, D.E., et al. (1978). *Theory development: What, why, how?* (Publication No. 15–1708). New York: National League for Nursing.

Jonas-Simpson, C. (1997). Living the art of the human becoming theory. *Nursing Science Quarterly*, 10(4), 175–179.

Kahneman, D. (2011). *Thinking fast and slow*. New York: Farrar, Straus and Giroux.

Kahn-John, M. (2016). The path to development of the Hozho Resilience Model for nursing research and practice. *Applied Nursing Research*, 29, 144–147.

Kaplan, A. (1964). *The conduct of inquiry: Methodology for behavioral science*. San Francisco, CA: Chandler.

Kearney, M.H. (1998). Ready-to-wear: Discovering grounded formal theory. *Research in Nursing and Health*, 21(2), 170–186.

Kelley, L.S. (1999). Evaluating change in quality of life from the perspective of the person: Advanced practice nursing and Parse's goal of nursing. *Holistic Nursing Practice*, 13(4), 61–70.

Ketefian, S. (1987). A case study of theory development: Moral behavior in nursing. *Advances in Nursing Science*, 9(2), 10–19.

Ketefian, S. and Redman, R.W. (1997). Nursing science in the global community. *Image: Journal of Nursing Scholarship*, 29(1), 11–15.

Kidd, P. and Morrison, E.F. (1988). The progression of knowledge in nursing: A search for meaning. *Image: Journal of Nursing Scholarship*, 20(4), 222–224.

Kim, H.S. (1987). Structuring the nursing knowledge system: A typology of four domains. *Scholarly Inquiry for Nursing Practice*, 1(2), 111–114.

Kim, H.S. (1999). Critical reflective inquiry for knowledge development in nursing practice. *Journal of Advanced Nursing*, 29(5), 1205–1212.

Kim, H.S. (2001). Directions for theory development in nursing. In N.L. Chaska (Ed.), *The nursing profession—Tomorrow and beyond* (pp. 272–285). Thousand Oaks, CA: Sage.

Kim, M.S., Shin, K.R., and Shin, S.R. (1998). Korean adolescents' experiences of smoking cessation: A prelude to research with the human becoming perspective. *Nursing Science Quarterly*, 11(3), 105–109.

King, I.M. (1964). Nursing theory: Problems and prospect. *Nursing Science*, 10, 394–403.

King, I.M. (1971). *Toward a theory for nursing*. New York: John Wiley & Sons.

King, I.M. (1978). The "why" of theory development. In J. G. Paterson (Ed.), *Theory development: What, why, how?* (Publication No. 15–1708, pp. 11–16). New York: National League for Nursing.

Kirkevold, M. (1997). Integrative nursing research—An important strategy to further the development of nursing science and nursing practice. *Journal of Advanced Nursing*, 25(5), 977–984.

Klein, J.F. (1978). Theory development in nursing. In N.L. Chaska (Ed.), *The nursing profession: Views through the mist*. New York: McGraw-Hill.

Knight, M.M. (2000). Cognitive ability and functional status. *Journal of Advanced Nursing*, 31(6), 1459–1468.

Kramer, M.K. (1993). Concept clarification and critical thinking: Integrated processes. *Journal of Nursing Education*, 32(9), 406–414.

Krawczyk, R.M. (1997). Teaching ethics: Effect on moral development. *Nursing Ethics*, 4(1), 57–65.

Kristjanson, L.J., Tamblyn, R., and Kuypers, J.A. (1987). A model to guide development and application of multiple nursing theories. *Journal of Advanced Nursing*, 12, 523–529.

*Kritek, P.B. (1978). The generation and classification of nursing diagnoses: Toward a theory of nursing. *Image: Journal of Nursing Scholarship*, 10(3), 33–40.

Kulbok, P.A., Gates, M.F., Vicenzi, A.E., and Schultz, P.R. (1999). Focus on community: Directions for nursing knowledge development. *Journal of Advanced Nursing*, 29(5), 1188–1196.

Kulig, J.C. (2000). Community resiliency: The potential for community health nursing theory development. *Public Health Nursing*, 17(5), 374–385.

Kuss, T., Proulx-Girouard, L., Lovitt. S., and Katz, C.B. (1997). A public health nursing model. *Kennelly P. Public Health Nursing*, 14(2), 81–91.

Lancaster, W. and Lancaster, J. (1980). Models and model building in nursing. *Advances in Nursing Science*, 3(1), 1–7.

Lauder, W. (2001). The utility of self-care theory as a theoretical basis for self-neglect. *Journal of Advanced Nursing*, 34(4), 545–551. Comment in *Journal of Advanced Nursing* (2001), 34(4), 552–553.

Lee, P. (1998). An analysis and evaluation of Casey's conceptual framework. *International Journal of Nursing Studies*, 35(4), 204–209.

Leenerts, M.H. and Magilvy, J.K. (2000). Investing in self-care: A midrange theory of self-care grounded in the lived experience of low-income HIV-positive white women. *Advances in Nursing Science*, 22(3), 58–75.

Legault, F. and Ferguson-Pare, M. (1999). Advancing nursing practice: An evaluation study of Parse's theory of human becoming. *Canadian Journal of Nursing Leadership*, 12(1), 30–35.

*Leininger, M.M. (1969). Introduction: Nature of science in nursing. *Nursing Research*, 18(5), 388–389.

Lerdal, A. (1998). A concept analysis of energy: Its meaning in the lives of three individuals with chronic illness. *Scandinavian Journal of Caring Sciences*, 12(1), 3–10.

Levesque, L., Ricard, N., Ducharme, F., Duquette, A., and Bonin, J.P. (1998). Empirical verification of a theoretical model derived from the Roy adaptation model: Findings from five studies. *Nursing Science Quarterly*, 11(1), 31–39.

Levine, M.E. (1988). Antecedent from adjunctive discipline: Creative of nursing theory. *Nursing Science Quarterly*, 1(1), 16–21.

Liehr, P. and Smith, M.J. (1999). Middle range theory: Spinning research and practice to create knowledge for the new millennium. *Advances in Nursing Science*, 21(4), 81–91.

Luntley, M. (2010). What do nurses know? *Nursing Philosophy*, 12(1), 22–33.

MacGregor, J. and Dewar, K. (1997). Opening up the options: Making the inflexible into a flexible framework. *Nurse Education Today*, 17(5), 502–507.

Madden, B.P. (1990). The hybrid model for concept development: Its value for the study of therapeutic alliance. *Advances in Nursing Science*, 12(3), 75–87.

Mantzorou, M. and Mastrogiannis, D. (2011). The value and significance of knowing the patient for professional practice, according to the Carper's patterns of knowing. *Health Science Journal*, 5(4), 251–261

Marineau, M. (2005). Health/Illness transition and telehealth: A concept analysis using the evolutionary method. *Nursing Forum*, 40(3), 96–106.

Markovic, M. (1997). From theory to perioperative practice with Parse. *Canadian Operating Room Nursing Journal*, 15(1), 13–19.

Martin, P.J. (2000). Hearing voices and listening to those that hear them. *Journal of Psychiatric and Mental Health Nursing*, 7(2),135–141.

Matas, K.E. (1997). Human patterning and chronic pain. *Nursing Science Quarterly*, 10(2), 88–96.

Mathwig, G. (1971). Nursing science: The theoretical core of nursing knowledge. *Image: Journal of Nursing Scholarship*, 4(1), 20–23.

McCance, T.V., McKenna, H.P., and Boore, J.R. (1997). Caring: Dealing with a difficult concept. *International Journal of Nursing Studies*, 34(4), 241–248.

McCance, T.V., McKenna, H.P., and Boore, J.R. (1999). Caring: Theoretical perspectives of relevance to nursing. *Journal of Advanced Nursing*, 30(6), 1388–1395.

*McCarthy, R.T. (1972). A practice theory of nursing care. *Nursing Research*, 21(5), 406–410.

McHolm, F.A. and Geib, K.M. (1998). Application of the Neuman Systems Model to teaching health assessment and nursing process. *Nursing Diagnosis*, 9(1), 23–33.

*McKay, R. (1969). Theories, models, and systems for nursing. *Nursing Research*, 18(5), 393–400.

*McKay, R.C. (1977). What is the relationship between the development and utilization of a taxonomy and nursing theory? *Nursing Research*, 26(3), 222–224.

McKenna, H. (1999). The role of reflection in the development of practice theory: A case study. *Journal of Psychiatric and Mental Health Nursing*, 6(2), 147–151.

McKenna, B. and Roberts R. (1999). Bridging the theory-practice gap. *Nursing New Zealand*, 5(2), 14–16.

McMahon, S. and Fleury, J. (2012). Wellness in older adults: A concept analysis. *Nursing Forum*, 47(1), 39–51.

McMurry, P.H. (1982). Toward a unique knowledge base in nursing. *Image: Journal of Nursing Scholarship*, 14(1), 12–15.

McNeill, C. (2014). Risk: A multidisciplinary concept analysis. *Nursing Forum*, 49(1), 11–17.

Meleis, A.I. (1985). International nursing for knowledge development. *Nursing Outlook*, 33(3), 144–147.

Meleis, A.I. (1987). ReVisions in knowledge development: A passion for substance. *Scholarly Inquiry for Nursing Practice*, 1(1), 5–19.

Meleis, A.I. (1987). Theoretical nursing: Today's challenges, tomorrow's bridges. Nursing papers: Perspectives in nursing. *Canadian Journal of Nursing Research*, 19(1), 45–56.

Meleis, A.I. (1992). Theoretical thinking progress in the discipline of nursing. In K. Kraus and P. Astedt-Kurki (Eds.), *International Perspectives on Nursing* (pp. 1–12). Tampere, Finland: University of Tampere Department of Nursing.

Meleis, A.I. (1998). ReVisions in knowledge development: A passion for substance. *Scholarly Inquiry in Nursing Practice*, 12(1), 65–77.

Meleis, A.I., Sawyer, L.M., Im, E.O., Hilfinger -Messias, D.K., and Schumacher, K. (2000). Experiencing transitions: An emerging middle-range theory. *Advances in Nursing Science*, 23(1), 12–28.

*Menke, E.M. (1978). Theory development: A challenge for nursing. In N.L. Chaska (Ed.), *The nursing profession: Views through the mist*. New York: McGraw-Hill.

Meredith, P., Ownsworth, T., and Strong J. (2008). A review of the evidence linking adult attachment theory and chronic pain: Presenting a conceptual model. *Clinical Psychology Review*, 28(3), 407–429.

Miller, M.E. and Dzurec, L.C. (1993). The power of the name. *Advances in Nursing Science*, 15(3), 15–22.

Miller, S.K. (1999). Nurse practitioners in the county correctional facility setting: Unique challenges and suggestions for effective health promotion. *Clinical Excellence in Nurse Practice*, 3(5), 268–272.

Moccia, P. (1986). *New approaches to theory development*. New York: National League for Nursing.

Mohr, W.K. (1999). Beyond cause and effect: Some thoughts on research and practice in child psychiatric nursing. *Journal of Child and Adolescent Psychiatric Nursing*, 12(3), 118–127.

Mohr, W.K. and Naylor, M.D. (1998). Creating a curriculum for the 21st century. *Nursing Outlook*, 46(5), 206–212.

Monti, E.J. and Tingen, M.S. (1999). Multiple paradigms of nursing science. *Advances in Nursing Science*, 21(4), 64–80.

*Moore, M. (1968). Nursing: A scientific discipline. *Forum*, 7(4), 340–348.

Morse, J.M. (1995). Exploring the theoretical basis of nursing using advanced techniques of concept analysis. *Advances in Nursing Science*, 17, 31–46.

Murphy, J.D. (1978). Toward a philosophy of nursing. In N.L. Chaska (Ed.), *The nursing profession: Views through the mist*. New York: McGraw-Hill.

Murphy, J.F. (Ed.). (1971). *Theoretical issues in professional nursing*. New York: Appleton-Century-Crofts. (Note especially Chapters 1, 2, and 3.)

*Murphy, S.A. and Hoeffer, B. (1983). Role of the specialties in nursing science. *Advances in Nursing Science*, 5(4), 31–39.

Neal, L.J. (1999). Facilitating the growth of nursing staff case management in PPS. *Caring*, 18(10), 46–48.

Neill, S.J. (1998). Developing children's nursing through action research. *Journal of Child Health Care*, 2(1), 11–15.

Nelson, S. (1997). Reading nursing history. *Nursing Inquiry*, 4(4), 229–236.

Newman, M. (1977). *Theory development in nursing*. Philadelphia, PA: F.A. Davis.

*Newman, M.A. (1972). Nursing's theoretical evolution. *Nursing Outlook*, 20(7), 449–453.

Nicoll, L. (1992). *Perspectives on nursing theory* (2nd ed.). Philadelphia, PA: J.B. Lippincott.

Noble-Adams, R. (1999). Ethics and nursing research. 1: Development, theories and principles. *British Journal of Nursing*, 8(13), 888–892.

Nolan, M., Lundh, U., and Tishelman, C. (1998). Nursing's knowledge base: Does it have to be unique? *British Journal of Nursing*, 7(5), 270–276.

Norris, C.M. (Ed.). (1969, 1970). *Proceedings, first, second, and third nursing theory conference*. Kansas City. MO: University of Kansas Medical Center, Department of Nursing Education.

Norris, C.M. (1982). *Concept classification in nursing*. Rockville, MD: Aspen Systems.

Northrup, D.T. and Cody, W.K. (1998). Evaluation of the human becoming theory in practice in an acute care psychiatric setting. *Nursing Science Quarterly*, 11(1), 23–30.

*Notter, L.E. (1975). The case for nursing research. *Nursing Outlook*, 23(12), 760–763.

Nursing Development Conference Group. (1979). *Concept formalization in nursing: Process and product*. Boston, MA: Little, Brown.

Nyamathi, A., Koniak-Griffin, D., and Greengold, B.A. (2007). Development of nursing theory and science in vulnerable populations research. *Annual Review of Nursing Research*, 25, 3–25.

O'Brien, B. and Pearson, A. (1993). Unwritten knowledge in nursing: Consider the spoken as well as the written word. *Scholarly Inquiry for Nursing Practice*, 7, 111–127.

O'Connell, B., Rapley, P., and Tibbett, P. (1999). Does the nursing diagnosis form the basis for patient care? *Collegian*, 6(3), 29–34.

Ohashi, J.P. (1985). The contributions of Dickoff and James to theory development in nursing. *Image: Journal of Nursing Scholarship*, 17(1), 17–20.

Olson, J. and Hanchett, E. (1997). Nurse-expressed empathy, patient outcomes, and development of a middle-range theory. *Image: Journal of Nursing Scholarship*, 29(1), 71–76.

Panel Discussion. (1968). Theory development in nursing. *Nursing Research*, 17(3), 223–227.

Parse, R.R. (1997). Transforming research and practice with the human becoming theory. *Nursing Science Quarterly*, 10(4), 171–174.

Parse, R.R. (1999). Nursing science: The transformation of practice. *Journal of Advanced Nursing*, 30(6), 1383–1387.

Paul, R.W. and Heaslip, P. (1995). Critical thinking and intuitive nursing practice. *Journal of Advanced Nursing*, 22, 40–47.

*Payne, L. (1983). Health: A basic concept in nursing theory. *Journal of Advanced Nursing*, 8(5), 393–395.

Peden, A.R. (1998). The evolution of an intervention—The use of Peplau's process of practice-based theory development. *Journal of Psychiatric and Mental Health Nursing*, 5(3), 173–178.

Perry, J. (1985). Has the discipline of nursing developed to the stage where nurses do "think nursing?" *Journal of Advanced Nursing*, 10(1), 31–37.

*Peterson, C.J. (1977). Questions frequently asked about the development of a conceptual framework. *Journal of Nursing Education*, 16(4), 22–23.

*Phillips, J.R. (1977). Nursing systems and nursing models. *Image: Journal of Nursing Scholarship*, 9(1), 4–7.

Piccinato, J.M. and Rosenbaum, J.N. (1997). Caregiver hardiness explored within Watson's theory of human caring in nursing. *Journal of Gerontological Nursing*, 23(10), 32–39.

Polk, L.V. (1997). Toward a middle-range theory of resilience. *Advances in Nursing Science*, 19(3), 1–13.

Priest, H. and Roberts, P. (1998). Assessing students' clinical performance. *Nursing Standard*, 12(48), 37–41.

*Putnam, P. (1965). A conceptual approach to nursing theory. *Nursing Science*, 3, 430–442.

*Quint, J.C. (1967). The case for theories generated from empirical data. *Nursing Research*, 16(2), 109–114.

Ramos, M. (1987). Adopting an evolutionary lens: An optimistic approach in discovering strength in nursing. *Advances in Nursing Science*, 10(1), 19–26.

Rankin, S.H. (2000). Life-span development: Refreshing a theoretical and practice perspective. *Scholarly Inquiry in Nursing Practice*, 14(4), 379–388.

Rankin, S.H. and Weekes, D.P. (2000). Life-span development: A review of theory and practice for families with chronically ill members. *Scholarly Inquiry in Nursing Practice*, 14(4), 355–373.

Rask, M. and Hallberg, I.R. (2000). Forensic psychiatric nursing care—Nurses apprehension of their responsibility and work content: A Swedish survey. *Journal of Psychiatric and Mental Health Nursing*, 7(2), 163–177.

Ravelin, T., Kylma, J., and Korhonen, T. (2006). Dance in mental health nursing: A hybrid concept analysis. *Issues in Mental Health Nursing*, 27(3), 307–317.

Ream, E. and Richardson. A. (1999). From theory to practice: Designing interventions to reduce fatigue in patients with cancer. *Oncology Nursing Forum*, 26(8), 1295–1303. Comment in *Oncology Nursing Forum* (2000), 27(3), 425–426.

Reed, P.G. (1989). Nursing theorizing as an ethical endeavor. *Advances in Nursing Science*, 11(3), 1–9.

Reed, P.G. (1998). A holistic view of nursing concepts and theories in practice. *Journal of Holistic Nursing*, 16(4), 415–419.

Reed, P.G. (2006). The dialogue within nursing theory-guided practice: A frontier of knowledge and development. *Nursing Science Quarterly*, 19(4), 328–329.

Relf, M.V. (1997). Illuminating meaning and transforming issues of spirituality in HIV disease and AIDS: An application of Parse's theory of human becoming. *Holistic Nursing Practice*, 12(1), 1–8.

Revell, S.M.H. (2012). Concept maps and nursing theory: A pedagogical approach. *Nurse Educator*, 37(3), 131–135.

Rew, L. and Barrow, E. (2007). State of the science: Intuition in nursing, a generation of studying the phenomenon. *Advances in Nursing Science*, 30(1), 15–25.

Richardson, L. (1994). Writing: A method of inquiry. In N.K. Denzin and Y.S. Lincoln (Eds.), *Handbook of qualitative research*. Thousand Oaks, CA: Sage.

Rinehart, J.M. (1978). The "how" of theory development in nursing. In J.G. Paterson (Ed.), *Theory development: What, why, how?* (Publication No. 15–1708, pp. 67–74). New York: National League for Nursing.

Roberts, D. (1997). Liaison mental health nursing: Origins, definition and prospects. *Journal of Advanced Nursing*, 25(1), 101–108.

Rodgers, B.L. (1989). Concepts, analysis, and the development of nursing knowledge: The evolutionary cycle. *Journal of Advanced Nursing*, 14, 330–335.

Rodgers, B.L. (1991). Using concept analysis to enhance clinical practice and research. *Applied Research*, 10, 28–34.

Rodgers, B.L. and Knafl, K.A. (1993). *Concept development in nursing: Foundations, techniques, and applications*. Philadelphia, PA: W.B. Saunders.

*Rogers, M.E. (1963). Some comments on the theoretical basis of nursing practice. *Nursing Science*, 1, 11–13, 60.

Rothrock, J.C. and Smith, D.A. (2000). Selecting the perioperative patient focused model. *Journal of the Association of PeriOperative Registered Nurses*, 71(5), 1030–1034.

*Rubin, R. (1968). A theory of clinical nursing. *Nursing Research*, 17(3), 210–212.

Running, A. (1997). Snapshots of experience: Vignettes from a nursing home. *Journal of Advanced Nursing*, 25(1), 117–122.

Ryles, S.M. (1999). A concept analysis of empowerment: Its relationship to mental health nursing. *Journal of Advanced Nursing*, 29(3), 600–607.

Sachse, D. (2007). Hope: More than a refuge in a storm. A concept analysis using the Wilson method and the Norris method. *International Journal of Psychiatric Nursing Research*, 13(1), 1546–1553.

Sanford, R.C. (2000). Caring through relation and dialogue: A nursing perspective for patient education. *Advances in Nursing Science*, 22(3), 1–15.

Sasmor, J.L. (1968). Toward developing theory in nursing. *Nursing Forum*, 7(2), 191–200.

Scanlan, J.M. and Chernomas, W.M. (1997). Developing the reflective teacher. *Journal of Advanced Nursing*, 25(6), 1138–1143.

Schafer, P.J. (1987). Philosophic analysis of a theory of clinical nursing. *Maternal-Child Nursing Journal*, 16(4), 289–368.

Schlotfeldt, R.M. (1988). Structuring nursing knowledge: A priority for creating nursing's future. *Nursing Science Quarterly*, 1(1), 35–38.

Schlotzhauer, M. and Farnham, R. (1997). Newman's theory and insulin dependent diabetes mellitus in adolescence. *Journal of Scholarly Nursing*, 13(3), 20–23.

Schultz, P. (1987). Toward holistic inquiry in nursing: A proposal for synthesis of patterns and methods. *Scholarly Inquiry for Nursing Practice*, 1(2), 135–146.

Schultz, P.R. (1987). When client means more than one: Extending the foundational concept of person. *Advances in Nursing Science*, 10(1), 71–80.

Schultz, P. and Meleis, A.I. (1988). Nursing epistemology: Traditions, insights, questions. *Image: Journal of Nursing Scholarship*, 20(4), 217–221.

Schwartz-Barcott, D. and Kim, H.S. (1993). An expansion and elaboration of the hybrid model of concept development. In B.L. Rodgers and K.A. Knafl (Eds.), *Concept development in nursing* (pp. 107–133). Philadelphia, PA: W.B. Saunders.

Severinsson, E.I. (1999). Ethics in clinical nursing supervision—An introduction to the theory and practice of different supervision models. *Collegian*, 6(3), 23–28.

Severinsson, E.I. (1998). Bridging the gap between theory and practice: A supervision programme for nursing students. *Journal of Advanced Nursing*, 27(6), 1269–1277.

Shih, F.J. (1998). Triangulation in nursing research: Issues of conceptual clarity and purpose. *Journal of Advanced Nursing*, 28(3), 631–641. Comment in *Journal of Advanced Nursing* (1999), 30(3), 775.

*Silva, M.C. and Rothbart, D. (1984). An analysis of changing trends in philosophies of science on nursing theory development and testing. *Advances in Nursing Science*, 6(2), 1–13.

Simko, L.C. (1999). Adults with congenital heart disease: Utilizing quality of life and Husted's nursing theory as a conceptual framework. *Critical Care Nursing Quarterly*, 22(3), 1–11.

Simon, H. (1971). Logical, empirical approach to developing a body of knowledge. In J. Murphy (Ed.), *Theoretical issues in professional nursing*. New York: Appleton-Century-Crofts.

Skaggs, B.G. and Barron, C.R. (2006). Searching for meaning in negative events: Concept analysis. *Journal of Advanced Nursing*, 53(5), 559–570.

Smith, L.S. (1998). Concept analysis: Cultural competence. *Journal of Cultural Diversity*, 5(1), 4–10.

Smith, M.J. and Liehr, P. (1999). Attentively embracing story: A middle-range theory with practice and research implications. *Scholarly Inquiry in Nursing Practice*, 13(3), 187–204.

Smoyak, S.A. (1969). Toward understanding nursing situation: A transaction paradigm. *Nursing Research*, 18(5), 405–411.

Sorenson, G. (Ed.). (1986). *Setting the agenda for the year (2000): Knowledge development in nursing*. Kansas City, MO: American Academy of Nursing.

Sorrell, J.M. (1994). Remembrance of things past through writing: Esthetic patterns of knowing in nursing. *Advances in Nursing Science*, 17(1), 60–70.

Spear, S.W. (2007). Nursing theory and knowledge development: A descriptive review of doctoral dissertations, 2000–2004. *Advances in Nursing Science*, 30(10), E1–E14.

Spouse, J. (2001). Bridging theory and practice in the supervisory relationship: A sociocultural perspective. *Journal of Advanced Nursing*, 33(4), 512–522.

*Stainton, M.C. (1982). The birth of nursing science. *Canadian Nurse*, 78(10), 24–28.

Stark, S., Cooke, P., and Stronach, I. (2000). Minding the gap: Some theory-practice disjunctions in nursing education research. *Nurse Education Today*, 20(2), 155–163.

Stein, K.F., Corte, C., Colling, K.B., and Whall, A. (1998). A theoretical analysis of Carper's ways of knowing using a model of social cognition. *Scholarly Inquiry in Nursing Practice*, 12(1), 43–60.

Stember, M.L. (1986). Model building as a strategy for theory development. In P.L. Chinn (Ed.), *Nursing research methodology* (pp. 103–117). Rockville, MD: Aspen Systems.

Stevenson, J.S. and Woods, N.F. (1986). Nursing science and contemporary science: Emerging paradigms. In G. Sorenson (Ed.), *Setting the agenda for the year (2000): Knowledge development in nursing*. Kansas City, MO: American Academy of Nursing.

Stoltz, P., Andersson, E.P., and Willman, A. (2007). Support in nursing–an evolutionary concept analysis. *International Journal of Nursing Studies*, 44(8), 1478–1489.

Suppe, F. and Jacox, A. (1985). Philosophy of science and the development of nursing theory. *Annual Review Nursing Research*, 3, 241–267.

Sykes, S., Wills, J., Rowlands, G., and Popple, K. (2013). Understanding critical health literacy: A concept analysis. *BMC Public Health*, 13(1), 150.

Thorne, S.E., Kirkham, S.R., and Henderson. A. (1999). Ideological implications of paradigm discourse. *Nursing Inquiry*, 6(2), 123–131.

*Tinkle, M.B. and Beaton, J.L. (1983). Toward a new view of science: Implications for nursing research. *Advances in Nursing Science*, 5(2), 27–36.

Tracy, J.P. (1997). Growing up with chronic illness: The experience of growing up with cystic fibrosis. *Holistic Nursing Practice*, 12(1), 27–35.

Tritsch, J.M. (1998). Application of King's theory of goal attainment and the Carondelet St. Mary's case management model. *Nursing Science Quarterly*, 11(2), 69–73.

*Tucker, R.W. (1979). The value decisions we know as science. *Advances in Nursing Science*, 1(2), 1–12.

Turner, S.L. and Bentley, G.W. (1998). A meaningful health assessment course for baccalaureate nursing students. *Nursing Connections*, 11(2), 5–12.

Verran, J.A. (1997). The value of theory-driven (rather than problem-driven) research. *Seminars for Nurse Managers*, 5(4), 169–172.

Villarruel, A.M. and Denyes, M.J. (1997). Testing Orem's theory with Mexican Americans. *Image: Journal of Nursing Scholarship*, 29(3), 283–288.

Visintainer, M.A. (1986). The nature of knowledge and theory in nursing. *Image: Journal of Nursing Scholarship*, 18(2), 32–38.

Wainwright, P. (2000). Towards an aesthetics of nursing. *Journal of Advanced Nursing*, 32(3), 750–756.

*Wald, F.S. and Leonard, R.C. (1964). Toward development of nursing practice theory. *Nursing Research*, 13(4), 309–313.

Walker, L.O. (1971). Toward a clearer understanding of the concept of nursing theory. *Nursing Research*, 20(5), 428–435.

Walker, L.O. (1972). Rejoinder to commentary: Toward a clearer understanding of the concept of nursing theory. *Nursing Research*, 21(1), 59–62.

Walker, L.O. and Avant, K.C. (2010). *Strategies for theory construction in nursing* (5th ed.). Upper Saddle River, NJ: Pearson/Prentice Hall.

*Weatherston, L. (1979). Theory of nursing: Creating effective care. *Journal of Advanced Nursing*, 4(7), 365–375.

Weaver, K., Morse, J., and Mitcham, C. (2008). Ethical sensitivity in professional practice: Concept analysis. *Journal of Advanced Nursing*, 62(5), 607–618.

Wellard, S. (1997). Constructions of family nursing: A critical exploration. *Contemporary Nurse*, 6(2), 78–84.

Wenzel, L.S., Briggs, K.L., and Puryear, B.L. (1998). Portfolio: Authentic assessment in the age of the curriculum revolution. *Journal of Nursing Education*, 37(5), 208–212.

West, P. and Isenberg, M. (1997). Instrument development: The Mental Health-Related Self-Care Agency Scale. *Archives of Psychiatric Nursing*, 11(3), 126–132.

Westbrook, L.O. and Schultz, P.R. (2000). From theory to practice: Community health nursing in a public health neighborhood team. *Advances in Nursing Science*, 23(2), 50–61.

White, L. (2014). Mindfulness in nursing: An evolutionary concept analysis. *Journal of Advanced Nursing*, 70(2), 282–294.

Whitener, L.M., Cox, K.R., and Maglich, S.A. (1998). Use of theory to guide nurses in the design of health messages for children. *Advances in Nursing Science*, 20(3), 21–35.

Whittemore, R. and Roy, C. (2002). Adapting to diabetes mellitus: A theory synthesis. *Nursing Science Quarterly*, 15(4), 311–317.

Wikberg, I. (2007). Imagining nursing practice 2050: The caritative caring theory. *Nursing Science Quarterly*, 20(4), 333–335.

Wilde, M.H. (1999). Why embodiment now? *Advances in Nursing Science*, 22(2), 25–38. Comment in *Advances in Nursing Science* (2000), 23(1), vi–vii.

Williams, A.M. (1998). The delivery of quality nursing care: A grounded theory study of the nurse's perspective. *Journal of Advanced Nursing*, 27(4), 808–816.

Willis, D.G., Grace, P.J., and Roy C. (2008). A central unifying focus for the discipline: Facilitating humanization, meaning, choice, quality of life, and healing in living and dying. *Advances in Nursing Science*, 31(1), E28–E40.

Wilshaw, G. (1999). Perspectives on surviving childhood sexual abuse. *Journal of Advanced Nursing*, 30(2), 303–309.

Wilson, J. (1963). *Thinking with concepts*. Cambridge, England: Cambridge University Press.

Wuest, J. (1994). A feminist approach to concept analysis. *Western Journal of Nursing Research*, 16(5), 577–586.

Wynne, N., Brand, S., and Smith, R. (1997). Incomplete holism in pre-registration nurse education: The position of the biological sciences. *Journal of Advanced Nursing*, 26(3), 470–474.

Yamashita, M. and Tall, F.D. (1998). A commentary on Newman's theory of health as expanding consciousness. *Advances in Nursing Science*, 21(1), 65–75. Comment in *Advances in Nursing Science*, (1999), 21(3), vii–viii; *Advances in Nursing Science*, (1999), 21(3), viii–ix; *Advances in Nursing Science*, (1999), 22(1), vi–vii.

Yegdich, T. (1998). How not to do clinical supervision in nursing. *Journal of Advanced Nursing*, 28(1), 193–202.

Younger, J.B. (1990). Literary works as a mode of knowing. *Image: Journal of Nursing Scholarship*, 22, 39–43.

4. Forces and Constraints in Theory Development: Women as Scientists

Abramson, J. (1975). *The invisible woman: Discrimination in the academic profession*. San Francisco, CA: Jossey-Bass.

Allen, D. (2014). Re-conceptualising holism in the contemporary nursing mandate: From individual to organisational relationships. *Social Science & Medicine*, 119; 131–138.

Andreoli, K. (1977). The status of nursing in academia. *Image: Journal of Nursing Scholarship*, 9(3), 52–58.

Arditti, R, Brennan, P., and Cavrak, S. (1980). *Science and liberation*. Boston, MA: South End Press.

Armeger, B. (1974). Scholarship in nursing. *Nursing Outlook*, 22(3), 162–163.

Astin, H.S. (1967). Factors associated with the participation of women doctorates in the labor force. *Personnel and Guidance Journal*, 46(3), 240–246.

Bachtold, L.M. and Werner, E.E. (1972). Personality characteristics of women scientists. *Psychological Reports*, 31, 391–396.

Benoliel, J. (1975). Scholarship—A women's perspective. *Image: Journal of Nursing Scholarship*, 7(2), 22–27.

Bissel, M. (1978). Equality for women scientists. *Grants Magazine*, 4, 331–334.

Blankenship, V. (1973). The scientist as a "political man." *British Journal of Sociology*, 24(3), 269–287.

Briscoe, A.M. and Pfafflin, S.M. (Eds.). (1979). Expanding the role of women in the sciences. *Annals of New York Academy of Science*, 323.

*Brown, C. (1975). Women workers in the health service industry. *International Journal of Health Services*, 5(2), 173–184.

Bullough, B. (1975). Barriers to the nurse practitioner movement: Problems of women in a woman's field. *International Journal of Health Services*, 5(2), 225–233.

Bullough, B. (1978). The struggle for women's rights in Denver: A personal account. *Nursing Outlook*, 26(9), 566–567.

Chafetz, J.S. (1978). *Masculine/feminine or human? An overview of the sociology of sex roles*. Itasca, IL: F.E. Peacock Publisher.

Cleland, V. (1974). To end sex discrimination. *Nursing Clinics of North America*, 9(3), 563–571.

Cole, J.R. (1979). *Fair science: Women in the scientific community*. New York: Free Press.

Cole, J.R. (1981). Women in science. *American Scientist*, 69(4), 385–391.

Conant, L.H. (1968). On becoming a nurse researcher. *Nursing Research*, 17(1), 68–71.

Croft, R.K. and Cash, P.A. (2012). Deconstructing contributing factors to bullying and lateral violence in nursing using a postcolonial feminist lens. *Contemporary Nurse*, 42(2), 226–242.

Curran, L. (1980). Science education: Did she drop out or was she pushed? In L. Birke et al. (Eds.), *Alice through the microscope*. London, UK: Virgo.

Epstein, C.F. (1973). Positive effects of the multiple negative: Explaining the success of black professional women. *American Journal of Sociology*, 78(4), 912–935.

Fausto-Sterling, A. (1981). Women in science. *Women Science International Forum*, 4, 41–50.

Feulner, P.A. (1979). *Women in the professions: A social psychological study*. Palo Alto, CA: R & E Research Association.

Fitzpatrick, M.L. (1977). Nursing: Review essay. *Signs: Journal of Women in Culture and Society*, 2(4), 818–833.

Grier, M.R. and Schnitzler, C.P. (1979). Nurses' propensity to risk. *Nursing Research*, 28(3), 186–191.

Grissum, M. and Spengler, C. (1976). *Woman power and health care*. Boston, MA: Little, Brown.

Hodges, A.J. and Park, B. (2013). Oppositional identities: Dissimilarities in how women and men experience parent versus professional roles. *Journal of Personality and Social Psychology*, 105(2), 193–216.

Humphreys, S.M. (1982). *Women and minorities in science: Strategies for increasing participation*. Boulder, CO: Westview Press.

Ibarra, H., Ely, R., and Kolb, D. (2013). Women rising: The unseen barriers. *Harvard Business Review*, 91(9), 60–66.

Jaquette, J.S. (1976). Political science: Review essay. *Signs: Journal of Women in Culture and Society*, 2(1), 147–176.

Keller, M.C. (1979). The effect of sexual stereotyping on the development of nursing theory. *American Journal of Nursing*, 79(9), 1584–1586.

Loomis, M.E. (1974). Collegiate nursing education: An ambivalent profession. *Journal of Nursing Education*, 39–48.

MacDonald, M.R. (1977). How do men and women students rate in empathy? *American Journal of Nursing*, 77(6), 998.

Martin, B.R. and Irvine, J. (1982). Women in science: The astronomical brain drain. *Women's Studies International Forum*, 5, 41–68.

May, K.M., Meleis, A.I., and Winstead-Fry, P. (1982). Mentorship for scholarliness: Opportunities and dilemmas. *Nursing Outlook*, 30, 22–28.

McCain, G. and Segal, E.M. (1977). *The game of science*. Monterey, CA: Brooks/Cole. (Note especially pp. 74–78.)

Meleis, A.I. and Dagenais, F. (1981). Sex role identity and perception of professional self in graduates of three programs. *Nursing Research*, 30(3), 162–167.

Meleis, A.I. and May, K. (1981). Nursing theory and scholarliness in the doctoral program. *Advances in Nursing Science*, 4(2), 31–41.

Meleis, A.I. and May, K. (1982). *Mentorship for scholarliness*. In Proceedings for Doctoral Forum (held in Seattle, Washington, 1981). Seattle, WA: University of Washington.

Meleis, A.I., Wilson, H.S., and Chater, S. (1980). Toward the socialization of a scholar: A model. *Research in Nursing and Health*, 3, 115–124.

Merchant, C. (1980). *The death of nature: Women, ecology and the scientific revolution*. San Francisco, CA: Harper & Row.

Moore, D., Decker, S., and Down, M.W. (1978). Baccalaureate nursing students' identification with the women's movement. *Nursing Research*, 27(5), 291–295.

Muench, U., Sindelar, J., Busch, S, and Buerhaus, P. (2015). Salary differences between male and female registered nurses in the United States. *Journal of the American Medical Association*, 313(12), 1265–1267.

Neusner, J. (1977, May 31). *The scholars' apprentice*. The Chronicle of Higher Education Point of View, p. 40.

Nowak, M.J. and Bonner, D. (2013). Juggling work and family demands: Lifestyle career anchors for female healthcare professionals. *International Journal of Healthcare Management*, 6(1), 3–11.

Roe, A. (1951). A psychological study of eminent biologists. *Psychological Monographs*, 65, 1–67.

Roe, A. (1963). *The making of a scientist*. New York: Dodd Mead.

Roe, A. (1966). Women in science. *Personnel and Guidance Journal*, 54, 784–787.

Rossi, A. (1972). Women in science: Why so few? In C. Safilios-Rothchild (Ed.), *Toward a sociology of women* (pp. 141–153). New York: Xerox Corp.

Rossiter, M.W. (1982). *Women scientists in America: Struggles and strategies in 1940*. Baltimore, MD: Johns Hopkins Press.

Seiden, A. (1976). Overview: Research on the psychology of women. I and II. Gender differences and sexual and reproductive life. *American Journal of Psychiatry*, 133(10), 1111–1118.

Shambaugh, R. (2016). The time-consuming activities that stall women's careers. *Harvard Business Review*. Retrieved from https://hbr.org/2016/03/the-time-consuming-activities-that-stall-womens-careers.

Speizer, J.J. (1981). Role models, mentors and sponsors: The elusive concepts. *Signs: Journal of Women in Culture and Society*, 6, 692–712.

Stroller, E.P. (1978). Perceptions of the nursing role: A case study of an entering class. *Journal of Nursing Education*, 17(6), 2–14.

Stromborg, M.F. (1976). Relationship of sex-role identity to occupational image of female nursing students. *Nursing Research*, 25(5), 363–369.

Vaughter, R. (1976, Autumn). Psychology: Review essay. *Signs: Journal of Women in Culture and Society*, 2(1), 120–146.

Wallsgrove, R. (1980). The masculine face of science. In L. Birke et al. (Eds.), *Alice through the microscope*. London, UK: Virgo.

Watson, J.D. (1968). *The double helix*. New York: New American Library.

White, M.S. (1972). Psychological and social barriers to women in science. In C. Safilios-Rothchild (Ed.), *Toward a sociology of women*. New York: Xerox Corp.

5. Forces and Constraints in Theory Development: Nursing Profession

American Nurses Association. (2010). *Nursing's social policy statement*. Washington, DC: Author.

Ashley, J.A. (1980). Power in structured misogyny: Implications for the politics of care. *Advances in Nursing Science*, 2(3), 3–22.

Ashley, J. (1976). *Hospital paternalism and the role of the nurse*. New York: Teachers' College Press.

Aydelotte, M.K. (1968). Issues of professional nursing: The need for clinical excellence. *Nursing Forum*, 7(1), 72–86.

Babich, K.S. (1968). The perception of professionalism: Equality. *Nursing Forum*, 7(1), 14–20.

Barber, B. (1963, Fall). Some problems in the sociology of professions. *Daedalus*, 92(4), 669–688.

Bixler, G. and Bixler, R.W. (1959). The professional status of nursing. *American Journal of Nursing*, 59(8), 1142–1147.

Brown, E.L. (1948). *Nursing for the future*. New York: Russel Sage Foundation. (Especially note pp. 669–688.)

*Brown, M.I. (1964). Research in the development of nursing theory. *Nursing Research*, 13(2), 109–112.

Caplow, T. (1954). *The sociology of work*. Minneapolis, MN: University of Minnesota Press. (Especially note p. 139.)

Cipriano, P.F. (2015). Nurses at the table: in the United States and around the world. *American Nurse*, 47(5), 3.

Cogan, M.L. (1955, January). The problem of defining a profession. *Annals of the American Academy of Political and Social Sciences*, 297, 105–111.

Colodarci, A. (1963). What about the word "profession?" *American Journal of Nursing*, 63(10), 116–118.

Conant, L.H. (1968). On becoming a nurse researcher. *Nursing Research*, 17(1), 68–72.

Conrad, P.I. and Pape, T.T. (2014). Roles and responsibilities of the nursing scholar. *Pediatric Nursing*. 40(2):87–90.

Cox, C. (1979). Who cares? Nursing and sociology: The development of symbiotic relationship. *Journal of Advanced Nursing*, 4, 237–252.

Devereux, G. and Weiner, F. (1950, October). The occupational status of nurses. *American Sociological Review*, 15, 628–634.

Dilworth, A. (1963, May). Goals in nursing. *Nursing Outlook*, 11, 336–340.

Ellison, M., Diers, D., and Leonard, R. (1965). The use of the behavioral sciences in nursing: Further comment. *Nursing Research*, 14, 71–72.

Feldman, H.R. (1980). Nursing research in the 1980s: Issues and implications. *Advances in Nursing Science*, 3(1), 85–92.

Feldman, H.R. (1981). A science of nursing—To be or not to be? *Image: Journal of Nursing Scholarship*, 13, 63–66.

Fox, D. (1964, Winter). A proposed model for identifying research areas in nursing. *Nursing Research*, 13, 29–36.

Goode, W.J. (1959). Community within a community: The professions. *American Sociological Review*, 194–200. (Bobbs-Merrill Reprint S-99.)

Goode, W.J. (1960, December). Encroachment, charlatanism, and the emerging profession: Psychology, sociology, and medicine. *American Sociological Review*, 25, 902–914.

Gouldner, A. (1961). Theoretical requirements of the applied social sciences. In W.G. Bennis, K.D. Benne, and R. Chin (Eds.), *The planning of change*. New York: Holt, Rinehart & Winston.

Hughes, E.C. (1958). *Men and their work*. Glencoe, IL: Free Press. (Especially note p. 133.)

Hughes, E.C. (1963, Fall). Professions. *Daedalus*, 655–668.

Hurley, B.A. (1979). Why a theoretical framework in nursing research. *Western Journal of Nursing Research*, 1(1), 28–41.

International Council of Nursing. (2015). *Definition of professional nursing*. Available online at http://www.icn.ch/who-we-are/icn-definition-of-nursing

Johnson, M. and Martin, H. (1958). A sociological analysis of the nurse role. *American Journal of Nursing*, 58(3), 373–377.

Lipton, N. (1968). Nursing education as a challenge to the professionalization of nursing. *Nursing Forum*, 7(2), 201–214.

Martin, H.W. (1958, October). The behavioral sciences and nursing education. *Social Forces*, 37, 61–67.

Masipa, A.L. (1996). Nursing theory development. *Curationis: South African Journal of Nursing*, 19(1), 61–64.

McGlothlin, W.J. (1960). *Patterns of professional education*. New York: G.P. Putnam's Sons. (Especially note pp. 1–25.)

McGlothlin, W.J. (1961, April). The place of nursing among the professions. *Nursing Outlook*, 9, 216.

Mead, M. (1956). Nursing—Primitive and civilized. *American Journal of Nursing*, 56(8), 948–950.

Meleis, A.I. and May, K. (1981). Nursing theory and scholarliness in the doctoral program. *Advances in Nursing Science*, 4(1), 31–41.

Nolan, M., Lundh, U., and Tishelman, C. (1998). Nursing's knowledge base: Does it have to be unique? *British Journal of Nursing*, 7(5), 270–276.

Montag, M. (1959). *Community college education for nursing*. New York: McGraw-Hill.

Parsons, T. (1939). *The professions and social structure*. Social Forces (S-219). The College Book Co. (Especially note pp. 457–467.)

Parsons, T. (1965). *Essays in sociological theory*. New York: Free Press.

Pierson, W. (1999). Considering the nature of intersubjectivity within professional nursing. *Journal of Advanced Nursing*, 30(2), 294–302.

Reissman, L. and Rorher, J.H. (Eds.). (1957). *Change and dilemma in the nursing profession.* New York: G.P. Putnam's Sons.

Rogers, M. (1975). Euphemisms in nursing's future. *Image: Journal of Nursing Scholarship,* 7(2), 3–9.

Royal College of Nurses (2014). *Defining nursing.* Retrieved from https://www.rcn.org.uk/professional-development/publications/pub-004768

Rutty, J.E. (1998). The nature of philosophy of science, theory and knowledge relating to nursing and professionalism. *Journal of Advanced Nursing,* 28(2), 243–250.

Sills, G.M. (1998). Peplau and professionalism: The emergence of the paradigm of professionalization. *Journal of Psychiatric and Mental Health Nursing,* 5(3), 167–171.

Tyler, R. (1952, April). Distinctive attributes of education for the professions. *Social Work Journal,* 33, 55–62.

Van Maanen, J.M.T., Mussallen, H.K., McGilloway, F.A., Cormack, D., Clarke, M., Bergman, R., and King, P. (1979). Janforum: The nursing profession: Ritualized, routinized or research-based? *Journal of Advanced Nursing,* 1, 87–89.

Willetts, G. and Clarke, D. (2014). Constructing nurses' professional identity through social identity theory. *International Journal of Nursing Practice,* 20, 164–169.

Wolensky, R.P. (1981). The graduate student's double bind: A professional socialization problem in sociology. *Sociological Spectrum,* 1, 393–414.

6. Theory and Science

*Abdellah, F.G. (1969). The nature of nursing science. *Nursing Research,* 18(5), 390–393.

*Andreoli, K.G. and Thompson, C.E. (1977). The nature of science in nursing. *Image: Journal of Nursing Scholarship,* 9(2), 32–37.

Barber, B. and Hirsch, W. (Eds.). (1962). *The sociology of science.* New York: Free Press of Glencoe.

Bernstein, J. (1978). *Experiencing science.* New York: Basic Books. (Especially note p. 87.)

Bilitski, J.S. (1981). Nursing science and the laws of health: The test of substance as a step in the process of theory development. *Advances in Nursing Science,* 4(1), 15–29.

Blume, S. (Ed.). (1977). *Perspectives in the sociology of science.* New York: John Wiley & Sons.

Bohny, B. (1980). Theory development for a nursing science. *Nursing Forum,* 19(1), 50–67.

Cody, W.K. (1994). The language of nursing science: If not now, when? *Nursing Science Quarterly,* 7, 98–99.

*Colaizzi, J. (1975). The proper object of nursing science. *International Journal of Nursing Studies,* 12(4), 197–200.

Crowley, D.M. (1968). Perspective of pure science. *Nursing Research,* 17(6), 497–501.

Danto, A. and Morgenbesser, S. (Eds.). (1966). Laws and theories. In *Philosophy of science.* New York: World Publishing (Especially note pp. 177–287.)

Eldridge, C.R. (2013). Nursing science and theory: Scientific underpinnings for practice. In M. Zaccagnini and K. White (Eds.), *The doctor of nursing practice: A new model for advanced practice nursing.* Burlington, MA: Jones and Bartlett.

Fawcett, J. (2008). On 'evidence-based practice': Purpose of research is to develop theory. *Nursing Science Quarterly,* 21(1), 89; Author reply 90–81.

Fawcett, J. (2008). The added value of nursing conceptual model-based research. *Journal of Advanced Nursing,* 61(6), 583.

Fawcett, J., Watson, J., Neuman, B., Walker, P.H., and Fitzpatrick, J.J. (2001). On nursing theories and evidence. *Journal of Nursing Scholarship,* 33(2), 115–119.

Gortner, S.R. (1980). Nursing science in transition. *Nursing Research,* 29(3), 180–183.

Grady, P.A. and Gough, L.L. (2015). Nursing science: Claiming the future. *Journal of Nursing Scholarship,* 47(6), 512–521.

*Green, J.A. (1979). Science, nursing and nursing science: A conceptual analysis. *Advances in Nursing Science,* 2(1), 57–64.

Huch, M.H. (1995). Nursing science as a basis for advanced practice. *Nursing Science Quarterly,* 8, 6–7.

*Johnson, D.E. (1959). The nature of a science of nursing. *Nursing Outlook,* 7(5), 291–294.

*Leininger, M.M. (1969). Introduction: Nature of science in nursing. *Nursing Research,* 18(5), 388–389.

Longino, H.E. (1981). Scientific objectivity and feminist theorizing. *Liberal Education,* 67, 187–195.

Mathwig, G. (1971). Nursing science: The theoretical core of nursing knowledge. *Image: Journal of Nursing Scholarship,* 4(1), 20–23.

McCrae, N. (2012). Whither nursing models? The value of nursing theory in the context of evidence-based practice and multidisciplinary health care. *Journal of Advanced Nursing,* 68(1), 222–229.

O'Brien, B.O. and Pearson, A. (1993). Unwritten knowledge in nursing: Consider the spoken as well as the written word. *Scholarly Inquiry for Nursing Practice,* 7(2), 111–127.

Phillips, J.R. (2001). Beyond a decade of research: Moving to the while hole of unitary science. *Nursing Science Quarterly,* 10(1), 6–7.

Ravetz, J.R. (1971). *Scientific knowledge and its social problems.* New York: Oxford University Press. (Especially note pp. 152, 162.)

*Rogers, M.E. (1963). Some comments on the theoretical basis of nursing practice. *Nursing Science,* 1, 11–13, 60.

Sarvimki A. (1994). Science and tradition in the nursing discipline. *Scandinavian Journal of Caring Sciences,* 8, 137–142.

Schrag, C. (1968). Science and the helping professions. *Nursing Research,* 17(6), 486–496.

Schumacher, K.L. and Gortner, S.R. (1992). (Mis)conceptions and reconceptions about traditional science. *Advances in Nursing Science,* 14(4), 1–11.

Schwab, J.J. (1966). The teaching of science as inquiry. In P.F. Brandwern (Ed.), *Elements in a strategy for teaching science in the elementary school.* Cambridge, MA: Harvard University Press. (Especially note pp. 12, 15, 17.)

Shermis, S.S. (1962, November). On becoming an intellectual discipline. *Phi Delta Kappa,* 84–86.

*Tucker, R.W. (1979). The value decisions we know as science. *Advances in Nursing Science,* 1(2), 1–12.

What is nursing science? An international dialogue. (1997). *Nursing Science Quarterly,* 10(1), 10–3.

Younger, J.B. (1990). Literary works as a mode of knowing. *Image: Journal of Nursing Scholarship,* 22(1), 39–43.

7. Theory and Research

Ader, R. (1980). Psychosomatic and psychoimmunologic research. *Psychosomatic Medicine,* 42(3), 307–321.

Allan, J.D. (1988). Knowing what to weigh: Women's self care activities related to weight. *Advances in Nursing Science,* 11(1), 47–60.

Backman, K. and Kyngas, H.A. (1999). Challenges of the grounded theory approach to a novice researcher. *Nursing and Health Sciences*, 1(3), 147–153.

*Batey, M. (1972). Values relative to research and to science in nursing as influenced by a sociological perspective. *Nursing Research*, 21(6), 504–508.

*Benoliel, J.Q. (1977). The interaction between theory and research. *Nursing Outlook*, 25(2), 108–113.

*Brown, M.I. (1964). Research on the development of nursing theory. *Nursing Research*, 13(2), 109–112.

Cheek, J. and Porter, S. (1997). Reviewing Foucault: Possibilities and problems for nursing and health care. *Nursing Inquiry*, 4(2), 108–119.

Chinn, P. (1985). Debunking myths in nursing theory and research. *Image: Journal of Nursing Scholarship*, 17(2), 45–49.

Clarke, P.N. (1998). Nursing theory as a guide for inquiry in family and community health nursing. *Nursing Science Quarterly*, 11(2), 47–48.

Compton, P. (1989). Drug abuse. A self-care deficit. *Journal of Psychosocial Nursing and Mental Health Services*, 27(3), 22–26.

Cressler, D.L. and Tomlinson, P.S. (1988). Nursing research and the discipline of etiological science. *Western Journal of Nursing Research*, 10(6), 743–756.

Curtin, L.L. (1984). Who or why or which or what? . . . is nursing. *Nursing Management*, 15(11), 7–8.

*Dickoff, J. and James, P. (1968). Researching research's role in theory development. *Nursing Research*, 17(3), 204–205.

Dierckx de Casterle, B., Roelens, A., and Gastmans, C. (1998). An adjusted version of Kohlberg's moral theory: Discussion of its validity for research in nursing ethics. *Journal of Advanced Nursing*, 27(4), 829–835.

Dobratz, M.C. (2006). Enriching the portrait: Methodological triangulation of life-closing theory. *Advances in Nursing Science*, 29(3), 260–270.

Duffy, J.R., Hoskins, L., and Seifert, R.F. (2007). Dimensions of caring: Psychometric evaluation of the caring assessment tool. *Advances in Nursing Science*, 30(3), 235–245.

Fawcett, J. (1978). The relationship between theory and research: A double helix. *Advances in Nursing Science*, 1(1), 49–62.

Fawcett, J. (1988). Conceptual models and theory development. *Journal of Obstetric, Gynecologic, and Neonatal Nursing*, 17(6), 400–403.

Fawcett, J. and Downs, F.S. (1986). *The relationship of theory and research*. Norwalk, CT: Appleton-Century-Crofts.

Fawcett, J. and Gigliotti, E. (2001). Using conceptual models of nursing to guide nursing research: The case of the Neuman systems model. *Nursing Science Quarterly*, 14(4), 339–345.

Feldman, H.R. (1980). Nursing research in the 1980s: Issues and implications. *Advances in Nursing Science*, 3(1), 85–92.

Fitzpatrick, J.J. (1988). How can we enhance nursing knowledge and practice? *Nursing and Health Care*, 9(9), 517–521.

Ford-Gilboe, M., Campbell, J., and Berman, H. (1995). Stories and numbers: Coexistence without compromise. *Advances in Nursing Science*, 18(1), 14–26.

Gunter, L.J. (1962). Notes on a theoretical framework for nursing research. *Nursing Research*, 11(4), 219–222.

Haller, K.B. (1988). Beyond idle speculation. *MCN, The American Journal of Maternal Child Nursing*, 13(5), 386.

Hardy, L.K. (1982). Nursing models and research: A restrictive view? *Journal of Advanced Nursing*, 7, 447–451.

Henderson, D.J. (1995). Consciousness-raising in participatory research: Method and methodology for emancipatory nursing inquiry. *Advances in Nursing Science*, 17(3), 58–69.

Hupcey, J.E. (1998). Clarifying the social support theory-research linkage. *Journal of Advanced Nursing*, 27(6), 1231–1241.

Hurley, B.A. (1979). Why a theoretical framework in nursing research? *Western Journal of Nursing Research*, 1(1), 28–41.

Hyrkas, K., Koivula, M., and Paunonen, M. (1999). Clinical supervision in nursing in the 1990s—Current state of concepts, theory and research. *Journal of Nursing Management*, 7(3), 177–187.

Ingram, M.R. (1988). Origins of nursing knowledge. *Image: Journal of Nursing Scholarship*, 20(4), 233.

Jezewski, M.A. (1995). Evolution of a grounded theory: Conflict resolution through culture brokering. *Advances in Nursing Science*, 17(3), 14–30.

Johnson, M. (1983). Some aspects of the relation between theory and research in nursing. *Journal of Advanced Nursing*, 8, 21–28.

Kidd, P. and Morrison, E.F. (1988). Comment. The progression of knowledge in nursing: A search for meaning. *Image: Journal of Nursing Scholarship*, 20(4), 222–224.

Kirkevold, M. (1997). Integrative nursing research—An important strategy to further the development of nursing science and nursing practice. *Journal of Advanced Nursing*, 25(5), 977–984.

Lindeman, C.A. (1985). *Theory and research as basic to nursing practice* [pamphlet]. (Publication. No. NP-68C, pp. 1–19). Kansas City, MO: American Nurses Association.

Lowenberg, J.S. (1994). The nurse-patient relationship reconsidered: An expanded research agenda. *Scholarly Inquiry for Nursing Practice*, 8, 167–190.

Ludemann, R. (1979). Editorial comment: The paradoxical nature of nursing research. *Image: Journal of Nursing Scholarship*, 11(1), 2–8.

MacPherson, K.I. (1983). Feminist methods: A new paradigm for nursing research. *Advances in Nursing Science*, 5, 17–26.

Magee, T., Lee, S.M., Giuliano, K.K., and Munro, B. (2006). Generating new knowledge from existing data: The use of large data sets for nursing research. *Nursing Research*, 55(2S), S50–S56.

McBride, A.B. (1986). Theory and research. *Journal of Psychological Nursing*, 24(9), 27–32.

McCourt, C. (2005). Research and theory for nursing and midwifery: Rethinking the nature of evidence. *Worldviews on Evidence-Based Nursing*, 2(2), 75–83.

McElmurry, B.J. (1995). Theory in nursing research . . . Editorial on theory in nursing research. *Research in Nursing and Health*, 18(4), 377.

McFarlane, J.K. (1976). Role of research in the development of nursing. *Journal of Advanced Nursing*, 1, 443–451.

McQuiston, C.M. and Campbell, J.C. (1997). Theoretical substruction: A guide for theory testing research. *Nursing Science Quarterly*, 10(3), 117–123.

Mischel, M.H. (1990). Reconceptualizing of the uncertainty in illness theory. *Image: Journal of Nursing Scholarship*, 22, 256–262.

Mitchell, G.J. (1994). Discipline-specific inquiry: The hermeneutics of theory-guided nursing research. *Nursing Outlook*, 42, 224–228.

Moch, S.D. (1990). Personal knowing: Evolving research and practice. *Scholarly Inquiry for Nursing Practice*, 4(2), 155–170.

Moody, L.E., Wilson, M.E., Smith, K., Schwartz, R., Tittle, M., and Van Cott, M.L. (1988). Analysis of a decade of nursing practice research: 1977–1986. *Nursing Research*, 37(6), 374–379.

Morse, J.M. (2005). The ramifications of perspective: How theory focuses research, data, and practice. *Journal of Wound, Ostomy, and Continence Nursing*, 32(2), 93–100.

Munhall, P.L. (1989). Philosophical pondering on qualitative research methods in nursing. *Nursing Science Quarterly*, 2(1), 20–28.

Murdaugh, C.L. (1989). Nursing research. The use of grounded theory methodology to study the process of lifestyle changes. *Journal of Cardiovascular Nursing*, 3(2), 56–58.

Nagle, L.M. and Mitchell, G.J. (1991). Theoretic diversity: Evolving paradigmatic issues in research and practice. *Advances in Nursing Science*, 14(1), 17–25.

Newshan, G. (1999). Nursing theory and nursing research: What's in it for me? *ASPMN-Pathways*, 8(4), 7, 10.

*Notter, L.E. (1975). The case for nursing research. *Nursing Outlook*, 23(12), 760–763.

Oiler, C. (1982). The phenomenological approach in nursing research. *Nursing Research*, 31(3), 178–181.

Orcutt, J. (1972). Toward a sociological theory of drug effects: A comparison of marijuana and alcohol. *Sociology and Social Research*, 56(2), 243–253.

Parse, R.R. (1989). Qualitative research: Publishing and funding [Editorial]. *Nursing Science Quarterly*, 2(1), 1–2.

*Payne, G. (1973). Comparative sociology: Some problems of theory and method. *British Journal of Sociology*, 24(1), 13–29.

Phillips, J.R. (1989). Qualitative research: A process of discovery. *Nursing Science Quarterly*, 2(1), 5–6.

Phillips, J.R. (1989). Science of unitary human beings: Changing research perspectives. *Nursing Science Quarterly*, 2(2), 57–60.

Phillips, J.R. (1995). Nursing theory-based research for advanced nursing practice. *Nursing Science Quarterly*, 8, 4–5.

*Quint, J.C. (1967). The case for theories generated from empirical data. *Nursing Research*, 16(2), 109–114.

Roberts, K.L. (1999). Through a looking glass: Nursing theory and clinical nursing research. *Clinical Nursing Research*, 8(4), 299–301.

Rubin, R. and Erickson, F. (1978). Research in clinical nursing. *Journal of Advanced Nursing*, 3(2), 131–144.

Salsberry, P.J., Smith, M.C., and Boyd, C.O. (1989). Phenomenological research in nursing: Commentary and responses. *Nursing Science Quarterly*, 2(1), 9–19.

Santopinto, M.D. (1989). The relentless drive to be ever thinner: A study using the phenomenological method. *Nursing Science Quarterly*, 2(1), 29–36.

Schlotfeldt, R.M. (1975). The conceptual framework of nursing research: The need for a conceptual framework. In P.J. Verhonick (Ed.), *Nursing research*. Boston, MA: Little, Brown.

Seng, J.S. (1998). Praxis as a conceptual framework for participatory research in nursing. *Advances in Nursing Science*, 20(4), 37–48.

*Silva, M.C. (1977). Philosophy, science, theory: Interrelationships and implications for nursing research. *Image: Journal of Nursing Scholarship*, 9(3), 59–63.

Smaldone, A.M. and Connor, J.A. (2003). The use of large administrative data sets in nursing research. *Applied Nursing Research*, 16(3), 205–207.

Tanner, C.A., Benner, P., Chesla, C., and Gordon, D.R. (1993). The phenomenology of knowing the patient. *Journal on Nursing Scholarship*, 25(4), 273–280.

Treece, E.W. and Treece, J.W. (1977). Theory and method. In *Elements of research in nursing* (2nd ed.). St. Louis, MO: C.V. Mosby.

Verran, J.A. (1997). The value of theory-driven (rather than problem-driven) research. *Seminars for Nurse Managers*, 5(4), 169–172.

Whitney, J.D. (1999). Spotlight on research. Thoughts on theory. *Journal of Wound, Ostomy, and Continence Nursing*, 26(5), 228–229.

Williamson, G.J. (2000). The test of a nursing theory: A personal view. *Nursing Science Quarterly*, 13(2), 124–128.

Willman, A. (2000). Nursing theory in education, practice, and research in Sweden. *Nursing Science Quarterly*, 13(3), 263–265.

Zelauskas, B.A., Howes, D.G., Christmyer, C.S., and Dennis, K.E. (1988). Bridging the gap: Theory to practice-Part II, Research applications. *Nursing Management*, 19(9), 50–52.

8. Theory and Practice

Adam, E. (1983). Frontiers of nursing in the 21st century: Development of models and theories on the concept of nursing. *Journal of Advanced Nursing*, 8, 41–45.

Aggleton, P. and Chalmers, H. (1987). Models of nursing, nursing practice and nursing education. *Journal of Advanced Nursing*, 12(5), 573–581.

Alligood, M.R. (1997). Models and theories: Critical thinking structures. In M.R. Alligood et al. (Eds.), *Nursing theory: Utilization and application* (pp. 31–45). St. Louis, MO: Mosby Year Book.

Alligood, M.R. (1997). Models and theories in nursing practice. In M.R. Alligood et al. (Eds.), *Nursing theory: Utilization and application* (pp. 15–30). St. Louis, MO: Mosby Year Book.

Anderson, K.H. (2000). The Family Health System approach to family systems nursing. *Journal of Family Nursing*, 6(2), 103–119.

Arndt, C. and Huckabay, L.M.D. (1975). Administrative theory within a systems' frame of reference. In *Nursing administration: Theory for practice with a systems approach* (pp. 18–44). St. Louis, MO: C.V. Mosby.

Arthur, D., Chan, H.K., Fung, W.Y., Wong, K.Y., and Yeung, K.W. (1999). Therapeutic communication strategies used by Hong Kong mental health nurses with their Chinese clients. *Journal of Psychiatric Mental Health Nursing*, 6(1), 29–36.

Aveyard, H. (2000). Is there a concept of autonomy that can usefully inform nursing practice? *Journal of Advanced Nursing*, 32(2), 352–358.

Baer, E.D. (1987). "A cooperative venture" in pursuit of professional status: A research journal for nursing. *Nursing Research*, 36(1), 18–25.

Baines, L. (1998). Researchers must reach across the practice-theory divide. *Nursing Times*, 94(38), 21.

Barker, P.J., Reynolds, W., and Stevenson, C. (1997). The human science basis of psychiatric nursing: Theory and practice. *Journal of Advanced Nursing*, 25, 660–667.

Barnard, K.E. (1980). Knowledge for practice: Directions for the future. *Nursing Research*, 29(4), 208–212.

Barton, J.A. and Brown, N.J. (1995). Home visitation to migrant farm worker families: An application of Zerwekh's family caregiving model for public health nursing. *Holistic Nursing Practice*, 9(4), 34–40.

Baumann, S.L. and Carroll, K. (2001). Human becoming practice with children. *Nursing Science Quarterly*, 14(2), 120–125.

*Beckstrand, J. (1978). The notion of a practice theory and the relationship of scientific and ethical knowledge to practice. *Research in Nursing and Health*, 1(3), 131–136.

*Beckstrand, J. (1978). The need for a practice theory as indicated by the knowledge used in the conduct of practice. *Research in Nursing and Health*, 1(4), 175–180.

*Beckstrand, J. (1980). A critique of several conceptions of practice theory in nursing. *Research in Nursing and Health*, 3, 69–79.

Bellin, C., Gagnon, M., Mich, M., Plemmons, S., and Watanabe-Hayami, C. (1997). Ecologic health nursing for community health: Applied chaos theory. *Complexity and Chaos in Nursing*, 3, 13–22.

Bender, M. and Feldman, M.S. (2015). A practice theory approach to understanding the interdependency of nursing practice and the environment. *Advances in Nursing Science*, 38(2), 96–109.

Bergen, A. (1995). Clinical notes. Theory and practice: Maintaining and facilitating the links after qualifying—The lecturer's view. *Journal of Clinical Nursing*, 4(1), 4.

Berragan, L. (1998). Nursing practice draws upon several different ways of knowing. *Journal of Clinical Nursing*, 7(3), 209–217.

Billings, J.R. (1995). Bonding theory-tying mothers in knots? A critical review of the application of a theory to nursing. *Journal of Clinical Nursing*, 4, 207–211.

Bottorff, J.L. (1991). Nursing: A practical science of caring. *Advances in Nursing Science*, 14(1), 26–39.

Boykin, A. and Schoenhofer, S. (1990). Caring in nursing: Analysis of extant theory. *Nursing Science Quarterly*, 3, 149–155.

Boykin, A. and Schoenhofer, S. (1994). Nursing as caring: A model for transforming practice. *Nursing Science Quarterly*, 7, 183–185.

Boykin, A. and Schoenhofer, S.O. (1991). Story as link between nursing practice, ontology, epistemology. *Image: Journal of Nursing Scholarship*, 23, 245–248.

Bradshaw, A. (1995). What are nurses doing to patients? A review of theories or nursing past and present. *Journal of Clinical Nursing*, 4, 81–92.

Brasell-Brian, R. and Wong, R.Y. (2002). Fears and worries associated with hypoglycaemia and diabetes complications: Perceptions and experience of Hong Kong Chinese clients. *Journal of Advanced Nursing*, 39(2), 155–163.

Brophy, M.S.S. (2001). Nurse advocacy in the neonatal unit: Putting theory into practice. *Journal of Neonatal Nursing*, 7(1), 10–12.

Buchanam, B.F. (1987). Conceptual models: An assessment framework. *Journal of Nursing Administration*, 17(10), 22–26.

Buchmann, W.F. (1997). Adherence: A matter of self-efficacy and power. *Journal of Advanced Nursing*, 26(1), 132–137.

Burns, C., Archbold, P., Stewart, B., and Shelton, K. (1993). New diagnosis: Caregiver role strain. *Nursing Diagnosis*, 4(2), 70–76.

Byers, J.F. and Smyth, K.A. (1997). Application of a transactional model of stress and coping with critically ill patients. *Dimensions of Critical Care Nursing*, 16(6), 292–300.

Carr, E.C.J. (1996). Reflecting on clinical practice: Hectoring talk or reality? *Journal of Clinical Nursing*, 5(5), 289–295.

Cassidy, C.A. (1999). Using the transtheoeretical model to facilitate behavior change in patients with chronic illness. *Journal of the American Academy of Nurse Practitioners*, 11(7), 281–287.

Chapman, J.S., Mitchell, G.J., and Forchuk C. (1994). A glimpse of nursing theory-based practice in Canada. *Nursing Science Quarterly*, 7, 104–112.

Christmyer, C.S., Catanzariti, P.M., Langford, A.M., and Reitz, J.A. (1988). Bridging the gap: Theory to practice—Part I, Clinical applications. *Nursing Management*, 19(8), 42–43, 46–48, 50.

Clarke, M. (1986). Action and reflection: Practice and theory in nursing. *Journal of Advanced Nursing*, 11, 3–11.

Clarke, P.N. and Cody, W.K. (1994). Nursing theory-based practice in the home and community: The crux of professional nursing education. *Advances in Nursing Science*, 17, 41–53.

Clifford, C. (1995). Caring: Fitting the concept to nursing practice. *Journal of Clinical Nursing*, 4, 37–41.

Cody, W.K. (1994). Nursing theory-guided practice: What it is and what it is not. *Nursing Science Quarterly*, 7, 144–145.

Cody, W.K. (2001). Bearing witness-not bearing witness as a synergistic individual-community becoming. *Nursing Science Quarterly*, 14(2), 94–100.

Cohen, J.A. (1991). Two portraits of caring: A comparison of the artists, Leininger and Watson. *Journal of Advanced Nursing*, 16(8), 899–909.

Craig, S.L. (1980). Theory development and its relevance for nursing. *Journal of Advanced Nursing*, 5, 349–355.

Creamer, E. (2000). Examining the care of patients with peripheral venous cannulas. *British Journal of Nursing*, 9(20), 2128, 2130, 2132.

Crossan, F. and Robb, A. (1998). Role of the nurse: Introducing theories and concepts. *British Journal of Nursing*, 7(10), 608–612.

Curtin, L.L. (1988). Thought-full nursing practice [Editorial]. *Nursing Management*, 19(10), 7–8.

Daly, J. and Jackson, D. (1999). On the use of nursing theory in nurse education, nursing practice, and nursing research in Australia. *Nursing Science Quarterly*, 12(4), 342–345.

Davhana-Maselesele, M., Tjallinks, J.E., and Norval, M.S. (2001). Theory-practice integration in selected clinical situations. *Curationis: South African Journal of Nursing*, 24(4), 4–9.

Davies, B. and Hughes, A.M. (1995). Clarification of advanced nursing practice: Characteristics and competencies. *Clinical Nurse Specialist*, 9(3), 156–160.

Davies, C., Welham, V., Glover, A., Jones, L., and Murphy F. (1999). Teaching in practice. *Nursing Standard*, 13(35), 33–38.

Davis, A.J. (1978). The phenomenological approach. In N.L. Chaska (Ed.), *The nursing profession: Views through the mist*. New York: McGraw-Hill.

DeGroot, H.A., Ferketich, S.L., and Larson, P.J. (1987). Theory development in a non-university service setting. *Journal of Nursing Administration*, 17(4), 38–44.

Derstine, J.B. (1989). The development of theory-based practice by graduate students in rehabilitation nursing. *Rehabilitation Nursing*, 14(2), 88–89.

DeSocio, J. and Sebastian, L. (1988). Towards a theoretical model for clinical nursing practice at Menningers. *Kansas Nurse*, 63(12), 4–5.

Dhasaradhan, I. (2001). Application of nursing theory into practice. *Nursing Journal of India*, 92(10), 224, 236.

Dickinson, J.K. (1999). A critical social theory approach to nursing care of adolescents with diabetes. *Issues in Comprehensive Pediatric Nursing*, 22(4), 143–152.

*Dickoff, J., James, P., and Wiedenbach, E. (1968). Theory in a practice discipline: Part I. Practice oriented theory. *Nursing Research*, 17(5), 415–435.

*Dickoff, J., James, P, and Wiedenbach, E. (1968). Theory in a practice discipline: Part II. Practice oriented research. *Nursing Research*, 17(6), 545–554.

Dodd, M.J. and Miaskowski, C. (2000). The PRO-SELF program: A self-care intervention program for patients receiving cancer treatment. *Seminars in Oncology Nursing*, 16(4), 300–314.

Doucet, T.J. and Merlin, M.D. (2014). Conceptualizations of health in nursing practice. *Nursing Science Quarterly*, 27(2), 118–125.

Duffy, K. and Scott, P.A. (1998). Viewing an old issue through a new lens: A critical theory insight into the education-practice gap. *Nurse Education Today*, 18(3), 183–189.

Edwards, S.D., Benner, P., and Wrubel, J. (2001). Benner and Wrubel on caring in nursing. *Journal of Advanced Nursing*, 33(2), 167–174.

Emblen, J. and Pesut, B. (2001). Strengthening transcendent meaning: A model for the spiritual nursing care of patients experiencing suffering. *Journal of Holistic Nursing*, 19(1), 42–56.

Fawcett, J. (1980). A declaration of nursing independence: The relation of theory and research to nursing practice. *Journal of Nursing Administration*, 10(6), 36–39.

Fawcett, J., Bekel, G., Biley, F.C., and Fragemann, K. (2007). Nursing, healthcare, and culture: A view of the year 2050 from Germany and the United Kingdom. *Nursing Science Quarterly*, 20(3), 232–236.

Fawcett, J. and Graham, I. (2005). Advanced practice nursing: Continuation of the dialogue. *Nursing Science Quarterly*, 18(1), 37–41.

Fawcett, J., Watson, J., Neuman, B., Walker, P.H., and Fitzpatrick, J.J. (2001). On nursing theories and evidence. *Journal of Nursing Scholarship*, 33(2), 115–119.

Fealy, G. (1997). The theory-practice relationship in nursing: An exploration of contemporary discourse. *Journal of Advanced Nursing*, 25, 1061–1069.

Fealy, G. (1999). The theory-practice relationship in nursing: The practitioners' perspective. *Journal of Advanced Nursing*, 30(1), 74–82.

Feldman, M.E. (1993). Uncovering clinical knowledge and caring practices. *Journal of Post Anesthesia Nursing*, 8(3), 159–162.

Fielding, R.G. and Llewelyn, S.P. (1987). Communication in nursing may damage your health and enthusiasm: Some warnings. *Journal of Advanced Nursing Science*, 12(3), 281–290.

Field, L. and Winslow, E.H. (1985). Moving to a nursing model. *American Journal of Nursing*, 85(10), 1100–1101.

Field, P.A. (1987). The impact of nursing theory on the clinical decision making process. *Journal of Advanced Nursing*, 12(5), 563–571.

Fisher, M.A. and Mitchell, G.J. (1998). Patients' view of quality of life: Transforming the knowledge base of nursing. *Clinical Nursing Specialist*, 12(3), 99–105.

Fitzpatrick, J.J. (1988). How can we enhance nursing knowledge and practice? *Nursing and Health Care*, 9(9), 517–521.

Flaskerud, J.H. (2000). Building excellence and scholarship with vulnerable populations: Overview . . . 33rd Annual Communicating Nursing Research Conference/14th Annual WIN Assembly, "Building on a Legacy of Excellence in Nursing Research," held April 13–15, 2000 at the Adam's Mark Hotel, Denver, Colorado. *Communicating Nursing Research*, 33, 102.

Forbes, D.A., King, K.M., Kushner, K.E., Letourneau, N.L., Myrick, A.F., and Profetto-McGrath, J. (1999). Warrantable evidence in nursing science. *Journal of Advanced Nursing*, 29(2), 373–379.

Friedmann, M.L. (1989). Closing the gap between grand theory and mental health practice with families. Part I: The framework of systemic organization for nursing of families and family members. *Archives of Psychiatric Nursing*, 3(1), 10–19.

Friedmann, M.L. (1989). The concept of family nursing. *Journal of Advanced Nursing*, 14(3), 211–216.

Frissell, S. (1988). So many models, so much confusion. *Nursing Administration Quarterly*, 12(2), 13–17.

Gaudine, A.P. (2001). Demonstrating theory in practice: Examples of the McGill Model of Nursing. *Journal of Continuing Education in Nursing*, 32(2), 77–85.

Geden, E.A, Isaramalai, S., and Taylor, S.G. (2001). Self-care deficit nursing theory and the nurse practitioner's practice in primary care settings. *Nursing Science Quarterly*, 14(1), 29–33.

Gendron, D. (1994). The tapestry of care. *Advances in Nursing Science*, 17(1), 25–30.

Georges, J.M. (2005). Linking nursing theory and practice: A critical-feminist approach. *Advances in Nursing Science*, 28(1), 50–57.

Goode, H. (1998). The theory-practice gap and student nurses. *Journal of Child Health Care*, 2(2), 86–90.

Gordon, M., Murphy, C.P., Candee, D., and Hiltunen, E. (1994). Clinical judgment: An integrated model. *Advances in Nursing Science*, 16(4), 55–70.

Gottlieb, L. and Lowat, K. (1987). The McGill model of nursing: A practice-derived model. *Advances in Nursing Science*, 9(4), 51–61.

Gottlieb, L.N. and Feeley, N. (1996). The McGill Model of Nursing and children with a chronic condition: "Who benefits, and why?" *Canadian Journal of Nursing Research*, 28(3), 29–48.

Green-Hernandez, C. (1997). Application of caring theory in primary care: A challenge for advanced practice. *Nursing Administration Quarterly*, 21(4), 77–82.

Greenwood, E. (1961). The practice of science and the science of practice. In W.G. Bennis, K.D. Benne, and R. Chin (Eds.), *The planning of change*. New York: Holt, Rinehart & Winston.

Griffiths, B. and Andrews, C.M. (2007). Nursing perspective. Putting nursing theory into practice. *Gastroenterology Nursing*, 30(6), 440–442.

Gruending, D.L. (1986). Nursing theory: A vehicle of professionalization. *Journal of Advanced Nursing Science*, 10(6), 553–558.

Hampton, D.C. (1994). Expertise: The true essence of nursing art. *Advances in Nursing Science*, 17(1), 15–24.

Hanchett, E.S. and Clark, P.N. (1988). Nursing theory and public health science: Is synthesis possible? *Public Health Nursing*, 5(1), 2–6.

Harbison J. (2001). Clinical decision making in nursing: Theoretical perspectives and their relevance to practice. *Journal of Advanced Nursing*, 35(1), 126–133.

Harrell, J.S. (1986). Needed nurse engineers to link theory and practice. *Nursing Outlook*, 34(4), 196–198.

Harrison, J., Saunders, M.E., and Sims, A. (1977). Integrating theory and practice in modular schemes for basic nurse education. *Journal of Advanced Nursing*, 2, 503–519.

Hartrick Doane, G. and Varcoe, C. (2005). Toward compassionate action: Pragmatism and the inseparability of theory/practice. *Advances in Nursing Science*, 28(1), 81–90.

Hathaway, D. and Strong, M. (1988). Theory, practice, and research in transplant nursing. *American Nephrology Nurses Association Journal*, 15(1), 9–12.

Hatlevik, I.K.R. (2012). The theory-practice relationship: Reflective skills and theoretical knowledge as key factors in bridging the gap between theory and practice in initial nursing education. *Journal of Advanced Nursing*, 68(4), 868–877.

Henderson, B. (1978). Nursing diagnosis: Theory and practice. *Advances in Nursing Science*, 1(1), 75–82.

Hinshaw, A.S. (1987). Response to "Structuring the nursing knowledge system: A typology of four domains." *Scholarly Inquiry for Nursing Practice*, 1(2), 111–114.

Holmes, C.A. and Warelow, P.J. (2000). Some implications of postmodernism for nursing theory, research, and practice. *Canadian Journal of Nursing Research*, 32(2), 89–101.

Hopkins, S. and McSherry, R. (2000). Is there a great divide between nursing theory and practice? *Nursing Times*, 96(17), 16.

Horsfall, J. (1997). Women's depression: Nursing theory and practice. *Contemporary Nurse*, 6(3–4), 129–135.

Hsieh, H. (2001). Letter to the editor . . . "The role of nursing theory in standards of practice: A Canadian perspective." *Nursing Science Quarterly*, 14(4), 367–368.

Huggins, E.A. and Scalzi, C.C. (1988). Limitations and alternatives: Ethical practice theory in nursing. *Advances in Nursing Science*, 10(4), 43–47.

Jacobs, B.B. (2001). Respect for human dignity: A central phenomenon to philosophically unite nursing theory and practice through consilience of knowledge. *Advances in Nursing Science*, 24(1), 17–35.

*Jacobs, M.K. and Huether, S.E. (1978). Nursing science: The theory-practice linkage. *Advances in Nursing Science*, 1(1), 63–73.

Jameton, A. and Fowler, M.D. (1989). Ethical inquiry and concept of research. *Advanced Nursing Science*, 11(3), 11–24.

Jennings, B.M. and Meleis, A.I. (1988). Nursing theory and administrative practice: Agenda for the 1990s. *Advances in Nursing Science*, 10(3), 56–69.

Jenny, J. and Logan, J. (1992). Knowing the patient: One aspect of clinical knowledge. *Image: Journal of Nursing Scholarship*, 24, 254–258.

Johnson, D. (1987). Evaluating conceptual models for use in critical care nursing practice. *Dimensions of Critical Care Nursing*, 6(4), 195–197.

Johnson, J.L. (1994). A dialectical examination of nursing art. *Advances in Nursing Science*, 17(1), 1–14.

Johnson, S.E. (1989). A picture is worth a thousand words: Helping students visualize a conceptual model. *Nurse Educator*, 14(3), 21–24.

Jones, S. (1989). Practice and theory. Is unity possible? *Nursing Standard*, 3(18), 22–23.

Kasch, C. (1984). Interpersonal competence and communication in the delivery of nursing care. *Advances in Nursing Science*, 6(2), 71–88.

Kathol, D.D., Geiger, M.L., and Hartig, J.L. (1998). Clinical correlation map. A tool for linking theory and practice. *Nurse Educator*, 23(4), 31–34.

Ketefian, S. (1987). A case study of theory development: Moral behavior in nursing. *Advances in Nursing Science*, 9(2), 10–19.

Khatib, H.M. and Ford, S. (1999). The theory-practice gap receives much attention in the press and in discussions—What does it mean? *Journal of Child Health Care*, 3(2), 36–38.

Kim, H.S. (1987). Response to "Structuring the nursing knowledge system: A typology of four domains." *Scholarly Inquiry for Nursing Practice*, 1(2), 111–114.

Kim, H.S. (1993). Putting theory into practice: Problems and prospects. *Journal of Advanced Nursing*, 18, 1632–1639.

Kim, H.S. (1994). Action science as an approach to develop knowledge for nursing practice. *Nursing Science Quarterly*, 7, 134–140.

Kim, H.S. (1999). Critical reflective inquiry for knowledge development in nursing practice. *Journal of Advanced Nursing*, 29(5), 1205–1212.

Kite, K. and Pearson, L. (1995). A rationale for mouth care: The integration of theory with practice. *Intensive and Critical Care Nursing*, 11(2), 71–76.

Kristjanson, L.J., Tamblyn, R., and Kuypers, J.A. (1987). A model to guide development and application of multiple nursing theories. *Journal of Advanced Nursing*, 12(4), 523–529.

Landers, M. (2001). The theory/practice gap in nursing: The views of the students. *All Ireland Journal Nursing Midwifery*, 1(4), 142–147.

Laurent, C.L. (2000). A nursing theory for nursing leadership. *Journal of Nursing Management*, 8(2), 83–87.

Lee, P. (1998). An analysis and evaluation of Casey's conceptual framework. *International Journal of Nursing Studies*, 35(4), 204–209.

Lego, S. (1998). The application of Peplau's theory to group psychotherapy. *Journal of Psychiatric Mental Health Nursing*, 5(3), 193–196.

Lewis, T. (1988). Leaping the chasm between nursing theory and practice. *Journal of Advanced Nursing*, 13(3), 345–351.

Litchfield, M. (1999). Practice wisdom. *Advances in Nursing Science*, 22(2), 62–73.

Lo, R. and Brown, R. (1999). The importance of theory in student nurses' psychiatric practicum. *International Journal of Psychiatric Nursing Research*, 5(1), 542–552.

Long, G.E. (1985). Professional advancement: Theory development through practice and research. *ANA Journal*, 12(1), 35–38.

Mahoney, J.S. and Engebretson, J. (2000). The interface of anthropology and nursing guiding culturally competent care in psychiatric nursing. *Archives of Psychiatric Nursing*, 14(4), 183–190.

Mason, D.J., Jones, D.A., Roy, C., Sullivan, C.G., and Wood, L.J. (2015). Commonalities of nurse-designed models of health care. *Nursing Outlook*, 63(5), 540–553.

Mathwig, G. (1971). Nursing science: The theoretical core of nursing knowledge. *Image: Journal of Nursing Scholarship*, 4(1), 20–23.

McAiney, C.A., Haughton, D., Jennings, J., Farr, D., et al. (2008). A unique practice model for nurse practitioners in long-term care homes. *Journal of Advanced Nursing*, 62(5), 562–571.

McBride, A.B. and McBride, W.L. (1981). Theoretical underpinnings for women's health. *Women and Health*, 6, 37–55.

*McCarthy, R.T. (1972). A practice theory of nursing care. *Nursing Research*, 21(5), 406–410.

McCluskey, K. (2007). Learning to care: A new graduate's perspective on applying nursing theory in practice. *International Journal for Human Caring*, 11(1), 47–48.

McFarlane, J.K. (1977). Developing a theory of nursing: The relationship of theory to practice, education, and research. *Journal of Advanced Nursing*, 2(3), 261–270.

McHolm, F.A. and Geib, K.M. (1998). Application of the Neuman systems model to teaching health assessment and nursing process. *Nursing Diagnosis*, 9(1), 23–33.

McIver, M. (1987). Putting theory into practice. *Canadian Nurse*, 83(10), 36–38.

McKenna, B. and Roberts, R. (1999). Bridging the theory-practice gap. *Nursing New Zealand*, 5(2), 14–16.

Meleis, A.I., Isenberg, M., Koerner, J.E., Lacey, B., and Stern, P. (1995). *Diversity, marginalization, and culturally competent health care issues in knowledge development*. Washington, DC: American Academy of Nursing.

Miller, S.R. (1978). Have we dichotomized theory and practice in nursing? *Nursing Leadership*, 1(1), 34–36.

Mitchell, G.J., Closson, T., Coulis, N., Flint, F., and Gray, B. (2000). Patient-focused care and human becoming thought: Connecting the right stuff. *Nursing Science Quarterly*, 13(3), 216–224.

Moch, S.D. (1990). Personal knowing: Evolving research and practice. *Scholarly Inquiry for Nursing Practice*, 4, 155–165.

Moody, L.E., Wilson, M.E., Smith, K., Schwartz, R., Tittle, M., and Van Cott, M.L. (1988). Analysis of a decade of nursing practice research: 1977–1986. *Nursing Research*, 37(6), 374–379.

Moore, M.A. (1968). Nursing: A scientific discipline? *Nursing Forum*, 7(4), 340–348.

Morse, J.M., Bottorff, J., Neander, W., and Solberg, S. (1991). Comparative analysis of conceptualizations and theories of caring. *Image: Journal of Nursing Scholarship*, 23, 119–126.

Morse, J.M., Solberg, S.M., Neander, W.L., Bottorff, J.L., and Johnson, J.L. (1990). Concepts of caring and caring as concept. *Advances in Nursing Science*, 13(1), 1–14.

Mulhall, A. (1997). Nursing research: Our world not theirs? *Journal of Advanced Nursing*, 25(5), 969–976.

Munhall, P.L. (1989). Philosophical pondering on qualitative research methods in nursing. *Nursing Science Quarterly*, 2(1), 20–28.

Munhall, P.L. (1993). Unknowing: Toward another pattern of knowing in nursing. *Nursing Outlook*, 41, 125–128.

Munnukka, T., Pukuri, T., Linnainmaa, P., and Kilkku, N. (2002). Integration of theory and practice in learning mental health nursing. *Journal of Psychiatric and Mental Health Nursing*, 9(1), 5–14.

Neal, J.E. (2001). Patient outcomes: A matter of perspective. *Nursing Outlook*, 49(2), 93–99.

Newman, M.A. (1994). Theory for nursing practice. *Nursing Science Quarterly*, 7(4), 153–157.

O'Brien, B. and Pearson, A. (1993). Unwritten knowledge in nursing: Consider the spoken as well as the written word. *Scholarly Inquiry for Nursing Practice*, 7, 111–127.

Olson, T.C. (1993). Laying claim to caring: Nursing and the language of training, 1915–1937. *Nursing Outlook*, 41, 68–72.

Ousey, K. and Gallagher, P. (2007). The theory-practice relationship in nursing: A debate. *Nurse Education in Practice*, 7(4), 199–205.

Parse, R.R. (2006). Research findings evince benefits of nursing theory-guided practice. *Nursing Science Quarterly*, 19(2), 87.

Patistea, E. (1999). Nurses' perceptions of caring as documented in theory and research. *Journal of Clinical Nursing*, 8(5), 487–495.

Pearson, A. (2002). Nursing in theory and in practice. *International Journal of Nursing Practice*, 8(3), 117.

Phillips, R., Donald, A., Mousseau-Gershman, Y., and Powell, T. (1998). Applying theory to practice—The use of "ripple effect" plans in continuing education. *Nurse Education Today*, 18(1), 12–19.

Pipe, T.B. (2007). Optimizing nursing care by integrating theory-driven evidence-based practice. *Journal of Nursing Care Quality*, 22(3), 234–238.

Piper, S. (2008). A qualitative study exploring the relationship between nursing and health promotion language, theory and practice. *Nurse Education Today*, 28(2), 186–193.

Scherer, Z.A., Scherer, E.A., and Pimenta -Carvalho, A.M. (2007). Group therapy with nursing students during the theory-practice transition. *Revista Latino-Americana de Enfermagem*, 15(2), 214–223.

Raudonis, B.M. and Acton, G.J. (1997). Theory-based nursing practice. *Journal of Advanced Nursing*, 26(1), 138–145.

Rawnsley, M. (1990). Of human bonding: The context of nursing as caring. *Advances in Nursing Science*, 13(1), 41–48.

Raymond, D.P. (1995). Esthetic and personal knowledge through humanistic nursing. *N&HC Perspectives on Community*, 16(6), 332–336.

Reed, P.G. (2006). The force of nursing theory-guided practice. *Nursing Science Quarterly*, 19(3), 225.

Reed, P.G. and Lawrence, L.A. (2008). A paradigm for the production of practice-based knowledge. *Journal of Nursing Management*, 16(4), 422–432.

Rew, L., Stuppy, D., and Becker, H. (1988). Construct validity in instrument development: A vital link between nursing practice, research, and theory. *Advances in Nursing Science*, 10(4), 10–22.

Robb, Y.A. (1997). Have nursing models a place in intensive care units? *Intensive and Critical Care Nursing*, 13(2), 93–98.

Rodgers, J.A. (1976). Today's preparation for tomorrow's practice. The Lehman College nursing program. *Journal of Advanced Nursing*, 1(4), 311–322.

Rodgers, S.J. (2000). The role of nursing theory in standards of practice: A Canadian perspective. *Nursing Science Quarterly*, 13(3), 260–262.

Rolfe, G. (1997). Beyond expertise: Theory, practice and the reflexive practitioner. *Journal of Clinical Nursing*, 6(2), 93–97.

Rolfe, G. (1998). The theory-practice gap in nursing: From research-based practice to practitioner-based research. *Journal of Advanced Nursing*, 28(3), 672–679.

Romeo, J.H. (2000). Comprehensive versus holistic care: Case studies of chronic disease. *Journal of Holistic Nursing*, 18(4), 352–361.

Roper, N. (1966). A model for nursing and nursology. *Journal of Advanced Nursing*, 1(2), 219–227.

Rosswurm, M.A. and Larrabee, J.H. (1999). A model for change to evidence-based practice. *Image: Journal of Nursing Scholarship*, 31(4), 317–322.

Roy, C. and Obby, S.M. (1978). The practitioner movement: Toward a science of nursing. *American Journal of Nursing*, 78(10), 1698–1702.

Saba, V.K. and Taylor, S.L. (2007). Moving past theory: Use of standardized, coded nursing terminology to enhance nursing visibility. *Computers Informatics Nursing*, 25(6), 324–331; quiz 332–323.

Saewyc, E.M. (2000). Nursing theories of caring: A paradigm for adolescent nursing practice. *Journal of Holistic Nursing*, 18(2), 114–128.

Santopinto, M.D. (1989). The relentless drive to be ever thinner: A study using the phenomenological method. *Nursing Science Quarterly*, 2(1), 29–36.

Sarter, B. (1987). Evolutionary idealism: A philosophical foundation for holistic nursing theory. *Advances in Nursing Science*, 9(2), 1–9.

Schafer, P.J. (1987). Philosophic analysis of a theory of clinical nursing. *Maternal-Child Nursing Journal*, 16(4), 289–363.

Schultz, P.R. (1987). When client means more than one: Extending the foundational concept of person. *Advances in Nursing Science*, 10(1), 71–86.

Schutzenhofer, K.K. (1991). Scholarly pursuit in the clinical setting: An obligation of professional nursing. *Journal of Professional Nursing*, 7, 10–15.

Schwartz-Barcott, D., Patterson, B.J., Lusardi, P., and Farmer, B.C. (2002). From practice to theory: Tightening the link via three fieldwork strategies. *Journal of Advanced Nursing*, 39(3), 281–289.

Severinsson, E.I. (1998). Bridging the gap between theory and practice: A supervision programme for nursing students. *Journal of Advanced Nursing*, 27(6), 1269–1277.

Shouli, C. (2001). Letter to the editor . . . "Nursing theory-guided practice: What it is and what is it not" by William K. Cody (1994). *Nursing Science Quarterly*, 14(2), 175.

Simpson, P., Chan, M.C., Cheung, L.Y., Hui, T.S., Li, K.Y., Tang, H.T., Tong, N.H., Wong, S.K., and Wong, P.M. (2002). Primary health care theory to practice: Experience of first-year nursing students in Hong Kong. *Journal of Nursing Education*, 41(7), 302–309.

Slatyer, S., Coventry, L.L., Twigg, D., and Davis, S. (2015). Professional practice models for nursing: A review of the literature and synthesis of key components. *Journal of Nursing Management*, 24(2):139–150.

Smith, C. (2006). From theory to practice: Capturing the uniqueness of nursing. *Nursing Older People*, 18(1), 16–20.

Smith, M.C. (1995). The core of advanced practice nursing. *Nursing Science Quarterly*, 8, 2–3.

Smith, M.C. and Parker, M.E. (2015). *Nursing theories and nursing practice* (4th ed.). Philadelphia, PA: F.A. Davis.

Spouse, J. (2001). Bridging theory and practice in the supervisory relationship: A sociocultural perspective. *Journal of Advanced Nursing*, 33(4), 512–522.

Stark, S., Cooke, P., and Stronach, I. (2000). Minding the gap: Some theory-practice disjunctions in nursing education research. *Nurse Education Today*, 20(2), 155–163.

Street, A.F. (1992). *Inside nursing: A critical ethnography of clinical nursing practice*. Albany, NY: State University of New York Press.

Taylor-Piliae, R.E. (1998). Establishing evidence-based practice: Issues and implications in critical care nursing. *Intensive and Critical Care Nursing*, 14(1), 30–37.

Timpson, J. (1996). Nursing theory: Everything the artist spits is art? *Journal of Advanced Nursing*, 23(5), 1030–1036.

Titler, M.G., Buckwalter, K.C., and Maas, M.L. (1993). Critical issues for the development of clinical nursing knowledge. *Advances in Clinical Nursing Research*, 28(2), 475–477.

Topham, D.L. and DeSilva, P. (1988). Evaluating congruency between steps in the research process. A critique guide for use in clinical nursing practice. *Clinical Nurse Specialist*, 2(2), 97–102.

Upton, D.J. (1999). How can we achieve evidence-based practice if we have a theory-practice gap in nursing today? *Journal of Advanced Nursing*, 29(3), 549–555.

Visintainer, M.A. (1986). The nature of nursing and theory in nursing. *Image: Journal of Nursing Scholarship*, 18(2), 32–38.

Von Krough, G. and Naden, D. (2008). Implementation of a documentation model comprising nursing terminologies—theoretical and methodological issues. *Journal of Nursing Management*, 16(3), 275–283.

Wald, F.S. and Leonard, R.C. (1971). Toward development of nursing practice theory. *Nursing Research*, 20(5), 428–435.

Welch, J.L., Jeffries, P.R., Lyon, B.L., Boland, D.L., and Backer, J.H. (2001). Experiential learning: Integrating theory and research into practice. *Nurse Educator*, 26(5), 240–243.

Welford, C. (2002). Transformational leadership in nursing: Matching theory to practice. *Nursing Management*, 9(4), 7–11.

Westbrook, L.O. and Schultz, P.R. (2000). From theory to practice: Community health nursing in a public health neighborhood team. *Advances in Nursing Science*, 23(2), 50–61.

Whittemore, R. (2005). Analysis of integration in nursing science and practice. *Journal of Nursing Scholarship*, 37(3), 261–267.

Widdershoven, G.A. (1999). Care, cure and interpersonal understanding. *Journal of Advanced Nursing*, 29(5), 1163–1169.

Wiest, D.A. (2006). Impact of conceptual nursing models in a professional environment. *Topics in Emergency Medicine*, 28(2), 161–166.

Wikberg, I. (2007). Imagining nursing practice 2050: The caritative caring theory. *Nursing Science Quarterly*, 20(4), 333–335.

Wilcox, V. (1995). Theory and practice: Maintaining and facilitating the links after qualifying-the practitioner's view. *Journal of Clinical Nursing*, 4, 3–4.

Yian, L.G. (2002). Theory-practice quandary. *Singapore Nursing Journal*, 29(1), 21–26.

Young, J. (1995). Bridging the theory-practice gap: Strategies to reduce the gap between research and practice in neonatal intensive care. *Journal of Neonatal Nursing*, 1(2), 16–20.

Zelauskas, B.A., Howes, D.G., Christmyer, C.S., and Dennis, K.E. (1988). Bridging the gap: Theory to practice—Part II, Research applications. *Nursing Management*, 19(8), 42–43, 46–48, 50.

Zoucha, R. and Husted, G.L. (2000). The ethical dimensions of delivering culturally congruent nursing and health care. *Issues in Mental Health Nursing*, 21(3), 325–340.

9. Theory and Nursing Taxonomies: Diagnosis and Intervention

Auvil-Novak, S.E. (1997). A middle-range theory of chronotherapeutic intervention for postsurgical pain. *Nursing Research*, 46(2), 66–71.

Barker, P.J., Keady, J., Croom, S., Stevenson, C., Adams, T., and Reynolds, W. (1998). The concept of serious mental illness: Modern myths and grim realities. *Journal of Psychiatric and Mental Health Nursing*, 5(4), 247–254.

Barker, P.J., Reynolds, W., and Stevenson, C. (1997). The human science basis of psychiatric nursing: Theory and practice. *Journal of Advanced Nursing*, 25(4), 660–667.

Barry, P. (1996). Integrating the Barry holistic system an the NANDA nursing diagnosis models. In P.D. Barry (Ed.), *Psychological nursing: Care of the physically ill patients and their families* (3rd ed.). Philadelphia, PA: Lippincott.

Batra, C. (1996). Nursing theory and nursing process in the community. In J.M. Cookfair (Ed.), *Nursing care in the community* (pp. 85–124). St. Louis, MO: Mosby Year Book.

Bianchi, M.T. and Alexander, B.M. (2006). Evidence based diagnosis: Does the language reflect the theory? *BMJ Journals*, 333(7565), 442–445.

Blegen, M.A. and Tripp-Reimer, T. (1997). Implications of nursing taxonomies for middle-range theory development. *Advances in Nursing Science*, 19(3), 37–49.

Bliss-Holtz, J. (1996). Using Orem's theory to generate nursing diagnoses for electronic documentation. *Nursing Science Quarterly*, 9(3), 121–125.

Brown, R. (2000). Describing a model of nursing as a focus for psychiatric nursing care. *International Journal of Psychiatric Nursing Research*, 6(1), 670–682.

Buckingham, C.D. and Adams, A. (2000). Classifying clinical decision making: Interpreting nursing intuition, heuristics and medical diagnosis. *Journal of Advanced Nursing*, 32(4), 990–998.

Burns, C., Archbold, P., Stewart, B., and Shelton, K. (1993). New diagnosis: Caregiver role strain. *Nursing Diagnosis*, 4(2), 70–76.

Burrell, M. and Hurm, R. (1999). Care of the patient with interstitial cystitis: Current theories and management. *Journal of PeriAnesthesia Nursing*, 14(1), 17–22.

Canuso, R. (1997). Rethinking behavior disorders: Whose attention has a deficit? *Journal of Psychosocial Nursing and Mental Health Services*, 35(4), 24–29.

Carlson-Catalano, J. (1997). Nursing diagnoses and interventions for post-acute phase battered women. In M.J. Rantz et al. (Eds.), *Classification of nursing diagnoses: Proceedings of the twelfth conference, North American Nursing Diagnosis Association* (p. 209). Glendale, CA: CINAHL Information Systems.

Carpenito, L.J. (1997). Defining nursing expertise in a multi-discipline health care arena. In M.J. Rantz et al. (Eds.), *Classification of nursing diagnoses: Proceedings of the twelfth conference, North American Nursing Diagnosis Association* (pp. 48–56). Glendale, CA: CINAHL Information Systems.

Cavendish, R., Luise, B.K., Horne, K., Bauer, M., Medefindt, J., Gallo, M.A., Calvino, C., and Kutza, T. (2000). Opportunities for enhanced spirituality relevant to well adults. *Nursing Diagnosis*, 11(4), 151–163.

Chambers, M. (1998). Interpersonal mental health nursing: Research issues and challenges. *Journal of Psychiatric and Mental Health Nursing*, 5(3), 203–211.

Chater, K. (1999). Risk and representation: Older people and noncompliance. *Nursing Inquiry*, 6(2), 132–138.

Clark, D.J. (1997). The international classification for nursing practice: A progress report. *Studies in Health Technologies and Informatics*, 46, 62–68.

Conley, V.M. (1998). Beyond knowledge deficit to a proposal for information-seeking behaviors. *Nursing Diagnosis*, 9(4), 129–135.

Cutler, L. (2000). Reflection on diagnosing as a nurse in ITU, including commentary by Johns, C. (2000). *Nursing in Critical Care*, 5(1), 22–30.

Daly, J.M. (1997). How nursing interventions classification fits in the patient information system Patient Core Data Set. *Computers in Nursing*, 15(Suppl 2), S77–S81.

Daly, J.M., Maas, M.L., and Johnson, M. (1997). Nursing outcomes classification. An essential -element in data sets for nursing and health care effectiveness. *Computers in Nursing*, 15(Suppl 2), S82–S86.

Davis, P. (1999). Using models and theories in orthopaedic nursing. *Journal of Orthopaedic Nursing*, 3(Suppl 1), 3–8.

Davis, R. (2000). Holographic community: Reconceptualizing the meaning of community in an era of health care reform. *Nursing Outlook*, 48(6), 294–301.

de Oliveira Lopes, M.V., Silva, V.M., and Herdman, T.H. (2015). Causation and validation of nursing diagnoses: A middle range theory. *International Journal of Nursing Knowledge*. doi: 10.1111/2047-3095.12104.

Dijkstra, A., Buist, G., and Dassen, T. (1998). Operationalization of the concept of "nursing care dependency" for use in long-term care facilities. *Australian and New Zealand Journal of Mental Health Nursing*, 7(4), 142–151.

Dougherty, C.M., Jankin, J.K., Lunney, M.R., and Whitley, G.G. (1993). Conceptual and research based validation of nursing diagnoses: 1950 to 1993. *Nursing Diagnosis*, 4(4), 156–165.

Durand, M. and Prince, R. (1966). Nursing diagnostics: Process and decision. *Nursing Forum*, 5(4), 50–64.

Eisenhauer, L.A. (1994). A typology of nursing therapeutics. *Image: Journal of Nursing Scholarship*, 26, 261–264.

Elliot, T. (1995). Impaired adjustment related to inappropriate utilization of resources: A down under diagnosis . . . "Implementation strategies and use of nursing diagnosis in tertiary institutions and major teaching hospitals throughout Australia." In M.J. Rantz et al. (Eds.), *Classification of nursing diagnoses: Proceedings of the eleventh conference, North American Nursing Diagnosis Association* (pp. 189–198). Glendale, CA: CINAHL Information Systems.

Fagerstrom, L. and Engberg, I.B. (1998). Measuring the unmeasurable: A caring science perspective on patient classification. *Journal of Nursing Management*, 6(3), 165–172.

Fagerstrom, L, Rainio, A.K., Rauhala, A., and Nojonen, K. (2000). Validation of a new method for patient classification, the Oulu Patient Classification. *Journal of Advanced Nursing*, 31(2), 481–490.

Fishel, A.H. (1998). Nursing management of anxiety and panic. *Nursing Clinics of North America*, 33(1), 135–151.

Fitzpatrick, J.J. and Zanotti, R. (1995). Where are we now? Nursing diagnosis internationally. *Nursing Diagnosis*, 6(1), 42–47.

Fredericks, D.W. and Williams, W.L. (1998). New definition of mental retardation for the American Association of Mental Retardation. *Image: Journal of Nursing Scholarship*, 30(1), 53–56.

Frisch, N. (1995). Nursing diagnosis and nursing theory—What does it really mean to combine the two? *Nursing Diagnosis*, 6(2), 51.

Frisch, N.C. (2001). Nursing as a context for alternative/complementary modalities. *Online Journal of Issues in Nursing*, 6(2), 2.

Frisch, N.C. and Kelley, J.H. (2002). Nursing diagnosis and nursing theory: Exploration of factors inhibiting and supporting simultaneous use. *Nursing Diagnosis*, 13(2), 53–61.

Gaberson, K.B. (1997). What's the answer? What's the question? *Journal of the Association of periOperative Registered Nurses*, 66(1), 148–151.

Gagan, M.J., Badger, T.A., and de Leon Baker, M. (1999). Nurse practitioner interventions for domestic violence. *Clinical Excellence in Nurse Practice*, 3(5), 273–278.

Gigliotti, E. (1998). You make the diagnosis. Case study: Integration of the Neuman Systems Model with the theory of nursing symptom in postpartum nursing, including commentary by Lunney, M. *Nursing Diagnosis*, 9(1), 14, 34–38.

Gill, J., Hopwood-Jones, L., Tyndall, J., Gregoroff, S., LeBlanc, P., Lovett, C., Rasco, L., and Ross, A. (1995). Incorporating nursing diagnosis and King's theory in the O.R. documentation. *Canadian Operating Room Nursing Journal*, 13(1), 10–14.

Gordon, M. (1979). The concept of nursing diagnosis. *Nursing Clinics of North America*, 14(3), 487–496.

Gordon, M. (1998, September 30). Nursing nomenclature and classification system development. *Online Journal of Issues in Nursing*. Retrieved from http://www.nursingworld.org/MainMenuCategories/ANAMarketplace/ANAPeriodicals/OJIN/TableofContents/Vol31998/No2Sept1998/NomenclatureandClassification.html

Gordon, M. (1998). President's reflection. *Nursing Diagnosis*, 9(Suppl 2), 5–6.

Gordon, M.D. (1985). Nursing diagnosis. *Annual Review of Nursing Research*, 3, 127–146.

Gordon, M., Murphy, C.P., Candee, D., and Hiltunen, E. (1994). Clinical judgment: An integrated model. *Advances in Nursing Science*, 16(4), 55–70.

Gordon, M. and Sweeny, M.A. (1979). Methodological problems and issues in identifying and standardizing nursing diagnosis. *Advances in Nursing Science*, 2(1), 1–15.

Gordon, M., Sweeny, M.A., and McKeehan, K. (1980). Nursing diagnosis: Looking at its use in the clinical area. *American Journal of Nursing*, 80, 672–674.

Grant, J., Kinney, M., and Guzzetta, C. (1990). A methodology for validating nursing diagnoses. *Advances in Nursing Science*, 12(3), 65–74.

Griffiths, P. (1998). An investigation into the description of patients' problems by nurses using two different needs-based nursing models. *Journal of Advanced Nursing*, 28(5), 969–977.

Grobe, S.J. (1990). Nursing intervention lexicon and taxonomy study: Language classification methods. *Advances in Nursing Science*, 13 (2), 22–33.

Grobe, S.J., Hughes, L.C., Robinson, L., Adler, D.C., Nuamah, I., and McCorkle, R. (1997). Nursing intervention intensity and focus: Indicators of process for outcomes studies. *Studies in Health Technologies and Informatics*, 46, 8–14.

Guzzetta, C.E. and Dossey, B.M. (1983). Nursing diagnosis: Framework, process, and problems. *Heart and Lung*, 12(3), 281–291.

Haas, B.K. (1999). Clarification and integration of similar quality of life concepts. *Image: The Journal of Nursing Scholarship*, 31(3), 215–220.

Harbison, J. (2001). Clinical decision making in nursing: Theoretical perspectives and their relevance to practice. *Journal of Advanced Nursing*, 35(1), 126–133.

Hardiker, N. and Kirby, J. (1997). A compositional approach to nursing terminology. *Studies in Health Technologies and Informatics*, 46, 3–7.

Hassell, J.S. (1996). Improvement management of depression through nursing model application and critical thinking. *Journal of the American Academy of Nurse Practitioners*, 8(4), 161–166.

Henderson, B. (1978). Nursing diagnosis: Theory and practice. *Advances in Nursing Science*, 1(1), 75–83.

Henry, S.B. and Mead, C.N. (1997). Evaluating standardized coding and classification systems for clinical practice: A critical review of the nursing literature in the United States. *Studies in Health Technologies and Informatics*, 446, 15–20.

Herdman, T.H. (2008). Nursing diagnosis: Is it time for a new definition? *International Journal of Nursing Terminologies and Classifications*, 19(1), 2–13.

Higuchi, K.A., Dulberg, C., and Duff, V. (1999). Factors associated with nursing diagnosis utilization in Canada. *Nursing Diagnosis*, 10(4), 134–147.

Hogston, R. (1997). Nursing diagnosis and classification systems: A positive paper. *Journal of Advanced Nursing*, 26(3), 496–500.

Hoskins, L.M. (1999). Sailing the course to advance professional practice with nursing diagnosis: The tenth and eleventh conferences. In M.J. Rantz et al. (Eds.), *Classification of nursing diagnoses: Proceedings of the thirteenth conference, North American Nursing Diagnosis Association (pp. 53–58)*. Celebrating the 25th anniversary of NANDA. Glendale, CA: CINAHL Information Systems.

Idvall, E., Rooke, L., and Hamrin, E. (1997). Quality indicators in clinical nursing: A review of the literature. *Journal of Advanced Nursing*, 25(1), 6–17.

Iowa Intervention Project. (1993). The NIC taxonomy structure. *Image: Journal of Nursing Scholarship*, 25(3), 187–192.

Iowa Intervention Project. (1995). Validation and coding of the NIC taxonomy structure. *Image: Journal of Nursing Scholarship*, 27(1), 43–49.

Irvin, S.M. and Harrison, S.A. (1996). Case study: High acuity to long term. *SCI Nursing*, 13(4), 88–95.

Jennings-Dozier, K. (1999). Predicting intentions to obtain a Pap smear among African American and Latina women: Testing the theory of planned behavior. *Nursing Research*, 48(4), 198–205.

Jenny, J. (1995). Advancing the science of nursing. In M.J. Rantz et al. (Eds.), *Classification of nursing diagnoses: Proceedings of the eleventh conference, North American Nursing Diagnosis Association* (pp. 73–81). Glendale, CA: CINAHL Information Systems.

Johnstone, M.J. (1999). Reflective topical autobiography: An under utilised interpretive research method in nursing. *Collegian*, 6(1), 24–29.

Kajbjer, K. (1997). European standardization in healthcare informatics and the need for increased involvement of healthcare professionals. *Studies in Health Technologies and Informatics*, 46, 269–274.

Kathol, D.D., Geiger, M.L., and Hartig, J.L. (1998). Clinical correlation map: A tool for linking theory and practice. *Nurse Educator*, 23(4), 31–34.

Kerr, M.E., Hoskins, L.M., Fitzpatrick, J.J., Warren, J.J., Avant, K.C., Carpenito, L.J., Hurley, M.E., Jakob, D., Lunney, M., Mills, W.C., and Rottkamp, B.C. (1992).

Development of definitions for taxonomy II. *Nursing Diagnosis*, 3(2), 65–71.

Kim, M. (1998). Physiologic nursing diagnosis: Its role and place in nursing taxonomy . . . from Classification of Nursing Diagnoses: Proceedings of the Fifth National Conference (placed on the page in an organized way, 60–62). Copyright 1984 by C.V. Mosby. Reprinted with permission. *Nursing Diagnosis*, 9 (Suppl 2), 32–38.

Kim, M.J. (1989). Nursing diagnosis. *Annual Review of Nursing Research*, 7, 117–142.

Kleinbeck, S.V. (2000). Dimensions of perioperative nursing for a national specialty nomenclature. *Journal of Advanced Nursing*, 31(3), 529–535.

Klemm, P.R. and Guarnieri, C. (1996). Cervical cancer: A developmental perspective. *Journal of Obstetric, Gynecologic and Neonatal Nursing*, 25(7), 629–634.

Knight, M.M. (2000). Cognitive ability and functional status. *Journal of Advanced Nursing*, 31(6), 1459–1468.

Kolcaba, K.Y. (1991). A taxonomic structure for the concept comfort. *Image: Journal of Nursing Scholarship*, 23, 237–244.

Kritek, P.B. (1978). The generation and classification of nursing diagnosis: Toward a theory of nursing. *Image: Journal of Nursing Scholarship*, 10(2), 33–40.

Kritek, P.B. (1985). Nursing diagnosis in perspective: Response to a critique. *Image: Journal of Nursing Scholarship*, 17(1), 3–8.

Kritek, P.B. (1985). Nursing diagnosis: Theoretical foundations. *Occupational Health Nursing*, 33(8), 393–396.

Lacko, L., Bryan, Y., Dellasega, C., and Salerno, F. (1999). Changing clinical practice through research: The case of delirium. *Clinical Nursing Research*, 8(3), 235–250.

Langford, C.P., Bowsher, J., Maloney, J.P., and Lillis, P.P. (1997). Social support: A conceptual analysis. *Journal of Advanced Nursing*, 25(1), 95–100.

Logue, G.A. (1997). An application of Orem's theory to the nursing management of pertussis. *Journal of School Nursing*, 13(4), 20–25.

Lunney, M. (2008). The need for international nursing diagnosis research and a theoretical framework. *International Journal of Nursing Terminologies and Classifications*, 19(1), 28–34.

Mackenzie, S.J. and Laschinger, H.K.S. (1995). Correlates of nursing diagnosis quality in public health nursing. *Journal of Advanced Nursing*, 21(4), 800–808.

Madsen, I. and Jytte Burgaard, S.A. (1997). The Danish Health Classification system—Nursing Interventions Classification—A part of a common Danish Health Care Classification. *Studies in Health Technologies and Informatics*, 46, 32–36.

Mason, G.M.C. and Attree, M. (1997). The relationship between research and the nursing process in clinical practice. *Journal of Advanced Nursing*, 26(5), 1045–1049.

McHolm, F.A. and Geib, K.M. (1998). Application of the Neuman Systems Model to teaching health assessment and nursing process. *Nursing Diagnosis*, 9(1), 23–33.

Mitchell, G.J. (1991). Nursing diagnosis: An ethical analysis. *Image: Journal of Nursing Scholarship*, 23, 99–103.

Modrcin-McCarthy, M.A., McCue, S., and Walker, J. (1997). Preterm infants and STRESS: A tool for the neonatal nurse. *Journal of Perinatal and Neonatal Nursing*, 10(4), 62–71.

Moen, A., Henry, S.B., and Warren, J.J. (1999). Representing nursing judgments in the electronic health record. *Journal of Advanced Nursing*, 30(4), 990–997.

Moorhead, S., Head, B., Johnson, M., and Maas, M. (1998). The nursing outcomes taxonomy: Development and coding. *Journal of Nursing Care Quality*, 12(6), 56–63.

Moreira, A.S.P. (1997). Nursing diagnoses and social representation: A methodological approach. In M.J. Rantz et al. (Eds.), *Classification of nursing diagnoses: Proceedings of the twelfth conference, North American Nursing Diagnosis Association* (p. 377). Glendale, CA: CINAHL Information Systems.

Nolan, M., Lundh, U., and Tishelman, C. (1998). Nursing's knowledge base: Does it have to be unique? *British Journal of Nursing*, 7(5), 270–276.

Nuamah, I.F., Cooley, M.E., Fawcett, J., and McCorkle, R. (1999). Testing a theory for health-related quality of life in cancer patients: A structural equation approach. *Research in Nursing and Health*, 22(3), 231–242.

O'Connell, B. (1998). The clinical application of the nursing process in selected acute care settings: A professional mirage. *Australian Journal of Advanced Nursing*, 15(4), 22–32.

O'Connell, B., Rapley, P., and Tibbett, P. (1999). Does the nursing diagnosis form the basis for patient care? *Collegian*, 6(3), 29–34.

Paredes, A.S., Furegato, A.R., and Coler, M.S. (1999). Nursing diagnosis and social representation: A methodology of diagnostic formulation. In M.J. Rantz et al. (Eds.), *Classification of nursing diagnoses: Proceedings of the thirteenth conference, North American Nursing Diagnosis Association* (p. 591). Celebrating the 25th anniversary of NANDA. Glendale, CA: CINAHL Information Systems.

Peck, S.D. (1998). The efficacy of therapeutic touch for improving functional ability in elders with degenerative arthritis. *Nursing Science Quarterly*, 11(3), 123–132.

Pollack, L.E. and Cramer, R.D. (1999). Patient satisfaction with two models of group therapy for people hospitalized with bipolar disorder. *Applied Nursing Research*, 12(3), 143–152.

Porter, E.J. (1985). Validating a diagnostic label. *Nursing Clinics in North America*, 20(4), 641–655.

Porter, E.J. (1986). Critical analysis of NANDA nursing diagnosis taxonomy I. *Image: Journal of Nursing Scholarship*, 18(4), 136–139.

Potter, M.L. and Bockenhauer, B.J. (2000). Implementing Orlando's nursing theory: A pilot study. *Journal of Psychosocial Nursing and Mental Health Services*, 38(3), 14–21.

Redes, S. and Lunney, M. (1997). Validation by school nurses of the Nursing Intervention Classification for computer software. *Computers in Nursing*, 15(6), 333–338.

Roberts, S.L., Johnson, L.H., and Keely, B. (1999). Fostering hope in the elderly congestive heart failure patient in critical care. *Geriatric Nursing*, 20(4), 195–199.

Scahill, L. (1991). Nursing diagnosis vs goal-oriented treatment planning in inpatient child psychiatry. *Image: Journal of Nursing Scholarship*, 23, 95–98.

Shamansky, S.L. and Yanni, C.R. (1983). In opposition to nursing diagnosis: A minority opinion. *Image: Journal of Nursing Scholarship*, 19(4), 184–185.

Sieleman, J. (1999). Utilization of nursing diagnoses in Iowa child health specialty clinics. *Nursing Diagnosis*, 10(3), 113–120.

Simon, J.M. (1998). Nursing theories and nursing diagnoses: How are they related? *Nursing Diagnosis*, 9(1), 3–4.

Sundin-Huard, D. and Fahy, K. (1999). Moral distress, advocacy and burnout: Theorizing the relationships. *International Journal of Nursing Practice*, 5(1), 8–13.

Taylor, S.G. (1991). The structure of nursing diagnosis from Orem's theory. *Nursing Science Quarterly*, 4(1), 24–32.

Thompson, C. (1999). A conceptual treadmill: The need for "middle ground" in clinical decision making theory in nursing. *Journal of Advanced Nursing*, 30(5), 1222–1229.

Tilley, J.D., Gregor, F.M., and Thieson, V. (1987). The nurses' role in patient education: Incongruent perceptions among nurses and patients. *Journal of Advanced Nursing*, 12, 291–391.

Titler, M.G., Bulechek, G.M., and McCloskey, J.C. (1996). Use of the nursing interventions classification by critical care nurses. *Critical Care Nurse*, 16(4), 45–54.

Tribotti, S., Lyons, N., Blackburn, S., Stein, M., and Withers, J. (1988). Nursing diagnosis for the postpartum woman. *Journal of Obstetric, Gynecologic, and Neonatal Nursing*, 17, 410–416.

Tripp-Reimer, T., Woodworth, G., McCloskey, J.C., and Bulechek, G. (1996). The dimensional structure of nursing interventions. *Nursing Research*, 45(1), 10–17.

Turkoski, B. (1988). Nursing diagnosis in print, 1950–1985. *Nursing Outlook*, 36(3), 142–144.

Turley, J.P. (1997). Developing informatics as a discipline. *Studies in Health Technologies and Informatics*, 46, 69–74.

Walker, K.M. and Alligood, M.R. (2001). Empathy from a nursing perspective: Moving beyond borrowed theory. *Archives of Psychiatric Nursing*, 15(3), 140–147.

Watson, R. and Lea, A. (1997). The Caring Dimensions Inventory (CDI): Content validity, reliability and scaling. *Journal of Advanced Nursing*, 25(1), 87–94.

Weber, P., Lovis, C.C., Michel, P.A., and Baud, R. (1997). Collection of nursing minimum data set (NMDS) could benefit from medical encoding experiences. *Studies in Health Technologies and Informatics*, 46, 263–268.

Wesorick, B. (1995). Moving nursing diagnosis from theory to reality. In M.J. Rantz et al. (Eds.), *Classification of nursing diagnoses: Proceedings of the eleventh conference, North American Nursing Diagnosis Association* (p. 249). Glendale, CA: CINAHL Information Systems.

White, S.J. (1997). Empathy: A literature review and concept analysis. *Journal of Clinical Nursing*, 6(4), 253–257.

Whitley, G.G. (1997). Three phases of research in validating nursing diagnoses. *Western Journal of Nursing Research*, 19(3), 379–399.

Woodtli, A. (1995). Mixed incontinence: A new nursing diagnosis? *Nursing Diagnosis*, 6(4), 135–142.

Wooldridge, J.B., Brown, O.F., and Herman, J. (1993). Nursing diagnosis: The central theme in nursing knowledge. *Nursing Diagnosis*, 4, 50–55.

10. Theory and Education

Aggleton, P. and Chalmers, H. (1987). Models of nursing, nursing practice and nursing education. *Journal of Advanced Nursing*, 12(5), 573–581.

Algase, D.L., Newton, S.E., and Higgins, P.A. (2001). Nursing theory across curricula: A status report from midwest nursing schools. *Journal of Professional Nursing*, 17(5), 248–255.

Allen, D. (1997). Nursing, knowledge and practice. *Journal of Health Services Research and Policy*, 2(3), 190–193.

Anderko, L., Uscian, M., and Robertson, J.F. (1999). Improving client outcomes through differentiated practice: A rural nursing center model. *Public Health Nursing*, 16(3), 168–175.

Armitage, G. (1998). Analysing childhood: A nursing perspective. *Journal of Child Health Care*, 2(2), 66–71.

Arthur, D., Chan, H.K., Fung, W.Y., Wong, K.Y., and Yeung, K.W. (1999). Therapeutic communication strategies used by Hong Kong mental health nurses with their Chinese clients. *Journal of Psychiatric and Mental Health Nursing*, 6(1), 29–36.

Arvay, M., Banister, E., Hoskins, M., and Snell A. (1999). Women's lived experience of conceptualizing the self: Implications for health care practice. *Health Care for Women International*, 20(4), 363–380.

Ashmore, R. and Banks, D. (1997). Student nurses perceptions of their interpersonal skills: A re-examination of Burnard and Morrison's findings. *International Journal of Nursing Studies*, 34(5), 335–345.

Attewell, A. (1998). Florence Nightingale's relevance to nurses. *Journal of Holistic Nursing*, 16(2), 281–291.

Backman, K. and Kyngas, H.A. (1999). Challenges of the grounded theory approach to a novice researcher. *Nursing and Health Sciences*, 1(3), 147–153.

Baer, E.D. (1987). "A cooperative venture" in pursuit of professional status: A research journal for nursing. *Nursing Research*, 36(1), 18–25.

Baker, C. (1999). From chaos to order: A nursing-based psycho-education program for parents of children with attention-deficit hyperactivity disorder. *Canadian Journal of Nursing Research*, 31(2), 71–75.

Banks, J.A. (2006). Improving race relations in schools: From theory and research to practice. *Journal of Social Issues*, 62(3), 607–614.

Barker, P., Jackson, S., and Stevenson, C. (1999). The need for psychiatric nursing: Towards a multidimensional theory of caring. *Nursing Inquiry*, 6(2), 103–111.

Barker, P., Jackson, S., and Stevenson, C. (1999). What are psychiatric nurses needed for? Developing a theory of essential nursing practice. *Journal of Psychiatric and Mental Health Nursing*, 6(4), 273–282.

Barkley, T.W., Jr., Rhodes, R.S., and Dufour, C.A. (1998). Predictors of success on the NCLEX-RN among baccalaureate nursing students. *Nursing and Health Care Perspectives*, 19(3), 132–137.

Barnes, M. (1999). Research in midwifery—The relevance of a feminist theoretical framework. *Journal of the Australian College of Midwives*, 12(2), 6–10.

Basuray, J. (1997). Nurse Miss Sahib: Colonial culture-bound education in India and transcultural nursing. *Journal of Transcultural Nursing*, 9(1), 14–19.

Batra, C. (1987). Nursing theory for undergraduates. *Nursing Outlook*, 35(4), 189–192.

Benson, A. and Latter, S. (1998). Implementing health promoting nursing: The integration of interpersonal skills and health promotion. *Journal of Advanced Nursing*, 27(1), 100–107.

Berragan, L. (1998). Nursing practice draws upon several different ways of knowing. *Journal of Clinical Nursing*, 7(3), 209–217.

Bevis, E.O. (1989, February). *Curriculum building in nursing: A process* (Publication No. 15–227, pp. i–xx, 1–282). New York: National League for Nursing.

Booth, K., Kenrick, M., and Woods, S. (1997). Nursing knowledge, theory and method revisited. *Journal of Advanced Nursing*, 26(4), 804–811.

Boykin, A. and Schoenhofer. S. (1997). Reframing outcomes: Enhancing personhood. *Advanced Practice Nursing Quarterly*, 3(1), 60–65.

Brooks, E.M. and Thomas, S. (1997). The perception and judgment of senior baccalaureate student nurses in clinical decision making. *Advances in Nursing Science*, 19(3), 50–69.

Brown, R. (2000). Describing a model of nursing as a focus for psychiatric nursing care. *International Journal of Psychiatric Nursing Research*, 6(1), 670–682.

Brown, S.J. (1999). Student nurses' perceptions of elderly care. *Journal of the National Black Nurses Association*, 10(2), 29–36.

Buerhaus, P.I. and Norman, L. (2001). It's time to require theory and methods of quality improvement in basic and graduate nursing education. *Nursing Outlook*, 49(2), 67–69.

Bunkers, S.S. (2001). Teaching-learning processes. On global health and justice: A nursing theory-guided perspective. *Nursing Science Quarterly*, 14(4), 297.

Bunkers, S.S. (2002). Teaching-learning processes. Nursing theory-guided models for teaching-learning. *Nursing Science Quarterly*, 15(2), 117.

*Burgess, G. (1978). The personal development of the nursing student as a conceptual framework. *Nursing Forum*, 17(1), 96–102.

Burks, K.J. (2001). Intentional action. *Journal of Advanced Nursing*, 34(5), 668–675.

Cain, P. (1999). Respecting and breaking confidences: Conceptual, ethical and educational issues. *Nurse Education Today*, 19(3), 175–181.

Cash, K. (1997). Social epistemology, gender and nursing theory. *International Journal of Nursing Studies*, 34(2), 137–143.

Cave, P. (1998). Nursing knowledge: The role of Plato in wound care. *Nursing Standard*, 13(11), 40–43.

Cessario, L. (1987). Utilization of board gaming for conceptual models of nursing. *Journal of Nursing Education*, 26(4), 167–169.

Chick, N. and Paull, D. (1988). Collaboration between nurse educators in Australia and New Zealand extends educational opportunities for nurses. *International Journal of Nursing Studies*, 25(4), 279–286.

Chinn, P.L. (1988). Knowing and doing [Editorial]. *Advances in Nursing Science*, 10(3), vii–viii.

Christmyer, C.S., Catanzariti, P.M., Langford, A.M., and Reitz, J.A. (1988). Bridging the gap: Theory to practice—Part I, Clinical applications. *Nursing Management*, 19(8), 42–43, 46–48, 50.

Clarke, D.J. and Holt, J. (2001). Philosophy: A key to open the door to critical thinking. *Nurse Education Today*, 21(1), 71–78.

Clifford, C. (1997). Nurse teachers and research. *Nurse Education Today*, 17(2), 115–120.

Cohen, S.S. and Milone-Nuzzo, P. (2001). Advancing health policy in nursing education through service learning. *Advances in Nursing Science*, 23(3), 28–40.

Colodny, A. (1997). Spinal cord injury nurses in action: Partners in practice. *SCI Nursing*, 14(3), 79–82.

Conley, V.M. (1998). Beyond knowledge deficit to a proposal for information-seeking behaviors. *Nursing Diagnosis*, 9(4), 129–135.

Cudmore. J. (1998). Keep with it. *Nursing Times*, 94(23), 78–79.

Curtin, L.L. (1987). Education and licensure: Once more into the breach [Editorial]. *Nursing Management*, 18(5), 9–10.

Cutcliffe, J.R. and Goward, P. (2000). Mental health nurses and qualitative research methods: A mutual attraction? *Journal of Advanced Nursing*, 31(3), 590–598.

Davies, C., Welham, V., Glover, A., Jones, L., and Murphy, F. (1999). Teaching in practice. *Nursing Standard*, 13(35), 33–38.

Dawson, P.J. (1997). Comment on: Journal of Psychiatric and Mental Health Nursing (1996), 3(1), 7–12. A reply to Kevin Gournay's "Schizophrenia: A review of the contemporary literature and implications for mental health nursing theory, practice and education." *Journal of Psychiatric and Mental Health Nursing*, 4(1), 1–7.

Dawson, P.J. (1997). Is there anyone in there? Psychiatric nursing meets biological psychiatry. *Nursing Inquiry*, 4(3), 167–175.

Dean, J.M. and Mountford, B. (1998). Innovation in the assessment of nursing theory and its evaluation: A team approach. *Journal of Advanced Nursing*, 28(2), 409–418.

DeGroot, H.A., Ferketich, S.L., and Larson, P.J. (1987). Theory development in a non-university service setting. *Journal of Nursing Administration*, 17(4), 38–44.

DeMong, N.C. and Assie-Lussier, L.L. (1999). Continuing education: An aspect of staff development relating to the nurse manager's role. *Journal for Nurses in Staff Development*, 15(1), 19–22.

Derdiarian, A. (1979). Education: A way to theory construction in nursing. *Journal of Nursing Education*, 18(2), 36–47.

Derstine, J.B. (1989). The development of theory-based practice by graduate students in rehabilitative nursing. *Rehabilitation Nursing*, 14(2), 88–89.

DeSanto-Madeya, S. (2007). Using case studies based on a nursing conceptual model to teach medical-surgical nursing. *Nursing Science Quarterly*, 20(4), 324–329.

DiBartolo, M.C. (1998). Philosophy of science in doctoral nursing education revisited. *Journal of Professional Nursing*, 14(6), 350–360.

Dickoff, J. and James, P. (1970). Beliefs and values: Bases for curriculum design. *Nursing Research*, 19(5), 415–427.

Diekelmann, N. (1988). *Curriculum revolution: A theoretical and philosophical mandate for change* (Publication No. 15–2224, pp. 137–157). New York: National League for Nursing.

Dougal, J. and Gonterman, R. (1999). A comparison of three teaching methods on learning and retention. *Journal for Nurses in Staff Development*, 15(5), 205–209.

Dowie, S. and Park, C. (1988). Relating nursing theory to students' life experiences. *Nurse Education Today*, 8(4), 191–196.

Downs, F.S. (1988). Doctoral education: Our claim to the future. *Nursing Outlook*, 36(1), 18–20.

Driver, J. and Campbell, J. (2000). An evaluation of the impact of lecturer practitioners on learning. *British Journal of Nursing*, 9(5), 292–300.

Dudley-Brown, S.L. (1997). The evaluation of nursing theory: A method for our madness. *International Journal of Nursing Studies*, 34(1), 76–83.

Duff, V. (1989). Perspective transformation: The challenge for the RN in the baccalaureate program. *Journal of Nursing Education*, 28(1), 38–39.

Duffy, K. and Scott, P.A. (1998). Viewing an old issue through a new lens: A critical theory insight into the education-practice gap. *Nurse Education Today*, 18(3), 183–189.

Duldt, B.W. (1995). Nursing process: The science of nursing in the curriculum. *Nurse Educator*, 20, 24–29.

Durgahee, T. (1998). Facilitating reflection: From a sage on stage to a guide on the side. *Nurse Education Today*, 18(2), 158–164.

Edmond, C.B. (2001). A new paradigm for practice education. *Nurse Education Today*, 21(4), 251–259.

Edwards, S.D. (1998). The art of nursing. *Nursing Ethics*, 5(5), 393–400.

Elcock. K. (1998). Lecturer practitioner: A concept analysis. *Journal of Advanced Nursing*, 28(5), 1092–1098.

Emden, C. (1998). Conducting a narrative analysis. *Collegian*, 5(3), 34–39.

Emden, C. and Young, W. (1987). Theory development in nursing: Australian nurses advance global debate. *Australian Journal of Advanced Nursing*, 4(3), 22–40.

Fawcett, J. (1985). Theory: Basis for the study and practice of nursing education. *Journal of Nursing Education*, 24(6), 226–229.

Fealy, G.M. (1997). The theory-practice relationship in nursing: An exploration of contemporary discourse. *Journal of Advanced Nursing*, 25(5), 1061–1069.

Fernandez, E. (1997). Just "doing the observations": Reflective practice in nursing. *British Journal of Nursing*, 6(16), 939–943.

Fielding, R.G. and Llewelyn, S.P. (1987). Communication in nursing may damage your health and enthusiasm: Some warnings. *Journal of Advanced Nursing Science*, 12(3), 281–290.

Fishel, A.H. (1998). Nursing management of anxiety and panic. *Nursing Clinics of North America*, 33(1), 135–151.

Fitzpatrick, J.J. (1987). Use of existing nursing models. *Journal of Gerontological Nursing*, 13(9), 8–9.

Fletcher, J. (1997). Do nurses really care? Some unwelcome findings from recent research and inquiry. *Journal of Nursing Management*, 5(1), 43–50.

Ford-Gilboe, M., Campbell, J., and Berman, H. (1995). Stories and numbers: Coexistence without compromise. *Advances in Nursing Science*, 18(1), 14–26.

Fowler, J. and Chevannes, M. (1998). Evaluating the efficacy of reflective practice within the context of clinical supervision. *Journal of Advanced Nursing*, 27(2), 379–382.

Francis, D., Owens, J., and Tollefson, J. (1998). "It comes together at the end": The impact of a one-year subject in Nursing Inquiry on philosophies of nursing. *Nursing Inquiry*, 5(4), 268–278.

Frank, B. (1994). Teaching nursing theory: A walk around the golf course. *Nurse Educator*, 19, 26–27.

Funnell. C. (1999). Empathy in the clinical context. *Contemporary Nurse*, 8(4), 142–145.

Gagan, M.J., Badger, T.A., and de Leon Baker, M. (1999). Nurse practitioner interventions for domestic violence. *Clinical Excellence in Nurse Practice*, 3(5), 273–278.

Gaines, C. (1999). Clearing up the "concept fog." *Journal of the Association of Black Nursing Faculty in Higher Education*,10(2), 52–53.

Gassner, L.A, Wotton, K., Clare, J., Hofmeyer, A., and Buckman, J. (1999). Evaluation of a model of collaboration: Academic and clinician partnership in the development and implementation of undergraduate teaching. *Collegian*, 6(3), 14–21.

Geanellos, R. (1998). Hermeneutic philosophy. Part II: A nursing research example of the hermeneutic imperative to address forestructures/pre-understandings. *Nursing Inquiry*, 5(4), 238–247.

Goode, H. (1998). The theory-practice gap and student nurses. *Journal of Child Health Care*, 2(2), 86–90.

Gordon, N.S. (1998). Influencing mental health nursing practice through the teaching of research and theory: A personal critical review. *Journal of Psychiatric and Mental Health Nursing*, 5(2), 119–128.

Gormley, K.J. (1997). Practice write-ups: An assessment instrument that contributes to bridging the differences between theory and practice for student nurses through the development of core skills. *Nurse Education Today*, 17(1), 53–57.

Graham, L. (1979). The development of a useful conceptual framework in curriculum design. *Nursing Papers Perspective in Nursing*, 9(3), 84–92.

Greenwood, J. (1988). More considerations concerning the application of nursing models to curricula: A reply to Lorraine Smith. *Nurse Education Today*, 8(4), 187–190.

Greenwood, J. (1998). Establishing an international network on nurses' clinical reasoning. *Journal of Advanced Nursing*, 27(4), 843–847.

Greenwood, J. (2000). Critical thinking and nursing scripts: The case for the development of both. *Journal of Advanced Nursing*, 31(2), 428–436.

Haddock. J. (1997). Reflection in groups: Contextual and theoretical considerations within nurse education and practice. *Nurse Education Today*, 17(5), 381–385.

Hagey, R. and MacKay RW. (2000). Qualitative research to identify racialist discourse: Towards equity in nursing curricula. *International Journal of Nursing Studies*, 37(1), 45–56.

Haggerty, L.A. (1987). An analysis of senior nursing students' immediate responses to distressed patients. *Journal of Advanced Nursing*, 12(4), 451–461.

Hall, K.V. (1979, April). Current trends in the use of conceptual frameworks in nursing education. *Journal of Nursing Education*, 18(4), 26–29.

Hallett, C.E. (1997). Learning through reflection in the community: The relevance of Schon's theories of coaching to nursing education. *International Journal of Nursing Studies*, 34(2), 103–110.

Hallett, C.E. (1997). The helping relationship in the community setting: The relevance of Rogerian theory to the supervision of Project (2000) students. *International Journal of Nursing Studies*, 34(6), 415–419.

Hams, S. (1998). Intuition and the coronary care nurse. *Nursing in Critical Care*, 3(3), 130–133.

Hancock, P. (1999). Reflective practice—Using a learning journal. *Nursing Standard*, 13(17), 37–40.

Happell, B. (1998). Psychiatric nursing: Has it been forgotten in contemporary nursing education? *Nurse Educator*, 23(6), 9–10.

Happell, B. (2007). Conference presentations: Developing nursing knowledge by disseminating research findings. *Nursing Research*, 15(1), 70–77.

Harrison, J., Saunders, M.E., and Sims, A. (1977). Integrating theory and practice in modular schemes for basic nursing education. *Journal of Advanced Nursing*, 2, 503–519.

Hartley, L.A. (1988). Congruence between teaching and learning self-care: A pilot study. *Nursing Science Quarterly*, 1(4), 161–167.

Hart, M.A. and Foster, S.N. (1998). Self-care agency in two groups of pregnant women. *Nursing Science Quarterly*, 11(4), 167–171.

Hartrick, G. (1998). A critical pedagogy for family nursing. *Journal of Nursing Education*, 37(2), 80–84.

Heinrich, K. (1989). Growing pains: Faculty stages in adopting a nursing model. *Nurse Educator*, 14(1), 3–4, 29.

Heinrich, K.T., Robinson, C.M., and Scales, M.E. (1998). Support groups: An empowering, experiential strategy. *Nurse Educator*, 23(4), 8–10.

Heslop, L. (1998). A discursive exploration of nursing work in the hospital emergency setting. *Nursing Inquiry*, 5(2), 87–95.

Heye, M.L. and Goddard. L. (1999). Teaching pain management: How to make it work. *Journal for Nurses in Staff Development*, 15(1), 27–36.

Higgins, A., Barker, P., and Begley, C.M. (2005). Neuroleptic medication and sexuality: The forgotten aspect of education and care. *Journal of Psychiatric and Mental Health Nursing*, 12(4), 439–446.

Hill, P.F. (1998). Assessing the competence of student nurses. *Journal of Child Health Care*, 2(1), 25–30.

Hilz, L.M. (2000). The informatics nurse specialist as change agent. Application of innovation-diffusion theory. *Computers in Nursing*, 18(6), 272–278.

Hisama, K.K. (1999). Towards an international theory of nursing. *Nursing and Health Sciences*, 1(2), 77–81.

Holland, S. (1999). Teaching nursing ethics by cases: A personal perspective. *Nursing Ethics*, 6(5), 434–436.

Hurlock-Chorostecki, C. (1999). Holistic care in the critical care setting: Application of a concept through Watson's and Orem's theories of nursing. *Official Journal of the Canadian Association of Critical Care Nurses/CACCN*, 10(4), 20–25.

Hyrkas, K., Koivula, M., and Paunonen, M. (1999). Clinical supervision in nursing in the 1990s—Current state of concepts, theory and research. *Journal of Nursing Management*, 7(3), 177–187.

Jaarsma, T., Halfens, R., Senten, M., Abu Saad, H.H., and Dracup, K. (1998). Developing a supportive-educative program for patients with advanced heart failure within Orem's general theory of nursing. *Nursing Science Quarterly*, 11(2), 79–85.

Jacobs-Kramer, M.K. and Huether, S.E. (1988). Curricular considerations for teaching nursing theory. *Journal of Professional Nursing*, 4(5), 373–380.

Jacobson, S. (1987). Studying and using conceptual models of nursing. *Image: Journal of Nursing Scholarship*, 19(2), 78–82.

Jameton, A. and Fowler, M.D. (1989). Ethical inquiry and the concept of research. *Advances in Nursing Science*, 11(3), 11–24.

Jansen, M.P.M. and Zwygart-Stauffacher, M. (2006). *Advanced practice nursing: Core concepts for professional role development* (3rd ed.). New York: Springer Publishing Company.

Johnson, S.E. (1989). A picture is worth a thousand words: Helping students visualize a conceptual model. *Nurse Educator*, 14(3), 21–24.

Johnstone, M.J. (1999). Reflective topical autobiography: An under utilised interpretive research method in nursing. *Collegian*, 6(1), 24–29.

Jones, K.N. (1999). Reflection: An alternative to nursing models. *Professional Nurse*, 14(12), 853–855.

Jordan, S. (1998). From classroom theory to clinical practice: Evaluating the impact of a post--registration course. *Nurse Education Today*, 18(4), 293–302.

Karmels, P. (1993). Conundrum game for nursing theorists Neuman, King, and Johnson. *Nurse Educator*, 18(6), 8–9.

Kathol, D.D., Geiger. M.L., and Hartig, J.L. (1998). Clinical correlation map. A tool for linking theory and practice. *Nurse Educator*, 23(4), 31–34.

Kennedy, D. and Barloon, L.F. (1997). Managing burnout in pediatric critical care: The human care commitment. *Critical Care Nursing Quarterly*, 20(2), 63–71.

Ketefian, S. and Redman, R.W. (1997). Nursing science in the global community. *Image: Journal of Nursing Scholarship*, 29(1), 11–15.

Khatib, H.M. and Ford, S. (1999). The virtual theory-practice gap. *Journal of Child Health Care*, 3(2), 36–38.

Kim, H.S. (1999). Critical reflective inquiry for knowledge development in nursing practice. *Journal of Advanced Nursing*, 29(5), 1205–1212.

King, I.M. (1997). King's theory of goal attainment in practice. *Nursing Science Quarterly*, 10(4), 180–185.

Krawczyk, R.M. (1997). Teaching ethics: Effect on moral development. *Nursing Ethics*, 4(1), 57–65.

Kristjanson, L.J., Tamblyn, R., and Kuypers, J.A. (1987). A model to guide development and application of multiple nursing theories. *Journal of Advanced Nursing*, 12(4), 523–529.

Kuss, T., Proulx-Girouard, L., Lovitt, S., Katz, C.B., and Kennelly, P. (1997). A public health nursing model. *Public Health Nursing*, 14(2), 81–91.

Lacko, L., Bryan, Y., Dellasega, C., and Salerno, F. (1999). Changing clinical practice through research: The case of delirium. *Clinical Nursing Research*, 8(3), 235–250.

Lait, M.E. (2000). The place of nursing history in an undergraduate curriculum. *Nurse Education Today*, 20(5), 395–400.

Landers, M.G. (2000). The theory-practice gap in nursing: The role of the nurse teacher. *Journal of Advanced Nursing*, 32(6), 1550–1556.

Landrum, B.J. (1998). Marketing innovations to nurses. Part 1: How people adopt innovations. *Journal of Wound, Ostomy, and Continence Nursing*, 25(4), 194–199.

Lauder, W. (1994). Beyond reflection: Practical wisdom and the practical syllogism. *Nurse Education Today*, 14(2), 91–98.

Lauder, W., Reynolds, W., and Angus, N. (1999). Transfer of knowledge and skills: Some implications for nursing and nurse education. *Nurse Education Today*, 19(6), 480–487.

Lawrence, S.A. and Lawrence, R.M. (1983). Curriculum development: Philosophy, objectives, and conceptual framework. *Nursing Outlook*, 31(3), 160–163.

Leininger, M. (1997). Transcultural nursing research to transform nursing education and practice: 40 years. *Image: Journal of Nursing Scholarship*, 29(4), 341–347.

Leininger, M.M. (1997). Transcultural nursing as a global care humanizer, diversifier, and unifier. *Hoitotiede*, 9(5), 219–225.

Liaschenko, J. and Fisher, A. (1999). Theorizing the knowledge that nurses use in the conduct of their work. *Scholarly Inquiry for Nursing Practice*, 13(1), 29–41.

Linscott, J., Spee, R., Flint, F., and Fisher, A. (1999). Creating a culture of patient-focused care through a learner-centered philosophy. *Canadian Journal of Nursing Leadership*, 12(4), 5–10.

Logsdon, M.C. and Ford, D. (1998). Service-learning for graduate students. *Nurse Educator*, 23(2), 34–37.

Long, G., Grandis, S., and Glasper, E.A. (1999). Investing in practice: Enquiry- and problem-based learning. *British Journal of Nursing*, 8(17), 1171–1174.

Lo, R. and Brown, R. (1999). The importance of theory in student nurses' psychiatric practicum. *International Journal of Psychiatric Nursing Research*, 5(1), 542–552.

Lott, J.W. and Hoath, S.B. (1998). Neonatal skin: The ideal nursing interface. *Journal of Pediatric Nursing*, 13(5), 302–306.

Luna, L. (1998). Culturally competent health care: A challenge for nurses in Saudi Arabia. *Journal of Transcultural Nursing*, 9(2), 8–14.

MacGregor, J. and Dewar, K. (1997). Opening up the options: Making the inflexible into a flexible framework. *Nurse Education Today*, 17(5), 502–507.

Mariano, C. (2002). Crisis theory and intervention: A critical component of nursing education. *Journal of the New York State Nurses Association*, 33(1), 19–24.

Markovic, M. (1997). From theory to perioperative practice with Parse. *Canadian Operating Room Nursing Journal*, 15(1), 13–19.

Martin, S.R. (1997). Agricultural safety and health: Principles and possibilities for nursing education. *Journal of Nursing Education*, 36(2), 74–78.

Masters, M. (1988). Nursing theory: An electric approach in baccalaureate education. *Kansas Nurse*, 63(12), 1–2.

Mavundla, T.R. (2000). Professional nurses' perception of nursing mentally ill people in a general hospital setting. *Journal of Advanced Nursing*, 32(6), 1569–1578.

McCance, T.V., McKenna, H.P., and Boore, J.R. (1999). Caring: Theoretical perspectives of relevance to nursing. *Journal of Advanced Nursing*, 30(6), 1388–1395.

McEwen, M. (2000). Teaching theory at the master's level: Report of a national survey of theory instructors. *Journal of Professional Nursing*, 16(6), 354–361.

McGrath, B.B. (1998). Illness as a problem of meaning: Moving culture from the classroom to the clinic. *Advances in Nursing Science*, 21(2), 17–29.

McHolm, F.A. and Geib, K.M. (1998). Application of the Neuman Systems Model to teaching health assessment and nursing process. *Nursing Diagnosis*, 9(1), 23–33.

McKenna, H.P. (1997). Theory and research: A linkage to benefit practice. *International Journal of Nursing Studies*, 34(6), 431–437.

McLaughlin, C. (1997). The effect of classroom theory and contact with patients on the attitudes of student nurses towards mentally ill people. *Journal of Advanced Nursing*, 26(6), 1221–1228.

McLoughlin, A. (1997). The "F" factor: Feminism forsaken? *Nurse Education Today*, 17(2), 111–114.

McMahon, R. (1988). The "24-hour reality orientation" type of approach to the confused elderly: A minimum standard for care. *Journal of Advanced Nursing*, 13(6), 693–700.

McVicar, A. and Clancy, J. (1998). Homeostasis: A framework for integrating the life sciences. *British Journal of Nursing*, 7(10), 601–607.

Meleis, A.I. and May, K.M. (1981). Nursing theory and scholarliness in the doctoral program. *Advances in Nursing Science*, 4(1), 31–41.

Meleis, A.I. and Price, M. (1988). Strategies and conditions for teaching theoretical nursing: An international perspective. *Journal of Advanced Nursing*, 13, 592–604.

Meleis, A.I., Wilson, H.S., and Chater, S. (1980). Toward scholarliness in doctoral dissertations: An analytical model. *Journal of Research in Nursing and Health*, 3, 115–124.

Miller, S.K. (1999). Nurse practitioners in the county correctional facility setting: Unique challenges and suggestions for effective health promotion. *Clinical Excellence in Nurse Practice*, 3(5), 268–272.

Minicucci, D.S. (1998). A review and synthesis of the literature: The use of presence in the nursing care of families. *Journal of the New York State Nurses Association*, 29(3–4), 9–15.

Mohr, W.K. and Naylor, M.D. (1998). Creating a curriculum for the 21st century. *Nursing Outlook*, 46(5), 206–212.

Mulholland, J. (1997). Assimilating sociology: Critical reflections on the "sociology in nursing" debate. *Journal of Advanced Nursing*, 25(4), 844–852.

Neal, L.J. (1997). The rehabilitation nursing paradigm: Implications for home care. *Caring*, 16(2), 66–68.

Neal, L.J. (1999). Facilitating the growth of nursing staff case management in PPS. *Caring*, 18(10), 46–48.

Nolan, M., Lundh, U., and Tishelman, C. (1998). Nursing's knowledge base: Does it have to be unique? *British Journal of Nursing*, 7(5), 270–276.

Nolan, M. and Tolson, D. (2000). Gerontological nursing. 1: Challenges nursing older people in acute care. *British Journal of Nursing*, 9(1), 39–42.

Nolan, M. and Tolson, D. (2000). Gerontological nursing. 5: Realizing the future potential. *British Journal of Nursing*, 9(5), 272–274.

Northrup, D.T. and Cody, W.K. (1998). Evaluation of the human becoming theory in practice in an acute care psychiatric setting. *Nursing Science Quarterly*, 11(1), 23–30.

Olsson, H.M. and Gullberg, M.T. (1987). Nursing education: A valuation of theoretical and practical sections of the education. Expectations and knowledge of the nurse role. *Vardi i Norden*, 7(13), 412–416.

Padgett, S.M. (2000). Benner and the critics: Promoting scholarly dialogue. *Scholarly Inquiry for Nursing Practice*, 14(3), 249–266.

Penney, W. and Warelow, P.J. (1999). Understanding the prattle of praxis. *Nursing Inquiry*, 6(4), 259–268.

Peplau, H.E. (1997). Peplau's theory of interpersonal relations. *Nursing Science Quarterly*, 10(4), 162–167.

Pepler, C. (1977). The practical aspects of using a conceptual framework. *Nursing Papers*, 9(3), 93–101.

Perry, B. (1998). Beliefs of eight exemplary oncology nurses related to Watson's nursing theory. *Canadian Oncology Nursing Journal*, 8(2), 97–107.

Phillips, R., Donald, A., Mousseau-Gershman, Y., and Powell, T. (1998). Applying theory to practice—The use of "ripple effect" plans in continuing education. *Nurse Education Today*, 18(1), 12–19.

Pierson, W. (1998). Reflection and nursing education. *Journal of Advanced Nursing*, 27(1), 165–170.

Potter, M.L. and Bockenhauer, B.J. (2000). Implementing Orlando's nursing theory: A pilot study. *Journal of Psychosocial Nursing and Mental Health Services*, 38(3), 14–21.

Priest, H. and Roberts, P. (1998). Assessing students' clinical performance. *Nursing Standard*, 12(48), 37–41.

Punton, S. (1989). King's fund nursing development. The Oxford experience. *Nursing Standard*, 3(22), 27–28.

Purdy. M. (1997). Humanist ideology and nurse education. I. Humanist educational theory. *Nurse Education Today*, 17(3), 192–195.

Rafael, A.R. (2000). Watson's philosophy, science, and theory of human caring as a conceptual framework for guiding community health nursing practice. *Advances in Nursing Science*, 23(2), 34–49.

Rajabally, M. (1977). Frankly speaking. Nursing education: Another tower of Babel. *Canadian Nurse*, 73(9), 30–31.

Ray, M.A. (1997). Consciousness and the moral ideal: A transcultural analysis of Watson's theory of transpersonal caring. *Advanced Practice Nursing Quarterly*, 3(1), 25–31.

Ream, E. and Richardson, A. (1999). Comment in Oncology Nursing Forum (2000), 27(3), 425–426. From theory to practice: Designing interventions to reduce fatigue in patients with cancer. *Oncology Nursing Forum*, 26(8), 1295–1303.

Reid, B., Allen, A.F., Gauthier, T., and Campbell, H. (1989). Solving the Orem mystery: An educational strategy. *Journal of Continuing Education in Nursing*, 20(3), 108–110.

Rogers, M.E. (1989). Creating a climate for the implementation of a nursing conceptual framework. *Journal of Continuing Education in Nursing*, 20(3), 112–116.

Rolfe, G. (1997). Beyond expertise: Theory, practice and the reflexive practitioner. *Journal of Clinical Nursing*, 6(2), 93–97.

Rosanoff, N. (1999). Intuition comes of age: Workplace applications of intuitive skill for occupational and environmental health nurses. *Official Journal of the American Association of Occupational Health Nurses*, 47(4), 156–162.

Ross, M.M., Bourbonnais, F.F., and Carroll, G. (1987). Curricular design and the Betty Neuman systems model: A new approach to learning. *International Nursing Review*, 34(3), 75–79.

Roy, C. (1979). Relating nursing theory to education: A new era. *Nurse Educator*, 4(2), 16–21.

Rutty, J.E. (1998). The nature of philosophy of science, theory and knowledge relating to nursing and professionalism. *Journal of Advanced Nursing*, 28(2), 243–250.

Sadala, M.L. (1999). Taking care as a relationship: A phenomenological view. *Journal of Advanced Nursing*, 30(4), 808–817.

Sakalys, J.A. (2002). Literary pedagogy in nursing: A theory-based perspective. *Journal of Nursing Education*, 41(9), 386–392.

Sanford, R.C. (2000). Caring through relation and dialogue: A nursing perspective for patient education. *Advances in Nursing Science*, 22(3), 1–15.

Scammell, J. and Miller, S. (1999). Back to basics: Exploring the conceptual basis of nursing. *Nurse Education Today*, 19(7), 570–577.

Scanlan, J.M. and Chernomas, W.M. (1997). Developing the reflective teacher. *Journal of Advanced Nursing*, 25(6), 1138–1143.

Scherer, Z.A. and Scherer, E.A. (2007). Reflections on nursing teaching in the post-modernity era and the metaphor of a theory-practice gap. *Revista Latino-Americana de Enfermagem*, 15(3), 498–501.

Schmieding, N.J. and Waldman, R.C. (1997). Gastric decompression in adult patients. Survey of nursing practice. *Clinical Nursing Research*, 6(2), 142–155.

Schultz, E.D. (1998). Academic advising from a nursing theory perspective. *Nurse Educator*, 23(2), 22–25.

Selanders, L.C. (1998). Florence Nightingale: The evolution and social impact of feminist values in nursing. *Journal of Holistic Nursing*, 16(2), 227–243.

Severinsson, E.I. (1998). Bridging the gap between theory and practice: A supervision programme for nursing students. *Journal of Advanced Nursing*, 27(6), 1269–1277.

Shriver, C.B. and Scott-Stiles, A. (2000). Health habits of nursing versus non-nursing students: A longitudinal study. *Journal of Nursing Education*, 39(7), 308–314.

Sills, G.M. (1998). Peplau and professionalism: The emergence of the paradigm of professionalization. *Journal of Psychiatric and Mental Health Nursing*, 5(3), 167–171.

Slaninka, S.C. (1999). Nursing theories: Creative teaching strategies make this course come alive. *Nurse Educator*, 24(3), 40–43.

Smith, A. (1998). Learning about reflection. *Journal of Advanced Nursing*, 28(4), 891–898.

Smith, L.S. (1998). Concept analysis: Cultural competence. *Journal of Cultural Diversity*, 5(1), 4–10.

Sorrell, J.M. and Redmond, G.M. (1997). The lived experiences of students in nursing: Voices of caring speak of the tact of teaching. *Journal of Professional Nursing*, 13(4), 228–235.

Sortet, J.P. (1989). Incongruence in the nursing profession. *Nursing Management*, 20(5), 64–66, 68.

Spouse, J. (2001). Bridging theory and practice in the supervisory relationship: A sociocultural perspective. *Journal of Advanced Nursing*, 33(4), 512–522.

Stark, S., Cooke, P., and Stronach, I. (2000). Minding the gap: Some theory-practice disjunctions in nursing education research. *Nurse Education Today*, 20(2), 155–163.

Stein, K.F., Corte, C., Colling, K.B., and Whall, A. (1998). A theoretical analysis of Carper's ways of knowing using a model of social cognition. *Scholarly Inquiry for Nursing Practice*, 12(1), 43–60.

Stewart, K.E., DiClemente, R.J., and Ross, D. (1999). Adolescents and HIV: Theory-based approaches to education of nurses. *Journal of Advanced Nursing*, 30(3), 687–696.

Tanner, J. (1999). Problem based learning: An opportunity for theatre nurse education. *British Journal of Theatre Nursing*, 9(11), 531–536.

Thompson, J.M. (2001). Teaching tools. An icebreaker to introduce nursing theory. *Nurse Educator*, 26(1), 13–14.

Thorne, S.E., Kirkham, S.R., and Henderson, A. (1999). Ideological implications of paradigm discourse. *Nursing Inquiry*, 6(2), 123–131.

Tilley, S. (1999). Altschul's legacy in mediating British and American psychiatric nursing discourses: Common sense and the "absence" of the accountable practitioner. *Journal of Psychiatric and Mental Health Nursing*, 6(4), 283–295.

Timpka, T. (2000). The patient and the primary care team: A small-scale critical theory. *Journal of Advanced Nursing*, 31(3), 558–564.

Torres, G. and Yura, H. (1974). *Today's conceptual framework: Its relationship to the curriculum development process* (Publication No. 15–1529). New York: National League for Nursing.

Turnbull, J. (1999). Intuition in nursing relationships: The result of "skills" or "qualities?" *British Journal of Nursing*, 8(5), 302–306.

Turner, S.L. and Bentley, G.W. (1998). A meaningful health assessment course for baccalaureate nursing students. *Nursing Connections*, 11(2), 5–12.

Upton, D.J. (1999). How can we achieve evidence-based practice if we have a theory-practice gap in nursing today? *Journal of Advanced Nursing*, 29(3), 549–555.

Vandermark, L.M. (2006). Awareness of self and expanding consciousness: Using nursing theories to prepare nurse-therapists. *Issues in Mental Health Nursing*, 27(6), 605–615.

Wainwright, P. (2000). Towards an aesthetics of nursing. *Journal of Advanced Nursing*, 32(3), 750–756.

Walker, M.K. and Norby, R.B. (1987–1988). An essay on friendships of utility: Resolving the disalignment between nursing education and nursing service. *Nursing Forum*, 23(1), 30–35.

Warelow, P.J. (1997). A nursing journey through discursive praxis. *Journal of Advanced Nursing*, 26(5), 1020–1027.

Weingourt, R. (1998). Using Margaret A. Newman's theory of health with elderly nursing home residents. *Perspectives in Psychiatric Care*, 34(3), 25–30.

Wenzel, L.S., Briggs, K.L., and Puryear, B.L. (1998). Portfolio: Authentic assessment in the age of the curriculum revolution. *Journal of Nursing Education*, 37(5), 208–212.

Westbrook, L.O. and Schultz, P.R. (2000). From theory to practice: Community health nursing in a public health neighborhood team. *Advances in Nursing Science*, 23(2), 50–61.

White, S.J. (1997). Empathy: A literature review and concept analysis. *Journal of Clinical Nursing*, 6(4), 253–257.

Whitener, L.M., Cox, K.R., and Maglich, S.A. (1998). Use of theory to guide nurses in the design of health messages for children. *Advances in Nursing Science*, 20(3), 21–35.

Wilkinson, C., Peters, L., Mitchell, K., Irwin, T., McCorrie, K., and MacLeod, M. (1998). "Being there": Learning through active participation. *Nurse Education Today*, 18(3), 226–230.

Wilkinson, R.A. (1999). Triage in accident and emergency. 2: Educational requirements. *British Journal of Nursing*, 8(3), 165–168.

Williams, A.M. (1998). The delivery of quality nursing care: A grounded theory study of the nurse's perspective. *Journal of Advanced Nursing*, 27(4), 808–816.

Williams, R. (1999). Cultural safety—What does it mean for our work practice? Australian and New Zealand Journal of Public Health, 23(2), 213–214. *Comment in: Australian and New Zealand Journal of Public Health*, 23(5), 552–553.

Willis, W.O. (1999). Culturally competent nursing care during the perinatal period. *Journal of Perinatal and Neonatal Nursing*, 13(3), 45–59.

Wilshaw, G. (1999). Perspectives on surviving childhood sexual abuse. *Journal of Advanced Nursing*, 30(2), 303–309.

Wissmann, J.L. (1994). Teaching nursing theory through an election campaign framework. *Nurse Educator*, 9, 21–23.

Wood, I. (1998). The effects of continuing professional education on the clinical practice of nurses: A review of the literature. *International Journal of Nursing Studies*, 35(3), 125–131.

Wynne, N., Brand, S., and Smith, R. (1997). Incomplete holism in pre-registration nurse education: The position of the biological sciences. *Journal of Advanced Nursing*, 26(3), 470–474.

Zoucha, R. and Husted, G.L. (2000). The ethical dimensions of delivering culturally congruent nursing and health care. *Issues in Mental Health Nursing*, 21(3), 325–340.

11. Theory and Administration

Allen, D. (1997). Nursing, knowledge and practice. *Journal of Health Services Research and Policy*, 2(3), 190–193.

Anderson, J.M. (1991). Reflexivity in fieldwork: Toward a feminist epistemology. *Image: Journal of Nursing Scholarship*, 23, 115–118.

Anderson, R.A., Dobal, M.T., and Blessing, B. (1992). Theory-based approach to computer skill development in nursing administration. *Computers in Nursing*, 10(4), 152–157.

August-Brady, M. (2000). Prevention as intervention. *Journal of Advanced Nursing*, 31(6), 1304–1308.

Barker, P. (1998). The future of the theory of interpersonal relations? A personal reflection on Peplau's legacy. *Journal of Psychiatric and Mental Health Nursing*, 5(3), 213–220.

Barker, P., Jackson, S., and Stevenson C. (1999). The need for psychiatric nursing: Towards a multidimensional theory of caring. *Nursing Inquiry*, 6(2), 103–111.

Barker, P., Jackson, S., and Stevenson C. (1999). What are psychiatric nurses needed for? Developing a theory of essential nursing practice. *Journal of Psychiatric and Mental Health Nursing*, 6(4), 273–282.

Barnes, M. (1999). Research in midwifery—The relevance of a feminist theoretical framework. *Journal of the Australian College of Midwives*, 12(2), 6–10.

Beck, C.T. (1982). The conceptualization of power. *Advances in Nursing Science*, 1, 1–17.

Beeber, L.S. (1998). Treating depression through the therapeutic nurse-client relationship. *Nursing Clinics of North America*, 33(1), 153–172.

Biley, F.C. and Freshwater, D. (1999). Trends in nursing and midwifery research and the need for change in complementary therapy research. *Complementary Therapies in Nursing and Midwifery*, 5(4), 99–102.

Blix, A. (1999). Integrating occupational health protection and health promotion: Theory and program application. *Journal of the American Association of Occupational Health Nurses*, 47(4), 168–171.

Bondas-Salonen, T. (1998). New mothers' experiences of postpartum care—A phenomenological follow-up study. *Journal of Clinical Nursing*, 7(2), 165–174.

Booth, K., Kenrick, M., and Woods, S. (1997). Nursing knowledge, theory and method revisited. *Journal of Advanced Nursing*, 26(4), 804–811.

Brennan, P.F. and Anthony, M.K. (2000). Measuring nursing practice models using Multi-Attribute Utility Theory. *Research in Nursing and Health*, 23(5), 372–382.

Brown, R. (2000). Describing a model of nursing as a focus for psychiatric nursing care. *International Journal of Psychiatric Nursing Research*, 6(1), 670–682.

Cash, K. (1997). Social epistemology, gender and nursing theory. *International Journal of Nursing Studies*, 34(2), 137–143.

Chambers, M. (1998). Interpersonal mental health nursing: Research issues and challenges. *Journal of Psychiatric and Mental Health Nursing*, 5(3), 203–211.

Clark, J. (1998). The unique function of the nurse. *Nursing Standard*, 12(16), 39–42.

Clifford, C. (1997). Nurse teachers and research. *Nurse Education Today*, 17(2), 115–120.

Colodny, A. (1997). Spinal cord injury nurses in action: Partners in practice. *SCI Nursing*, 14(3), 79–82.

Crossan, F. and Robb, A. (1998). Role of the nurse: Introducing theories and concepts. *British Journal of Nursing*, 7(10), 608–612.

Cutcliffe, J.R. (2000). Methodological issues in grounded theory. *Journal of Advanced Nursing*, 31(6), 1476–1484.

DeGroot, H.A., Ferketich, S.L., and Larson, P.J. (1987). Theory development in a non-university service setting. *Journal of Nursing Administration*, 17(4), 38–44.

DeMong, N.C. and Assie-Lussier. L.L. (1999). Continuing education: An aspect of staff development relating to the nurse manager's role. *Journal of Nursing Staff Development*, 15(1), 19–22.

Dixon, E.L. (1999). Community health nursing practice and the Roy Adaptation Model. *Public Health Nursing*, 16(4), 290–300.

Dorsey, K. and Purcell, S. (1987). Translating a nursing theory into a nursing system. *Geriatric Nursing*, 8(3), 136–137.

Driver, J. and Campbell, J. (2000). An evaluation of the impact of lecturer practitioners on learning. *British Journal of Nursing*, 9(5), 292–300.

Dunlap, K. (1998). The practice of nursing theory in the operating room. *Today's Surgical Nurse*, 20(5), 18–22.

Dyson, M. (1999). Intensive care unit psychosis, the therapeutic nurse-patient relationship and the influence of the intensive care setting: Analyses of interrelating factors. *Journal of Clinical Nursing*, 8(3), 284–290.

Engebretson, J. (1997). A multiparadigm approach to nursing. *Advances in Nursing Science*, 20(1), 21–33.

Fagerstrom, L. and Engberg, I.B. (1998). Measuring the unmeasurable: A caring science perspective on patient classification. *Journal of Nursing Management*, 6(3), 165–172.

Fawcett, J., Botter, M., Burritt, J., Crossly, J., and Frink, B. (1989). Conceptual models of nursing and organization theories. In B. Henry, C. Arndt, M. DiVincenti, and A. Marriner-Tomey (Eds.), *Dimensions of nursing administration: Theory, research, education, practice*. Boston, MA: Blackwell Scientific Publications.

Fealy, G.M. (1999). The theory-practice relationship in nursing: The practitioners' perspective. *Journal of Advanced Nursing*, 30(1), 74–82.

Fielding, R.G. and Llewelyn, S.P. (1987). Communication training in nursing may damage your health and enthusiasm: Some warnings. *Journal of Advanced Nursing*, 12(3), 281–290.

Fishel, A.H. (1998). Nursing management of anxiety and panic. *Nursing Clinics of North America*, 33(1), 135–151.

Fisher, M.A. and Mitchell, G.J. (1998). Patients' views of quality of life: Transforming the knowledge base of nursing. *Clinical Nurse Specialist*, 12(3), 99–105. Comment in *Clinical Nurse Specialist* (1998) 12(3), 98.

Forchuk, C., Jewell, J., Schofield, R., Sircelj, M., and Valledor, T. (1998). From hospital to community: Bridging therapeutic relationships. *Journal of Psychiatric and Mental Health Nursing*, 5(3),197–202.

Fowler, J. and Chevannes, M. (1998). Evaluating the efficacy of reflective practice within the context of clinical supervision. *Journal of Advanced Nursing*, 27(2), 379–382.

Francis, D., Owens, J., and Tollefson, J. (1998). "It comes together at the end": The impact of a one-year subject in Nursing Inquiry on philosophies of nursing. *Nursing Inquiry*, 5(4), 268–278.

Fry, S.T. (1999). The philosophy of nursing. *Scholarly Inquiry in Nursing Practice*, 13(1), 5–15.

Gagan, M.J., Badger, T.A., and de Leon Baker, M. (1999). Nurse practitioner interventions for domestic violence. *Clinical Excellence in Nurse Practice*, 3(5), 273–278.

Gordon, N.S. (1998). Influencing mental health nursing practice through the teaching of research and theory: A personal critical review. *Journal of Psychiatric and Mental Health Nursing*, 5(2), 119–128.

Gottlieb, L.N. and Gottlieb, B. (1998). Evolutionary principles can guide nursing's future development. *Journal of Advanced Nursing*, 28(5), 1099–1105.

Griffith, K.A. (1999). Holism in the care of the allogeneic bone marrow transplant population: Role of the nurse practitioner. *Holistic Nursing Practice*, 13(2), 20–27.

Hallett, C.E. (1997). The helping relationship in the community setting: The relevance of Rogerian theory to the supervision of Project (2000) students. *International Journal of Nursing Studies*, 34(6), 415–419.

Hays, B.J., Norris, J., Martin, K.S., and Androwich, I. (1994). Informatics issues for nursing's future. *Advances in Nursing Science*, 16, 71–81.

Henry, B., Arndt, C., DiVincenti, M., and Marriner-Tomey, A. (Eds.). (1989). *Dimensions of nursing administration: Theory, research, education, practice*. Boston, MA: Blackwell Scientific Publications.

Heslop, L. (1998). A discursive exploration of nursing work in the hospital emergency setting. *Nursing Inquiry*, 5(2), 87–95.

Hickey, G. and Kipping, C. (1998). Exploring the concept of user involvement in mental health through a participation continuum. *Journal of Clinical Nursing*, 7(1), 83–88.

Hicks, C. (1998). Barriers to evidence-based care in nursing: Historical legacies and conflicting cultures. *Journal of the Association of University Programs in Health Administration*, 11(3), 137–147.

Hilz, L.M. (2000). The informatics nurse specialist as change agent. Application of innovation-diffusion theory. *Computers in Nursing*, 18(6), 272–278.

Holland, S. (1999). Teaching nursing ethics by cases: A personal perspective. *Nursing Ethics*, 6(5), 434–436.

Hopkinson, J.B. and Hallett, C.E. (2001). Patients' perceptions of hospice day care: A phenomenological study. *International Journal of Nursing Studies*, 38(1), 117–125.

Hopton, J. (1997). Towards a critical theory of mental health nursing. *Journal of Advanced Nursing*, 25(3), 492–500.

Horrocks, S. (2000). Hunting for Heidegger: Questioning the sources in the Benner/Cash debate. *International Journal of Nursing Studies*, 37(3), 237–243.

Hyrkas, K., Koivula, M., and Paunonen, M. (1999). Clinical supervision in nursing in the 1990s—Current state of concepts, theory and research. *Journal of Nursing Management*, 7(3), 177–187.

Jaarsma, T., Halfens, R., Senten, M., Abu Saad, H.H., and Dracup, K. (1998). Developing a supportive-educative program for patients with advanced heart failure within Orem's general theory of nursing. *Nursing Science Quarterly*, 11(2), 79–85.

Jennings, B.M. and Meleis, A.I. (1988). Nursing theory and administrative practice: Agenda for the 1990s. *Advances in Nursing Science*, 10(3), 56–69.

Jorgenson, J. (1997). Therapeutic use of companion animals in health care. *Image: Journal of Nursing Scholarship*, 29(3), 249–254.

Keddy, B., Gregor, F., Foster, S., and Denney, D. (1999). Theorizing about nurses' work lives: The personal and professional aftermath of living with health care "reform." *Nursing Inquiry*, 6(1), 58–64.

King, I.M. (1997). King's theory of goal attainment in practice. *Nursing Science Quarterly*, 10(4), 180–185.

Kleinbeck, S.V. (2000). Dimensions of perioperative nursing for a national specialty nomenclature. *Journal of Advanced Nursing*, 31(3), 529–535.

Kulbok, P.A., Gates, M.F., Vicenzi, A.E., and Schultz, P.R. (1999). Focus on community: Directions for nursing knowledge development. *Journal of Advanced Nursing*, 29(5), 1188–1196.

Landers, M.G. (2000). The theory-practice gap in nursing: The role of the nurse teacher. *Journal of Advanced Nursing*, 32(6), 1550–1556.

Laurent, C.L. (2000). A nursing theory for nursing leadership. *Journal of Nursing Management*, 8(2), 83–87.

Lego, S. (1998). The application of Peplau's theory to group psychotherapy. *Journal of Psychiatric and Mental Health Nursing*, 5(3), 193–196.

LeVasseur, J.J. (1999). Toward an understanding of art in nursing. *Advances in Nursing Science*, 21(4), 48–63.

Linscott, J., Spee, R., Flint, F., and Fisher, A. (1999). Creating a culture of patient-focused care through a learner-centered philosophy. *Canadian Journal of Nursing Leadership*, 12(4), 5–10.

Machin, T. and Stevenson, C. (1997). Towards a framework for clarifying psychiatric nursing roles. *Journal of Psychiatric and Mental Health Nursing*, 4(2), 81–87.

Mackintosh, C. (2000). "Is there a place for 'care' within nursing?" *International Journal of Nursing Studies*, 37(4), 321–327.

Marck, P. (2000). Nursing in a technological world: Searching for healing communities. *Advances in Nursing Science*, 23(2), 62–81.

McGuire, E. (1999). Chaos theory. Learning a new science. *Journal of Nursing Administration*, 29(2), 8–9.

McKenna, B. and Roberts, R. (1999). Bridging the theory-practice gap. *Nursing New Zealand*, 5(2), 14–16.

McKenna, H. (1999). The role of reflection in the development of practice theory: A case study. *Journal of Psychiatric and Mental Health Nursing*, 6(2), 147–151.

McKenna, H.P. (1997). Theory and research: A linkage to benefit practice. *International Journal of Nursing Studies*, 34(6), 431–437.

Meleis, A.I. (1998). ReVisions in knowledge development: A passion for substance. *Scholarly Inquiry in Nursing Practice*, 12(1), 65–77.

Meleis, A.I. and Jennings, B.M. (1989). Theoretical nursing administration: Today's challenges, tomorrow's bridges. In B. Henry, C. Arndt, M. DiVincenti, and A. Marriner-Tomey (Eds.), *Dimensions of nursing administration: Theory, research, education, practice*. Boston, MA: Blackwell Scientific Publications.

Miller, S.K. (1999). Nurse practitioners in the county correctional facility setting: Unique challenges and suggestions for effective health promotion. *Clinical Excellence in Nurse Practice*, 3(5), 268–272.

Minicucci, D.S. (1998). A review and synthesis of the literature: The use of presence in the nursing care of families. *Journal of the New York State Nurses Association*, 29(3–4), 9–15.

Mohr, W.K. and Naylor, M.D. (1998). Creating a curriculum for the 21st century. *Nursing Outlook*, 46(5), 206–212.

Monti, E.J. and Tingen, M.S. (1999). Multiple paradigms of nursing science. *Advances in Nursing Science*, 21(4), 64–80.

Mulholland, J. (1997). Assimilating sociology: Critical reflections on the "sociology in nursing" debate. *Journal of Advanced Nursing*, 25(4), 844–852.

Neal, L.J. (1999). Facilitating the growth of nursing staff case management in PPS. *Caring*, 18(10), 46–48.

Neill, S.J. (1998). Developing children's nursing through action research. *Journal of Child Health Care*, 2(1), 11–15.

Nelson, S. (1997). Reading nursing history. *Nursing Inquiry*, 4(4), 229–236.

Nolan, M. and Tolson, D. (2000). Gerontological nursing. 1: Challenges nursing older people in acute care. *British Journal of Nursing*, 9(1), 39–42.

Northrup, D.T. and Cody, W.K. (1998). Evaluation of the human becoming theory in practice in an acute care psychiatric setting. *Nursing Science Quarterly*, 11(1), 23–30.

Nyberg, J. (1990). Theoretic explorations of human care and economics: Foundations of nursing administration practice. *Advances in Nursing Science*, 13(1), 74–84.

O'Connell, B., Rapley, P., and Tibbett, P. (1999). Does the nursing diagnosis form the basis for patient care? *Collegian*, 6(3), 29–34.

Parse, R.R. (1999). Nursing science: The transformation of practice. *Journal of Advanced Nursing*, 30(6), 1383–1387.

Penney, W. and Warelow, P.J. (1999). Understanding the prattle of praxis. *Nursing Inquiry*, 6(4), 259–268.

Peplau, H.E. (1997), Peplau's theory of interpersonal relations. *Nursing Science Quarterly*, 10(4), 162–167.

Phillips, R., Donald, A., Mousseau-Gershman, Y., and Powell, T. (1998). Applying theory to practice—The use of "ripple effect" plans in continuing education. *Nurse Education Today*, 18(1), 12–19.

Pierson, W. (1999). Considering the nature of intersubjectivity within professional nursing. *Journal of Advanced Nursing*, 30(2), 294–302.

Ray, M.A. (1997). The ethical theory of existential authenticity: The lived experience of the art of caring in nursing administration. *Canadian Journal of Nursing Research*, 29(1), 111–126.

Rogers, M.E. (1989). Creating a climate for the implementation of a nursing conceptual framework. *Journal of Continuing Education in Nursing*, 20(3), 112–116.

Rolfe, G. (1998). The theory-practice gap in nursing: From research-based practice to practitioner-based research. *Journal of Advanced Nursing*, 28(3), 672–679.

Rosanoff, N. (1999). Intuition comes of age: Workplace applications of intuitive skill for occupational and environmental health nurses. *Journal of the American Association of Occupational Health Nurses*, 47(4), 156–162.

Rosswurm, M.A. and Larrabee, J.H. (1999). A model for change to evidence-based practice. *Image: Journal of Nursing Scholarship*, 31(4), 317–322.

Rothrock, J.C. and Smith, D.A. (2000). Selecting the perioperative patient focused model. *Journal of the Association of periOperative Registered Nurses*, 71(5), 1030–1034.

Roy, C. (2000). A theorist envisions the future and speaks to nursing administrators. *Nursing Administration Quarterly*, 24(2), 1–12.

Rutty, J.E. (1998). The nature of philosophy of science, theory and knowledge relating to nursing and professionalism. *Journal of Advanced Nursing*, 28(2), 243–250.

Sanford, R.C. (2000). Caring through relation and dialogue: A nursing perspective for patient education. *Advances in Nursing Science*, 22(3), 1–15.

Scammell, J. and Miller, S. (1999). Back to basics: Exploring the conceptual basis of nursing. *Nurse Education Today*, 19(7), 570–577.

Scherer, P. (1988). Hospitals that attract (and keep) nurses. *American Journal of Nursing*, 88(1), 34–40.

Schmieding, N.J. (1988). Action process of nurse administrators to problematic situations based on Orlando's theory. *Journal of Advanced Nursing*, 13(1), 99–107.

Severinsson, E.I. (1999). Ethics in clinical nursing supervision—An introduction to the theory and practice of different supervision models. *Collegian*, 6(3), 23–28.

Sharp, K. (1998). The case for case studies in nursing research: The problem of generalization. *Journal of Advanced Nursing*, 27(4), 785–789.

Sheafor, M. (1991). Productive work groups in complex hospital units: Proposed contributions of the nurse executive. *Journal of Nursing Administration*, 21(5), 25–30.

Sills, G.M. (1998). Peplau and professionalism: The emergence of the paradigm of professionalization. *Journal of Psychiatric and Mental Health Nursing*, 5(3), 167–171.

Smith, M. and Cusack, L. (2000). The Ottawa Charter—From nursing theory to practice: Insights from the area of alcohol and other drugs. *International Journal of Nursing Practice*, 6(4), 168–173.

Smith, M.C. (1993). The contribution of nursing theory to nursing administration practice. *Image: Journal of Nursing Scholarship*, 25, 63–67.

Spouse, J. (2001). Bridging theory and practice in the supervisory relationship: A sociocultural perspective. *Journal of Advanced Nursing*, 33(4), 512–522.

Taylor, J.S. (1997). Nursing ideology: Identification and legitimation. *Journal of Advanced Nursing*, 25(3), 442–446.

Thorne, S.E., Kirkham, S.R., and Henderson, A. (1999). Ideological implications of paradigm discourse. *Nursing Inquiry*, 6(2), 123–131.

Tilley, S. (1999). Altschul's legacy in mediating British and American psychiatric nursing discourses: Common sense and the "absence" of the accountable practitioner. *Journal of Psychiatric and Mental Health Nursing*, 6(4), 283–295.

Traynor, M. (1997). Postmodern research: No grounding or privilege, just free-floating trouble making. *Nursing Inquiry*, 4(2), 99–107.

Turner, S.L. and Bentley, G.W. (1998). A meaningful health assessment course for baccalaureate nursing students. *Nursing Connections*, 11(2), 5–12.

Upton, D.J. (1999). How can we achieve evidence-based practice if we have a theory-practice gap in nursing today? *Journal of Advanced Nursing*, 29(3), 549–555.

Verran, J.A. (1997). The value of theory-driven (rather than problem-driven) research. *Seminars for Nurse Managers*, 5(4), 169–172.

Verran, J.A. and Reid, P.J. (1987). Replicated testing of the nursing technology model. *Nursing Research*, 36(3), 190–194.

Ward, S.L. (1998). Caring and healing in the 21st century. *MCN, The American Journal of Maternal Child Nursing*, 23(4), 210–215.

Webster, J. and Cowart, P. (1999). An innovative professional nursing practice model. *Nursing Administration Quarterly*, 23(3), 11–16.

Westbrook, L.O. and Schultz, P.R. (2000). From theory to practice: Community health nursing in a public health neighborhood team. *Advances in Nursing Science*, 23(2), 50–61.

Wewers, M.E. and Lenz, E.R. (1987). Relapse among ex-smokers: An example of theory derivation. *Advances in Nursing Science*, 9(2), 44–53.

Williams, A.M. (1998). The delivery of quality nursing care: A grounded theory study of the nurse's perspective. *Journal of Advanced Nursing*, 27(4), 808–816.

Williams, R. (1999). Cultural safety—What does it mean for our work practice? *Australia and New Zealand Journal of Public Health*, 23(2), 213–214. Comment in *Australia New Zealand Journal of Public Health* (1999), 23(5), 552–553.

Wilshaw, G. (1999). Perspectives on surviving childhood sexual abuse. *Journal of Advanced Nursing*, 30(2), 303–309.

Wimpenny, P. and Gass, J. (2000). Interviewing in phenomenology and grounded theory: Is there a difference? *Journal of Advanced Nursing*, 31(6), 1485–1492.

Wood, I. (1998). The effects of continuing professional education on the clinical practice of nurses: A review of the literature. *International Journal of Nursing Studies*, 35(3), 125–131.

Woods, S. (1998). A theory of holism for nursing. *Medical Health Care Philosophy*, 1(3), 255–261.

Wuest, J. (2000). Negotiating with helping systems: An example of grounded theory evolving through emergent fit. *Qualitative Health Research*, 10(1), 51–70.

Yegdich, T. (1998). How not to do clinical supervision in nursing. *Journal of Advanced Nursing*, 28(1), 193–202.

Yegdich, T. (1999). Clinical supervision and managerial supervision: Some historical and conceptual considerations. *Journal of Advanced Nursing*, 30(5), 1195–1204.

Zerwekh, J.V. (2000). Caring on the ragged edge: Nursing persons who are disenfranchised. *Advances in Nursing Science*, 22(4), 47–61.

12. Theory Analysis and Critique: Factors Affecting the Acceptance of Scientific Theories

Acton, G.J., Irvin, B.L., and Hopkins, B.A. (1991). Theory-testing research: Building the science. *Advances in Nursing Science*, 14(1), 52–61.

Acton, G.J., Irvin, B.L., Jensen, B.A., Hopkins, B.A., and Miller, E.W. (1997). Explicating middle-range theory through methodological diversity. *Advances in Nursing Science*, 19(3), 78–85.

Allan, J. and Hall, B. (1988). Challenging the focus on technology: A critique of the medical model in a changing health care system. *Advances in Nursing Science*, 10(3), 22–34.

Anderko, L., Uscian, M., and Robertson, J.F. (1999). Improving client outcomes through differentiated practice: A rural nursing center model. *Public Health Nursing*, 16(3), 168–175.

Andershed, B. and Ternestedt, B.M. (2001). Development of a theoretical framework describing relatives' involvement in palliative care. *Journal of Advanced Nursing*, 34(4), 554–562.

Annells, M. (1997). Grounded theory method, Part I: Within the five moments of qualitative research. *Nursing Inquiry*, 4(2), 120–129.

Arthur, D., Chan, H.K., Fung, W.Y., Wong, K.Y., and Yeung, K.W. (1999). Therapeutic communication strategies used by Hong Kong mental health nurses with their Chinese clients. *Journal of Psychiatric/Mental Health Nursing*, 6(1), 29–36.

Ashley, J.A. (1978). Foundations for scholarship: Historical research in nursing. *Advances in Nursing Science*, 1, 25–36.

Ashore, R. and Banks, D. (1997). Student nurses perceptions of their interpersonal skills: A re-examination of Burnard and Morrison's findings. *International Journal of Nursing Studies*, 34(5), 335–345.

Auvil-Novak, S.E. (1997). A middle-range theory of chronotherapeutic intervention for postsurgical pain. *Nursing Research*, 46(2), 66–71.

Baas, L.S., Fontana, J.A., and Bhat, G. (1997). Relationships between self-care resources and the quality of life of persons with heart failure: A comparison of treatment groups. *Progress in Cardiovascular Nursing*, 12(1), 25–38.

Backman, K. and Kyngas, H.A. (1999). Challenges of the grounded theory approach to a novice researcher. *Nursing and Health Sciences*, 1(3), 147–153.

Baker, C. (1999). From chaos to order: A nursing-based psycho-education program for parents of children with attention-deficit hyperactivity disorder. *Canadian Journal of Nursing Research*, 31(2), 71–75.

Barkley, T.W., Jr., Rhodes, R.S., and Dufour, C.A. (1998). Predictors of success on the NCLEX-RN among baccalaureate nursing students. *Nursing and Health Care Perspectives*, 19(3),132–137.

Barnum, B.J.S. (1994). Criteria for evaluating theories. In B.J.S. Barnum (Ed.), *Nursing theory: Analysis, application and evaluation* (4th ed.). Philadelphia, PA: J.B. Lippincott.

Barrett, E.A. and Caroselli, C. (1998). Methodological ponderings related to the power as knowing participation in change tool. *Nursing Science Quarterly*, 11(1), 17–22.

Baumann, S.L. (1997). Contrasting two approaches in a community-based nursing practice with older adults: The medical model and Parse's nursing theory. *Nursing Science Quarterly*, 10(3), 124–130.

Beeman, P.B. and Waterhouse, J.K. (2001). NCLEX-RN performance: Predicting success on the computerized examination. *Journal of Professional Nursing*, 17(4), 158–165.

Bell, A., Horsfall, J., and Goodin. W. (1998). The Mental Health Nursing Clinical Confidence Scale: A tool for measuring undergraduate learning on mental health clinical placements. *Australian and New Zealand Journal of Mental Health Nursing*, 7(4), 184–190.

Bennett, J.A. (1997). A case for theory triangulation. *Nursing Science Quarterly*, 10(2), 97–102.

Bent, K.N. (1999). Seeking the both/and of a nursing research proposal. *Advances in Nursing Science*, 21(3), 76–89.

Berragan, L. (1998). Nursing practice draws upon several different ways of knowing. *Journal of Clinical Nursing*, 7(3), 209–217.

Blix, A. (1999). Integrating occupational health protection and health promotion: Theory and program application. *Journal of the American Association of Occupational Health Nurses*, 47(4), 168–171.

Bott, M. (1997). Embedded nursing practice: A case study. *Journal of the Canadian Association of Nephrology Nurses and Technicians*, 7(4), 25–26.

Boychuk Duchscher, J.E. (1999). Catching the wave: Understanding the concept of critical thinking. *Journal of Advanced Nursing*, 29(3), 577–583.

Bradshaw, A. (1995). What are nurses doing to patients? A review of theories of nursing past and present. *Journal of Clinical Nursing*, 4(2), 81–92.

Brennan, P.F. and Anthony, M. (2000). Measuring nursing practice models using Multi-Attribute Utility theory. *Research in Nursing and Health*, 23(5), 372–382.

Brooks, E.M. and Thomas, S. (1997). The perception and judgment of senior baccalaureate student nurses in clinical decision making. *Advances in Nursing Science*, 19(3), 50–69.

Brown, S.J. (1999). Student nurses' perceptions of elderly care. *Journal of National Black Nurses Association*, 10(2), 29–36.

Buchanan, B. (1987). Conceptual models: An assessment framework. *Journal of Nursing Administration*, 17(10), 22–26.

Burks, K.J. (2001). Intentional action. *Journal of Advanced Nursing*, 34(5), 668–675.

Cain, P. (1999). Respecting and breaking confidences: Conceptual, ethical and educational issues. *Nurse Education Today*, 19(3), 175–181.

Caris-Verhallen, W.M., Kerkstra, A., and Bensing, J.M. (1997). The role of communication in nursing care for elderly people: A review of the literature. *Journal of Advanced Nursing*, 25(5), 915–933.

Carson, M.G. and Mitchell, G.J. (1998). The experience of living with persistent pain. *Journal of Advanced Nursing*, 28(6), 1242–1248.

Chafetz, J.S. (1979). *A primer on the construction and testing of theories in sociology*. Itasca, IL: F.E. Peacock Publisher. (Especially note Chapter 8.)

Chinn, P.L. and Jacobs, M.K. (1987). *Theory and nursing: A systematic approach*. St. Louis, MO: C.V. Mosby.

Chinn, P.L. and Jacobs, M.K. (1983). The evaluation of theory. In P.L. Chinn and M.K. Jacobs (Eds.), *Theory and nursing: A systematic approach*. St. Louis: C.V. Mosby.

Clift, J. and Barrett, E. (1998). Testing nursing theory cross-culturally. *International Nursing Review*, 45(4), 123–126.

Conley, V.M. (1998). Beyond knowledge deficit to a proposal for information-seeking behaviors. *Nursing Diagnosis*, 9(4), 129–135.

Cooley, M.E. (1999). Analysis and evaluation of the Trajectory Theory of Chronic Illness Management. *Scholarly Inquiry for Nursing Practice*, 13(2), 75–95.

Copnell, B. (1998). Synthesis in nursing knowledge: An analysis of two approaches. *Journal of Advanced Nursing*, 27(4), 870–874.

Corner, J. (1997). Beyond survival rates and side effects: Cancer nursing as therapy. The Robert Tiffany Lecture. 9th International Conference on Cancer Nursing, Brighton, UK, August 1996. *Cancer Nursing*, 20(1), 3–11.

Cowley, S. and Billings, J.R. (1999). Resources revisited: Salutogenesis from a lay perspective. *Journal of Advanced Nursing*, 29(4), 994–1004.

Croom, S., Procter, S., and Couteur, A.L. (2000). Developing a concept analysis of control for use in child and adolescent mental health nursing. *Journal of Advanced Nursing*, 31(6), 1324–1332.

Crossan, F. and Robb, A. (1998). Role of the nurse: Introducing theories and concepts. *British Journal of Nursing*, 7(10), 608–612.

Davis, K. and Glass, N. (1999). Contemporary theories and contemporary nursing—Advancing nursing care for those who are marginalized. *Contemporary Nurse*, 8(2), 32–38.

Dawson, P.J. (1997). Is there anyone in there? Psychiatric nursing meets biological psychiatry. *Nursing Inquiry*, 4(3), 167–175.

Dean, J.M. and Mountfourd, B. (1998). Innovation in the assessment of nursing theory and its evaluation: A team approach. *Journal of Advanced Nursing*, 28(2), 409–418.

Deatrick, J.A., Knafl, K.A., and Murphy-Moore, C. (1999). Clarifying the concept of normalization. *Image: Journal of Nursing Scholarship*, 31(3), 209–214.

DeSantis, L. and Ugarriza, D.N. (2000). The concept of theme as used in qualitative nursing research. *Western Journal of Nursing Research*, 22(3), 351–372.

Dewey, J. (1958). *Experience and nature* (Rev. ed.). New York: Dover Publications.

Dierckx de Casterle, B., Roelens, A., and Gastmans, C. (1998). An adjusted version of Kohlberg's moral theory: Discussion of its validity for research in nursing ethics. *Journal of Advanced Nursing*, 27(4), 829–835.

Dijkstra, A., Buist, G., and Dassen, T. (1998). Operationalization of the concept of "nursing care dependency" for use in long-term care facilities. *Australian and New Zealand Journal of Mental Health Nursing*, 7(4), 142–151.

Dolan, K. (1997). Children in accident and emergency. *Accident and Emergency Nursing*, 5(2), 88–91.

Draper, P. (1993). A critique of Fawcett's "Conceptual models and nursing practice: The reciprocal relationship." *Journal of Advanced Nursing*, 18, 558–564.

Driver, J. and Campbell, J. (2000). An evaluation of the impact of lecturer practitioners on learning. *British Journal of Nursing*, 9(5), 292–300.

Dubos, R. (1963). *The cultural roots and social fruits of science*. Eugene, OR: University of Oregon Books.

Dudley-Brown, S.L. (1997). The evaluation of nursing theory: A method for our madness. *International Journal of Nursing Studies*, 34, 76–83.

Duffey, M. and Muhlenkamp, A.F. (1974). A framework for theory analysis. *Nursing Outlook*, 22(9), 570–574.

Duffy, M.E. (1994). Testing the theory of transcending options: Health behaviors of single parents. *Scholarly Inquiry for Nursing Practice*, 8, 191–282.

Eakes, G.G., Burke, M.L., and Hainsworth, M.A. (1998). Middle-range theory of chronic sorrow. *Image: Journal of Nursing Scholarship*, 30(2), 179–184.

Edwards, P. (Editor in Chief). (1967). *Pragmatic theory of truth: Pragmatism. The encyclopedia of philosophy* (Vol. 6). New York: Macmillan and Free Press.

Elcock, K. (1998). Lecturer practitioner: A concept analysis. *Journal of Advanced Nursing*, 28(5), 1092–1098.

*Ellis, R. (1968). Characteristics of significant theories. *Nursing Research*, 17(3), 217–222.

Emden, C. (1998). Conducting a narrative analysis. *Collegian*, 5(3), 34–39.

Evangelista, L.S. (1999). Compliance: A concept analysis. *Nursing Forum*, 34(1), 5–11.

Facione, N.C., Facione, P.A., and Sanchez, C.A. (1994). Critical thinking disposition as a measure of competent clinical judgment. The development of the "California Critical Thinking Disposition Inventory." *Journal of Nursing Education*, 33(8), 345–350.

Fagerstrom, L. and Engberg, I.B. (1998). Measuring the unmeasurable: A caring science perspective on patient classification. *Journal of Nursing Management*, 6(3), 165–172.

*Fawcett, J. (1980). A framework for analysis and evaluation of conceptual models of nursing. *Nurse Educator*, 5(6), 10–14.

Fawcett, J. (1989). *Analysis and evaluation of conceptual models of nursing* (2nd ed.). Philadelphia, PA: F.A. Davis.

Fawcett, J. (2006). The state of nursing science: Where is the nursing in the science? Theoria, *Journal of Nursing Theory*, 15(4), 3–10.

Fawcett, J. (2012). Thoughts on concept analysis: Multiple approaches, one result. *Nursing Science Quarterly*, 25(3), 285–287.

Fawcett, J. (2013). Thoughts about conceptual models and measurement validity. *Nursing Science Quarterly*, 26(2), 189–191.

Fawcett, J. and Desanto-Madeya, S. (2013). *Contemporary nursing knowledge: Analysis and evaluation of nursing models and theories* (3rd ed.). Philadelphia, PA: F.A. Davis.

Fawcett, J., Watson, J,. Neuman, B., Walker, P.H., and Fitzpatrick, J.J. (2001). On nursing theories and evidence. *Journal of Nursing Scholarship*, 33(2), 115–119.

Fealy, G.M. (1997). The theory-practice relationship in nursing: An exploration of contemporary discourse. *Journal of Advanced Nursing*, 25(5), 1061–1069.

Fernandez, E. (1997). Just "doing the observations": Reflective practice in nursing. *British Journal of Nursing*, 6(16), 939–943.

Fisher, M.A. and Mitchell, G.J. (1998). Patients' views of quality of life: Transforming the knowledge base of nursing. *Clinical Nurse Specialist*, 12(3), 99–105. Comment in *Clinical Nurse Specialist* (1998), 12(3), 98.

Fitzpatrick, J. and Whall, A. (1989). *Conceptual models of nursing: Analysis and application* (2nd ed.). Bowie, MD: Robert J. Brady Co.

Forbes, D.A., King, K.M., Kushner, K.E., Letourneau, N.L., Myrick, A.F., and Profetto-McGrath, J. (1999). Warrantable evidence in nursing science. *Journal of Advanced Nursing*, 29(2), 373–379.

Forbes, M.A. (1999). Hope in the older adult with chronic illness: A comparison of two research methods in theory building. *Advances in Nursing Science*, 22(2), 74–87.

Forchuk, C., Jewell, J., Schofield, R., Sirceljm, M., and Valledor, T. (1998). From hospital to community: Bridging therapeutic relationships. *Journal of Psychiatric/Mental Health Nursing*, 5(3), 197–202.

Frank, P.G. (1954). The variety of reasons for the acceptance of scientific theories. Scientific Monthly, 79(3), 139–145.

Frank, P.G. (1956). The variety of reasons for the acceptance of scientific theories. In P.G. Frank (Ed.), *The validation of scientific theories*. Boston, MA: Beacon Press.

Freeman, M., Baumann, A., Blythe, J., Fisher, A. and Akhtar-Danesh, N. (2012). Migration: A concept analysis from a nursing perspective. *Journal of Advanced Nursing*, 68(5), 1176–1186.

Freshwater, D. (1998). From acorn to oak tree: A neoplatonic perspective of reflection and caring. *Australian Journal of Holistic Nursing*, 5(2), 14–19.

Gagan, M.J., Badger, T.A., and de Leon Baker, M. (1999), Nurse practitioner interventions for domestic violence. *Clinical Excellence in Nurse Practice*, 3(5), 273–278.

Gastaldo, D. and Holmes D. (1999). Foucault and nursing: A history of the present. *Nursing Inquiry*, 6(4), 231–240.

Geanellos, R. (2000). Exploring Ricoeur's hermeneutic theory of interpretation as a method of analysing research texts. *Nursing Inquiry*, 7(2), 112–119.

Giles, M., McClenahan, C., Armour, C., Millar, S., Rae, G., Mallet, J., and Stewart-Knox, B. (2014). Evaluation of a theory of planned behavior-based breastfeeding intervention in Northern Irish schools using a randomized cluster design. *British Journal of Health Psychology*, 19(1), 16–35.

Goulet, C., Bell, L., St-Cyr, D., Paul, D., and Lang, A. (1998). A concept analysis of parent-infant attachment. *Journal of Advanced Nursing*, 28(5), 1071–1081.

Gramling, L.F., Lambert, V.A., and Pursley-Crotteau, S. (1998). Coping in young women: Theoretical retroduction. *Journal of Advanced Nursing*, 28(5), 1082–1091.

Greenwood. J. (1998). Establishing an international network on nurses' clinical reasoning. *Journal of Advanced Nursing*, 27(4), 843–847.

Gulzar, L. (1999). Access to health care. *Image: Journal of Nursing Scholarship*, 31(1), 13–19.

Gustafsson, G. and Andersson, L. (2001). "The Nine-Field Model" for evaluation of theoretical constructs in nursing. Part I: Development of a new model for nursing theory evaluation and application of this model to theory description of the SAUC model. *Theoria Journal of Nursing Theory*, 10(1), 10–33.

Gustafsson, G. and Andersson, L. (2001). "The Nine-Field Model" for evaluation of theoretical constructs in nursing. Part II: Application of the evaluation model to theory analysis, theory critique and theory support of the SAUC model. *Theoria Journal of Nursing Theory*, 10(2), 19–38.

Haas, B.K. (1999). Clarification and integration of similar quality of life concepts. *Image: Journal of Nursing Scholarship*, 31(3), 215–220.

Hall, B.A. (1997). Spirituality in terminal illness: An alternative view of theory. *Journal of Holistic Nursing*, 15(1), 82–96.

Hams, S.P. (1997). Concept analysis of trust: A coronary care perspective. *Intensive and Critical Care Nursing*, 13(6), 351–356.

Harden, J. (2000). Language, discourse and the chronotope: Applying literary theory to the narratives in health care. *Journal of Advanced Nursing*, 31(3), 506–512.

Hart, M.A. and Foster, S.N. (1998). Self-care agency in two groups of pregnant women. *Nursing Science Quarterly*, 11(4), 167–171.

Hartrick, G. (1998). A critical pedagogy for family nursing. *Journal of Nursing Education*, 37(2), 80–84.

Hawley, P., Young, S., and Pasco, A.C. (2000). Reductionism in the pursuit of nursing science: (In)congruent with nursing's core values? *Canadian Journal of Nursing Research*, 32(2), 75–88.

Heinrich, K.T., Robinson, C.M., and Scales, M.E. (1998). Support groups: An empowering, experiential strategy. *Nurse Educator*, 23(4), 8–10.

Henly, S.J., Vermeersch, P.E., and Duckett, L.J. (1998). Model selection for covariance structures analysis in nursing research. *Western Journal of Nursing Research*, 20(3), 344–355.

Herth, K. (1998). Hope as seen through the eyes of homeless children. *Journal of Advanced Nursing*, 28(5), 1053–1062.

Heslop, L. (1997). The (im)possibilities of poststructuralist and critical social nursing inquiry. *Nursing Inquiry*, 4(1), 48–56.

Holmes, C.A. and Warelow, P.J. (1997). Culture, needs and nursing: A critical theory approach. *Journal of Advanced Nursing*, 25(3), 463–470.

Horsburgh, M.E. (1999). Self-care of well adult Canadians and adult Canadians with end stage renal disease. *International Journal of Nursing Studies*, 36(6), 443–453.

Hunk, M. (1981, November 16). Taking it: The scandal that rocked science. *This World, San Francisco Chronicle*, 16–19, 21.

Hyrkas, K., Koivula, M., and Paunonen, M. (1999). Clinical supervision in nursing in the 1990s—Current state of concepts, theory and research. *Journal of Nursing Management*, 7(3), 177–187.

Im, E.O. (2015). The current status of theory evaluation in nursing. *Journal of Advanced Nursing*. 71(10), 2268–2278.

Im, E.O. and Meleis, A.I. (1999). A situation-specific theory of Korean immigrant women's menopausal transition. *Image: Journal of Nursing Scholarship*, 31(4), 333–338.

Jacobs, M.K. (1986). Can nursing theory be tested? In P.L. Chinn (Ed.), *Nursing research methodology: Issues and implementation* (pp. 39–54). Rockville, MD: Aspen Systems.

Jacobson, S.F. (1987). Studying and using conceptual models of nursing. *Image: Journal of Nursing Scholarship*, 19(2), 78–82.

Johnstone, M.J. (1999). Reflective topical autobiography: An under utilised interpretive research method in nursing. *Collegian*, 6(1), 24–29.

Kaariainen, M., Kanste, O., Elo, S., Polkki, T., Miettunen, J., and Kyngas, H. (2011). Testing and verifying nursing theory by confirmatory factor analysis. *Journal of Advanced Nursing*, 67(5), 1163–1172.

Kaba, E., Thompson, D.R., and Burnard, P. (2000). Coping after heart transplantation: A descriptive study of heart transplant recipients' methods of coping. *Journal of Advanced Nursing*, 32(4), 930–936.

Kaplan, A. (1964). *The conduct of inquiry: Methodology of behavioral science*. San Francisco, CA: Chandler.

Kathol, D.D., Geiger, M.L., and Hartig, J.L. (1998). Clinical correlation map: A tool for linking theory and practice. *Nurse Educator*, 23(4), 31–34.

Kearney, M.H. (1998). Ready-to-wear: Discovering grounded formal theory. *Research in Nursing and Health*, 21(2), 179–186.

Keddy, B., Gregor, F., Foster, S., and Denney, D. (1999). Theorizing about nurses' work lives: The personal and professional aftermath of living with healthcare "reform." *Nursing Inquiry*, 6(1), 58–64.

Kelley, L.S. (1999). Evaluating change in quality of life from the perspective of the person: Advanced practice nursing and Parse's goal of nursing. *Holistic Nursing Practice*, 13(4), 61–70.

Kim, H.S. (1999). Critical reflective inquiry for knowledge development in nursing practice. *Journal of Advanced Nursing*, 29(5), 1205–1212.

Kleinbeck, S.V. (2000). Dimensions of perioperative nursing for a national specialty nomenclature. *Journal of Advanced Nursing*, 31(3), 529–535.

Knight, M.M. (2000). Cognitive ability and functional status. *Journal of Advanced Nursing*, 31(6), 1459–1468.

Kuhn, T. (1977). *The essential tension: Selected studies in scientific tradition and change*. Chicago, IL: University of Chicago Press. (Especially note Chapter 13.)

Langford, C.P., Bowsher, J., Maloney, J.P., and Lillis, P.P. (1997). Social support: A conceptual analysis. *Journal of Advanced Nursing*, 25(1), 95–100.

Laudan, L. (1977). *Progress and its problems: Toward a theory of scientific growth*. Berkeley, CA: University of California Press.

LeBlanc, R.G. (1997). Definitions of oppression. *Nursing Inquiry*, 4(4), 257–261.

Lee, M.B. (1999). Power, self-care and health in women living in urban squatter settlements in Karachi, Pakistan: A test of Orem's theory. *Journal of Advanced Nursing*, 30(1), 248–259.

Lee, P. (1998). An analysis and evaluation of Casey's conceptual framework. *International Journal of Nursing Studies*, 35(4), 204–209.

Lego, S. (1998). The application of Peplau's theory to group psychotherapy. *Journal of Psychiatric/Mental Health Nursing*, 5(3), 193–196.

Lerdal, A. (1998). A concept analysis of energy: Its meaning in the lives of three individuals with chronic illness. *Scandinavian Journal of Caring Sciences*, 12(1), 3–10.

Levesque, L., Ricard, N., Ducharme, F., Duquette, A., and Bonin, J.P. (1998). Empirical verification of a theoretical model derived from the Roy adaptation model: Findings from five studies. *Nursing Science Quarterly*, 11(1), 31–39.

Levine, M.E. (1995). The rhetoric of nursing theory. *Image: Journal of Nursing Scholarship*, 27(1), 11–14.

Liehr, P. and Smith, M.J. (1999). Middle range theory: Spinning research and practice to create knowledge for the new millennium. *Advances in Nursing Science*, 21(4), 81–91.

Linscott, J., Spee, R., Flint, F., and Fisher A. (1999). Creating a culture of patient-focused care through a learner-centered philosophy. *Canadian Journal of Nursing Leadership*, 12(4), 5–10.

Logan, J. and Jenny, J. (1997). Qualitative analysis of patients' work during mechanical ventilation and weaning. *Heart and Lung*, 26(2), 140–147.

Long, A. and Slevin, E. (1999). Living with dementia: Communicating with an older person and her family. *Nursing Ethics*, 6(1), 23–36.

Lukkarinen, H. and Hentinen, M. (1997). Self-care agency and factors related to this agency among patients with coronary heart disease. *International Journal of Nursing Studies*, 34(4), 295–304.

Maggs-Rapport, F. (2000). Combining methodological approaches in research: Ethnography and interpretive phenomenology. *Journal of Advanced Nursing*, 31(1), 219–225.

Mahoney, J.S. and Engebretson, J. (2000). The interface of anthropology and nursing guiding culturally competent care in psychiatric nursing. *Archives of Psychiatric Nursing*, 14(4), 183–190.

Matas, K.E. (1997). Human patterning and chronic pain. *Nursing Science Quarterly*, 10(2), 88–96.

Mavundla, T.R. (2000). Professional nurses' perception of nursing mentally ill people in a general hospital setting. *Journal of Advanced Nursing*, 32(6), 1569–1578.

McCance, T.V., McKenna, H.P., and Boore, J.R. (1997). Caring: Dealing with a difficult concept. *International Journal of Nursing Studies*, 34(4), 241–248.

McCance, T.V., McKenna, H.P., and Boore, J.R. (1999). Caring: Theoretical perspectives of relevance to nursing. *Journal of Advanced Nursing*, 30(6), 1388–1395.

McCance, T.V., McKenna, H.P., and Boore, J.R. (2001). Exploring caring using narrative methodology: An analysis of the approach. *Journal of Advanced Nursing*, 33(3), 350–356.

McGrath, B.B. (1998). Illness as a problem of meaning: Moving culture from the classroom to the clinic. *Advances in Nursing Science*, 21(2), 17–29.

McHolm, F.A. and Geib, K.M. (1998). Application of the Neuman Systems Model to teaching health assessment and nursing process. *Nursing Diagnosis*, 9(1), 23–33.

McLaughlin C. (1997). The effect of classroom theory and contact with patients on the attitudes of student nurses towards mentally ill people. *Journal of Advanced Nursing*, 26(6), 1221–1228.

McQuiston, C.M. and Campbell, J.C. (1997). Theoretical substruction: A guide for theory testing research. *Nursing Science Quarterly*, 10(3), 117–123.

Meleis, A.I. (1983). A model for theory description, analysis, and critique. In N.L. Chaska (Ed.), *The nursing profession: A time to speak*. New York: McGraw-Hill.

Meleis, A.I. (1994). Theory testing and theory support: Principles, challenges, and a sojourn into the future. In B. Neuman (Ed.), *The Neuman systems model* (pp. 447–457). East Norwalk, CT: Appleton & Lange.

Meleis, A.I., Sawyer, L.M., Im, E.O., Hilfinger Messias, D.K., and Schumacher, K. (2000). Experiencing transitions: An emerging middle-range theory. *Advances in Nursing Science*, 23(1), 12–28.

Moore, B. (1954). Influence of political creeds on the acceptance of theories. *Scientific Monthly*, 79(3), 146–148.

Neill, S.J. (1998). Developing children's nursing through action research. *Journal of Child Health Care*, 2(1), 11–15.

Nuamah, I.F., Cooley, M.E., Fawcett, J., and McCorkle, R. (1999). Testing a theory for health-related quality of life in cancer patients: A structural equation approach. *Research in Nursing and Health*, 22(3), 231–242.

Olson, J. and Hanchett, E. (1997). Nurse-expressed empathy, patient outcomes, and development of a middle-range theory. *Image: Journal of Nursing Scholarship*, 29(1), 71–76.

Parse, R.R. (1987). *Nursing science: Major paradigms, theories, and critiques*. Philadelphia, PA: W.B. Saunders.

Phillips, R., Donald, A., Mousseau-Gershman, Y., and Powell, T. (1998). Applying theory to practice—The use of "ripple effect" plans in continuing education. *Nurse Education Today*, 18(1), 12–19.

Pilkington, F.B. (1999). A qualitative study of life after stroke. *Journal of Neuroscience Nursing*, 31(6), 336–347.

Polk, L.V. (1997). Toward a middle-range theory of resilience. *Advances in Nursing Science*, 19(3), 1–13.

Rankin, S.H. and Weekes, D.P. (2000). Life-span development: A review of theory and practice for families with chronically ill members. *Scholarly Inquiry for Nursing Practice*, 14(4), 355–373.

Ray, M.A. (1997). Consciousness and the moral ideal: A transcultural analysis of Watson's theory of transpersonal caring. *Advanced Practice Nursing Quarterly*, 3(1), 25–31.

Reimer, A.P., Clochesy, J.M. and Moore, S.M. (2013). Early examination of the middle-range theory of flight nursing expertise. *Applied Nursing Research*, 26(4), 276–279.

Reynolds, P.D. (1971). *A primer in theory construction*. Indianapolis, IN: Bobbs-Merrill.

Reynolds, W.J. (1997). Peplau's theory in practice. *Nursing Science Quarterly*, 10(4), 168–170.

Richer, M.C. and Ezer, H. (2000). Understanding beliefs and meanings in the experience of cancer: A concept analysis. *Journal of Advanced Nursing*, 32(5), 1108–1115.

Riehl-Sisca, J.P. (1989). *Conceptual models for nursing practice* (3rd ed.). East Norwalk, CT: Appleton & Lange.

Rogan, F., Shmied, V., Barclay, L., Everitt, L., and Wyllie, A. (1997). "Becoming a mother"—Developing a new theory of early motherhood. *Journal of Advanced Nursing*, 25(5), 877–885.

Rolfe, G. (1998). The theory-practice gap in nursing: From research-based practice to practitioner-based research. *Journal of Advanced Nursing*, 28(3), 672–679.

Rolfe, G. (1999). The pleasure of the bottomless: Postmodernism, chaos and paradigm shifts. *Nurse Education Today*, 19(8), 668–672.

Rudner, R. (1954). Remarks on value judgments in scientific validation. *Scientific Monthly*, 79(3), 1951–1953.

Ryles, S.M. (1999). A concept analysis of empowerment: Its relationship to mental health nursing. *Journal of Advanced Nursing*, 29(3), 600–607.

Scammell, J. and Miller, S. (1999). Back to basics: Exploring the conceptual basis of nursing. *Nurse Education Today*, 19(7), 570–577.

Schrag, C. (1967). Elements of theoretical analysis in sociology. In L. Gross (Ed.), *Sociological theory: Inquiries and paradigms*. New York: Harper & Row.

Severinsson, E.I. (1998). Bridging the gap between theory and practice: A supervision programme for nursing students. *Journal of Advanced Nursing*, 27(6), 1269–1277.

Sharp, K. (1998). The case for case studies in nursing research: The problem of generalization. *Journal of Advanced Nursing*, 27(4), 785–789.

Silva, M.C. (1986). Research testing nursing theory: State of the art. *Advances in Nursing Science*, 9(1), 1–11.

Silva, M.C. and Sorrell, J.M. (1992). Testing of nursing theory: Critique and philosophical expansion. *Advances in Nursing Science*, 14(4), 12–23.

Sim, J. (1998). Collecting and analysing qualitative data: Issues raised by the focus group. *Journal of Advanced Nursing*, 28(2), 345–352.

Sim, J. and Sharp, K. (1998). A critical appraisal of the role of triangulation in nursing research. *International Journal of Nursing Studies*, 35(1–2), 23–31.

Simko, L.C. (1999). Adults with congenital heart disease: Utilizing quality of life and Husted's nursing theory as a conceptual framework. *Critical Care Nursing Quarterly*, 22(3), 1–11.

Slaninka, S.C. (1999). Nursing theories: Creative teaching strategies make this course come alive. *Nurse Educator*, 24(3), 40–43.

Slusher, I.L. (1999). Self-care agency and self-care practice of adolescents. *Issues in Comprehensive Pediatric Nursing*, 22(1), 49–58.

Smith, L.S. (1998). Concept analysis: Cultural competence. *Journal of Cultural Diversity*, 5(1), 4–10.

Smith, M. and Cusack, L. (2000). The Ottawa Charter— From nursing theory to practice: Insights from the area of alcohol and other drugs. *International Journal of Nursing Practice*, 6(4), 168–173.

Spearman, S.A., Duldt, B.W., and Brown, S. (1993). Research testing theory: A selective review of Orem's self-care theory, 1986–1991. *Journal of Advanced Nursing*, 18, 1626–1631.

Stein, K.F., Corte, C., Colling, K.B., and Whall, A. (1998). A theoretical analysis of Carper's ways of knowing using a model of social cognition. *Scholarly Inquiry for Nursing Practice*, 12(1), 43–60.

Stewart, K.E., DiClemente, R.J., and Ross, D. (1999). Adolescents and HIV: Theory-based approaches to education of nurses. *Journal of Advanced Nursing*, 30(3), 687–696.

Thelander, B.L. (1997). The psychotherapy of Hildegard Peplau in the treatment of people with serious mental illness. *Perspectives in Psychiatric Care*, 33(3), 24–32.

Thibodeau, J. and MacRae, J. (1997). Breast cancer survival: A phenomenological inquiry. *Advances in Nursing Science*, 19(4), 65–74.

Thorne, S.E., Kirkham, S.R., and Henderson, A. (1999). Ideological implications of paradigm discourse. *Nursing Inquiry*, 6(2), 123–131.

Timpka, T. (2000). The patient and the primary care team: A small-scale critical theory. *Journal of Advanced Nursing*, 31(3), 558–564.

Torres, G. (1986). *Theoretical foundations of nursing*. Norwalk, CT: Appleton-Century-Crofts.

Upton, D.J. (1999). How can we achieve evidence-based practice if we have a theory-practice gap in nursing today? *Journal of Advanced Nursing*, 29(3), 549–555.

Vellone, E., Riegel, B., D'Agostino, F., Fida, R., Rocco, G., Cocchieri, A., and Alvaro, R. (2013). Structural equation model testing the situation-specific theory of heart failure self-care. *Journal of Advanced Nursing*, 2481–2492.

Villarruel, A.M. and Denyes, M.J. (1997). Testing Orem's theory with Mexican Americans. *Image: Journal of Nursing Scholarship*, 29(3), 283–288.

Walker, K.M. and Alligood, M.R. (2001). Empathy from a nursing perspective: Moving beyond borrowed theory. *Archives of Psychiatric Nursing*, 15(3), 140–147.

Watson, J. (1981, July). Nursing's scientific quest. *Nursing Outlook*, 29(7), 413–416.

Webb, C. (1999). Analysing qualitative data: Computerized and other approaches. *Journal of Advanced Nursing*, 29(2), 323–330.

Webster, G., Jacox, A., and Baldwin, B. (1981). Nursing theory and the ghost of the received view. In M. Grace and N. McCloskey (Eds.), *Current issues in nursing*. Scranton, PA: Blackwell Scientific Publications.

West, P. and Isenberg, M. (1997). Instrument development: The Mental Health-Related Self-Care Agency Scale. *Archives of Psychiatric Nursing*, 11(3), 126–132.

Westbrook, L.O. and Schultz, P.R. (2000). From theory to practice: Community health nursing in a public health neighborhood team. *Advances in Nursing Science*, 23(2), 50–61.

White, S.J. (1997). Empathy: A literature review and concept analysis. *Journal of Clinical Nursing*, 6(4), 253–257.

Whitley, G.G. (1997). Three phases of research in validating nursing diagnoses. *Western Journal of Nursing Research*, 19(3), 379–399.

Widdershoven, G.A. (1999). Care, cure and interpersonal understanding. *Journal of Advanced Nursing*, 29(5), 1163–1169.

Wilkinson, C., Peters, L., Mitchell, K., Irwin, T., McCorrie, K., and MacLeod, M. (1998). "Being there": Learning through active participation. *Nurse Education Today*, 18(3), 226–230.

Wimpenny, P. and Gass, J. (2000). Interviewing in phenomenology and grounded theory: Is there a difference? *Journal of Advanced Nursing*, 31(6), 1485–1492.

Winstead-Fry, P. (Ed.). (1986). *Case studies in nursing theory*. New York: National League for Nursing.

Zetterberg, H.L. (1965). *On theory verification in sociology* (3rd ed.). New York: Bedminister Press.

Zoucha, R. and Husted, G.L. (2000). The ethical dimensions of delivering culturally congruent nursing and health care. *Issues in Mental Health Nursing*, 21(3), 325–340.

Zulkowski, K. (1998). Construct validity of minimum data set items within the context of the Braden conceptual schema. *Ostomy/Wound Management*, 44(10), 36–40.

NURSING THEORY AND THEORISTS

13. Faye Abdellah

Abdellah, F.G. (1969). The nature of nursing science. *Nursing Research*, 18, 390–393.

*Abdellah, F.G. (1970). Overview of nursing research 1955–1968, Part 1. *Nursing Research*, 19, 6–17.

Abdellah, F.G. (1970). Overview of nursing research 1955–1968, Part 2. *Nursing Research*, 19, 151–162.

Abdellah, F.G. (1970). Overview of nursing research 1955–1968, Part 3. *Nursing Research*, 19, 239–252.

Abdellah, F.G. (1971). Evolution of nursing as a profession: Perspective on manpower development. *International Nursing Review*, 19, 119–235.

Abdellah, F.G. (1972). The physician-nurse team approach to coronary care. *Nursing Clinics of North America*, 7, 423–430.

Abdellah, F.G. (1976). Nurse practitioners and nursing practice. *American Journal of Public Health*, 66, 245–246.

Abdellah, F.G. (1976). Nursing's role in future health care. *AORN Journal*, 24(2), 236–240.

Abdellah, F.G. (1978). Long term care policy issues. *Annals of the American Academy of Political and Social Science*, 438, 22.

Abdellah, F.G. (1981). Nursing care of the aged in the United States of America. *Journal of Gerontological Nursing*, 7(11), 657–663.

Abdellah, F.G. (1982). The nurse practitioner 17 years later: Present and emerging issues. *Inquiry*, 19, 105–116.

Abdellah, F.G., Beland, I.L., Martin, A., and Matheney, R.V. (1973). *New directions in patient centered nursing: Guidelines for systems of service, education and research.* New York: Macmillan.

Abdellah, F.G., Foerst, H.V., and Chow, R.K. (1979). PACE: An approach to improving care to the elderly. *American Journal of Nursing*, 79, 1109–1110.

Abdellah, F.G. and Levine, R. (1957). Developing a measure of patient and personnel satisfaction with nursing care. *Nursing Research*, 5, 100–108.

Abdellah, F.G. and Levine, R. (1965). Aims of nursing research. *Nursing Research*, 14, 29–32.

Abdellah, F.G. and Levine, R. (1965). *Better patient care through nursing research.* New York: Macmillan.

Abdellah, F.G. and Levine, R. (1979). *Better patient care through nursing research* (2nd ed.). New York: Macmillan.

Alward, R.R. (1983). Patient classification systems: The ideal vs. reality. *Journal of Nursing Administration*, 13(2), 14–19.

Anderson, M.A., Pena, R.A., and Helms, L.B. (1998). Home care utilization by congestive heart failure patients: A pilot study. *Public Health Nursing*, 15(2), 146–162.

Avis, M. (1995). Valid arguments—A consideration of the concept of validity in establishing the credibility of research findings. *Journal of Advanced Nursing*, 22(6), 1203–1209.

Bergman, R., Stockler, R.A., Shavit, N., Sharon, R., Feinberg, D., and Danon, A. (1981). Role, selection and preparation of head nurses—I. *International Journal of Nursing Studies*, 18(2), 123–152.

Bergman, R., Stockler, R.A., Shavit, N., Sharon, R., Feinberg, D., and Danon, A. (1981). Role, selection and preparation of head nurses—III. *International Journal of Nursing Studies*, 18(4), 237–250.

Blegan, M.A., Goode, C.J., and Reed, L. (1998). Nurse staffing and patient outcomes. *Nursing Research*, 47(1), 43–50.

Brown, G.D. (1995). Understanding barriers to basing nursing practice upon research—A communication model approach. *Journal of Advanced Nursing*, 21(1), 154–157.

Chang, K. (1997). Dimensions and indicators of patients' perceived nursing care quality in the hospital setting. *Journal of Nursing Care Quality*, 11(6), 26–37.

Chow, R. (1969). Postoperative cardiac nursing research: A method for identifying and categorizing nursing action. *Nursing Research*, 18(1), 4–13.

Clarke, P.N., Pendry, N.C., and Kim, Y.S. (1997). Patterns of violence in homeless women. *Western Journal of Nursing Research*, 19(4), 490–500.

Copp, L.A. (1973). Professional change: Which trends do nurses endorse? *International Journal of Nursing Studies*, 10, 55–63.

Cornell, S.A. (1974). Development of an instrument for measuring quality of nursing care. *Nursing Research*, 23, 108–117.

Craig, S.L. (1980). Theory development and its relevance for nursing. *Journal of Advanced Nursing*, 5, 349–355.

Dickoff, J. and James, P. (1970). Beliefs and values: Bases for curriculum design. *Nursing Research*, 19, 415–427.

Ditzengerber, G.R., Collins, S.D., and Bantawright, S.A. (1995). Combining the roles of clinical nurse specialist and neonatal nurse practitioner—The experience in one academic tertiary care setting. *Journal of Perinatal and Neonatal Nursing*, 9(3), 45–52.

Downs, F.S. and Fitzpatrick, J.J. (1976). Preliminary investigation of the reliability and validity of a tool for the assessment of body position and motor activity. *Nursing Research*, 25, 404–408.

Dycus, D., Schmeiser, D., Taggart, F., and Yancey, R. (1989). Faye Glenn Abdellah: Twenty-one nursing problems. In A. Marriner-Tomey (Ed.), *Nursing theorists and their work* (2nd ed.). St. Louis, MO: C.V. Mosby.

Elms, R.R. (1972). Recovery room behavior and post-operative convalescence. *Nursing Research*, 21, 390–397.

Fairman, J. (2000). Economically practical and critically necessary? The development of intensive care at Chestnut Hill Hospital. *Bulletin of the History of Medicine*, 74(1), 80–106.

Fairman, J. and Kagan, S. (1999). Creating critical care: The case of the Hospital of the University of Pennsylvania, 1950–1965. *Advances in Nursing Science*, 22(1), 63–77.

Fiedler, I.G., Laud, P.W., Maiman, D.J., et al. (1999). Economics of managed care in spinal cord injury. *Archives of Physical Medicine and Rehabilitation*, 80(11), 1441–1449.

Fortinsky, R.H., Granger, C.V., and Seltzer, G.B. (1981). The use of functional assessment in understanding home care needs. *Medical Care*, 19(5), 489–497.

Goodwin, J.O. and Edwards, B.S. (1975). Developing a computer program to assist the nursing process: Phase I—From systems analysis to an expandable program. *Nursing Research*, 24, 299–305.

Gordon, M. (1980). Determining study topics. *Nursing Research*, 29, 83–87.

Gordon, M. and Sweeney, M.A. (1979). Methodological problems and issues in identifying and standardizing nursing diagnosis. *Advances in Nursing Science*, 2(1), 1–15.

Greaves, F. (1980). Objectively toward curriculum improvement in nursing education in England and Wales. *Journal of Advanced Nursing*, 5, 591–599.

Green, J.A. (1979). Science, nursing, and nursing science: A conceptual analysis. *Advances in Nursing Science*, 2(1), 57–64.

Grier, M.R. and Schnitzler, C.P. (1979). Nurses' propensity to risk. *Nursing Research*, 28(3), 186–190.

Hardy, L.K. (1982). Nursing models and research—A restricting view? *Journal of Advanced Nursing*, 7, 447–451.

Hill, J. (1997). Patient satisfaction in a nurse-led rheumatology clinic. *Journal of Advanced Nursing*, 25(2), 347–354.

Hisama, K.K. (2001). The acceptance of nursing theory in Japan: A cultural perspective. *Nursing Science Quarterly*, 14(3), 255–259.

Hlusko, D.L. and Nichols, B.S. (1996). Can you depend on your patient classification system? *Journal of Nursing Administration*, 26(4), 39–44.

Hunt, J. (2001). Research into practice: The foundation for evidence-based care. *Cancer Nursing*, 24(2), 78–87.

Jacob, G. and Bengel, J. (2000). The construct "patient satisfaction": A critical review. *Zeitschrift fur Klinische Psychologie Psychiatrie und Psychotherapie*, 48(3), 280–301.

Jennings, C.P. and Jennings, T.F. (1977). Containing costs through prospective reimbursement. *American Journal of Nursing*, 77, 1155–1159.

Jhandler, M.C. and Mason, W.H. (1995). Solution-focused therapy—An alternative approach to addictions nursing. *Perspectives in Psychiatric Care*, 31(1), 8–13.

Jones, P.E. (1979). A terminology for nursing diagnosis. *Advances in Nursing Science*, 2(1), 65–72.

Karimi, M., and Clark, A.M. (2016). How do patients' values influence heart failure self-care decision-making?: A mixed-methods systematic review. *International Journal of Nursing Studies*, 59, 89–104.

King, I.M. (1968). A conceptual frame of reference for nursing. *Nursing Research*, 17, 27–31.

LaMontagne, L.L., Pressler, J.L., and Salisbury, M.H. (1996). Scholarly mission: Fostering scholarship in research, theory and practice. *N&HC Perspectives on Community*, 17(6), 298–302.

Lanara, V.A. (1976). Philosophy of nursing and current nursing problems. *International Nursing Review*, 23(2), 48–54.

Landi, F., Zuccala, G., Bernabei, R., et al. (1997). Physiotherapy and occupational therapy—A geriatric experience in the acute care hospital. *American Journal of Physical Medicine and Rehabilitation*, 76(1), 38–42.

Leke, J.T. (1978). Nigerian patients' perception of their nursing care needs. *Journal of Advanced Nursing*, 3, 181–187.

Majesky, S.J., Brester, M.H., and Nishio, K.T. (1978). Development of a research tool: Patient indicators of nursing care. *Nursing Research*, 27, 365–371.

McAuliffe, M.S. (1998). Interview with Faye G. Abdellah on nursing research and health policy. *Image: Journal of Nursing Scholarship*, 30(3), 215–219.

McGilloway, F.A. (1980). The nursing process: A problem solving approach to patient care. *International Nursing Studies*, 17(2), 79–90.

McLane, A.M. (1978). Core competencies of masters-prepared nurses. *Nursing Research*, 27(1), 43–58.

McSherry, R. (1997). What do registered nurses and midwives feel and know about research? *Journal of Advanced Nursing*, 25(5), 985–976.

Minckley, B.B. (1974). Physiological and psychological responses of elective surgical patients. *Nursing Research*, 23(5), 392–401.

Mulhall, A. (1996). Anthropology, nursing and midwifery: A natural alliance? *International Journal of Nursing Studies*, 33(6), 629–637.

Mulhall, A. (1997). Nursing research: Our world not theirs? *Journal of Advanced Nursing*, 25(5), 969–976.

Muntinga, M.E., Mokkink, L.B., Knol, D.L., Nijpels, G., and Jansen, A.P.D. (2014). Measurement properties of the Client-centered Care Questionnaire (CCCQ): factor structure, reliability and validity of a questionnaire to assess self-reported client-centeredness of home care services in a population of frail, older people. *Quality of Life Research*, 23(7), 2063–2072.

Price, M.R. (1980). Nursing diagnosis: Making a concept come alive. *American Journal of Nursing*, 80(4), 668–671.

Regan, J.A. (1998). Will current clinical effectiveness initiatives encourage and facilitate practitioners to use evidence-based practice for the benefit of their clients? *Journal of Clinical Nursing*, 7(3), 244–250.

Riddlesperger, K.L., Beard, M., Flowers, D.L., et al. (1996). CINAHL: An exploratory analysis of the current status of nursing theory construction as reflected by the electronic domain. *Journal of Advanced Nursing*, 24(3), 599–606.

Rubenstein, L.Z. (1981). Specialized geriatric assessment units and their clinical implications. *Western Journal of Medicine*, 135(6), 497–502.

See, E.M. (1989). Abdellah's model for nursing: Twenty-one nursing problems. In J. Fitzpatrick and A. Whall (Eds.), *Conceptual models of nursing: Analysis and application* (2nd ed.). East Norwalk, CT: Appleton & Lange.

Sitzia, J. and Wood, N. (1997). Patient satisfaction: A review of issues and concepts. *Social Science and Medicine*, 45(12), 1829–1843.

Shi, L.Y., Samuels, M.E., Ricketts, T.C., et al. (1994). A rural-urban comparative-study of nonphysician providers in community and migrant health centers. *Public Health Reports*, 109(6), 809–815.

Stevens, B.J. (1971). Analysis of structural forms used in nursing curricula. *Nursing Research*, 20(5), 388–397.

Walker, C. and Deuble, H. (1968). A schema for analysis of accident prevention activities in public health nurses' records. *Nursing Research*, 17(5), 408–414.

Walker, L.O. (1971). Toward a clearer understanding of the concept of nursing theory. *Nursing Research*, 20(5), 428–435.

Wright, J. (1998). Female nurses' perceptions of acceptable female body size: An exploratory study. *Journal of Clinical Nursing*, 7(4), 307–315.

Ziff, M.A., Conrad, P., and Lachman, M.E. (1995). The relative effects of perceived personal control and responsibility on health and health-related behaviors in young and middle-aged adults. *Health Education Quarterly*, 22(1), 127–142.

14. Patricia Benner

Benner, P. (1991). The role of experience, narrative, and community in skilled ethical comportment. *Advances in Nursing Science*, 14(2), 13–28.

Benner, P. (1996). A response by P. Benner to K. Cash, "Benner and expertise in nursing: A critique." *International Journal of Nursing Studies*, 33(6), 669–674.

Benner, P. (1997). A dialogue between virtue ethics and care ethics. *Theoretical Medicine*, 18(1–2), 47–61.

Benner, P. (1997). Developing a language for nursing. [Article in German]. *Pflege*, 10(2), 67–71.

Benner, P.A. (1985). Quality of life: A phenomenological perspective on explanation, prediction, and understanding in nursing science. *Advances in Nursing Science*, 8(1), 1–14.

Benner, P., Tanner, C., and Chesla, C. (1991). From beginner to expert: Gaining a differentiated clinical world in critical care nursing. *Advances in Nursing Science*, 14(3), 13–28.

Benner, R. and Benner, P. (1991). Stories from the front lines. *Healthcare Forum Journal*, 34(4), 68–74.

Bowen, K., and Prentice, D. (2016). Are Benner's expert nurses near extinction? *Nursing Philosophy*, 17(2), 144–148.

Gentile, D.L. (2012). Applying the novice-to-expert model to infusion nursing. *Journal of Infusion Nursing*, 35(2), 101–107.

Heyes, C.J., and Thachuk, A. (2015). Queering know-how: Clinical skill acquisition as ethical practice. *Journal of bioethical inquiry*, 12(2), 331–341.

Hofrocks, S. (2000). Hunting for Heidegger: Questioning the sources in the Benner/Cash debate. *International Journal of Nursing Studies*, 37(3), 237–243. Padgett, S.M. (2000). Benner and the critics: Promoting scholarly dialogue. *Scholarly Inquiry for Nursing Practice*, 14(3), 249–271.

Paley, J. (2000). Asthma and dualism. *Journal of Advanced Nursing*, 31(6), 1293–1299.

Tanner, C.A., Benner, P., Chesla, C., and Gordon, D.R. (1993). The phenomenology of knowing the patient. *Image: Journal of Nursing Scholarship*, 25(4), 273–280.

Thompson, C. (1999). A conceptual treadmill: The need for "middle ground" in clinical decision making theory in nursing. *Journal of Advanced Nursing*, 30(5), 1222–1229.

Weidman, N.A. (2013). The lived experience of the transition of the clinical nurse expert to the novice nurse educator. *Teaching and Learning in Nursing*, 8(3), 102–109.

15. Betty Jo Hadley

Hadley, B.J. (1967, April). The dynamic interactionist concept of role. *Journal of Nursing Education*, 6(2), 5–10, 24–25.

Hadley, B.J. (1969). Evolution of a conception of nursing. *Nursing Research*, 18(5), 400–406.

16. Beverly Hall

Artinian, B.M. (1983). Implementation of the intersystem patient-care model in clinical practice. *Journal of Advanced Nursing*, 8, 117–124.

Hall, B.A. (1975). Mutual withdrawal: The nonparticipant in a therapeutic community. *Perspectives in Psychiatric Care*, 14(2), 75–77.

Hall, B.A. (1975). Socializing patients into the psychiatric sick role. *Perspectives in Psychiatric Care*, 13, 123–129.

Hall, B.A. (1977). The effect of interpersonal attraction on the therapeutic relationship: A review and suggestion for further study. *Journal of Psychiatric Nursing*, 15(9), 18–23.

Hall, B.A. (1977). Occupational values and family perspectives: A comparison of pre-nursing and pre-medical women. *Communicating Nursing Research*, 8, 124–132.

*Hall, B.A. (1981). The change paradigm in nursing: Growth versus persistence. *Advances in Nursing Science*, 3(4), 1–6.

Hall, B.A., McKay, R.P., and Mitsunaga, B.K. (1971). Dimensions of role commitment: Career patterns of deans of nursing. *Communicating Nursing Research*, 4, 84–98.

Hall, B.A. and Mitsunaga, B.K. (1979). Education of the nurse to promote interpersonal attraction. *Journal of Nursing Education*, 18(5), 16–21.

Hall, B.A., Mitsunaga, B.K., and DeTornyay, R. (1981). Deans of nursing: Changing socialization patterns. *Nursing Outlook*, 29, 92–95.

Hall, B.A., von Endt, B., and Parker, G. (1981). A framework for measuring satisfaction of nursing staff. *Nursing Leadership*, 4(4), 29–33.

Mitsunaga, B.K. and Hall, B.A. (1979). Interpersonal attraction and perceived quality of medical-surgical care. *Western Journal of Nursing Research*, 1(1), 5–26.

*Murphy, S.A. and Hoeffer, B. (1983). Role of the specialties in nursing science. *Advances in Nursing Science*, 5(4), 31–39.

17. Mary Harms and Fred McDonald

Bailey, J.T., McDonald, F.J., and Harms, M.T. (1966). A new approach to curriculum development. *Nursing Outlook*, 14(7), 33–36.

Harms, M.T. and McDonald, F.J. (1966). A new curriculum design, Part III. *Nursing Outlook*, 14(9), 50–53.

Harms, M.T. and McDonald, F.J. (1966). The teaching-learning process, Part IV. *Nursing Outlook*, 14(10), 54–58.

McDonald, F.J. and Harms, M.T. (1966). A theoretical model for an experimental curriculum, Part II. *Nursing Outlook*, 14(8), 48–51.

18. Virginia Henderson

Ahtisham, Y., and Jacoline, S. (2015). Integrating Nursing Theory and Process into Practice; Virginia's Henderson Need Theory. *International Journal of Caring Sciences*, 8(2), 443–450.

DeMeester, D., Lauer, T., Neal, S., and Williams, S. (1989). Virginia Henderson: Definition of nursing. In A. Marriner-Tomey (Ed.), *Nursing theorists and their work* (2nd ed.). St. Louis, MO: C.V. Mosby.

Dijkstra, A., Yönt, G.H., Korhan, E.A., Muszalik, M., Kędziora-Kornatowska, K., and Suzuki, M. (2012). The Care Dependency Scale for measuring basic human needs: An international comparison. *Journal of Advanced Nursing*, 68(10), 2341–2348.

Fulton, J.S. (1987). Virginia Henderson: Theorist, prophet, poet. *Advances in Nursing Science*, 10(1), 1–17.

Furukawa, C.Y. and Howe, J.K. (1980). Virginia Henderson. In The Nursing Theories Conference Group (Eds.), *Nursing theories: The base for professional nursing practice*. Englewood Cliffs, NJ: Prentice-Hall.

Henderson, V. (1964). The nature of nursing. *American Journal of Nursing*, 64(8), 62–68.

Henderson, V. (1966). *The nature of nursing*. New York: Macmillan.

Henderson, V. (1969). Excellence in nursing. *American Journal of Nursing*, 69(9), 2133–2137.

Henderson, V. (1978). The concept of nursing. *Journal of Advanced Nursing*, 3, 113–130.

Henderson, V. (1980). Preserving the essence of nursing in a technological age. *Journal of Advanced Nursing*, 5, 245–260.

Lazenby, M. (2013). On the humanities of nursing. *Nursing Outlook*, 61(1), e9–e14.

Nicely, B. and DeLario, G. (2011). Virginia Henderson's principles and practice of nursing applied to organ donation after brain death. *Progress in Transplantation*, 21(1), 72–77.

Runk, J.A. and Quillin, S.I.M. (1989). Henderson's definition of nursing. In J.J. Fitzpatrick and A.L. Whall (Eds.), *Conceptual models of nursing: Analysis and application* (2nd ed.). Bowie, MD: Robert J. Brady Co.

19. Douglas Howland

Howland, D. (1963). Approaches to the systems problem, Part I. *Nursing Research*, 13, 172–174.

Howland, D. (1963). A hospital system model, Part II. *Nursing Research*, 12(4), 232–236.

Howland, D. (1966). Approach to nurse-monitor research. *American Journal of Nursing*, 66(3), 566–588.

Howland, D. and McDowell, W.E. (1964). The measurement of patient care: A conceptual framework. *Nursing Research*, 13(1), 4–7.

20. Dorothy Johnson

Adam, E. (1987). Nursing theory: What it is and what it is not. *Nursing Papers/Perspectives on Nursing*, 19(1), 5–14.

Ainsworth, M. (1972). Attachment and dependency: A comparison. In J. Gewirtz (Ed.), *Attachment and dependency*. Englewood Cliffs, NJ: Prentice-Hall.

Alligood, M.R. (2002). Philosophies, models, theories: Critical thinking structures. In M.R. Alligood and A. Marriner Tomey (Eds.), *Nursing theory utilization and applications* (2nd ed., pp. 41–61). St. Louis, MO: C.V. Mosby.

Alligood, M.R. (2014). Philosophies, models and theories: Critical thinking structures. In M.R. Alligood (Ed.) *Nursing theory: Utilization and application* (5th ed., pp. 40–62). St. Louis: C.V. Mosby

Auger, J.R. (1976). *Behavioral systems and nursing*. Englewood Cliffs, NJ: Prentice-Hall.

†Auger, J.R. and Dee, V. (1983). A patient classification system based on the behavioral system model of nursing: Part 1. *Journal of Nursing Administration*, 13, 38–43.

Bluhm, R.L. (2014). The (dis)unity of nursing science. *Nursing Philosophy*, 15(4), 250–260.

Botha, M.E. (1989). Theory development in perspective: The role of conceptual frameworks and models in theory development. *Journal of Advanced Nursing*, 14(1), 49–55.

†Broncatello, K.F. (1980). Auger in action: Application of the model. *Advances in Nursing Science*, 2(2), 13–23.

Bruce, G.L., Hinds, P., Hudak, J., Mucha, A., Taylor, M.C., and Thompson, C.R. (1980). Implementation of ANA's quality assurance program for clients with end-stage renal disease. *Advances in Nursing Science*, 2(2), 79–95.

Buckley, W. (1968). *Modern systems research for the behavioral scientist*. Chicago, IL: Aldine.

Chen, C.J., Chen, Y.C., Sung, H.C., Kuo, P.C., and Wang, C.H. (2011). Perinatal attachment in naturally pregnant and infertility-treated pregnant women in Taiwan. *Journal of Advanced Nursing*, 67(10), 2200–2208.

Chin, R. (1961). The utility of system models and developmental models for practitioners. In W.G. Bennis, K.D. Beene, and R. Chin (Eds.), *The planning of change* (pp. 201–215). New York: Holt, Rinehart and Winston.

Clough, D.H. and Derdiarian, A. (1980). A behavioral checklist to measure dependence and independence. *Nursing Research*, 29(1), 55–58.

Colling, J., Owen, T.R., McCreedy, M., and Newman, D. (2003). The effects of a continence program on frail community-dwelling elderly persons. *Urologic Nursing*, 23(2), 117–127.

Conner, S., Magers, J., and Watt, J. (1989). Dorothy E. Johnson: Behavioral system model. In A. Marriner-Tomey (Ed.), *Nursing theorists and their work* (2nd ed.). St. Louis, MO: C.V. Mosby.

Cormack, D.F. and Reynolds, W. (1992). Criteria for evaluating the clinical and practical utility of models used by nurses. *Journal of Advanced Nursing*, 17(12), 1472–1478.

Coward, D.D. and Wilkie, D.J. (2000). Metastatic bone pain: Meanings associated with self-report and self-management decision making. *Cancer Nursing*, 23(2), 101–108.

Damus, K. (1980). An application of the Johnson behavioral system model for nursing practice. In J.P. Riehl and C. Roy (Eds.), *Conceptual models for nursing practice*. New York: Appleton-Century-Crofts.

Dee, V. (1986). *Validation of a patient classification instrument for psychiatric patients based on the Johnson model for nursing*. Unpublished doctoral dissertation. University of California, San Francisco.

Dee, V. (1990). Implementation of the Johnson model: One hospital's experience. In M.E. Parker (Ed.), *Nursing theories in practice* (pp. 33–44). New York: National League for Nursing.

†Dee, V. and Auger, J.R. (1983). A patient classification system based on the behavioral system model of nursing: Part 2. *Journal of Nursing Administration*, 13, 18–23.

Dee. V. and Poster, E.C. (1995). Applying Kanter's theory of innovative change: The transition from a primary to attending model of nursing care delivery. *Journal of American Psychiatric Nurses Association*, 1(4), 112–119.

Dee, V. and van Servellen, G. (1998). Managed behavioral health care patients and their nursing care problems, level of functioning, and impairment at discharge. *Journal of American Psychiatric Nurses Association*, 4(2), 57–66.

Derdiarian, A. (1984). *An investigation of the variables and boundaries of cancer nursing: A pioneering approach using Johnson's behavioral systems model for nursing*. In Proceedings of the 3rd International Conference on Cancer Nursing. Melbourne, Australia: The Cancer Institute/Peter MacCallum Hospital and the Royal Melbourne Hospital.

Derdiarian, A.K. (1981). Nursing conceptual frameworks: Implications for education, practice, and research. In D.L. Vredevoe et al. (Eds.), *Concepts of oncology nursing* (pp. 369–386). Englewood Cliffs, NJ: Prentice-Hall.

†Derdiarian, A.K. (1983). An instrument for theory and research development using the behavioral systems model for nursing: The cancer patient. Part I. *Nursing Research*, 32(4), 196–201.

Derdiarian, A.K. (1990). Effects of using systematic assessment instruments on patient and nurse satisfaction with nursing care. *Oncology Nursing Forum*, 17, 95–101.

Derdiarian, A.K. (1990). The relationships among the subsystems of Johnson's behavioral system model. *Image: Journal of Nursing Scholarship*, 22, 219–225.

Derdiarian, A.K. (1991). Effects of using a nursing model-based assessment instrument on quality of nursing care. *Nursing Administration Quarterly*, 15(3), 1–16.

Derdiarian, A.K. (1993). Application of the Johnson Behavioral System Model in nursing practice. In M.E. Parker (Ed.), *Patterns of nursing theories in practice* (pp. 285–298). New York: National League for Nursing.

Derdiarian, A.K. (1993). The Johnson Behavioral System Model: Perspectives for nursing practice. In M.E. Parker (Ed.), *Patterns of nursing theories in practice* (pp. 267–284). New York: National League for Nursing.

Derdiarian, A.K. and Clough, D. (1980). A behavioral checklist to measure dependence and independence. *Nursing Research*, 28, 55–58.

†Derdiarian, A. and Forsythe, A.B. (1983). An instrument for theory and research development using the behavioral systems model for nursing: The cancer patient, Part II. *Nursing Research*, 32(4), 260–267.

Dickerson, S.S., Alqaissi, N., Underhill, M., and Lally, R.M. (2011). Surviving the wait: Defining support while awaiting breast cancer surgery. *Journal of Advanced Medicine*, 67(7), 1468–1479.

Dickoff, J., James, P., and Wiedenbach, E. (1968). Theory in a practice discipline, Part 1. Practice oriented theory. *Nursing Research*, 17(5), 415–435.

Draucker, C.B., Martsolf, D. and Stephenson, P.S. (2012). Ambiguity and violence in adolescent dating relationships. *Journal of Child and Adolescent Psychiatric Nursing*, 25(3), 149–157.

Fawcett, J. (1989). Johnson's behavioral system model. In J. Fawcett (Ed.), *Analysis and evaluation of conceptual models of nursing* (2nd ed.). Philadelphia, PA: F.A. Davis.

Feshback, S. (1970). Aggression. In P. Mussen (Ed.), *Carmichael's manual of child psychology* (3rd ed.). New York: John Wiley & Sons.

Frey, M.A., Rooke, L., Sieloff, C., Messmer, P.R., and Kameoka, T. (1995). King's framework theory in Japan, Sweden, and the United States. *Image: Journal of Nursing Scholarship*, 27, 127–130.

Fruehwirth, S. (1989). An application of Johnson's behavioral model: A case study. *Journal of Community Health Nursing*, 6(2), 61–71.

†Grubbs, J. (1980). An interpretation of the Johnson behavioral system model for nursing practice. In J.P. Riehl and C. Roy (Eds.), *Conceptual models for nursing practice*. New York: Appleton-Century-Crofts.

Hadley, B.J. (1970, March). *The utility of theoretical frameworks for curriculum development in nursing: The happening at Colorado*. Paper presented at WICHEN General Session, Honolulu, Hawaii.

Harris, R.B. (1986). Introduction of a conceptual model into a fundamental baccalaureate course. *Journal of Nursing Education*, 25, 66–69.

Holaday, B. (1974). Achievement behavior in chronically ill children. *Nursing Research*, 23, 25–30.

†Holaday, B. (1980). Implementing the Johnson model for nursing practice. In J.P. Riehl and C. Roy (Eds.), *Conceptual models for nursing practice* (2nd ed.). New York: Appleton-Century-Crofts.

Holaday, B. (1981). Maternal response to their chronically ill infants' attachment behavior of crying. *Nursing Research*, 30(6), 343–347.

Holaday, B. (1981). The Johnson behavioral system model for nursing and the pursuit of quality health care. In G.E. Lasker (Ed.), *Applied systems and cybernetics* (Vol. 4). New York: Pergamon Press.

Holaday, B. (1982). Maternal conceptual set development: Identifying patterns of maternal response to chronically ill infant crying. *Maternal-Child Nursing Journal*, 11(1), 47–58.

Holaday, B. (1987). Patterns of interaction between mothers and their chronically ill infants. *Maternal-Child Nursing Journal*, 16, 29–45.

Holaday, B. (1997). Johnson's behavioral system model in nursing practice. In M.R. Alligood et al. (Eds.), *Nursing theory: Utilization and application* (pp. 49–70). St. Louis, MO: Mosby Year Book.

Holaday, B. (2002). Johnson's behavioral system model in nursing practice. In M.R. Alligood and A. Marriner-Tomey (Eds.), *Nursing theory: Utilization and application* (2nd ed., pp. 149–171.) St. Louis, MO: C.V. Mosby.

Holaday, B. (2014). Dorothy E. Johnson's behavioral system model. In M.R. Alligood (Ed.), *Nursing theorists and their work* (8th ed., pp. 332–355). St. Louis, MO: C.V. Mosby

Holaday, B. (2015). Dorothy Johnson's behavioral system model and its application. In M.C. Smith and M.E. Parker (Eds.), *Nursing theories and nursing practice* (4th ed., pp. 89–104). Philadelphia, PA: F.A. Davis

Holaday, B. and Turner-Henson, A. (1987). Chronically ill school-age children's use of time. *Pediatric Nursing*, 13, 410–414.

Holaday, B., Turner-Henson, A., and Swan, J. (1996). The Johnson behavioral system model: Explaining activities of chronically ill children. In P.H. Walker and B. Neuman (Eds.), *Blueprint for use of nursing models* (pp. 33–63). New York: NLN Press.

*Johnson, D.E. (1959). The nature of a science of nursing. *Nursing Outlook*, 7(5), 291–294.

†Johnson, D.E. (1959). A philosophy of nursing. *Nursing Outlook*, 7(4), 198–200.

†Johnson, D.E. (1961). The significance of nursing care. *Nursing Outlook*, 61(11), 63–66.

Johnson, D.E. (1964). *Is there an identifiable body of knowledge essential to the development of a generic professional nursing program?* Paper presented at First Interuniversity Faculty Work Conference Nursing Council, NEBHE, Stowe, VT.

Johnson, D.E. (1968). *One conceptual model of nursing.* Paper presented at Vanderbilt University, Nashville, TN.

*Johnson, D.E. (1968). Theory in nursing: Borrowed or unique. *Nursing Research*, 17(3), 206–209.

Johnson, D.E. (1974). Development of theory: A requisite for nursing as a primary health profession. *Nursing Research*, 23(5), 372–377.

Johnson, D.E. (1978). State of the art of theory development in nursing. In *Theory development: What, why, how?* New York: National League for Nursing.

†Johnson, D.E. (1980). The behavioral system model for nursing. In J.P. Riehl and C. Roy (Eds.), *Conceptual models for nursing practice* (2nd ed.). New York: Appleton-Century-Crofts.

Johnson, D.E. (1987). Evaluating conceptual models for use in critical care nursing practice. *Dimensions of Critical Care Nursing*, 6(4), 195–197.

Johnson, D.E. (1989). Some thoughts on nursing. *Clinical Nurse Specialist*, 3(1), 1–4.

Johnson, D.E. (1990). The behavioral system model for nursing. In M.E. Parker (Ed.), *Nursing theories in practice* (pp. 23–32). New York: National League for Nursing.

Johnson, D.E. (1992). The origins of the behavioral system model. In F.N. Nightingale (Ed.), *Notes on nursing: What it is, and what it is not* (Commemorative edition, pp. 23–27). Philadelphia, PA: J.B. Lippincott.

Johnson, D.E. (1996). Introduction to the Johnson behavioral system model: Explaining activities of chronically ill children. In P. Hinton Walker and B. Neuman (Eds.), *Blueprint for use of nursing models* (pp, 33–34). New York: NLN Press.

Karmels, P. (1993). Conundrum game for nursing theorists Neuman, King, and Johnson. *Nurse Educator*, 18(6), 8–9.

Kaya, N. (2012). Effect of attachment styles of individuals discharged from an intensive care unit on intensive care experience. *Journal of Critical Care*, 27(1), 103e7–103e14.

Lachicotte, J.L. and Alexander, J.W. (1990). Management attitudes and nurse impairment. *Nursing Management*, 21, 102–104, 106, 108, 110.

Lobo, M.L. (2002). Behavioral system model: Dorothy E. Johnson. In J.B. George (Ed.), *Nursing theories: The base for professional nursing practice* (5th ed., pp. 155–169). Upper Saddle River, NJ: Prentice Hall.

†Lovejoy, N.C. (1983). The leukemic child's perceptions of family behaviors. *Oncology Nursing Forum*, 10(4), 20–25.

Lovejoy, N. (1985). *Needs of vigil and nonvigil visitors in cancer research units*. In Fourth Cancer Nursing Research Conference Proceedings. Honolulu, HI: American Cancer Society.

Loveland-Cherry, C. and Wilkerson, S.A. (1989). Dorothy Johnson's behavioral system model. In J.J. Fitzpatrick and A.L. Whall (Eds.), *Conceptual methods of nursing: Analysis to application* (2nd ed.). Bowie, MD: Robert J. Brady Co.

Majesky, S.J., Brester, M.H., and Nishio, K.T. (1978). Development of a research tool: Patient indicators of nursing care. *Nursing Research*, 27, 365–371.

McCauley, K., Choromanski, J., and Liu, K. (1984). Learning to live with controlled ventricular tachycardia: Utilizing the Johnson model. *Heart and Lung*, 13(6), 633–638.

Naguib, H.H. (1988). *Physicians,' nurses,' and patients' perceptions of the surgical patients' educational rights*. Unpublished doctoral dissertation. University of Alexandria, United Republic of Egypt.

Newman, M.A. (1994). Theory for nursing practice. *Nursing Science Quarterly*, 7(4), 153–157.

Oyedele, O.A., Wright, S.C.D., and Maja, T.M.M. (2013). Prevention of teenage pregnancies in Soshanguve, South Africa: Using the Johnson behavioral system model. *Journal of Nursing and Midwifery*, 15(1), 95–108.

Parsons, T. (1951). *The social system*. New York: Free Press.

†Porter, L.S. (1972). The impact of physical-physiological activity on infants' growth and development. *Nursing Research*, 21(3), 210–219.

Poster, E.C. and Beliz, L. (1988). Behavioral category ratings of adolescents in an inpatient psychiatric unit. *International Journal of Adolescence and Youth*, 1, 293–303.

Poster, E.C. and Beliz, L. (1992). The use of the Johnson behavioral system model to measure changes during adolescent hospitalization. *International Journal of Adolescence and Youth*, 4, 73–84.

Poster, E.C., Dee, V., and Randell, B.P. (1997). The Johnson behavioral system model as framework for patient outcome evaluation. *Journal of the American Psychiatric Nurses Association*, 3, 73–80.

Randell, B.P. (1991). NANDA versus the Johnson behavioral systems model: Is there a diagnostic difference? In R.M. Carroll-Johnson (Ed.), *Classification of nursing diagnoses: Proceedings of the ninth conference, North American Nursing Diagnosis Association* (pp. 154–160). Philadelphia, PA: Lippincott.

Randell, B.P. (1992). Nursing theory: The 21st century. *Nursing Science Quarterly*, 5(4), 176–184.

Rapaport, A. (1968). Forward. In W. Buckley (Ed.), *Modern systems research for the behavioral scientist* (pp. xiii–xxii). Chicago, IL: Aldine.

†Rawls, A.C. (1980). Evaluation of the Johnson behavioral model in clinical practice. Report of a test and evaluation of the Johnson theory. *Image: Journal of Nursing Scholarship*, 12, 13–16.

Reynolds, W. and Cormack, D.F. (1991). An evaluation of the Johnson Behavioral System Model of Nursing. *Journal of Advanced Nursing*, 16(9), 1122–1130.

Roy, C. (1980). A case study viewed according to different models. In J.P. Riehl and C. Roy (Eds.), *Conceptual models for nursing practice*. New York: Appleton-Century-Crofts.

Sears, R.R., Maccoby, E.E., and Levin, H. (1957). Patterns of child rearing. Evanston, IL: Row & Peterson.

†Small, B. (1980). Nursing visually impaired children with Johnson's model as a conceptual framework. In J.P. Riehl and C. Roy (Eds.), *Conceptual models for nursing practice* (2nd ed.). New York: Appleton-Century-Crofts.

Stamler, C. and Palmer, J.O. (1971). Dependency and repetitive visits to the nurse's office in elementary school children. *Nursing Research*, 20(3), 254–255.

von Bertalanffy, L. (1968). *General systems theory: Foundations, development, application*. New York: George Braziller.

Wilkie, D. (1990). Cancer pain management: State-of-the-art care. *Nursing Clinics of North America*, 25, 331–343.

Wilkie, D.J., Lovejoy, N., Dodd, M., and Tesler, M. (1988). Cancer pain control behaviors: Description and correlation with pain intensity. *Oncology Nursing Forum*, 15(6), 723–731.

Wilkie, D.J., Lovejoy, N., Dodd, M., and Tesler, M. (1989). Pain control behaviors of patients with cancer. In S.G. Funk, E.M. Tornquist, M.T. Champagne, L.A. Copp, and R.A. Wiese (Eds.), *Key aspects of comfort: Management of pain, fatigue, and nausea*. New York: Springer-Verlag.

Wu, R. (1973). *Behavior and illness*. Englewood Cliffs, NJ: Prentice-Hall.

Zetterberg, H.L. (1963). *On theory verification in sociology* (Rev. ed.). Totowa, NJ: Bedminster Press.

21. Imogene King

Ackermann, M., Brink, S., Clanton, J., Jones, C., Moody, S., Perlich, G., Price, D., and Prusinski, B. (1989). Imogene King: Theory of goal attainment. In A. Marriner-Tomey (Ed.), *Nursing theorists and their work* (2nd ed.). St. Louis, MO: C.V. Mosby.

Aggleton, P. and Chalmers, H. (1990). Nursing models. King's model. *Nursing Times*, 86(1), 38–39.

Allan, N. (1999). Imogene King's goal attainment theory as the framework for nursing research. *Perspectives*, 23(2), 15–19.

Alligood, M.R. (2001). A theory of nursing empathy in King's Interacting Systems. *Tennessee Nurse*, 64(2), 18.

Alligood, M.R. (2014). Philosophies, models, and theories: Critical thinking structure. In M.A. Alligood (Ed.), *Nursing theory utilization and application* (5th ed., pp. 40–62). St Louis, MO: Mosby Company.

Alligood, M.R. and May, B.A. (2000). A nursing theory of personal system empathy: Interpreting a conceptualizing of empathy in King's interacting systems. *Nursing Science Quarterly*, 13(3), 243–247.

Alligood, M.R. and May, B.A. (2000). A nursing theory of personal system empathy: Interpreting a conceptualization of empathy in King's interacting systems. *Nursing Science Quarterly*, 13(2), 243–247.

Archibong, U.E. (1999). Evaluating the impact of primary nursing practice on the quality of nursing care: A Nigerian study. *Journal of Advanced Nursing*, 29(3), 680–689.

Asay, M.K. and Osler, C.C. (Eds.). (1984). *Conceptual models of nursing. Applications in community health nursing*. In Proceedings of the Eighth Annual Community Health Nursing Conference. Chapel Hill, NC: Department of Public Health Nursing, School of Public Health, University of North Carolina.

Astedt-Kurki, P., Friedemann, M.L., Paavilainen, E., et al. (2001). Assessment of strategies in families tested by Finnish families. *International Journal of Nursing Studies*, 38(1), 17–24.

Austin, J.K. and Champion, V.L. (1983). King's theory for nursing: Explication and evaluation. In P. Chinn (Ed.), *Advances in nursing theory development* (pp. 49–61). Rockville, MD: Aspen Systems.

Barnum, B.J.S. (1994). *Nursing theory: Analysis, application, and evaluation* (4th ed.). Philadelphia, PA: Lippincott.

Bauer, R. (1998). A dialectic reflection on the psychotherapeutic efficacy of nursing interventions [Article in German]. *Pflege*, 11(6), 305–311.

Bauer, R. (1999). A dialectic view of the efficacy of nursing interventions. Connections between interventions and effects of psychotherapy [Article in German]. *Pflege*, 12(1), 5–10.

Baumann, S.L. (2000). Family nursing: Theory-anemic, nursing theory-deprived. *Nursing Science Quarterly*, 13(4), 285–290.

Bello, I.T.R. (2000). Imogene King's theory as the foundation for the set of a teaching-learning process with undergraduation [sic] students [Portuguese]. *Texto & Contexto Enfermagem*, 9(2 part 2), 646–657.

Berggren, I., Barbosa sa Silva, A., and Severinsson, E. (2005). Core ethical issues of clinical nursing supervision. *Nursing and Health Sciences*, 7(1), 21–28.

Bradshaw, A. (1995). What are nurses doing to patients—A review of theories of nursing past and present. *Journal of Clinical Nursing*, 4(2), 81–92.

Bramlett, M.H., Gueldner, S.H., and Sowell, R.L. (1990). Consumer-centric advocacy: Its connection to nursing frameworks. *Nursing Science Quarterly*, 3(4), 156–161.

Brillhart, B. (2004). Studying the quality of life and life satisfaction among persons with spinal cord injury undergoing urinary management. *Rehabilitation Nursing*, 29(4), 122–126.

Brooks, E.M. and Thomas S. (1997). The perception and judgment of senior baccalaureate student nurses in clinical decision making. *Advances in Nursing Science*, 19(3), 50–69.

Brower, H.T. (1981). Social organization and nurses' attitudes toward older persons. *Journal of Gerontological Nursing*, 7, 293–298.

Brown, S.J. (1999). Student nurses' perceptions of elderly care. *Journal of the National Black Nurses Association*, 10(2), 29–36.

Brown, S.T. and Lee, B.T. (1980). Imogene King's conceptual framework: A proposed model for continuing nursing education. *Journal of Advanced Nursing*, 5(5), 467–473.

Bunting, S.M. (1988). The concept of perception in selected nursing theories. *Nursing Science Quarterly*, 1(4), 168–174.

Burney, M.A. (1992). King and Neuman: In search of the nursing paradigm. *Journal of Advanced Nursing*, 17(5), 601–603.

Byrne-Coker, E. and Schreiber, R. (1990). King at the bedside. *Canadian Nurse*, 86(1), 24–26.

Caceres, B.A. (2015). King's theory of goal attainment: Exploring functional status. *Nursing Science Quarterly*, 28(2), 151–155.

Carter, K.F. and Dufour, L.I. (1994). King's theory: A critique of the critiques. *Nursing Science Quarterly*, 7(3), 128–133.

Cho, M.K. (2013). Effect of health contract intervention on renal dialysis patients in Korea. *Nursing and Health Sciences*, 15(1), 86–93.

Clarke, P.N., Killeen, M.B., Messmer, P.R., and Sieloff, C.L. (2009). Imogene M. King's scholars reflect on her wisdom and influence on nursing science. *Nursing Science Quarterly*, 22(2), 128–133.

Clements, H. and Melby, V. (1998). An investigation into the information obtained by patients undergoing gastroscopy investigations. *Journal of Clinical Nursing*, 7(4), 333–342.

Daniel, J.M. (2002). Young adults' perceptions of living with chronic inflammatory bowel disease. *Gastroenterology Nursing*, 25(3), 83–94.

Daubenmire, M.J. (1989). A baccalaureate nursing curriculum based on King's conceptual framework. In J. Riehl-Sisca (Ed.), *Conceptual models for nursing practice* (3rd ed.). Norwalk, CT: Appleton & Lange.

Daubenmire, M.J. and King, I.M. (1973). Nursing process models: A systems approach. *Nursing Outlook*, 21(8), 512–517.

de Witte, L., Schoot, T., and Proot, I. (2006). Development of the client-centered care questionnaire. *Journal of Advanced Nursing*, 56(1), 62–68.

DiNardo, P.B. (1989). Evaluation of the nursing theory of Imogene M. King. In J. Riehl-Sisca (Ed.), *Conceptual models for nursing practice* (3rd ed.). Norwalk, CT: Appleton & Lange.

Doornbos, M.M. (1995). Using King's systems framework to explore family health in the families of the young chronically mentally ill. In M.A. Frey and C.L. Sieloff (Eds.), *Advancing King's systems framework and theory of nursing* (pp. 192–205). Thousand Oaks, CA: Sage.

Doornbos, M.M. (2000). King's systems framework and family health: The derivation and testing of a theory. *Journal of Theory Construction and Testing*, 4(1), 20–26.

Doornbos, M.M. (2007). King's conceptual system and family health theory in the families of adults with persistent mental illnesses–An evolving conceptualization. In C.L. Sieloff, M.A. Frey, and I.M. King (Eds.), *Middle range theory development using King's conceptual system*. New York: Springer Publishing Company.

Dougal, J. and Gonterman, R. (1999). A comparison of three teaching methods on learning and retention. *Journal For Nurses in Staff Development*, 15(5), 205–209.

Douglas, T.S., Mann, N.H., and Hodge, A.L. (1998). Evaluation of preoperative patient education and computer-assisted patient instruction. *Journal of Spinal Disorders*, 11(1), 29–35.

Draaistra, H., Singh, M.D., Ireland, S, and Harper, T. (2012). Patients' perceptions of their roles in goal setting in a spinal cord injury regional rehabilitation program. *Canadian Journal of Neuroscience Nursing*, 34(3), 22–30.

Duldt, B.W. (1995). Integrating nursing theory and ethics. *Perspectives in Psychiatric Care*, 31(2), 4–10.

du Mont, P. (2007). A theory of asynchronous development. In C.L. Sieloff, M.A. Frey, and I.M. King (Eds.), *Middle range theory development using King's conceptual system*. New York: Springer Publishing Company.

Ehrenberger, H.E., Alligood, M.R., Thomas, S.P., Wallace, D.C., and Licavoli, C.M. (2002). Testing a theory of decision-making derived from King's systems framework in women eligible for a cancer clinical trial. *Nursing Science Quarterly*, 15(2), 156–163.

Elberson, K. (1989). Applying King's model to nursing administration. In B. Henry, C. Arndt, M. DiVincenti, and A. Marriner-Tomey (Eds.), *Dimensions of nursing administration: Theory, research, education, practice*. Boston, MA: Blackwell Scientific Publications.

Erci, B. (2005). Nursing theories applied to vulnerable populations: Examples from Turkey. In M. de Chesnay (Ed.), *Caring for the vulnerable: Perspectives in nursing theory, practice, and research*. Sudbury, MA: Jones & Bartlett Publishers.

Fairfax, J. (2007). Development of a middle range theory of quality of life of stroke survivors derived from King's conceptual system. In C.L. Sieloff, M.A. Frey, and I.M. King (Eds.), *Middle range theory development using King's conceptual system*. New York: Springer Publishing Company.

Fawcett, J. (1989). King's interacting systems framework. In J. Fawcett (Ed.), *Analysis and evaluation of conceptual models of nursing* (2nd ed.). Philadelphia, PA: F.A. Davis.

Fawcett, J. (2001). The nurse theorists: 21st-century updates—Imogene M. King. *Nursing Science Quarterly*, 14(4), 311–315.

Fawcett, J. and DeSanto-Madeya, S. (2013). *Contemporary nursing knowledge: Analysis and evaluation of nursing models and theories* (3rd ed.). Philadelphia, PA: F.A. Davis.

Fawcett, J.M., Vaillancourt, V.H., and Watson, C.A. (1995). Integration of King's framework into nursing practice. In. M.A. Frey and C.L. Sieloff (Eds.), *Advancing King's system framework and theory of goal attainment* (p. 176). Thousand Oaks, CA: Sage Publications.

Fewster-Thuente, L. and Velsor-Friedrich, B. (2008). Interdisciplinary collaboration for healthcare professionals. *Nursing Administration Quarterly*, 32(1), 40–48.

Fontana, J.A. (1996). The emergence of the person-environment interaction in a descriptive study of vigor in heart failure. *Advances in Nursing Science*, 18(4), 70–82.

Franca, I.S.X. and Pagliuca, L.M.F. (2002). Usefulness and the social significance of the theory of goal attainment by King [Portuguese]. *Revista Brasileira De Enfermagem*, 55(1), 44–51.

Frey, M.A. (1989). Social support and health: A theoretical formulation derived from King's conceptual framework. *Nursing Science Quarterly*, 138–148.

Frey, M.A. and Norris, D. (1997). King's systems framework and theory in nursing practice. In M.R. Alligood (Ed.), *Nursing theory: Utilization and application* (pp. 71–88). St. Louis, MO: Mosby Year Book.

Frey, M.A., Rooke, L., Sieloff, C., Messmer, P.R., and Kameoka, T. (1995). King's framework and theory in Japan, Sweden, and the United States. *Image: Journal of Nursing Scholarship*, 27(2), 127–130.

Frey, M.A. and Sieloff, C. (Eds.). (1995). *Advancing King's systems framework and theory of nursing*. Thousand Oaks, CA: Sage.

Frey, M.A., Sieloff, C.L., and Norris, D.M. (2002). King's conceptual system and theory of goal attainment: Past, present, and future. *Nursing Science Quarterly*, 15(2), 107–112.

Friedmann, M.L. (1989). The concept of family nursing. *Journal of Advanced Nursing*, 14, 211–216.

George, J.B. (1980). Imogene King. In The Nursing Theories Conference Group (Eds.), *Nursing theories: The base for professional nursing practice*. Englewood Cliffs, NJ: Prentice-Hall.

George, J.B. (2002). Systems framework and theory of goal attainment—Imogene M. King. In J.B. George (Ed.), *Nursing theories: The base for professional nursing practice* (5th ed., pp. 241–267). Upper Saddle River, NJ: Prentice Hall.

Gold, C., Haas, S., and King, I. (2000). Conceptual frameworks. Putting the nursing focus into care curricula. *Nurse Educator*, 25(2), 95–98.

Gonot, P.J. (1983). Imogene M. King: A theory for nursing. In J.J. Fitzpatrick and A.L. Whall (Eds.), *Conceptual models of nursing: Analysis and application*. Bowie, MD: Robert J. Brady Co.

Gonot, P.J. (1986). Family therapy as derived from King's conceptual model. In A.L. Whall (Ed.), *Family therapy for nursing. Four approaches*. Norwalk, CT: Appleton-Century-Crofts.

Gonot, P.J. (1989). Imogene M. King's conceptual framework of nursing. In J.J. Fitzpatrick and A.L. Whall (Eds.), *Conceptual models of nursing: Analysis and application* (2nd ed.). Bowie, MD: Robert J. Brady Co.

Goodwin, Z., Kiehl, E.M., and Peterson, J.Z. (2002). King's theory as foundation for an advance directive decision-making model. *Nursing Science Quarterly*, 15(3), 237–241.

Gulitz, E.A. and King, I.M. (1988). King's general systems model: Application to curriculum development. *Nursing Science Quarterly*, 1(3), 128–132.

Hampton, D.C. (1994). King's theory of goal attainment as a framework for managed care implementation in a hospital setting. *Nursing Science Quarterly*, 7(4), 170–173.

Hanchett, E.S. (1990). Nursing models and community as client. *Nursing Science Quarterly*, 3(2), 67–72.

Hanna, K.M. (1997). An oral contraceptive perception scale for female adolescents. *Western Journal of Nursing Research*, 19(4), 519–529.

Hanna, K.M. (1999). Commentary on "An adolescent and young adult condom perception scale"—Response by Hanna. *Western Journal of Nursing Research*, 21(5), 633–634.

Hanucharurnkui, S. (1989). Comparative analysis of Orem's and King's theories. *Journal of Advanced Nursing*, 14, 365–372.

Hanucharurnkui, S. and Vinya-nguag, P. (1991). Effects of promoting patients' participation in self-care on postoperative recovery and satisfaction with care. *Nursing Science Quarterly*, 4(1), 14–20.

Hawks, J.H. (1991). Power: A concept analysis. *Journal of Advanced Nursing*, 16(6), 754–762.

Heikkila, K., Sarvimaki, A., and Ekman, S.L. (2007). Culturally congruent care for older people: Finnish care in Sweden. *Scandinavian Journal of Caring Sciences*, 21(3), 354–361.

Hilton, P.A. (1997). Theoretical perspectives of nursing: A review of the literature. *Journal of Advanced Nursing*, 26(6), 1211–1220.

Huch, M.H. (1991). Perspectives on health. *Nursing Science Quarterly*, 4(1), 33–40.

Huch, M.H. (1995). Nursing and the next millennium. *Nursing Science Quarterly*, 8(1), 38–44.

Hupcey, J.E. and Penrod, J. (2005). Concept analysis: Examining the state of the science. *Research and Theory in Nursing Practice*, 19(2), 197–208.

Husband, A. (1988). Application of King's theory of nursing to the care of the adult with diabetes. *Journal of Advanced Nursing*, 13(4), 484–488.

Husting, P.M. (1997). A transcultural critique of Imogene King's theory of global attainment. *Journal of Multicultural Nursing and Health*, 3(3), 15–20.

Isac, C., Ezhilarau, P. and Chacko, R.T. (2012). Information: A priceless gift in chronic care management of cancer patients. *International Journal of Biosciences*, 2(1), 80–85.

Janzen, S.K., Nelson, A., Nodhturft, V., and Quigley, P. (2001). James A. Haley's dedication to Dr. Imogene King, our link between theory and nursing services. *Florida Nurse*, 49(3), 21.

Jones, A. (2005). Perceptions on individualized approaches to mental health care. *Journal of Psychiatric and Mental Health Nursing*, 12(4), 396–404.

Jones, A. and Bugge, C. (2006). Improving understanding and rigour through triangulation: An exemplar based on patient participation in interaction. *Journal of Advanced Nursing*, 55(5), 612–621.

Karmels, P. (1993). Conundrum game for nursing theorists Neuman, King, and Johnson. *Nurse Educator*, 18(6), 8–9.

Kemppainen, J.K. (1990). Imogene King's theory: A nursing case study of a psychotic client with human immunodeficiency virus infection. *Archives of Psychiatric Nursing*, 4(6), 384–388.

Kenny, T. (1990). Erosion of individuality in care of elderly people in hospital—An alternative approach. *Journal of Advanced Nursing*, 15(5), 571–576.

Khowaja, K. (2006). Utilization of King's interacting systems framework and theory of goal attainment with new multidisciplinary model: Clinical pathway. *Australian Journal of Advanced Nursing*, 24(2), 44–50.

Killeen, M.B. (2007). Development and initial testing of a theory of patient satisfaction with nursing care. In C.L. Sieloff, M.A. Frey, and I.M. King (Eds.), *Middle range theory development using King's conceptual system*. New York: Springer Publishing Company.

Killeen, M.B. and King, I.M. (2007). Viewpoint: Use of King's conceptual system, nursing informatics, and nursing classification systems for global communication. *International Journal of Nursing Terminologies and Classifications*, 18(2), 51–57.

Kim, I.M. and Whelton, B.J.B. (2001). Letters to the editor . . . "A nursing theory of personal system empathy: Interpreting a conceptualization of empathy in King's Interacting Systems." *Nursing Science Quarterly*, 14(1), 80–82.

King, I.M. (1964). Nursing theory: Problems and prospects. *Nursing Science*, 2, 394–403.

King, I.M. (1968). A conceptual frame of reference for nursing. *Nursing Research*, 17(1), 27–31.

King, I.M. (1971). *Toward a theory for nursing: General concepts of human behavior*. New York: John Wiley & Sons.

King, I.M. (1975). A process for developing concepts for nursing through research. In P.J. Verhonick (Ed.), *Nursing research* (Vol. 1). Boston, MA: Little, Brown.

King, I.M. (1976). The health care system: Nursing intervention subsystem. In W.H. Werley et al. (Eds.), *Health research: The systems approach*. New York: Springer-Verlag.

King, I.M. (1978). USA: Loyola University of Chicago School of Nursing. *Journal of Advanced Nursing*, 3, 390.

King, I.M. (1981). *A theory for nursing: Systems, concepts, process*. New York: John Wiley & Sons.

King, I.M. (1983). The family coping with a medical illness. Analysis and application of King's theory of goal attainment. In I.W. Clements and F.B. Roberts (Eds.), *Family health: A theoretical approach to nursing care*. New York: John Wiley & Sons.

King, I.M. (1983). King's theory of nursing. In I.W. Clements and F.B. Roberts (Eds.), *Family health: A theoretical approach to nursing*. New York: John Wiley & Sons.

King, I.M. (1984). Effectiveness of nursing care: Use of a goal oriented nursing record in end stage renal disease. *American Association of Nephrology Nurses and Technicians Journal*, 11(2), 11–17, 60.

King, I.M. (1984). Philosophy of nursing education: A national survey. *Western Journal of Nursing Research*, 6(4), 387–406.

King, I.M. (1986). King's theory of goal attainment. In P. Winstead-Fry (Ed.), *Case studies in nursing theory*. New York: National League for Nursing.

King, I.M. (1986). *Curriculum and instruction in nursing*. Norwalk, CT: Appleton-Century-Crofts.

King, I.M. (1987). Translating research into practice. *Journal of Neuroscience Nursing*, 19(1), 44–48.

King, I.M. (1987). King's theory of goal attainment. In R.R. Parse (Ed.), *Nursing science: Major paradigms, theories, and critiques*. Philadelphia, PA: W.B. Saunders.

King, I.M. (1988). Concepts: Essential elements of theories. *Nursing Science Quarterly*, 1(1), 22–25.

King, I.M. (1988). Measuring health goal attainment in patients. In C.F. Waltz and O. Strickland (Eds.), *Measurement of nursing outcomes: Measuring client outcomes*. New York: Springer Publishing Company.

King, I.M. (1989). King's systems framework and theory. In J. Riehl-Sisca (Ed.), *Conceptual models for nursing practice* (3rd ed.). Norwalk, CT: Appleton & Lange.

King, I.M. (1989). King's system framework for nursing administration. In B. Henry, C. Arndt, M. DiVincenti, and A. Marriner-Tomey (Eds.), *Dimensions of nursing administration: Theory, research, education, practice*. Boston, MA: Blackwell Scientific Publications.

King, I.M. (1990). Health as the goal for nursing. *Nursing Science Quarterly*, 3(3), 123–128.

King, I.M. (1990). King's conceptual framework and theory of goal attainment. In M.E. Parker (Ed.), *Nursing theories in practice* (pp. 73–84). New York: National League for Nursing.

King, I.M. (1992). King's theory of goal attainment. *Nursing Science Quarterly*, 5(1), 19–26.

King, I.M. (1992). Window on general systems framework and theory of goal attainment. In M. O'Toole (Ed.). *Miller Keane encyclopedia and dictionary of medicine, nursing, and allied health* (p. 604). Philadelphia, PA: W.B. Saunders.

King, I.M. (1994). Quality of life and goal attainment. *Nursing Science Quarterly*, 7(1), 29–32.

King, I.M. (1996). The theory of goal attainment in research and practice. *Nursing Science Quarterly*, 9(2), 61–66.

King, I.M. (1996). A systems framework for nursing. In M.A. Frey and C.L. Sieloff (Eds.), *Advancing King's systems framework and theory of nursing* (pp. 14–22). Los Angeles, CA: Sage Publications.

King, I.M. (1996). The theory of goal attainment. In M.A. Frey and C.L. Sieloff (Eds.), *Advancing King's systems framework and theory of nursing* (pp. 23–32). Los Angeles, CA: Sage Publications.

King, I.M. (1997). King's theory of goal attainment in practice. *Nursing Science Quarterly*, 10(4), 180–185.

King, I.M. (1997). Reflections of the past and a vision for the future. *Nursing Science Quarterly*, 10(1), 15–17.

King, I.M. (1997). Knowledge development for nursing: A process. In I.M. King and J. Fawcett (Eds.), *The language of nursing theory and metatheory* (pp. 19–25). Indianapolis, IN: Sigma Theta Tau International Center Nursing Press.

King, I.M. (1999). A theory of goal attainment: Philosophical and ethical implications. *Nursing Science Quarterly*, 12(4), 292–296.

King, I.M. (2000). Evidence-based nursing practice. *Theoria: Journal of Nursing Theory*, 9(2), 4–9.

King, I.M. (2001). Imogene M. King: Theory of goal attainment. In M.E. Parker (Ed.), *Nursing theories and nursing practice* (pp. 275–286). Philadelphia, PA: F.A. Davis.

King, I.M. (2006). A systems approach in nursing administration: Structure, process, and outcome. *Nursing Administration Quarterly*, 30(2), 100–104.

King, I.M. (2007). King's conceptual system, theory of goal attainment, and transaction process in the 21st century. *Nursing Science Quarterly*, 20(2), 109–111.

King, I.M. (2007). King's structure, process, and outcome in the 21st century. In C.L. Sieloff, M.A. Frey, and I.M. King (Eds.), *Middle range theory development using King's conceptual system*. New York: Springer Publishing Company.

King, I.M. (2008). Adversity and theory development. *Nursing Science Quarterly*, 21(2), 137–138.

Kline, K.S., Scott, L.D., and Britton, A.S. (2007). The use of supportive-educative and mutual goal-setting strategies to improve self-management for patients with heart failure. *Home Healthcare Nurse*, 25(8), 502–510.

Laben, J.K., Dodd, D., and Sneed, L. (1991). King's theory of goal attainment applied in group therapy for inpatient juvenile sexual offenders, maximum security state offenders, and community parolees, using visual aids. *Issues in Mental Health Nursing*, 12(1), 51–64.

Laitinen, P. and Isola, A. (1996). Promoting participation and informal caregivers in the hospital care of the elderly patient: Informal caregivers' perceptions. *Journal of Advanced Nursing*, 23(5), 942–947.

Larrabee, J.H., Engle, V.F., and Tolley, E.A. (1995). Predictors of patient-perceived quality. *Scandinavian Journal of Caring Sciences*, 9(3), 153–164.

Lawler, J., Dowswell, G., Hearn, J., et al. (1999). Recovering from stroke: A qualitative investigation of the role of goal setting in late stroke recovery. *Journal of Advanced Nursing*, 30(2), 401–409.

Lehna, C., Pfoutz, S., Peterson, T.G., et al. (1999). Nursing attire: Indicators of professionalism? *Journal of Professional Nursing*, 15(3), 192–199.

Leinonen, T.A., Leini-Kilpi, H. and Jouko, K. (1996). The quality of intraoperative nursing care: The patient's perspective. *Journal of Advanced Nursing*, 24(4), 843–852.

Lither, M. and Zilling, T. (2000). Pre- and postoperative information needs. *Patient Education and Counseling*, 40(1), 29–37.

Lockart, J.S. (2000). Nurses' perceptions of head and neck oncology patients after surgery: Severity of facial disfigurement and patient gender. *Plastic Surgical Nursing*, 20(2), 68–80.

Lowry, D.A. (1998). Issues of non-compliance in mental health. *Journal of Advanced Nursing*, 28(2), 280–287.

Magan, S. (1987). A critique of King's theory. In R.R. Parse (Ed.), *Nursing science: Major paradigms, theories, and critiques*. Philadelphia, PA: W.B. Saunders.

Martin, J.P. (1990). Male cancer awareness: Impact of an employee education program. *Oncology Nursing Forum*, 17, 59–64.

Masters, K. (2005). Framework for professional nursing practice. In K. Masters (Ed.), *Role development in professional nursing practice*. Sudbury, MA: Jones & Bartlett Publishers.

McKinney, N.L. and Dean, P.R. (2000). Application of King's theory of dynamic interacting systems to the study of child abuse and the development of alcohol use/dependence in adult females. *Journal of Addictions Nursing*, 12(2), 73–82.

Meleis, A.I. (1985). International nursing for knowledge development. *Nursing Outlook*, 33(3), 144–147.

Meleis, A.I. and Jones, A. (1983). Ethical crises and cultural differences. *Western Journal of Medicine*, 138(6), 889–893.

Messmer, P. (1995). Implementation of theory-based nursing practice. In M.A. Frey and C.L. Sieloff (Eds.), *Advancing King's systems framework and theory of nursing* (p. 294). Thousand Oaks, CA: Sage Publications.

Messmer, P.R. (2006). Professional model of care: Using King's theory of goal attainment. *Nursing Science Quarterly*, 19(3), 227–229.

Meyer, G. and Lavin, M.A. (2005). Vigilance: The essence of nursing. *Online Journal of Issues in Nursing*, 10(3), 8.

Michota, S. (1995). A hospital-based skilled nursing facility— A special place to care for the elderly. *Geriatric Nursing*, 16(2), 64–66.

Miller, T., Kanai, T., Kebritchi, M., Grendell, R., and Howard, T. (2015). Hiring nurses re-entering the workforce after chemical dependence. *Journal of Nursing Education and Practice*, 5(11), 65–72.

Moreira, T.M.M. and Araujo, T.L. (2002). The conceptual model of interactive open systems and the theory of goal attainment by Imogene King [Portuguese]. *Revista Latino-Americana de Enfermagem*, 10(1), 97–103.

Moreira, T.M.M. and Araujo, T.L. (2002). Interpersonal system of Imogene King: The relationships among patients with no-compliance to the treatment of the hypertension and professionals of health [Portuguese]. *Acta Paulista de Enfermagem*, 15(3), 35–43.

Moreira, T.M.M., Araujo, T.L., and Pagliuca, L.M.F. (2001). King's theory reach to families of persons with systemic arterial hypertension [Portuguese]. *Revista Gaucha de Enfermagem*, 22(2), 74–89.

Munhall, P.L. (2006). Epistemology in nursing. In P.L. Munhall (Ed.), *Nursing research: A qualitative perspective* (4th ed.). Sudbury, MA: Jones & Bartlett Publishers.

Murray, R.L.E. and Baier, M. (1996). King's conceptual framework applied to a transitional living program. *Perspectives in Psychiatric Care*, 32(1), 15–19.

Norgan, G.H., Ettipio, A.M., and Lasome, C.E. (1995). A program plan addressing carpal tunnel syndrome: The utility of King's goal attainment theory. *Journal of the American Association of Occupational Health Nurses*, 43(8), 407–411.

Norris, D.M. and Frey, M.A. (2002). King's interacting systems framework and theory in nursing practice. In M.R. Alligood and A. Mariner-Tomey (Eds.), *Nursing theory utilization and application* (2nd ed., pp. 173–196). St. Louis, MO: C.V. Mosby.

Norris, D.M. and Hoyer, P.J. (1993). Dynamism in practice: Parenting within King's framework. *Nursing Science Quarterly*, 6(2), 79–85.

Omnibus Budget Reconciliation Act. (1990), Pub. L. No. 101–508 and 4206, 4751 (From Goodwin, Kiehl, and Patterson, 2002).

Paavilainen, E. and Astedt-Kurki, P. (1997). The client-nurse relationship as experienced by public health nurses: Toward better collaboration. *Public Health Nursing*, 14(3), 137–142.

Parse, R.R. (2008). Nursing knowledge development: Who's to say how? *Nursing Science Quarterly*, 21(2), 101.

Patistea, E. (1999). Nurses' perceptions of caring as documented in theory and research. *Journal of Clinical Nursing*, 8(5), 487–495.

Pierce, S., Grodal, K., Smith, L.S., Elia-Tyvoll, S., Miller, A., and Tallman, C. (2002). Image of the nurse on Internet greeting cards. *Journal of Undergraduate Nursing Scholarship*, 4(1), 10.

Pilkington, F.B. (2007). Envisioning nursing in 2050 through the eyes of nurse theorists: King, Neuman, and Roy. *Nursing Science Quarterly*, 20(2), 108.

Plummer, M. and Molzahn, A.E. (2009). Quality of life in contemporary nursing theory: A concept analysis. *Nursing Science Quarterly*, 22(2), 134–140.

Poroch, D. (1995). The effect of preparatory patient education on the anxiety and satisfaction of cancer patients receiving radiation therapy. *Cancer Nursing*, 18(3), 206–214.

Richard-Hughes, S. (1997). Attitudes and beliefs of Afro-Americans related to organ and tissue donation. *International Journal of Trauma Nursing*, 119–123.

Rooke, L. (1995). Focusing on King's theory and systems framework in education by using an experiential learning model: A challenge to improve the quality of nursing care. In M.A. Frey and C. Sieloff (Eds.), *Advancing King's framework and theory for nursing* (pp. 278–293). Newbury Park, CA: Sage.

Rooda, L.A. (1992). The development of a conceptual model for multicultural nursing. *Journal of Holistic Nursing*, 10(4), 337–347.

Rooke, L. and Norberg, A. (1988). Problematic and meaningful situations in nursing interpreted by concepts from King's nursing theory and four additional concepts. *Scandinavian Journal of Caring Sciences*, 2(2), 80–87.

Rosendahl, P.B. and Ross, V. (1982). Does your behavior affect your patient's response? *Journal of Gerontological Nursing*, 8, 572–575.

Ross, M.M., Hoff, L.A., and Coutu-Wakulczyk, G. (1998). Nursing curricula and violence issues. *Journal of Nursing Education*, 37(2), 53–60.

Ryle, S. (2008). Current evidence on anticoagulant management and outcomes for postpolypectomy: An integrative literature review to assist advanced practice nurses. *Gastroenterology Nursing*, 31(5), 354–364.

Schreiber, R. (1991). Psychiatric assessment "a la King." *Nursing Management*, 22(5), 90, 92, 94.

Shanta, L.L., and Connolly, M. (2013). Using King's interacting systems theory to link emotional intelligence and nursing practice. *Journal of Professional Nursing*, 29(3), 174–180.

Sheldon, L.K. (2005). *Communication for nurses: Talking with patients*. Sudbury, MA: Jones & Bartlett Publishers.

Shuldham, C. (1999). Pre-operative education—A review of the research design. *International Journal of Nursing Studies*, 36(2), 179–187.

Sieloff, C.L. (2003). Measuring nursing power within organizations. *Journal of Nursing Scholarship*, 35(2), 183–187.

Sieloff, C.L. (2007). The theory of group power within organizations evaluating conceptualization within King's conceptual system. In C.L. Sieloff and M.A. Frey (Eds.), *Middle-Range theory development using King's conceptual system* (pp. 196–214). New York: Springer Publishing Company.

Sieloff, C.L. (2010). Improving work environment through the use of research instrument: An example. *Nursing Administration Quarterly*, 34(1), 56–60.

Sieloff, C.L., Frey, M.A., and King, I.M. (2007). *Middle range theory development using King's conceptual system*. New York: Springer Publishing Company.

Smith, M. (1988). King's theory in practice. *Nursing Science Quarterly*, 1(4), 145–146.

Sowell, R.L. and Lowenstein, A. (1994). King's theory as a framework for quality: Linking theory to practice. *Nursing Connections*, 7(2), 19–31.

Stevens, K.R. and Messmer, P.R. (2008). In remembrance of Imogene M. King, January 30, 1923–December 24, 2007: Imogene, a pioneer and dear colleague. *Nursing Outlook*, 56(3), 100–101.

Takahashi, T. (1992). Perspectives on nursing knowledge. *Nursing Science Quarterly*, 5(2), 86–91.

Temple, A. and Fawdry, K. (1992). King's theory of goal attainment. Resolving filial caregiver role strain. *Journal of Gerontological Nursing*, 18(3), 11–15.

Topps, C., Lopez, L., Messmer, P.R., and Franco, M. (2005). Perceptions of pediatric nurses toward bar-code point-of-care medication administration. *Nursing Administration Quarterly*, 29(1), 102–107.

Tritsch, J.M. (1998). Application of King's theory of goal attainment and the Carondelet St. Mary's case management model. *Nursing Science Quarterly*, 11(2), 69–73.

Uys, L. (1987). Foundational studies in nursing. *Journal of Advanced Nursing*, 12(3), 275–280.

Viera, C.S. and Rossi, L. (2000). Nursing diagnoses from NANDA's taxonomy in women with a hospitalized preterm child and King's conceptual system [Portuguese]. *Revista Latino-Americana de Enfermagem*, 8(6), 110–116.

von Bertalanffy, L. (1968). *General systems theory: Foundations, development, application*. New York: George Braziller.

Wadensten, B. (2005). The content of morning time conversations between nursing home staff and residents. *Journal of Clinical Nursing*, 14(8B), 84–89.

Wadensten, B. (2006). An analysis of psychosocial theories of aging and their relevance to practical gerontological nursing in Sweden. *Scandinavian Journal of Caring Sciences*, 20(3), 347–354.

Walker, K.M. and Alligood, M.R. (2001). Empathy from a nursing perspective: Moving beyond borrowed theory. *Archives of Psychiatric Nursing*, 15(3), 140–147.

Weed, L.L. (1969). *Medical records, medical education, and patient care*. Cleveland, OH: Case Western Reserve University Press.

West, P. (1991). Theory implementation: A challenging journey. *Canadian Journal of Nursing Administration*, 4(1), 29–30.

Whelton, B.J.B. (1999). The philosophical core of King's conceptual system. *Nursing Science Quarterly*, 12(2), 158–163.

Whelton, B.J.B. (2007). The nursing act is an excellent human act. In C.L. Sieloff, M.A. Frey, and I.M. King (Eds.), *Middle range theory development using King's conceptual system*. New York: Springer Publishing Company.

Whelton, B.J.B. (2008). Human nature: A foundation for palliative care. *Nursing Philosophy*, 9(2), 77–88.

Wicks, M.N., Rice, M.C., and Talley, C.H. (2007). Further exploration of family health within the context of chronic obstructive pulmonary disease. In C.L. Sieloff, M.A. Frey, and I.M. King (Eds.), *Middle range theory development using King's conceptual system*. New York: Springer Publishing Company.

Williams, C. (1996). Patient-controlled analgesia: A review of the literature. *Journal of Clinical Nursing*, 5(3), 139–147.

Williams, L.A. (2001). Imogene King's interacting systems theory: Application in emergency and rural nursing. *Online Journal of Rural Nursing and Health Care*, 2(1), 6.

Woods, E.C. (1994). King's theory in practice with elders. *Nursing Science Quarterly*, 7(2), 65–69.

Zetterberg, H.L. (1963). *On theory and verification in sociology* (Rev. ed.). Totowa, NJ: Bedminster Press.

Zoffmann, V., Harder, I., and Kirkevold, M. (2008). A person-centered communication and reflection model: Sharing decision-making in chronic care. *Qualitative Health Research*, 18(5), 670–685.

Zoffmann, V. and Kirkevold, M. (2005). Life versus disease in difficult diabetes care: Conflicting perspectives disempower patients and professionals in problem solving. *Qualitative Health Research*, 15(6), 750–765.

22. Madeleine Leininger

Basuray, J. (1997). Nurse Miss Sahib: Colonial culture-bound education in India and transcultural nursing. *Journal of Transcultural Nursing*, 9(1), 14–19.

Blackman, R. (2011). Understanding culture in practice: Reflections of an Australian Indigenous nurse. *Contemporary Nurse*, 37(1), 31–34.

Bodner, A. and Leininger, M. (1992). Transcultural nursing care values, beliefs, and practices of American (USA) gypsies. *Journal of Transcultural Nursing*, 4(1), 17–28.

Carr, J.M. (1998). Vigilance as a caring expression and Leininger's theory of cultural care diversity and universality. *Nursing Science Quarterly*, 11(2), 74–78.

Chmielarczyk, V. (1991). Transcultural nursing: Providing culturally congruent care to the Hausa of Northwest Africa. *Journal of Transcultural Nursing*, 3(1), 15–19.

Cohen, J.A. (1991). Two portraits of caring: A comparison of the artists, Leininger and Watson. *Journal of Advanced Nursing*, 16, 899–909.

Fawcett, J. (2002). The nurse theorists: 21st century updates—Madeleine M. Leininger. *Nursing Science Quarterly*, 15(2), 131–136.

Horsburgh, M.E., and Foley, D.M. (1990). The phenomena of care in Sicilian-Canadian culture: An ethnonursing case study. *Nursing Forum*, 25(3), 14–22.

Johnstone, M.J. (2015). Decolonizing nursing ethics. *International Nursing Review*, 62(2), 141–142.

Leininger, M. (1990). Leininger clarifies transcultural nursing [Letter; comment]. *International Nursing Review*, 37(6), 356.

Leininger, M. (1997). Transcultural nursing research to transform nursing education and practice: 40 years. *Image: Journal of Nursing Scholarship*, 29(4), 341–347.

Leininger, M. (2001). Response and reflections on Bruni's 1988 critique of Leininger's theory. *Collegian*, 8(1). 37–38.

Leininger, M. (2002). Culture care theory: A major contribution to advance transcultural nursing and practices. *Journal of Transcultural Nursing*, 13(3), 189–192.

Leininger, M.M. (1997). Transcultural nursing as a global care humanizer, diversifier, and unifier. *Hoitotiede*, 9(5), 219–225.

Luna, L. (1998). Culturally competent health care: A challenge for nurses in Saudi Arabia. *Journal of Transcultural Nursing*, 9(2), 8–14.

Luna, L.J. (1989). Transcultural nursing care of Arab Muslims. *Journal of Transcultural Nursing*, 1(1), 22–26.

McFarland, M.R. (1997). Use of cultural care theory with Anglo- and African-American elders in a long-term care setting. *Nursing Science Quarterly*, 10(4), 186–192.

McFarland, M.R., Mixer, S.J., Webhe-Alamah, H., and Burk, R. (2012). Ethnonursing: A qualitative research method for studying culturally competent care across disciplines. *International Journal of Qualitative Methods*, 11(3), 259–279.

Miller, J. (1997). Politics and care: A study of Czech Americans within Leininger's theory of culture care diversity and universality. *Journal of Transcultural Nursing*, 9(1), 3–13.

Milton, C.L. (2016). Ethics and defining cultural competence an alternative view. *Nursing Science Quarterly*, 29(1), 21–23.

Morgan, M.G. (1992). Pregnancy and childbirth beliefs and practices of American Hare Krishna devotees within transcultural nursing. *Journal of Transcultural Nursing*, 4(1), 5–10.

Pilkington, F.B. (2007). Envisioning nursing in 2050 through the eyes of nurse theorists: Leininger and Watson. *Nursing Science Quarterly*, 20(1), 8.

Polaschek, N.R. (1998). Cultural safety: A new concept in nursing people of different ethnicities. *Journal of Advanced Nursing*, 27(3), 452–457.

Queiroz, M.V.O. and Pagliuca, L.M.F. (2001). The concept of transcultural nursing: The analysis of its development in a master's degree dissertation [Portuguese]. *Revista Brasileira de Enfermagem*, 54(4), 630–637.

Rosenbaum, J.N. (1989). Depression: Viewed from a transcultural nursing theoretical perspective. *Journal of Advanced Nursing*, 14(1), 7–12.

Spangler, Z. (1992). Transcultural care values and nursing practices of Philippine-American nurses. *Journal of Transcultural Nursing*, 4(2), 28–37.

Zoucha, R. and Husted, G.L. (2000). The ethical dimensions of delivering culturally competent congruent nursing and health care. *Issues in Mental Health Nursing*, 21(3), 325–340.

23. Myra Levine

Abdellah, F.G. and Levine, E. (1986). *Better patient care through nursing research* (3rd ed.). New York: Macmillan.

Abumaria, I.M., Hastings-Tolsma, M., and Sakraida, T.J. (2015). Levine's conservation model: A framework for advanced gerontology nursing practice. *Nursing Forum*, 50(3), 179–188.

Allvin, R., Berg, K., Idvall, E., and Nilsson, U. (2007). Postoperative recovery: A concept analysis. *Journal of Advanced Nursing*, 57(5), 552–558.

Andrews, G.J. and Moon, G. (2005). Space, place, and the evidence base: Part II-Rereading nursing environment through geographical research. *Worldviews on Evidence-Based Nursing*, 2(3), 142–156.

Artigue, G.S., Foli, K.J., Johnson, T., Marriner-Tomey, A., Poat, M.C., Poppa, L.D., Woeste, R., and Zoretich, S.T. (1994). Myra Levine: Four conservation principles. In A. Marriner-Tomey (Ed.), *Nursing theorists and their work* (4th ed., pp. 199–210). St. Louis, MO: C.V. Mosby.

Bao, Y., Vedina, R., Moodie, S., and Dolan, S. (2013). The relationship between value incongruence and individual and organizational well-being outcomes: an exploratory study among Catalan nurses. *Journal of Advanced Nursing*, 69(3), 631–641.

Barnum, B.J.S. (1994). *Nursing theory: Analysis, application, and evaluation* (4th ed.). Philadelphia, PA: Lippincott.

Bates, M. (1967). A naturalist at large. *Natural History*, 76(6), 8–16.

Bernard, C. (1957). *An introduction to the study of experimental medicine*. New York: Dover.

Bertalanffy, L. (1968). *General system theory*. New York: George Braziller.

Buber, M. (1967). *Between man and man*. New York: Macmillan.

Bunting, S.M. (1988). The concept of perception in selected nursing theories. *Nursing Science Quarterly*, 1(4), 168–174.

Burd, C., Langemo, D.K., Olson, B., Hanson, D., Hunter, S., and Sauvage, T. (1992). Skin problems: Epidemiology of pressure ulcers in a skilled care facility. *Journal of Gerontological Nursing*, 18(9), 29–39.

Burd, C., Olson, B., Langemo, D., Hunter, S., Hanson, D., Osowski, K.F., and Sauvage, T. (1994). Skin care strategies in a skilled nursing home. *Journal of Gerontological Nursing*, 20(1), 28–34.

Cader, R., Campbell, S., and Watson, D. (2005). Cognitive continuum theory in nursing decision-making. *Journal of Advanced Nursing*, 49(4), 397–405.

Cannon, W.B. (1939). *The wisdom of the body*. New York: W.W. Norton.

Cox, R.A., Sr. (1991). A tradition of caring: Use of Levine's model in long-term care. In K.M. Schaefer and J.B. Pond (Eds.), *Levine's conservation model: A framework for nursing practice* (pp. 179–197). Philadelphia, PA: F.A. Davis.

Delmore, B.A. (2006). Levine's framework in long-term ventilated patients during the weaning course. *Nursing Science Quarterly*, 19(3), 247–258.

Donaldson, S.K. and Crowley, D.M. (1978). The discipline of nursing. *Nursing Outlook*, 26(2), 113–120.

Dubos, R. (1966). *Man adapting*. New Haven, CT: Yale University Press.

Erikson, E. (1968). *Identity, youth and crisis*. New York: W.W. Norton.

†Esposito, C.H. and Leonard, M.K. (1980). Myra Estrin Levine. In The Nursing Theories Conference Group (Eds.), *Nursing theories: The base for professional nursing practice* (pp. 150–163). Englewood Cliffs, NJ: Prentice-Hall.

Fawcett, J. (1989). Levine's conservation model. In J. Fawcett (Ed.), *Analysis and evaluation of conceptual models of nursing* (2nd ed.). Philadelphia, PA: F.A. Davis.

Fawcett, J. (2005). *Contemporary nursing knowledge: Analysis and evaluation of nursing models and theories* (2nd ed.). Philadelphia, PA: F.A. Davis.

Fawcett, J. (2014). Thoughts about conceptual models, theories, and quality improvement projects. *Nursing Science Quarterly*, 17(4), 336–339.

Feynman, R. (1965). *The character of physical law*. Cambridge, MA: MIT Press.

Fjellstrom, R. (2005). Respect for persons, respect for integrity: Remarks for the conceptualization of integrity in social ethics. *Medicine, Health Care and Philosophy*, 8(2), 231–242.

Flaskerud, J.H. and Halloran, E.J. (1980). Areas of agreement in nursing theory development. *Advances in Nursing Science*, 3(1), 1–7.

Gagner-Tjellesen, D., Yurkovich, E.E., and Gragert, M. (2001). Use of music therapy and other ITNIs in acute care. *Journal of Psychosocial Nursing and Mental Health Services*, 39(10), 26–37, 52–53.

Foli, K., Johnson, T., Marriner-Tomey, A., Poat, M., Poppa, L., Woeste, R., and Zoretich, S. (1989). Myra Estrin Levine: Four conservation principles. In A. Marriner-Tomey (Ed.), *Nursing theorists and their work* (2nd ed.). St. Louis, MO: C.V. Mosby.

Glass, J.L. (1989). Levine's theory of nursing: A critique. In J. Riehl-Sisca (Ed.), *Conceptual models for nursing practice* (3rd ed.). Norwalk, CT: Appleton & Lange.

Grindley, J. and Paradowski, M. (1991). Developing an undergraduate program using Levine's model. In K.M. Schaefer and J.B. Pond (Eds.), *Levine's conservation model: A framework for nursing practice* (pp. 199–208). Philadelphia, PA: F.A. Davis.

Hall, K.V. (1979). Current trends in the use of conceptual frameworks in nursing education. *Journal of Nursing Education*, 18(4), 26–29.

†Hirschfeld, M.J. (1976). The cognitively impaired older adult. *American Journal of Nursing*, 76(12), 1981–1984.

Irvin, S.M. (2007). Sensorineural hearing changes after myelogram. *Journal of Perianesthesia Nursing*, 22(1), 27–39.

Laustsen, G. (2006). Environment, ecosystems, and ecological behavior: A dialogue toward developing nursing ecological theory. *Advances in Nursing Science*, 29(1), 43–54.

Leach, M.J. (2006). Wound management: Using Levine's conservation model to guide practice. *Ostomy Wound Management*, 52(8), 74–80

Levine, M. (1969). *Introduction to clinical nursing*. Philadelphia, PA: F.A. Davis.

†Levine, M.E. (1966). Adaptation and assessment: A rationale for nursing intervention. *American Journal of Nursing*, 66(11), 2450–2454.

Levine, M.E. (1966). Trophicognosis: An alternative to nursing diagnosis. In *Exploring progress in medical-surgical nursing practice* (pp. 55–70). New York: American Nurses' Association.

†Levine, M.E. (1967). The four conservation principles of nursing. *Nursing Forum*, 6(1), 45–59.

†Levine, M.E. (1969). The pursuit of wholeness. *American Journal of Nursing*, 69(1), 93–98.

†Levine, M.E. (1971). Holistic nursing. *Nursing Clinics of North America*, 6(2), 253–264.

†Levine, M.E. (1971). Time has come to speak of . . . health care. *AORN Journal*, 13, 37–43.

Levine, M.E. (1973). *Introduction to clinical nursing* (2nd ed.). Philadelphia, PA: F.A. Davis.

Levine, M.E. (1977). Nursing ethics and the ethical nurse. *American Journal of Nursing*, 77(5), 845–849.

Levine, M.E. (1979). The science is spurious. *American Journal of Nursing*, 79(8), 1379–1383.

Levine, M.E. (1988). Antecedents from adjunctive disciplines: Creation of nursing theory. *Nursing Science Quarterly*, 1(1), 16–21.

Levine, M.E. (1988). Rationing health care [Letter]. *Nursing Outlook*, 36(6), 265.

Levine, M.E. (1989). Beyond dilemma. *Seminars in Oncology Nursing*, 5(2), 124–128.

Levine, M.E. (1989). The ethics of nursing rhetoric. *Image: Journal of Nursing Scholarship*, 21(1), 4–6.

Levine, M.E. (1989). Ethical issues in cancer care: Beyond dilemma. *Seminars in Oncology Nursing*, 5(2), 124–128.

Levine, M.E. (1989). The ethics of nursing rhetoric. *Image: Journal of Nursing Scholarship*, 21(1), 4–6.

Levine, M.E. (1989). The four conservation principles: Twenty years later. In J.P. Riehl-Sisca (Ed.), *Conceptual models for nursing practice* (3rd ed.). Norwalk, CT: Appleton & Lange.

Levine, M.E. (1989). Ration or rescue: The elderly patient in critical care. *Critical Care Nursing Quarterly*, 12(1), 82–89.

Levine, M.E. (1990). Conservation and integrity. In M.E. Parker (Ed.), *Nursing theories in practice* (pp. 189–202). New York: National League for Nursing.

Levine, M.E. (1991). The conservation principles: A model for health. In K.M. Schaefer and J.B. Pond (Eds.), *Levine's conservation model: A framework for nursing practice* (pp. 1–11). Philadelphia, PA: F.A. Davis.

Levine, M.E. (1995). The rhetoric of nursing theory. *Image: The Journal of Nursing Scholarship*, 27(1), 11–14.

Levine, M.E. (1996). The conservation principles: A retrospective. *Nursing Science Quarterly*, 9(1), 38–41.

Levine, M.E. (1999). On the humanities in nursing . . . originally published as a discourse in *Canadian Journal of Nursing Research*, 1995, 27(2), 19–23. *Canadian Journal of Nursing Research*, 30(4), 213–217.

Lyon, B. (2005). Getting back on track: Nursing's autonomous scope of practice. *Clinical Nursing Specialist*, 19(1), 28–33.

Mantle, F. (2001). Complementary therapies and nursing models . . . originally published in D. Rankin-Box (Ed.), 2001 Nurse's handbook of complementary therapies. *Complementary Therapies in Nursing and Midwifery*, 7(3), 142–145.

Marriner-Tomey, A. and Alligood, M.R. (2005). *Nursing theorists and their work* (6th ed.). St. Louis, MO: Mosby/Elsevier.

Mefford, L.C. and Alligood, M.R. (2011). Evaluating nurse staffing patterns and neonatal intensive care unit outcomes using Levine's conservation model of nursing. *Journal of Nursing Management*, 19(8), 998–1011.

Melancon, B. and Miller, L.H. (2005). Massage therapy versus traditional therapy for low back pain relief: Implications for holistic nursing practice. *Holistic Nursing Practice*, 19(3), 116–121.

Mock, V., Pickett, M., Ropka, M.E., Lin, E.M., Steward, K.J., Rhodes, V.A., McDaniel, R., Grimm, P.M., Krumm, S., and McCorkle, R. (2001). Fatigue and quality of life outcomes of exercise during cancer treatment. *Cancer Practice*, 9(3), 119–127.

Mock, V., Ropka, M.E., Rhodes, V.A., Pickett, M., Grimm, P.M., McDaniel, R., Lin, E.M., Allocca, P., Dienemann, J.A., Haisfield-Wolfe, M.E., Steward, K.J., and McCorkle, R. (1998). Establishing mechanisms to conduct multi-institutional research—fatigue in patients with cancer: An exercise intervention. *Oncology Nursing Forum*, 25(8), 1391–1397.

Mock, V., St. Ours, C., Hall, S., Bositis, A., Tillery, M., Belcher, A., et al. (2007). Using a conceptual model in nursing research–mitigating fatigue in cancer patients. *Journal of Advanced Nursing*, 58(5), 503–512.

Netto, L., Moura, M.A., Queiroz, A.B., Tyrrell, M.A., and Bravo, M. (2014). Violence against women and its consequences. *Acta Paulista de Enfermagem*, 27(5), 458–464.

Newport, M.A. (1984). Conserving thermal energy and social integrity in the newborn. *Western Journal of Nursing Research*, 6(2), 175–199.

Nightingale, F. (1969). *Notes on nursing. What it is and what it is not.* New York: Dover Publications.

Piccoli, M. and Galvao, C.M. (2001). Perioperative nursing: Identification of the nursing diagnosis infection risk based on Levine's conceptual model [Portuguese]. *Revista Latino-Americana de Enfermagem*, 9(4), 37–43.

Pieper, B.A. (1989). Levine's nursing model: The conservation principles. In J.J. Fitzpatrick and A.L. Whall (Eds.), *Conceptual models of nursing: Analysis and application* (2nd ed.). Bowie, MD: Robert J. Brady Co.

Pond, J.B. (1990). Application of Levine's conservation model to nursing the homeless community. In M.E. Parker (Ed.), *Nursing theories in practice* (pp. 203–216). New York: National League for Nursing.

Pond, J.B. (1991). Ambulatory care of the homeless. In K.M. Schaefer and J.B. Pond (Eds.), *Levine's conservation model: A framework for nursing practice* (pp. 167–178). Philadelphia, PA: F.A. Davis.

Pond, J.B. and Taney, S.G. (1991). Emergency care in a large university emergency department. In K.M. Schaefer and J.B. Pond (Eds.), *Levine's conservation model: A framework for nursing practice* (pp. 151–166). Philadelphia, PA: F.A. Davis.

Riehl, J.P. (1980). Nursing models in current use. In J.P. Riehl and C. Roy (Eds.), *Conceptual models for nursing practice* (2nd ed., pp. 393–398). New York: Appleton-Century-Crofts.

Rogers, C.R. (1961). *On becoming a person*. Boston, MA: Houghton-Mifflin.

Rogers, M.E. (1964). *Reveille in nursing*. Philadelphia, PA: F.A. Davis.

Rogers, M.E. (1970). *An introduction to the theoretical basis of nursing*. Philadelphia, PA: F.A. Davis.

Schaefer, K.M. (1997). Levine's conservation model in nursing practice. In M.R. Alligood et al. (Eds.), *Nursing theory: Utilization and application* (pp. 89–107). St. Louis, MO: Mosby Year Book.

Selye, H. (1956). *The stress of life*. New York: McGraw-Hill.

Taylor, J.W. (1974). Measuring the outcomes of nursing care. *Nursing Clinics of North America*, 9, 337–348.

Taylor, J.W. (1989). Levine's conservation principles: Using the model for nursing diagnosis in a neurological setting. In J. Riehl-Sisca (Ed.), *Conceptual models for nursing practice* (3rd ed.). Norwalk, CT: Appleton & Lange.

Teeri, S., Valimaki, M., Katajisto, J., and Leino–Kilpi, H. (2007). Nurses perceptions of older patients integrity in long-term institutions. *Scandinavian Journal of Caring Sciences*, 21(4), 490–499.

Tillich, P. (1961). The meaning of health. *Perspectives in Biology and Medicine*, 5, 92–100.

Todero-Franceschi, V. (2001). Energy: A bridging concept for nursing science. *Nursing Science Quarterly*, 14(2), 132–140.

Tompkins, E.S. (1980). Effect of restricted mobility and dominance on perceived duration. *Nursing Research*, 29(6), 333–338.

Webster's Third New International Dictionary. (1986). Springfield, MA: Merriam-Webster.

24. Afaf Ibrahim Meleis

Baird, M.B. (2012). Well-being in refugee women experiencing cultural transition. ANS. *Advances in Nursing Science*, 35(3), 249–263.

Baird, M.B. and Reed, P.G. (2015). Liminality in cultural transition: Applying ID-EA to advance a concept into theory-based practice. *Research and Theory for Nursing Practice: An International Journal*, 29(1), 25–37.

Bull, M.J. and McShane, R.E. (2008). Seeking what's best during the transition to adult day health services. *Qualitative Health Research*, 18(5), 597–605.

Cooley, W.C. and Sagerman, P.J. (2011). Supporting the health care transition from adolescence to adulthood in the medical home. *Pediatrics*, 128(1), 182–200.

Dagenais, F. and Meleis, A.I. (1982). Professionalism, work ethic, and empathy in nursing: The nurse self-description form. *Western Journal of Nursing Research*, 4(4), 407–422.

Davidson, P.M., Dracup, K., Phillips, J., Padilla, G., and Daly, J. (2007). Maintaining hope in transition: a theoretical framework to guide interventions for people with heart failure. *The Journal of Cardiovascular Nursing*, 22(1), 58–64.

Dracup, K., Meleis, A.I., Baker, C., and Edlefsen, P. (1984). Family-focused cardiac rehabilitation: A role supplementation program for cardiac patients and spouses. *Nursing Clinics of North America*, 19, 112–124.

Fegran, L., Hall, E.O., Uhrenfeldt, L., Aagaard, H., and Ludvigsen, M.S. (2014). Adolescents' and young adults' transition experiences when transferring from paediatric to adult care: a qualitative metasynthesis. *International Journal of Nursing Studies*, 51(1), 123–135.

Gaffney, K.F. (1992). Nursing practice model for maternal role sufficiency. *Advances in Nursing Science*, 15(2), 76–84.

Geary, C.R. and Schumacher, K.L. (2012). Care transitions: Integrating transition theory and complexity science concepts. *Advances in Nursing Science*, 35(3), 236–248.

Hall, J.M., Stevens, P.E., and Meleis, A.I. (1994). Marginalization: A guiding concept for valuing diversity in nursing knowledge development. *Advances in Nursing Science*, 16(4), 23–41.

Im, E.O. (2011). Transitions theory: A trajectory of theoretical development in nursing. *Nursing Outlook*, 59(5), 278–285.

Im, E.O. (2013). Chapter 20, Afaf Ibrahim Meleis: Transition theory. In M.R. Alligood (Eds.), *Nursing theorists and their work*. St. Louis: Elsevier Health Sciences.

Im, E.O. (2013). Theory in transitions. In M.J. Smith and P. Liehr (Eds.), *Middle range theory for nursing* (3rd ed., pp. 253–277). New York: Springer.

Im, E.O. (2014). Situation-specific theories from the middle-range transitions theory. *Advances in Nursing Science*, 37(1), 19–31.

Im, E.O. and Meleis, A.I. (1999). A situation-specific theory of Korean immigrant women's menopausal transition. *Image: Journal of Nursing Scholarship*, 31(4), 333–338.

Jones, P.S. and Meleis, A.I. (1993). Health is empowerment. *Advances in Nursing Science*, 15(3), 1–14.

Koniak-Griffin, D. (1993). Maternal role attainment. *Image: Journal of Nursing Scholarship*, 25, 257–262.

Lindgren, E., Söderberg, S., and Skär, L. (2013). The gap in transition between child and adolescent psychiatry and general adult psychiatry. *Journal of Child and Adolescent Psychiatric Nursing*, 26(2), 103–109.

Lindgren, E., Söderberg, S., and Skär, L. (2015). Swedish young adults' experiences of psychiatric care during transition to adulthood. *Issues in Mental Health Nursing*, 36(3), 182–189.

Malley, A., Kenner, C., Kim, T., and Blakeney, B. (2015). The role of the nurse and the preoperative assessment in patient transitions. *AORN Journal*, 102(2), 181.e1–181.e9.

Mansell, D.M. and Porter-Chantemerle, K. (1979). *Conceptualization and measurement of a role supplementation program: The effect of role supplementation on career success of neophyte nurses*. MINH undergraduate psychiatric nursing training and demonstration project. Tempe, AZ: Arizona State University, College of Nursing.

Maten-Speksnijder, A.T., Pool, A., Grypdonck, M., Meurs, P., and Staa, A. (2015). Driven by ambitions: The nurse practitioner's role transition in Dutch Hospital Care. *Journal of Nursing Scholarship*, 47(6), 544–554.

Meleis, A.I. (1971). Self-concept and family planning. *Nursing Research*, 20, 229–236.

Meleis, A.I. (1974). Self-concept photographs: A research tool. *Videosociology*, 2(2), 46–62.

Meleis, A.I. (1975). Role insufficiency and role supplementation: A conceptual framework. *Nursing Research*, 24, 264–271.

Meleis, A.I. (1979). The graduate dilemma: The Kuwaiti experience. *International Journal of Nursing Studies*, 16, 337–343.

Meleis, A.I. (1986). Theory development and domain concepts. In P. Moccia (Ed.), *New approaches to theory development*. New York: National League for Nursing.

Meleis, A.I. (1990). Being and becoming healthy: The core of nursing knowledge. *Nursing Science Quarterly*, 3(3), 107–114.

Meleis, A.I. (1992). On the way to scholarship: From master's to doctorate. *Journal of Professional Nursing*, 8(6), 328 334.

Meleis, A.I. (1995). Theory testing and theory support: Principles, challenges, and a sojourn into the future. In B. Neuman (Ed.), *The Neuman systems model* (pp. 447–457). Norwalk, CT: Appleton-Lange.

Meleis, A.I. (1998). ReVisions in knowledge development: A passion for substance. *Scholarly Inquiry in Nursing Practice*, 12(1), 65–77.

Meleis, A.I. (2010). *Transitions theory: Middle range and situation specific theories in research and practice*. New York: Springer Publishing Company.

Meleis, A.I. (2015). The undeaning transition: Toward becoming a former dean. *Nursing Outlook*, 64(2), 186–196.

Meleis, A.I. (2015). Chapter 1, Transition to retirement: A life cycle transition. In H. Loureiro (Ed.), *Transição para a Reforma: Um programa a implementar em Cuidados de Saúde Primários* (1st ed.). REATIVA.

Meleis, A.I. (2015). Chapter 20, Transitions theory. In M.E. Parker and M.C. Smith (Eds.), *Nursing theories & nursing practice* (4th ed.). Philadelphia, PA: F.A. Davis.

Meleis, A.I. and Burton, P. (1981). Educational innovations: A model. *International Journal of Nursing Studies*, 33–39.

Meleis, A.I. and Dagenais, F. (1981). Sex role identity and perception of professional self in graduates of three nursing programs. *Nursing Research*, 30, 162–167.

Meleis, A.I. and Schumacher, K.L. (2011). Transitions and health. In J.J. Fitzpatrick and M. Wallace (Eds.), *Encyclopedia of nursing research* (3rd ed.). New York: Springer Publishing Company.

Meleis, A.I., Sawyer, L.M., Im, E.O., Hilfinger Messias, D.K., and Schumacher, K. (2000). Experiencing transitions: An emerging middle-range theory. *Advances in Nursing Science*, 23(1), 12–28.

Meleis, A.I. and Swendsen, L. (1975). Role supplementation: An empirical test of nursing intervention. *Nursing Research*, 24, 264–271.

Meleis, A.I., Swendsen, L., and Jones, D. (1980). Preventive role supplementation: A grounded conceptual framework. In M.H. Miller and B. Flynn (Eds.), *Current perspectives in nursing: Social issues and trends* (Vol. 2). St. Louis, MO: C.V. Mosby.

Meleis, A.I. and Trangenstein, P.A. (1994). Facilitating transitions: Redefinition of the nursing mission. *Nursing Outlook*, 42, 255–259.

Neves-Arruda, E.N., Larson, P.J., and Meleis, A.I. (1992). Comfort. Immigrant Hispanic cancer patients' views. *Cancer Nursing*, 15(6), 387–394.

Ramsay, P., Huby, G., Thompson, A., and Walsh, T. (2014). Intensive care survivors' experiences of ward-based care: Meleis' theory of nursing transitions and role development among critical care outreach services. *Journal of Clinical Nursing*, 23(5–6), 605–615.

Schumacher, K. and Meleis, A.I. (1994). Transitions: A central concept in nursing. *Image: Journal of Nursing Scholarship*, 26(2), 119–127.

Suva, G., Sager, S., Mina, E.S., Sinclair, N., Lloyd, M., Bajnok, I., and Xiao, S. (2015). Systematic review: Bridging the gap in RPN-to-RN transitions. *Journal of Nursing Scholarship*, 47(4), 363–370.

Swendsen, L., Meleis, A.I., and Jones, D. (1978). Role supplementation for new parents: A role mastery plan. *MCN, The American Journal of Maternal Child Nursing*, 3(2), 84–91.

Thomet, C., Schwerzmann, M., and Greutmann, M. (2015). Transition from adolescence to adulthood in congenital heart disease—Many roads lead to Rome. *Progress in Pediatric Cardiology*, 39(2), 119–124.

25. Betty Neuman

Aggleton, P. and Chalmers, H. (1989). Nursing models. Neuman's systems model. *Nursing Times*, 85(51), 27–29.

Angosta, A.D., Ceria-Ulep, C.D., and Tse, A.M. (2014). Care delivery for Filipino Americans using the Neuman systems model. *Nursing Science Quarterly*, 27(2), 142–148.

August-Brady, M. (2000). Prevention as intervention. *Journal of Advances in Nursing*, 31(6), 1304–1308.

Barnum, B.J.S. (1994). *Nursing theory: Analysis, application, and evaluation* (4th ed.). Philadelphia, PA: J.B. Lippincott.

Barnum, B.J.S. (1998). *Nursing theory: Analysis, application, evaluation* (5th ed.). Philadelphia, PA: Lippincott Williams & Wilkins.

Baumann, S.L. (2012). What's wrong with the concept of self-management? *Nursing Science Quarterly*, 25(4), 362–363.

Beck, C.T. (1983). Parturients' temporal experiences during the phases of labor. *Western Journal of Nursing Research*, 5, 283–295.

Beckman, S., Bruick–Sorge, C., Boxley–Harges, S., and Salmon, B. (2009, May). *The evolution of student nurses' concepts of spirituality*. Powerpoint presented at the 12th International Biennial Neuman Systems Model Symposium, Las Vegas, NV.

Beckman, S.J., Boxley-Harges, S.L., and Kaskel, B.L. (2012). Experience informs: Spanning three decades with the Neuman systems model. *Nursing Science Quarterly*, 25(4), 341–346.

Beddome, G. (1989). Application of the Neuman systems model to the assessment of community-as-client. In B. Neuman (Ed.), *The Neuman systems model* (2nd ed.). Norwalk, CT: Appleton & Lange.

Beitler, B., Tkachuck, B., and Aamodt, D. (1980). The Neuman model applied to health, mental health and medical-surgical nursing. In J.P. Riehl and C. Roy (Eds.), *Conceptual models of nursing practice*. New York: Appleton-Century-Crofts.

Benedict, M.B. and Sproles, J.B. (1982). Application of the Neuman model to public health nursing practice. In B. Neuman (Ed.), *The Neuman systems model. Application to nursing education and practice*. Norwalk, CT: Appleton-Century-Crofts.

Bergstrom, D. (1992). Hypermetabolism in multisystem organ failure: A Neuman systems perspective. *Critical Care Nursing Quarterly*, 15(3), 63–70.

Bertalanffy, L. (1968). *General system theory*. New York: George Braziller.

Biley, F. (1990). The Neuman model: An analysis. *Nursing*, 4(14), 25–28.

Binhosen, V., Panuthai, S., Srisuphun, W., Chang, E., Sucamvang, K., and Cioffi, J. (2003). Physical activity and health related quality of life among the urban Thai elderly. *Thai Journal of Nursing Research*, 7(4), 231–243.

Black, P., Deeny, P., and McKenna, H. (1997). Sensoristrain: An exploration of nursing interventions in the context of the Neuman systems theory. *Intensive and Critical Care Nursing*, 13(5), 249–258.

Blank, J.J., Clark, L., Longman, A.J., and Atwood, J.R. (1989). Perceived home care needs of cancer patients and their caregivers. *Cancer Nursing*, 12(2), 78–84.

Bourbonnais, F.F. and Ross, M.M. (1985). The Neuman systems model in nursing. Course development and implementation. *Journal of Advanced Nursing*, 10(2), 117–123.

Bourdeanu, L. and Dee, V. (2013). Assessment of chemotherapy-induced nausea and vomiting in women with breast cancer: A Neuman systems model framework. *Research and Theory for Nursing Practice: An International Journal*, 27(4), 296–304.

Bowman, A.M. (1997). Sleep satisfaction, perceived pain and acute confusion in elderly clients undergoing orthopaedic procedures. *Journal of Advanced Nursing*, 26(3), 550–564.

Breckenridge, D. (1989). Primary prevention as an intervention modality for the renal client. In B. Neuman (Ed.), *The Neuman systems model* (2nd ed.). Norwalk, CT: Appleton & Lange.

Breckenridge, D. (2010). The Neuman systems model and evidence-based nursing practice. In B. Neuman and J. Fawcett (Eds.). *The Neuman systems model* (5th ed., pp. 245–252). Upper Saddle River, NJ: Pearson Education Press.

Breckenridge, D.M. (2002). Using the Neuman systems model to guide nursing research in the United States. In B. Neuman and J. Fawcett (Eds.), *The Neuman systems model* (4th ed., pp. 176–182). Upper Saddle River, NJ: Prentice Hall.

Brink, L.W., Neuman, B., and Wynn, J. (1992). Transport of the critically ill patient with upper airway obstruction. *Critical Care Clinics*, 8(3), 633–647.

Buchanan, B.R. (1987). Human environment interaction: A modification of the Neuman systems model for aggregates, families, and the community. *Public Health Nursing*, 4(1), 52–64.

Bunkers, S.S., Petardi, L.A., Pilkington, F.B., et al. (1996). Challenging the myths surrounding qualitative research in nursing. *Nursing Science Quarterly*, 9(1), 33–37.

Burke, M.E., Capers, C., O'Connell, R., Quinn, R., and Sinnott, M. (1989). Neuman-based nursing practice in a hospital setting. In B. Neuman (Ed.), *The Neuman systems model* (2nd ed.). Norwalk, CT: Appleton & Lange.

Burkley, J.L. (2009, May). *Using Neuman's metaparadigm of environment to explore the caste system of healthcare*. Poster session presented at the 12th International Biennial Neuman Systems Model Symposium, Las Vegas, NV.

Burney, M.A. (1992). King and Neuman: In search of the nursing paradigm. *Journal of Advanced Nursing*, 17(5), 601–603.

Cammuso, B.S. and Wallen, A.J. (2002). Using the Neuman systems model to guide nursing education in the United States. In B. Neuman and J. Fawcett (Eds.), *The Neuman systems model* (4th ed., pp. 244–253). Upper Saddle River, NJ: Prentice Hall.

Campbell, V. and Keller, K. (1989). The Betty Neuman health care systems model: An analysis. In J. Riehl-Sisca (Ed.), *Conceptual models for nursing practice* (3rd ed.). Norwalk, CT: Appleton & Lange.

Capers, C.F. and Kelly, R. (1987). Neuman's nursing process: A model of holistic care. *Holistic Nursing Practice*, 1(3), 19–26.

Capers, C.F., O'Brien, C., Quinn, R., Kelly, R., and Fenerty, A. (1985). The Neuman systems model in practice. Planning phase. *Journal of Nursing Administration*, 15(5), 29–39.

Caplan, G. (1964). Principles of preventive psychiatry. New York: Basic Books.

Caris-Verhallen, W.M.C.M., Kerkstra, A., and Bensing, J.M. (1997). The role of communication in nursing care for elderly people: A review of the literature. *Journal of Advanced Nursing*, 25(5), 915–933.

Casalenuovo, G.A. (2002). Fatigue in diabetes mellitus: Testing a middle range theory of well-being derived from the Neuman theory of optimal client system stability and the Neuman systems model. *Dissertation Abstracts International*, 63, 2301B.

Chan, C.W.H. and Chang, A.M. (1999). Stress associated with tasks for family caregivers of patients with cancer in Hong Kong. *Cancer Nursing*, 22(4), 260–265.

Chardin, P.T. (1955). *The phenomena of man*. London, UK: Collins.

Clark, J. (1982). Development of models and theories on the concept of nursing. *Journal of Advanced Nursing*, 7, 129–134.

Clarke, P.N. and Lowry, L. (2012). Dialogue with Lois Lowry: Development of the Neuman systems model. *Nursing Science Quarterly*, 25(4), 332–335.

Cobb, R.K. (2012). How well does spirituality predict health status in adults living with HIV-disease: A Neuman systems model study. *Nursing Science Quarterly*, 25(4), 347–355.

Cody, A. (1996). Helping the vulnerable or condoning control within the family: Where is nursing? *Journal of Advanced Nursing*, 23(5), 882–886.

Cody, W.K. (1997). The many faces of change: Discomfort with the new. *Nursing Science Quarterly*, 10(2), 65–67.

Cody, W.K. (1998). Response: The threat of drowning in eclecticism. *Nursing Science Quarterly*, 11(3), 102–104.

Cornu, A. (1957). *The origins of Marxian thought*. Springfield, IL: Charles C. Thomas.

Craddock, R.B. and Stanhope, M.K. (1980). The Neuman health-care systems model: Recommended adaptation. In J.P. Riehl and C. Roy (Eds.), *Conceptual models of nursing practice*. New York: Appleton-Century-Crofts.

Cutcliffe, J.R. (1997). The nature of expert psychiatric nurse practice: A grounded theory study. *Journal of Clinical Nursing*, 6(4), 325–332.

Dale, M.L. and Savala, S.M. (1990). A new approach to the senior practicum. *Nursing Connections*, 3(1), 45–51.

Deloughery, G.W., Gebbie, K.M., and Neuman, B.M. (1974). Teaching organizational concepts to nurses in community mental health. *Journal of Nursing Education*, 13, 8–14.

Deloughery, G.W., Neuman, B.M., and Gebbie, K.M. (1970). Change in problem-solving ability among nurses receiving mental health consultation. *Communicating Nursing Research*, 3(3), 41–53.

Delunas, L.R. (1990). Prevention of elder abuse: Betty Neuman health care systems approach. *Clinical Nurse Specialist*, 4(1), 54–58.

de Munck, R. and Murk, A. (2002). Using the Neuman systems model to guide administration of nursing services in Holland: The case of Emergis, Institute for Mental Health Care. In B. Neuman and J. Fawcett (Eds.), *The Neuman systems model* (4th ed., pp. 300–316). Upper Saddle River, NJ: Prentice Hall.

Denyes, M.J., Neuman, B.M., and Villarruel, A.M. (1991). Nursing actions to prevent and alleviate pain in hospitalized children. *Issues in Comprehensive Pediatric Nursing*, 14(1), 31–48.

Drevdahl, D. (1999). Sailing beyond: Nursing theory and the person. *Advances in Nursing Science*, 21(4), 1–13.

Drew, L., Craig, D., and Beynon, C. (1989). The Neuman systems model for community health administration and practice: Provinces of Manitoba and Ontario, Canada. In B. Neuman (Ed.), *The Neuman systems model* (2nd ed.). Norwalk, CT: Appleton & Lange.

Dunn, S. and Trepanier, M. (1989). Application of the Neuman systems model to perinatal nursing. In B. Neuman (Ed.), *The Neuman systems model* (2nd ed.). Norwalk, CT: Appleton & Lange.

Easom, A. and Allbritton, G. (2000). Advanced practice nurses in nephrology. *Advances in Renal Replacement Therapy*, 7(3), 247–260.

Edelman, M. and Lunney, M. (2000). You make the diagnosis. Case study: A diabetic educator's use of the Neuman Systems Model. *Nursing Diagnosis*, 11(4), 179–182.

Edelson, M. (1970). *Sociotherapy and psychotherapy*. Chicago, IL: University of Chicago Press.

Edwards, N., Bunn, H., Mei, W.C., et al. (1999). Building community health nursing in the People's Republic of China: A partnership between schools of nursing in Ottawa, Canada, and Tianjin, China. *Public Health Nursing*, 16(2), 140–145.

Eilert-Petersson, E. and Olsson, H. (2003). Humour and slimming related to the Neuman systems model: A study of slimming women in Sweden. *Theoria Journal of Nursing Theory*, 12(3), 4–18.

England, M. (1997). Self-coherence, emotional arousal and perceived health of adult children -caring for a brain-impaired parent. *Journal of Advanced Nursing*, 26(4), 672–682.

Fagerstrom, L., Eriksson, K., and Engberg, I.B. (1998). The patient's perceived caring needs as a message of suffering. *Journal of Advanced Nursing*, 28(5), 978–987.

Falk-Rafael, A. (2005. Advancing nursing theory through theory-guided practice: The emergence of a critical caring perspective. *Advances in Nursing Science*, 28(1), 38–49.

Fawcett, J. (1984). Neuman's systems model. In J. Fawcett (Ed.), *Analysis and evaluation of conceptual models of nursing*. Philadelphia, PA: F.A. Davis.

Fawcett, J. (1989). Neuman's systems model. In J. Fawcett (Ed.), *Analysis and evaluation of conceptual models of nursing* (2nd ed.). Philadelphia, PA: F.A. Davis.

Fawcett, J. (2001). The nurse theorists: 21st century updates—Betty Neuman. *Nursing Science Quarterly*, 14(3), 211–214.

Fawcett, J. (2004). Conceptual models of nursing: International in scope and substance? The case of the Neuman systems model. *Nursing Science Quarterly*, 17(1), 50–54.

Fawcett, J. (2005). *Contemporary nursing knowledge: Analysis and evaluation of nursing models and theories* (2nd ed.). Philadelphia, PA: F.A. Davis.

Fawcett, J. (2006). Commentary: Finding patterns of knowing in the work of Florence Nightingale. *Nursing Outlook*, 54(5), 275–277.

Fawcett, J. (2008). A comment on integrating nursing and health policy. *Nursing Outlook*, 56(1), 41–43.

Fawcett, J. and DeSanto-Madeya (2013). *Contemporary nursing knowledge: Analysis and evaluation of nursing models and theories* (3rd ed.). Philadelphia, PA: F.A. Davis.

Fawcett, J. and Giangrande, S.K. (2001). Neuman systems model-based research: An integrative review project. *Nursing Science Quarterly*, 14(3), 231–238.

Fawcett, J. and Giangrande, S.K. (2002). The Neuman systems model and research: An integrative review. In B. Neuman and J. Fawcett (Eds.), *The Neuman systems model* (4th ed., pp. 120–149). Upper Saddle River, NJ: Prentice Hall.

Fawcett, J. and Gigliotti, E. (2001). Using conceptual models of nursing to guide nursing research: The case of Neuman systems model. *Nursing Science Quarterly*, 14(4), 339–345.

Fawcett, J., Watson, J., Neuman, B., Walker, P.H., and Fitzpatrick, J.J. (2001). On nursing theories and evidence. *Journal of Nursing Scholarship*, 33(2), 115–119.

Ferguson, L. and Day, R.A. (2005). Evidence-based nursing education: Myth or reality? *Journal of Nursing Education*, 44(3), 107–115.

Field, P.A. (1987). The impact of nursing theory on the clinical decision making process. *Journal of Advanced Nursing*, 12(5), 563–571.

Flaskerud, J.H. and Halloran, E.J. (1980). Areas of agreement in nursing theory development. *Advances in Nursing Science*, 3(1), 1–7.

Florczak, K., Poradzisz, M., and Hampson, S. (2012). Nursing in a complex world: A case for grand theory. *Nursing Science Quarterly*, 25(4), 307–312.

Fontana, J.A. (1996). The emergence of the person-environment interaction in a descriptive study of vigor in health failure. *Advances in Nursing Science*, 18(4), 70–82.

Foote, A.W., Piazza, D., and Schultz, M. (1990). The Neuman systems model: Application to a patient with a cervical spinal cord injury. *Journal of Neuroscience Nursing*, 22, 302–306.

Freshwater, D. (1999). Polarity and unity in caring: The healing power of symptoms. *Complementary Therapies in Nursing and Midwifery*, 5(5), 136–139.

Fuller, C.C. and Hartley, B. (2000). Linear scleroderma: A Neuman nursing perspective. *Journal of Pediatric Nursing*, 15(3), 168–174.

Gebbie, K.M., Deloughery, G.W., and Neuman, B.M. (1970). Levels of utilization: Nursing specialists in community mental health. *Journal of Psychiatric Nursing*, 8, 37–39.

Gehrling, K.R. and Memmott, R.J. (2008). Adversity in the context of the Neuman systems model. *Nursing Science Quarterly*, 21(2), 135–137.

Gerrish, K., Ashworth, P., Lacey, A., Bailey, J., et al. (2007). Factors influencing the development of evidence-based practice: A research tool. *Journal of Advanced Nursing*, 57(3), 328–338.

Gigliotti, E. (1997). Use of Neuman's lines of defense and resistance in nursing research: Conceptual and empirical considerations. *Nursing Science Quarterly*, 10(3), 136–143.

Gigliotti, E. (1999). Women's multiple role stress: Testing Neuman's flexible line of defense. *Nursing Science Quarterly*, 12(1), 36–44.

Gigliotti, E. (2001). Empirical tests of the Neuman systems model: Relational statement analysis. *Nursing Science Quarterly*, 14(2), 149–157.

Gigliotti, E. (2002). A theory-based clinical nurse specialist practice exemplar using Neuman's Systems Model and nursing's taxonomies. *Clinical Nurse Specialist*, 16(1), 10–16.

Gigliotti, E. (2003). The Neuman systems model institute: Testing middle-range theories. *Nursing Science Quarterly*, 16(3), 201–206.

Gigliotti, E. (2007). Improving external and internal validity of a model of midlife women's maternal-student role stress. *Nursing Science Quarterly*, 20(2), 161–170.

Gigliotti, E. (2011). Deriving middle range theories from the Neuman systems model. In B. Neuman and J. Fawcett (eds.). *The Neuman systems model* (5th ed., pp. 283–298). Upper Saddle River, NJ: Prentice-Hall Publications.

Gilgun, J.F. (2005). The four cornerstones of evidence-based practice in social work. *Research on Social Work Practice*, 15(1), 52–61.

Giuliano, K.K., Tyer-Viola, L., and Lopez, R.P. (2005). Unity of knowledge in the advancement of nursing knowledge. *Nursing Science Quarterly*, 18(3), 243–248.

Gomez-Tovar, L.O., Diaz-Suarez, L., and Cortes-Munoz, F. (2016). Evidence and Betty Neuman's model-based nursing care to prevent delirium in the intensive care unit. *Enfermeria Global*, 41, 64–77.

Goulet, C., Polomeno, V., and Harel, F. (1996). Canadian cross-cultural comparison of the High-Risk Pregnancy Stress Scale. *Stress Medicine*, 12(3), 145–154.

Haggart, M. (1993). A critical analysis of Neuman's systems model in relation to public health nursing. *Journal of Advanced Nursing*, 18, 1917–1922.

Hamilton, P. (1983). Community nursing diagnosis. *Advances in Nursing Science*, 5(3), 21–36.

Hanson, M.J.S. (1999). Cross-cultural study of beliefs about smoking among teenaged females. *Western Journal of Nursing Research*, 21(5), 635–647.

Harris, S., Hermiz, M., Meininger, M., and Steinkeler, S. (1989). Betty Neuman: Systems model. In A. Marriner-Tomey (Ed.), *Nursing theorists and their work* (2nd ed.). St. Louis, MO: C.V. Mosby.

Hassell, J.S. (1996). Improved management of depression through nursing model application and critical thinking. *Journal of the American Academy of Nurse Practitioners*, 8(4), 161–166.

Hathaway, D., Jacob, S., Stegbauer, C., Thompson, C., and Graff, C. (2006). The practice doctorate: Perspectives of early adopters. *Journal of Nursing Education*, 45(12), 487–496.

Heffline, M.S. (1991). A comparative study of pharmacological versus nursing interventions in the treatment of postanesthesia shivering. *Journal of Post Anesthesia Nursing*, 6(5), 311–320.

Henderson, B. (1978). Nursing diagnosis: Theory and practice. *Advances in Nursing Science*, 1(1), 75–83.

Herrick, C.A. and Goodykoontz, L. (1989). Neuman's systems model for nursing practice as a conceptual framework for a family assessment. *Journal of Child and Adolescent Psychiatric and Mental Health*, 2(2), 61–67.

Higgins, P.A. and Moore, S.M. (2000). Levels of theoretical thinking in nursing. *Nursing Outlook*, 48(4), 179–183.

Hilton, P.A. (1997). Theoretical perspectives of nursing: A review of the literature. *Journal of Advanced Nursing*, 26(6), 1211–1220.

Hinds, C. (1990). Personal and contextual factors predicting patients' reported quality of life: Exploring congruency with Betty Neuman's assumptions. *Journal of Advanced Nursing*, 15(4), 456–462.

Hinton-Walker, P. and Raborn, M. (1989). Application of the Neuman model in nursing administration and practice. In B. Henry, C. Arndt, M. DiVincenti, and A. Marriner-Tomey (Eds.), *Dimensions of nursing administration: Theory, research, education, practice*. Boston, MA: Blackwell Scientific Publications.

Hisama, K.K. (2001). The acceptance of nursing theory in Japan: A cultural perspective. *Nursing Science Quarterly*, 14(3), 255–259.

Hoeman, S. and Winters, D.M. (1990). Theory based case management: High cervical spinal cord injury. *Home Health Care Nurse*, 8, 25–33.

Holtslander, L.F. (2008). Ways of knowing hope: Carper's fundamental patterns as guide for hope research with bereaved palliative caregivers. *Nursing Outlook*, 56(1), 25–30.

Huch, M.H. (1991). Perspectives on health. *Nursing Science Quarterly*, 4(1), 33–40.

Hungelmann, J., Kenkel-Rossi, E., Klaasen, L., et al. (1996). Focus on spiritual well-being: Harmonious interconnectedness of mind-body-spirit—Use of the JAREL Spiritual Well-Being Scale—Assessment of spiritual well-being is essential to the health of individuals. *Geriatric Nursing*, 17(6), 262–266.

John, W.S. (1998). Just what do we mean by community? Conceptualization from the field. *Health and Social Care in the Community*, 6(2), 63–70.

Johnson, E.D. (1989). In search of applications of nursing theories: The Nursing Citation Index. *Bulletin of the Medical Library Association*, 77(2), 176–184.

Johnson, M. (1983). Some aspects of the relation between theory and practice in nursing. *Journal of Advanced Nursing*, 8, 21–28.

Johnson, S.E. (1989). A picture is worth a thousand words: Helping students visualize a conceptual model. *Nurse Educator*, 14(3), 21–24.

Jones, P.S. (1978). An adaptation model for nursing practice. *American Journal of Nursing*, 78, 1900–1906.

Jones-Cannon, S. and Davis, B.L. (2005). Coping among African-American daughters caring for aging parents. *The ABNF Journal*, 16(6), 118–123.

Julliard, K., Klimenko, E., and Jacob, M.S. (2006). Definitions of health among healthcare providers. *Nursing Science Quarterly*, 19(3), 265–271.

Karmels, P. (1993). Conundrum game for nursing theorists Neuman, King, and Johnson. *Nurse Educator*, 18(6), 8–9.

Kaufman, J.E. (1996). Personal definitions of health among elderly people: A link to effective health promotion. *Family and Community Health*, 19(2), 58–68.

Kelley, J., Sanders, N., and Pierce, J. (1989). A systems approach to the role of the nurse administrator. In B. Neuman (Ed.), *The Neuman systems model* (2nd ed.). Norwalk, CT: Appleton & Lange.

Kim, H.S. (2000). An integrative framework for conceptualizing clients: A proposal for a nursing perspective in the new century. *Nursing Science Quarterly*, 13(1), 37–40.

Kirkham, S.R., Baumbusch, J.L., Schultz, A.S.H., and Anderson, J.M. (2007). Knowledge development and evidence-based practice: Insights and opportunities from a postcolonial feminist perspective for transformative nursing practice. *Advances in Nursing Science*, 30(1), 26–40.

Knight, J.B. (1990). The Betty Neuman Systems Model applied to practice: A client with multiple sclerosis. *Journal of Advanced Nursing*, 15(4), 447–455.

Kottwitz, D. and Bowling, S. (2003). A pilot study of the elder abuse questionnaire. *Kansas Nurse*, 78(7), 4–6.

Kubsch, S., Linton, S.M., Hankerson, C., and Wichowski, H. (2008). Holistic interventions protocol for interstitial cystitis symptom control. *Holistic Nursing Practice*, 22(4), 183–190; quiz 191–192.

Lamb, K.A. (1999). Baccalaureate nursing students' perception of empathy and stress in their interactions with clinical instructors testing a theory of optimum student system stability according to the Neuman systems model. *Dissertation Abstracts International*, 60, 1028B.

Lancaster, D. and Whall, A. (1989). The Neuman systems model. In J.J. Fitzpatrick and A.L. Whall (Eds.), *Conceptual models of nursing: Analysis and application* (2nd ed.). Norwalk, CT: Appleton & Lange.

Laschinger, H.K. and Duff, V. (1991). Attitudes of practicing nurses towards theory-based nursing practice. *Canadian Journal of Nursing Administration*, 4(1), 6–10.

Lebold, M. and Davis, L. (1980). A baccalaureate nursing curriculum based on the Neuman health-systems model. In J.P. Riehl and C. Roy (Eds.), *Conceptual models of nursing practice*. New York: Appleton-Century-Crofts.

Lillis, P. and Cora, V. (1989). A case study analysis using the Neuman nursing process format: An abstract. In B. Neuman (Ed.), *The Neuman systems model* (2nd ed.). Norwalk, CT: Appleton & Lange.

Lindell, M. and Olsson, H. (1991). Can combined oral contraceptives be made more effective by means of a nursing care model? *Journal of Advanced Nursing*, 16(4), 475–479.

Louis, M. (1989). An intervention to reduce anxiety levels for nurses working with long-term care clients using Neuman's model. In J. Riehl-Sisca (Ed.), *Conceptual models for nursing practice* (3rd ed.). Norwalk, CT: Appleton & Lange.

Louis, M. (1995). The Neuman model in nursing research: An update. In B. Neuman (Ed.), *The Neuman systems model* (pp. 473–495). Norwalk, CT: Appleton & Lange.

Louis, M. and Koertvelyessy, A. (1989). The Neuman model in nursing research. In B. Neuman (Ed.), *The Neuman systems model* (2nd ed.). Norwalk, CT: Appleton & Lange.

Lowry, L., Beckman, S., Gehrling, K.R., and Fawcett, J. (2007). Imagining nursing practice: The Neuman systems model in 2050. *Nursing Science Quarterly*, 20(3), 226–231.

Lowry, L. and Jopp, M. (1989). An evaluation instrument for assessing an associate degree nursing curriculum based on the Neuman systems model. In J. Riehl-Sisca (Ed.), *Conceptual models for nursing practice* (3rd ed.). Norwalk, CT: Appleton & Lange.

Lowry, L.W. (2002). The Neuman systems model and education: An integrative review. In B. Neuman and J. Fawcett (Eds.), *The Neuman systems model* (4th ed., pp. 216–237). Upper Saddle River, NJ: Prentice Hall.

Lowry, L.W. (2009, May). *A fresh look at the Neuman Systems Model.* Powerpoint presented at the 12th International Biennial Neuman Systems Model Symposium, Las Vegas, NV.

Lowry, L.W. (2012). A qualitative descriptive study of spirituality guided by the Neuman systems model. *Nursing Science Quarterly*, 25(4), 356–361.

Lowry, L.W. and Anderson, B. (1993). Neuman's framework and ventilator dependency: A pilot study. *Nursing Science Quarterly*, 6(4), 195–200.

Lowry, L.W., Burns, C.M., Smith, A.A., et al. (2000). Compete or complement? An interdisciplinary approach to training health professionals. *Nursing and Health Care Perspectives*, 21(2), 76–80.

Luker, K.A., Beaver, K., Leinster, S.J., et al. (1996). Meaning of illness for women with breast cancer. *Journal of Advanced Nursing*, 23(6), 1194–1201.

Malinski, V.M. (2003). Nursing research and nursing conceptual models: Betty Neuman's systems model. *Nursing Science Quarterly*, 16(3), 201–206.

Marett, K.M., Gibbons, W.E., Memmott, R.J., et al. (1998). The organizational role of the clinical practice models in interdisciplinary collaborative practice. *Clinic Social Work Journal*, 26(2), 217–225.

Martins, C.L., Echevarria-Guanilo, M.E., Silveira, D.T., Gonzales, R.I.C., and Pai, D.D. (2015). Risk perception of work-related burn injuries from the workers perspective. *Texto Contexto Enferm, Florianopolis*, 24(4), 1148–1156.

May, K.M. and Hu, J. (2000). Caregiving and help seeking by mothers of low birthweight infants and mothers of normal birthweight infants. *Public Health Nursing*, 17(4), 273–279.

McClure, M. and Gigliotti, E. (2012). A medieval metaphor to aid use of the Neuman systems model in simulation debriefing. *Nursing Science Quarterly*, 25(4), 318–324.

McDowell, B.M., Chang, N.J., and Choi, S.S. (2003). Children's health retention in South Korea and the United States: A cross-cultural comparison. *Journal of Pediatric Nursing*, 18(6), 409–415.

McHolm, F.A. and Geib, K.M. (1998). Application of the Neuman Systems Model to teaching health assessment and nursing process. *Nursing Diagnosis*, 9(1), 23–33.

McRae-Bergeron, C.E., May, L., Foulks, R.W., et al. (1999). A medical readiness model of health assessment or well-being in first-increment Air Combat Command medical personnel. *Military Medicine*, 164(6), 379–388.

Merks, A., Verberk, F., de Kuiper, M., and Lowry, L.W. (2012). Neuman systems model in Holland: An update. *Nursing Science Quarterly*, 25(4), 364–368.

Meyer, T. and Xu, Y. (2005). Academic and clinical dissonance in nursing education: Are we guilty of failure to rescue? *Nurse Educator*, 30(2), 76–79.

Mirenda, R.M. (1986). The Neuman systems model: Description and application. In P. Winstead-Fry (Ed.), *Case studies in nursing theory*. New York: National League for Nursing.

Mohr, W.K. (1995). Multiple ideologies and their proposed roles in the outcomes of nurse practice settings—The for-profit psychiatric-hospital scandal as a paradigm case. *Nursing Outlook*, 43(5), 215–223.

Molassiotis, A. (1997). A conceptual mode of adaptation to illness and quality of life for cancer patients treated with bone marrow transplants. *Journal of Advanced Nursing*, 26(3), 572–579.

Moore, D. (2009, May). *Expanding the least restrictive continuum in mental health practice.* Powerpoint presented at the 12th International Biennial Neuman Systems Model Symposium, Las Vegas, NV.

Moore, S.L. and Munro, M.F. (1990). The Neuman Systems Model applied to mental health nursing of older adults. *Journal of Advanced Nursing*, 15(3), 293–299.

Morales-Mann, E.T. and Kaitell, C.A. (2001). Problem-based learning in a new Canadian curriculum. *Journal of Advanced Nursing*, 33(1), 13–19.

Moscaritolo, L.M. (2009). Interventional strategies to decrease nursing student anxiety in the clinical learning environment. *Journal of Nursing Education*, 48(1), 17–23.

Mrkonich, D., Miller, M., and Hessian, M. (1989). Cooperative baccalaureate education: The Minnesota intercollegiate nursing consortium. In B. Neuman (Ed.), *The Neuman systems model* (2nd ed.). Norwalk, CT: Appleton & Lange.

Mrkonich, D.E., Hessian, M., and Miller, M. (1989). A cooperative process in curriculum development using the Neuman health care systems model. In J. Riehl-Sisca (Ed.), *Conceptual models for nursing practice* (3rd ed.). Norwalk, CT: Appleton & Lange.

Mulhall, A. (1996). Cultural discourse and the myth of stress in nursing and medicine. *International Journal of Nursing Studies*, 33(5), 455–468.

Neal, J.E. (2001). Patient outcomes: A matter of perspective. *Nursing Outlook*, 49(2), 93–99.

Nelson, A.M. (2008). Addressing the threat of evidence-based practice to qualitative inquiry through increasing attention to quality: A discussion paper. *International Journal of Nursing Studies*, 45(2), 316–322.

Nelson, L., Hansen, M., and McCullagh, M. (1989). A new baccalaureate North Dakota-Minnesota nursing education consortium. In B. Neuman (Ed.), *The Neuman systems model* (2nd ed.). Norwalk, CT: Appleton & Lange.

Neufeld, A. (1983). Curriculum revision: Making the process work. *Journal of Advanced Nursing*, 8, 213–220.

Neuman, B. (1989). In conclusion-in transition. In B. Neuman (Ed.), *The Neuman systems model* (2nd ed.). Norwalk, CT: Appleton & Lange.

Neuman, B. (1995). *The Neuman systems model.* Norwalk, CT: Appleton & Lange.

Neuman, B. (1996). The Neuman systems model in research and practice. *Nursing Science Quarterly*, 9(2), 67–70.

Neuman, B.M. (1974). The Betty Neuman health-care systems model: A total person approach to patient problems. In J.P. Riehl and C. Roy (Eds.), *Conceptual models for nursing practice*. New York: Appleton-Century-Crofts.

Neuman, B.M. (1980). The Betty Neuman health care systems model: A total person approach to patient problems. In J.P. Riehl and C. Roy (Eds.), *Conceptual models for nursing practice*. New York: Appleton-Century-Crofts.

Neuman, B.M. (1982). *The Neuman systems model. Application to nursing education and practice.* Norwalk, CT: Appleton-Century-Crofts.

Neuman, B.M. (1989). The Neuman systems model. In B. Neuman (Ed.), *The Neuman systems model* (2nd ed.). Norwalk, CT: Appleton & Lange.

Neuman, B.M. (1989). The Neuman nursing process format: Family case study. In J. Riehl-Sisca (Ed.), *Conceptual models for nursing practice* (3rd ed.). Norwalk, CT: Appleton & Lange.

Neuman, B.M. (1990). Health as a continuum based on the Neuman systems model. *Nursing Science Quarterly*, 3(3), 129–135.

Neuman, B. and Fawcett, J. (Eds.) (2011). *The Neuman systems model* (5th ed). Upper Saddle River, NJ: Pearson.

Neuman, B. and Fawcett, J. (2012). Thoughts about the Neuman systems model: A Dialogue. *Nursing Science Quarterly*, 25(4), 374–376.

Neuman, B. and Reed, K.S. (2007). A Neuman systems model perspective on nursing in 2050. *Nursing Science Quarterly*, 20(2), 111–113.

Neuman, B., Chadwick, P.L., Beynon, C.E., et al. (1997). The Neuman systems model: Reflections and projections. *Nursing Science Quarterly*, 10(1), 18–21.

Neuman, B., Newman, D.M.L., and Holder, P. (2000). Leadership-scholarship integration: Using the Neuman systems model for 21st century professional nursing practice. *Nursing Science Quarterly*, 13(1), 60–63.

Neuman, B.M. and Reed, K.S. (2007). A Neuman systems model perspective on nursing in 2050. *Nursing Science Quarterly*, 20(2), 111–113.

Neuman, B.M. and Wyatt, M. (1980). The Neuman stress/adaptation systems approach to education for nurse administrators. In J.P. Riehl and C. Roy (Eds.), *Conceptual models of nursing practice*. New York: Appleton-Century-Crofts.

Neuman, B.M. and Wyatt, M. (1981). Prospects for change: Some evaluative reflections from one articulated baccalaureate program. *Journal of Nursing Education*, 20(1), 40–46.

Neuman, B.M. and Young, R.J. (1972). A model for teaching a total person approach to patient problems. *Nursing Research*, 21, 264–269.

Newman, D.M.L. (2005). A community nursing center for the health promotion of senior citizens based on the Neuman systems model. *Nursing Education Perspectives*, 26(4), 221–223.

Newman, D.M.L., Neuman, B., and Fawcett, J. (2002). Guidelines for Neuman systems model-based education for the health professions. In B. Neuman and J. Fawcett (Eds.), *The Neuman systems model* (4th ed., pp. 193–215). Upper Saddle River, NJ: Prentice Hall.

Newman, M.A. (2003). A world of no boundaries. *Advances in Nursing Science*, 26(4), 240–245.

Norrish, M.E. and Jooste, K. (2001). Nursing care of the patient undergoing alcohol detoxification. *Curationis*, 24(3), 36–48.

Nosek, M.A. (1996). Wellness among women with physical disabilities. *Sexuality and Disability*, 14(3), 165–181.

Paley, J. (2006). Evidence and expertise. *Nursing Inquiry*, 13(2), 82–93.

Paley, J., Cheyne, H., Dalgleish, L., Duncan, E.A.S., and Niven, C.A. (2007). Nursing's ways of knowing and dual process theories of cognition. *Journal of Advanced Nursing*, 60(6), 692–701.

Peternelj-Taylor, C.A. and Johnson, R. (1996). Custody and caring: Clinical placement of student nurses in a forensic setting. *Perspectives in Psychiatric Care*, 32(4), 23–29.

Philpin, S. (2007). Managing ambiguity and danger in an intensive therapy unit: Ritual practices and sequestration. *Nursing Inquiry*, 14(1), 51–59.

Picard, C. and Jones, D.A. (2005). *Giving voice to what we know: Margaret Newman's theory of health as expanding consciousness in nursing practice, research, and education*. Sudbury, MA: Jones & Bartlett Publishers.

Pierce, J.D. and Hutton, E. (1992). Applying the new concepts of the Neuman Systems Model. *Nursing Forum*, 27(1), 15–18.

Pilkington, F.B. (2007). Envisioning nursing in 2050 through the eyes of nurse theorists: King, Neuman, and Roy. *Nursing Science Quarterly*, 20(2), 108.

Poe, A.H. (2002). *Predictors of spontaneous lacerations in primigravidae*. In Proceedings of the 26th Triennial Congress of Midwives. Vienna, Austria, Europe: International Confederation of Midwives.

Polivka, B.J. (1996). Rural sex education: Assessment of programs and interagency collaboration. *Public Health Nursing*, 13(6), 425–433.

Pothiban, L. (2002). Using the Neuman systems model to guide nursing research in Thailand. In B. Neuman and J. Fawcett (Eds.), *The Neuman systems model* (4th ed., pp. 183–190). Upper Saddle River, NJ: Prentice Hall.

Potter, M.L. and Zauszniewski, J.A. (2000). Spirituality, resourcefulness, and arthritis impact on health perception of elders with rheumatoid arthritis. *Journal of Holistic Nursing*, 18(4), 311–336.

Putt, A. (1972). Entropy, evolution and equifinality in nursing. In J. Smith (Ed.), *Five years of cooperation to improve curricula in Western schools of nursing*. Boulder, CO: Western Interstate Commission for Higher Education.

Rafael, A.R.F. (2000). Watson's philosophy, science, and theory of human caring as a conceptual framework for guiding community health nursing practice. *Advances in Nursing Science*, 23(2), 34–49.

Randell, B.P. (1992). Nursing theory: The 21st century. *Nursing Science Quarterly*, 5(4), 176–184.

Reed, K. (1989). Family theory related to the Neuman systems model. In B. Neuman (Ed.), *The Neuman systems model* (2nd ed.). Norwalk, CT: Appleton & Lange.

Reed, K.S. (2002). The Neuman systems model and educational tools. In B. Neuman and J. Fawcett (Eds.), *The Neuman systems model* (4th ed., pp. 238–243). Upper Saddle River, NJ: Prentice Hall.

Reed, K.S. (2003). Grief is more than tears. *Nursing Science Quarterly*, 16(1), 77–81.

Reed, P.G. (2006). Commentary on neomodernism and evidence-based nursing: Implications for the production of nursing knowledge. *Nursing Outlook*, 54(1), 36–38.

Reed, P.G. and Rolfe, G. (2006). Nursing knowledge and nurses' knowledge: A reply to Mitchell and Bournes. *Nursing Science Quarterly*, 19(2), 120–122.

Robichaud-Ekstrand, S. and Delisle, L. (1989). The Neuman model in medical-surgical settings. *Canadian Nurse*, 85(6), 32–35.

Ross, M. and Bourbonnais, F. (1985). The Betty Neuman systems model in nursing practice: A nursing study approach. *Journal of Advanced Nursing*, 10(3), 199–207.

Ross, M.M., Bourbonnais, F.F., and Carroll, G. (1987). Curricular design and the Betty Neuman systems model: A new approach to learning. *International Nursing Review*, 34(3), 75–79.

Roy, C. (2007). Update from the future: Thinking of theorist Callista Roy. *Nursing Science Quarterly*, 20(2), 113–116.

Roy, C. (2008). Adversity and theory: The broad picture. *Nursing Science Quarterly*, 21(2), 138–139.

Sabo, C.E. and Michael, S.R. (1996). The influence of personal message with music on anxiety and side effects associated with chemotherapy. *Cancer Nursing*, 19(4), 283–289.

Sanders, N.F. and Kelley, J.A. (2002). The Neuman systems model and administration of nursing services: An integrative review. In B. Neuman and J. Fawcett (Eds.), *The Neuman systems model* (4th ed., pp. 271–187). Upper Saddle River, NJ: Prentice Hall.

Selye, H. (1950). *The physiology and pathology of exposure to stress*. Montreal, Canada: Acta.

Skalski, C.A., DiGerolamo, L., and Gigliotti, E. (2006). Stressors in five client populations: Neuman systems model-based literature review. *Journal of Advanced Nursing*, 56(1), 69–78.

Shamsudin, N. (2002). Can the Neuman systems model be adapted to the Malaysian nursing context? *International Journal of Nursing Practice*, 8(2), 99–105.

Sipple, J. and Freese, B. (1989). Transition from technical to professional-level nursing education. In B. Neuman (Ed.), *The Neuman systems model* (2nd ed.). Norwalk, CT: Appleton & Lange.

Skillen, D.L., Anderson, M.C., and Knight, C.L. (2001). The created environment for physical assessment by case managers. *Western Journal of Nursing Research*, 23(1), 72–89.

Smith, M.C. (1989). Neuman's model in practice. *Nursing Science Quarterly*, 2(3), 116–117.

Sohier, R. (1989). Nursing care for the people of a small planet: Culture and the Neuman systems model. In B. Neuman (Ed.), *The Neuman systems model* (2nd ed.). Norwalk, CT: Appleton & Lange.

Sohier, R. (1997). Neuman's systems model in nursing practice. In M.R. Alligood et al. (Eds.), *Nursing theory: Utilization and application* (pp. 109–127). St. Louis, MO: Mosby Year Book.

Spencer, P. (2002). Support system. *Learning Disability Practice*, 5(7), 16–20.

Stepans, M.B.F. and Knight, J.R. (2002). Application of Neuman's framework: Infant exposure to environmental tobacco smoke. *Nursing Science Quarterly*, 15(4), 327–334.

Stevens, K.R. and Staley, J.M. (2006). The Quality Chasm reports, evidence-based practice, and nursing's response to improve healthcare. *Nursing Outlook*, 54(2), 94–101.

Stewart, M., Brown, J.B., Donner, A., et al. (2000). The impact of patient-centered care on outcomes. *Journal of Family Practice*, 49(9), 796–804.

Story, E.L. and Ross, M.M. (1986). Family centered community health nursing and the Betty Neuman systems model. *Nursing Papers*, 18(2), 77–88.

Stranahan, S. (2001). Spiritual perception, attitudes about spiritual care, and spiritual care practices among nurse practitioners. *Western Journal of Nursing Research*, 23(1), 90–104.

Sullivan, J. (1986). Using Neuman's model in the acute phase of spinal cord injury. *Focus on Critical Care*, 13(5), 34–41.

Taylor, S.G., Renpenning, K.E., Geden, E.A., Neuman, B.M., and Hart, M.A. (2001). A theory of dependent-care: A corollary to Orem's theory of self-care. *Nursing Science Quarterly*, 14(1), 39–47.

Thorellekstrand, I. and Bjorvell, H. (1994). The VIPS-Model used by nursing students—Review of educational care plans. *Scandinavian Journal of Caring Sciences*, 8(4), 195–205.

Tierney, K., Facione, N., Padilla, G., and Dodd, M. (2007). Response shift – A theoretical exploration of quality of life following hematopoietic cell transplantation. *Cancer Nursing*, 30(2), 125–138.

Timmermans, O., van Linge, R., van Petergem, P., van Rompaey, B. and Denekens, J. (2013). A contingency perspective on team learning and innovation in nursing. *Journal of Advanced Nursing*, 69(2), 363–373.

Torakis, M.L. and Smigielski, C.M. (2000). Documentation of model-based practice: One hospital's experience. *Pediatric Nursing*, 26(4), 394–399, 428.

Tough, S.C., Johnston, D.W., Siever, J.E., Jorgenson, G., et al. (2006). Does supplementary prenatal nursing and home visitation support improve resource use in a universal healthcare system? A randomized controlled trial in Canada. *Birth-Issues in Perinatal Care*, 33(3), 183–194.

Trepanier, M.J. (1989). Application of the Neuman systems model to perinatal nursing. In B. Neuman (Ed.), *The Neuman systems model* (2nd ed.). Norwalk, CT: Appleton & Lange.

Turner, S.B. and Kaylor, S.D. (2015). Neuman systems model as a conceptual framework for nurse resilience. *Nursing Science Quarterly*, 28(3), 213–217.

Tusaie, K.R. and Patterson, K. (2006). Relationships among trait, situational, and comparative optimism: Clarifying concepts for a theoretically consistent and evidence-based intervention to maximize resilience. *Archives of Psychiatric Nursing*, 20(3), 144–150.

Ume–Nwagbo, P.N., DeWan, S.A., and Lowry, L.W. (2006). Using the Neuman systems model for best practices. *Nursing Science Quarterly*, 19(1), 31–35.

Venable, J.F. (1980). The Neuman health-care systems model: An analysis. In J.P. Riehl and C. Roy (Eds.), *Conceptual models of nursing practice*. New York: Appleton-Century-Crofts.

Villarruel, A.M., Bishop, T.L., Simpson, E.M., et al. (2001). Borrowed theories, shared theories, and the advancement of nursing knowledge. *Nursing Science Quarterly*, 14(2), 158–163.

Weaver, K. and Olson, J.K. (2006). Understanding paradigms used for nursing research. *Journal of Advanced Nursing*, 53(4), 459–469.

Whall, A.L. (1983). The Betty Neuman health care system model. In J.J. Fitzpatrick and A.L. Whall (Eds.), *Conceptual models of nursing: Analysis and application*. Bowie, MD: Robert J. Brady Co.

Whall, A.L., Sinclair, M., and Parahoo, K. (2006). A philosophic analysis of evidence-based nursing: Recurrent themes, metanarratives, and exemplar cases. *Nursing Outlook*, 54(1), 30–35.

Wilson, L.C. (2000). Implementation and evaluation of church-based health fairs. *Journal of Community Health Nursing*, 17(1), 39–48.

Wright, P.S., Piazza, D., Holcombe, J., and Foote, A. (1994). A comparison of three theories of nursing used as a guide for the nursing care of an 8–year-old with leukemia. *Journal of Pediatric Oncology Nursing*, 11(1), 14–19.

Ziemer, M.M. (1983). Effects of information on postsurgical coping. *Nursing Research*, 32, 282–287.

26. Margaret Newman

Aita, M., Richer, M.C., and Heon, M. (2007). Illuminating the processes of knowledge transfer in nursing. *Worldviews on Evidence-Based Nursing*, 4(3), 146–155.

August-Brady, M. (2000). Prevention as intervention. *Journal of Advanced Nursing*, 31(6), 1304–1308.

Averill, J.B. and Clements, P.T. (2007). Patterns of knowing as a foundation for action-sensitive pedagogy. *Qualitative Health Research*, 17(3), 386–399.

Banks-Wallace, J., Despins, L., Adams-Leander, S., McBroom, L., and Tandy, L. (2008). Reaffirming and reconceptualizing disciplinary knowledge as the foundation for doctoral education. *Advances in Nursing Science*, 31(1), 67–78.

Bateman, G.C., and Merryfeather, L. (2014). Newman's Theory of health as expanding consciousness a personal evolution. *Nursing Science Quarterly*, 27(1), 57–61.

Bekemeier, B. and Butterfield, P. (2005). Unreconciled inconsistencies – A critical review of the concept of social justice in 3 national nursing documents. *Advances in Nursing Science*, 28(2), 152–162.

Biley, F.C. and Galvin, K.T. (2007). Lifeworld, the arts and mental health nursing. *Journal of Psychiatric and Mental Health Nursing*, 14(8), 800–807.

Brown, J.W. (2011). Health as expanding consciousness a nursing perspective for grounded theory research. *Nursing Science Quarterly*, 24(3), 197–201.

Clarke, P.N., and Jones, D.A. (2011). Expanding consciousness in nursing education and practice. *Nursing Science Quarterly*, 24(3), 223–226.

Connor, M.J. (1998). Expanding the dialogue on praxis in nursing research and practice. *Nursing Science Quarterly*, 11(2), 51–55.

Daly, J., Speedy, S., Jackson, D., Lambert, V.A., and Lambert, C.E. (2005). *Professional nursing: Concepts, issues, and challenges*. New York: Springer Publishing Company.

de Jong, A.E.E., Middelkoop, E., Faber, A.W., and Van Loey, N.E.E. (2007). Non-pharmacological nursing interventions for procedural pain relief in adults with burns: A systematic literature review. *Burns*, 33(7), 811–827.

Dyess, S.M. (2011). Faith: a concept analysis. *Journal of Advanced Nursing*, 67(12), 2723–2731.

Endo, E. (1999). Comment in Advances in Nursing Science, 21(3), vii–viii. Pattern recognition as a nursing intervention with Japanese women with ovarian cancer. *Advances in Nursing Science* (1998), 20(4), 49–61.

Engle, V. (1989). Newman's model of health. In J.J. Fitzpatrick and A.L. Whall (Eds.), *Conceptual models of nursing: Analysis and application* (2nd ed.). Norwalk, CT: Appleton & Lange.

Field, L. and Newman, M. (1982). Clinical application of the unitary man framework: Case study analysis. In M.J. Kim and D.A. Moritz (Eds.), *Classification of nursing diagnosis* (pp. 249–263). New York: McGraw-Hill.

Ford-Gilboe, M.V. (1994). A comparison of two nursing models: Allen's developmental health model and Newman's theory of health as expanding consciousness. *Nursing Science Quarterly*, 7(3), 113–118.

Hall, B. (1980). Book review of Theory Development in Nursing by Margaret Newman. *Nursing Research*, 29(5), 311.

Hall, E.O.C. (1996). Husserlian phenomenology and nursing in a unitary-transformative program. *Vard I Norden Nursing Science and Research in the Nordic Countries*, 16(3), 4–8.

Hensley, D., Keffer, M., Kilgore-Keever, K., Langfitt, J., and Peterson, L. (1989). Margaret A. Newman: Model of health. In A. Marriner-Tomey (Ed.), *Nursing theorists and their work* (2nd ed.). St. Louis, MO: C.V. Mosby.

Lindsay, G., Cross, N., and Ives-Baine, L. (2012). Narratives of neonatal intensive care unit nurses: Experience with end-of-life care. *Illness, Crisis & Loss*, 20(3), 239–253.

Macharia, K.S., Jelagat, R.R., and Juma, M.D. (2015). Applying Margaret Newman's theory of health as expanding consciousness to psychosocial nursing care of HIV infected patients in Kenya. *American Journal of Nursing*, 4(1), 6–11.

Musker, K.M., and Kagan, P.N. (2011). Health as expanding consciousness: Implications for health policy as praxis. *Nursing Science Quarterly*, 24(3), 279–286.

Newman, M. (1984). Nursing diagnosis. *American Journal of Nursing*, 84(12), 1496–1499.

Newman, M. (1986). *Health as expanding consciousness*. St. Louis, MO: C.V. Mosby.

Newman, M. (1987). Aging as increasing complexity [Survey]. *Journal of Gerontological Nursing*, 13(9), 16–18.

Newman, M. (1987). Perception of time among Japanese inpatients. *Western Journal of Nursing Research*, 9(20), 299–300.

Newman, M. (1989). The spirit of nursing. *Holistic Nursing Practice*, 3(3), 1–6.

Newman, M.A. (1972). Time estimation in relation to gait tempo. *Perceptual Motor Skills*, 34, 359–366.

Newman, M.A. (1972). Nursing's theoretical evolution. *Nursing Outlook*, 20, 449–453.

Newman, M.A. (1976). Movement tempo and the experience of time. *Nursing Research*, 25(4), 273–279.

Newman, M.A. (1979). *Theory development in nursing*. Philadelphia, PA: F.A. Davis.

Newman, M.A. (1981). The meaning of health. In G.E. Lasker (Ed.), *Applied systems research and cybernetics*: *Systems research in health care, biocybernetics and ecology* (Vol. 4, pp. 1739–1743). New York: Pergamon.

Newman, M.A. (1982). *Thoughts on Bohm's concept of implicate order and its meaning for nursing science*. Presented at the Nursing Theory Think Tank, Dallas, TX.

Newman, M.A. (1982). Time as an index of consciousness with age. *Nursing Research*, 31, 290–293.

Newman, M.A. (1982). What differentiates clinical research? *Image: Journal of Nursing Scholarship*, 14(3), 86–88.

Newman, M.A. (1983). *Health as expanding consciousness*. In Proceedings of Seventh International Conference on Human Functioning. Wichita, KS: Biomedical Synergistics Institute.

Newman, M.A. (1983). Newman's health theory. In I. Clements and F. Roberts (Eds.), *Family health: A theoretical approach to nursing care* (pp. 161–175). New York: John Wiley & Sons.

Newman, M.A. (1995). Retrospective: Theory for nursing practice. In *A developing discipline: Selected works of Margaret Newman* (Publication No. 14–2671, pp. 273–285). New York: National League for Nursing.

Newman, M.A. (1994). Theory for nursing practice. *Nursing Science Quarterly*, 7, 153–157.

Newman, M.A. (1997). Experiencing the whole. *Advances in Nursing Science*, 20(1), 34–39.

Newman, M.A. and Gaudiano, J.K. (1984). Depression as an explanation for decreased subjective time in the elderly. *Nursing Research*, 33(3), 137–139.

Newman, M.A., Sime, A.M., and Corcoran-Perry, S.A. (1991). The focus of the discipline of nursing. *Advances in Nursing Science*, 14(1), 1–6.

Newman, M.A., Tompkins, E.S., Isenberg, M.A., Fitzpatrick, J.J., and Scott, D.W. (1980). *Movement, time and consciousness: Parameters of health* [Symposium]. Proceedings of Western Society for Research.

Nojima, Y., Oda, A., Nishii, H., Fukui, M., Seo, K., and Akiyoshi, H. (1987). Perception of time among Japanese inpatients. *Western Journal of Nursing Research*, 9(3), 288–300.

Picard, C. and Mariolis, T. (2002). Praxis as a mirroring process: Teaching psychiatric nursing grounded in Newman's health as expanding consciousness. *Nursing Science Quarterly*, 15(2), 1181–122.

Pilkington, F.B. (2007). Envisioning nursing in 2050 through the eyes of nurse theorists: Katie Eriksson and Margaret Newman. *Nursing Science Quarterly*, 20(3), 200.

Roy, C., Rogers, M.E., Fitzpatrick, J.J., Newman, M., and Orem, D.E. (1982). Nursing diagnosis and nursing theory. In M.J. Kim and D.A. Moritz (Eds.), *Classification of nursing diagnosis* (pp. 215–231). New York: McGraw-Hill.

Sarter, B. (1988). Philosophical sources of nursing theory. *Nursing Science Quarterly*, 1(2), 52–59.

Schlotzhauer, M. and Farnham, R. (1997). Newman's theory and insulin dependent diabetes mellitus in adolescence. *Journal of School Nursing*, 13(3), 20–23.

Smith, M.C. (2011). Integrative review of research related to Margaret Newman's theory of health as expanding consciousness. *Nursing Science Quarterly*, 24(3), 256–272.

Weingourt, R. (1998). Using Margaret A. Newman's theory of health with elderly nursing home residents. *Perspectives in Psychiatric Care*, 34(3), 25–30.

Yamashita, M. (1997). Family caregiving: Application of Newman's and Peplau's theories. *Journal of Psychiatric and Mental Health Nursing*, 4(6), 401–405.

Yamashita, M. (1998). Family coping with mental illness: A comparative study. *Journal of Psychiatric and Mental Health Nursing*, 5(6), 515–523.

Yamashita. M. (1998). Newman's theory of health as expanding consciousness: Research on family caregiving in mental illness in Japan. *Nursing Science Quarterly*, 11(3), 110–115.

Yamashita, M. and Tall, F.D. (1998). A commentary on Newman's theory of health as expanding consciousness. *Advances in Nursing Science*, 21(1), 65–75.

27. Florence Nightingale

Anderson, R.J. (2011). Florence Nightingale: The Biostatistician. *Molecular Interventions*, 11(2), 63.

Armstrong, D. (1983). The fabrication of nurse-patient relationships. *Social Science and Medicine*, 17(8), 457–460.

Attewell, A. (1998). Florence Nightingale's relevance to nurses. *Journal of Holistic Nursing*, 16(2), 281–291.

Barnard, K. and Neal, M.U. (1977). Maternal-child nursing research: Review of the past and strategies for the future. *Nursing Research*, 26, 193–200.

Beck, D.M., Dossey, B.M., and Rushton, C.H. (2013). Building the Nightingale Initiative for Global Health—NIGH Can we engage and empower the public voices of nurses worldwide? *Nursing Science Quarterly*, 26(4), 366–371.

Boland, L. (1988). Five Nightingale theories spell success. *Today's Nurse*, 10(12), 18–21.

Bourgeois, M.J. (1975). The special nurse research fellow: Characteristics and trends. *Nursing Research*, 24, 184–188.

Brynes, M.A. (1982). Non-nursing functions: Nurses state their case. *American Journal of Nursing*, 82, 1089–1093.

Chinn, P.L. (1983). Editorial. *Advances in Nursing Science*, 6(1), ix–x.

Christoffel, T. (1976). Medical care evaluation: An old idea. *Journal of Medical Education*, 51(2), 83–88.

Cohen, I.B. (1984). Florence Nightingale. *Scientific America*, 250, 128–137.

Crow, R. (1982). How nursing and the community can benefit from nursing research. *International Journal of Nursing Studies*, 19(1), 37–45.

deGraaf, K., Marriner-Tomey, A., Mossman, C., and Slebodnik, M. (1989). Florence Nightingale: Modern nursing. In A. Marriner-Tomey (Ed.), *Nursing theorists and their work* (2nd ed.). St. Louis, MO: C.V. Mosby.

Dennis, K.E. and Prescott, P.A. (1985). Florence Nightingale: Yesterday, today and tomorrow. *Advances in Nursing Science*, 7(2), 66–81.

Dinc, G., Naderi, S., and Kanpolat, Y. (2013). Florence Nightingale: Light to illuminate the world from the woman with the lantern. *World Neurosurgery*, 79(1), 198–206.

Dominiczak, M.H. (2014). Florence Nightingale: Nurse, writer, and consummate politician. *Clinical Chemistry*, 60(1), 284–285.

Dunphy, L. (2010). Florence Nightingale's legacy of caring and its application. In M. Parker and M. Smith (Eds), *Nursing theories and nursing practice* (pp. 35–51). Philadelphia, PA: FA Davis.

Francis, G. (1980). Gesellschaft and the hospital: Is total care a misnomer? *Advances in Nursing Science*, 2(4), 9–13.

Francis, H.W. (1982). On gossips, eavesdroppers and peeping toms. *Journal of Medical Ethics*, 8, 134–143.

Goldwater, M. (1987). Like Florence Nightingale, we use the political system. *The American Nurse*, 19(2), 15.

Grier, B. and Grier, M. (1978). Contributions of the passionate statistician. *Research in Nursing and Health*, 1(3), 103–109.

Hays, J.D. (1989). Florence Nightingale and the India sanitary reforms. *Public Health Nursing*, 6(3), 152–154.

Hegge, M. (2011). The empty carriage lessons in leadership from Florence Nightingale. *Nursing Science Quarterly*, 24(1), 21–25.

Hegge, M. (2013). Nightingale's Environmental Theory. *Nursing Science Quarterly*, 26(3), 211–219.

Hegge, M.J. (2011). The lingering presence of the Nightingale legacy. *Nursing Science Quarterly*, 24(2), 152–162.

Heistand, W.C. (1982). Nursing, the family and the "new" social history. *Advances in Nursing Science*, 4(3), 1–12.

Henderson, V.A. (1978). The concept of nursing. *Journal of Advanced Nursing*, 3, 113–130.

Henderson, V.A. (1980). Preserving the essence of nursing in a technological age. *Journal of Advanced Nursing*, 5, 245–260.

Hughes, L. (1980). The public image of the nurse. *Advances in Nursing Science*, 2, 55–72.

Johnson, D.E. (1974). Development of theory: A requisite for nursing as a primary health profession. *Nursing Research*, 23(5), 372–377.

Kagan, S.H. (2014). Florence Nightingale's notes on nursing and the determinants of health. *Cancer Nursing*, 37(6), 478.

Kalish, B.J. and Kalish, P.A. (1983). Heroine out of focus: Media images of Florence Nightingale. Part I: Popular biographies and stage productions. *Nursing and Health Care*, 4, 181–187.

Kalish, P.A. and Kalish, B.J. (1982). The image of nurses in novels. *American Journal of Nursing*, 82, 1220–1224.

Keith, J.M. (1988). Florence Nightingale: Statistician and consultant epidemiologist. *International Nursing Review*, 35(5), 147–151.

Kelly, L.Y. (1976). Our nursing heritage: Have we renounced it? *Image: Journal of Nursing Scholarship*, 8(3), 43–48.

Kopf, E.W. (1978). Florence Nightingale as statistician. *Research in Nursing and Health*, 1(3), 93–102.

Kovacs, A.R. (1978). The personality of Florence Nightingale. *International Nursing Review*, 20, 78–81.

Lee, G., Clark, A.M., and Thompson, D.R. (2013). Florence Nightingale–never more relevant than today. *Journal of Advanced Nursing*, 69(2), 245–246.

Lim, F.A., and Shi, T. (2013). Florence Nightingale: A pioneer of self-reflection. *Nursing*, 43(5), 1–3.

Macrae, J. (1995). Nightingale's spiritual philosophy and its significance for modern nursing. *Image: Journal of Nursing Scholarship*, 27, 8–10.

Matthews, C.A. and Gaul, A.L. (1979). Nursing diagnosis from the perspective of concept attainment and critical thinking. *Advances in Nursing Science*, 2(1), 17–26.

McDonald, L. (2014). Florence Nightingale, statistics and the Crimean War. *Journal of the Royal Statistical Society: Series A (Statistics in Society)*, 177(3), 569–586.

Monteiro, L. (1972). Research into things past: Tracking down one of Miss Nightingale's correspondents. *Nursing Research*, 21(5), 526–529.

Nightingale, F. (1992). *Notes on nursing* [Reprint of 1859 edition]. Philadelphia, PA: J.B. Lippincott.

Novak, J.C. (1988). The social mandate and historical basis for nursing's role in health promotion. *Journal of Professional Nursing*, 4(2), 80–87.

Palmer, I.S. (1977). Florence Nightingale: Reformer, reactionary, researcher. *Nursing Research*, 26(2), 84–89.

Palmer, I.S. (1981). Florence Nightingale and international origins of modern nursing. *Image Journal of Nursing Scholarship*, 13, 28–31.

Palmer, I.S. (1983). Nightingale revisited. *Nursing Outlook*, 31(4), 229–233.

Palmer, I.S. (1983). Origins of education for nurses. *Nursing Forum*, 22(3), 102–110.

Parker, P. (1977). Florence Nightingale: First lady of administrative nursing. *Supervisor Nurse*, 8(3), 24–25.

Reed, P.G. and Zurakowski, T.L. (1983). Nightingale: A visionary model for nursing. In J.J. Fitzpatrick and A.L. Whall (Eds.), *Conceptual models of nursing: Analysis and application*. Bowie, MD: Robert J. Brady Co.

Reed, P.G. and Zurakowski, T.L. (1989). Nightingale revisited: A visionary model for nursing. In J.J. Fitzpatrick and A.L. Whall (Eds.), *Conceptual models of nursing: Analysis and application* (2nd ed.). Norwalk, CT: Appleton & Lange.

Rogers, P.S. (1972). Design for patient care. *International Nursing Review*, 19(3), 267–282.

Romano, C., McCormick, L.D., and McNeely, L.D. (1982). Nursing documentation: A model for a computerized data base. *Advances in Nursing Science*, 1(2), 43–56.

Schlotfeldt, R.M. (1977). Nursing research: Reflection of values. *Nursing Research*, 26(1), 4–9.

Schrock, R.A. (1977). On political consciousness in nurses. *Journal of Advanced Nursing*, 2, 41–50.

Seelye, A. (1982). Hospital ward layout and nurse staffing. *Journal of Advanced Nursing*, 7, 195–201.

Selanders, L.C. (1998). Florence Nightingale. The evolution and social impact of feminist values in nursing. *Journal of Holistic Nursing*, 16(2), 227–243.

Selanders, L.C. (1998). The power of environmental adaptation. Florence Nightingale's original theory for nursing practice. *Journal of Holistic Nursing*, 16(2), 247–263.

Selanders, L. and Crane, P. (2012). The voice of Florence Nightingale on advocacy. *Online Journal of Issues in Nursing*, 17(1), 1.

Seymer, L.R. (1960). One hundred years ago. *American Journal of Nursing*, 60, 658–661.

Smith, F.T. (1981). Florence Nightingale: Early feminist. *American Journal of Nursing*, 81, 1021–1024.

Tebbe, S. (1988). Nightingale's environmental theory—A 20th century reality. *Today's Nurse*, 10(8), 8–15.

Thompson, J.D. (1980). The passionate humanist: From Nightingale to the new nurse. *Nursing Outlook*, 28(5), 290–295.

Torres, G. (1981). The nursing education administrator: Accountable, vulnerable and oppressed. *Advances in Nursing Science*, 3(3), 1–16.

Weiler, P.G. (1975). Health manpower dialectic: Physician, nurse, physician assistant. *American Journal of Public Health*, 65(8), 858–863.

Whittaker, E.W. and Olesen, V.L. (1967). Why Florence Nightingale? *American Journal of Nursing*, 67, 2338–2341.

Williams, B. (1965). Back to Florence Nightingale and Lawson Tait. *The Practitioner*, 194, 800–804.

Wolstenholme, G.E.W. (1970). Florence Nightingale: New lamps for old. *Proceedings of the Royal Society of Medicine*, 63, 1282–1288.

Zborowsky, T. (2014). The legacy of Florence Nightingale's environmental theory: Nursing research focusing on the impact of healthcare environments. *HERD: Health Environments Research & Design Journal*, 7(4), 19–34.

28. Dorothea Orem

Abdellah, G.F., Beland, I.L., Martin, A., and Matheney, R.V. (1961). *Patient-centered approaches to nursing*. New York: Macmillan.

Ageborg, M., Allenius, B.L., and Cederfjall, C. (2005, October). Quality of life, self-care ability, and sense of coherence in hemodialysis patients: A comparative study. *Hemodialysis International*, 9(Suppl 1), S8–14.

Aggleton, P. and Chalmers, H. (1985). Models and theories: Orem's self care model (part 5). *Nursing Times*, 81(1), 36–39.

Ailinger, R.L., Braun, M.A., Lasus, H., and Whitt, K. (2005). Factors influencing osteoporosis knowledge: A community study. *Journal of Community Health Nursing*, 22(3), 135–142.

Ailinger, R.L. and Dear, M.R. (1993). Self-care agency in persons with rheumatoid arthritis. *Arthritis Care and Research*, 6(3), 134–140.

Ailinger, R.L. and Dear, M.R. (1997). An examination of the self-care needs of clients with rheumatoid arthritis. *Rehabilitation Nursing*, 22(3), 135–140.

Ailinger, R.L., Lasus, H., and Braun, M.A. (2003). Revision of the facts on osteoporosis quiz. *Nursing Research*, 52(3), 198–201.

Ailinger, R.L., Moore, J.B., Nguyen, N., and Lasus, H. (2006). Adherence to latent tuberculosis infection therapy among Laotian immigrants. *Public Health Nursing*, 23(4), 307–313.

Aish, A.E. and Isenberg, M. (1996). Effects of Orem-based nursing intervention on nutritional self-care of myocardial infarction patients. *International Journal of Nursing Studies*, 33(3), 259–270.

Akyol, A.D., Cetinkaya, Y., Bakan, G., Yarali, S., and Akkus, S. (2007). Self-care agency and factors related to this agency among patients with hypertension. *Journal of Clinical Nursing*, 16(4), 679–687.

Ali, A.J.I, Sayej, S., and Fashafsheh, I.H. (2014). Evaluating self-care practices of children with type 1 diabetes mellitus in Northern West Bank: A controlled randomized study utilizing Orem Self-Care theory. *Journal of Education and Practice*, 5(11), 53–63.

Allan, J. (1988). Knowing what to weigh: Women's self care activities related to weight. *Advances in Nursing Science*, 11(1), 47–60

Allen, D. (2000). Negotiating the role of expert carers on an adult hospital ward. *Sociology of Health and Illness*, 22(2), 149–171.

†Allison, S.E. (1973). A framework for nursing action in a nurse-conducted diabetic management clinic. *Journal of Nursing Administration*, 3(4), 53–60.

Allison, S.E. (2007). Self-care requirements for activity and rest: An Orem nursing focus. *Nursing Science Quarterly*, 20(1), 68–76.

Altay, N. and Cavusoglu, H. (2013). Using Orem's self-care model for asthmatic adolescents. *Journal for Specialists in Pediatric Nursing*, 18(3), 233–242.

Alteneder, R.R. (1998). Conceptualizing sexual health in cancer care—Commentary. *Western Journal of Nursing Research*, 20(6), 701–703.

Anastasio, C., McMahan, T., Daniels, A., Nicholas, P.K., and Paul-Simon, A. (1995). Self-care burden in women with human immunodeficiency virus. *Journal of the Association of Nurses in AIDS Care*, 6(3), 31–42.

Anderson, J.A. (2001). Understanding homeless adults by testing the theory of self-care. *Nursing Science Quarterly*, 14(1), 59–67.

Anderson, J.A. and Olnhausen, K.S. (1999). Adolescent self-esteem: A foundational disposition. *Nursing Science Quarterly*, 12(1), 61–67.

Anderson, S.B. (1992). Guillain-Barré syndrome: Giving the patient control. *Journal of Neuroscience Nursing*, 24(3), 158–162.

†Anna, D.J., Christensen, D.G., Hohn, S.A., Ord, L., and Wells, S.R. (1978). Implementing Orem's conceptual framework. *Journal of Nursing Administration*, 8(11), 8–11.

Aponte, J. and Nickitas, D.M. (2007). Community as client: Reaching an underserved urban community and meeting unmet primary health care needs. *Journal of Community Health Nursing*, 24(3), 177–190.

Arevian, M. (2005). The significance of a collaborative practice model in delivering care to chronically ill patients; A case study of managing diabetes mellitus in a primary health care center. *Journal of Interprofessional Care*, 19(5), 444–451.

Arman, M. and Hok, J. (2015, Sept 22). Self-care follows from compassionate care – Chronic pain patients' experience of integrative rehabilitation. *Scandinavian Journal of Caring Sciences*. doi: 10.1111/scs.12258.

Arpanantikul, M. (2006). Self-care process as experienced by middle-aged Thai women. *Health Care Women International*, 27(10), 893–907.

Artinian, N.T., Magnan, M., Sloan, M., and Lange, M.P. (2002). Self-care behaviors among patients with heart failure. *Heart and Lung*, 31(3), 161–172.

Arts, S., Kersten, H., and Kerkstra, A. (1996). The daily practice in home help services in the Netherlands: Instrument development. *Health and Social Care in the Community*, 4(5), 280–289.

Ashcraft, P.F. and Gatto, S.L. (2015). Care-of-self in undergraduate nursing students: A pilot study. *Nursing Education Perspectives*, 36(4), 255–256.

Astedt-Kurki, P., Friedemann, M.L., Paavilainen, E., et al. (2001). Assessment of strategies in families tested by Finnish families. *International Journal of Nursing Studies*, 38(1), 17–24.

Autar, R. (1996). Nursing assessment of clients at risk of deep vein thrombosis (DVT): The Autar DVT scale. *Journal of Advanced Nursing*, 23(4), 763–770.

Backman, K. and Hentinen, M. (1999). Model for the self-care of home-dwelling elderly. *Journal of Advanced Nursing*, 30(3), 564–572.

Backscheider, J. (1971). The use of self as the essence of clinical supervision in ambulatory patient care. *Nursing Clinics of North America*, 6(4), 785–794.

†Backscheider, J.E. (1974). Self-care requirements, self-care capabilities, and nursing systems in the diabetic nurse management clinic. *American Journal of Public Health*, 64(12), 1138–1146.

Baker, L.K. and Denyes, M.J. (2008). Predictors of self-care in adolescents with cystic fibrosis: A test of Orem's theories of self-care and self-care deficit. *Journal of Pediatric Nursing*, 23(1), 37–48.

Banfield, B.E. (1997). *A philosophical inquiry of Orem's self-care deficit theory*. Unpublished doctoral dissertation. Wayne State University, Ann Arbor, MI.

Banfield, B.E. (2001). Philosophic foundations of Orem's work. In D. Orem (Ed.), *Nursing: Concepts of practice* (pp. xi–xvi). St. Louis, MO: C.V. Mosby.

Barnard, A. (1996). Technology and nursing: An anatomy of definition. *International Journal of Nursing Studies*, 33(4), 433–441.

Barnard, A. (1997). A critical review of the belief that technology is a neutral object and nurses are its master. *Journal of Advanced Nursing*, 16(1), 126–131.

Barnes, C.R. and Adamson-Macedo, E.N. (2007). Perceived maternal parenting self-efficacy (PMP S-E) tool: Development and validation with mothers of hospitalized preterm neonates. *Journal of Advanced Nursing*, 60(5), 550–560.

Barnum, B.J.S. (1994). *Nursing theory: Analysis, application, and evaluation*. Philadelphia, PA: Lippincott.

Bartle, J. (1991). Nursing models: Caring in relation to Orem's theory. *Nursing Standard*, 5(37), 33–36.

Beach, E.K., Smith, A., Luthringer, L., et al. (1996). Self-care limitations of persons after acute myocardial infarction. *Applied Nursing Research*, 9(1), 24–28.

Behi, R. (1986). Look after yourself: Orem's self-care model. *Nursing Times*, 82(37), 35–37.

Bennett, J.A. (1995). Nurses' attitudes about acquired-immunodeficiency-syndrome care—What research tells us. *Journal of Professional Nursing*, 11(6), 339–350.

Bennett, J.A. (1997). A case for theory triangulation. *Nursing Science Quarterly*, 10(2), 97–102.

Bennett, J.G. (1980). Forward to the symposium on the self-care concept in nursing. *Nursing Clinics of North America*, 15(1), 129–130.

Berbiglia, V.A. (1991). A case study: Perspectives on a self-care deficit nursing theory-based curriculum. *Journal of Advanced Nursing*, 16(10), 1158–1163.

Berbiglia, V.A. (1997). Orem's self-care deficit theory in nursing practice. In M.R. Alligood et al. (Eds.), *Nursing theory: Utilization and application* (pp. 129–152). St. Louis, MO: Mosby Year Book.

Berbiglia, V.A. (2011). The self-care deficit nursing theory as a curriculum conceptual framework in baccalaureate education. *Nursing Science Quarterly*, 24(2), 137–145.

Berbiglia, V.A. and Banfield, B. (2014). Self-care deficit theory of nursing. In M.R. Aligood (Ed.), *Nursing theorists and their work*. St. Louis, MO: Elsevier.

Berhe, K.K., Demissie, A., Kahsay, A.B., and Gebru, H.B. (2012). Diabetes self-care practices and associated factors among type 2 diabetic patients in Tikur Anbessa Specialized Hospital, Addis Ababa, Ethiopia – A cross-sectional study. *International Journal of Pharmaceutical Sciences and Research*, 3(11), 4219–4229.

Berndtsson, I., Lindholm, E., and Ekman, I. (2005). Thirty years of experience living with a continent ileostomy: Bad restrooms–not my reservoir–decide my life. *Journal of Wound, Ostomy Continence Nursing*, 32(5), 321–328.

Bernhard, L. (1997). Self-care strategies of menopausal women. *Journal of Women and Aging*, 9(1–2), 77–89.

Betz, C.L. (2000). California healthy and ready to work transition health care guide: Developmental guidelines for teaching health care self-care skills to children. *Issues in Comprehensive Pediatric Nursing*, 23(4), 203–244.

Bevan, M.T. (2000). Dialysis as "deus ex machina": A critical analysis of haemodialysis. *Journal of Advanced Nursing*, 31(2), 437–443.

Bhanji, S.M. (2012). Comparison and contrast of Orem's self-care theory and Roy's adaptation model. *Journal of Nursing*, 1(1), 48–53.

Biehler, B.A. (1992). Impact of role-sets on implementing self-care theory with children. *Pediatric Nursing*, 18(1), 30–34.

Biggs, A. (2008). Orem's self-care deficit nursing theory: Update on the state of the art and science. *Nursing Science Quarterly*, 21(3), 200–206.

Biley, F. and Dennerley, M. (1990). Orem's model: A critical analysis. *Nursing*, 4(13), 19–22.

Bliss-Holtz, J. (1996). Using Orem's theory to generate nursing diagnoses for electronic documentation. *Nursing Science Quarterly*, 9(3), 121–125.

Bliss-Holtz, J., Taylor, S.G., and McLaughlin, K. (1992). Nursing theory as a base for a computerized nursing information system. *Nursing Science Quarterly*, 5(3), 124–128.

Bonamy, C., Schultz, P., Graham, K., and Hampton, M. (1995). The use of theory-based nursing practice in the Department of Veterans' Affairs Medical Centers. *Journal of Nursing Staff Development*, 11(1), 27–30.

Bowles, K.H., Ratcliffe, S.J., Holmes, J.H., Liberatore, M., Nydick, R., and Naylor, M.D. (2008). Post-acute referral decisions made by multidisciplinary experts compared to hospital clinicians and the patients' 12–week outcomes. *Medical Care*, 46(2), 158–166.

Bradshaw, A. (1995). What are nurses doing to patients—A review of theories of nursing past and present. *Journal of Clinical Nursing*, 4(2), 81–92

Bramlett, M.H., Gueldner, S.H., and Sowell, R.L. (1990). Consumer-centric advocacy: Its connection to nursing frameworks. *Nursing Science Quarterly*, 3(4), 156–161.

Brillhart, B. (2005). Pressure sore and skin tear prevention and treatment during a 10–month program. *Rehabilitation Nursing*, 30(3), 85–91.

†Bromley, B. (1980). Applying Orem's self-care theory in enterostomal therapy. *American Journal of Nursing*, 80(2), 245–249.

Brown, B. (2015). Towards a critical understanding of mutuality in mental healthcare: Relationships, power and social capital. *Journal of Psychiatric and Mental Health Nursing*, 22(10), 829–835.

†Buckwalter, K.C. and Kerfoot, K.M. (1982). Teaching patients self-care: A critical aspect of psychiatric discharge planning. *Journal of Psychiatric Nursing and Mental Health Services*, 20(5), 15–20.

Budinger, J.M. (2007). A patient education tool for nonoperative management of blunt abdominal trauma. *Journal of Trauma Nursing*, 14(1), 19–23.

Bunn, M.H., O'Connor, A.M., Tansey, M.S., et al. (1997). Characteristics of clients with schizophrenia who express certainty or uncertainty about continuing treatment with depot neuroleptic medication. *Archives of Psychiatric Nursing*, 11(5), 238–248.

Burks, K.J. (1999). A nursing practice model for chronic illness. *Rehabilitation Nursing*, 24(5), 197–200.

Burks, K.J. (2001). Intentional action. *Journal of Advanced Nursing*, 34(5), 668–675.

Bussing, A. and Herbig, B. (1998). The challenges of a care information system reflecting holistic nursing care. *Computers in Nursing*, 16(6), 311–317.

Caetano, J.A. and Pagliuca, L.M. (2006). Self-care and HIV/AIDS patients: Nursing care systematization. *Revista Latino-Americana de Enfermagem*, 14(3), 336–345.

Cade, N.V. (2001). Orem's self-care deficit theory applied to hypertensive people (Portuguese). *Revista Latino-Americana de Enfermagem*, 9(3), 43–50.

†Caley, J.M., Dirkensen, M., Engally, M., and Hennrich, M.L. (1980). The Orem self-care model. In J.P. Riehl and C. Roy (Eds.), *Conceptual models for nursing practice* (2nd ed.). New York: Appleton-Century-Crofts.

Callaghan, D. (2005). Healthy behaviors, self-efficacy, self-care, and basic conditioning factors in older adults. *Journal of Community Healthy Nursing*, 22(3), 169–178.

Callaghan, D. (2006). Basic conditioning factors' influences on adolescents' healthy behaviors, self-efficacy, and self-care. *Issues in Comprehensive Pediatric Nursing*, 29(4), 191–204.

Callaghan, D. (2006). The influence of basic conditioning factors on healthy behaviors, self-efficacy, and self-care in adults. *Journal of Holistic Nursing*, 24(3), 178–185.

Callaghan, D.M. (2003). Health-promoting self-care behaviors, self-care, self-efficacy, and self-care agency. *Nursing Science Quarterly*, 16(3), 247–254.

Callaghan, D.M. (2005). The influence of spiritual growth on adolescents' initiative and responsibility for self-care. *Pediatric Nursing*, 31(2), 91–95, 115.

Cammermeyer, M. (1983). Growth model of self-care for neurologically impaired people. *Journal of Neurosurgical Nursing*, 15, 299–305.

Campbell, J.C. (1986). Nursing assessment for risk of homicide with battered women. *Advances in Nursing Science*, 8(4), 36–51.

Campbell, J.C. and Soeken, K.L. (1999). Women's responses to battering: A test of the model. *Research in Nursing and Health*, 22(1), 49–58.

Campbell, J.C. and Weber, N. (2000). An empirical test of a self-care model of women's responses to battering. *Nursing Science Quarterly*, 13(1), 45–53.

Campuzano, M. (1982). Self-care following coronary artery bypass surgery. *Focus on Critical Care*, 9(1), 55–56.

Canty-Mitchell, J. (2001). Life change events, hope and self-care agency in inner-city adolescents. *Journal of Child and Adolescent Psychiatric Nursing*, 14(1), 18–31.

Caris-Verhallen, W.M.C.M., Kerkstra, A. and Bensing, J.M. (1997). The role of communication in nursing care for elderly people: A review of the literature. *Journal of Advanced Nursing*, 25(5), 915–933.

Carper, B.A. (1978). Fundamental patterns of knowing in nursing. *Advances in Nursing Science*, 1(1), 13–23.

Carter, P.A. (1998). Self-care agency: The concept and how it is measured. *Journal of Nursing Measurement*, 6(2), 195–207.

Cebeci, F. and Celik, S.S. (2008). Discharge training and counselling increase self-care ability and reduce post-discharge, 6(2), 195–207. problems in CABG patients. *Journal of Clinical Nursing*, 17(3), 412–420.

†Chang, B.L. (1980). Evaluation of health care professionals in facilitating self-care: Review of the literature and a conceptual model. *Advances in Nursing Science*, 3(1), 43–58.

Chan, M.F. and Zang, Y.L. (2007). Nurses' perceived and actual level of diabetes mellitus knowledge: Results of a cluster analysis. *Journal of Clinical Nursing*, 16(7B), 234–242.

Chapman, P. (1984). Specifics and generalities: A critical examination of two nursing models . . . Orem's and Preisner's. *Nurse Educator Today*, 4(6), 141–144.

Chen, A.M.H., Yehle, K.S., Albert, N.M., Ferraro, K.F., et al (2014). Relationships between health literacy and heart failure knowledge, self-efficacy, and self-care adherence. *Research in Social and Administrative Pharmacy*, 10(2), 378–386.

Chen, M.Y., James, K., Hsu, L.L., Chang, S.W., Huang, L.H., and Wang, E.K. (2005). Health-related behavior and adolescent mothers. *Public Health Nursing*, 22(4), 280–288.

Chernecky, C., Macklin, D., and Walter, J. (2006). Internet design preferences of patients with cancer. *Oncology Nursing Forum*, 33(4), 787–792.

Chevannes, M. (1997). Nurses caring for families—Issues in a multiracial society. *Journal of Clinical Nursing*, 6(2), 161–167.

Clark, M. (1986). Application of Orem's theory of self-care: A case study. *Journal of Community Health Nursing*, 3(3), 127–135.

Clarke, P.N., Allison, S.E., Berbiglia, V.A., and Taylor, S.G. (2009). The impact of Dorothea E. Orem's life and work: An interview with Orem Scholars. *Nursing Science Quarterly*, 22(1), 41–46.

Clinton, J.F., Denyes, M.J., Goodwin, J.O., and Koto, E.M. (1977). Developing criterion measures of nursing care: Case study of a process. *Journal of Nursing Administration*, 7(7), 41–45.

Closson, B.L., Mattingly, L.J., Finne, K.M., and Larson, J.A. (1994). Telephone follow-up program evaluation: Application of Orem's self-care model. *Rehabilitation Nursing*, 19(5), 287–292.

Cody, W.K. (1996). Drowning in eclecticism. *Nursing Science Quarterly*, 9(3), 86–88.

Cody, W.K. (1997). The many faces of change: Discomfort with the new. *Nursing Science Quarterly*, 10(2), 65–67.

Cody, W.K. (2000). Paradigm shift or paradigm drift? A meditation on commitment and transcendence. *Nursing Science Quarterly*, 13(2), 93–102.

†Coleman, L.J. (1980). Orem's self-care concept of nursing. In J.P. Riehl and C. Roy (Eds.), *Conceptual models for nursing practice* (2nd ed., pp. 315–328). New York: Appleton-Century-Crofts.

Comley, A.L. (1995). A comparative analysis of Orem's self-care model and Peplau's interpersonal theory. *Journal of Advanced Nursing*, 20(4), 755–760.

Compton, P. (1989). Drug abuse, a self-care deficit. *Journal of Psychosocial Nursing*, 27(3), 22–26.

Cox, K.R. and Taylor, S.G. (2005). Orem's self-care deficit nursing theory: Pediatric asthma as exemplar. *Nursing Science Quarterly*, 18(3), 249–257.

Coyle, M.K. and Martin, E.M. (2007). Reflecting on a self-care process in the home setting for traumatic brain injury survivors. *Journal of Neuroscience Nursing*, 39(5), 274–277.

Craddock, R.B., Adams, P.F., Usui, W.M., et al. (1999). An intervention to increase use and effectiveness of self-care measures for breast cancer chemotherapy patients. *Cancer Nursing*, 22(4), 312–319.

Cull, V.V. (1996). Exposure to violence and self-care practices of adolescents. *Family and Community Health*, 19(1), 31–41.

Cutler, C.G. (2001). Self-care agency and symptom management in patients treated for mood disorder. *Archives of Psychiatric Nursing*, 15(1), 24–31.

Dahn, M.L.L. (1998). An innovative approach to appropriate resource utilization. *Nursing Economics*, 16(6), 317–319.

Dashiff, C. (1988). Theory development in psychiatric mental health nursing: An analysis of Orem's theory. *Archives of Psychiatric Nursing*, 2(6), 366–372.

Dashiff, C.J. (1992). Self-care capabilities in black girls in anticipation of menarche. *Health Care for Women International*, 13(1), 67–76.

Davidhizar, R. and Cosgray, R. (1990). The use of Orem's model in psychiatric rehabilitation assessment. *Rehabilitation Nursing*, 15(1), 39–41.

Decramer, M. Gosselink, R., Troosters, T., et al. (1997). Muscle weakness is related to utilization of health care resources in COPD patients. *European Respiratory Journal*, 10(2), 417–423.

Decurvas, L.H.O. and Campo, J.H.L. (1995). A program for the home care of patients with a symptomatic malignant terminal disease. *Cancer Nursing*, 18(5), 368–373.

DeGeest, S., Borgermans, L., Gemoets, H., et al. (1995). Incidence, determinants, and consequences of subclinical noncompliance with immunosuppressive therapy in renal transplant recipients. *Transplantation*, 59, 340–347.

Delbar, V. and Benor, D.E. (2001). Impact of a nursing intervention on cancer patients' ability to cope. *Journal of Psychosocial Oncology*, 19(2), 57–75.

Deng, X. and Xie, X. (2001). Apply Orem theory and theory of holistic nursing care to set up a nursing model for the aged in community [Chinese]. *Chinese Nursing Research*, 15(3), 173–174.

Denyes, M.J. (1982). Measurement of self-care agency in adolescents [Abstract]. *Nursing Research*, 31, 63.

Denyes, M.J. (1988). Orem's model used for health promotion: Directions from research. *Advances in Nursing Science*, 11(1), 13–21.

Denyes, M.J., Neuman, B.M., and Villarruel, A.M. (1991). Nursing actions to prevent and alleviate pain in hospitalized children. *Issues in Comprehensive Pediatric Nursing*, 14(1), 31–48.

Denyes, M.J., O'Connor, N., Oakley, D., and Ferguson, S. (1989). Integrating nursing theory, practice and research through collaborative research. *Journal of Advanced Nursing*, 14, 141–145.

Denyes, M.J., Orem, D.E., and SozWiss, G. (2001). Self-care: A foundational science. *Nursing Science Quarterly*, 14(1), 48–54.

†Dickson, G.L. and Lee-Villasenor, H. (1982). Nursing theory and practice: A self-care approach. *Advances in Nursing Science*, 5, 29–40.

Dijkstra, A., Buist, G., Moorer, P., et al. (1999). Construct validity of the Nursing Care Dependency Scale. *Journal of Clinical Nursing*, 8(4), 380–388.

Dijkstra, A., Buist, G., Moorer, P., et al. (2000). A reliability and utility study of the Care Dependency Scale. *Scandinavian Journal of Caring Sciences*, 14(3), 155–161.

Dijkstra, A., Sipsma, D., and Dassen, T. (1999). Predictors of care dependency in Alzheimer's disease after a two-year period. *International Journal of Nursing Studies*, 36(6), 487–495.

Drevenhorn, E., Bengtson, A., Nyberg, P., and Kjellgren, K.I. (2015). Assessment of hypertensive patients' self-care agency after counseling training of nurses. *Journal of the American Association of Nurse Practitioners*, 27(11), 624–630.

Dropkin, M.J. (1981). Development of a self-care teaching program for postoperative head and neck patients. *Cancer Nursing*, 103–106.

Dumas, L. (1991). The Orem's conceptual framework as a self determinant for the nursing profession. *Arctic Medical Research*, Supplement, 207.

Easton, K.L. (1993). Defining the concept of self-care. *Rehabilitation Nursing*, 18(6), 384–387.

Eben, J., Gashti, N., Nation, M., Marriner-Tomey, A., and Nordmeyer, S. (1989). Dorothea E. Orem: Self-care deficit theory of nursing. In A. Marriner-Tomey (Ed.), *Nursing theorists and their work* (2nd ed.). St. Louis, MO: C.V. Mosby.

Emerson, J. and Enderby, P. (1996). Management of speech and language disorders in a mental illness unit. *European Journal of Disorders of Communication*, 31(3), 237–244.

England, M. (1996). Sense of relatedness and interpersonal network of adult offspring caregivers: Linkages with crisis, emotional arousal, and perceived health. *Archives of Psychiatric Nursing*, 10(2), 85–95.

England, M. (1997). Self-coherence, emotional arousal and perceived health of adult children caring for a brain-impaired parent. *Journal of Advanced Nursing*, 26(4), 672–682.

Erci, B. (2005). Nursing theories applied to vulnerable populations: Examples from Turkey. In M.D. Chesnay (Ed.), *Caring for the vulnerable: Perspectives in nursing theory, practice, and research* (pp. 45–60). Sudbury, MA: Jones & Bartlett Publishers.

Estes, S.D. and Hart, M. (1993). A model for the development of the CNS role in adolescent health promotion self-care. *Clinical Nurse Specialist*, 7(3), 111–115.

Evangelista, L.S. (2008). What do we know about adherence and self-care. *Journal of Cardiovascular Nursing*, 23(3), 250–257.

Evers, G.C.M. (1997). Pseudo-opioid resistant pain. *Supportive Care in Cancer*, 5(6), 457–460.

Evers, G., Viane, A., Sermeus, W., et al. (2000). Frequency of and indications for wholly compensatory nursing care related to enteral food intake: A secondary analysis of the Belgium National Nursing Minimum Data Set. *Journal of Advanced Nursing*, 32(1), 194–201.

Ewing, G. (1989). The nursing preparation of stoma patients for self-care. *Journal of Advanced Nursing*, 14, 41–420.

Fan, L. (2008). Self-care behaviors of school-age children with heart disease. *Pediatric Nursing*, 34(2), 131–138.

Faucett, J., Ellis, V., Underwood, P., Naqvi, A., and Wilson, D. (1990). The effect of Orem's self-care model on nursing care in a nursing home setting. *Journal of Advanced Nursing*, 15(6), 659–666.

Fawcett, J. (1984). Orem's self-care model. In J. Fawcett (Ed.), *Analysis and evaluation of conceptual models of nursing*. Philadelphia, PA: F.A. Davis.

Fawcett, J. (1989). Orem's self-care model. In J. Fawcett (Ed.), *Analysis and evaluation of conceptual models of nursing* (2nd ed.). Philadelphia, PA: F.A. Davis.

Fawcett, J. (2001). The nurse theorists: 21st-century updates— Dorothea E. Orem. *Nursing Science Quarterly*, 14(1), 34–38.

Fawcett, J. (2005). *Contemporary nursing knowledge: Analysis and evaluation of nursing models and theories* (2nd ed.). Philadelphia, PA: F.A. Davis.

Fawcett, J. (2006). The state of nursing science: Hallmarks of the 20th and 21st centuries. In W. K. Cody and J. W. Kenney (Eds.), *Philosophical and theoretical perspectives for advanced nursing practice* (4th ed., pp. 51–58). Sudbury, MA: Jones & Bartlett Publishers.

Fawcett, J., Bekel, G., Biley, F.C., and Fragemann, K. (2007). Nursing, healthcare, and culture: A view of the year 2050 from Germany and the United Kingdom. *Nursing Science Quarterly*, 20(3), 232–236.

Fawcett, J. and DeSanto-Madeya, S. (2013). *Contemporary nursing knowledge: Analysis and evaluation of nursing models and theories* (3rd ed.). Philadelphia, PA: F.A. Davis.

Fawdry, M.K., Berry, M.L., and Rajacich, D. (1996). The articulation of nursing systems with dependent care systems of intergenerational caregivers. *Nursing Science Quarterly*, 9(1), 22–26.

Feathers, R. (1989). Orem's self-care nursing theory. In J. Riehl-Sisca (Ed.), *Conceptual models for nursing practice* (3rd ed.). Norwalk, CT: Appleton & Lange.

Fenner, K. (1979). Developing a conceptual framework. *Nursing Outlook*, 27, 122–126.

Field, P.A. (1987). The impact of nursing theory on the clinical decision making process. *Journal of Advanced Nursing*, 12(5), 563–571.

Fitzgerald, S. (1980). Utilizing Orem's self-care nursing model in designing an educational program for the diabetic. *Topics in Clinical Nursing*, 2(2), 57–65.

Flensner, G. and Lindencrona, C. (2002). The cooling-suit: A study of ten multiple sclerosis patients' experiences in daily life. *Journal of Advanced Nursing*, 37(6), 541–550.

Fontana, J.A. (1996). The emergence of the person-environment interaction in a descriptive study of vigor in heart failure. *Advances in Nursing Science*, 18(4), 70–82.

Foster, P.C. and Janssens, N.P. (1980). Dorothea E. Orem. In The Nursing Theories Conference Group (Eds.), *Nursing theories: The base for professional nursing practice*. Englewood Cliffs, NJ: Prentice-Hall.

Franklin, A. (2001). Orem's self-care model in practice. *Vision*, 7(13), 24–26.

Frey, M.A. and Fox, M.A. (1990). Assessing and teaching self-care to youths with diabetes mellitus. *Pediatric Nursing*, 16, 597–800.

Furlong, S. (1996). Self-care: The application of a ward philosophy. *Journal of Clinical Nursing*, 5(2), 85–90.

Gaffney, K.F. and Moore, J.B. (1996). Testing Orem's theory of self-care deficit: Dependent care agent performance for children. *Nursing Science Quarterly*, 9(4), 160–164.

Garcia, M.A. and Castillo, L. (2000). Client categorization: A tool to assess nursing workloads. *Revista Medica de Chile*, 128(2), 177–183.

Gardulf, A., Bjorvell, H., Andersen, V., et al. (1995). Life-long treatment with gammaglobulin for primary antibody deficiencies: The patients' experiences of subcutaneous self-infusions and home therapy. *Journal of Advanced Nursing*, 21(5), 917–927.

Geden, B. (1997). Theory based research and defining populations ... Reprinted with permission from: Theory-based nursing process and produce: Using Orem's self-care deficit theory of nursing in practice, education, and research. *International Orem Society Newsletter*, 5(2), 6–9.

Geden, E. (1989). The relationship between self-care theory and empirical research. In J. Riehl-Sisca (Ed.), *Conceptual models for nursing practice* (3rd ed.). Norwalk, CT: Appleton & Lange.

Geden, E.A., Isaramalai, S.A., and Taylor, S.G. (2001). Self-care deficit nursing theory and the nurse practitioner's practice in primary care settings. *Nursing Science Quarterly*, 14(1), 29–33.

Glaven, K.A., Haynes, N., Jones, D.R., et al. (1998). A military application of a medical self-care program. *Military Medicine*, 163(10), 678–681.

Good, M. (1995). A comparison of the effects of jaw relaxation and music on postoperative pain. *Nursing Research*, 44(1), 51–57.

Good, M. (1996). Effects of relaxation and music on postoperative pain: A review. *Journal of Advanced Nursing*, 24(5), 905–914.

Gormley, K.J. (1997). Practice write-ups: An assessment instrument that contributes to bridging the differences between theory and practice for student nurses through the development of core skills. *Nursing Education Today*, 17(1), 53–57.

Grant, M. and Hezekiah, J. (1996). Knowledge and beliefs about hypertension among Jamaican female clients. *International Journal of Nursing Studies*, 33(1), 58–66.

Greenfield, E. and Pace, J. (1985). Orem's self-care theory of nursing: Practical application to the end stage renal disease (ESRD) patient. *Journal of Nephrology Nursing*, 2(4), 187–193.

Griffiths, P. (1998). An investigation into the description of patients' problems by nurses using two different needs-based nursing models. *Journal of Advanced Nursing*, 28(5), 969–977.

Gulick, E.E. (2001). Emotional distress and activities of daily living functions in persons with multiple sclerosis. *Nursing Research*, 50(3), 147–154.

Haas, D.L. (1990). Application of Orem's Self-Care Deficit Theory to the pediatric chronically ill population. *Issues in Comprehensive Pediatric Nursing*, 13(4), 253–264.

Hagopian, G.A. (1996). The effects of informational audiotapes on knowledge and self-care behaviors of patients undergoing radiation therapy. *Oncology Nursing Forum*, 23(4), 697–700.

Halfens, R.J.G., van Alphen, A., Hasman, A., et al. (1999). The effect of item observability, clarity and wording on patient/nurse ratings when using the ASA scale. *Scandinavian Journal of Caring Sciences*, 13(3), 159–164.

Hanchett, E.S. (1990). Nursing models and community as client. *Nursing Science Quarterly*, 3(2), 67–72.

Hanson, B.R. and Bickel, L. (1985). Development and testing of the questionnaire on perception of self-care agency. In J. Riehl-Sisca (Ed.), *The science and art of self-care*. Norwalk, CT: Appleton-Century-Crofts.

Hanucharurnkui, S. and Vinya-nguag, P. (1991). Effects of promoting patients' participation in self-care on postoperative recovery and satisfaction with care. *Nursing Science Quarterly*, 4(1), 14–20.

Harris, J.K. (1980). Self-care is possible after delivery. *Nursing Clinics of North America*, 15(1), 191–194.

Harrison-Raines, K. (1993). Nursing and self-care theory applied to utilization review: Concepts and cases. *American Journal of Medical Quality*, 8(4), 197–199.

Hart, M.A. (1995). Orem's self-care deficit theory: Research with pregnant women. *Nursing Science Quarterly*, 8(3), 120–126.

Hartley, L. (1988). Congruence between teaching and learning self care: A pilot study. *Nursing Science Quarterly*, 1(4), 161–167.

Hart, M.A. and Foster, S.N. (1998). Self-care agency in two groups of pregnant women. *Nursing Science Quarterly*, 11(4), 167–171.

Hartweg, D.L. (1993). Self-care actions of healthy middle-aged women to promote well-being. *Nursing Research*, 42(4), 221–227.

Hashemi, F., Dolatabad, F.R., Yektatalab, S., Ayaz, M., Zare, N., and Mansouri, P. (2014). Effect of Orem self-care program on the life quality of burn patients referred to Ghotb-al-Din-e-Shirazi Burn Center, Shiraz, Iran: A randomized controlled trial. *International Journal of Community Based Nursing and Midwifery*, 2(1), 40–50.

Hecker, E.J. (2000). Feria de Salud: Implementation and evaluation of a communitywide health fair. *Public Health Nursing*, 17(4), 247–256.

Henderson, V. (1991). *The nature of nursing* (2nd ed.). New York: Harry N. Abrams.

Herber, O.R., Schnepp, W., and Rieger, M.A. (2008). Developing a nurse-led education program to enhance self-care agency in leg ulcer patients. *Nursing Science Quarterly*, 21(2), 150–155.

Higgins, P.A. and Moore, S.M. (2000). Levels of theoretical thinking in nursing. *Nursing Outlook*, 48(4), 179–183.

Hildebrandt, E. and Robertson, B. (1995). Self-care of older black adults in a South African community. *N&HC Perspectives on Community*, 16(3), 136–143.

Hines, S.H., Sampselle, C.M., Ronis, D.L., Yeo, S., et al. (2007). Women's self-care agency to manage urinary incontinence: The impact of nursing agency and body experience. *Advances in Nursing Science*, 30(2), 175–188.

Hintze, A. (2011). Orem-based nursing education in Germany. *Nursing Science Quarterly*, 24(1), 66–70.

Hiromoto, B.M. and Dungan, J. (1991). Contract learning for self-care activities. A protocol study among chemotherapy outpatients. *Cancer Nursing*, 14(3), 148–154.

Hisama, K.K. (2001). The acceptance of nursing theory in Japan: A cultural perspective. *Nursing Science Quarterly*, 14(3), 255–259.

Holzemer, W.L. (1992). Linking primary health care and self-care through case management. *International Nursing Review*, 39(3), 83–89.

Horsburgh, M.E. (1999). Self-care of well adult Canadians and adult Canadians with end stage renal disease. *International Journal of Nursing Studies*, 36(6), 443–453.

Horsburgh, M.E., Beanlands, H., Locking-Cusolito, H., et al. (2000). Personality traits and self-care in adults awaiting renal transplant. *Western Journal of Nursing Research*, 22(4), 407–430.

Hoy, B., Wagner, L., and Hall, E.O.C. (2007). Self-care as a health source of elders: An integrative review of the concept. *Scandinavian Journal of Caring Science*, 21(4), 456–466.

Hsieh, C.H., Wang, C.Y., McCubbin, M., Zhang, S., and Inouye, J. (2008). Factors influencing osteoporosis preventive behaviours: Testing a path model. *Journal of Advanced Nursing*, 62(3), 336–345.

Huch, M.H. (1999). Welcome and introduction. *Nursing Science Quarterly*, 12(1), 80–83.

Hurlock-Chorostecki, C. (1999). Holistic care in the critical care setting: Application of a concept through Watson's and Orem's theories of nursing. *Official Journal of the Canadian Association of Critical Care Nurses*, 10(4), 20–25.

Huss, K., Salerno, M., and Huss, R.W. (1991). Computer-assisted reinforcement of instruction: Effects on adherence in adult atopic asthmatics. *Research in Nursing and Health*, 14(4) 259–267.

Jaarsma, T., Abu-Saad, H.H., Dracup, K., et al. (2000). Self-care behaviour of patients with heart failure. *Scandinavian Journal of Caring Sciences*, 14(2), 112–119.

Jaarsma, T., Halfens, R., Senten, M., Abu-Saad, H.H., and Dracup, K. (1998). Developing a supportive-educative program for patients with advanced heart failure within Orem's general theory of nursing. *Nursing Science Quarterly*, 11(2), 79–85.

Jacobs, C.J. (1990). Orem's self-care model: Is it relevant to patients in intensive care? *Intensive Care Nursing*, 6(2), 100–103.

Jenny, J. (1991). Self-care deficit theory and nursing diagnosis: A test of conceptual fit. *Journal of Nursing Education*, 30(5), 227–232.

Jirovec, M.M. and Kasno, J. (1990). Self-care agency as a function of patient-environmental factors among nursing home residents. *Research in Nursing and Health*, 13(5), 303–309.

Johnston, R.L. (1983). Orem self-care model of nursing. In J.J. Fitzpatrick and A.L. Whall (Eds.), *Conceptual models of nursing: Analysis and application*. Bowie, MD: Robert J. Brady Co.

Johnston, R.L. (1989). Orem's self care model of nursing. In J.J. Fitzpatrick and A.L. Whall (Eds.), *Conceptual models of nursing: Analysis and application* (2nd ed.). Norwalk, CT: Appleton & Lange.

Jopp, M., Carroll, M.C., and Waters, L. (1993). Using self-care theory to guide nursing management of the older adult after hospitalization. *Rehabilitation Nursing*, 18(2), 91–94.

Joseph, L.S. (1980). Self-care and the nursing process. *Nursing Clinics of North America*, 15(1), 131–143.

†Karl, C.A. (1982). The effect of an exercise program on self-care activities for the institutionalized elderly. *Journal of Gerontological Nursing*, 8, 282–285.

Kaul, V., Khurana, S., and Munoz, S. (2000). Management of medication noncompliance in solid-organ transplant recipients. *BioDrugs*, 13(5), 313–326.

Kearney, B.Y. and Fleischer, B.J. (1979). Development of an instrument to measure exercise of self-care agency. *Research in Nursing and Health*, 2(1), 25–34.

Kim, H.S. (2000). An integrative framework for conceptualizing clients: A proposal for a nursing perspective in the new century. *Nursing Science Quarterly*, 13(1), 37–40.

King, C. (1980). The self-care, self-help concept. *Nurse Practitioner*, 5, 34–35.

Kinlein, M.L. (1977). *Independent nursing practice with clients*. Philadelphia, PA: J.B. Lippincott.

Kinlein, M.L. (1977). Self-care concept. *American Journal of Nursing*, 77, 598–601.

Kinlein, M.L. (1978). Point of view on the front: Nursing and family and community health. *Family and Community Health*, 1, 57–68.

Kline, K.S., Scott, L.D., and Britton, A.S. (2007). The use of supportive-educative and mutual goal-setting strategies to improve self-management for patients with heart failure. *Home Holistic Nurse*, 25(8), 502–510.

Krishnasamy, M. (1996). Social support and the patient with cancer: A consideration of the literature. *Journal of Advanced Nursing*, 23(4), 757–762.

Kubricht, D. (1984). Therapeutic self-care demands expressed by outpatients receiving external radiation therapy. *Cancer Nursing*, 7, 43–52.

Kulig, J.C. (2000). Community resiliency: The potential for community health nursing theory development. *Public Health Nursing*, 17(5), 374–385.

Kumar, C.P. (2007). Application of Orem's self-care deficit theory and standardized nursing languages in a case study of a woman with diabetes. *International Journal of Nursing Terminologies and Classifications*, 18(3), 103–110.

Kuriansky, J., Gurland, B., Fleiss, J., and Cowan, D. (1976). The assessment of self-care capacity in geriatric psychiatric patients by objective and subjective methods. *Journal of Clinical Psychology*, 32, 95–102.

Landau, J., Cole, R.E., Tuttle, J., et al. (2000). Family connectedness and women's sexual risk behaviors: Implications for the prevention/intervention of STD/HIV infection. *Family Process*, 39(4), 461–475.

Lane, D.E. (1981). Self-medication of psychiatric patients. *Journal of Psychiatric Nursing and Mental Health Services*, 19, 27–28.

Langland, R.M. and Farrah, S.J. (1990). Using a self-care framework for continuing education in gerontological nursing. *Journal of Continuing Education in Nursing*, 21(6), 267–270.

Lanigan, T.L. (2000). The patient-family learning centre. *Canadian Nurse*, 96(3), 18–21.

Larrabee, J.H., Bolden, L.V., and Knight, M.R. (1998). The lived experience of patient prudence in health care. *Journal of Advanced Nursing*, 28(4), 802–808.

Laschinger, H.K. and Duff, V. (1991). Attitudes of practicing nurses towards theory-based nursing practice. *Canadian Journal of Nursing Administration*, 4(1), 6–10.

Lauder, W. (1999). A survey of self-neglect in patients living in the community. *Journal of Clinical Nursing*, 8(1), 95–102.

Lauder, W. (2001). The utility of self-care theory as a theoretical basis for self-neglect. *Journal of Advanced Nursing*, 34(4), 545–551.

Lauder, W., Kroll, T., and Jones M. (2007). Social determinants of mental health: The missing dimensions of mental health nursing? *Journal of Psychiatric and Mental Health Nursing*, 14(7), 661–669.

Laurent, C.L. (2000). A nursing theory for nursing leadership. *Journal of Nursing Management*, 8(2), 83–87.

Lee, M.B. (1999). Power, self-care and health in women living in urban squatter settlements in Karachi, Pakistan: A test of Orem's theory. *Journal of Advanced Nursing*, 30(1), 248–259.

Lee, P. (1998). An analysis and evaluation of Casey's conceptual framework. *International Journal of Nursing Studies*, 35(4), 204–209.

Leenerts, M.H., Teel, C.S., and Pendleton, M.K. (2002). Building a model of self-care for health promotion in aging. *Journal of Nursing Scholarship*, 34(4), 355–361.

Levin, L.S. (1976). *Self-care: Lay initiatives in health*. New York: Neale Watson Academic Publications.

Levin, L.S. (1977). Forces and issues in the revival of interest in self-care: Impetus for redirection for health. *Health Education Monographs*, 5, 115–120.

Levin, L.S. (1978). Patient education and self-care: How do they differ? *Nursing Outlook*, 26(3), 170–175.

Ljungberg, C., Hanson, E., and Lovgren, M. (2001). A home rehabilitation program for stroke patients—A pilot study. *Scandinavian Journal of Caring Sciences*, 15(1), 44–53.

Logue, G.A. (1997). An application of Orem's theory to the nursing management of pertussis. *Journal of School Nursing*, 13(4), 20–25.

Lorensen, M., Holter, I., Evers, G., Isenberg, M.A., and Van Achterberg, T. (1991). Cross-cultural testing of the appraisal of self-care agency scale. *International Journal of Nursing Studies*, 30(1), 15–23.

Lukkarinen, H. and Hentinen, M. (1997). Self-care agency and factors related to this agency among patients with coronary heart disease. *International Journal of Nursing Studies*, 34(4), 295–304.

Lundgren, A. and Wahren, L.K. (1999). Effect of education on evidence-based care and handling of peripheral intravenous lines. *Journal of Clinical Nursing*, 8(5), 577–585.

Lundh, U., Soder, M., and Waerness, K. (1987). Nursing theories: A critical review. *Image: Journal of Nursing Scholarship*, 20(1), 36–40.

Lyte, G. and Jones, K. (2001). Developing a unified language for children's nurses, children and their families in the United Kingdom. *Journal of Clinical Nursing*, 10(1), 79–85.

Malinski, V.M. (2008). Update on research framed in Orem's model. *Nursing Science Quarterly*, 21(3), 199–200.

Marland, G.R. (1999). Atypical neuroleptics: Autonomy and compliance? *Journal of Advanced Nursing*, 29(3), 615–622.

Maunz, E.R. and Woods, N.F. (1988). Self-care practices among young adult women: Influence of symptoms, employment, and sex-role orientation. *Health Care for Women International*, 9, 29–41.

McBride, S. (1987). Validation of an instrument to measure exercise of self-care agency. *Research in Nursing and Health*, 10, 311–316.

McBride, S.H. (1991). Comparative analysis of three instruments designed to measure self-care agency. *Nursing Research*, 40(1), 12–16.

McCaleb, A. and Edgil, A. (1994). Self-concept and self-care practices of healthy adolescents. *Journal of Pediatric Nursing*, 9(4), 233–238.

McCaughan, E.M. and Thompson, K.A. (2000). Information needs of cancer patients receiving chemotherapy at

a day-case unit in Northern Ireland. *Journal of Clinical Nursing*, 9, 851–858.

McDermott, M.A. (1993). Learned helplessness as an interacting variable with self-care agency: Testing a theoretical model. *Nursing Science Quarterly*, 6(1), 28–38.

McFarlane, E.A. (1980). Nursing theory: The comparison of four theoretical proposals. *Journal of Advanced Nursing*, 5, 3–9.

McGillivray, T. and Marland, G.R. (1999). Assisting demented patients with feeding: Problems in a ward environment. A review of the literature. *Journal of Advanced Nursing*, 29(3), 608–614.

McGraw, E., Barthel, H., and Arrington, M. (2000). A model for demand management in a managed care environment. *Military Medicine*, 165(4), 305–308.

McIntyre, K. (1980). The Perry model as a framework for self-care. *Nurse Practitioner*, 5(6), 34–37.

McLaughlin, C. (1997). The effect of classroom theory and contact with patients on the attitudes of student nurses towards mentally ill people. *Journal of Advanced Nursing*, 26(6), 1221–1228.

McLaughlin, K. (1993). Implementing self-care deficit nursing theory: A process of staff development. In M.E. Parker (Ed.), *Patterns of nursing theories in practice* (pp. 241–251). New York: National League for Nursing.

McQuiston, C.M. and Campbell, J.C. (1997). Theoretical substruction: A guide for theory testing research. *Nursing Science Quarterly*, 10(3), 117–123.

Melnyk, K.A.M. (1983). The process of theory analysis: An examination of the nursing theory of Dorothea E. Orem. *Nursing Research*, 32(3), 170–174.

Meriney, D.K. (1990). Application of Orem's conceptual framework to patients with hypercalcemia related to breast cancer. *Cancer Nursing*, 13(5), 316–323.

Michael, M.M. and Sewall, K.S. (1980). Use of the adolescent peer group to increase the self-care agency of adolescent alcohol abusers. *Nursing Clinics of North America*, 15, 157–176.

†Miller, J.F. (1980). The dynamic focus of nursing: A challenge to nursing administration. *Journal of Nursing Administration*, 10(1), 13–18.

†Miller, J.F. (1982). Categories of self-care needs of ambulatory patients with diabetes. *Journal of Advanced Nursing*, 7, 25–31.

Millio, N. (1977). Self-care in urban settings. *Health Education Monographs*, 5, 136–144.

Mitchell, G.J. (2001). Prescription, freedom, and participation: Drilling down into theory-based nursing practice. *Nursing Science Quarterly*, 14(3), 205–210.

Moore, J.B. (1987). Effects of assertion training and first aid instruction on children's autonomy and self-care agency. *Research in Nursing and Health*, 10, 101–109.

Moore, J.B. (1993). Predictors of children's self-care performance: Testing the theory of self-care deficit. *Scholarly Inquiry for Nursing Practice*, 7(3), 199–212.

Moore, J.B. (1995). Measuring self-care practice of children and adolescents: Instrument development. *Maternal-Child Nursing Journal*, 23(3), 101–108.

Moore, J.B. and Beckwitt, A.E. (2006). Self-care operations and nursing interventions for children with cancer and their parents. *Nursing Science Quarterly*, 19(2), 147–156.

Moore, J.B. and Pichler, V.H. (2000). Measurements of Orem's basic conditioning factors: A review of published research. *Nursing Science Quarterly*, 13(2), 137–142.

Morales-Mann, E.T. and Jiang, S.L. (1993). Applicability of Orem's conceptual framework: A cross cultural point of view. *Journal of Advanced Nursing*, 18(5), 737–741.

Morgan, S.A. and Dearduff, A. (1997). The cold clinic: A collaborative nursing effort to benefit students. *Journal of American College Health*, 46(1), 35–37.

Morse, W. and Werner, J. (1988). Individualization of patient care using Orem's theory. *Cancer Nursing*, 11(3), 195–202.

Moser, A., van der Bruggen, H., Widdershoven, G., and Spreeuwenberg, C. (2008). Self-management of type 2 diabetes mellitus: A qualitative investigation from the perspective of participants in a nurse-led, shared-care program in the Netherlands. *BMC Public Health*. 2008; 8(91).

Mosher, R.B. and Moore, J.B. (1998). The relationship of self-concept and self-care in children with cancer. *Nursing Science Quarterly*, 11(3), 116–122.

Mullin, V.I. (1980). Implementing the self-care concept in the acute care setting. *Nursing Clinics of North America*, 15(1), 177–190.

†Murphy, P.P. (1981). The hospice model and self-care theory. *Oncology Nursing Forum*, 8(2), 19–21.

Neal, J.E. (2001). Patient outcomes: A matter of perspective. *Nursing Outlook*, 49(2), 93–99.

Newell-Withrow, C. (2000). Health protecting and health promoting behaviors of African Americans living in Appalachia. *Public Health Nursing*, 17(5), 392–397.

Nilsson, U.B. and Willman, A. (2000). Evaluation of nursing documentation—A comparative study using the instruments NoGA(c) and Cat-ch-ing(c) after an educational intervention. *Scandinavian Journal of Caring Sciences*, 14(3), 199–206.

Noone, J. (1995). Acute pancreatitis: An Orem approach to nursing assessment and care. *Critical Care Nurse*, 15(4), 27–35.

Norris, C.M. (1979). Self-care. *American Journal of Nursing*, 79(3), 486–489.

Norris, M.K. (1991). Applying Orem's theory to the long-term care of adolescent transplant recipients. *American Nephrology Nurses Association Journal*, 18(1), 45–47, 53.

Nowakowski, L. (1980). Health promotion/self-care programs for the community. *Topics in Clinical Nursing*, 2, 21–27.

Nowicki, J.S. (1996). Health behaviors and the great depression. *Geriatric Nursing*, 17(5), 247–250.

Nursing Development Conference Group. (1973). *Concept formalization in nursing: Process and product*. Boston, MA: Little, Brown.

Nursing Development Conference Group. (1979). *Concept formalization in nursing: Process and product* (2nd ed.). Boston, MA: Little, Brown.

Oberle, K. and Allen, M. (2001). The nature of advanced practice nursing. *Nursing Outlook*, 49(3), 148–153.

Orem, D.E. (1959). *Guides for developing curriculae for the education of practical nurses*. Washington, DC: U.S. Department of Health, Education, and Welfare, Office of Education.

Orem, D.E. (1971). *Nursing: Concepts of practice*. New York: McGraw-Hill.

Orem, D.E. (1980). *Nursing: Concepts of practice* (2nd ed.). New York: McGraw-Hill.

Orem, D.E. (1983). The self-care deficit theory of nursing: A general theory. In I.W. Clements and F.B. Roberts (Eds.), *Family health: A theoretical approach to nursing care* (pp. 205–217). New York: John Wiley & Sons.

Orem, D.E. (1985). *Nursing: Concepts of practice* (3rd ed.). New York: McGraw-Hill.

Orem, D.E. (1987). Orem's general theory of nursing. In R.R. Parse (Ed.), *Nursing science: Major paradigms, theories, and critiques*. Philadelphia, PA: W.B. Saunders.

Orem, D.E. (1988). The form of nursing science. *Nursing Science Quarterly*, 1(2), 75–79.

Orem, D.E. (1989). Theories and hypotheses for nursing administration. In B. Henry, M. Di Vincenti, C. Arndt, and A. Marriner (Eds.), *Dimensions of nursing administration. Theory, research, education, and practice*. Boston, MA: Blackwell Scientific Publications.

Orem, D.E. (1991). *Nursing: Concepts of practice* (4th ed.). St. Louis, MO: C.V. Mosby.

Orem, D.E. (1995). *Nursing: Concepts of practice* (5th ed.). St. Louis, MO: C.V. Mosby.

Orem, D.E. (1997). Views of human beings specific to nursing. *Nursing Science Quarterly*, 10(1), 26–31.

Orem, D.E. (2001). *Nursing concepts of practice* (6th ed.). St. Louis, MO: C.V. Mosby.

Orem, D.E. (2001). Response to: Lauder, W. (2001). Comment: The utility of self-care theory as a theoretical basis for self-neglect. *Journal of Advanced Nursing*, 34(4), 545–551, 552–553.

Orem, D.E. (2001). The utility of self-care theory as a theoretical basis for self-neglect. Response. *Journal of Advanced Nursing*, 34(4), 552–553.

Orem, D.E. (2004). Reflections on nursing practice science: Then nature, the structure and the foundation of nursing sciences. *Self-Care, Dependent-Care, and Nursing*, 12(3), 4–11

Orem, D.E. and Taylor, S.G. (1986). Orem's general theory of nursing. In P. Winstead-Fry (Ed.), *Case studies in nursing theory*. New York: National League for Nursing.

Orem, D.E. and Taylor, S.G. (2011). Reflections on nursing practice science: The nature, the structure, and the foundation of nursing science. *Nursing Science Quarterly*, 24(1), 35–41.

Orem, D.E. and Vardiman, E.M. (1995). Orem's nursing theory and positive mental health: Practical considerations. *Nursing Science Quarterly*, 8(4), 165–173.

Pagels, A., Wang, M., and Wengstrom, Y. (2008). The impact of a nurse-led clinic on self-care ability, disease-specific knowledge, and home dialysis modality. *Nephrology Nursing Journal*, 35(3), 242–248.

Parse, R.R. (2000). Paradigms: A reprise. *Nursing Science Quarterly*, 13(4), 275–276.

Patton, J.G., Conrad, M.A., and Kreidler, M.C. (1995). Interdisciplinary faculty and student practice in a nurse-managed campus wellness program. *Nursing Connections*, 8(1), 27–35.

Payne, S., Hardey, M., and Coleman, P. (2000). Interactions between nurses during handovers in elderly care. *Journal of Advanced Nursing*, 32(2), 277–285.

Pearson, A. (2008). Dead poets, nursing theorists and contemporary nursing practice. *International Journal of Nursing Practice*, 14(1), 1–2.

Peltzer, J. and Leenerts, M.H. (2007). Spirituality as a component of holistic self-care practices in human immunodeficiency virus – positive women with histories of abuse. *Holistic Nursing Practice*, 21(3), 105–112.

Perrson, K., Svensson, P.G., and Ek, A.C. (1997). Breast self-examination: An analysis of self-reported practice. *Journal of Advanced Nursing*, 25(5), 886–892.

†Petrlik, J.C. (1976). Diabetic peripheral neuropathy. *American Journal of Nursing*, 76, 1794–1797.

Phillips, K.D. and Morris, J.H. (1998). Nursing management of anxiety in HIV infection. *Issues in Mental Health Nursing*, 19(4), 375–397.

Pickens, J.M. (1999). Living with serious mental illness: The desire for normalcy. *Nursing Science Quarterly*, 12(3), 233–239.

†Porter, D. and Shamian, J. (1983). Self-care in theory and practice. *Canadian Nurse*, 79(8), 21–23.

Priest, H.M. (1999). Psychological care in nursing education and practice: A search for definition and dimensions. *Nursing Education Today*, 19(1), 71–78.

Proot, I.M., Abu-Saad, H.H., de Esch-Janssen, W.P., et al. (2000). Patient autonomy during rehabilitation: The experiences of stroke patients in nursing homes. *International Journal of Nursing Studies*, 37(3), 267–276.

Rabie, T., Klopper, H.C., and Watson, M.J. (2015). *Effect of socio-economic status on self-care of the older person in the Potchefstroom district, South Africa*. Health SA Gesondheid. doi: 10.1016/j.hsag.2015.02.007.

Ramfelt, E., Langius, A., Bjorvell, H., et al. (2000). Treatment decision-making and its relation to the sense of coherence and the meaning of the disease in a group of patients with colorectal cancer. *European Journal of Cancer Care*, 9(3), 158–165.

Randell, B.P. (1992). Nursing theory: The 21st century. *Nursing Science Quarterly*, 5(4), 176–184.

Ranjani, S. (2013). Compare and contrast of Roy and Orem's nursing theory. *International Journal of Innovative Research and Development*, 2(8), 237–240.

Raven, M. (1988–1989). Application of Orem's self-care model to nursing practice in developmental disability. *Australian Journal of Advanced Nursing*, 6(2), 16–23.

Rawnsley, M.M. (1997). A case for theory triangulation—Response. *Nursing Science Quarterly*, 10(2), 103–106.

Reed, P.G. (1995). A treatise on nursing knowledge development for the 21st century—Beyond postmodernism. *Advances in Nursing Science*, 17(3), 70–84.

Rehwaldt, M., Wickham, R., Purl, S., Tariman, J., et al. (2009). Self-care strategies to cope with taste changes after chemotherapy. *Oncology Nursing Forum*, 36(2), E47–E56.

Reid, B., Allen, A.F., Gauthier, T., and Campbell, H. (1989). Solving the Orem mystery: An educational strategy. *Journal of Continuing Education in Nursing*, 20(3), 108–110.

Renpenning, K.M., SozWiss, G.B., Denyes, M.J., Orem, D.E., and Taylor, S.G. (2011). Exlication of the nature and meaning of nursing diagnosis. *Nursing Science Quarterly*, 24(2), 130–136.

Rew, L. (2003). A theory of taking care of oneself grounded in experiences of homeless youth. *Nursing Research*, 52(4), 234–241.

Richardson, A. (1992). Studies exploring self-care for the person coping with cancer treatment: A review. *International Journal of Nursing Studies*, 29(2), 191–204.

Richardson, A. and Ream, E.K. (1997). Self-care behaviours initiated by chemotherapy patients in response to fatigue. *International Journal of Nursing Studies*, 34(1), 35–43.

Ricka, R., Vanrenterghem, Y., and Evers, G.C.M. (2002). Adequate self-care of dialysed patients: A review of the literature. *International Journal of Nursing Studies*, 39(3), 329–339.

Riegel, B. and Dickson, V.V. (2008). A situation-specific theory of heart failure self-care. *Journal of Cardiovascular Nursing*, 23(3), 190–196.

Riehl-Sisca, J. (1989). Orem's general theory of nursing: An interpretation. In J. Riehl-Sisca (Ed.), *Conceptual models for nursing practice* (3rd ed.). Norwalk, CT: Appleton & Lange.

Riehl-Sisca, J.P. (1989). *Conceptual models for nursing practice* (3rd ed.). East Norwalk, CT: Appleton & Lange.

Roberts, C.S. (1982). Identifying the real patient problems. *Nursing Clinics of North America*, 17(3), 481–489.

Roldan-Merino, J., Lluch-Canut, T., Menarguez-Alcaina, M., Foix-Sanjuan, A., Abad, J.M., and QuestERA Working Group. (2012). Psychometric evaluation of a new instrument in Spanish to measure self-care requisites in patients with schizophrenia. *Perspectives in Psychiatric Care*, 50(2), 93–101.

Roldan-Merino, J., Miguel-Ruiz, D., Lluch-Canut, M.T., Puig-Llobet, M., Feria-Raposo, I., and QuestERA Working Group. (2015, August 13). Psychometric properties of self-care requisites scale (SCRS-h) in hospitalized patients diagnosed with schizophrenia. *Perspectives in Psychiatric Care*. doi: 10.1111/ppc.12133.

Romine, S. (1986). Applying Orem's self-care to staff development. *Journal of Nursing Staff Development*, 2(2), 77–79.

Rosenbaum, J.N. (1986). Comparison of two theorists on care: Orem and Leininger. *Journal of Advanced Nursing*, 11, 409–419.

Ross, M.M., Carswell, A., Hing, M., et al. (2001). Seniors' decision making about pain management. *Journal of Advanced Nursing*, 35(3), 442–451.

Rothlis, J. (1984). The effect of a self-help group on feelings of hopelessness and helplessness. *Western Journal of Nursing Research*, 6, 157–173.

Roy, C. (1980). A case study viewed according to different models. In J.P. Riehl and C. Roy (Eds.), *Conceptual models for nursing practice* (2nd ed.). New York: Appleton-Century-Crofts.

Roy, C. (1995). Developing nursing knowledge—Practice issues raised from four philosophical perspectives. *Nursing Science Quarterly*, 8(2), 79–85.

Ruland, C.M. (1999). Decision support for patient preference-based care planning: Effects on nursing care and patient outcomes. *Journal of the American Medical Informatics Association*, 6(4), 304–312.

Russell, C.K., Bunting, S.M., and Gregory, D.M. (1997). Protective care-receiving: The active role of care-recipients. *Journal of Advanced Nursing*, 25(3), 532–540.

Sandman, P.O., Norberg, A., Adolfsson, R., Axelsson, K., and Hedly, V. (1986). Morning care of patients with Alzheimer-type dementia. A theoretical model based on direct observations. *Journal of Advanced Nursing*, 11, 369–378.

Sanford, R.C. (2000). Caring through relation and dialogue: A nursing perspective for patient education. *Advances in Nursing Science*, 22(3), 1–15.

Scammell, J. and Miller, S. (1999). Back to basics: Exploring the conceptual basis of nursing. *Nursing Education Today*, 19(7), 570–577.

Schottbaer, D., Fisher, L., and Gregory, C. (1995). Dependent care, caregiver burden, hardiness, and self-care agency of caregivers. *Cancer Nursing*, 18(4), 299–305.

Schreiber, R., MacDonald, M. (2010). Keeping vigil over the patient: A grounded theory of nurse anesthesia practice. *Journal of Advanced Nursing*, 66(3), 552–561.

Schuller, A. (1999). Aspects of autonomy-promoting elder care between individuals and organization. *Gruppendynamik*, 30(4), 353–363.

Schumacher, K.L. (1996). Reconceptualizing family caregiving: Family-based illness care during chemotherapy. *Research in Nursing and Health*, 19(4), 261–271.

Shah, M., Abdullah, A., and Khan, H. (2013). Compare and contrast of grand theories: Orem's self-care deficit theory and Roy's adaptation model. *International Journal of Science and Research*, 4(1), 1834–1837. Retrieved from www.ijsr.net

Shuldham, C., Theaker, C., Jaarsma, T., and Cowie, M.R. (2007). Evaluation of the European heart failure self-care behaviour scale in a United Kingdom population. *Journal of Advanced Nursing*, 60(1), 87–95.

Silva, M.C. (1986). Research testing nursing theory: State of the art. *Advances in Nursing Science*, 9(1), 1–11.

Silva, M.C., Sorrell, J.M., and Sorrell, C.D. (1995). From Carper patterns of knowing to ways of being—An ontological philosophical shift in nursing. *Advances in Nursing Science*, 18(1), 1–13.

Simmons, L. (2009). Dorthea Orem's self care theory as related to nursing practice in hemodialysis. *Nephrology Nursing Journal*, 36(4), 419–421.

Slusher, I.L. (1999). Self-care agency and self-care practice of adolescents. *Issues in Comprehensive Pediatric Nursing*, 22(1), 49–58.

†Smith, M.C. (1979). Proposed metaparadigm for nursing research and theory development: An analysis of Orem's self-care theory. *Image: Journal of Nursing Scholarship*, 11(3), 75–79.

Smith, M.C. (1987). A critique of Orem's theory. In R.R. Parse (Ed.), *Nursing science: Major paradigms, theories, and critiques*. Philadelphia, PA: W.B. Saunders.

Soderhamn, O. (1998). Self-care ability in a group of elderly Swedish people: A phenomenological study. *Journal of Advanced Nursing*, 28(4), 745–753.

Söderhamn, O. and Cliffordson, C. (2001). The structure of self-care in a group of elderly people. *Nursing Science Quarterly*, 14(1), 55–58.

Soderhamn, O., Evers, G., and Hamrin, E. (1996). A Swedish version of the Appraisal of Self-Care Agency (ASA) scale. *Scandinavian Journal of Caring Sciences*, 10(1), 3–9.

Soderhamn, O., Lindencrona, C., and Ek, A.C. (2000). Ability for self-care among home dwelling elderly people in a health district in Sweden. *International Journal of Nursing Studies*, 37(4), 361–368.

Söderhamn, U., Bachrach-Lindström, M., and Ek, A-C. (2008). Self-care ability and sense of coherence in older nutritional at-risk patients. *European Journal of Clinical Nutrition*, 62, 96–103.

Sousa, V.D., Zauszniewski, J.A., Zeller, R.A., and Neese, J.B. (2008). Factor analysis of the appraisal of self-care agency scale in American adults with diabetes. *The Diabetes Educator*, 34(1), 98–108.

Spearman, S.A., Duldt, B.W., and Brown, S. (1993). Research testing theory: A selective review of Orem's self-care theory, 1986–1991. *Journal of Advanced Nursing*, 18(10), 1626–1631.

Storm, D. and Baumgartner, R. (1987). Achieving self care in the ventilator-dependent patient: A critical analysis of a case study. *International Journal of Nursing Studies*, 24(2), 95–106.

†Sullivan, T.J. (1980). Self-care model for nursing. In *New directions for nursing in the '80s*. Kansas City, MO: American Nurses Association.

Taylor, S.G. (1988). Nursing theory and nursing process: Orem's theory in practice. *Nursing Science Quarterly*, 1(3), 111–119.

Taylor, S.G. (1990). Practical applications of Orem's theory of self-care deficit nursing theory. In M.E. Parker (Ed.), *Nursing theories in practice* (pp. 61–70). New York: National League for Nursing.

Taylor, S.G. (1991). The structure of nursing diagnosis from Orem's theory. *Nursing Science Quarterly*, 4(1), 24–32.

Taylor, S.G. (2001). A theory of dependent-care: A corollary theory to Orem's theory of self-care. *Nursing Science Quarterly*, 14(1), 39–47.

Taylor, S.G. (2001). Orem's general theory of nursing and families. *Nursing Science Quarterly*, 14(1), 7–9.

Taylor, S.G., Geden, E., Isaramalai, S., et al. (2000). Orem's self-car deficit nursing theory: Its philosophic foundation and the state of the science. *Nursing Science Quarterly*, 13(2), 104–110.

Taylor, S.G. and Godfrey, N.S. (1999). The ethics of Orem's theory. *Nursing Science Quarterly*, 12(3), 202–207.

Taylor, S.G. and McLaughlin, K. (1991). Orem's general theory of nursing and community nursing. *Nursing Science Quarterly*, 4(4), 153–160.

Taylor, S.G. and Renpenning, K.M. (2001). The practice of nursing in multiperson situations, family and community. In D. Orem (Ed.), *Nursing: Concepts of practice* (pp. 394–433). St. Louis, MO: C.V. Mosby.

Taylor, S.G., Renpenning, K.E., Geden, E.A., et al. (2001). A theory of dependent-care: A corollary theory to Orem's theory of self-care. *Nursing Science Quarterly*, 14(1), 39–47.

Timmins, F. (2008). A critical review of appropriate conceptual models for use by coronary care nurses. *International Nursing Review*, 55(1), 117–124.

Timmins, F. and Horan, P. (2007). A critical analysis of the potential contribution of Orem's (2001) self-care deficit nursing theory to contemporary coronary care nursing practice. *European Journal of Cardiovascular Nursing*, 6(1), 32–39.

Titus, S. and Porter, P. (1989). Orem's theory applied to pediatric residential treatment. *Pediatric Nursing*, 15(5), 465–468.

Tokem, Y., Akyol, A.D., and Argon, G. (2007). The relationship between disability and self-care agency of Turkish people with rheumatoid arthritis. *Journal of Clinical Nursing*, 16(3a), 44–50.

Toth, J.C. (1980). Effect of structured preparation for transfer on patient anxiety on leaving coronary care unit. *Nursing Research*, 29(1), 28–34.

Tsai, Y.F. (2007). Self-care management and risk factors for depressive symptoms among Taiwanese institutionalized older persons. *Nursing Research*, 56(2), 124–131.

Tsai, Y-F., Wong, T.K.S., and Ku, Y-C. (2008). Self-care management of sleep disturbances and risk factors for poor sleep among older residents of Taiwanese nursing homes. *Journal of Clinical Nursing*, 17, 1219–1226.

Ulbrich, S.L. (1999). Nursing practice theory of exercise as self-care. *Image: Journal of Nursing Scholarship*, 31(1), 65–70.

Underwood, P.R. (1980). Facilitating self-care. In P. Pothier (Ed.), *Psychiatric nursing* (pp. 115–144). Boston, MA: Little, Brown.

Urbancic, J.C. (1992). Empowerment support with female survivors of childhood incest: Part I—Theories and research. *Archives of Psychiatric Nursing*, 6(5), 275–281.

Urbancic, J.C. (1992). Empowerment support with adult female survivors of childhood incest: Part II—Application of Orem's methods of helping. *Archives of Psychiatric Nursing*, 6(5), 282–286.

Utz, S.W. and Ramos, M.C. (1993). Mitral valve prolapse and its effects: A programme of inquiry within Orem's Self-Care Deficit Theory of Nursing. *Journal of Advanced Nursing*, 18(5), 742–751.

Utz, S.W., Shuster, G.F., 3rd, Merwin, E., and Williams, B. (1994). A community-based smoking-cessation program: Self-care behaviors and success. *Public Health Nursing*, 11(5), 291–299.

Uys, L. (1987). Foundational studies in nursing. *Journal of Advanced Nursing*, 12(3), 275–280.

Van Achterberg, T., Lorensen, M., Isenberg, M., Evers, G., Levin, E., and Philipsen, H. (1991). The Norwegian, Danish, and Dutch version of the appraisal of self-care agency scale: Comparing reliability aspects. *Scandinavian Journal of Caring Sciences*, 5(1), 1–8.

van der Scheuren, E., Kesteloot, K., and Cleemput, I. (2000). Federation of European Cancer Societies. Full Report. Economic evaluation in cancer care: Questions and answers on how to alleviate conflicts between rising needs and expectations and tightening budgets. *European Journal of Cancer*, 36(1), 13–36.

Vasquez, M.A. (1992). From theory to practice: Orem's self-care nursing model and ambulatory care. *Journal of Post Anesthesia Nursing*, 7(4), 251–255.

Villarruel, A.M. (1995). Mexican-American cultural meanings, expressions, self-care and dependent-care actions associated with experiences of pain. *Research in Nursing and Health*, 18(5), 427–436.

Villarruel, A.M., Bishop, T.L., Simpson, E.M., et al. (2001). Borrowed theories, shared theories, and the advancement of nursing knowledge. *Nursing Science Quarterly*, 14(2), 158–163.

Villarruel, A.M. and Denyes, M.J. (1991). Pain assessment in children: Theoretical and empirical validity. *Advances in Nursing Science*, 14(2), 32–41.

Villarruel, A.M. and Denyes, M.J. (1997). Testing Orem's theory with Mexican Americans. *Image: Journal of Nursing Scholarship*, 29(3), 283–288.

Walborn, K.A. (1980). A nursing model for hospice, primary and self-care. *Nursing Clinics of North America*, 15(1), 205–217.

Walker, D.M. (1993). A nursing administration perspective on use of Orem's Self-Care Deficit Nursing theory. In M.E. Parker (Ed.), *Patterns of nursing theories in practice* (pp. 252–263). New York: National League for Nursing.

Walker, L.O. and Grobe, S.J. (1999). The construct of thriving in pregnancy and postpartum. *Nursing Science Quarterly*, 12(2), 151–157.

Walker, L.O. and Sterling, B.S. (2006). The structure of thriving/distress among low-income women at 3 months after giving birth. *Family and Community Health*, 30(Suppl 1), S95–S103.

Wallace, W.A. (1996). *The modeling of nature: Philosophy of science and philosophy of nature in synthesis*. Washington, DC: The Catholic University of America Press.

Walton, J. (1985). An overview: Orem's self care deficit theory of nursing. *Focus Critical Care*, 12(1), 54–58.

Wang, C.Y. (1997). The cross-cultural applicability of Orem's conceptual framework. *Journal of Cultural Diversity*, 4(2), 44–48.

Wang, H.H. (2001). A comparison of two models of health-promoting lifestyle in rural elderly Taiwanese women. *Public Health Nursing*, 18(3), 204–211.

Wang, H.H. and Laffrey, S.C. (2001). A predictive model of well-being and self-care for rural elderly women in Taiwan. *Research in Nursing and Health*, 24(2), 122–132.

Watkins, G.R. (1995). Patient comprehension of gastroenterology (GI). Educational materials. *Gastroenterology Nursing*, 18(4), 123–127.

Weaver, M.T. (1987). Perceived self-care agency: A LISREL, factor analysis of Bickel and Hanson's questionnaire. *Nursing Research*, 36, 381–387.

Webb, M. (2001). Integration of nursing theorists in community care practice. *Vision*, 7(13), 27–28.

Weinrich, S.P. (1990). Predictors of older adults' participation in fecal occult blood screening. *Oncology Nursing Forum*, 17(5), 715–720.

Wengstrom, Y., Haggmark, C., Strander, H., et al. (1999). Effects of a nursing intervention on subjective distress, side effects and quality of life of breast cancer patients receiving curative radiation therapy—A randomized study. *Acta Oncologica*, 38(6), 763–770.

Werlin, S.H., Schauffler, H.H., and Avery, C.H. (1977). Research and demonstration issues in self-care: Measuring the decline of medicocentricism. *Health Education Monographs*, 5(2), 161–181.

West, P. and Isenberg, M. (1997). Instrument development: The mental health-related self-care agency scale. *Archives of Psychiatric Nursing*, 11(3), 126–132.

Westerbotn, M., Fahlström, J, Agüero-Torres, H., and Hilleras, P. (2008). How do older people experience their management of medicines? *Journal of Clinical Nursing*, 17(5a), 106–115.

Whelan, E. (1984). Analysis and application of Dorothea Orem's self-care practice model. *Journal of Nursing Education*, 24(6), 226–229.

Whitener, L.M., Cox, K.R., and Maglich, S.A. (1998). Use of theory to guide nurses in the design of health messages for children. *Advances in Nursing Science*, 20(3), 21–35.

Wilkinson, A. and Whitehead, L. (2009). Evolution of the concept of self–care and implications for nurses: A literature review. *International Journal of Nursing Studies*, 46, 1143–1147.

Williams, P.D., Ducey, K.A., Sears, A.M., et al. (2001). Treatment type and symptom severity among oncology patients by self-report. *International Journal of Nursing Studies*, 38(3), 359–367.

Williams, S. and Ramos, M.C. (1993). Mitral valve prolapse and its effects: A program of inquiry within Orem's self-care deficit theory of nursing. *Journal of Advanced Nursing*, 18, 242–251.

Williams, S., Shuster, G.F. III, Merwin, E., and Williams, B. (1994). A community-based smoking cessation program: Self-care behaviors and success. *Public Health Nursing*, 11(5), 291–299.

Wilson, F.L., Baker, L.M., and Nordstrom, C.K. (2008). Using the teach-back and Orem's self-care deficit nursing theory to increase childhood immunization communication among low-income mothers. *Issues in Comprehensive Pediatric Nursing*, 31, 7–22.

Wilson, F.L., Mood, D.W., Risk, J., and Kershaw, T. (2003). Evaluation of education materials using Orem's self-care deficit theory. *Nursing Science Quarterly*, 16(1), 68–76.

Womack, S. (1997). The elderly in nursing homes: A special population. *Nurse Practitioner Forum*, 8(1), 32–35.

Wong, C.L., Ip, W.Y. and Lam, L.W. (2015). Examining self-care behaviors and their associated factors among adolescent girls with dysmenorrhea: An application of Orem's self-care deficit nursing theory. *Journal of Nursing Scholarship*, 47(3), 219–227.

Woods, N. (1989). Conceptualizations of self-care: Toward health-oriented models. *Advances in Nursing Science*, 12(1), 1–13.

Wright, P.S., Piazza, D., Holcombe, J., and Foote, A. (1994). A comparison of three theories of nursing used as a guide for the nursing care of an 8–year-old child with leukemia. *Journal of Pediatric Oncology Nursing*, 11(1), 14–19.

Young, L. (1996). Spaces for famine: A comparative geographical analysis of famine in Ireland and the Highlands in the 1840s. *Transactions (Institute of British Geographers)*, 21(4), 666–680.

Zerull, L.M. (1999). Community nurse case management: Evolving over time to meet new demands. *Family and Community Health*, 22(3), 12–29.

29. Ida Orlando

Allen, D.E., Bockenhauer, B., Egan, C., and Kinnaird, L.S. (2006). Relating outcomes to excellent nursing practice. *Journal of Nursing Administration*, 36(3), 140–147.

Anderson, B.J., Mertz, H., and Leonard, R.C. (1965). Two experimental tests of a patient-centered admission process. *Nursing Research*, 14, 151–157.

Andrews, C.M. (1983). Ida Orlando's model of nursing. In J.J. Fitzpatrick and A.L. Whall (Eds.), *Conceptual models of nursing: Analysis and application*. Bowie, MD: Robert J. Brady Co.

Andrews, C.M. (1989). Ida Orlando's model of nursing practice. In J.J. Fitzpatrick and A.L. Whall (Eds.), *Conceptual models of nursing: Analysis and application* (2nd ed.). Norwalk, CT: Appleton & Lange.

Andrews, G.J. and Moon, G. (2005). Space, place, and the evidence base: Part II—rereading nursing environment through geographical research. *Worldviews on Evidence-Based Nursing*, 2(3), 142–156.

Arevian, M. (2005). The significance of a collaborative practice model in delivering care to chronically ill patients: A case study of managing diabetes mellitus in a primary health care center. *Journal of Interprofessional Care*, 19(5), 444–451.

Artinian, B.M. (1995). Risking involvement with cancer patients. *Western Journal of Nursing Research*, 17(3), 292–304.

Aseratie, M., Murugan, R., and Molla, M. (2014). Assessment of factors affecting implementation of nursing process among nurses in selected governmental hospitals, Adis Ababa, Ethiopia; Cross-sectional study. *Journal of Nursing Care*, 3(3), 1–8.

Barnard, K.E. (1980). Knowledge for practice: Directions for the future. *Nursing Research*, 29(4), 208.

Barnum, B.J.S. (1994). *Nursing theory: Analysis, application, and evaluation* (4th ed.). Philadelphia, PA: Lippincott.

Barnum, B.J.S. (1998). *Nursing theory: Analysis, application, evaluation* (5th ed.). Philadelphia, PA: Lippincott Williams & Wilkins.

Barron, M.A. (1966). The effects varied nursing approaches have on patients' complaints of pain [Abstract]. *Nursing Research*, 15(1), 90–91.

Bauer, M.S., McBride, L., Williford, W.O., Glick, H., Kinosian, B., Altshuler, L., et al. (2006). Collaborative care for bipolar disorder: Part I. Intervention and implementation in a randomized effectiveness trial. *Psychiatric Services*, 57(7), 927–936.

Benoliel, J.Q. (1995). Multiple meanings of pain and complexities of pain management. *Nursing Clinics of North America*, 30(4), 583–596.

Blomqvist, K. and Hallberg, I.R. (2001). Recognising pain in order adults living in sheltered accommodations: The views of nurses and older adults. *International Journal of Nursing Studies*, 38(3), 305–318.

Bochnak, M.A. (1963). The effect of an automatic and deliberative process of nursing activity on the relief of patients' pain: A clinical experiment. *Nursing Research*, 12, 191–192.

Burssen, B. and Diers, D.K. (1964). Pseudo-patient centered orientations. *Nursing Forum*, 3(2), 38–50.

Cameron, J. (1963). An exploratory study of the verbal responses of the nurse-patient interactions. *Nursing Research*, 12, 192.

Caris Verhallen, W.M.C.M., Kerkstra, A., and Bensing, J.M. (1997). The role of communication in nursing care for elderly people. A review of the literature. *Journal of Advanced Nursing*, 25(5), 915–933.

Cody, W.K. (1996). Drowning in eclecticism. *Nursing Science Quarterly*, 9(3), 86–88.

Crane, M.D. (1980). Ida Jean Orlando. In The Nursing Theories Conference Group (Eds.), *Nursing theories: The base for professional nursing practice*. Englewood Cliffs, NJ: Prentice-Hall.

Crigger, N.J. (1997). The trouble with caring: A review of eight arguments against an ethic of care. *Journal of Professional Nursing*, 13(4), 217–221.

Cutcliffe, J.R. and Goward, P. (2000). Mental health nurses and qualitative research methods: A mutual attraction? *Journal of Advanced Nursing*, 31(3), 590–598.

Diers, D. (1970). Faculty research development at Yale. *Nursing Research*, 19(1), 64–71.

Diers, D.K. (1966). The nurse orientation system: A method for analyzing the nurse-patient interactions [Abstract]. *Nursing Research*, 15(1), 91.

Dracup, K.A. and Breu, C.S. (1978). Using nursing research findings to meet the needs of grieving spouses. *Nursing Research*, 27(4), 212–216.

Dumas, R.G. (1963). Psychological preparation for surgery. *American Journal of Nursing*, 63(8), 52–55.

Dumas, R.G. and Leonard, R.C. (1963). The effect of nursing on the incidence of postoperative vomiting. *Nursing Research*, 12(1), 12–15.

Dune, L. (2006). Integrating tuina acupressure and traditional Chinese medicine concepts into a holistic nursing practice. *Explore: The Journal of Science and Healing*, 2(6), 543–546.

Dye, M.C. (1963). A descriptive study of conditions conductive to an effective process of nursing activity. *Nursing Research*, 12, 194.

Dye, M.C. (1963). Clarifying patients' communication. *American Journal of Nursing*, 63(8), 56–59.

Dye, M., Orlando, I.J., and Dumas, R.G. (1963). Validating a theory of nursing practice. *American Journal of Nursing*, 63(8), 52–59.

Eisler, J., Wolfer, J., and Diers, D. (1972). Relationship between the need for social approval and postoperative recovery and welfare. *Nursing Research*, 21(5), 520–525.

Elder, R.G. (1963). What is the patient saying? *Nursing Forum*, 2(1), 25–37.

Elms, R.R. and Leonard, R.C. (1966). Effects of nursing approaches during admission. *Nursing Research*, 15(1), 39–48.

England, M. (2005). Analysis of nurse conversation: Methodology of the process recording. *Journal of Psychiatric and Mental Health Nursing*, 12(6), 661–671.

Fagerberg, I. and Ekman, S.L. (1997). First-year Swedish nursing students' experiences with elderly patients. *Western Journal of Nursing Research*, 19(2), 177–189.

Fairman, J. (2008). Context and contingency in the history of post World War II nursing scholarship in the United States. *Journal of Nursing Scholarship*, 40(1), 4–11.

Faust, C. (2002). Clinical outlook. Orlando's Deliberative Nursing Process Theory: A practice application in an extended care facility. *Journal of Gerontological Nursing*, 28(7), 14–18.

Fawcett, J. (2005). Middle-range nursing theories are necessary for the advancement of the discipline. *Revista Aquichan*, 5(1), 32–43.

Forchuk, C. (1991). A comparison of the works of Peplau and Orlando. *Archives of Psychiatric Nursing*, 5(1), 38–45.

Forchuk, C. (1995). Uniqueness within the nurse-client relationship. *Archives of Psychiatric Nursing*, 9(1), 34–39.

Forchuk, C. and Dorsay, J.P. (1995). Hildegard-Peplau meets family systems nursing—Innovation in theory-based practice. *Journal of Advanced Nursing*, 21(1), 110–115.

Fitzpatrick, J. and Whall, A. (1983). *Conceptual models of nursing: Analysis and application.* Bowie, MD: Robert J. Brady Co.

Georges, J.M. (2005). Linking nursing theory and practice: A critical-feminist approach. *Advances in Nursing Science*, 28(1), 50–57.

Gilliss, S.L. (1976). Sleeplessness—Can you help? *Canadian Nurse*, 72(7), 32–34.

Gowan, N.I. and Morris, M. (1964). Nurses' responses to expressed patient needs. *Nursing Research*, 13, 68–71.

Graham, I. (1996). A presentation of a conceptual framework and its use in the definition of nursing development within a number of nursing development units. *Journal of Advanced Nursing*, 23(2), 260–266.

Griffiths, B. and Andrews, C.M. (2007). Nursing perspective. Putting nursing theory into practice. *Gastroenterology Nursing*, 30(6), 440–442.

Hage, J. (1972). *Techniques and problems of theory construction in sociology.* New York: John Wiley & Sons.

Haggerty, L.A. (1985). A theoretical model for developing students' communication skills. *Journal of Nursing Education*, 24(7), 296–298.

Haggerty, L.A. (1987). An analysis of senior nursing students' immediate response to distressed patients. *Journal of Advanced Nursing*, 12, 451–461.

Halloran, E.J. (1995). Guiding principles for nurse executives. *Journal of Nursing Administration*, 25(12), 5–6.

Hall-Lord, M. and Larsson, B.W. (2005). Experiences of pain, distress, and quality of care in relation to different perspectives. In K.V. Oxington (Ed.), *Psychology of stress* (pp. 207–254). New York: Nova Science Publishers, Inc.

Hampe, S.O. (1975). Needs of grieving spouses in a hospital setting. *Nursing Research*, 24(2), 113.

Heikkila, K., Sarvimaki, A., and Ekman, S.L. (2007). Culturally congruent care for older people: Finnish care in Sweden. *Scandinavian Journal of Caring Sciences*, 21(3), 354–361.

Henderson, V. (2006). The concept of nursing. 1977. *Journal of Advanced Nursing*, 53(1), 21–31; discussion 32–34.

Hines-Martin, V. and Robinson, K. (2006). Supervision as professional development for psychiatric mental health nurses. *Clinical Nurse Specialist*, 20(6), 293–297.

Hunter, L.P. and Hunter, L.A. (2006). Storytelling as an educational strategy for midwifery students. *Journal of Midwifery & Women's Health*, 51(4), 273–278.

Johnson, D.E. (1974). Development of theory: A requisite for nursing as a primary health profession. *Nursing Research*, 23(5), 372.

Johnson, J.E. (1999). Self-regulation theory and coping with physical illness. *Research in Nursing and Health*, 22(6), 435–448.

King, I.M. (1997). Reflections on the past and a vision for the future. *Nursing Science Quarterly*, 10(1), 15–17.

Kolcaba, K. (2001). Evolution of mid range theory of comfort for outcomes research. *Nursing Outlook*, 49(2), 86–92.

Kubsch, S.M. (1996). Conflict, enactment, empowerment: Conditions of independent therapeutic nursing intervention. *Journal of Advanced Nursing*, 23(1), 192–200.

Larson, P.A. (1977). Influence of patient status and health condition on nurse perceptions of patient characteristics. *Nursing Research*, 26(6), 416.

Laurent, C.L. (2000). A nursing theory for nursing leadership. *Journal of Nursing Management*, 8(2), 83–87.

Leenerts, M.H. and Teel, C.S. (2006). Relational conversation as method for creating partnerships: Pilot study. *Journal of Advanced Nursing*, 54(4), 467–476.

Lego, S. (1999). The one-to-one nurse-patient relationship. *Perspectives in Psychiatric Care*, 35(4), 4–23.

Leonard, R.C., Skipper, J.K., Jr., and Wodridge, P.J. (1967). Small sample field experiments for evaluating patient care. *Health Services Research*, 2(1), 47–60.

Lipson, J. and Meleis, A.I. (1983). Issues in health care of Middle-Eastern patients. *The Western Journal of Medicine*, 139, 854–861.

Marriner-Tomey, A., Mills, D., and Sauter, M. (1989). Ida Jean Orlando (Pelletier): Nursing process theory. In A. Marriner-Tomey (Ed.), *Nursing theorists and their work* (2nd ed.). St. Louis, MO: C.V. Mosby.

McCann, T.V. and Baker, H. (2001). Mutual relating: Developing interpersonal relationships in the community. *Journal of Advanced Nursing*, 34(4), 530–537.

McNaughton, D.B. (2000). A synthesis of qualitative home visiting research. *Public Health Nursing*, 17(6), 405–414.

Mertz, H. (1962). Nurse actions that reduce stress in patients. In *Emergency intervention by the nurse* (Monograph No. 1, pp. 10–14). New York: American Nurses Association.

Mohr, W.K. (1999). Deconstructing the language of psychiatric hospitalization. *Journal of Advanced Nursing*, 29(5), 1052–1059.

Morse, J.M., Bottorff, J.L., and Hutchinson, S. (1995). The paradox of comfort. *Nursing Research*, 44(1), 14–19.

Nagle, L.M. (1999). A matter of extinction or distinction. *Western Journal of Nursing Research*, 21(1), 71–82.

New England Board of Higher Education. (1977). *Mental health continuing education for associate degree nursing faculties: Project report.* Wellesley, MA: New England Board of Higher Education. NIH Training Grant No. 715 MH13182.

Nordby, H. (2007). Meaning and normativity in nurse-patient interaction. *Nursing Philosophy*, 8(1), 16–27.

Olson, J. and Hanchett, E. (1997). Nurse-expressed empathy, patient outcomes, and development of a middle-range theory. *Image: The Journal of Nursing Scholarship*, 29(1), 71–76.

Orlando, I. (1961). *The dynamic nurse-patient relationship.* New York: G.P. Putnam's Sons.

Orlando, I. (1972). *The discipline and teaching of nursing process.* New York: G.P. Putnam's Sons.

Orlando, I. (1987). Nursing in the 21st century . . . alternate paths. *Journal of Advanced Nursing*, 12(4), 405–412.

Orlando, I. and Dugan, A.B. (1989). Independent and dependent path: The fundamental issue for the nursing profession. *Nursing and Health Care*, 10(2), 76–80.

Orlando-Pelletier, I.J. (1990). Preface to the NLN edition. In I.J. Orlando (Ed.), *The dynamic nurse patient relationship: Function, process, and principles* (pp. vii–viii). New York: National League for Nursing.

Pascoe, E. (1996). The value to nursing research of Gadamer's hermeneutic philosophy. *Journal of Advanced Nursing*, 24(6), 1309–1314.

Peitchinis, J.A. (1972). Therapeutic effectiveness of counseling by nursing personnel. *Nursing Research*, 21(2), 138–148.

Peplau, H.E. (1991). *Interpersonal relations in nursing: A conceptual frame of reference for psychodynamic nursing.* New York: Springer Publishing Company. (Original work published 1952).

Pienschke, D. (1973). Guardedness or openness on the cancer unit. *Nursing Research*, 22(6), 484–490.

Potter, M. and Dawson, A. (2001). From safety contract to safety agreement. *Journal of Psychosocial Nursing and Mental Health Services*, 39(8), 38–45.

Potter, M.L. and Bockenhauer, B.J. (2000). Implementing Orlando's nursing theory: A pilot study. *Journal of Psychosocial Nursing and Mental Health Services*, 39(3), 14–21.

Potter, M. and Tinker, S. (2000). Put power in nurses' hands: Orlando's nursing theory supports nurses—simply. *Nursing Management*, 31(7 Part 1), 40–41.

Potter, M.L., Vitale-Nolen, R., and Dawson, A.M. (2005). Implementation of safety agreements in an acute psychiatric facility. *Journal of the American Psychiatric Nurses Association*, 11(3), 144–155.

Rawnsley, M.M. (2000). Response to Kim's human living concept as a unifying perspective for nursing. *Nursing Science Quarterly*, 13(1), 41–44.

Reynolds, W.J. and Scott, B. (2000). Do nurses and other professional helpers normally display much empathy? *Journal of Advanced Nursing*, 31(1), 226–234.

Rhymes, J. (1964). A description of nurse-patient interaction in effective nursing activity [abstract]. *Nursing Research*, 13(4), 365.

Rosenthal, B.C. (1996). An interactionist's approach to perioperative nursing. *Journal of the Association of peri-Operative Registered Nurses*, 64(2), 254–260.

Sahlsten, M.J., Larsson, I.E., Lindencrona, C.S., and Plos, K.A. (2005). Patient participation in nursing care: An interpretation by Swedish registered nurses. *Journal of Clinical Nursing*, 14(1), 35–42.

Schmieding, N.J. (1983). An analysis of Orlando's nursing theory based on Kuhn's theory of science. In P.L. Chinn (Ed.), *Advances in nursing theory development* (pp. 63–87). Rockville, MD: Aspen Systems.

Schmieding, N.J. (1984). Putting Orlando's theory into practice. *American Journal of Nursing*, 84(6), 759–761.

Schmieding, N.J. (1986). Orlando's theory. In P. Winstead-Fry (Ed.), *Case studies in nursing theory.* New York: National League for Nursing.

Schmieding, N.J. (1987). Face-to-face contacts: Exploring their meaning. *Nursing Management*, 18, 83–86.

Schmieding, N.J. (1987). Problematic situations in nursing: Analysis of Orlando's theory based on Dewey's theory of inquiry. *Journal of Advanced Nursing*, 12(4), 431–440.

Schmieding, N.J. (1988). Action process of nurse administrators to problematic situations based on Orlando's theory. *Journal of Advanced Nursing*, 13(1), 99–107.

Schmieding, N.J. (1990). Do head nurses include staff nurses in problem-solving? *Nursing Management*, 21(3), 58–60.

Schmieding, N.J. (1990). An integrative nursing theoretical framework. *Journal of Advanced Nursing*, 15(4), 463–467.

Schmieding, N.J. (1990). A model for assessing nurse administrators' actions. *Western Journal of Nursing Research*, 12(3), 293–306.

Schmieding, N.J. (1999). Reflective inquiry framework for nurse administrators. *Journal of Advanced Nursing*, 30(3), 631–639.

Schmieding, N.J. (2002). Ida Jean Orlando (Pelletier): Nursing process theory. In A.M. Tomey and M.R. Alligood (Eds.), *Nurse theorists and their work* (5th ed., pp. 399–417). St. Louis, MO: C.V. Mosby.

Sellers, S.C. (1991). A philosophical analysis of conceptual models of nursing. *Dissertation Abstracts International*, 52, 1937B. (University Microfilms No. AAC91–26248)

Sheafor, M. (1991). Productive work groups in complex hospital units: Proposed contributions of the nurse-executive. *Journal of Nursing Administration*, 21(5), 25–30.

Shea, N., McBride, L., Gavin, C., and Bauer, M.S. (1997). The effects of an ambulatory collaborative practice model on process outcomes of care for bipolar disorder. *Journal of the American Psychiatric Nurses Association*, 3(2), 49–57.

Sieger, M., Fritz, E. and Them, C. (2012). In discourse: Bourdieu's theory of practice and habitus in the context of a communication-oriented nursing interaction model. *Journal of Advanced Nursing*, 68(2), 480–489.

Stevens, B.J. (1971). Analysis of structural forms used in nursing curricula. *Nursing Research*, 20(5), 388–397.

Theis, E.C. (1973). Book review of Ida J. Orlando's The discipline and teaching of nursing process. *Nursing Research*, 22(1), 73.

Thorellekstrand, I. and Bjorvell, H. (1994). The VIPS-Model used by nursing student—Review of educational care plans. *Scandinavian Journal of Caring Sciences*, 8(4), 195–204.

Toniolli, A.C. and Pagliuca, L.M. (2002). Analysis of the applicability of Orlando's theory in Brazilian nursing journals [Portuguese]. *Revista Brasileira de Enfermagem*, 55(5), 489–494.

Tryon, P.A. (1962). The effect of patient participation in decision making on the outcome of a nursing procedure.

In *Nursing and the patients' motivation* (Clinical Paper No. 19, pp. 14–18). New York: American Nurses Association.

Tryon, P.A. (1963). An experiment of the effect of patients' participation in planning the administration of a nursing procedure. *Nursing Research*, 12, 262–265.

Tryon, P.A. and Leonard, R.C. (1964). The effect of patients' participation on the outcome of a nursing procedure. *Nursing Forum*, 3(2), 79–89.

Tutton, E. and Seers, K. (2003). An exploration of the concept of comfort. *Journal of Clinical Nursing*, 12(5), 689–696.

Varcoe, C. (1996). Disparagement of the nursing process: The new dogma? *Journal of Advanced Nursing*, 23(1), 120–125.

Vatne, S. and Fagermoen, M.S. (2007). To correct and to acknowledge: Two simultaneous and conflicting perspectives of limit-setting in mental health nursing. *Journal of Psychiatric and Mental Health Nursing*, 14(1), 41–48.

Vaughan, B. (1998). Developing nursing practice. *Journal of Clinical Nursing*, 7(3), 199–200.

von Krogh, G., Dale, C., and Naden, D. (2005). A framework for integrating NANDA, NIC, and NOC terminology in electronic patient records. *Journal of Nursing Scholarship*, 37(3), 275–281.

Wadensten, B. (2005). The content of morning time conversations between nursing home staff and residents. *Journal of Clinical Nursing*, 14(8B), 84–89.

Wadensten, B. and Carlsson, M. (2003). Nursing theory views on how to support the process of ageing. *Journal of Advanced Nursing*, 42(2), 118–124.

Williamson, K.M. (2007). Home health care nurses' perceptions of empowerment. *Journal of Community Health Nursing*, 24(3), 133–153.

Williamson, Y. (1978). Methodologic dilemmas in tapping the concept of patient needs. *Nursing Research*, 27(3), 172.

Wolfer, J. and Visintainer, M.A. (1975). Pediatric surgical patients' and parents' stress response and adjustment as a function of psychological preparation and stress-point nursing care. *Nursing Research*, 24(4), 244–255.

Wurzbach, M.E. (1996). Comfort and nurses' moral choices. *Journal of Advanced Nursing*, 24(2), 260–264.

Zoffmann, V., Harder, I., and Kirkevold, M. (2008). A person-centered communication and reflection model: Sharing decision-making in chronic care. *Qualitative Health Research*, 18(5), 670–685.

Zoffmann, V. and Kirkevold, M. (2005). Life versus disease in difficult diabetes care: Conflicting perspectives disempower patients and professionals in problem solving. *Qualitative Health Research*, 15(6), 750–765.

30. Rosemarie Parse

Allchin-Petardi, L. (1998). Weathering the storm: Persevering through a difficult time. *Nursing Science Quarterly*, 11(4), 172–177.

Aquino-Russell, C., Strüby, F.V.M., and Reviczky, K. (2007). Living attentive presence and changing perspectives with a web-based nursing theory course. *Nursing Science Quarterly*, 20(2), 128–134.

Banonis, B. (1989). The lived experience of recovering from addiction: A phenomenological study. *Nursing Science Quarterly*, 2(1), 37–43.

Baumann, S.L. (1997). Contrasting two approaches in a community-based nursing practice with older adults: The medical model and Parse's nursing theory. *Nursing Science Quarterly*, 10(3), 124–130.

Bunkers, S.S. (1998). Considering tomorrow: Parse's theory-guided research. *Nursing Science Quarterly*, 11(2), 56–63.

Bunkers, S.S. (2015). Awakening to Becoming. *Nursing Science Quarterly*, 28(3), 183–187.

Bunkers, S.S., Michaels, C., and Ethridge, P. (1997). Advanced practice nursing in community: Nursing's opportunity. *Advanced Practice Nursing Quarterly*, 2(4), 79–84.

Butler, M. (1988). Family transformation: Parse's theory in practice. *Nursing Science Quarterly*, 1(2), 68–74.

Butler, M.J. and Snodgrass, F.G. (1991). Beyond abuse: Parse's theory in practice. *Nursing Science Quarterly*, 4(2), 76–82.

Chrisman, M. and Riehl-Sisca, J. (1989). The systems-developmental-stress model. In J. Riehl-Sisca (Ed.), *Conceptual models for nursing practice* (3rd ed.). Norwalk, CT: Appleton & Lange.

Cody, W.K. and Mitchell, G.J. (1992). Parse's theory as a model for practice: The cutting edge. *Advances in Nursing Science*, 15(2), 52–65.

Cody, W.K. (2000). Parse's human becoming school of thought and families. *Nursing Science Quarterly*, 13(4). 281–284.

Condon, B.B. (2012). Celebrating now in teaching-learning. *Nursing Science Quarterly*, 25(1), 28–33.

Condon, B.B. (2014). The Living Experience of Feeling Overwhelmed A Parse Research Study. *Nursing Science Quarterly*, 27(3), 216–225.

Cowling, W.R. (1989). Parse's theory of nursing. In J.J. Fitzpatrick and A.L. Whall (Eds.), *Conceptual models of nursing: Analysis and application* (2nd ed.). Norwalk, CT: Appleton & Lange.

Daly, J., Mitchell, G.J., and Jonas-Simpson, C.M. (1996). The quality of life and the human becoming theory: Exploring discipline-specific contributions. *Nursing Science Quarterly*, 9(4), 170–174.

English, J. (1989). The systems-developmental-stress model in psychiatric nursing. In J. Riehl-Sisca (Ed.), *Conceptual models for nursing practice* (3rd ed.). Norwalk, CT: Appleton & Lange.

Freshwater, D. (1998). From acorn to oak tree: A neoplatonic perspective of reflection and caring. *Australian Journal of Holistic Nursing*, 5(2), 14–19.

Gunson, J. and Chawngthu, L. (2012). Health economics and informatics the gap-fit of current healthcare and parse practice. *Nursing Science Quarterly*, 25(2), 176–181.

Hart, J.D. (2015). Evaluating long-term care through the humanbecoming lens. *Nursing Science Quarterly*, 28(4), 280–283.

Janes, N.M. and Wells, D.L. (1997). Elderly patients' experiences with nurses guided by Parse's theory of human becoming. *Clinical Nursing Research*, 6(3), 205–222.

Jonas-Simpson, C. (1997). Living the art of the human becoming theory. *Nursing Science Quarterly*, 10(4), 175–179.

Kelley, L.S. (1995). Parse's theory in practice with a group in the community. *Nursing Science Quarterly*, 8(3), 127–132.

Kim, M.S., Shin, K.R., and Shin, S.R. (1998). Korean adolescents' experiences of smoking cessation: A prelude to research with the human becoming perspective. *Nursing Science Quarterly*, 11(3), 105–109.

Laschinger, H.K. and Duff, V. (1991). Attitudes of practicing nurses towards theory-based nursing practice. *Canadian Journal of Nursing Administration*, 4(1), 6–10.

Lee, R. and Schumacher, L. (1989). Rosemarie Rizzo Parse: Man-living-health. In A. Marriner-Tomey (Ed.),

Nursing theorists and their work (2nd ed.). St. Louis, MO: C.V. Mosby.

Legault, F. and Ferguson-Pare, M. (1999). Advancing nursing practice: An evaluation study of Parse's theory of human becoming. *Canadian Journal of Nursing Leadership*, 12(1), 30–35.

Letcher, D.C. (2014). Imagination Innovating the Could Be. *Nursing Science Quarterly*, 27(4), 287–291.

Limandri, B.J. (1982). Review of "Man-living-health: A theory of nursing." *Western Journal of Nursing Research*, 4(1), 105–106.

Markovic, M. (1997). From theory to perioperative practice with Parse. *Canadian Operating Room Nursing Journal*, 15(1), 13–19.

Martin, M.L., Forchuk, C., Santopinto, M., and Butcher, H.K. (1992). Alternative approaches to nursing practice: Application of Peplau, Rogers, and Parse. *Nursing Science Quarterly*, 5(2), 80–85.

Martin, P.J. (2000). Hearing voices and listening to those that hear them. *Journal of Psychiatric and Mental Health Nursing*, 7(2), 135–141.

Mattice, M. (1991). Parse's theory of nursing in practice: A manager's perspective. *Canadian Journal of Nursing Administration*, 4(1), 11–13.

Melnechenko, K.L. (1995). Parse's theory of human becoming: An alternative guide to nursing practice for pediatric oncology nurses. *Journal of Pediatric Oncology Nursing*, 12(3), 122–127.

Michell, G.J. (1988). Man-living-health: The theory in practice. *Nursing Science Quarterly*, 1(3), 120–127.

Mitchell, G.J. (1990). The lived experience of taking life day-by-day in later life: Research guided by Parse's emergent method. *Nursing Science Quarterly*, 3(1), 29–36.

Mitchell, G.J. (1990). Struggling in change: From the traditional approach to Parse's theory-based practice. *Nursing Science Quarterly*, 3(4), 170–176.

Mitchell, G.J. (1992). Parse's theory and the multidisciplinary team: Clarifying scientific values. *Nursing Science Quarterly*, 5(3), 104–106.

Mitchell, G.J. (1994). Discipline-specific inquiry: The hermeneutics of theory-guided nursing research. *Nursing Outlook*, 42(5), 224–228.

Mitchell, G.J. and Cody, W.K. (1992). Nursing knowledge and human science: Ontological and epistemological considerations. *Nursing Science Quarterly*, 5(2), 54–61.

Mitchell, G.J. and Heidt, P. (1994). The lived experience of wanting to help another: Research with Parse's method. *Nursing Science Quarterly*, 7(3), 119–127.

Mitchell, G.J. and Pilkington, B. (1990). Theoretical approaches in nursing practice: A comparison of Roy and Parse. *Nursing Science Quarterly*, 3(2), 81–87.

Norris, J.R. (2002). One-to-one teleapprenticeship as a means for nurses teaching and learning Parse' theory of human becoming. *Nursing Science Quarterly*, 15(2), 143–149.

Northrup, D.T. and Cody, W.K. (1998). Evaluation of the human becoming theory in practice in an acute care psychiatric setting. *Nursing Science Quarterly*, 11(1), 23–30.

Parse, R.R. (1974). *Nursing fundamentals*. Flushing, NY: Medical Examination Publishers.

Parse, R.R. (1981). *Man-living-health: A theory of nursing*. New York: John Wiley & Sons.

Parse, R.R. (1987). *Nursing science: Major paradigms, theories, and critiques*. Philadelphia, PA: W.B. Saunders.

Parse, R.R. (1987). Parse's man-living-health theory of nursing. In R.R. Parse (Ed.), *Nursing science: Major paradigms, theories, and critiques*. Philadelphia, PA: W.B. Saunders.

Parse, R.R. (1987). The simultaneity paradigm. In R.R. Parse (Ed.), *Nursing science: Major paradigms, theories, and critiques*. Philadelphia, PA: W.B. Saunders.

Parse, R.R. (1989). Man-living-health: A theory of nursing. In J. Riehl-Sisca (Ed.), *Conceptual models for nursing practice* (3rd ed.). Norwalk, CT: Appleton & Lange.

Parse, R.R. (1989). Essentials for practicing the art of nursing [Editorial]. *Nursing Science Quarterly*, 2(3), 111.

Parse, R.R. (1989). Making more out of less [Editorial]. *Nursing Science Quarterly*, 2(4), 155.

Parse, R.R. (1989). Parse's man-living-health model and administration of nursing service. In B. Henry, C. Arndt, M. DiVincenti, and A. Marriner-Tomey (Eds.), *Dimensions of nursing administration: Theory, research, education, practice*. Boston, MA: Blackwell Scientific Publications.

Parse, R.R. (1989). Qualitative research: Publishing and funding [Editorial]. *Nursing Science Quarterly*, 2(1), 1–2.

Parse, R.R. (1990). Health: A personal commitment. *Nursing Science Quarterly*, 3(3), 136–140.

Parse, R.R. (1990). Nursing theory-based practice: A challenge for the 90s [Editorial]. *Nursing Science Quarterly*, 3(2), 53.

Parse, R.R. (1990). Parse's research methodology with an illustration of the lived experience of hope. *Nursing Science Quarterly*, 3, 9–17.

Parse, R.R. (1990). Promotion and prevention: Two distinct cosmologies [Editorial]. *Nursing Science Quarterly*, 3(3), 101.

Parse, R.R. (1991). Electronic publishing: Beyond browsing [Editorial]. *Nursing Science Quarterly*, 4(1), 1.

Parse, R.R. (1991). Growing the discipline of nursing [Editorial]. *Nursing Science Quarterly*, 4(4), 139.

Parse, R.R. (1991). Mysteries of health and healing: Two perspectives [Editorial]. *Nursing Science Quarterly*, 4(3), 93.

Parse, R.R. (1991). The right soil, the right stuff [Editorial]. *Nursing Science Quarterly*, 4(2), 47.

Parse, R.R. (1992). Nursing knowledge for the 21st century: An international commitment. *Nursing Science Quarterly*, 5(1), 8–12.

Parse, R.R. (1992). Human becoming: Parse's theory of nursing. *Nursing Science Quarterly*, 5(1), 35–42.

Parse, R.R. (1992). Moving beyond the barrier reef [Editorial]. *Nursing Science Quarterly*, 5(3), 97.

Parse, R.R. (1992). The performing art of nursing [Editorial]. *Nursing Science Quarterly*, 5(4), 147.

Parse, R.R. (1992). The unsung shapers of nursing science [Editorial]. *Nursing Science Quarterly*, 5(2), 47.

Parse, R.R. (1995). Building the realm of nursing knowledge. *Nursing Science Quarterly*, 8, 51.

Parse, R.R. (1996). The human becoming theory: Challenges in practice and research. *Nursing Science Quarterly*, 9(2), 55–60.

Parse, R.R. (1997). Transforming research and practice with the human becoming theory. *Nursing Science Quarterly*, 10(4), 171–174.

Parse, R.R. (1999). Nursing science: The transformation of practice. *Journal of Advanced Nursing*, 30(6), 1383–1387.

Parse, R.R. (2008). Nursing knowledge development: Who's to say how? *Nursing Science Quarterly*, 21(2), 101.

Parse, R.R. (2011). Humanbecoming leading-following the meaning of holding up the mirror. *Nursing Science Quarterly*, 24(2), 169–171.

Parse, R.R. (2012). New humanbecoming conceptualizations and the humanbecoming community model expansions with sciencing and living the art. *Nursing Science Quarterly*, 25(1), 44–52.

Parse, R.R. (2013). Living quality a humanbecoming phenomenon. *Nursing Science Quarterly*, 26(2), 111–115.

Parse, R.R. (2016). Humanbecoming hermeneutic sciencing: Reverence, awe, betrayal, and shame in the lives of others. *Nursing Science Quarterly*, 29(2), 128.

Parse, R.R., Coyne, A.B., and Smith, M.J. (1985). Nursing research: Qualitative methods. Bowie, MD: Robert J. Brady Co.

Phillips, J.R. (1987). A critique of Parse's man-living-health theory. In R.R. Parse (Ed.), *Nursing science: Major paradigms, theories, and critiques*. Philadelphia, PA: W.B. Saunders.

Pilkington, F.B. (1999). A qualitative study of life after stroke. *Journal of Neuroscience Nursing*, 31(6), 336–347.

Pilkington, F.B. (2007). Envisioning nursing in 2050 through the eyes of nurse theorists: Rosemarie Rizzo Parse and Martha E. Rogers. *Nursing Science Quarterly*, 20(4), 307–308.

Pugliese, L. (1989). The theory of man-living-health: An analysis. In J. Riehl-Sisca (Ed.), *Conceptual models for nursing practice* (3rd ed.). Norwalk, CT: Appleton & Lange.

Quiquero, A., Knights, D., and Meo, C.O. (1991). Theory as a guide to practice: Staff nurses choose Parse's theory. *Canadian Journal of Nursing Administration*, 4(1), 14–16.

Reed, P.G. (1983). Implications of the life-span developmental framework for well-being in adulthood and aging. *Advances in Nursing Science*, 6(1), 18–25.

Relf, M.V. (1997). Illuminating meaning and transforming issues of spirituality in HIV disease and AIDS: An application of Parse's theory of human becoming. *Holistic Nursing Practice*, 12(1), 1–8.

Sarter, B. (1988). Philosophy sources of nursing theory. *Nursing Science Quarterly*, 1(2), 52–59.

Smith, M.J. (1989). Research and practice application related to man-living-health. In J. Riehl-Sisca (Ed.), *Conceptual models for nursing practice* (3rd ed.). Norwalk, CT: Appleton & Lange.

Stanley, G.D. and Meghani, S.H. (2001). Reflections on using Parse's theory of human becoming in a palliative care setting in Pakistan. *Canadian Nurse*, 97(7), 23–25.

Walker, C.A. (1996). Coalescing the theories of two nurse visionaries: Parse and Watson. *Journal of Advanced Nursing*, 24(5), 988–996.

Winkler, S.J. (1983). Parse's theory of nursing. In J.J. Fitzpatrick and A.L. Whall (Eds.), *Conceptual models of nursing: Analysis and application*. Bowie, MD: Robert J. Brady Co.

31. Josephine Paterson and Loretta Zderad

Anderson, C. and Adamsen, L. (2001). Continuous video recording: A new clinical research tool for studying the nursing care of cancer patients. *Journal of Advanced Nursing*, 35(2), 257–267.

Andrews, G.J. and Moon, G. (2005). Space, place, and the evidence base: Part II–Rereading nursing environment through geographical research. *Worldviews on Evidence-Based Nursing*, 2(3), 142–156.

Annells, M. (2006). The experience of flatus incontinence from a bowel ostomy: A hermeneutic phenomenology. *Journal of WOCN*, 33(5), 518–524.

Azevedo, N.A., Kantorski, L.P., and Ornellas, C.P. (2000). Families of patients undergoing chemotherapy, based on Paterson and Zderad's theory [Portuguese]. *Texto & Contexto Enfermagem*, 9(2 Part 1), 17–27.

Baillie, L. (1996). A phenomenological study of the nature of empathy. *Journal of Advanced Nursing*, 24(6), 1300–1308.

Barker, P.J., Buchanan–Barker, P., and Whitehill, I. (2005). *The tidal model: A guide for mental health professionals*. New York: Psychology Press.

Barnum, B.J.S. (1994). *Nursing theory: Analysis, application, and evaluation* (4th ed.). Philadelphia, PA: Lippincott.

Barnum, B.J.S. (1998). *Nursing theory: Analysis, application, evaluation* (5th ed.). Philadelphia, PA: Lippincott.

Bauer, R. (1998). A dialectic reflection on the psychotherapeutic efficacy of nursing interventions. *Nursing interventions and effectiveness of psychotherapy* [German]. *Pflege*, 11(6), 305–311.

Bauer, R. (1999). A dialectic view of the efficacy of nursing interventions. Connections between nursing interventions and effects of psychotherapy [German]. *Pflege*, 12(1), 5–10.

Beeber, L.S., Cooper, C., Van Noy, B.E., Schwartz, T.A., Blanchard, H.C., Canuso, R., et al. (2007). Flying under the radar: Engagement and retention of depressed low-income mothers in a mental health intervention. *Advances in Nursing Science*, 30(3), 221–234.

Berg, M. (2005). A midwifery model of care for childbearing women at high risk: Genuine caring in caring for the genuine. *Journal of Perinatal Education*, 14(1), 9–21.

Billay, D., Myrick, F., Luhanga, F., and Yonge, O. (2007). A pragmatic view of intuitive knowledge in nursing practice. *Nursing Forum*, 42(3), 147–155.

Brouse, S.H. and Laffrey, S.C. (1989). Paterson and Zderad's humanistic nursing framework. In J.J. Fitzpatrick and A.L. Whall (Ed.), *Conceptual models of nursing: Analysis and application* (2nd ed.). Norwalk, CT: Appleton & Lange.

Bruce, A. and Davies, B. (2005). Mindfulness in hospice care: Practicing meditation-in-action. *Qualitative Health Research*, 15(10), 1329–1344.

Callister, L.C. and Cox, A.H. (2006). Opening our hearts and minds: The meaning of international clinical nursing electives in the personal and professional lives of nurses. *Nursing and Health Sciences*, 8(2), 95–102.

Carlen, P. and Bengtsson, A. (2007). Suicidal patients as experienced by psychiatric nurses in inpatient care. *International Journal of Mental Health Nursing*, 16(4), 257–265.

Chan, M.F., Lou, F.L., Arthur, D.G., Cao, F.L., Wu, L.H, Li, P., et al. (2008). Investigating factors associate to nurses' attitudes towards perinatal bereavement care. *Journal of Clinical Nursing*, 17(4), 509–518.

Cotton, A.H. and Roden, J. (2006). Using patterns of knowing in nursing as a possible framework for nursing care of homeless families with children. *Contemporary Nurse*, 23(2), 331–341.

Covington, H. (2005). Caring presence: Providing a safe space for patients. *Holistic Nursing Practice*, 19(4), 169–172.

Cutcliffe, J.R. and Cassedy, P. (1999). The development of empathy in students on a short, skill based counselling course: A pilot study. *Nursing Education Today*, 19(3), 250–257.

Dariel, O.P.D. (2009). Nursing education: In pursuit of cosmopolitanism. *Nurse Education Today*, 29(5), 566–569.

Davis, L.A. (2005). A phenomenological study of patient expectations concerning nursing care. *Holistic Nursing Practice*, 19(3), 126–133.

Davis, L.A. (2006). Hospitalized patients' expectations of spiritual care from nurses. In S.D. Ambrose (Ed.), *Religion and psychology: New research* (pp. 1–38). New York: Nova Publishers.

de Witte, L., Schoot, T., and Proot, I. (2006). Development of the client-centered care questionnaire. *Journal of Advanced Nursing*, 56(1), 62–68.

Donaldson, S.K. (1983). Let us not abandon the humanities. *Nursing Outlook*, 31(1), 40–43.

doNascimento, E.R. and Trentini, M. (2004). Nursing care at the intensive care unit (ICU): Going beyond objectivity [Portuguese]. *Revista Latino-Americana de Enfermagem*, 12(2), 250–257.

Finfgeld-Connett, D. (2005). Telephone social support or nursing presence? Analysis of a nursing intervention. *Qualitative Health Research*, 15(1), 19–29.

Finfgeld-Connett, D. (2006). Meta-synthesis of presence in nursing. *Journal of Advanced Nursing*, 55(6), 708–714.

Finfgeld-Connett, D. (2008). Qualitative comparison and synthesis of nursing presence and caring. *International Journal of Nursing Terminologies & Classifications*, 19(3), 111–119.

Frisch, N.C. (2005). Nursing as a context for alternative/complementary modalities. In L.C. Andrist, P.K. Nicholas, and K. Wolf (Eds.), *A history of nursing ideas*. Sudbury, MA: Jones & Bartlett Publishers.

Grevin, F. (1996). Posttraumatic stress disorder, ego defense mechanisms, and empathy among urban paramedics. *Psychological Reports*, 79(2), 483–495.

Hall, E.O.C. and Brinchmann, B.S. (2009). Mothers of preterm infants: Experiences of space, tone and transfer in the neonatal care unit. *Journal of Neonatal Nursing*, 15(4), 129–136.

Hanley, M.A. and Fenton, M.V. (2007). Exploring improvisation in nursing. *Journal of Holistic Nursing*, 25(2), 126–133.

Hartrick, G. (1997). Relational capacity: The foundation for interpersonal nursing practice. *Journal of Advanced Nursing*, 26(3), 523–528.

Hartrick, G. (1999). Transcending behaviorism in communication education. *Journal of Nursing Education*, 38(1), 17–22.

Hasegawa, H. (1987). On "humanistic nursing" by J. Paterson and L. Zderad [Japanese]. *Kangogaku Zasshi—Japanese Journal of Nursing*, 51(12), 158–1159.

Hopkinson, J.B. (2007). How people with advanced cancer manage changing eating habits. *Journal of Advanced Nursing*, 59(5), 454–462.

Hopkinson, J.B. and Hallett, C.E. (2001). Patients' perceptions of hospice day care: A phenomenology study. *International Journal of Nursing Studies*, 38(1), 117–125.

Hopkinson, J., Wright, D., and Corner, J. (2006). Exploring the experience of weight loss in people with advanced cancer. *Journal of Advanced Nursing*, 54(3), 304–312.

Jacob, J.D., Holmes, D., and Buus, N. (2008). Humanism in forensic psychiatry: The use of the tidal nursing model. *Nursing Inquiry*, 15(3), 224–230.

Kant, I. (1953). *Prolegomena to any future metaphysics*. P.G. Lucas (Trans.). Manchester, England: University of Manchester Press.

Kawano, M. (1987). Nursing theory. On "Humanistic Nursing" by J. Paterson and L. Zderad. *Kangogaku Zasshi—Japanese Journal of Nursing*, 51(10), 950–951.

Kleiman, S. (1986). Humanistic nursing: The phenomenological theory of Paterson and Zderad. In P. Winstead-Fry (Ed.), *Case studies in nursing theory*. New York: National League for Nursing.

Kleiman, S. (1993). Reflections on knowing Josephine Paterson and Loretta Zderad. *NLN Publications*, (15–2548), 15–19.

Kleiman, S. (2002). *The essences of the lived experiences of nurse practitioners interacting with their patients*. Adelphi University, PhD.

Kleiman, S. (2004). What is the nature of nurse practitioners' lived experiences interacting with patients? *Journal of the American Academy of Nurse Practitioners*, 16(6), 263–269.

Kleiman, S. (2008). *Human centered nursing: The foundation of quality care*. Philadelphia, PA: F.A. Davis.

Kleinman, S. (2008). *Instructor's guide for human centered nursing: The foundation of quality care*. New York: Institute for Human Centered Caring.

Kleiman, S. (2009). On the way to learning. *MEDSURG Nursing*, 18(1), 33–37.

Kleiman, S. (2010). Josephine Paterson and Loretta Zderad's humanistic nursing theory. In M.E. Parker and M.C. Smith (Eds), *Nursing theories and nursing practice* (3rd ed., pp. 337–350). Philadelphia, PA: F.A. Davis.

Kolcaba, K.Y. and Kolcaba, R.J. (1991). An analysis of the concept of comfort. *Journal of Advanced Nursing*, 16(11), 1301–1310.

Kostovich, C.T. (2002). *Development of a scale to measure nursing presence*. Loyola University of Chicago, PhD.

Kostovich, C.T. (2012). Development and psychometric assessment of the presence of nursing scale. *Nursing Science Quarterly*, 25(2), 167–175.

Krug, S.B. and Somavilla Vda, C. (2004). A reflexive analysis on professional nursing actions involving work accident victims in view of the theory of Paterson and Zderad. *Revista Latino-Americana de Enfermagem*, 12(2), 277–279.

Larson, S.G. (2002). *Contemplative spirituality: Towards phenomenological understanding*. University of Kansas, PhD.

Lavoie, M., DeKoninck, T., and Blondeau, D. (2006). The nature of care in light of Emmanuel Levinas. *Nursing Philosophy*, 7(4), 225–234.

Leenerts, M.H. and Teel, C.S. (2006). Relational conversation as method for creating partnerships: Pilot study. *Journal of Advanced Nursing*, 54(4), 467–476.

Lego, S. (1999). The one-to-one nurse-patient relationship. *Perspectives in Psychiatric Care*, 35(4), 4–23.

Lobchuk, M. (1996). Humanistic care—A vital dialog with myself as a nurse [German]. *Pflege*, 9(2), 120–126.

Lobchuk, M. (1999). Humanistic reflections of a research nurse in a longitudinal study: A personal essay. *Canadian Oncology Nursing Journal*, 9(2), 71–73.

Mason, T. and Patterson, R. (1990). A critical review of the use of Rogers' model within a special hospital: A single case study. *Journal of Advanced Nursing*, 15, 130–141.

McCamant, K.L. (2006). Humanistic nursing, interpersonal relations theory, and the empathy-altruism hypothesis. *Nursing Science Quarterly*, 19(4), 334–338.

McCance, C., Paterson, J.G., Nommo, A.W., and Hunter, D. (1987). Psychiatric geography: Where patients live and their use of services—A study of computerized mapping of case register data. *Health Bulletin*, 45(4), 197–210.

McQueen, A. (1997). The emotional work of caring, with a focus on gynaecological nursing. *Journal of Clinical Nursing*, 6(3), 233–240.

Medina, R.F. and Backes, V.M. (2002). Humanism in the care of surgery patients [Portuguese]. *Revista Brasileira de Enfermagem*, 55(5), 522–527.

Menke, E.M. (1978). Theory development: A challenge for nursing. In N.L. Chaska (Ed.), *The nursing profession: Views through the mist.* New York: McGraw-Hill.

Merryfeather, L. (2015). Passionate scholarship or academic safety: An ethical issue. *Journal of Holistic Nursing,* 33(1), 60–67.

Mitchell, G.J. and Cody, W.K. (2006). Nursing knowledge and human science: Ontological and epistemological considerations. In W.K. Cody and J.W. Kenney (Eds.), *Philosophical and theoretical perspectives for advanced nursing practice* (4th ed., pp. 241–256). Sudbury, MA: Jones & Bartlett Publishers.

Mitchell, S.G., Peterson, J.A., Latkin, C.A., and Coffey, S. (2006). The nurse-patient relationship in cancer care as a shared covenant: A concept analysis. *Advances in Nursing Science,* 29(4), 308–323.

Morse, J.M., Bottorff, J., Anderson, G., O'Brien, B., and Solberg, S. (2006). Beyond empathy: Expanding expressions of caring. 1991. *Journal of Advanced Nursing,* 53(1), 75–87; discussion 87–90.

Munhall, P.L. (1982). Nursing philosophy and nursing research: In apposition or opposition? *Nursing Research,* 31(3), 776–786.

Munhall, P.L. (2006). Epistemology in nursing. In P.L. Munhall (Ed.), *Nursing research: A qualitative perspective* (4th ed.). Sudbury, MA: Jones & Bartlett Publishers.

Munhall, P.L. (2006). Language and nursing research: The evolution. In P.L. Munhall (Ed.), *Nursing research: A qualitative perspective.* Sudbury, MA: Jones & Bartlett Publishers.

Munhall, P.L. (2007). The landscape of qualitative research in nursing. In P.L. Munhall (Ed.), *Nursing research: A qualitative perspective.* Sudbury, MA: Jones & Bartlett Publishers.

Muniz, R.M., Santana, M.G., and Serqueira, H.C. (2000). Nursing care tuned to the young adult human being who is the carrier of a chronic disease, under the light of Paterson and Zderad's humanistic nursing theory [Portuguese]. *Texto & Contexto Enfermagem,* 9(2 Part 1), 158–168.

Nystrom, M. (2007). A patient-oriented perspective in existential issues: A theoretical argument for applying Peplau's interpersonal relation model in healthcare science and practice. *Scandinavian Journal of Caring Sciences,* 21(2), 282–288.

Ohlen, J., Andershed, B., Berg, C., Frid, I., Palm, C.A., Ternestedt, B.M., et al. (2007). Relatives in end-of-life care—Part 2: A theory for enabling safety. *Journal of Clinical Nursing,* 16(2), 382–390.

Oiler, C. (1982). The phenomenological approach in nursing research. *Nursing Research,* 31(3), 178–181.

Olsen, D.P. (1997). When the patient causes the problem: The effect of patient responsibility on the nurse-patient relationship. *Journal of Advanced Nursing,* 26(3), 515–522.

Paini, J.P. (2000). Dialogues as care: A humanistic approach next to nursing academicians [Portuguese]. *Texto & Contexto Enfermagem,* 9(2 Part 2), 632–645.

Paterson, J.G. (1971). From a philosophy of clinical nursing to a method of nursology. *Nursing Research,* 20(2), 143–146.

Paterson, J.G. (1978). The tortuous way toward nursing theory. In J.G. Paterson (Ed.), *Theory development: What, why, how?* (Publication No. 15–1708, pp. 49–65). New York: National League for Nursing.

Paterson, J.G. and Zderad, L.T. (1970–1971). All together through complementary syntheses the worlds of the many. *Image: Journal of Nursing Scholarship,* 4(3), 13–16.

Paterson, J.G. and Zderad, L.T. (1976). *Humanistic nursing.* New York: John Wiley & Sons.

Paterson, J.G. and Zderad, L.T. (1976). *Humanistic nursing.* New York: John Wiley & Sons. Retrieved from Project Gutenberg http://www.gutenberg.org/files/25020/25020–8.txt

Paterson, J.G. and Zderad, L.T. (1988). *Humanistic nursing* (Publication No. 41–2218, pp. i–iv, 1–129). New York: National League for Nursing.

Paula, C.C., Padoin, S.M., Vernier, E.T., and Moota Mda, G. (2003). Reflections on the child being and on the nursing care in AIDS context [Portuguese]. *Revista Guacha de Enfermagem,* 24(2), 189–195.

Peltomaki, P. (1997). Goodness in nurse's heart matters. What is goodness in nursing practice? [Finnish]. *Sairaanhoitaja* (Helsinki), 70(7), 10–12.

Pilkington, F.B., and Bournes, D.A. (2005). Nursing theory. In J. Daly, S. Speedy, and D. Jackson (Eds.), *Professional nursing: Concepts, issues, and challenges* (pp. 133–152). New York: Springer Publishing Company.

Reed, P.G. (2006). Nursing: The ontology of the discipline. In W.K. Cody and J.W. Kenney (Eds.), *Philosophical and theoretical perspectives for advanced nursing practice* (pp. 123–130). Sudbury, MA: Jones & Bartlett Publishers.

Reed, P.G. (2006). The practice turn in nursing epistemology. *Nursing Science Quarterly,* 19(1), 36–38.

Rich, K.L. (2005). Ethics in psychiatric and mental health nursing. In J. Butts and K. Rich (Eds.), *Nursing ethics: Across the curriculum and into practice* (pp. 147–174). Sudbury, MA: Jones & Bartlett Publishers.

Risjord, M. (2014). Nursing and human freedom. *Nursing Philosophy,* 15(1), 35–45.

Sahlsten, M.J., Larsson, I.E., Lindencrona, C.S., and Plos, K.A. (2005). Patient participation in nursing care: An interpretation by Swedish registered nurses. *Journal of Clinical Nursing,* 14(1), 35–42.

Sahlsten, M.J., Larsson, I.E., Sjostrom, B., Lindencrona, C.S.C., and Plos, K.A.E. (2007). Patient participation in nursing care: Towards a concept clarification from a nurse perspective. *Journal of Clinical Nursing,* 16(4), 630–637.

Schofield, I., Tolson, D., Arthur, D., Davies, S., and Nolan, M. (2005). An exploration of the caring attributes and perceptions of work place change among gerontological nursing staff in England, Scotland and China (Hong Kong). *International Journal of Nursing Studies,* 42(2), 197–209.

Silva, T.N. (2013). Paterson and Zderad's humanistic theory: Entering the between through being when called upon. *Nursing Science Quarterly,* 26(2), 132–135.

Smyth, T. (1996). Reinstating the person in the professional: Reflections on empathy and aesthetic experience. *Journal of Advanced Nursing,* 24(5), 932–937.

Soares, M.C., Santana, M.G., and Serqueira, H.C.H. (2000). Nursing care in the daily living of autonomous nurses under the light of some of Paterson and Zderad's humanistic theory concepts [Portuguese]. *Texto & Contexto Enfermagem,* 9(2 Part 1), 106–117.

Sousa, A.S., Kantorski, L.P., Bielemann, V.L.M., and Ornellas, C.P. (2000). The human being with AIDS coexisting within a family [Portuguese]. *Texto & Contexto Enfermagem,* 9(2 Part 1), 186–196.

Souza, L.N.A., and Padilha, M.I.C. (2000). Humanization in critical care: A way under construction [Portuguese]. *Texto & Contexto Enfermagem,* 9(2 Part 1), 324–335.

Starr, S.S. (2008). Authenticity: A concept analysis. *Nursing Forum,* 43(2), 55–62.

Stern, P.N. (1980). Grounded theory methodology: Its uses and processes. *Image*, 12, 20–23.

Stevens, B.J.S. (1984). *Nursing theory: Analysis, application, and evaluation* (2nd ed.). Boston, MA: Little, Brown.

Stoltz, P., Lindholm, M., Uden, G., and Willman, A. (2006). The meaning of being supportive for family caregivers as narrated by registered nurses working in palliative homecare. *Nursing Science Quarterly*, 19(2), 163–173.

Taggart, L. and Slevin, E. (2006). Care planning in mental health settings. In B. Gates (Ed.), *Care planning and delivery in intellectual disability nursing* (pp. 158–194). Malden, MA: Blackwell Publishing.

Thomas, S.P. (2005). Through the lens of Merleau-Ponty: Advancing the phenomenological approach to nursing research. *Nursing Philosophy*, 6(1), 63–76.

Tuckett, A.G. (2005). The care encounter: Pondering caring, honest communication and control. *International Journal of Nursing Practice*, 11(2), 77–84.

Tuckett, A.G. (2007). Stepping across the line: Information sharing, truth telling, and the role of the personal carer in the Australian nursing home. *Qualitative Health Research*, 17(4), 489–500.

Tutton, E. and Seers, K. (2003). An exploration of the concept of comfort. *Journal of Clinical Nursing*, 12(5), 689–696.

Wagner, A.L. (2000). Connecting to nurse-self through reflective poetic story. *International Journal for Human Caring*, 4(2), 7–12.

Westin, L. and Danielson, E. (2007). Encounters in Swedish nursing homes: A hermeneutic study of residents' experiences. *Journal of Advanced Nursing*, 60(2), 172–180.

White, S.J. (1997). Empathy: A literature review and concept analysis. *Journal of Clinical Nursing*, 6(4), 253–257.

Willis, D.G., Grace, P.J., and Roy, C. (2008). A central unifying focus for the discipline: Facilitating humanization, meaning, choice, quality of life, and healing in living and dying. *Advances in Nursing Science*, 31(1), E28–E40.

Wilson, H.S. (1977). Limiting intrusion: Social control of outsiders in a healing community. *Nursing Research*, 26(2), 103–111.

Wu, H.L. and Volker, D.L. (2012). Humanistic nursing theory: Application to hospice and palliative care. *Journal of Advanced Nursing*, 68(2), 471–479.

Yegdich, T. (1999). On the phenomenology of empathy in nursing: Empathy or sympathy? *Journal of Advanced Nursing*, 30(1), 83–93.

Zderad, L.T. (1968). *A concept of empathy*. Unpublished doctoral dissertation. Georgetown University, Washington, DC.

Zderad, L.T. (1969). Empathetic nursing: Realization of a human capacity. *Nursing Clinics of North America*, 4, 655–662.

Zderad, L.T. (1970). *Empathy: From cliche to construct*. In Proceedings of the Third Nursing Theory Conference (pp. 46–75). University of Kansas Medical Center Department of Nursing.

Zderad, L.T. (1978). From here and now to theory: Reflections on "how." In J.G. Paterson (Ed.), *Theory development: What, why, how?* (Publication No. 15–1708, pp. 35–48). New York: National League for Nursing.

32. Hildegard Peplau

Barker, P. (1998). The future of the theory of interpersonal relations? A personal reflection on Peplau's legacy. *Journal of Psychiatric and Mental Health Nursing*, 5(3), 213–220.

Beeber, L.S. (1998). Treating depression through the therapeutic nurse-client relationship. *Nursing Clinics of North America*, 33(1), 153–172.

Beeber, L.S. and Bourbonniere, M. (1998). The concept of interpersonal pattern in Peplau's theory of nursing. *Journal of Psychiatric and Mental Health Nursing*, 5(3), 187–192.

Carey, E.T., Noll, J., Rasmussen, L., Searcy, B., and Stark, N. (1989). Hildegard E. Peplau: Psychodynamic nursing. In A. Marriner-Tomey (Ed.), *Nursing theorists and their work* (2nd ed.). St. Louis, MO: C.V. Mosby.

Chambers, M. (1998). Interpersonal mental health nursing: Research issues and challenges. *Journal of Psychiatric and Mental Health Nursing*, 5(3), 203–211.

Deane, W.H. and Fain, J.A. (2015, April 8). Incorporating Peplau's theory of interpersonal relations to promote holistic communication between older adults and nursing students. *Journal of Holistic Nursing*. doi: 10.1177/0898010115577975.

Feely, M. (1997). Using Peplau's theory in nurse-patient relations. *International Nursing Review*, 44(4), 115–120.

Forchuk, C. (1989). Establish a nurse-client relationship. *Journal of Psychosocial Nursing*, 27(2), 30–34.

Forchuk, C. (1991). A comparison of the works of Peplau and Orlando. *Archives of Psychiatric Nursing*, 5(1), 38–45.

Forchuk, C., Beaton, S., Crawford, L., Ide, L., Voorberg, N., and Bethune, J. (1989). Incorporating Peplau's theory and case management. *Journal of Psychosocial Nursing and Mental Health Services*, 27(2), 35–38.

Forchuk, C. and Dorsay, J.P. (1995). Hildegard Peplau meets family system nursing: Innovation in theory-based practice. *Journal of Advanced Nursing*, 21(1), 110–115.

Forchuk, C., Jewell, J., Schofield, R., Sircelj, M. and Valledor, T. (1998). From hospital to community: Bridging therapeutic relationships. *Journal of Psychiatric and Mental Health Nursing*, 5(3), 197–202.

Gregg, D.E. (1978). Hildegard E. Peplau: Her contributions. *Perspectives in Psychiatric Care*, 16(3), 118–121.

Haber, J. (2000). Hildegarde E. Peplau: The psychiatric nursing legacy of a legend. *Journal of the American Psychiatric Nurses Association*, 6(2), 56–62.

Lego, S. (1998). The application of Peplau's theory to group psychotherapy. *Journal of Psychiatric and Mental Health Nursing*, 5(3), 193–196.

Mahoney, J.S. and Engebretson, J. (2000). The interface of anthropology and nursing guiding culturally competent care in psychiatric nursing. *Archives of Psychiatric Nursing*, 14(4), 183–190.

Peden, A.R. (1998). The evolution of an intervention—The use of Peplau's process of practice-based theory development. *Journal of Psychiatric and Mental Health Nursing*, 5(3), 173–178.

Peplau, H. (1962). Interpersonal techniques: The crux of psychiatric nursing. *American Journal of Nursing*, 62(6), 50–54.

Peplau, H. (1963). Interpersonal relations and the process of adaptation. *Nursing Science*, 3, 272–279.

Peplau, H. (1964). *Basic principles of patient counseling*. Philadelphia, PA: Smith Kline & French Laboratory.

Peplau, H. (1967). Interpersonal relations and the work of the industrial nurse. *American Association of Industrial Nurses*, 15(11), 7–12.

Peplau, H. (1968). Operational definitions and nursing science. In L.T. Zderad and H.C. Belcher (Eds.), *Developing behavioral concepts in nursing*. Atlanta, GA: Southern Regional Education Board.

Peplau, H. (1968). Psychotherapeutic strategies. *Perspectives in Psychiatric Care*, 6(6), 264–270.

Peplau, H. (1969). Professional closeness . . as a special kind of involvement with a patient, client, or family group. *Nursing Forum*, 8(4), 342.

Peplau, H. (1970). Changed patterns of practice. *Washington Street Journal of Nursing*, 42, 4–6.

Peplau, H. (1971). Communication in crisis intervention. *Psychiatric Forum*, 2, 1–7.

Peplau, H. (1974). Biography. *Nursing '74*, 4(2), 13.

Peplau, H. (1978). Psychiatric nursing: Role of nurses and psychiatric nurses. *International Nursing Review*, 25(2), 41–47.

Peplau, H. (1986). *Credentialing in nursing: Contemporary developments and trends: Internal vs. external regulation* [Pamphlet] (Publication No. G-172B, pp. 1–10). Kansas City, MO: American Nurses Association.

Peplau, H. (1987). Nursing science: A historical perspective. In R.R. Parse (Ed.), *Nursing science: Major paradigms, theories, and critiques*. Philadelphia, PA: W.B. Saunders.

Peplau, H. (1988). The art and science of nursing: Similarities, differences, and relations. *Nursing Science Quarterly*, 1(1), 8–15.

Peplau, H. (1988). Future directions in psychiatric nursing from the perspective of history. *Journal of Psychosocial Nursing and Mental Health Services*, 27(2), 18–21, 25–28.

Peplau, H.E. (1991). *Interpersonal relations in nursing: A conceptual frame of reference for psychodynamic nursing*. New York: Springer Publishing Company. (Original work published 1952).

Peplau, H.E. (1997). Peplau's theory of interpersonal relations. *Nursing Science Quarterly*, 10(4), 162–167.

Price, B. (1998). Explorations in body image care: Peplau and practice knowledge. *Journal of Psychiatric and Mental Health Nursing*, 5(3), 179–186.

Reed, P.G. and Johnston, R.L. (1983). Peplau's nursing model: The interpersonal process. In J.J. Fitzpatrick and A.L. Whall (Eds.), *Conceptual models of nursing: Analysis and application*. Bowie, MD: Robert J. Brady Co.

Reed, P.G. and Johnston, R.L. (1989). Peplau's nursing model: The interpersonal process. In J.J. Fitzpatrick and A.L. Whall (Eds.), *Conceptual models of nursing: Analysis and application* (2nd ed.). Norwalk, CT: Appleton & Lange.

Reynolds, W.J. (1997). Peplau's theory in practice. *Nursing Science Quarterly*, 10(4), 168–170.

Roy, C. (1980). A case study viewed according to different models. In J.P. Riehl and C. Roy (Eds.), *Conceptual models for nursing practice* (2nd ed.). New York: Appleton-Century-Crofts.

Schafer, P. (1999). Working with Dave. Application of Peplau's interpersonal nursing theory in the correctional environment. *Journal of Psychosocial Nursing and Mental Health Services*, 37(9), 18–24.

Senn, J.F. (2013). Peplau's theory of interpersonal relations: Application in emergency and rural nursing. *Nursing Science Quarterly*, 26(1), 31–35.

Sills, G.M. (1978). Hildegard E. Peplau: Leader, practitioner, academician, scholar, theorist. *Perspectives in Psychiatric Care*, 16(3), 122–128.

Sills, G.M. (1998). Peplau and professionalism: The emergence of the paradigm of professionalization. *Journal of Psychiatric and Mental Health Nursing*, 5(3), 167–171.

Thelander, B.L. (1997). The psychotherapy of Hildegard Peplau in the treatment of people with serious mental illness. *Perspectives in Psychiatric Care*, 33(3), 24–32.

Thompson, L. (1986). Peplau's theory: An application to short-term individual therapy. *Journal of Psychological Nursing and Mental Health Service*, 24(8), 26–31.

Yamashita, M. (1997). Family caregiving: Application of Newman's and Peplau's theories. *Journal of Psychiatric and Mental Health Nursing*, 4(6), 401–405.

Zarea, K., Maghsoudi, S., Dashtebozorgi, B., Hghighizadeh, M.H., and Javadi, M. (2014). The impact of Peplau's therapeutic communication model on anxiety and depression in patients candidate for coronary artery bypass. *Clinical Practice and Epidemiology in Mental Health*, 10, 159–165.

33. Martha Rogers

Aggleton, P. and Chalmers, H. (1984). Rogers' unitary field model. *Nursing Times*, 80(50), 35–39.

Alligood, M. (1989). Rogers's theory and nursing administration: A perspective on health and environment. In B. Henry, C. Arndt, M. DiVincenti, and A. Marriner-Tomey (Eds.), *Dimensions of nursing administration: Theory, research, education, practice*. Boston, MA: Blackwell Scientific Publications.

Alligood, M.R. (1990). Rogers' theory: Research to practice. *Rogerian Nursing Science News*, 2(3), 2–3.

Alligood, M.R. (2002). A theory of the art of nursing discovered in Rogers' science of unitary human beings. *International Journal for Human Caring*, 6(2), 55–60.

Andrews, G.J. and Moon, G. (2005). Space, place, and the evidence base: Part II—rereading nursing environment through geographical research. *Worldviews on Evidence-Based Nursing*, 2(3), 142–156.

Andrist, L.C., Nicholas, P.K., and Wolf, K. (2005). *A history of nursing ideas*. Sudbury, MA: Jones & Bartlett Publishers.

Aquino-Russell, C., Struby, F.V.M., and Reviczky, K. (2007). Living attentive presence and changing perspectives with a web-based nursing theory course. *Nursing Science Quarterly*, 20(2), 128–134.

Armstrong, M.A. and Kelly, A.E. (1995). More than the sum of their parts: Martha Rogers and Hildegard Peplau. *Archives of Psychiatric Nursing*, 9(1), 40–44.

Banonis, B. (1989). The lived experience of recovering from addiction: A phenomenological study. *Nursing Science Quarterly*, 2(1), 37–43.

Barnes, S.J. and Adair, B. (2002). The cognition-sensitive approach to dementia parallels with the science of unitary human beings. *Journal of Psychosocial Nursing and Mental Health Services*, 40(11), 30–37.

Barnum, B.J.S. (1994). *Nursing theory: Analysis, application, and evaluation* (4th ed.). Philadelphia, PA: Lippincott.

Barrett, E.A. (1986). Investigation of the principle of helicy: The relationship of human field motion and power. In V.M. Malinski (Ed.), *Explorations on Martha Rogers' science of unitary human beings* (pp. 173–187). Norwalk, CT: Appleton-Century-Crofts.

Barrett, E.A. (1989). A nursing theory of power for nursing practice: Derivation from Rogers' paradigm. In J. Riehl-Sisca (Ed.), *Conceptual models for nursing practice* (3rd ed.). Norwalk, CT: Appleton & Lange.

Barrett, E.A. (1990). The continuing revolution of Rogers' science-based nursing education. In E.A. Barrett (Ed.), *Visions of Rogers' science-based nursing* (pp. 303–317). New York: National League for Nursing.

Barrett, E.A. (1990). Visions of Rogers' science-based nursing. In E.A. Barrett (Ed.), *Visions of Rogers' science-based nursing* (pp. 31–44). New York: National League for Nursing.

Barrett, E.A. (1991). Space nursing. *Cutis*, 48(4), 299–303.

Barrett, E.A. (2002). What is nursing science? *Nursing Science Quarterly*, 15(1), 51–60.

Barrett, E.A. (2003). A measure of power as knowing participation in change. In O.L. Strickland and C.Diloria (Eds.), *Measurement in nursing outcomes* (2nd ed., Vol. 3), New York: Springer.

Barrett. E.A. (2010). Power as knowing participation in change: What's new and what is next. *Nursing Science Quarterly*, 23(1), 47–54.

Barrett, E.A. and Caroselli, C. (1998). Methodological ponderings related to the power as knowing participation in change tool. *Nursing Science Quarterly*, 11(1), 17–22.

Barrett, E.A., Paletta, J., and Winstead-Fry, P. (1991). Transcultural exploration of measurement scales for the study of Rogers' science of unitary human beings. *Rogerian Nursing Science News*, 4(1), 6.

Barrett, K. (1972). Theoretical construct of the concepts of touch as they relate to nursing. *Nursing Research*, 21, 102–110.

Baumann, S.L. (2005). Exploring being: An international dialogue. *Nursing Science Quarterly*, 18(2), 171–175.

Baumann, S.L., Wright, S.G. and Settecase-Wu, C. (2014). A science of unitary human beings perspective of global health nursing. *Nursing Science Quarterly*, 27(4), 324–328.

Benedict, S.C. and Burge, J.M. (1990). The relationship between human field motion and preferred visible wavelengths. *Nursing Science Quarterly*, 3(2), 73–80.

Benonis, B.C. (1989). The lived experience of recovering from addiction: A phenomenological study. *Nursing Science Quarterly*, 2(1), 37–43.

Berg, M. (2005). A midwifery model of care for childbearing women at high risk: Genuine caring in caring for the genuine. *Journal of Perinatal Education*, 14(1), 9–21.

Biley, F. (1990). Rogers' model: An analysis. *Nursing*, 4(15), 31–33.

Biley, F.C. (1992). The perception of time as a factor in Rogers' science of unitary human beings: A literature review. *Journal of Advanced Nursing*, 17(9), 1141–1145.

Biley, F.C. (1993). Energy fields nursing: A brief encounter of a unitary kind. *International Journal of Nursing Studies*, 30(6), 519–525.

Blair, C. (1979). Hyperactivity in children: Viewed within the framework of synergistic man. *Nursing Forum*, 18, 293–303.

Botha, M.E. (1989). Theory development in perspective: The role of conceptual frameworks and models in theory development. *Journal of Advanced Nursing*, 14(1), 49–55.

Bradshaw, A. (1995). What are nurses doing to patients—A review of theories of nursing past and present. *Journal of Clinical Nursing*, 4(2), 81–92.

Bramlett, M.H., Gueldner, S.H., and Sowell, R.L. (1990). Consumer-centric advocacy: Its connection to nursing frameworks. *Nursing Science Quarterly*, 3(4), 156–161.

Bultemeier, K. (1997). Rogers' science of unitary human beings in nursing practice. In M.R. Alligood et al. (Eds.), *Nursing theory: Utilization and application* (pp. 153–174). St. Louis, MO: Mosby Year Book.

Bultemeier, K. (2002). Rogers' science of unitary human beings in nursing practice. In M.R. Alligood and A. Marriner-Tomey (Eds.), *Nursing theory: Utilization and application* (2nd ed., pp. 267–288). St. Louis, MO: C.V. Mosby.

Burr, H.S. and Northrop, F.S.C. (1935). The electrodynamic theory of life. *The Quarterly Review of Biology*, 10, 322–333.

Butcher, H.K. (1993). Kaleidoscoping in life's turbulence: From Seurat's art to Rogers' nursing science. In M.E. Parker (Ed.), *Patterns of nursing theories in practice* (pp. 183–198). New York: National League for Nursing.

Butcher, H.K. (1994). The unitary field pattern portrait method: Development of a research method for Rogers' science of unitary human beings. In M. Madrid and E.A. Barrett (Eds.), *Rogers' scientific art of nursing practice* (pp. 397–429, 430–435). New York: National League for Nursing.

Butcher, H.K. (2002). Living in the heart of helicy: An inquiry into the meaning of compassion and unpredictability within Rogers' nursing science. *Visions: The Journal of Rogerian Nursing Science*, 10(1), 6–22.

Butcher, H.K. and Forchuk, C. (1992). The overview effect: The impact of space exploration on the evolution of nursing science. *Nursing Science Quarterly*, 5(3), 118–123.

Butcher, H.K. and Malinski, V.M. (2010). Martha Rogers' science of unitary human beings. In M.E. Parker and M.C. Smith (Eds.), *Nursing theories and nursing practice* (3rd ed., pp. 253–276). Philadelphia, PA: F.A. Davis.

Butcher, H.K. and McGonigal-Kenney, M. (2005). Depression and dispiritedness in later life: A 'gray drizzle of horror' isn't inevitable. *American Journal of Nursing*, 105(12), 52–61; quiz 61–62.

Butcher, H.K. and McGonigal-Kenney, M. (2005). Depression and dispiritedness in later life. *American Journal of Nursing*, 105(12), 52–61.

Butcher, H.K. and Parker, N. (1988). Guided imagery within Rogers' science of unitary human beings: An experimental study. *Nursing Science Quarterly*, 1(3), 103–110.

Caggins, R.P. (1991). The Caggins Synergy Nursing Model. *ABNF Journal*, 2(1), 15–18.

Caratao-Mojica, R. (2015). The science of unitary human beings in a creative perspective. *Nursing Science Quarterly*, 28(4), 297–299.

Carboni, J.T. (1991). A Rogerian theoretical tapestry. *Nursing Science Quarterly*, 4(3), 130–136.

Carboni, J.T. (1995). Enfolding health-as-wholeness-and-harmony: A theory of Rogerian nursing practice. *Nursing Science Quarterly*, 8(2), 71–78.

Carboni, J.T. (1995). The Rogerian process of inquiry. *Nursing Science Quarterly*, 8(1), 22–37.

Caroselli, C. (1995). Power and feminism: A nursing science perspective. *Nursing Science Quarterly*, 8(3), 115–119.

Caroselli, C. and Barrett, E.A.M. (1998). A review of the power as knowing participation in change literature. *Nursing Science Quarterly*, 11(1), 9–16.

Cerilli, K. and Burd, S. (1989). An analysis of Martha Rogers' nursing as a science of unitary human beings. In J. Riehl-Sisca (Ed.), *Conceptual models for nursing practice* (3rd ed.). Norwalk, CT: Appleton & Lange.

Chardin, T. (1961). *The phenomenon of man*. New York: Harper Torchbooks.

Clarke, P.N. (1986). Theoretical and measurement issues in the study of field phenomena. The human field and self actualization in healthy women. *Advances in Nursing Science*, 9(1), 29–39.

Cody, W.K. (2003). Theoretical concerns. Paternalism in nursing and healthcare: Central issues and their relation to theory. *Nursing Science Quarterly*, 16(4), 288–296.

Cody, W.K. and Kenney, J.W. (2006). *Philosophical and theoretical perspectives for advanced nursing practice* (4th ed.). Sudbury, MA: Jones & Bartlett Publishers.

Compton, M.A. (1989). A Rogerian view of drug abuse: Implications for nursing. *Nursing Science Quarterly*, 2(2), 98–105.

Coulter, M.A. (1990). A review of two theories of learning and their application in the practice of nurse education. *Nurse Education Today*, 10(5), 333–338.

Covington, H. (2001). Therapeutic music for patients with psychiatric disorders. *Holistic Nursing Practice*, 15(2), 59–69.

Cowling, W.R. (1986). The science of unitary human beings: Theoretical issues, methodological challenges, and research realities. In V. Malinski (Ed.), *Explorations on Martha Rogers' science of unitary human beings*. Norwalk, CT: Appleton-Century-Crofts.

Cowling, W.R. III. (2005). Despairing women and healing outcomes: A unitary appreciative nursing perspective. *Advances in Nursing Science*, 28(2), 94–106.

Cowling, W.R. III. (2006). A unitary healing praxis model for women in despair. *Nursing Science Quarterly*, 19(2), 123–132.

Cowling, W.R. III, Shattell, M.M., and Todd, M. (2006). Hall's authentic meaning of medicalization: An extended discourse. *Advances in Nursing Science*, 29(4), 291–304; discussion 305–307.

Cox, T. (2003). Theory and exemplars of advanced practice spiritual intervention. *Complementary Therapies in Nursing and Midwifery*, 9(1), 30–34.

Dailey, J., Maupin, J., Satterly, M., Schnell, D., and Wallace, T. (1989). Martha E. Rogers: Unitary human beings. In A. Marriner-Tomey (Ed.), *Nursing theorists and their work* (2nd ed.). St. Louis, MO: C.V. Mosby.

Davis, B. (2005). Mediators of the relationship between hope and well-being in older adults. *Clinical Nursing Research*, 14(3), 253–272.

de Jong, A.E., Middelkoop, E., Faber, A.W., and Van Loey, N.E. (2007). Non-pharmacological nursing interventions for procedural pain relief in adults with burns: A systematic literature review. *Burns*, 33(7), 811–827.

Delaney, C. (2005). The spirituality scale: Development and psychometric testing of a holistic instrument to assess the human spiritual dimension. *Journal of Holistic Nursing*, 23(2), 145–167; discussion 168–171.

Delgado, C. (2005). A discussion of the concept of spirituality. *Nursing Science Quarterly*, 18(2), 157–162.

Denison, B. (2004). Touch the pain away: New research on therapeutic touch and persons with fibromyalgia syndrome. *Holistic Nursing Practice*, 18(3), 142–151.

Dijoseph, J. and Cavendish, R. (2005). Expanding the dialogue on prayer relevant to holistic care. *Holistic Nursing Practice*, 19(4), 147–154; quiz 154–155.

Duffey, M. and Muhlenkamp, A.F. (1974). A framework for theory analysis. *Nursing Outlook*, 22(9), 570–574.

Edvardsson, J.D., Sandman, P.O., and Rasmussen, B.H. (2005). Sensing an atmosphere of ease: A tentative theory of supportive care settings. *Scandinavian Journal of Caring Sciences*, 19(4), 344–353.

Egan, M. and Kadushin, G. (1997). Rural hospital social work: Views of physicians and social workers. *Social Work in Health Care*, 26(1), 1–23.

†Egbert, E. (1980, January). Concept of wellness. *Journal of Psychosocial Nursing and Mental Health Services*, 18(1), 9–12.

†Falco, S.M. and Lobo, M.L. (1980). Martha E. Rogers. In The Nursing Theories Conference Group (Eds.), *Nursing theories: The base for professional nursing practice*. Englewood Cliffs, NJ: Prentice-Hall.

Farren, A.T. (2009). An oncology case study demonstrating the use of Roger's science of unitary human beings and standardized nursing languages. *International Journal of Nursing Terminologies and Classifications*, 20(1), 34–39.

Fawcett, J. (1977). The relationship between identification and patterns of change in spouses' body image during and after pregnancy. *International Journal of Nursing Studies*, 14, 199–213.

Fawcett, J. (1984). Rogers' life process model. In J. Fawcett (Ed.), *Analysis and evaluation of conceptual models of nursing*. Philadelphia, PA: F.A. Davis.

Fawcett, J. (2003). The science of unitary human beings: Analysis of qualitative research approaches. *Visions: The Journal of Rogerian Nursing Science*, 11(1), 7–20.

Fawcett, J. (2003). The nurse theorists: 21st century updates—Martha E. Rogers. *Nursing Science Quarterly*, 16(1), 44–51.

Fawcett, J. (2004). The theory of human becoming in action. *Nursing Science Quarterly*, 17(3), 226.

Fawcett, J., Bekel, G., Biley, F.C., and Fragemann, K. (2007). Nursing, healthcare, and culture: A view of the year 2050 from Germany and the United Kingdom. *Nursing Science Quarterly*, 20(3), 232–236.

Fawcett, J. and DeSanto-Madeya (2013). Rogers' science of unitary human beings. In J. Fawcett and S. DeSanto-Madeya (Eds.), *Contemporary nursing knowledge: Analysis and evaluation of nursing models and theories* (3rd ed). Philadelphia, PA: F.A. Davis.

Ference, H. (1986). The relationship of time experience, creativity traits, differentiation, and human field motion. In V. Malinski (Ed.), *Explorations on Martha Rogers' science of unitary human beings*. Norwalk, CT: Appleton-Century-Crofts.

Ference, H. (1989). Comforting the dying: Nursing practice according to the Rogerian model. In J. Riehl-Sisca (Ed.), *Conceptual models for nursing practice* (3rd ed.). Norwalk, CT: Appleton & Lange.

Ference, H. (1989). Nursing science theories and administration. In B. Henry, C. Arndt, M. DiVincenti, and A. Marriner-Tomey (Eds.), *Dimensions of nursing administration: Theory, research, education, practice*. Boston, MA: Blackwell Scientific Publications.

Field, L. and Newman, M. (1982). Clinical application of the unitary man framework: Case study analysis (1980). In M.J. Kim and D.A. Moritz (Eds.), *Classification of nursing diagnosis: Proceedings of the third and fourth national conference*. New York: McGraw-Hill.

Finfgeld-Connett, D. (2006). Meta-synthesis of presence in nursing. *Journal of Advanced Nursing*, 55(6), 708–714.

Fisher, L. and Reichenbach, M. (1987–1988). From Tinkerbell to Rogers (how a fairy tale facilitated an understanding of Rogers' theory of unitary being). *Nursing Forum*, 13(1), 5–9.

Fitzpatrick, J.J. (1980). Patient's perception of time: Current research. *International Nursing Review*, 27, 148–153, 160.

Fitzpatrick, J.J. (1988). Theory based on Rogers' conceptual model. *Journal of Gerontological Nursing*, 14(9), 14–16.

Floyd, J.A. (1983). Research using Rogers' conceptual system: Development of a testable theorem. *Advances in Nursing Science*, 5(2), 37–48.

Forker, J.E. and Billing, C.V. (1989). Nursing therapeutics in a group encounter. *Archives of Psychiatric Nursing*, 3(2), 108–112.

Garon, M. (1992). Contributions of Martha Rogers to the development of nursing knowledge. *Nursing Outlook*, 40(2), 67–72.

Gill, B.P. and Atwood, J.R. (1981). Reciprocity and helicy used to relate mEGF and wound healing. *Nursing Research*, 30(2), 68–72.

Gioiella, E. (1989). Professionalizing nursing: A Rogers legacy. *Nursing Science Quarterly*, 2(2), 61–62.

Gjerberg, E. and Kjolsrod, L. (2001). The doctor-nurse relationship: How easy is it to be a female doctor co-operating with a female nurse? *Social Science and Medicine*, 52(2), 189–202.

Goldberg, W.G. and Fitzpatrick, J.J. (1980). Movement therapy with the aged. *Nursing Research*, 29(6), 339–346.

Graham, I.W., Andrewes, T., and Clark, L. (2005). Mutual suffering: A nurse's story of caring for the living as they are dying. *International Journal of Nursing Practice*, 11(6), 277–285.

Green, C.A. (1998). Critically exploring the use of Rogers' nursing theory of unitary human beings as a framework to underpin therapeutic touch practice. *European Nurse*, 3(3), 158–169.

Gudmunsen, A.M. (1995). Personal reflections on Martha E. Rogers. *Nursing and Healthcare Perspectives on Community*, 16(1), 36–37.

Gueldner, S. (1989). Applying Rogers's model to nursing administration: Emphasis on client and nursing. In B. Henry, C. Arndt, M. DiVincenti, and A. Marriner-Tomey (Eds.), *Dimensions of nursing administration: Theory, research, education, practice*. Boston, MA: Blackwell Scientific Publications.

Gueldner, S.H. (1994). Now she belongs to the ages . . . A pandimensional tribute to the extraordinary life of Martha E. Rogers. *Reflections*, 20(2), 25.

Gueldner, S.H. and Britton, G. (2005). Giving voice to vulnerable persons: Rogerian theory. In M.D. Chesnay (Ed.), *Caring for the vulnerable: Perspectives in nursing theory, practice, and research* (pp. 111–118). Sudbury, MA: Jones & Bartlett Publishers.

Gueldner, S.H., Michel, Y., Bramlett, M.H., Liu, C.F., Johnston, L.W., Endo, E., et al. (2005). The well-being picture scale: A revision of the index of field energy. *Nursing Science Quarterly*, 18(1), 42–50.

Guinane, C.S., McCanless, J., and Giles, D. (2006). What makes our hospitals different: The nursing role in a specialty hospital. *American Heart Hospital Journal*, 4(2), 113–119.

Hagedorn, M.E. and Zahourek, R.P. (2007). Research paradigms and methods for investigating holistic nursing concerns. *Nursing Clinics of North America*, 42(2), 335–353, viii.

Hallett, C.E. (1997). The helping relationship in the community setting: The relevance of Rogerian theory to the supervision of Project 2000 students. *International Journal of Nursing Studies*, 34(6), 415–419.

Hanchett, E.S. (1990). Nursing models and community as client. *Nursing Science Quarterly*, 3(2), 67–72.

Hanchett, E.S. (1992). Concepts from eastern philosophy and Rogers' science of unitary human beings. *Nursing Science Quarterly*, 5(4), 164–170.

Hanley, M.A. and Fenton, M.V. (2007). Exploring improvisation in nursing. *Journal of Holistic Nursing*, 25(2), 126–133.

Hardin, S.R. (2003). Spirituality as integrality among chronic heart failure patients: A pilot study. *Visions: The Journal of Rogerian Nursing Science*, 11(1), 43–53.

Heggie, J., Schoenmehl, P., Chang, M., and Grieco, C. (1989). Selection and implementation of Dr. Martha Rogers' nursing conceptual model in an acute care setting. *Clinical Nurse Specialist*, 3(3), 143–147.

Heidt, P. (1981). Effect of therapeutic touch on anxiety level of hospitalized patients. *Nursing Research*, 30(1), 32–37.

Heise, J.L. (1993). The valuing process. A vehicle for creating reality. *Journal of Holistic Nursing*, 11(1), 56–63.

Hektor, L.M. (1989). Martha E. Rogers: A life history. *Nursing Science Quarterly*, 2(2), 63–73.

Herdtner, S. (2000). Using therapeutic touch in nursing practice. *Orthopedic Nursing*, 19(5), 77–82.

Hill, L. and Oliver, N. (1993). Technique integration. Therapeutic touch and theory-based mental health nursing. *Journal of Psychosocial Nursing and Mental Health Services*, 31(2), 18–22.

Hills, R.G.S. and Hanchett, E. (2001). Human change and individuation in pivotal life situations: Development and testing the theory of enlightenment. *Visions: The Journal of Rogerian Nursing Science*, 9(1), 6–19.

Hosking, P. (1993). Utilizing Rogers' theory of self-concept in mental health nursing. *Journal of Advanced Nursing*, 18(6), 980–984.

Huch, M.H. (1995). Nursing and the next millennium. *Nursing Science Quarterly*, 8(1), 38–44.

Huch, M.H. (1991). Perspectives on health. *Nursing Science Quarterly*, 4(1), 33–40.

Jacono, J. and Jacono, B. (2008). The use of puppetry for health promotion and suicide prevention among Mi'Kmaq youth. *Journal of Holistic Nursing*, 26(1), 50–55.

Johnston, N., Rogers, M., Cross, N., and Sochan, A. (2005). Teaching as if the future matters. *Nursing Education Perspectives*, 26(3), 152–156.

Johnston, R.L., Fitzpatrick, J.J., and Donovan, M.J. (1982). Developmental stage: Relationship to temporal dimensions [Abstract]. *Nursing Research*, 31, 120.

Kao, H.F., Reeder, F.M, Hsu, M.T., and Cheng, S.F. (2006). A Chinese view of the western nursing metaparadigm. *Journal of Holistic Nursing*, 24(2), 92–101.

Karnick, P.M. (2014). The science of unitary human beings continues to flourish. *Nursing Science Quarterly*, 27(1), 29.

†Katz, V. (1971). Auditory stimulation and developmental behavior of the premature infant. *Nursing Research*, 20(3), 196–201.

Kelly, A.E., Sullivan, P., Fawcett, J., and Samarel, N. (2004). Therapeutic touch, quiet time, and dialogue: Perceptions of women with breast cancer. *Oncology Nursing Forum*, 31(3), 625–631.

Kim, M.J. and Moritz, D.A. (Eds.). (1982). *Classification of nursing diagnosis: Proceedings of the third and fourth national conference*. New York: McGraw-Hill.

Kim, H.S. (1983). Use of Rogers' conceptual system in research: Comments. *Nursing Research*, 32(2), 89–91.

Kim, T.S. (2001). Relation of magnetic field therapy to pain and power over time in persons with chronic primary headache: A pilot study. *Visions: The Journal of Rogerian Nursing Science*, 9(1), 27–42.

Kim, T.S. (2008). Science of unitary human beings: An update on research. *Nursing Science Quarterly*, 21(4), 294–299.

Kim, T.S., Kim, C., Park, K.M., Park, Y.S., and Lee, B.S. (2008). The relation of power and well-being in Korean adults. *Nursing Science Quarterly*, 21(3), 247–254.

Kim, T.S., Park, J.S., and Kim, M.A. (2008). The relation of meditation to power and well-being. *Nursing Science Quarterly*, 21(1), 49–58.

King, M.O. and Gates, M.F. (2006). Perceived barriers to holistic nursing in undergraduate nursing programs. *Explore: The Journal of Science and Healing*, 2(4), 334–338.

Kranzman, J. (1993). Use of computer technology in enterostomal therapy nursing. *Journal of Enterostomal Therapy Nursing*, 20(3), 116–120.

Krieger, D. (1975). Therapeutic touch: The imprimatur of nursing. *American Journal of Nursing*, 75(5), 784–787.

Krieger, D. (1976). Healing by the laying on of hands as a facilitator of bioenergetic change: The response of in-vivo human hemoglobin. *International Journal of Psychoenergetic Systems*, 1, 121–129.

Krieger, D. (1979). *Therapeutic touch: How to use your hands to help and heal*. Englewood Cliffs, NJ: Prentice-Hall.

Krieger, D., Peper, E., and Ancoli, S. (1979). Therapeutic touch: Searching for evidence of physiological change. *American Journal of Nursing*, 79, 660–662.

Larkin, D.M. (2007). Ericksonian hypnosis in chronic care support groups: A Rogerian exploration of power and self-defined health-promoting goals. *Nursing Science Quarterly*, 20(4), 357–369.

Laschinger, H.K. and Duff, V. (1991). Attitudes of practicing nurses towards theory-based nursing practice. *Canadian Journal of Nursing Administration*, 4(1), 6–10.

Laurent, C.L. (2000). A nursing theory for nursing leadership. *Journal of Nursing Management*, 8(2), 83–87.

Leddy, S.K. (1995). Measuring mutual process: Development and psychometric testing of the Person-Environment Participation Scale. *Visions: Journal of Rogerian Nursing Science*, 3(1), 20–31.

Leddy, S.K. (2003). A unitary energy-based nursing practice theory: Theory and application. *Visions: The Journal of Rogerian Nursing Science*, 11(1), 21–28.

Leksell, J.K., Johansson, I., Wibell, L.B., and Wikblad, K.F. (2001). Power and self-perceived health in blind diabetic and nondiabetic individuals. *Journal of Advanced Nursing*, 34(4), 511–519.

Lewandowski, W.A. (2002). Patterning of pain and power with guided imagery: An experimental study with persons experiencing chronic pain. *Case Western Reserve University*, March 8.

Lewandowski, W.A. (2004). Patterning of pain and power with guided imagery. *Nursing Science Quarterly*, 17(3), 233–241.

Lewandowski, W. and Good, M. (2007). Chronic pain: A nursing perspective. In S. Kreitler and D. Beltrutti (Eds.), *Handbook of chronic pain* (pp. 361–378). New York: Nova Publishers.

Lewandowski, W, Good, M., and Draucker, C.B. (2005). Changes in the meaning of pain with the use of guided imagery. *Pain Management Nursing*, 6(2), 58–67.

Lewin, K. (1964). *Field theory in the social sciences*. New York: Harper Torchbooks.

Lipp, A. (1998). An enquiry into a combined approach for nursing ethics. *Nursing Ethics*, 5(2), 122–138.

Lowry, R.C. (2002). The effect of an educational intervention on willingness to receive therapeutic touch. *Journal of Holistic Nursing*, 20(1), 48–60.

Macrae, J. (1979). Therapeutic touch in practice. *American Journal of Nursing*, 79, 664–665.

Madrid, M. and Winstead-Fry, P. (1986). Rogers's conceptual model. In P. Winstead-Fry (Ed.), *Case studies in nursing theory*. New York: National League for Nursing.

Magan, S.J., Gibbon, E.J. and Mrozek, R. (1990). Nursing theory applications: A practice model. *Issues in Mental Health Nursing*, 11(3), 297–312.

Malinski, V.M. (1986). *Explorations on Martha Rogers' science of unitary human beings*. Norwalk, CT: Appleton-Century-Crofts.

Malinski, V.M. (1991). The experience of laughing at oneself in older couples. *Nursing Science Quarterly*, 4(2), 69–75.

Malinski, V.M. (2002). Research issues. Developing a nursing perspective on spirituality and healing. *Nursing Science Quarterly*, 15(4), 281–287.

Malinski, V.M. (2006). Dying and grieving seen through a unitary lens. *Nursing Science Quarterly*, 19(4), 296–297.

Malinski, V.M. (2006). Rogerian science-based nursing theories. *Nursing Science Quarterly*, 19(1), 7–12; discussion 16.

Malinski, V.M. (2007). Martha E. Rogers over the years. *Nursing Science Quarterly*, 20(1), 6.

Malinski, V.M. (2008). Research diversity from the perspective of the science of unitary human beings. *Nursing Science Quarterly*, 21(4), 291–293.

Malinski, V.M. (2009). Intentionality, consciousness, and creating community. *Nursing Science Quarterly*, 22(1), 13–14.

Malinski, V.M. (2012). Meditations on the unitary rhythm of dying-grieving. *Nursing Science Quarterly*, 25(3), 239–244.

Manhart, E.A. (1988). Using Rogers' science of unitary human beings in nursing practice. *Nursing Science Quarterly*, 50–51.

Manias, E. and Street, A. (2001). The interplay of knowledge and decision making between nurses and doctors in critical care. *International Journal of Nursing Studies*, 38(2), 129–140.

Marrs, J.A. and Lowry, L.W. (2006). Nursing theory and practice: Connecting the dots. *Nursing Science Quarterly*, 19(1), 44–50.

Martell, L.K. (1999). Maternity care during the post-World War II baby boom: The experience of general duty nurses. *Western Journal of Nursing Research*, 21(3), 387–404.

Mason, T. and Patterson, R. (1990). A critical review of the use of Rogers' model within a special hospital: A single case study. *Journal of Advanced Nursing*, 15(2), 130–141.

Matas, K.E. (1997). Human patterning and chronic pain. *Nursing Science Quarterly*, 10(2), 88–96.

Maville, J.A., Bowen, J.E., and Benham, G. (2008). Effect of healing touch on stress perception and biological correlates. *Holistic Nursing Practice*, 22(2), 103–110.

McSherry, W. and Draper, P. (1998). The debates emerging from the literature surrounding the concept of spirituality as applied to nursing. *Journal of Advanced Nursing*, 27(4), 683–691.

Meleis, A.I. (1988). Book reviews (Malinski, V.M. [1986] Explorations on Martha Rogers' science of unitary human beings). *Research in Nursing and Health*, 11, 59–63.

Mitchell, G.J. and Cody, W.K. (2006). Nursing knowledge and human science: Ontological and epistemological considerations. In W.K. Cody and J.W. Kenney (Eds.), *Philosophical and theoretical perspectives for advanced nursing practice* (pp. 241–256). Sudbury, MA: Jones & Bartlett Publishers.

Moccia, P. (1985). A further investigation of "Dialectical thinking as a means of understanding systems in development: Relevance to Rogers's Principles" [Commentary]. *Advances in Nursing Science*, 7(4), 33–38.

Morse, J.M. (2005). The ramifications of perspective: How theory focuses research, data, and practice. *Journal of Wound, Ostomy & Continence Nursing*, 32(2), 93–100.

Naef, R. (2006). Bearing witness: A moral way of engaging in the nurse-person relationship. *Nursing Philosophy*, 7(3), 146–156.

Newbold, D. and Roberts, J. (2007). An analysis of the demarcation problem in science and its application to therapeutic touch theory. *International Journal of Nursing Practice*, 13(6), 324–330.

Newman, M.A. (1976). Movement, tempo, and the experience of time. *Nursing Research*, 25(4), 273–279.

Newman, M.A. (1979). *Theory development in nursing.* Philadelphia, PA: F.A. Davis.

Newman, M.A. (1986). *Health as expanding consciousness.* St. Louis, MO: C.V. Mosby.

Newman, M.A. (1989). The spirit of nursing. *Holistic Nursing Practice*, 3(3), 1–6.

Newman, M.A. (1994). Theory for nursing practice. *Nursing Science Quarterly*, 7(4), 153–157.

Newman, M.A. (1994). *Health as expanding consciousness.* New York: National League for Nursing

Newman, M.A. (2003). A world of no boundaries. *Advances in Nursing Science*, 26(4), 240–245.

Newman, M.A., Sime, A.M., and Corcoran-Perry, S.A. (1991). The focus of the discipline of nursing. *Advances in Nursing Science*, 14(1), 1–6.

O'Mathuna, D.P., Pryjmachuk, S., Spencer, W., Stanwick, M., and Matthiesen, S. (2002). A critical evaluation of the theory and practice of therapeutic touch. *Nursing Philosophy*, 3(2), 163–176.

Onieva-Zafra, M.D., Garcia, L.H. and del Valle, M.G. (2015). Effectiveness of guided imagery relaxation on levels of pain and depression in patients diagnosed with fibromyalgia. *Holistic Nursing Practice*, 29(1), 13–21.

Overman, B. (1994). Lessons from the Tao for birthing practice. *Journal of Holistic Nursing*, 12(2), 142–147.

Parker, M. and Barry, C. (1999). Community practice guided by a nursing model. *Nursing Science Quarterly*, 12(2), 125–131.

Parse, R.R. (2000). Enjoy your flight: Health in the new millennium. *Visions: The Journal of Rogerian Nursing Science*, 8(1), 26–31.

Parse, R.R. (2002). Transforming healthcare with unitary view of the human. *Nursing Science Quarterly*, 15(1), 46–50.

Perkins, J.B. (2003). Healing through spirit: The experience of the eternal in the everyday. *Visions: The Journal of Rogerian Nursing Science*, 11(1), 29–42.

Pesut, D.J. (1998). Matters of the mind, heart and soul. *Nursing Outlook*, 46(4), 154.

Phillips, J.R. (1989). Science of unitary human being: Changing research perspective. *Nursing Science Quarterly*, 2(2), 57–60.

Phillips, J.R. (1994). Martha E. Rogers' clarion call for global nursing research. *Nursing Science Quarterly*, 7(3), 100–101.

Phillips, J.R. (2000). Rogerian nursing science and research: A healing process for nursing. *Nursing Science Quarterly*, 13(3), 196–201.

Phillips, J.R. (2013). Creating an epiphany with Martha E. Rogers. *Nursing Science Quarterly*, 26(3), 241–246.

Phillips. J.R. (2015). Martha E. Rogers: Heretic and heroine. *Nursing Science Quarterly*, 28(1), 42–48.

Picard, C. and Jones, D.A. (2005). *Giving voice to what we know: Margaret Newman's theory of health as expanding consciousness in nursing practice, research, and education.* Sudbury, MA: Jones & Bartlett Publishers.

Pilkington, F.B. (2005). The concept of intentionality in human science nursing theories. *Nursing Science Quarterly*, 18(2), 98–104.

Pilkington, F.B. (2005). Myth and symbol in nursing theories. *Nursing Science Quarterly*, 18(3), 198–203.

Pilkington, F.B. (2007). Envisioning nursing in 2050 through the eyes of nurse theorists: Rosemarie Rizzo Parse and Martha E. Rogers. *Nursing Science Quarterly*, 20(4), 307–308.

Plummer, M. and Molzahn, A.E. (2009). Quality of life in contemporary nursing theory: A concept analysis. *Nursing Science Quarterly*, 22(2), 134–140.

Polanyi, M. (1958). *Personal knowledge.* Chicago, IL: University of Chicago Press.

†Porter, L.S. (1972). The impact of physical-physiological activity on infant growth and development. *Nursing Research*, 21(3), 210–219.

Powers, C.P., Hart, V.A., Shattell, M. and MacCulloch, T. (2012). The concept of "the will to thrive" in mental health. *Issues in Mental Health Nursing*, 33(11), 805–807.

Proctor, S., Wilcockson, J., Pearson, P., et al. (2001). Going home from hospital: The carer/patient dyad. *Journal of Advanced Nursing*, 35(2), 206–217.

Reis, P.J. and Alligood, M.R. (2014). Prenatal yoga in late pregnancy and optimism, power, and well-being. *Nursing Science Quarterly*, 27(1), 30–36.

Quillin, S.I.M. and Runk, J.A. (1983). Martha Rogers' model. In J.J. Fitzpatrick and A.L. Whall (Eds.), *Conceptual models of nursing: Analysis and application.* Bowie, MD: Robert J. Brady Co.

Quillin, S.I.M. and Runk, J.A. (1989). Martha Rogers' unitary person model. In J.J. Fitzpatrick and A.L. Whall (Eds.), *Conceptual models of nursing: Analysis and application* (2nd ed.). Norwalk, CT: Appleton & Lange.

Quinn, J.F. (1979). One nurse's evolution as a healer. *American Journal of Nursing*, 79, 662–664.

Quinn, J.F. (1989). Therapeutic touch as energy exchange: Replication and extension. *Nursing Science Quarterly*, 2(2), 74–78.

Randell, B.P. (1992). Nursing theory: The 21st century. *Nursing Science Quarterly*, 5(4), 176–184.

Rasmussen, B.H. and Edwardsson, D. (2007). The influence of environment in palliative care: Supporting or hindering experiences of 'at–homeness.' *Contemporary Nurse: A Journal for the Australian Nursing Profession*, 27(1), 119–131.

Reed, P.G. (1991). Toward a nursing theory of self-transcendence: Deductive reformulation using developmental theories. *Advances in Nursing Science*, 13(4), 64–77.

Reed, P.G. and Runquist, J.J. (2007). Reformulation of a methodological concept in grounded theory. *Nursing Science Quarterly*, 20(2), 118–122.

Reeder, F. (1984). Philosophical issues in the Rogerian science of unitary human beings. *Advances in Nursing Science*, 6(2), 14–23.

Reeder, F. (1993). The science of unitary human beings and interpretive human science. *Nursing Science Quarterly*, 6(1), 13–24.

Rew, L. (2005). *Adolescent health: A multidisciplinary approach to theory, research, and intervention*. Thousand Oaks, CA: Sage Publications, Inc.

Ring, M.E. (2009). An exploration of the perception of time from the perspective of the science of unitary human beings. *Nursing Science Quarterly*, 22(1), 8–12.

Ring, M.E. (2009). Reiki and changes in pattern manifestations. *Nursing Science Quarterly*, 22(3), 250–258.

Rogers, M.E. (1963). Building a strong educational foundation. *American Journal of Nursing*, 63(6), 94–95.

Rogers, M.E. (1963). Some comments on the theoretical basis for nursing practice. *Nursing Science*, 63(1), 11–13, 60–61.

Rogers, M.E. (1964). *Reveille in nursing*. Philadelphia, PA: F.A. Davis.

Rogers, M.E. (1969). *Nursing research: Relevant to practice?* In Fifth Annual Research Conference of the American Nurses Association (pp. 352–359). Kansas City, MO: ANA.

†Rogers, M.E. (1970). *An introduction to the theoretical basis of nursing*. Philadelphia, PA: F.A. Davis.

†Rogers, M.E. (1975). Euphemisms in nursing's future. *Image: Journal of Nursing Scholarship*, 7(2), 3–9.

†Rogers, M.E. (1980). Nursing: A science of unitary man. In J.P. Riehl and C. Roy (Eds.), *Conceptual models for nursing practice* (2nd ed.). New York: Appleton-Century-Crofts.

Rogers, M.E. (1980). *The science of unitary man* [Videotapes]. New York: Media for Nursing.

Rogers, M.E. (1981). Beyond the horizon. In N. Chaska (Ed.), *The nursing profession: A time to speak*. New York: McGraw-Hill.

Rogers, M.E. (1981). Science of unitary man: A paradigm for nursing. In G.E. Lasker (Ed.), *Applied systems and cybernetics* (Vol. IV, pp. 219–228). New York: Pergamon Press.

Rogers, M.E. (1983). *Nursing science: A science of unitary human beings*. Paper presented at the First National Rogerian Conference, New York University.

Rogers, M.E. (1983). Science of unitary human being: A paradigm for nursing. In I.W. Clements and F.B. Roberts (Eds.), *Family health: A theoretical approach to nursing care*. New York: John Wiley & Sons.

Rogers, M.E. (1985). A paradigm for nursing. In R. Wood and J. Kekahbah (Eds.), *Examining the cultural implications of Martha E. Rogers' science of unitary human beings*. Lecampton, KS: Wood-Kekahbah Associates.

Rogers, M.E. (1986). Science of unitary human beings. In V. Malinski (Ed.), *Explorations on Martha Rogers' science of unitary human beings*. Norwalk, CT: Appleton-Century-Crofts.

Rogers, M.E. (1987). Rogers's science of unitary human beings. In R.R. Parse (Ed.), *Nursing science: Major paradigms, theories, and critiques*. Philadelphia, PA: W.B. Saunders.

Rogers, M.E. (1987). *Nursing research in the future* (Publication. No. 14–2203, pp. 121–123). New York: National League for Nursing.

Rogers, M.E. (1988). Nursing science and art: A prospective. *Nursing Science Quarterly*, 1(3), 99–102.

Rogers, M.E. (1989). Creating a climate for the implementation of a nursing conceptual framework. *Journal of Continuing Education in Nursing*, 20(3), 112–116.

Rogers, M.E. (1989). Nursing: A science of unitary human beings. In J. Riehl-Sisca (Ed.), *Conceptual models for nursing practice* (3rd ed.). Norwalk, CT: Appleton & Lange.

Rogers, M.E. (1990). Nursing: Science of unitary, irreducible, human beings: Update 1990. In E.A. Barrett (Ed.), *Visions of Rogers' science-based nursing* (pp. 5–11). New York: National League for Nursing.

Rogers, M.E. (1990). Space age paradigm for new frontiers in nursing. In M.E. Parker (Ed.), *Nursing theories in practice* (pp. 105–113). New York: NLN Press.

Rogers, M.E. (1991). Nursing: Science of irreducible human and environmental energy fields [Glossary]. *Rogerian Nursing Science News*, 4(2), 6–7.

Rogers, M.E. (1992). Nursing science and the space age. *Nursing Science Quarterly*, 5(1), 27–34.

Rogers, M.E. (1994). Nursing science evolves. In M. Madrid and E.A. Barrett (Eds.), *Rogers' scientific art of nursing practice* (pp. 3–9). New York: National League for Nursing.

Rogers, M.E. (1994). The science of unitary human beings: Current perspectives. *Nursing Science Quarterly*, 7(1), 33–35.

Rossi, L. and Krekeler, K. (1982). Small-group reactions to the theoretical framework "Unitary Man" (1980). In M.J. Kim and D.A. Moritz (Eds.), *Classification of nursing diagnosis: Proceedings of the third and fourth national conference*. New York: McGraw-Hill.

Roy, C. (1980). Rogers' theoretical basis of nursing. In J.P. Riehl and C. Roy (Eds.), *Conceptual models for nursing practice* (2nd ed.). New York: Appleton-Century-Crofts.

Safier, G. (1977). *Contemporary American leaders: An oral history*. New York: McGraw-Hill.

Salerno, E.M. (2002). Hope, power and perception of self in individuals recovering from schizophrenia: A Rogerian perspective. *Visions: The Journal of Rogerian Nursing Science*, 10(1), 23–36.

Sanchez, R. (1989). Empathy, diversity, and telepathy in mother-daughter dyads: An empirical investigation utilizing Rogers' conceptual framework. *Scholarly Inquiry for Nursing Practice*, 3(1), 29–51.

Sarter, B. (1988). *The stream of becoming: A study of Martha Rogers' theory*. New York: National League for Nursing.

Sarter, B. (1989). Some critical philosophical issues in the science of unitary human being. *Nursing Science Quarterly*, 3, 74–78.

Schneider, P.E. (1995). Focusing awareness: The process of extraordinary healing from a Rogerian perspective. *Visions: Journal of Rogerian Nursing Science*, 3(1), 32–43.

Schodt, C. (1989). Parental-fetal attachment and couvade: A study of patterns of human-environment integrality. *Nursing Science Quarterly*, 2(2), 88–97.

Schumacher, B. (2002). NICU (Neonatal intensive care unit): Staging a dance show [Portuguese]. *Texto & Contexto Enfermagem*, 11(3), 27–35.

Shanley, E., Jubb, M., and Latter, P. (2003). Partnership in coping: An Australian system of mental health nursing. *Journal of Psychiatric and Mental Health Nursing*, 10(4), 431–441.

Shearer, N.B.C. (2009). Health empowerment theory as a guide for practice. *Geriatric Nursing*, 30(2), 4–10.

Shearer, N.B.C., Cisar, N., and Greenberg, E.A. (2007). A telephone-delivered empowerment intervention with patients diagnosed with heart failure. *Heart & Lung*, 36(3), 159–169.

Shearer, N.B.C. and Reed, P.G. (2004). Empowerment: Reformulation of a non-Rogerian concept. *Nursing Science Quarterly*, 17(3), 253–259.

Sherman, D.W. (1997). Rogerian science: Opening new frontiers of nursing knowledge through its application in quantitative research. *Nursing Science Quarterly*, 10(3), 131–135.

Siedliecki, S.L. and Good, M. (2006). Effect of music on power, pain, depression, and disability. *Journal of Advanced Nursing*, 54(5), 553–562.

Smith, D.W. (1995). Power and spirituality in polio survivors: A study based on Rogers' science. *Nursing Science Quarterly*, 8(3), 133–139.

Smith, D.W. and Broida, J.P. (2007). Pandimensional field pattern changes in healers and healees: Experiencing therapeutic touch. *Journal of Holistic Nursing*, 25(4), 217–225; discussion 226–227.

Smith, L.H. and Guthrie, B.J. (2005). Testing a model: A developmental perspective of adolescent male sexuality. *Journal for Specialists in Pediatric Nursing*, 10(3), 124–138.

Smith, M.C. and Kyle, L. (2008). Holistic foundations of aromatherapy for nursing. *Holistic Nursing Practice*, 22(1), 3–9; quiz 10–11.

Smith, M.J. (1986). Human-environment process: A test of Rogers' principle of integrality. *Advances in Nursing Science*, 9(1), 21–28.

Smith, M.J. (1988). Testing propositions derived from Rogers' conceptual system. *Nursing Science Quarterly*, 1(2), 60–67.

Snellman, I. and Wikblad, K. (2006). Health in patients with Type 2 diabetes: An interview study based on the Welfare Theory of Health. *Scandinavian Journal of Caring Services*, 20(4), 462–471.

Stilos, K., Moura, S.L., and Flint, F. (2007). Building comfort with ambiguity in nursing practice. *Clinical Journal of Oncology Nursing*, 11(2), 259–263.

Takahashi, T. (1992). Perspectives on nursing knowledge. *Nursing Science Quarterly*, 5(2), 86–91.

Tettero, I., Jackson, S., and Wilson, S. (1993). Theory to practice: Developing a Rogerian-based assessment tool. *Journal of Advanced Nursing*, 18(5), 776–782.

Timpka, T. (2000). The patient and the primary care team: A small-scale critical theory. *Journal of Advanced Nursing*, 31(3), 558–564.

Todaro-Franceschi, V. (2001). Energy: A bridging concept for nursing science. *Nursing Science Quarterly*, 14(2), 132–140.

Todaro-Franceschi, V. (2006). Studying synchronicity related to dead loved ones AKA after-death communication: Martha, what do you think? *Nursing Science Quarterly*, 19(4), 297–299.

Todaro-Franceschi, V. (2007). Imagining nursing practice in the year 2050: Looking through a Rogerian looking glass. *Nursing Science Quarterly*, 20(3), 229–231.

Todaro-Franceschi, V. (2008). Clarifying the enigma of energy, philosophically speaking. *Nursing Science Quarterly*, 21(4), 285–290.

Tourville, C. and Ingalls, K. (2003). The living tree of nursing theories. *Nursing Forum*, 38(3), 21–30, 36.

Tudor, C.A., Keegan-Jones, L. and Bens, E.M. (1994). Implementing Rogers' science-based nursing practice in a pediatric nursing service setting. In M. Madrid and E.A. Barrett (Eds.), *Rogers' scientific art of nursing practice* (pp. 305–322). New York: National League for Nursing.

Ugarriza, D.N. (2002). Intentionality: Applications within selected theories of nursing. *Holistic Nursing Practice*, 16(4), 41–50.

Uys, L.R. (1987). Foundational studies in nursing. *Journal of Advanced Nursing*, 12(3), 275–280.

Vitale, A. (2007). An integrative review of Reiki touch therapy research. *Holistic Nursing Practice*, 21(4), 167–179; quiz 180–181.

Vitale, A.T. and O'Connor, P.C. (2006). The effect of Reiki on pain and anxiety in women with abdominal hysterectomies: A quasi-experimental pilot study. *Holistic Nursing Practice*, 20(6), 263–272; quiz 273–274.

von Bertalanffy, L. (1968). *General systems theory: Foundations, development, application*. New York: George Braziller.

von Krogh, G., Dale, C., and Naden, D. (2005). A framework for integrating NANDA, NIC, and NOC terminology in electronic patient records. *Journal of Nursing Scholarship*, 37(3), 275–281.

Wadensten, B. and Carlsson, M. (2003). Nursing theory views on how to support the process of ageing. *Journal of Advanced Nursing*, 42(2), 118–124.

Wall, L.M. (2000). Changes in hope and power in lung cancer patients who exercise. *Nursing Science Quarterly*, 13(3), 234–242.

Walling, A. (2006). Therapeutic modulation of the psychoneuroimmune system by medical acupuncture creates enhanced feelings of well-being. *Journal of the American Academy of Nurse Practitioners*, 18(4), 135–143.

Watson, J. (2002). Changing paradigms in epidemiology: Catching up with Martha Rogers. *Visions: The Journal of Rogerian Nursing Science*, 10(1), 37–50.

Watson, J. (2006). Walking pilgrimage as caritas action in the world. *Journal of Holistic Nursing*, 24(4), 289–296.

Watson, J. and Smith, M.C. (2002). Caring science and the science of unitary human beings: A trans-theoretical discourse for nursing knowledge development. *Journal of Advanced Nursing*, 37(5), 452–461.

West, M.M. (2002). Early risk indicators of substance abuse among nurses. *Journal of Nursing Scholarship*, 34(2), 187–193.

Whall, A. (1987). A critique of Rogers's framework. In R.R. Parse (Ed.), *Nursing science: Major paradigms, theories, and critiques*. Philadelphia, PA: W.B. Saunders.

Whelan, K.M. and Wishnia, G.S. (2003). Reiki therapy: The benefits to a nurse/Reiki practitioner. *Holistic Nursing Practice*, 17(4), 209–217.

†Whelton, B.J. (1979). An operationalization of Martha Rogers' theory throughout the nursing process. *International Journal of Nursing Studies*, 16, 7–20.

Winstead-Fry, P. (2000). Rogers' conceptual system and family nursing. *Nursing Science Quarterly*, 13(4), 278–280.

Wright, B.W. (2004). Trust and power in adults: An investigation using Rogers' science of unitary human beings. *Nursing Science Quarterly*, 17(2), 139–146.

Wright, B.W. (2006). Rogers' science of unitary human beings. *Nursing Science Quarterly*, 19(3), 229–230.

Wright, B.W. (2007). The evolution of Roger's science of unitary human beings: 21st century reflections. *Nursing Science Quarterly*, 20(1), 64–67.

Yarcheski, A. and Mahon, N.E. (1991). An empirical test of Rogers' original and revised theory of correlates in adolescents. *Research in Nursing and Health*, 14(6), 447–455.

Yarcheski, A. and Mahon, N.E. (1995). Rogers' pattern manifestations and health in adolescents. *Western Journal of Nursing Research*, 17(4), 383–397.

Yarcheski, A., Mahon, N.E., and Yarcheski, T.J. (2002). Humor and health in early adolescents: Perceived field motion as a mediating variable. *Nursing Science Quarterly*, 15(2), 150–155.

Yarcheski, A., Mahon, N.E., and Yarcheski, T.J. (2004). Health and well-being in early adolescents using Rogers' science of unitary human beings. *Nursing Science Quarterly*, 17(1), 72–77.

Zust, B.L. (2006). Death as a transformation of wholeness: An "aha" experience of health as expanding consciousness. *Nursing Science Quarterly*, 19(1), 57–60.

In addition, the April 1979 volume of the American Journal of Nursing contains three articles on therapeutic touch based on Rogers' conceptual model.

34. Callista Roy

Aggleton, P. and Chalmers, H. (1984). The Roy adaptation model. *Nursing Times*, 80(40), 45–48.

Aktan, N.M. (2007). Functional status after childbirth: A review of the literature. *Clinical Nursing Research*, 16(3), 195–211.

Aktan, N.M. (2012). Social support and anxiety in pregnant and postpartum women: A secondary analysis. *Clinical Nursing Research*, 21(2), 183–194.

Akyil, R.C. and Erguney, S. (2013). Roy's adaptation model-guided education for adaptation to chronic obstructive pulmonary disease. *Journal of Advanced Nursing*, 69(5), 1063–1075.

Alimohammadi, N., Maleksi, B., Shahriari, M. and Chitsaz, A. (2015). Effect of a care plan based on Roy adaptation model biological dimension on stroke patients' physiologic adaptation level. *Iranian Journal of Nursing and Midwifery Research*, 20(2), 275–281.

Andrews, H. (1989). Implementation of the Roy adaptation model: An application of educational change research. In J. Riehl-Sisca (Ed.), *Conceptual models for nursing practice* (3rd ed.). Norwalk, CT: Appleton & Lange.

Andrews, H.A. (1991). Overview of the self-concept mode. In C. Roy and H.A. Andrews (Eds.), *The Roy adaptation model: The definitive statement* (pp. 269–279). Norwalk, CT: Appleton & Lange.

Andrews, H. and Roy, C. (1986). *Essentials of the Roy adaptation model*. Englewood Cliffs, NJ: Prentice-Hall.

Araich, M. (2001). Roy's Adaptive Model: Demonstration of theory integration into process of care in coronary care unit. *Icus and Nursing Web Journal*, (7), 12.

Arai, Y.C., Ito, H., Kandatsu, N., Kurokawa, S., -Kinugasa, S., and Komatsu, T. (2007). Parental presence during induction enhances the effect of oral midazolam on emergence behavior of children undergoing general anesthesia. *Acta Anaesthesiologica Scandinavica*, 51(7), 858–861.

Artinian, N.T. (1991). Stress experience of spouses of patients having coronary artery bypass during hospitalization and 6 weeks after discharge. *Heart and Lung*, 20, 52–59.

Artinian, N.T. (1992). Spouse adaptation to mate's CABG surgery: 1 year follow-up. *American Journal of Critical Care*, 1(2), 36–42.

Ashton, K.S. (2015). The orientation period: Essential for new registered nurses' adaptation. *Nursing Science Quarterly*, 28(2), 142–150.

Bakan, G. and Akyol, A.D. (2008). Theory-guided interventions for adaptation to heart failure. *Journal of Advanced Nursing*, 61(6), 596–608.

Barone, S.H., Roy C.L., and Frederickson, K.C. (2008). Instruments used in Roy adaptation model-based research. *Nursing Science Quarterly*, 21(4), 353–362.

Beeber, A.S. (2008). Interdependence: Building partnerships to continue older adult's residence in the community. *Journal of Gerontological Nursing*, 34(1), 19–25.

Bertalanffy, L. (1968). *General system theory*. New York: George Braziller.

Bhanji, S.M. (2012). Comparison and contrast of Orem's self-care theory and Roy's adaptation model. *Journal of Nursing*, 1(1), 48–53.

Black, K.D. (2007). Stress, symptoms, self-monitoring confidence, well-being, and social support in the progression of preeclampsia/gestational hypertension. *Journal of Obstetric, Gynecologic, and Neonatal Nursing*, 36(5), 419–429.

Blue, C., Brubaker, K., Fine, J., Kirsch, M., Papazian, K., and Riester, C. (1989). Sister Callista Roy: Adaptation model. In A. Marriner-Tomey (Ed.), *Nursing theorists and their work* (2nd ed.). St. Louis, MO: C.V. Mosby.

Boston-Based Adaptation Research in Nursing Society. (1999). *Roy Adaptation Model-Based Research: 25 Years of Contributions to Nursing Science*. Indianapolis, IN: Center Nursing Press.

†Brower, H.T. and Baker, D.J. (1976). Using the adaptation model in a practitioner curriculum. *Nursing Outlook*, 24(11), 686–689.

Buckner, E.B., Simmons, S., Brakefield, J.A., Hawkins, A.K., Feeley, C., Kilgore, L.A.F., et al. (2007). Maturing responsibility in young teens participating in an asthma camp: Adaptive mechanisms and outcomes. *Journal for Specialists in Pediatric Nursing*, 12(1), 24–36.

Bunting, S.M. (1988). The concept of perception in selected nursing theories. *Nursing Science Quarterly*, 1, 168–174.

Burns, D. (2004). Physical and psychosocial adaptation of blacks on hemodialysis. *Applied Nursing Research*, 17(2), 116–124.

Camooso, C., Green, M., and Reilly, P. (1981). Students' adaptation according to Roy. *Nursing Outlook*, 29, 108–109.

Chardin, P.T. (1965). *Hymn of the universe*. S. Bartholomew (Trans.). New York: Harper & Row.

Chayput, P. and Roy, C. (2007). Psychometric testing of the Thai version of coping and adaption processing scale–short form (TCAPS-SF). *Thai Journal of Nursing Council*, 22(3), 29–39.

Chen, C.C. (2005). A framework for studying the nutritional health of community-dwelling elders. *Nursing Research*, 54(1), 13–21.

Chen, C.C., Chang, C.K., Chyun, D.A., and McCorkle, R. (2005). Dynamics of nutritional health in a community sample of American elders: A multidimensional approach using Roy adaptation model. *Advances in Nursing Science*, 28(4), 376–389.

Chen, Y.J. and Narsavage, G.L. (2006). Factors related to chronic obstructive pulmonary disease readmission in Taiwan. *Western Journal of Nursing Research*, 28(1), 105–124.

Chiou, C. (2000). A meta-analysis of the interrelationships between the modes of Roy's adaptation model. *Nursing Science Quarterly*, 13(3), 252–258.

Chung, L.Y., Wong, F.K., and Chan, M.F. (2007). Relationship of nurses' spirituality to their understanding and practice of spiritual care. *Journal of Advanced Nursing*, 58(2), 158–170.

Chung, S.C. (2004). Conceptual models of nursing: International in scope and substance? The case of the Roy adaptation model. *Nursing Science Quarterly*, 17(3), 281–282.

Clements, I.W. and Roberts, F.B. (Eds.). (1983). *Family health: A theoretical approach to nursing care*. New York: John Wiley & Sons.

Coleman, E.A., Tulman, L., Samarel, N., Wilmoth, M.C., Rickel, L., Rickel, M., et al. (2005). The effect of telephone social support and education on adaptation to breast cancer during the year following diagnosis. *Oncology Nursing Forum*, 32(4), 822–829.

Cottrell, B. and Shannahan, M. (1986). Effect of the birth chair on duration of second stage labor and maternal outcome. *Nursing Research*, 35(6), 364–367.

Cottrell, B. and Shannahan, M. (1987). A comparison of fetal outcome in birth chair and delivery table births. *Nursing Research and Health*, 10, 239–243.

Craig, D.I. (1990). The adaptation to pregnancy of spinal cord injured women. *Rehabilitation Nursing*, 15(1), 6–9.

Cunningham, D.A. (2002). Application of Roy's adaptation model when caring for a group of women coping with menopause. *Journal of Community Health Nursing*, 19(1), 49–60.

Dahlen, R. (1980). *Analysis of selected factors related to the elderly person's ability to adapt to visual prostheses following senile cataract surgery*. Doctoral dissertation, University of Maryland.

DeSanto-Madeya, S.A. (2006). A secondary analysis of the meaning of living with spinal cord injury using Roy's adaptation model. *Nursing Science Quarterly*, 19(3), 240–246.

DeSanto-Madeya, S.A. (2009). Adaptation to spinal cord injury for families post-injury. *Nursing Science Quarterly*, 22(1), 57–66.

DiIorio, C. (1989). Application of the Roy model to nursing administration. In B. Henry, C. Arndt, M. DiVincenti, and A. Marriner-Tomey (Eds.), *Dimensions of nursing administration: Theory, research, education, practice*. Boston, MA: Blackwell Scientific Publications.

DiMattio, M.J. and Tulman, L. (2003). A longitudinal study of functional status and correlates following coronary artery bypass graft surgery in women. *Nursing Research*, 52(2), 98–107.

Dixon, E.L. (1999). Community health nursing practice and the Roy Adaptation Model. *Public Health Nursing*, 16(4), 290–300.

Dobratz M. C. (1984), Life closure. In S.C. Roy (Ed.), *Introduction to nursing: An adaptation model* (2nd ed., pp. 497–518). Englewood Cliffs, NJ: Prentice-Hall, Inc.

Dobratz, M.C. (2002). The pattern of the becoming-self in death and dying. *Nursing Science Quarterly*, 15(2), 137–142.

Dobratz, M.C. (2003). Putting the pieces together: Teaching undergraduate research from a theoretical perspective. *Journal of Advanced Nursing*, 41(4), 383–392.

Dobratz, M.C. (2004). Life-closing spirituality and the philosophic assumptions of the Roy adaptation model. *Nursing Science Quarterly*, 17(4), 335–338.

Dobratz, M.C. (2008). Moving nursing science forward within the framework of the Roy adaptation model. *Nursing Science Quarterly*, 21(3), 255–259.

Dobratz, M.C. (2014). Life closure with the Roy adaptation model. *Nursing Science Quarterly*, 27(1), 51–56.

Dobratz, M.C. and Pilkington, F.B. (2004). A dialogue about two nursing science traditions: The Roy adaptation model and the human becoming theory. *Nursing Science Quarterly*, 17(4), 301–307.

Dominiak, M.C. (2004). The concept of branding: Is it relevant to nursing? *Nursing Science Quarterly*, 17(4), 295–300.

Downey, C. (1974). Adaptation nursing applied to an obstetric patient. In J.P. Riehl and C. Roy (Eds.), *Conceptual models for nursing practice* (pp. 151–159). New York: Appleton-Century-Crofts.

Duffy, M.E. (1998). The concept of adaptation: Examining alternatives for the study of nursing phenomena. *Scholarly Inquiry in Nursing Practice*, 12(2), 163–176.

Dunn, H.C. and Dunn, D.G. (1997). The Roy Adaptation Model and its application to clinical nursing practice. *Journal of Ophthalmic Nursing and Technology*, 16(2), 74–78.

Dunn, K.S. (2004). Toward a middle-range theory of adaptation to chronic pain. *Nursing Science Quarterly*, 17(1), 78–84.

Duquette, A.M. (1997). Adaptation: A concept analysis. *Journal of School Nursing*, 13(3), 30–33.

†Farkas, L. (1981). Adaptation problems with nursing home application for elderly persons: An application of the Roy adaptation nursing model. *Journal of Advanced Nursing*, 6(5), 363–368.

Fawcett, J. (1981). Assessing and understanding the cesarean father. In C.F. Kehoe (Ed.), *The cesarean experience: Theoretical and clinical perspectives for nurses*. New York: Appleton-Century-Crofts.

Fawcett, J. (1981). Needs of cesarean birth parents. *Journal of Obstetric, Gynecologic, and Neonatal Nursing*, 10, 371–376.

Fawcett, J. (1984). Roy's adaptation model. In J. Fawcett (Ed.), *Analysis and evaluation of conceptual models of nursing*. Philadelphia: F.A. Davis.

Fawcett, J. (2002). The nurse theorists: 21st century updates—Callista Roy. *Nursing Science Quarterly*, 15(4), 308–310.

Fawcett, J. (2003). Conceptual models of nursing: International in scope and substance? The case of the Roy adaptation model. *Nursing Science Quarterly*, 16(4), 315–318.

Fawcett J. (2005). Using the Roy adaptation model to guide nursing research. *Nursing Science Quarterly*, 18(4), 320–323.

Fawcett, J., Aber, C., Weiss, M., Haussler, S., Myers, S.T., King, C., et al. (2005). Adaptation to cesarean birth: Implementation of an international multisite study. *Nursing Science Quarterly*, 18(3) 204–210.

Fawcett, J. and Henklein, J. (1987). Antenatal education for cesarean birth: Extension of a field test. *Journal of Obstetric, Gynecologic, and Neonatal Nursing*, 16, 61–65.

Field, P.A. (1987). The impact of nursing theory on the clinical decision making process. *Journal of Advanced Nursing*, 12(5), 563–571.

Flood, M. and Scharer, K. (2006). Creativity enhancement: Possibilities for successful aging. *Issues in Mental Health Nursing*, 27(9), 939–959.

Frame, K. (2003). Empowering preadolescents with ADHD: Demons or delights. *Advances in Nursing Science*, 26(2), 131–139.

Frame, K., Kelly, L., and Bayley, E. (2003). Increasing perceptions of self-worth in preadolescents diagnosed with ADHD. *Journal of Nursing Scholarship*, 35(3), 225–229.

Frederickson, K. (2000). Nursing knowledge development through research: Using the Roy adaptation model. *Nursing Science Quarterly*, 13(1), 12–17

Frederickson, K. (2000). Research issues. Nursing knowledge development through research: Using the Roy adaptation model . . . including commentary by Malinski, V.M. *Nursing Science Quarterly*, 13(1), 12–17.

Gagliardi, B.A. (2003). The experience of sexuality for individuals living with multiple sclerosis. *Journal of Clinical Nursing*, 12, 571–578.

Gagliardi, B.A., Frederickson, K., and Shanley, D.A. (2002). Living with multiple sclerosis: A Roy adaptation model-based study. *Nursing Science Quarterly*, 15(3), 230–236.

Galbreath, J.G. (1980). Sister Callista Roy. In The Nursing Theories Conference Group (Eds.), *Nursing theories: The base for professional nursing practice*. Englewood Cliffs, NJ: Prentice-Hall.

†Galligan, A.C. (1979). Using Roy's concept of adaptation to care for young children. *MCN, The American Journal of Maternal Child Nursing*, 4(1), 24–28.

Gless, P.A. (1995). Applying the Roy adaptation model to the care of clients with quadriplegia. *Rehabilitation Nursing*, 20(1), 11–16.

Goodall, D. (2006). Environmental changes increase hospital safety for dementia patients. *Holistic Nursing Practice*, 20(2), 80–84.

Goodwin, J.O. (1980). A cross-cultural approach to integrating nursing theory and practice. *Nurse Educator*, 5(6), 15–20.

Gordon, J. (1974). Nursing assessment and care plan for a cardiac patient. In J.P. Riehl and C. Roy (Eds.), *Conceptual models for nursing practice* (pp. 144–150). New York: Appleton-Century-Crofts.

Granero-Molina, J., Cortes, M.D., Membrive, J.M., Castro-Sanchez, A.M., Entrambasaguas, O.M.L., and Fernandez-Sola, C. (2014). Religious faith in coping with terminal cancer: What is the nursing experience? *European Journal of Cancer Care*, 23(3), 300–309.

Hallen, P. (1981). A holistic model of individual and family health based on a continuum of choice. *Advances in Nursing Science*, 3(4), 27–42.

Hamer, B.A. (1991). Music therapy: Harmony for change. *Journal of Psychosocial Nursing and Mental Health Services*, 29(12), 5–7.

Hamilton, R.J. and Bowers, B.J. (2007). The theory of genetic vulnerability: A Roy model exemplar. *Nursing Science Quarterly*, 20(3), 254–264.

Hanchett, E.S. (1990). Nursing models and community as client. *Nursing Science Quarterly*, 3, 67–72.

Hanna, D.R. (2005). The lived experience of moral distress: Nurses who assisted with elective abortions. *Research and Theory in Nursing Practice*, 19(1), 95–124.

Hanna, D.R. (2006). Using the Roy adaptation model in management of work groups. *Nursing Science Quarterly*, 19(3), 226–227.

Hanna, D.R. and Roy, C. (2001). Roy adaptation model and perspectives on the family. *Nursing Science Quarterly*, 14(1), 9–13.

Hannon-Engel, S.L. (2008). Knowledge development: The Roy adaptation model and bulimia nervosa. *Nursing Science Quarterly*, 21(2), 126–132.

Harrison, L.L., Leeper, J.D., and Yoon, M. (1990). Effects of early parent touch on preterm infants' heart rates and arterial oxygen saturation levels. *Journal of Advanced Nursing*, 15, 877–885.

Helson, H. (1964). *Adaptation-level theory: An experimental and systematic approach to behavior*. New York: Harper & Row.

Henderson, V. (1960). *Basic principles of nursing care*. London, UK: International Council of Nurses.

Hoch, C. (1987). Assessing delivery of nursing care. *Journal of Gerontological Nursing*, 13(1), 10–17.

Huch, M.H. (1987). A critique of the Roy adaptation model. In R.R. Parse (Ed.), *Nursing science: Major paradigms, theories, and critiques*. Philadelphia, PA: W.B. Saunders.

Idle, B.A. (1978). SPAL: A tool for measuring self-perceived adaptation level appropriate for an elderly population. In E.E. Bauwens (Ed.), *Clinical nursing research: Its strategies and findings* (Monograph series No. 2). Indianapolis, IN: Sigma Theta Tau.

Isbir, G.G. and Mete, S. (2013). Experiences with nausea and vomiting during pregnancy in Turkish women based on Roy adaptation model: A content analysis. *Asian Nursing Research*, 7(4), 175–181.

†Janelli, L.M. (1980). Utilizing Roy's adaptation model from a gerontological perspective. *Journal of Gerontological Nursing*, 6(3), 140–150.

†Jones, P.S. (1978). An adaptation model for nursing practice. *American Journal of Nursing*, 78(11), 1900–1906.

Kang, K.A., Miller, J.R., and Lee, W.H. (2006). Psychological responses to terminal illness and eventual death in Koreans with cancer. *Research and Theory in Nursing Practice*, 20(1), 29–47.

Kasemwatana, S. (1982). An application of Roy's adaptation model. *Thai Journal of Nursing*, 31(1), 25–46.

Kehoe, C.F. (1981). Identifying the nursing needs of the postpartum cesarean mother. In C.F. Kehoe (Ed.), *The cesarean experience: Theoretical and clinical perspectives for nurses*. New York: Appleton-Century-Crofts.

Kehoe, C.F. and Fawcett, J. (1981). An overview of the Roy adaptation model. In C.F. Kehoe (Ed.), *The cesarean experience: Theoretical and clinical perspectives for nurses*. New York: Appleton-Century-Crofts.

Keller, J.S. (2006). Implementation of a prechemotherapy educational intervention for women newly diagnosed with breast cancer. *Clinical Journal of Oncology Nursing*, 10(1), 57–60.

Kerr, M.E., Hoskins, L.M., Fitzpatrick, J.J., et al. (1992). Development of definitions for Taxonomy II. *Nursing Diagnosis*, 3(2), 65–71.

Kim, H.S. (1993). Putting theory into practice: Problems and prospects. *Journal of Advanced Nursing*, 18, 1632–1639.

Kurek-Ovshinsky, C. (1991). Group psychotherapy in an acute inpatient setting: Techniques that nourish self-esteem. *Issues in Mental Health Nursing*, 12, 81–88.

Laros, J. (1977). Deriving outcome criteria from a conceptual model. *Nursing Outlook*, 25, 333–336.

Laurent, C.L. (2000). A nursing theory for nursing leadership. *Journal of Nursing Management*, 8(2), 83–87.

Lee, L.Y.K., Tsang, A.Y.K., Wong, K.F., and Lee, J.K.L. (2011). Using the Roy adaptation model to develop an antenatal assessment instrument. *Nursing Science Quarterly*, 24(4), 363–369.

Lefaiver, C.A., Keough, V., Letizia, M., and Lanuza, D.M. (2007). Using the Roy adaptation model to explore the dynamics of quality of life and the relationship between lung transplant candidates and their caregivers. *Advances in Nursing Science*, 30(3), 266–274.

Leuze, M. and McKenzie, J. (1987). Preoperative assessment: Using the Roy's adaptation model. *AORN Journal*, 46(6), 1126–1129, 1131–1134.

Levesque, L. (1980, October 22–24). Rehabilitation of the chronically ill elderly: A method of operationalizing a conceptual model for nursing. In R.C. MacKay and E.G. Zilm (Eds.), *Research for practice: Proceedings of the National Nursing Research Conference*. Halifax, Nova Scotia.

Levesque, L., Ricard, N., Ducharme, F., Duquette, A. and Bonin, J. (1998). Empirical verification of a theoretical model derived from the Roy adaptation model: Findings from five studies. *Nursing Science Quarterly*, 11(1), 31–39.

Levine, M.E. (1966). Adaptation and assessment: A rationale for nursing intervention. *American Journal of Nursing*, 66, 2450–2453.

Lewis, F., et al. (1978). Measuring adaptation of chemotherapy patients. In J.C. Krueger, A.H. Nelson, and M. Opal (Eds.), *Nursing research: Development, collaboration, utilization*. Germantown, MD: Aspen Systems.

Lewis, F., Firsich, S.C., and Parsell, S. (1978). Development of reliable measures of patient health outcomes related to quality nursing care for chemotherapy patients. In J.C. Krueger, A.H. Nelson, and M.O. Wolanin (Eds.), *Nursing research: Development, collaboration, utilization*. Germantown, MD: Aspen.

Lewis, F.M., Firsich, S.C., and Parsell, S. (1979). Clinical tool development for adult chemotherapy patients: Process and content. *Cancer Nursing*, 2(2), 99–108.

Li, H.J. and Shyu, Y.I. (2007). Coping processes of Taiwanese families during the postdischarge period for an elderly family member with hip fracture. *Nursing Science Quarterly*, 20(3), 273–279.

Limandri, B.J. (1986). Research and practice with abused women: Use of the Roy adaptation model as an explanatory framework. *Advances in Nursing Science*, 8(4), 52–61.

Lin, L.L. (2005). Multiple role adaptation among women who have children and re-enter nursing school in Taiwan. *Journal of Nursing Education*. 44(3), 116–123.

Lopes, M.V., Pagliuca, L.M., and Araujo, T.L. (2006). Historical evolution of the concept environment proposed in the Roy adaptation model. *Revista Latino–Americana de Enfermagem*, 14(2), 259–265.

Magee, T. and Roy, C. (2008). Predicting school-age behavior problems: The role of early childhood risk factors. *Pediatric Nursing*, 34(1), 37–44.

Malinski, V.M. (2002). Developing a nursing perspective on spirituality and healing. *Nursing Science Quarterly*, 15(4), 281–287.

Malinski, V.M. (2004). Nursing research in the human science and natural science perspectives. *Nursing Science Quarterly*, 17, 301.

Martorella, G., Côté, J., and Choiniére, M. (2008). Pain catastrophizing: A dimensional concept analysis. *Journal of Advanced Nursing*, 63(4), 417–426.

†Mastal, M.F. and Hammond, H. (1980). Analysis and expansion of the Roy adaptation model: A contribution to holistic nursing. *Advances in Nursing Science*, 2(4), 71–81.

†Mastal, M., Hammond, H., and Roberts, M. (1982). Theory into hospital practice: A pilot implementation. *Journal of Nursing Administration*, 12(6), 9–15.

Maxwell, T., Givant, E., and Kowalski, M.O. (2001). Exploring the management of bone metastasis according to the Roy adaptation model. *Oncology Nursing Forum*, 28(7), 1173–1181.

Mengel, A., Sherman, S., Nahigian, E., and Coleman, I. (1989). Adaptation of the Roy model in an educational setting. In J. Riehl-Sisca (Ed.), *Conceptual models for nursing practice* (3rd ed.). Norwalk, CT: Appleton & Lange.

Modrcin-Talbott, M.A., Harrison, L.L., Groer, M.W., and Younger, M.S. (2003). The biobehavioral effects of gentle human touch on preterm infants. *Nursing Science Quarterly*, 16(1), 60–67.

Morales-Mann, E.T. and Logan, M. (1990). Implementing the Roy model: Challenges for nurse educators. *Journal of Advanced Nursing*, 15, 142–147.

Moreno, M.E., Duran, M.M., and Hernandez, A. (2009). Nursing care for adaptation. *Nursing Science Quarterly*, 22(1), 67–73.

Morgan, P.D., Gaston-Johansson, F., and Mock, V. (2006). Spiritual well-being, religious coping, and the quality of life of African-American breast cancer treatment: A pilot study. *The ABNF Journal*, 17(2), 73–77.

Morgillo-Freeman, S. and Roy, C. (2005). Cognitive behavior therapy and the Roy adaptation model: A discussion of theoretical integration. In S. Morgillo-Freeman and A. Freeman (Eds.), *Cognitive behavior therapy in nursing practice* (pp. 3–27). New York: Springer Publishing Company.

Munn, V.A. and Tichy, A.M. (1987). Nurses' perceptions of stressors in pediatric intensive care. *Journal of Pediatric Nursing*, 2, 405–411.

Nayback, A.M. (2009). PTSD in the combat veteran: Using Roy's adaptation model to examine the combat veteran as a human adaptive system. *Issues in Mental Health Nursing*, 30(5), 304–310.

Newman, D.M. (2005). Functional status, personal health, and self-esteem of caregivers of children in a body cast: A pilot study. *Orthopaedic Nursing*, 24(6), 416–423.

Nicholson Jr., N.R. (2009). Social isolation in older adults: An evolutionary concept analysis. *Journal of Advanced Nursing*, 65(6), 1342–1352.

Nightingale, F. (1859). *Notes on nursing: What it is and what it is not*. London, UK: Harrison. Reprinted 1995. Philadelphia, PA: J.B. Lippincott.

Norris, S., Campbell, L., and Brenkert, S. (1982). Nursing procedures and alterations in transcutaneous oxygen tension in premature infants. *Nursing Research*, 31(6), 330–336.

Nuamah, I.F., Cooley, M.E., Fawcett, J. and McCorkle, R. (1999). Testing a theory for health-related quality of life in cancer patients: A structural equation approach. *Research in Nursing and Health*, 22(3), 231–242.

Ordin, Y., Karayurt, O. and Wellard, S. (2013). Investigation of adaptation after liver transplantation using Roy's adaptation model. *Nursing and Health Sciences*, 15(1), 31–38.

Ospina, A.M., Munoz, L., and Ruiz, C.H. (2012). Coping and adaptation process during puerperium. *Colombia Medica*, 43(2), 167–174.

Perrett, S.E. (2007). Review of Roy adaptation model-based qualitative research. *Nursing Science Quarterly*, 20(4), 349–356.

Perrett, S.E. and Biley, F.C. (2013). A Roy model study of adapting to being HIV positive. *Nursing Science Quarterly*, 26(4), 337–343.

Petchprapai, N. and Winkelman, C. (2007). Mild traumatic brain injury: Determinants and subsequent quality of life. A review of the literature. *Journal of Neuroscience Nursing*, 39(5), 260–272.

Phillips, K.D. (1997). Roy's adaptation model in nursing practice. In M.R. Alligood et al. (Eds.), *Nursing theory: Utilization and application* (pp. 175–200). St. Louis, MO: Mosby Year Book.

Pilkington, F.B., Frederickson, K., and Welsasco-Whetsell, M. (2006). The glass menagerie as heuristic for explicating nursing theory. *Nursing Science Quarterly*, 19(3), 190–196.

Pioli, C. and Sandor, J. (1989). The Roy adaptation model: An analysis. In J. Riehl-Sisca (Ed.), *Conceptual models for nursing practice* (3rd ed.). Norwalk, CT: Appleton & Lange.

Pollock, S.E. (1986). Human responses to chronic illness: Physiologic and psychological adaptation. *Nursing Research*, 35(2), 90–95.

Pollock, S.E., Frederickson, K., Carson, M.A., Massey, V.H., and Roy, C. (1994). Contributions to nursing science: Synthesis of findings from adaptation model research. *Scholarly Inquiry for Nursing Practice*, 8(4), 361–372.

Porth, C.M. (1977). Physiological coping: A model for teaching pathophysiology. *Nursing Outlook*, 25, 781–784.

Rambo, B. (1984). *Adaptation nursing: Assessment and intervention*. Philadelphia, PA: W.B. Saunders.

Ramini, S.K., Brown, R., and Buckner, E.B. (2008). Embracing changes: Adaptations by adolescents with cancer. *Pediatric Nursing*, 34(1), 72–79.

Randell, B., Tedrow, M., and van Landingham, J. (1982). *Adaptation nursing: The Roy conceptual model applied*. St. Louis, MO: C.V. Mosby.

Ranjani, S. (2013). Compare and contrast of Roy and Orem's nursing theory. *International Journal of Innovative Research and Development*, 2(8), 237–240.

Read, C.Y., Perry, D.J., and Duffy, M.E. (2005). Design and psychometric evaluation of the psychological adaptation to genetic information scale. *Journal of Nursing Scholarship*, 37(3), 203–208.

Romino, S.L., Keatley, V.M., Secrest, J., and Good, K. (2005). Parental presence during anesthesia induction in children. *AORN Journal*, 81(4), 780–783, 785–789, 792; quiz 793–796.

Roy Adaptation Association. (2007). Cultural issues of the Roy adaptation model examined. *RAA Review*, 9(2), 2.

Roy, C. (1967). Role cues and mothers of hospitalized children. *Nursing Research*, 16(2), 178–182.

†Roy, C. (1970). Adaptation: A conceptual framework for nursing. *Nursing Outlook*, 18(3), 42–45.

†Roy, C. (1971). Adaptation: A basis for nursing practice. *Nursing Outlook*, 19(4), 254–257.

Roy, C. (1973). Adaptation: Implications for curriculum change. *Nursing Outlook*, 21(3), 163–168.

Roy, C. (1975). Adaptation framework. In *Curriculum innovation through framework application*. Loma Linda, CA: Loma Linda University.

Roy, C. (1975). The impact of nursing diagnosis. *AORN Journal*, 21(6), 1023–1030.

Roy, C. (1976). *Introduction to nursing: An adaptational model*. Englewood Cliffs, NJ: Prentice-Hall.

†Roy, C. (1976). The Roy adaptation model: Comment. *Nursing Outlook*, 24(11), 690–691.

Roy, C. (1977). *Decision-making by the physically ill and adaptation during illness*. Doctoral dissertation, University of California, Los Angeles.

Roy, C. (1978). The stress of hospital events: Measuring changes in level of stress. In M.V. Batey (Ed.), *Symposium on stress: Conference on communicating nursing research*. Boulder, CO: Western Interstate Commission on Higher Education.

Roy, C. (1979, December). Nursing diagnosis from the perspective of a nursing model. In *Nursing diagnosis newsletter* (Vol. 6). St. Louis, MO: St. Louis School of Nursing.

†Roy, C. (1979). Relating nursing theory to education: A new era. *Nurse Educator*, 4(2), 16–21.

†Roy, C. (1980). The Roy adaptation model. In J.P. Riehl and C. Roy (Eds.), *Conceptual models for nursing practice* (2nd ed.). New York: Appleton-Century-Crofts.

Roy, C. (1981). *Introduction to nursing: An adaptation model*. Englewood Cliffs, NJ: Prentice-Hall.

Roy, C. (1981). *A systems model of nursing care and its effect on the quality of human life*. In Proceedings of the International Congress on Applied Systems Research and Cybernetics. London, UK: Pergamon Press.

Roy, C. (1983). The expectant family: Analysis and application of the Roy adaptation model. In I.W. Clements and F.B. Roberts (Eds.), *Family health: A theoretical approach to nursing care*. New York: John Wiley & Sons.

Roy, C. (1983). Roy adaptation model. In I.W. Clements and F.B. Roberts (Eds.), *Family health: A theoretical approach to nursing care*. New York: John Wiley & Sons.

Roy, C. (1983). Theory development in nursing: A proposal for direction. In N. Chaska (Ed.), *The nursing profession: A time to speak*. New York: McGraw-Hill.

Roy, C. (1984). *Introduction to nursing: An adaptation model* (2nd ed.). Englewood Cliffs, NJ: Prentice-Hall.

Roy, C. (1987). Response to "Needs of spouses of surgical patients: A conceptualization within the Roy adaptation model." *Scholarly Inquiry for Nursing Practice*, 1(1), 45–50.

Roy, C. (1987). Roy's adaptation model. In R.R. Parse (Ed.), *Nursing science: Major paradigms, theories, and critiques*. Philadelphia, PA: W.B. Saunders.

Roy, C. (1988). Altered cognition: An information processing approach. In P.H. Mitchell, L.C. Hodges, M. Muwaswes, and C.A. Walleck (Eds.), *AANN's neuroscience nursing: Phenomenon and practice: Human responses to neurological health problems* (pp. 185–211). East Norwalk, CT: Appleton & Lange.

Roy, C. (1988). An explication of the philosophical assumptions of the Roy adaptation model. *Nursing Science Quarterly*, 1(1), 26–34.

Roy, C. (1988). Human information processing. *Annual Review of Nursing Research*, 6, 237–262.

Roy, C. (1989). The Roy adaptation model. In J. Riehl-Sisca (Ed.), *Conceptual models for nursing practice* (3rd ed.). Norwalk, CT: Appleton & Lange.

Roy, C. (1991). The Roy adaptation model in nursing research. In C. Roy and H.A. Andrews (Eds.), *The Roy adaptation model: The definitive statement* (pp. 445–458). Norwalk, CT: Appleton & Lange.

Roy, C. (2000). A theorist envisions the future and speaks to nursing administrators. *Nursing Administration Quarterly*, 24(2), 1–12.

Roy, C. (2000). The visible and invisible fields that shape the future of the nursing care system. *Nursing Administration Quarterly*, 25(1), 119–131.

Roy, C. (2005). A community of scholars. *Nursing Science Quarterly*, 18(2), 121–122.

Roy, C. (2007). *Coping and adaptation processing coping scale* (CAPS). Boston, MA: Boston College

Roy, C. (2007). Update from the future: Thinking of theorist Callista Roy. *Nursing Science Quarterly*, 20(2), 113–116.

Roy. C. (2008). Adversity and theory: The broad picture. *Nursing Science Quarterly*, 21(2), 138–139.

Roy, C. (2009). *The Roy adaptation model* (3rd ed.). Upper Saddle River, NJ: Prentice Hall Health

Roy, C. (2011). Extending the Roy adaptation model to meet changing global needs. *Nursing Science Quarterly*, 24(4), 345–351.

Roy, C. (2011). Research based on the Roy adaptation model: Last 25 years. *Nursing Science Quarterly*, 24(4), 312–320.

Roy, C. and Andrews, H.A. (1991). *The Roy adaptation model: The definitive statement*. Norwalk, CT: Appleton & Lange.

Roy, C. and Andrews, H.A. (1999). *The Roy adaptation model* (2nd ed.). Norwalk, CT: Appleton & Lange.

Roy, C. and Anway, J. (1989). Roy's adaptation model: Theories for nursing administration. In B. Henry, C. Arndt, M. DiVincenti, and A. Marriner-Tomey (Eds.), *Dimensions of nursing administration: Theory, research, education, practice*. Boston, MA: Blackwell Scientific Publications.

Roy, C. and Corliss, C.P. (1993). The Roy adaptation model: Theoretical update and knowledge for practice. In M.E. Parker (Ed.), *Patterns of nursing theory in practice* (pp. 215–229). New York: National League for Nursing.

Roy, C. and Jones, D. (2002). Knowledge Impact Conference 2001: Action plans linking nursing knowledge to practice outcomes. *Research and Theory for Nursing Practice*, 16(1), 63–66.

Roy, C. and Jones, D. (2007). *Nursing knowledge development and clinical practice*. New York: Springer Publishing Company.

Roy, C.L. (1995). Developing nursing knowledge: Practice issues raised from four philosophical perspectives. *Nursing Science Quarterly*, 8(2), 79–85.

Roy, C. and Linendoll, N.M. (2006). Deriving international consensus on mentorship in doctoral education. *Journal of Research in Nursing*, 11(4), 345–353.

Roy, C. and McLeod, D. (1981). Theory of the person as an adaptive system. In C. Roy and S.L. Roberts (Eds.), *Theory construction in nursing: An adaptation model* (pp. 49–69). Englewood Cliffs, NJ: Prentice-Hall.

Roy, C. and Obloy, M. (1978). The practitioner movement: Toward a science of nursing. *American Journal of Nursing*, 78, 1698–1701.

Roy, C. and Roberts, S. (1981). *Theory construction in nursing: An adaptation model*. Englewood Cliffs, NJ: Prentice-Hall.

Roy, C., Whetsell, M.V., and Frederickson, K. (2009). The Roy adaptation model and research: Global Perspective. *Nursing Science Quarterly*, 22(3), 209–211.

Roy, C. and Zhan, L. (2006). Sister Callista Roy's adaptation model and its applications. In M. Parker (Ed.), *Nursing theories and nursing practice* (2nd ed., pp. 268–280). Philadelphia, PA: F.A. Davis.

Samarel, N., Tulman, L., and Fawcett, J. (2002). Effects of two types of social support and education on adaptation to early-stage breast cancer. *Research in Nursing and Health*, 25, 459–470.

Sato, M. (1986). The Roy adaptation model. In P. Winstead-Fry (Ed.), *Case studies in nursing theory*. New York: National League for Nursing.

†Schmitz, M. (1980). The Roy adaptation model: Application in a community setting. In J.P. Riehl and C. Roy (Eds.), *Conceptual models for nursing practice* (2nd ed., pp. 193–206). New York: Appleton-Century-Crofts.

Scura, K.W., Budin, W., and Garfing, E. (2004). Telephone social support and education for adaptation to prostate cancer: A pilot study. *Oncology Nursing Forum*, 31(2), 335–338.

Senesac, P. and Roy, C. (2015). Sister Callista Roy's adaptation model. In M.C. Smith and M.E. Parker (Eds.), *Nursing theories and nursing practice* (4th ed.). Philadelphia, PA: F.A. Davis.

Shah, M., Abdullah, A., and Khan, H. (2013). Compare and contrast of grand theories: Orem's self-care deficit theory and Roy's adaptation model. *International Journal of Science and Research*, 4(1), 1834–1837. Retrieved from www.ijsr.net

Shyu, Y. (2000). Role tuning between caregiver and care receiver during discharge transition: An illustration of role function mode in Roy's adaptation theory. *Nursing Science Quarterly*, 13(4), 323–331.

Shyu, Y., Liang, J., Lu, J.R., and Wu, C. (2004). Environmental barriers and mobility in Taiwan: Is the Roy adaptation model applicable? *Nursing Science Quarterly*, 17(2), 165–170.

Silva, M.C. (1987). Needs of spouses of surgical patients: A conceptualization within the Roy adaptation model. *Scholarly Inquiry for Nursing Practice*, 1, 29–44.

Smith, C.E., Pace, K., Kochinda, C., Kleinbeck, S.V.M., Koehler, J., and Popkess-Vawter, S. (2002). Caregiving effectiveness model evolution to a midrange theory of home care: A process for critique and replication. *Advances in Nursing Science*, 25(1), 50–64.

Smith, M. (1988). Roy adaptation model in practice. *Nursing Science Quarterly*, 1(2), 97–98.

†Starr, S.L. (1980). Adaptation applied to the dying patient. In J.P. Riehl and C. Roy (Eds.), *Conceptual models for nursing practice* (2nd ed.). New York: Appleton-Century-Crofts.

Strohmyer, L.L., Noroian, E.L., Patterson, L.M., and Carlin, B.P. (1993). Adaptation six months after multiple trauma: A pilot study. *Journal of Neuroscience Nursing*, 25, 30–37.

Swimme, B. and Berry, T. (1992). *The universe story*. San Francisco, CA: Harper Collins.

Tanyi, R.A. and Werner, J.S. (2003). Adjustment, spirituality, and health in women on hemodialysis. *Clinical Nursing Research*, 12(3), 229–245.

Tiedman, M.E. (1983). The Roy adaptation model. In J.J. Fitzpatrick and A.L. Whall (Eds.), *Conceptual models of nursing: Analysis and application*. Bowie, MD: Robert J. Brady Co.

Tiedman, M.E. (1989). The Roy adaptation model. In J.J. Fitzpatrick and A.L. Whall (Eds.), *Conceptual models of nursing: Analysis and application* (2nd ed.). Norwalk, CT: Appleton & Lange.

Thomas, C.M. (2007). The influence of self-concept on adherence to recommended health regimens in adults with heart failure. *Journal of Cardiovascular Nursing*, 22(5), 405–416.

Tsai, P. (2003). A middle-range theory of caregiver stress. *Nursing Science Quarterly*, 16(2), 137–145.

Tsai, P.F. (2005). Predictors of distress and depression in elders with arthritic pain. *Journal of Advanced Nursing*, 51(2), 158–165.

Tsai, P.F., Tak, S., Moore, C., and Palencia, I. (2003). Testing a theory of chronic pain. *Journal of Advanced Nursing*, 43(2), 158–169.

Tulman, L. and Fawcett, J. (1988). Return of functional ability after childbirth. *Nursing Research*, 37(2), 77–81.

Tulman, L. and Fawcett, J. (2007). Development of the comprehensive inventory of functioning-cancer. *Cancer Nursing*, 30(3), 205–212.

Uding, J., Jackson, E., and Hart, A.L. (2002). Efficacy of a teaching intervention on nurses' knowledge regarding diabetes. *Journal of Nurses Staff Development*, 18(6), 297–303.

Villareal, E. (2003). Using Roy's adaptation model when caring for a group of young women contemplating quitting smoking. *Public Health Nursing*, 20(5), 377–384.

von Krogh, G. and Naden, D. (2008). A nursing-specific model of EPR documentation: Organizational and professional requirements. *Journal of Nursing Scholarship*, 40(1), 68–75.

Wadensten, B. and Carlsson, M. (2003). Nursing theory views on how to support the process of ageing. *Journal of Advanced Nursing*, 42(2), 118–124.

†Wagner, P. (1976). The Roy adaptation model: Testing the adaptation model in practice. *Nursing Outlook*, 24(11), 682–685.

Wallace, C.L. (1993). Resources for nursing theories in practice. In M.E. Parker (Ed.), *Patterns of nursing theories in practice* (pp. 301–311). New York: National League for Nursing.

Waweru, S.M., Reynolds, A., and Buckner, E.B. (2008). Perceptions of children with HIV/AIDS from the USA and Kenya: Self-concept and emotional indicators. *Pediatric Nursing*, 34(2), 117–124.

Weinert, C., Cudney, S., and Spring, A. (2008). Evolution of a conceptual model for adaptation to chronic illness. *Journal of Nursing Scholarship*, 40(4), 364–372.

Weiss, M., Fawcett, J., and Aber, C. (2009). Adaptation, postpartum concerns, and learning needs in the first two weeks after caesarean birth. *Journal of Clinical Nursing*, 18(21), 2938–2948.

Wendler, M.C. (2003). Effects of Tellington touch in healthy adults awaiting venipuncture. *Research in Nursing and Health*, 26(1), 40–52.

Whittemore, R., Chase, S., Mandle, C.L., and Roy, C. (2001). The content, integrity, and efficacy of a nurse coaching intervention in type 2 diabetes. *Diabetes Educator*, 27(6), 887–898.

Whittemore, R., Chase, S., Mandle, C.L., and Roy, C. (2002). Lifestyle changes in type 2 diabetes: A process model. *Nursing Research*, 51(1), 18–25.

Whittemore, R. and Roy, C. (2002). Adapting to diabetes mellitus: A theory synthesis. *Nursing Science Quarterly*, 15(4), 311–317.

Willis, D.G., DeSanto-Madeya, S., Ross, R., Sheehan, D.L., and Fawcett, J. (2015). Spiritual healing in the aftermath of childhood maltreatment: Translating men's lived experiences utilizing nursing conceptual models and theory. *Advances in Nursing Science*, 38(3), 162–174.

Woods, S.J. and Isenberg, M.A. (2001). Adaptation as a mediator of intimate abuse and traumatic stress in battered women. *Nursing Science Quarterly*, 14(3), 215–221.

Wright, P.S., Piazza, D., Holcombe, J., and Foote, A. (1994). A comparison of three theories of nursing used as a guide for the nursing care of an 8–year-old child with leukemia. *Journal of Pediatric Oncology*, 11(1), 14–19.

Yeh, C. (2002). Health-related quality of life in pediatric patients with cancer: A structural equation approach with the Roy adaptation model. *Cancer Nursing*, 25(1), 74–80.

Yeh, C. (2003). Psychosocial distress: Testing hypotheses based on Roy's adaptation model. *Nursing Science Quarterly*, 16(3), 255–263.

Yoder, L.H. (2005). Using the Roy adaptation model: A program of research in a military nursing research service. *Nursing Science Quarterly*, 18(4), 321–323; discussion 320.

Young-McCaughan, S., Mays, M.Z., Arzola, S.M., Yoder, L.H., Dramiga, S.A., Leclerc, K.M., et al. (2003). Change in exercise tolerance, activity and sleep patterns, and quality of life in patients with cancer participating in a structured exercise program. *Oncology Nursing Forum*, 30(3), 441–454.

Zeigler, L., Smith, P.A., and Fawcett, J. (2004). Breast cancer: Evaluation of the Common Journey Breast Cancer Support Group. *Journal of Clinical Nursing*, 13(4), 467–478.

35. Joyce Travelbee

Allen, D. (2007). What do you do at work? Profession building and doing nursing. *International Nursing Review*, 54(1), 41–48.

Barker, P. (2000). Reflections on caring as a virtue ethic within an evidence-based culture. *International Journal of Nursing Studies*, 37(4), 329–336.

Barker, P., Buchanan-Barker, P., and Whitehill, I. (2005). *The tidal model: A guide for mental health professionals*. New York: Psychology Press.

Barker, P.J., Reynolds, W., and Ward, T. (1995). The proper focus of nursing—A critique of the caring ideology. *International Journal of Nursing Studies*, 32(4), 386–397.

Barrett-Leonard, G.T. (1962). Dimensions of therapist responses as causal factors in therapeutic change. *Psychological Monographs*, 76(43, Whole No. 562), 1–33.

Begat, I.B.E. and Severinsson, E.I. (2001). Nurses' reflections on episodes occurring during their provision of care—An interview study. *International Journal of Nursing Studies*, 38(1), 71–77.

Bennett, J. (1998). Fear of contagion: A response to stress? *Advances in Nursing Science*, 21(1), 76–87.

Bennett, J.A. (1995). Nurses' attitudes about acquired-immunodeficiency-syndrome care—What research tells us. *Journal of Professional Nursing*, 11(6), 339–350.

Bennett, J.A. (1997). A case for theory triangulation. *Nursing Science Quarterly*, 10(2), 97–102.

Berg, G.V., Hedelin, B., and Sarvimaki, A. (2005). A holistic approach to the promotion of older hospital patients' health. *International Nursing Review*, 52(1), 73–80.

Berg, G.V., Sarvimaki, A., and Hedelin, B. (2006). Hospitalized older peoples' views of health and health promotion. *International Journal of Older People Nursing*, 1(1), 25–33.

Bergland, A. and Kirkevold, M. (2005). Resident-caregiver relationships and thriving among nursing home residents. *Research in Nursing & Health*, 28(5), 365–375.

Berg, M. (2005). A midwifery model of care for childbearing women at high risk: Genuine caring in caring for the genuine. *Journal of Perinatal Education*, 14(1), 9–21.

Bullough, V.L. and Bullough, B. (1997). Sex education in American nursing—A historical view. *Nursing History Review*, 5, 199–217.

Bunston, T., Mings, D., Mackie, A., et al. (1995). Facilitating hopefulness: The determinants of hope. *Journal of Psychosocial Oncology*, 13(4), 79–103.

Cartwright, R.D. and Lerner, B. (1963). Empathy, need to change, and improvement with psychotherapy. *Journal of Consulting Psychology*, 27, 138–144.

Chin, R. (1974). The utility of system models and developmental models for practitioners. In J. Riehl and C. Roy (Eds.), *Conceptual models in nursing practice*. New York: Appleton-Century-Crofts.

Chinsky, J.M. and Rappaport, J. (1970). Brief critique of the meaning and reliability of "accurate empathy" ratings. *Psychological Bulletin*, 73, 379–382.

Coffey, S. (2006). The nurse-patient relationship in cancer care as a shared covenant: A concept analysis. *Advances in Nursing Science*, 29(4), 308–323.

Cook, L. (1989). Nurses in crisis: A support group based on Travelbee's nursing theory. *Nursing and Health Care*, 10(4), 203–205.

Cutcliffe, J.R. and Goward, P. (2000). Mental health nurses and qualitative research methods: A mutual attraction? *Journal of Advanced Nursing*, 31(3), 590–598.

Davis, L.A. (2006). Hospitalized patients' expectations of spiritual care from nurses. In S.D. Ambrose (Ed.), *Religion and Psychology: New Research* (pp. 1–38). New York: Nova Publishers.

Delmar, C., Boje, T., Dylmer, D., Forup, L., Jakobsen, C., Moller, M., et al. (2005). Achieving harmony with oneself: Life with a chronic illness. *Scandinavian Journal of Caring Sciences*, 19(3), 204–212.

Dennison, S. (1995). An exploration of the communication that takes place between nurses and patients while cancer-chemotherapy is administered. *Journal of Clinical Nursing*, 4(4), 227–233.

Dewar, A.L. and Morse, J.M. (1995). Unbearable incidents— Failure to endure the experience of illness. *Journal of Advanced Nursing*, 22(5), 957–964.

Doona, M.E. (1979). *Travelbee's intervention in psychiatric nursing* (2nd ed.). Philadelphia, PA: F.A. Davis.

Duffey, M. and Muhlenkamp, A.F. (1974). A framework for theory analysis. *Nursing Outlook*, 22(9), 570–574.

Dutra, L.C.R. and Assuncao, A.N. (2000). Developing a practice on the nursing communication process under the light of Joyce Travelbee's theory [Portuguese]. *Texto & Contexto Enfermagem*, 9(2 Part 1), 211–225.

England, M. (2005). Analysis of nurse conversation: Methodology of the process recording. *Journal of Psychiatric and Mental Health Nursing*, 12(6), 661–671.

Farrell, G.A. (2001). From tall poppies to squashed weeds: Why don't nurses pull together more? *Journal of Advanced Nursing*, 35(1), 26–33.

Fochtman, D. (2006). The concept of suffering in children and adolescents with cancer. *Journal of Pediatric Oncology Nursing*, 23(2), 92–102.

Frankel, V. (1963). *Man's search for meaning: An introduction to logotherapy*. New York: Washington Square Press.

Freihofer, P. and Felton, G. (1976). Nursing behaviors in bereavement: An exploratory study. *Nursing Research*, 25(5), 332–337.

Fujieda, T. (1998). On interpersonal aspects of nursing by Joyce Travelbee [Japanese]. *Kangogaku Zasshi—Japanese Journal of Nursing*, 52(3), 222–223.

Gadow, S. (1980). Introduction. In Spickor and S. Gadow (Eds.), *Nursing: Images and ideals—Opening dialogue with the humanities*. New York: Springer-Verlag.

Hall-Lord, M. and Larsson, B.W. (2005). Experiences of pain, distress, and quality of care in relation to different perspectives. In K.V. Oxington (Ed.), *Psychology of stress* (pp. 207–254). New York: Nova Publishers.

Hasegawa, H. (1998). On interpersonal aspects of nursing by Joyce Travelbee [Japanese]. *Kangogaku Zasshi—Japanese Journal of Nursing*, 52(1), 14–15.

Haugan, G. (2013). Nurse-patient interaction is a resource for hope, meaning in life and self-transcendence in nursing home patients. *Scandinavian Journal of Caring Sciences*, 28(1), 74–88.

Haugan, G. (2013). The relationship between nurse-patient interaction and meaning-in-life in cognitively intact nursing home patients. *Journal of Advanced Nursing*, 70(1), 107–120.

Haugan, G., Innstrand, S.T., and Moksnes, U.K. (2013). The effect of nurse-patient interaction on anxiety and depression in cognitively intact nursing home patients. *Journal of Clinical Nursing*, 22, 2192–2205.

Haugan, G., Rannestad, T., Hanssen, B. and Espnes, G.A. (2012). Self-transcendence and nurse-patient interaction in cognitively intact nursing home patients. *Journal of Clinical Nursing*, 21, 3429–3441.

Hawley, G. (1998). Facing uncertainty and possible death: The Christian patients' experience. *Journal of Clinical Nursing*, 7(5), 467–478.

Herth, K. (2005). State of the science of hope in nursing practice: Hope, the nurse, and the patient. In J.A. Elliott (Ed.), *Interdisciplinary perspectives on hope* (pp. 169–211). New York: Nova Publishers.

Hertzberg, A. and Ekman, S.L. (2000). "We, not them and us?"—Views on the relationships and interactions between staff and relatives of older people permanently living in nursing homes. *Journal of Advanced Nursing*, 31(3), 614–622.

Hilton, P.A. (1997). Theoretical perspectives of nursing: A review of the literature. *Journal of Advanced Nursing*, 26(6), 1211–1220.

Hines-Martin, V. and Robinson, K. (2006). Supervision as professional development for psychiatric mental health nurses. *Clinical Nurse Specialist*, 20(6), 293–297.

Hisama, K.K. (2001). The acceptance of nursing theory in Japan: A cultural perspective. *Nursing Science Quarterly*, 14(3). 255–259.

Hobble, W., Lansinger, T., and Magers, J. (1989). Joyce Travelbee: Human-to-human relationship. In A. Marriner-Tomey (Ed.), *Nursing theorists and their work* (2nd ed.). St. Louis, MO: C.V. Mosby.

Jones, A. (2005). Perceptions on individualized approaches to mental health care. *Journal of Psychiatric and Mental Health Nursing*, 12(4), 396–404.

Kirby, C. (2006). The therapeutic relationship. In J. Cooper (Ed.), *Stepping into palliative care 1: Relationships and responses* (2nd ed., pp. 81–88). Abingdon: Radcliffe Publishing.

Kirk, T.W. (2007). Beyond empathy: Clinical intimacy in nursing practice. *Nursing Philosophy*, 8(4), 233–243.

Kitson, A.L. (1996). Does nursing have a future? *British Medical Journal*, 313(7072), 1647–1651.

Kurtz, R.R. and Grummon, D.L. (1972). Different approaches to the measurement of therapist empathy and their relationship to therapy outcomes. *Journal of Consulting and Clinical Psychology*, 30, 106–115.

Kylma, J. (2005). Dynamics of hope in adults living with HIV/AIDS: A substantive theory. *Journal of Advanced Nursing*, 52(6), 620–630.

Landmark, B.T., Strandmark, M., and Wahl, A.K. (2001). Living with newly diagnoses breast cancer: The meaning of existential issues—A qualitative study of 10 women with newly diagnosed breast cancer, based on grounded theory. *Cancer Nursing*, 24(3), 220–226.

Larsson, I.E., Sahlsten, M.J., Sjostrom, B., Lindencrona, C.S., and Plos, K.A. (2007). Patient participation in nursing care from a patient perspective: A grounded theory study. *Scandinavian Journal of Caring Sciences*, 21(3), 313–320.

Lego, S. (1999). The one-to-one nurse-patient relationship. *Perspectives in Psychiatric Care*, 35(4), 4–23.

Lohne, V. and Severinsson, E. (2006). The power of hope: Patients' experiences of hope a year after acute spinal cord injury. *Journal of Clinical Nursing*, 15(3), 315–323.

May, R. (1953). *Man's search for himself.* New York: W.W. Norton.

McBride, M.A. (1967). Nursing approach, pain, and relief: An exploratory experiment. *Nursing Research*, 16(4), 337–341.

McCann, T.V. and Baker, H. (2001). Mutual relating: Developing interpersonal relationships in the community. *Journal of Advanced Nursing*, 34(4), 530–537.

Morse, J.M. (2001). Toward a praxis theory of suffering. *Advances in Nursing Science*, 24(1), 47–59.

Morse, J.M. (2005). Towards a praxis theory of suffering. In J.R, Cutcliff and H.P. McKenna (Eds.), *The essential concepts of nursing* (pp. 257–272). New York: Elsevier, Churchill Livingstone.

Morse, J.M., Bottorff, J., Anderson, G., O'Brien, B., and Solberg, S. (2006). Beyond empathy: Expanding expressions of caring. *Journal of Advanced Nursing*, 53(1), 75–87.

Moses, M.M. (1994). Caring incidents: A gift to the present. *Journal of Holistic Nursing*, 12(2), 193–203.

Narayanasamy, A. (1999). Learning spiritual dimensions of care from a historical perspective. *Nursing Education Today*, 19(5), 386–395.

Nordby, H. (2006). Nurse-patient communication: Language mastery and concept possession. *Nursing Inquiry*, 13(1), 64–72.

Nordby, H. (2007). Meaning and normativity in nurse-patient interaction. *Nursing Philosophy*, 8(1), 16–27.

Nowak, K.B. and Wandel, J.C. (1998). The sharing of self in geriatric clinical practice: Case report and analysis. *Geriatric Nursing*, 19(1), 34–37.

Nystrom, M. (2007). A patient-oriented perspective in existential issues: A theoretical argument for applying Peplau's interpersonal relation model in healthcare science and practice. *Scandinavian Journal of Caring Sciences*, 21(2), 282–288.

O'Baugh, J., Wilkes, L.M., Luke, S., and George, A. (2008). Positive attitude in cancer: The nurse's perspective. *International Journal of Nursing Practice*, 14, 109–114.

Odling, G., Danielson, E., Christensen, S.B., et al. (1998). Living with breast cancer: Caregivers' perceptions in a surgical ward. *Cancer Nursing*, 21(3), 187–195.

O'Gorman, S.M. (1998). Death and dying in contemporary society: An evaluation of current attitudes and the rituals associated with death and dying and their relevance to recent understandings of health and healing. *Journal of Advanced Nursing*, 27(6), 1127–1135.

Olsen, D.P. (1997). When the patient causes the problem: The effect of patient responsibility on the nurse-patient relationship. *Journal of Advanced Nursing*, 26(3), 515–522.

Parrish, E., Peden, A., and Staten, R.T. (2008). Strategies used by advanced practice psychiatric nurses in treating adults with depression. *Perspectives in Psychiatric Care*, 44(4), 232–240.

Pascoe, E. (1996). The value to nursing research of Gadamer's hermeneutic philosophy. *Journal of Advanced Nursing*, 24(6), 1309–1314.

Patistea, E. (1999). Nurses' perceptions of caring as documented in theory and research. *Journal of Clinical Nursing*, 8(5), 487–495.

Pillon, S.C. and Laranjeira, R.R. (2005). Formal education and nurses' attitudes towards alcohol and alcoholism in a Brazilian sample. *Sao Paulo Medical Journal*, 123(4), 175–180.

Puchalski, C.M., Lunsford, B., Harris, M.H., and Miller, R.T. (2006). Interdisciplinary spiritual care for seriously ill and dying patients: A collaborative model. *Cancer Journal*, 12(5), 398–416.

Rawnsley, M.M. (1997). A case for theory triangulation—Response. *Nursing Science Quarterly*, 10(2), 103–106.

Repique, R.J. (2007). Computers and information technologies in psychiatric nursing. *Perspectives in Psychiatric Care*, 43(2), 77–83.

Rich, K.L. (2005). Ethics in geriatric and chronic illness nursing. In J.B. Butts and K. Rich (Eds.), *Nursing ethics: Across the curriculum and into practice* (pp. 175–202). Sudbury, MA: Jones & Bartlett Publishers.

Rich, K.L. (2005). Ethics in psychiatric and mental health nursing. In J.B. Butts and K. Rich (Eds.), *Nursing ethics: Across the curriculum and into practice* (pp. 147–174). Sudbury, MA: Jones & Bartlett Publishers.

Ross, L. (1995). The spiritual dimension—Its importance to patients' health, well-being and quality-of-life and its implications for nursing practice. *International Journal of Nursing Studies*, 32(5), 457–468.

Rustoen, T. (1995). Hope and quality-of-life, two central issues for cancer patients—A theoretical analysis. *Cancer Nursing*, 18(5), 355–361.

Rustoen, T. and Hanestad, B.R. (1998). Nursing intervention to increase hope in cancer patients. *Journal of Clinical Nursing*, 7(1), 19–27.

Rustoen, T. and Wiklund, I. (2000). Hope in newly diagnosed patients with cancer. *Cancer Nursing*, 23(3), 214–219.

Rusteon, T., Wiklund, I., Hanestad, B.R., et al. (1998). Nursing intervention to increase hope and quality of life in newly diagnosed cancer patients. *Cancer Nursing*, 21(4), 235–245.

Sadala, M.L.A. (1999). Taking care as a relationship: A phenomenological view. *Journal of Advanced Nursing*, 30(4), 808–817.

Saegrov, S. and Lorensen, M. (2006). Cancer patients' opinions concerning post-treatment follow-up. *European Journal of Cancer Care (Engl)*, 15(1), 56–64.

Sahlsten, M.J., Larsson, I.E., Lindencrona, C.S., and Plos, K.A. (2005). Patient participation in nursing care: An interpretation by Swedish registered nurses. *Journal of Clinical Nursing*, 14(1), 35–42.

Sahlsten, M.J., Larsson, I.E., Plos, K.A., and Lindencrona, C.S. (2005). Hindrance for patient participation in nursing care. *Scandinavian Journal of Caring Sciences*, 19(3), 223–229.

Sahlsten, M.J., Larsson, I.E., Sjostrom, B., Lindencrona, C.S., and Plos, K.A. (2007). Patient participation in nursing care: Towards a concept clarification from a nurse perspective. *Journal of Clinical Nursing*, 16(4), 630–637.

Sarlore, J.P. (1966). Existentialism. In W.V. Spanos (Ed.), *A casebook on existentialism.* New York: Thomas V. Crowell.

Scanlon, A. (2006). Psychiatric nurses' perceptions of the constituents of the therapeutic relationship: A grounded theory study. *Journal of Psychiatric and Mental Health Nursing,* 13(3), 319–329.

Scanlon, C. and Weir, W.S. (1997). Learning from practice? Mental health nurses' perceptions and experiences of clinical supervision. *Journal of Advanced Nursing,* 26(2), 295–303.

Shattell, M.M., Starr, S.S., and Thomas, S.P. (2007). 'Take my hand, help me out': mental health service recipients' experience of the therapeutic relationship. *International Journal of Mental Health Nursing,* 16(4), 274–284.

Sheldon, L.K. (2005). *Communication for nurses: Talking with patients.* Sudbury, MA: Jones & Bartlett Publishers.

Sloane, A. (1966). Review of "Interpersonal aspects of nursing" by J. Travelbee. *American Journal of Nursing,* 66(6), 77.

Smith, B.A. (1998). The problem drinker's lived experience of suffering: An exploration using hermeneutic phenomenology. *Journal of Advanced Nursing,* 27(1), 213–222.

Snowball, J. (1996). Asking nurses about advocating for patients: "Reactive" and "proactive" accounts. *Journal of Advanced Nursing,* 24(1), 67–75.

Stetler, C. (1977). Relationship of perceived empathy of nurses' communication. *Nursing Research,* 26(6), 432–438.

Timmins, F. and Kelly, J. (2008). Spiritual assessment in intensive and cardiac care nursing. *Nursing in Critical Care,* 13(3), 124–131.

Topaz, M., Troutman-Jordan, M. and MacKenzie, M. (2014). Construction, deconstruction, and reconstruction: The roots of successful aging theories. *Nursing Science Quarterly,* 27(3), 226–233.

Tranvag, O. and Kristoffersen, K. (2008). Experience of being the spouse/cohabitant of a person with bipolar affective disorder: A cumulative process over time. *Scandinavian Journal of Caring Sciences,* 22(1), 5–18.

†Travelbee, J. (1963). What do we mean by "rapport?" *American Journal of Nursing,* 63(2), 70–72.

Travelbee, J. (1964). What's wrong with sympathy? *American Journal of Nursing,* 64(1), 68–71.

Travelbee, J. (1969). *Intervention in psychiatric nursing.* New York: Springer-Verlag.

Travelbee, J. (1971). *Interpersonal aspects of nursing* (2nd ed.). Philadelphia: F.A. Davis.

Travelbee, J. (1971). The nature of nursing. In J. Travelbee (Ed.), *Interpersonal aspects of nursing* (2nd ed., pp. 7–21). Philadelphia, PA: F.A. Davis.

Truax, C. and Carkhuff, R.R. (1967). *Toward effective counseling and psychotherapy.* Chicago, IL: Aldine.

Tuck, I., Wallace, D., and Pullen, L. (2001). Spirituality and spiritual care provided by parish nurses. *Western Journal of Nursing Research,* 23(5), 441–453.

Turner, de S. and Stokes, L. (2006). Hope promoting strategies of registered nurses. *Journal of Advanced Nursing,* 56(4), 363–372.

Tutton, E., Seers, K., and Langstaff, D. (2009). An exploration of hope as a concept for nursing. *Journal of Orthopaedic Nursing,* 13, 119–127.

van Dover, L. and Pfeiffer, J.B. (2007). Spiritual care in Christian parish nursing. *Journal of Advanced Nursing,* 57(2), 213–221.

Vatne, S. and Fagermoen, M.S. (2007). To correct and to acknowledge: Two simultaneous and conflicting perspectives of limit-setting in mental health nursing. *Journal of Psychiatric and Mental Health Nursing,* 14(1), 41–48.

von Krogh, G. and Naden, D. (2008). A nursing-specific model of EPR documentation: Organizational and professional requirements. *Journal of Nursing Scholarship,* 40(1), 68–75.

von Krogh, G., Dale, C., and Naden, D. (2005). A framework for integrating NANDA, NIC, and NOC terminology in electronic patient records. *Journal of Nursing Scholarship,* 37(3), 275–281.

Wadensten, B. (2005). The content of morning time conversations between nursing home staff and residents. *Journal of Clinical Nursing,* 14(8B), 84–89.

Wadensten, B. and Carlsson, M. (2003). Nursing theory views on how to support the process of ageing. *Journal of Advanced Nursing,* 42(2), 118–124.

Wadensten, B., Engholm, R., Fahlström, G., and Hägglund, D. (2009). Nursing staff's description of a good encounter in nursing homes. *International Journal of Older People Nursing,* 4, 203–210.

Wallerstedt, B. and Andershed, B. (2007). Caring for dying patients outside special palliative care settings: Experiences from a nursing perspective. *Scandinavian Journal of Caring Sciences,* 21(1), 32–40.

Weaver, K., Morse, J., and Mitcham, C. (2008). Ethical sensitivity in professional practice: Concept analysis. *Journal of Advanced Nursing,* 62(5), 607–618.

Webb, C. and Hope, K. (1995). What kind of nurses do patients want. *Journal of Clinical Nursing,* 4(2), 101–108.

Welch, M. (2005). Pivotal moments in the therapeutic relationship. *International Journal of Mental Health Nursing,* 14(3), 161–165.

Wiklund, L. (2008). Existential aspects of living with addiction – Part II: Caring needs. A hermeneutic expansion of qualitative findings. *Journal of Clinical Nursing,* 17, 2435–2443.

Williams, A. (2001). A literature review on the concept of intimacy in nursing. *Journal of Advanced Nursing,* 33(5), 660–667.

Willis, W.O. (1999). Culturally competent nursing care during the perinatal period. *Journal of Perinatal and Neonatal Nursing,* 13(3), 45–59.

Wolff, I.S. (1966). Review of "Interpersonal aspects of nursing" by J. Travelbee. *Nursing Outlook,* 1504–1506.

Wright, K., Haigh, K., and McKeown, M. (2007). Reclaiming the humanity in personality disorder. *International Journal of Mental Health Nursing,* 16(4), 236–246.

36. Jean Watson

Arslan-Özkan, İ., Okumuş, H., and Buldukoğlu, K. (2014). A randomized controlled trial of the effects of nursing care based on Watson's Theory of Human Caring on distress, self-efficacy and adjustment in infertile women. *Journal of Advanced Nursing,* 70(8), 1801–1812.

Barker, P. and Reynolds, B. (1994). Watson's caring ideology: The proper focus of psychiatric nursing? *Journal of Psychosocial Nursing,* 32, 17–22.

Bennet, P., Porter, B., and Sloan, R. (1989). Jean -Watson: Philosophy and science of caring. In A. Marriner-Tomey (Ed.), *Nursing theorists and their work* (2nd ed.). St. Louis, MO: C.V. Mosby.

Bevis, E.O. and Watson, J. (1989). *Toward a caring curriculum: A new pedagogy for nursing* (pp. iii–xix, 1–394). New York: National League for Nursing.

Boyd, C. and Mast, D. (1989). Watson's model of human care. In J.J. Fitzpatrick and A.L. Whall (Eds.), *Conceptual models of nursing: Analysis and application* (2nd ed.). Norwalk, CT: Appleton & Lange.

Bunkers, S.S., Michaels, C., and Ethridge, P. (1997). Advanced practice nursing in community: Nursing's opportunity. *Advanced Practice Nursing Quarterly*, 2(4), 79–84.

Burns, P. (1991). *Elements of spirituality and Watson's theory of transpersonal caring: Expansion of focus* (pp. 141–153). New York: National League for Nursing.

Carson, M.G. (1992). An application of Watson's theory to group work with the elderly. *Perspectives*, 16(4), 7–13.

Chipman, Y. (1991). Caring: Its meaning and place in the practice of nursing. *Journal of Nursing Education*, 30(4), 171–175.

Clayton, G. (1989). Research testing Watson's theory: The phenomena of caring in an elderly population. In J. Riehl-Sisca (Ed.), *Conceptual models for nursing practice* (3rd ed.). Norwalk, CT: Appleton & Lange.

Cohen, J.A. (1991). Two portraits of caring: A comparison of the artists, Leininger and Watson. *Journal of Advanced Nursing*, 16(8), 899–909.

Cooper, M.C. (1989). Gilligan's different voice: A perspective for nursing. *Journal of Professional Nursing*, 5(1), 10–16.

Duffy, J.R., Hoskins, L., and Seifert, R.F. (2007). Dimensions of caring: Psychometric evaluation of the caring assessment tool. *Advances in Nursing Science*, 30(3), 235–245.

Fawcett, J. (2002). The nurse theorists: 21st century updates— Jean Watson. *Nursing Science Quarterly*, 15(3), 214–219.

Griffith, K.A. (1999). Holism in the care of the allogeneic bone marrow transplant population: Role of the nurse practitioner. *Holistic Nursing Practice*, 13(2), 20–27.

Jones, N., Kearins, J., and Watson, J. (1987). The human tongue show and observers willingness to interact: Replication and extensions. *Psychology Reports*, 60(3, Part 1), 759–764.

Kolcaba, K.Y. and Kolcaba, R.J. (1991). An analysis of the concept of comfort. *Journal of Advanced Nursing*, 16(11), 1301–1310.

Krysl, M. and Watson, J. (1988). Existential moments of caring: Facets of nursing and social support. *Advances in Nursing Science*, 10(2), 12–17.

Lachman, V.D. (2012). Applying the ethics of care to your nursing practice. *Medsurg Nursing*, 21(2), 112.

Lukose, A. (2011). Developing a practice model for Watson's theory of caring. *Nursing Science Quarterly*, 24(1), 27–30.

Marckx, B.B. (1995). Watson's theory of caring: A model for implementation in practice. *Journal of Nursing Care Quality*, 9, 43–54.

Martin, L.S. (1991). Using Watson's theory to explore the dimensions of adult polycystic kidney disease. *American Nephrology Nurses Association Journal*, 18(5), 493–496, 499.

Mathes, S. (2011). Implementing a caring model. *Creative Nursing*, 17(1), 36–42.

McCance, T.V., McKenna, H.P., and Boore, J.R. (1999). Caring: Theoretical perspectives of relevance to nursing. *Journal of Advanced Nursing*, 30(6), 1388–1395.

McKay, P., Rajacich, D., and Rosenbaum, J. (2002). Enhancing palliative care through Watson's carative factors. *Canadian Oncology Nursing Journal*, 12(1), 34–38.

Mendyka, B.E. (2000). Exploring culture in nursing: A theory-driven practice. *Holistic Nursing Practice*, 15(1), 32–41.

Mitchell, G.J. and Cody, W.K. (1992). Nursing knowledge and human science: Ontological and epistemological considerations. *Nursing Science Quarterly*, 5(2), 54–61.

Mullaney, J.A.B. (2000). The lived experience of using Watson's actual caring occasion to treat depressed women. *Journal of Holistic Nursing*, 18(2), 129–142.

Nelson-Marten, P., Hecomovich, K. and Pangle, M. (1998). Caring theory: A framework for advanced practice nursing. *Advanced Practice Nursing Quarterly*, 4(1), 70–77.

Norred, C.L. (2000). Minimizing preoperative anxiety with alternative caring-healing therapies. *Journal of the Association of periOperative Registered Nurses*, 72(5), 838–840.

Özkan, İ.A., Okumuş, H., Buldukoğlu, K., and Watson, J. (2013). A case study based on Watson's Theory of human caring being an infertile woman in Turkey. *Nursing Science Quarterly*, 26(4), 352–359.

Perry, B. (1998). Beliefs of eight exemplary oncology nurses related to Watson's nursing theory. *Canadian Oncology Nursing Journal*, 8(2), 97–107.

Piccinato, J.M. and Rosenbaum, J.N. (1997). Caregiver hardiness explored within Watson's Theory of Human Caring in Nursing. *Journal of Gerontological Nursing*, 23(10), 32–39.

Pilkington, F.B. (2007). Envisioning nursing in 2050 through the eyes of nurse theorists: Leininger and Watson. *Nursing Science Quarterly*, 20(1), 8.

Rafael, A.R. (2000). Watson's philosophy, science, and theory of human caring as a conceptual framework for guiding community health nursing practice. *Advances in Nursing Science*, 23(2), 34–49.

Ray, M.A. (1997). Consciousness and the moral ideal: A transcultural analysis of Watson's theory of transpersonal caring. *Advanced Practice Nursing Quarterly*, 3(1), 25–31.

Ryan, L. (1989). A critique of nursing: Human science and human care. In J. Riehl-Sisca (Ed.), *Conceptual models for nursing practice* (3rd ed.). Norwalk, CT: Appleton & Lange.

Santos, M.R.D., Bousso, R.S., Vendramim, P., Baliza, M.F., Misko, M.D., and Silva, L. (2014). The practice of nurses caring for families of pediatric inpatients in light of Jean Watson. *Revista da Escola de Enfermagem da USP*, 48(SPE), 80–86.

Shroeder, C. and Maeve, M.K. (1992). Nursing care partnerships at the Denver nursing project in human caring: An application and extension of caring theory in practice. *Advances in Nursing Science*, 15(2), 25–38.

Sithichoke-Rattan, N. (1989). A clinical application of Watson's theory. *Pediatric Nursing*, 15(5), 458–462.

Swanson, K.M. (1991). Empirical development of a middle range theory of caring. *Nursing Research*, 40(3), 161–166.

Vandenhouten, C., Kubsch, S., Peterson, M., Murdock, J., and Lehrer, L. (2012). Watson's theory of transpersonal caring: Factors impacting nurses professional caring. *Holistic Nursing Practice*, 26(6), 326–334.

Walker, C.A. (1996). Coalescing the theories of two nurse visionaries: Parse and Watson. *Journal of Advanced Nursing*, 24(5), 988–996.

Watson, J. (1979). *Nursing: The philosophy and science of caring*. Boston, MA: Little, Brown.

Watson, J. (1981). Conceptual systems of students, practitioners. *Western Journal of Nursing Research*, 3, 197–198.

Watson, J. (1981). The lost art of nursing. *Nursing Forum*, 20, 244–249.

Watson, J. (1981). Some issues related to a science of caring for nursing practice. In M. Leininger (Ed.), *Caring: An essential human need*. Thorofare, NJ: Charles Slack.

Watson, J. (1985). *Nursing: Human science and human care*. Norwalk, CT: Appleton-Century-Crofts.

Watson, J. (1987). *The dream curriculum* (Publication No. 15–2179, pp. 91–104.). New York: National League for Nursing.

Watson, J. (1987). Nursing on the caring edge: Metaphorical vignettes. *Advances in Nursing Science*, 10(1), 10–18.

Watson, J. (1987). *The professional doctorate as an entry level into practice* (Publication No. 41–2199, pp. 41–47). New York: National League for Nursing.

Watson, J. (1988). *An ethic of caring/curing/nursing qua nursing: Introduction* (Publication No. 15–2237, pp. 1–3). New York: National League for Nursing.

Watson, J. (1988). *A case study: Curriculum in transition* (Publication No. 15–2224, pp. 1–8). New York: National League for Nursing.

Watson, J. (1988). Human caring as moral context for nursing education. *Nursing and Health Care*, 9(8), 422–425.

Watson, J. (1988). New dimensions of human caring theory. *Nursing Science Quarterly*, 1(4), 175–181.

Watson, J. (1988). *Nursing: Human science and human care. A theory of nursing* (Publication No. 15–2236, pp. 1–104). New York: National League for Nursing.

Watson, J. (1989). Watson's philosophy and theory of human caring. In J. Riehl-Sisca (Ed.), *Conceptual models for nursing practice* (3rd ed.). Norwalk, CT: Appleton & Lange.

Watson, J. (1990). Caring knowledge and informed moral passion. *Advances in Nursing Science*, 13(1), 15–24.

Watson, J. (2002). Intentionality and caring-healing consciousness: A practice of transpersonal nursing. *Holistic Nursing Practice*, 16(4), 12–19.

Watson, J. (2002). Intentionality and care-healing consciousness: A practice of transpersonal nursing. *Holistic Nursing Practice*, 16(4), 12–19.

Watson, J. (2005). What, may I ask is happening to nursing knowledge and professional practices? What is nursing thinking at this turn in human history? *Journal of Clinical Nursing*, 14(8), 913–914.

Watson, J., and Brewer, B.B. (2015). Caring science research: Criteria, evidence, and measurement. *Journal of Nursing Administration*, 45(5), 235–236.

Watson, J. and Smith, M.C. (2002). Caring science and the science of unitary human beings: A transtheoretical discourse for nursing knowledge development. *Journal of Advanced Nursing*, 37(5), 452–461.

37. Ernestine Wiedenbach

Adamsen, L., Rasmussen, J.M., and Pedersen, L.S. (2001). "Brothers in arms": How men with cancer experience a sense of comradeship through group intervention which combines physical activity with information relay. *Journal of Clinical Nursing*, 10(4), 528–537.

Anderson, C. and Adamsen, L. (2001). Continuous video recording: A new clinical research tool for studying the nursing care of cancer patients. *Journal of Advanced Nursing*, 35(2), 257–267.

Barger, M., Faucher, M.A. and Murphy, P.A. (2015). Theorists and historical influences. *Journal of Midwifery and Women's Health*, 60(1), 89–98.

Barnum, B.J.S. (1998). *Nursing theory: Analysis, application, evaluation* (5th ed.). Philadelphia, PA: Lippincott.

Bennett, A.M. and Foster, P.C. (1980). Ernestine Wiedenbach. In The Nursing Theories Conference Group (Eds.), *Nursing theories: The base for professional nursing practice*. Englewood Cliffs, NJ: Prentice-Hall.

Burst, H.V. (1998). In memoriam—Ernestine Widenbach, DNM, MA, FACNM. *Journal of Nurse-Midwifery*, 43(5), 361–362.

Burst, H.V. (2000). The circle of safety: A tool for clinical preceptors. *Journal of Midwifery and Women's Health*, 45(5), 408–410.

Carper, B.A. (2006). Fundamental patterns of knowing in nursing. In W.K. Cody and J.W. Kenney (Eds.), *Philosophical and theoretical perspectives for advanced nursing practice* (4th ed.). Sudbury, MA: Jones & Bartlett Publishers.

Clausen, J., et al. (1977). *Maternity nursing today*. New York: McGraw-Hill.

Danko, M., Hunt, N., Marich, J., Marriner-Tomey, A., McCreary, C., and Stuart, M. (1989). Ernestine Wiedenbach: The helping art of clinical nursing. In A. Marriner-Tomey (Ed.), *Nursing theorists and their work* (2nd ed.). St. Louis, MO: C.V. Mosby.

Dickoff, J., James, P., and Wiedenbach, E. (1968). Theory in a practice discipline. *Nursing Research*, 19(5), 415–427.

Diers, D. (1966). The nurse orientation system: A method for analyzing nurse-patient interactions. *Nursing Research*, 15(1), 91.

Dracup, K. and Breu, C. (1978). Using nursing research findings to meet the needs of grieving spouses. *Nursing Research*, 27(4), 212–216.

Dumas, R. and Leonard, R. (1963). The effect of nursing on the incidence of postoperative vomiting. *Nursing Research*, 12(1), 12–15.

Eisler, J., Wolfer, J.A., and Diers, D. (1972). Relationship between the need for social approval and postoperative recovery welfare. *Nursing Research*, 21(5), 520–525.

Elms, R.R. and Leonard, R.C. (1966). Effects of nursing approaches during admission. *Nursing Research*, 15(1), 37–48.

Flannery, J. and Van Gaasbeek, D.E. (1998). Factors of job satisfaction of the psychiatric clinical nurse specialist. *Nursing Connections*, 11(4), 27–36.

Griffiths, B. and Andrews, C.M. (2007). Nursing perspective. Putting nursing theory into practice. *Gastroenterology Nursing*, 30(6), 440–442

Hickman, J.S. (2005). *Faith community nursing*. Philadelphia, PA: Lippincott Williams & Wilkins.

Hilton, P.A. (1997). Theoretical perspectives of nursing: A review of the literature. *Journal of Advanced Nursing*, 26(6), 1211–1220.

Hunter, L.P. and Hunter, L.A. (2006). Storytelling as an educational strategy for midwifery students. *Journal of Midwifery and Women's Health*, 51(4), 273–278.

Kielhofner, G. (2005). A scholarship of practice: Creating discourse between theory, research, and practice. *Occupational Therapy in Health Care*, 19(1/2), 7–16.

Klopper, H.C. (2002). A constructivist strategy for health science education. *South African Journal of Physiotherapy*, 58(4), 13–18.

Kolcaba, K. (2003). *Comfort theory and practice: A vision for holistic health care and research*. New York: Springer Publishing Company.

Larson, P.A. (1977). Nurse perception of client illness. *Nursing Research*, 26(6), 416–421.

Leonard, R.C., Skipper, J.K., and Woolridge, P.J. (1967). Small sample field experiments for evaluating patient care. *Health Services Research*, 2(1), 46–50.

Lyon, B. (2005). Getting back on track: Nursing's autonomous scope of practice. 1990. *Clinical Nurse Specialist*, 19(1), 28–33.

Nickel, S, Gesse, T., and MacLaren, A. (1992). Ernestine Wiedenbach: Her professional legacy. *Journal of Nurse-Midwifery*, 37(3), 161–167.

Powers, B.A. and Knapp, T.R. (2006). *Dictionary of nursing theory and research* (3rd ed.). New York: Springer Publishing Company.

Raleigh, E. (1983). Wiedenbach's model. In J.J. Fitzpatrick and A.L. Whall (Eds.), *Conceptual models of nursing: Analysis and application*. Bowie, MD: Robert J. Brady Co.

Raleigh, E. (1989). Wiedenbach's model of nursing practice. In J.J. Fitzpatrick and A.L. Whall (Eds.), *Conceptual models of nursing: Analysis and application* (2nd ed.). Norwalk, CT: Appleton & Lange.

Rickelman, B.L. (1971). Bio-psychosocial linguistics: A conceptual approach to nurse-patient interaction. *Nursing Research*, 20(5), 398–403.

Sharp, E.S. (1998). Ethics in reproductive health care: A midwifery perspective. *Journal of Nurse-Midwifery*, 43(3), 235–245.

Shields, D. (1978). Nursing care in labor and patient satisfaction. A descriptive study. *Journal of Advances in Nursing*, 3, 535–550.

Trivette, C.M., Dunst, C.J., Boyd, K., et al. (1996). Family-oriented program models, helpgiving practices, and parental control appraisals. *Exceptional Children*, 62(3), 237–248.

VandeVusse, L. (1997). Sculpting a nurse-midwifery philosophy—Ernestine Wiedenbach's influence. *Journal of Nurse-Midwifery*, 42(1), 43–48.

Villafuerte, A. (1996). Structured clinical preparation time for culturally diverse baccalaureate nursing students. *International Journal of Nursing Studies*, 33(2), 161–170.

von Krogh, G., Dale, C., and Naden, D. (2005). A framework for integrating NANDA, NIC, and NOC terminology in electronic patient records. *Journal of Nursing Scholarship*, 37(3), 275–281.

Wadensten, B. (2005). Nursing theories applied to vulnerable populations: Example from Sweden. In M.D. Chesnay (Ed.), *Caring for the vulnerable: Perspectives in nursing theory, practice, and research* (pp. 61–70). Sudbury, MA: Jones & Bartlett Publishers.

Walker, D.S. (2007). Midwifery models: Students' conceptualization of a midwifery philosophy in clay. *Journal of Midwifery and Women's Health*, 52(1), 63–66.

Wallace, C.L. and Appleton, C. (1995). Nursing as the promotion of well-being—The client's experience. *Journal of Advanced Nursing*, 22(2), 285–289.

White, J. (1995). Patterns of knowing—Review, critique and update. *Advances in Nursing Science*, 17(4), 73–86.

Wiedenbach, E. (1962, June). *A concept of dynamic nursing: Philosophy, purpose, practice, and process*. A Conference on Maternal and Child Nursing, University of Pittsburgh School of Nursing.

Wiedenbach, E. (1963). The helping art of nursing. *American Journal of Nursing*, 63(11), 54–57.

Wiedenbach, E. (1964). *Clinical nursing: A helping art*. New York: Springer-Verlag.

Wiedenbach, E. (1965). Family nurse practitioner for maternal and child care. *Nursing Outlook*, 13, 50–51.

Wiedenbach, E. (1968). Nurse's role in family planning: A conceptual base for practice. *Nursing Clinics of North America*, 3(2), 355–365.

Wiedenbach, E. (1969). *Meeting the realities in clinical teaching*. New York: Springer-Verlag.

Wiedenbach, E. (1970). Comment on beliefs and values: Basis for curriculum design. *Nursing Research*, 19(5), 427.

Wiedenbach, E. (1970). Nurses' wisdom in nursing theory. *American Journal of Nursing*, 70(5), 1057–1062.

Wiedenbach, E. (1973). The nursing process in maternity nursing. In J.P. Clausen et al. (Eds.), *Maternity nursing today*. New York: McGraw-Hill.

Wiedenbach, E. and Falls, C.E. (1978). *Communication: Key to effective nursing*. New York: Tiresias Press.

Williams, D.L. (2008). Safeguarding attitudes. *Journal of Forensic Nursing*, 4(1), 47–48.

Wilmoth, T.A. and Elder, J.P. (1995). An assessment of research on breast-feeding promotion strategies in developing countries. *Social Science and Medicine*, 41(4), 579–594.

Wolfer, J. and Visintainer, M. (1975). Pediatric surgical patients' and parents' stress responses and adjustment. *Nursing Research*, 24(4), 244–255.

PARADIGMS THAT HAVE INFLUENCED NURSING

38. Psychoanalytic Theory

Alexander, F. (1958). Unexplored areas in psychoanalytic theory and treatment. *Behavioral Sciences*, 3, 293–316.

Brams, J. (1968). From Freud to Fromm. *Psychology Today*, 1, 32–35, 64–65.

Brenner, C. (1973). *An elementary textbook of psychoanalysis*. Garden City, NY: International Universities Press.

Brill, A.A. (1922). *Psychoanalysis, its theories and practical application* (3rd ed.). Philadelphia, PA: W.B. Saunders.

Brill, A.A. (1969). *Basic principles of psychoanalysis (1921)*. Garden City, NY: Doubleday.

Burchard, E.M.L. (1960). Mystical and scientific aspects of the psychoanalytic theories of Freud, Adler, and Jung. *American Journal of Psychotherapy*, 15, 289–307.

Chertok, L. (1968). From Liebeault to Freud. *American Journal of Psychotherapy*, 22, 96–101.

Corsini, R. (1977). *Current personality theories*. Itasca, IL: F.A. Peacock Publisher.

Desmonde, W.H., Mead, G.H., and Freud, S. (1957). American social psychology and psychoanalysis. *Psychoanalysis*, 4 & 5, 31–50.

Engel, G.L. (1977, April). The need for a new medical model: A challenge for biomedicine. *Science*, 196, 129–135.

Engel, G.L. (1980). The clinical application of the biopsychosocial model. *American Journal of Psychiatry*, 137(5), 535–544.

Fenichel, O. (1945). *The psychoanalytic theory of neurosis* (pp. 3–13). New York: W.W. Norton.

Fine, R. (1962). *Freud: A critical re-evaluation of his theories*. New York: McKay.

Fine, R. (1979). *A history of psychoanalysis*. New York: Columbia University Press.

Ford, D.H. and Urban, H.B. (1963). *Systems of psychotherapy: A comparative study*. New York: John Wiley & Sons.

Freedman, A., Kaplan, H., and Sadock, B. (1976). *Modern synopsis of comprehensive psychiatry* (2nd ed.). Baltimore, MD: Williams & Wilkins.

Freud, S. (1924). *The complete introductory lectures on psychoanalysis*. New York: Pocket Books.

Freud, S. (1924). *A general introduction to psycho-analysis*. New York: Pocket Books.

Freud, S. (1925–1950). *Collected papers* (Vols. I–V). London, UK: Hogarth.

Freud, S. (1938). *The basic writings of Sigmund Freud*. A.A. Brill (Ed.). New York: Random House.

Freud, S. (1946). *An autobiographical study (1935)* (Rev. ed.). London, UK: Hogarth.

Freud, S. (1953–1955). *The standard edition of the complete psychological works* (24 Vols.). J. Strachey (Trans.). London, UK: Hogarth.

Freud, S. (1954). *The origin of psychoanalysis: Letters to Wilhelm Fleiss*. E. Mosbacher and J. Strachey (Trans.), M. Bonaparte, A. Freud, and E. Dris (Eds.). New York: Basic Books.

Freud, S. (1957). *A general selection of the works of Sigmund Freud*. J. Rickman (Ed.). New York: Liveright.

Freud, S. (1959). *Beyond the pleasure principle*. J. Strachey (Trans.). New York: Bantam Books.

Freud, S. (1959). *Collected papers*. New York: Basic Books.

Freud, S. (1962). *The ego and the id*. J. Riviere and J. Strachey (Trans.). New York: W.W. Norton.

Freud, S. (1963). *Dora: An analysis of a case of hysteria*. P. Reiff (Ed.). New York: Macmillan.

Freud, S. (1965). *The interpretation of dreams*. J. -Strachey (Ed.). New York: Avon Books.

Freud, S. (1965). *The psychopathology of everyday life*. New York: W.W. Norton.

Freud, S. (1966). *On the history of the psychoanalytic movement*. New York: W.W. Norton.

Freud, S. (1969). *An outline of psycho-analysis*. New York: W.W. Norton.

Glover, E. (1959). *Freud or Jung*. New York: W.W. Norton.

Goshen, C.E. (1952). The original case material of psycho-analysis. *American Journal of Psychiatry*, 108, 829–832.

Hall, C. (1954). *A primer of Freudian psychology*. New York: New American Library.

Hall, C.S. and Lindzey, G. (1970). *Theories of personality*. New York: John Wiley & Sons.

Janger, J. (1968). *Theories of development*. New York: Holt, Rinehart & Winston.

Johnstone, R.L. (1982). Individual psychotherapy: Relationship of theoretical approaches to nursing conceptual models. In J.J. Fitzpatrick, A.L. Whall, R.L. Johnstone, and J.S. Floyd (Eds.), *Nursing models and their psychiatric mental health applications*. Bowie, MD: Robert J. Brady.

Jones, E. (1953, 1955, 1957). *The life and work of Sigmund Freud* (3 Vols.). New York: Basic Books.

Kardinar, A., Karush, A., and Ovesey, L. (1966). A methodological study of Freudian theory. *International Journal of Psychiatry*, 2, 489–544.

Kolb, L.C. (1977). *Modern clinical psychiatry*. Philadelphia, PA: W.B. Saunders.

Krech, D. and Klein, G.S. (1966). *Theoretical models and personality theory*. New York: Greenwood Press.

Mahler, M., Pine, F., and Bergman, A. (1975). *The psychological birth of the human infant*. New York: Basic Books.

Mehrabian, A. (1968). *An analysis of personality theories*. Englewood Cliffs, NJ: Prentice-Hall.

Munroe, R.L. (1955). *Schools of psychoanalytic thought*. New York: Dryden Press.

Murphy, G. (1956). The current impact of Freud upon psychology. *American Psychologist*, 11, 663–672.

Pervin, L.A. (1975). *Personality: Theory, assessment, and research*. New York: John Wiley & Sons.

Reiser, M.F. (1979). Psychosomatic medicine: A meeting ground for oriental and occidental medical theory and practice. *Psychotherapy Psychosomatics*, 31, 315–323.

Schmid, F. (1952). Freud's sociological thinking. *Bulletin of the Menninger Clinic*, 16, 1–13.

Schmied, V. and Lupton, D. (2001). The externality of the inside: Body images of pregnancy. *Nursing Inquiry*, 8(1), 32–40.

Shakow, N. and Rapaport, D. (1964). The influence of Freud on American psychology. *Psychological Issues*, 4, 1–243.

Shaw, M.E. and Costanzo, P.R. (1982). *Theories of social psychology* (2nd ed.). New York: McGraw-Hill.

Sherman, M.H. (1966). *Psychoanalysis in America*. Springfield, IL: Charles C. Thomas.

Sherwood, M. (1969). *The logic of explanation in psychoanalysis*. New York: Academic Press.

Stafford-Clark, D. (1967). *What Freud really said*. New York: Schoken Books.

Stone, I. (1971). *The passions of the mind*. New York: Doubleday.

Toman, W. (1960). *An introduction to psychoanalytic theory of motivation*. New York: Pergamon Press.

Turiell, E. (1967). An historical analysis of the Freudian conception of the superego. *Psychoanalytical Review*, 54, 118–140.

Waelder, R. (1960). *Basic theory of psychoanalysis*. New York: International Universities Press.

West, R. (1967). The social significance of the uncompleted father analysis of Sigmund Freud. *Psychotherapy Psychosomatics*, 15, 69.

Wolff, P.H. (1960). *The developmental psychologies of Jean Piaget and psychoanalysis*. New York: International University Press.

39. Symbolic Interaction

Allport, G.W. (1955). *Becoming: Basic considerations for a psychology of personality*. New Haven, CT: Yale University Press.

Banton, M. (1965). *Roles: An introduction to the study of social relations*. New York: Basic Books.

Benzies, K.M. and Allen, M.N. (2001). Symbolic interactionism as a theoretical perspective for multiple method research. *Journal of Advanced Nursing*, 33(4), 541–547.

Biddle, B.J. and Thomas, E.J. (1966). *Role theory: Concepts and research*. New York: John Wiley & Sons.

Blasi, A. (1972). Symbolic interactions as theory. *Sociology and Social Research*, 56(4), 453–455.

Blumer, H. (1966). Sociological implications of the thought of George Herbert Mead. *American Journal of Sociology*, 71, 535–544.

Blumer, H. (1969). *Symbolic interactionism: Perspective and method*. Englewood Cliffs, NJ: Prentice-Hall.

Blumer, H. (1980). Mead and Blumer: The convergent methodological perspectives of social behaviorism and symbolic interactionism. *American Sociological Review*, 45, 409–419.

Bower, F. and Jacobson, M.J. (1979). Family theories: Frameworks for nursing practice. In S.E. Archer and R. Fleshman (Eds.), *Community health nursing: Patterns and practice* (2nd ed.). North Scituate, MA: Duxbury Press.

Burr, W.R., Leigh, G.K., Day, R.D., and Constantine, J. (1979). Symbolic interaction and the family. In W.R. Burr, R. Hill, F.I. Nye, and I.L. Reiss (Eds.), *Contemporary theories about the family, Vol. 2: General theories/theoretical orientations*. New York: Free Press.

Carlson, E. (2013). Precepting and symbolic interactionism–a theoretical look at preceptorship during clinical practice. *Journal of Advanced Nursing*, 69(2), 457–464.

Chamberlain-Salaun, J., Mills, J., and Usher, K. (2013). Linking symbolic interactionism and grounded theory methods in a research design. *Sage Open*, 3(3). doi:10.1177/2158244013505757.

Charon, J. (1979). *Symbolic interaction*. Englewood Cliffs, NJ: Prentice-Hall.

Coser, L.A. (1971). George Herbert Mead, 1863–1931. In *Masters of sociological thought* (pp. 333–355). New York: Harcourt Brace Jovanovich.

Cottrell, L.S., Jr. (1942). The adjustment of the individual to his age and sex roles. *American Sociological Review*, 7, 617–620.

Gordon, C. and Gerzen, K.J. (1968). *The self in social interaction (Vol. 1). Classic and contemporary perspectives.* New York: John Wiley & Sons.

Gordon, G. (1966). *Role theory and illness: A sociological perspective.* New Haven, CT: College and University Press.

Hammer, M.L. (1977). Symbols of aging as perceived by the young. *Journal of Gerontological Nursing*, 3(4), 17–18.

Handberg, C., Thorne, S., Midtgaard, J., Nielsen, C.V., and Lomborg, K. (2014). Revisiting symbolic interactionism as a theoretical framework beyond the grounded theory tradition. Qualitative health research. doi: 10.1177/1049732314554231.

Hewitt, J. (1983). *Self and society: A symbolic interactionist social psychology* (3rd ed.). Boston, MA: Allyn & Bacon.

Huber, J. (1973). Symbolic interaction as a pragmatic perspective: The bias of emergent theory. *American Sociological Review*, 38(2), 274–284.

Kuhn, M.H. (1964). Major trends in symbolic interaction theory in the past twenty-five years. *Sociological Quarterly*, 5, 61–84.

Laborde, J.M. (1979). Symbolism and gift-giving in family therapy. *Journal of Psychiatric Nursing*, 17(4), 32–35.

Linton, R. (1936). *The study of man*. New York: Appleton-Century-Crofts.

Manis, J.G. and Meltzer, B.N. (1972). *Symbolic interaction* (2nd ed.). Boston, MA: Allyn & Bacon.

Martins, D.C., and Burbank, P.M. (2011). Critical interactionism: An upstream-downstream approach to health care reform. *Advances in Nursing Science*, 34(4), 315–329.

McPhail, C. and Rexroth, C. (1979). The divergent methodological perspectives of social behaviorism and symbolic interactionism. *American Sociological Review*, 44, 449–467.

Mead, G.H. (1937). *Mind, self and society*. Introduction by C.W. Morris. Chicago, IL: University of Chicago Press.

Mead, G.H. (1956). *The social psychology of G.H. Mead*. Edited and with revised introduction by A. Strauss. Chicago, IL: University of Chicago Press.

Meltzer, B.N. (1972). Mead's social psychology. In J.G. Manis and B.N. Meltzer (Eds.), *Symbolic interaction: A reader in social psychology* (2nd ed.). Boston, MA: Allyn & Bacon.

Milliken, P.J. and Schreiber, R. (2012). Examining the nexus between grounded theory and symbolic interactionism. *International Journal of Qualitative Methods*, 11(5), 684–696.

Mowrer, O.H. (1960). *Learning theory and the symbolic process*. New York: John Wiley & Sons.

Nilsson, L., Hofflander, M., Eriksén, S., and Borg, C. (2012). The importance of interaction in the implementation of information technology in health care: A symbolic interactionism study on the meaning of accessibility. *Informatics for Health and Social Care*, 37(4), 277–290.

Porter, S.F. (1978). Interaction modeling: An educational strategy for new graduate leadership development. *Journal of Nursing Administration*, 8(4), 20–24.

Rickelman, B.L. (1971). Bio-psychosocial linguistics: A conceptual approach to nurse-patient interaction. *Nursing Research*, 20(5), 398–403.

Riehl, J.P. (1974). Application of interaction theory. In J.P. Riehl and C. Roy (Eds.), *Conceptual models for nursing practice*. New York: Appleton-Century-Crofts.

Rose, A. (1960). Incomplete socialization: Sociology and socialization. *Nursing Research*, 44, 244–250.

Rose, A. (Ed.). (1962). *Human behavior and social processes: An interactional approach*. Boston, MA: Houghton-Mifflin.

Rose, A. (1974). A systematic summary of symbolic interaction theory. In J.P. Riehl and C. Roy (Eds.), *Conceptual models for nursing practice* (pp. 34–46). New York: Appleton-Century-Crofts.

Sarbin, T. (1954). Role theory. In G. Lindzey (Ed.), *Handbook of social psychology* (Vol. 1, pp. 223–258). Cambridge, MA: Addison-Wesley.

Sarbin, T. (1968). Role theory. In G. Lindzey and E. Aronson (Eds.), *Handbook of social psychology* (Vol. 1, 2nd ed., pp. 488–567). Cambridge, MA: Addison-Wesley.

Schroeder, K.A. (1981). Symbolic interactionism: A conceptual framework useful for nurses working with obese persons. *Image: Journal of Nursing Scholarship*, 13(3), 78–81.

Shibutani, T. (1961). *Society and personality*. Englewood Cliffs, NJ: Prentice-Hall.

Shott, S. (1979). Emotion and social life: A symbolic interactionist analysis. *American Journal of Sociology*, 84(2), 1317–1334.

Simmel, G. (1964). *The sociology of Georg Simmel*. K.H. Wolff (Ed., Trans.). New York: Free Press.

Strauss, A. (Ed.). (1956). *The social psychology of George H. Mead*. Chicago, IL: University of Chicago Press.

Strauss, A. (1977). Sociological theories of personality. In R. Corsini (Ed.), *Current personality theories* (pp. 277–281). Itasca, IL: F.E. Peacock Publisher.

Strauss, A. and Fisher, B.M. (1978). *Interactionism (working paper)*. University of California San Francisco and New York University.

Stryker, S. (1959). Symbolic interaction as an approach to family research. *Marriage Family Living*, 21, 111–119.

Turner, R.H. (1956). Role taking, role standpoint, and reference group behavior. *American Journal of Sociology*, 61, 316–328.

Turner, R.H. (1962). Role taking: Process vs. conformity. In A. Rose (Ed.), *Human behavior and social processes* (pp. 20–40). Boston, MA: Houghton-Mifflin.

Turner, R.H. (1968). The self-conception in social interaction. In C. Gordon and K.J. Gergen (Eds.), *Self in social interaction*. New York: John Wiley & Sons.

Turner, R.H. (1978). *The structure of sociological theory* (2nd ed., Chap. 14–17). Homewood, IL: Dorsey Press.

40. Holism

Abbot, E.A. (1984). *Flatland: A romance of many dimensions*. New York: Signet.

Agan, R.D. (1987). Intuitive knowing as a dimension of nursing. *Advances in Nursing Science*, 10(1), 63–70.

Allen, D. (2014). Re-conceptualising holism in the contemporary nursing mandate: From individual to organisational relationships. *Social Science & Medicine*, 119, 131–138.

Archibald, M.M. (2012). The holism of aesthetic knowing in nursing. *Nursing Philosophy*, 13(3), 179–188.

Barnum, B.J.S. (1994). *Nursing theory: Analysis, application, and evaluation* (4th ed.). Philadelphia, PA: J.B. Lippincott.

Bollinger, E. (2001). Applied concepts of holistic nursing. *Journal of Holistic Nursing*, 19(2), 212–214.

Clark, C.S. (2012). Beyond holism: Incorporating an integral approach to support caring-healing-sustainable nursing practices. *Holistic Nursing Practice*, 26(2), 92–102.

Copeland, M. (2002). e-Community health nursing. *Journal of Holistic Nursing*, 20(2), 152–165.

Drevdahl. D. (1999). Sailing beyond: Nursing theory and the person. *Advances in Nursing Science*, 21(4), 1–13.

Duhl, L. (1986). Health and the inner and outer self. *Journal of Humanistic Psychology*, 26(3), 46–61.

Flynn, P. (1980). *Holistic health*. Bowie, MD: Robert J. Brady Co.

Fuller, G. (1978). Holistic man and the science and practice of nursing. *Nursing Outlook*, 26(11), 700–704.

Hall, B.A. and Allan, J.D. (1994). Self in relation: A prolegomenon for holistic nursing. *Nursing Outlook*, 42(3), 110–116.

Harmon, W. and Rheingold, H. (1984). *Higher creativity: Liberating the unconscious for breakthrough insights*. Los Angeles, CA: Jeremy P. Tarcher.

Holmes, C.A. (1990). Alternatives to natural science: Foundations for nursing. *International Journal of Nursing Studies*, 27, 187–198.

Kalischuk, R.G. and Davies, B. (2001). A theory of healing in the aftermath of youth suicide: Implications for holistic nursing practice. *Journal of Holistic Nursing*, 19(2), 163–186.

Kolcaba, R. (1997). The primary holisms in nursing. *Journal of Advanced Nursing*, 25(2), 290–296.

Mast, D. (1986). Effects of imagery. *Image: Journal of Nursing Scholarship*, 18(3), 118–120.

Morgan, A. (1998). Holism in nursing. *Australian Journal of Holistic Nursing*, 5(2), 32–35.

Mulholland, J. (1995). Nursing, humanism, and transcultural theory: The "bracketing-out" of reality. *Journal of Advanced Nursing*, 22, 442–449.

Papathanasiou, I., Sklavou, M., and Kourkouta, L. (2013). Holistic nursing care: Theories and perspectives. *American Journal of Nursing Science*, 2(1), 1–5.

Povlsen, L., and Borup, I.K. (2011). Holism in nursing and health promotion: distinct or related perspectives?–A literature review. *Scandinavian Journal of Caring Sciences*, 25(4), 798–805.

Reed, P.G. (1998). A holistic view of nursing concepts and theories in practice. *Journal of Holistic Nursing*, 16(4), 415–419.

Schnect, K. (1985). Convergence, energy and optimal health. *Journal of Holistic Medicine*, 7(2), 178–193.

Smith, M. (1984). Transformation: The key to shaping nursing. *Image: Journal of Nursing Scholarship*, 16(1), 28–30.

Stiles, K.A. (2011). Advancing nursing knowledge through complex holism. *Advances in Nursing Science*, 34(1), 39–50.

Woods, S. (1998). A theory of holism for nursing. *Medicine, Health Care, and Philosophy*, 1(3), 255–261.

Yorks, L. and Sharoff, L. (2001). An extended epistemology for fostering transformative learning in holistic nursing education and practice. *Holistic Nursing Practice*, 16(1), 21–29.

41. Organizational Theory

Astley, W.G. (1985). Administrative science as socially constructed truth. *Administrative Science Quarterly*, 30, 497–513.

Bechky, B.A. (2011). Making organizational theory work: Institutions, occupations, and negotiated orders. *Organization Science*, 22(5), 1157–1167.

Bellot, J. (2011, January). Defining and assessing organizational culture. *Nursing Forum*, 46, 1, 29–37. (Blackwell Publishing Inc)

Daffe, R.L. (1986). *Organization theory and design* (2nd ed.). St. Paul, MN: West Publishing.

Hegyvary, S., Duxbury, M., Hall, R., Krueger, J., Lindeman, C., Scott, J., and Scott, W. (1987). *The evolution of nursing professional organizations: Alternative models for the future*. Kansas City, MO: American Academy of Nursing.

Jennings, B.M. and Meleis, A.I. (1988). Nursing theory and administrative nursing practice: Agenda for the 1990s. *Advances in Nursing Science*, 10(3), 56–69.

Kast, F.E. and Rosenzweig, J.E. (1985). The subject is organizations. In *Organization and management: A systems and contingency approach* (pp. 3–22). New York: McGraw-Hill.

Rakich, J., Longest, B., and Darr, K. (1985). *Managing health services organization* (2nd ed.). Philadelphia, PA: W.B. Saunders.

Rowlinson, M., Hassard, J., and Decker, S. (2014). Research strategies for organizational history: A dialogue between historical theory and organization theory. *Academy of Management Review*, 39(3), 250–274.

Scott, W. (1987). The subject is organizations. In *Organizations: Rational, natural and open systems* (pp. 3–27). Englewood Cliffs, NJ: Prentice-Hall.

Suter, E., Goldman, J., Martimianakis, T., Chatalalsingh, C., DeMatteo, D.J., and Reeves, S. (2013). The use of systems and organizational theories in the interprofessional field: Findings from a scoping review. *Journal of interprofessional care*, 27(1), 57–64.

42. Developmental Theory

Almy, M. (Ed.). (1967). *Young children's thinking*. New York: Teachers' College Press.

Baltes, P.B. (1987). Theoretical propositions of life-span developmental psychology: On the dynamics between growth and decline. *Developmental Psychology*, 23(5), 611–626.

Buhler, C. (1935). The curve of life as studied in biographies. *Journal of Applied Psychology*, 19, 405–409.

Buhler, C. (1959). Theoretical observations about life's tendencies. *American Journal of Psychotherapy*, 13(3), 561–581.

Buhler, C. and Massarik, F. (1968). *The course of human life*. New York: Springer-Verlag.

Burnside, I.M., Ebersole, P., and Monea, H.E. (Eds.). (1979). *Psychosocial caring throughout the life span*. New York: McGraw-Hill.

Caldwell, B.M. and Richmond, J.B. (1962). The impact of theories of child development. *Children*, 9(2), 73–78.

Capps, D., Capps, W., and Bradford, M.G. (Eds.). (1977). *Encounter with Erikson*. Missoula, MT: Scholars Press.

Carroll, E. (1977). *Human emotions*. New York: Plenum Press.

Chin, R. (1980). Developmental models. In J. Riehl and C. Roy (Eds.), *Conceptual models for nursing practice* (2nd ed., pp. 55–59). New York: Appleton-Century-Crofts.

Coles, R. (1970). *Erik H. Erikson: The growth of his work*. Boston, MA: Little, Brown.

Davis, G. and Jones, A. (1980). Theories of personality development. In J. Lancaster (Ed.) *Adult psychiatric nursing: Current clinical nursing series*. Garden City, NY: Medical Examination Publishing.

Donabedian, A. (1966). Evaluating the quality of medical care. *Milbank Memorial Fund Quarterly*, 44(Suppl 3), 166–206.

Erikson, E.H. (1953). Growth and crises of the healthy personality. In C. Kluckhohn and H. Murray (Eds.), *Personality in nature, society and culture*. New York: Alfred Knopf.

Erikson, E.H. (1964). Inner and outer space: Reflections on womanhood. *Daedalus*, 93(2), 582–606.

Erikson, E.H. (1970). The quest for identity. Newsweek, December 21, 1976.

Erikson, E.H. (1978). *Adulthood*. New York: W.W. Norton.

Erikson, E.H. and Smelser, N. (Eds.). (1980). *Themes of work and love in adulthood*. Cambridge, MA: Harvard University Press.

Evans, R.I. (1967). *Dialogue with Erik Erikson* (pp. 11–58). New York: Harper & Row.

Flavel, J. (1963). *The developmental psychology of Jean Piaget*. Princeton, NJ: D. Nostrand.

Ford-Gilboe, M. (2002). Developing knowledge about family health promotion by testing the developmental model of health and nursing. *Journal of Family Nursing*, 8(2), 140–156.

Frenkel, E.B. (1968). Adjustments and reorientation in the course of the life span. In B.L. Neugarten (Ed.), *Middle age and aging* (pp. 77–84). Chicago, IL: University of Chicago Press.

Furth, H.G. (1981). *Piaget and knowledge* (2nd ed.). Chicago, IL: University of Chicago Press.

Goode, W. (1973). *Explorations in social theory*. London, UK: Oxford University Press.

Gould, R.L. (1972). The phases of adult life: A study in developmental psychology. *American Journal of Psychiatry*, 129(5), 521.

Gruen, W. (1964). Adult personality: An empirical study of Erikson's theory of ego development. In B.L. Neugarten (Ed.), *Personality in middle and late life*. New York: Atherton Press.

Haan, N. (1976). Personality organizations of well-functioning younger people and older adults. *International Aging and Human Development*, 7(2), 117–127.

Handel, A. (1987). Personal theories about the life-span development of one's self in autobiographical self-presentations of adults. *Human Development*, 30, 83–98.

Harris, D.B. (Ed.). (1957). *The concept of development: An issue in the study of human behavior*. Minneapolis, MN: University Press.

Harris, D.B. (1957). Problems in formulating a scientific concept of development. In *The concept of development* (pp. 3–14). Minneapolis, MN: University Press.

Harrison, K., Bost, K.K., McBride, B.A., Donovan, S.M., Grigsby-Toussaint, D.S., Kim, J., . . . and Jacobsohn, G.C. (2011). Toward a developmental conceptualization of contributors to overweight and obesity in childhood: The Six-Cs model. *Child Development Perspectives*, 5(1), 50–58.

Janosik, E. (1982). Aspects of group development: Stages and levels. In E.H. Janosik and L.B. Phipps (Eds.), *Life-cycle group work in nursing*. Monterey, CA: Wadsworth.

Josselyn, I.M. (1948). *Psychosocial development of children*. New York: Family Service Association of America.

Kimmel, D.C. (1980). *Adulthood and aging: An interdisciplinary developmental view* (2nd ed.). New York: John Wiley & Sons.

Kuhlen, R.G. (1968). Developmental changes in motivation during the adult years. In B.L. Neugarten (Ed.). *Middle age and aging*. Chicago, IL: University of Chicago Press.

Lazarus, R.S. (1966). *Psychological stress and the coping process*. New York: McGraw-Hill.

LeFrancois, G.R. (1972). *Psychological theories and human learning: Kongor's report*. Monterey, CA: Brooks/Cole.

Levinson, D.J. (1978). *The seasons of a man's life*. New York: Ballantine Books.

Lidz, T. (1976). *The life cycle. The person* (2nd ed.). New York: Basic Books.

Loft, W.R. and Svoboda, C.P. (1975). Structuralism in cognitive developmental psychology: Past, contemporary and future perspective. In K.F. Riegel and G.C. Rosenwals (Eds.), *Structure and transformation*. New York: John Wiley & Sons.

Lowenthal, M.F., Thurnber, M., and Chiriboga, D. (1976). *Four stages of life*. San Francisco, CA: Jossey-Bass.

Maier, H.W. (1963). *Three theories of child development*. New York: Harper & Row.

Maier, H.W. (1978). The psychoanalytic theory of Erik H. Erikson. In H.W. Maier (Ed.), *Three theories of child development* (Rev. ed.). New York: Harper & Row.

Neugarten, B. (Ed.). (1968). *Middle age and aging*. Chicago, IL: University of Chicago Press.

Papalia, D. and Wendkos Olds, S. (1981). The adolescent. In *Human development* (2nd ed.). New York: McGraw-Hill.

Peck, R.C. (1968). Psychological developments in the second half of life. In B.L. Neugarten (Ed.), *Middle age and aging* (pp. 88–92). Chicago, IL: University of Chicago Press.

Perry, D.G., and Pauletti, R.E. (2011). Gender and adolescent development. *Journal of Research on Adolescence*, 21(1), 61–74.

Pulaski, M. (1971). *Understanding Piaget*. New York: Harper & Row.

Reed, P.G. (1983). Implications of the life-span developmental framework for well-being in adulthood and aging. *Advances in Nursing Science*, 6(1), 18–25.

Riegel, K.F. (1969). History as a nomothetic science: Some generalizations from theory and research in developmental psychology. *Journal of Social Issues*, 4, 99–127.

Riegel, K.F. (1972). Influence of economic and political ideologies on the development of developmental psychology. *Psychological Bulletin*, 78(2), 129–141.

Roazen, P. (1976). *Erik H. Erikson: The power and limits of vision*. New York: Free Press.

Roberts, S. (1980). Piaget's theory reapplied to the critically ill. *Advances in Nursing Science*, 2(2), 61–79.

Rowe, G.P. (1966). The developmental conceptual framework to the study of the family. In F.I. Nye and F.M. Berardo (Eds.), *Emerging conceptual frameworks in family analysis*. New York: Praeger.

Sanford, N. (1966). *Self and society: Social change and individual development*. New York: Atherton Press.

Schaie, W.K. (1977–1978). Toward a stage theory of adult cognitive development. *International Journal of Aging and Human Development*, 8(2), 129–138.

Schuster, C. (1980). *The process of human development*. Boston, MA: Little, Brown.

Sheehy, G. (1976). *Passages: Predictable crises of adult life*. New York: E.P. Dutton.

Sullivan, C., Grant, M.Q., and Grant, J.D. (1957). The development of interpersonal maturity: Application to delinquency. *Psychiatry*, 20, 373–385.

Sullivan, H.S. (1953). *Interpersonal theory of psychiatry*. New York: W.W. Norton.

Thibaut, J.W. and Kelley, H.H. (1967). *The social psychology of groups, Part I: Dyadic Relationships*. New York: John Wiley & Sons.

Thomas, A. (1981). Current trends in development theory. *American Journal of Orthopsychiatry*, 51(4), 580–609.

Thomas, H. (1970). Theory of aging and cognitive theory of personality. *Human Development*, 13(1), 1–16.

Thompson, R.A. (2012). Whither the preconventional child? Toward a life-span moral development theory. *Child Development Perspectives*, 6(4), 423–429.

Toffler, A. (1971). *Future shock*. New York: Bantam/Random House.

Troll, L.E. (1975). *Early and middle adulthood: The best is yet to be—Maybe*. Monterey, CA: Brooks/Cole.

Ungar, M., Ghazinour, M., and Richter, J. (2013). Annual Research Review: What is resilience within the social ecology of human development? *Journal of Child Psychology and Psychiatry*, 54(4), 348–366.

Van Den Daele, L.D. (1975). Ego development and preferential judgment in life span perspective. In N. Datan and L.H. Ginsberg (Eds.), *Life-span developmental psychology*. New York: Academic Press.

Wadsworth, B.J. (1971). *Piaget's theory of cognitive development*. New York: David McKay Co.

Waechter, E.H. (1980). The developmental model. In M. Kalkman and A. Davis (Eds.). *New dimensions in mental health-psychiatric nursing* (2nd ed.). New York: McGraw-Hill.

Wahba, M. and Bridwell, L.G. (1976). Maslow reconsidered: A review of research on the need for hierarchy theory. *Organizational Behavior and Human Performance*, 15, 212–224.

Wolman, B.B. (Ed.). (1982). *Handbook of developmental psychology*. Englewood Cliffs, NJ: Prentice-Hall.

43. Systems Theory

Abbey, J.C. (1970). General system theory: A framework for nursing. In J. Smith (Ed.), *Improvement of curricula in schools of nursing through selection and application of care concepts of nursing: An interim report*. Boulder, CO: Western Interstate Commission for Higher Education.

Abdolvahab, B., Ghazal, T., and Yaser, B. (2012). Decision-making in Australia's healthcare system and insights from complex adaptive systems theory. *Health Scope*, 1(1), 29–38.

Allport, G.W. (1960). The open system in personality theory. *Journal of Abnormal and Social Psychology*, 61, 310–21.

Altschul, A.T. (1978). A systems' approach to the nursing process. *Journal of Advanced Nursing*, 3(4), 333–340.

Barnum, B.J.S. (1994). *Nursing theory: Analysis, application, and evaluation* (4th ed.). Philadelphia, PA: J.B. Lippincott.

Battista, J.R. (1977). The holistic paradigm and general systems theory. *General Systems Yearbook*, 22, 65–71.

Beavers, W.R. (1977). Systems theory, family systems, and the self. In *Psychotherapy and growth: A family perspective* (pp. 19–41). New York: Brunner-Mazel.

Becht G. (1974, October). Systems theory, the key to holism and reductionism. *Bio Science*, 24(10), 569–578.

Bertalanffy, L. von. (1967). *Robots, men and minds*. Part 2. New York: George Braziller.

Bertalanffy, L. von. (1968). *General systems theory: Foundations, development application* (Rev. ed.). New York: George Braziller.

Bertalanffy, L. von. (1969). General systems theory and psychiatry—An overview. In W. Gray et al. (Eds.). *General systems theory and psychiatry* (pp. 33–50). Boston, MA: Little, Brown.

Bertalanffy, L. von. (1975). *Perspectives on general systems theory*. New York: George Braziller.

Black, M. (1961). *The social theories of Talcott Parsons: A critical examination*. Englewood Cliffs, NJ: Prentice-Hall.

Boulding, K.E. (1956). General systems theory—The skeleton of science. *Management Science*, 2, 197–208.

Broderick, C. and Smith, J. (1979). The general systems approach to family. In W.R. Burr (Ed.), *Contemporary theories about the family* (pp. 112–129). New York: Free Press.

Brody, H. and Sobel, D.S. (1980). A systems view of health and disease. *Holistic Health Review*, 3(3), 163–178.

Buckley, W. (1967). *Sociology and modern systems theory*. Englewood Cliffs, NJ: Prentice-Hall.

Bunge, M. (1977). General systems and holism. *General Systems Yearbook*, 22, 87–90.

Bunge, M. (1979). A systems concept of society; beyond individualism and holism. *General Systems Yearbook*, 24, 27–44.

Chinn, P.L. (1979). Practice oriented theory: Part 2. *Advances in Nursing Science*, 1(2), 41–52.

Chin, R. (1961). The utility of system models and developmental models for practitioners. In W.G. Bennis, K.D. Benne, and R. Chin (Eds.), *The planning of change*. New York: Holt, Rinehart & Winston.

Chrisman, M. and Riehl, J. (1980). The system-developmental stress model. In J.P. Riehl and C. Roy (Eds.), *Conceptual models for nursing practice* (2nd ed.). New York: Appleton-Century-Crofts.

Churchman, C.W. (1968). *The systems approach*. New York: Dell.

Cummings, T.G. (Ed.). (1981). *Systems theory for organizational development*. New York: John Wiley & Sons.

Demerath, N.J. and Peterson, R.A. (Eds.). (1967). *System, change and conflict*. New York: Free Press.

Emery, F.E. (Ed.). (1969). *Systems thinking*. Middlesex, England: Penguin Books.

Ericson, R.F. (1979). Society for general systems research at twenty-five. What agenda for our second quarter century? *Behavioral Science*, 24(5), 225–237.

Founds, S.A. (2009). Introducing systems biology for nursing science. *Biological Research for Nursing*, 11(1), 73–80.

Glenister, D.A. (2011, September). *Towards a general systems theory of nursing: A literature review* (Vol. 55, No. 1). In Proceedings of the 55th Annual Meeting of the ISSS-2011. Hull, UK.

Gray, W. (1972). Bertalanffian principles as a basis for humanistic psychiatry. In E. Laszlo (Ed.), *The relevance of general systems theory*. New York: George Braziller.

Grinker, R.R. (Ed.). (1967). *Toward a unified theory of human behavior: An introduction to general systems theory* (Rev. ed.). New York: Basic Books.

Hall, A.D. and Fagen, R.E. (1956). Definition of system. *General Systems Yearbook*, 1, 18–28.

Hamilton, G.A. (1979, January). Miller's living systems: A theory critique. *Advances in Nursing Science*, 1(2), 41–52.

Hardin, P.K. (2003). Shape-shifting discourses of anorexia nervosa: Reconstituting psychopathology. *Nursing Inquiry*, 10(4), 209–217.

Hazzard, M.E. (1971). An overview of systems theory. *Nursing Clinics of North America*, 6(3), 385–393.

Jantsch, E. (1970). Inter- and transdisciplinary university: A systems approach to education and innovation. *Policy Sciences*, 1, 403–428.

Kalmus, H. (Ed.). (1966). *Regulation and control in living systems*. New York: John Wiley & Sons.

Laszlo, E. (Ed.). (1972). *The relevance of general systems theory*. New York: George Braziller.

Laszlo, E. (1972). *The systems view of the world*. New York: George Braziller.

Laszlo, E. (1975). The meaning and significance of general systems theory. *Behavioral Science*, 20(1), 9–24.

Lilienfeld, R. (1978). *The rise of systems theory: An ideological analysis*. New York: John Wiley & Sons.

Maslow, A.H. (1970). *Motivation and personality* (2nd ed.). New York: Harper & Row.

Miller, J. (1965). Living systems: Basic concepts. *Behavioral Science*, 10, 193–237.

Parsons, T. (1951). *The social system*. London, UK: Free Press of Glencoe.

Parsons. T. (1967). *Sociological theory and modern society*. New York: Free Press.

Pierce, L.M. (1972). Usefulness of a systems approach for problem conceptualization and investigation. *Nursing Research*, 21, 509–513.

Powers, P.S. and Girgenti, J.R. (1978). Analysis of a system. *Journal of Psychosocial Nursing and Mental Health Services*, 17–22.

Prigogine, I. and Stengers, I. (1984). *Order out of chaos*. New York: Bantam Books.

Rapoport, A. (1970). Modern systems theory—An outlook for coping with change. *General Systems Yearbook*, 15, 15–25.

Ritterman, M.K. (1977). Paradigmatic classification of family therapy theories. *Family Process*, 16(1), 29–48.

Rudolph, E. (1980). Defining the parameters of general living systems theory. *The Family*, 7(2), 83–91.

Shrode, W.A. and Voich, D. (1974). *Organization and management: Basic systems concepts*. Homewood, IL: R.D. Irwin.

Sills, G.M. and Hall, J.E. (1977). A general systems perspective for nursing. In J.E. Hall and B.R. Weaver (Eds.), *Distributive nursing practice: A systems approach to community health* (pp. 19–28). Philadelphia, PA: J.B. Lippincott.

Somers, J.B. (1977). Purpose and performance: A system analysis of nurse staffing. *Journal of Nursing Administration*, 7, 4–9.

Stephen, W.R. (1978). Toward a redefinition of action theory: Paying the cognitive element its due. *American Journal of Sociology*, 83(6), 1317–1349.

Suter, E., Goldman, J., Martimianakis, T., Chatalalsingh, C., DeMatteo, D.J., and Reeves, S. (2013). The use of systems and organizational theories in the interprofessional field: Findings from a scoping review. *Journal of Interprofessional Care*, 27(1), 57–64.

Sutherland, J.W. (1973). *A general systems philosophy for the social and behavioral sciences*. New York: George Braziller.

Tantsch, E. (1970). Inter- and transdisciplinary university: A systems approach to education and innovation. *Policy Sciences*, 1, 403–428.

Tashdjian, E. (1972). A systems approach to higher education with special reference to the core curriculum. *Policy Sciences*, 3, 219–33.

Weiner, N. (1948). *Cybernetics or control and communication in the animal and machine*. Paris: Herman and Cie.

Werley, H.H., et al. (Eds.). (1976). *Health research: The systems approach*. New York: Springer-Verlag.

44. Stress and Adaptation

Ambriz, M.G.J., Izal, M., and Montorio, I. (2012). Psychological and social factors that promote positive adaptation to stress and adversity in the adult life cycle. *Journal of Happiness Studies*, 13(5), 833–848.

Appley, M.H. (1971). *Adaptation-level theory: A symposium*. New York: Academic Press.

Auger, J.R. (1976). *Behavioral systems and nursing*. Englewood Cliffs, NJ: Prentice-Hall.

Bell, J.M. (1977). Stressful life events and coping methods in mental illness and wellness behaviors. *Nursing Research*, 26, 136–141.

Brower, H., Terri, F., and Baker, B.J. (1976). Using the adaptation model in a practitioner curriculum. *Nursing Outlook*, 24, 686–689.

Bruner, J., Olver, R.R, Greenfield, P.M., et al. (1966). *Studies in cognitive growth*. New York: John Wiley & Sons.

Coelho, G.V., Hamburg, D.A., and Adams, J.E. (1974). Introduction. In G.V. Coelho et al. (Eds.), *Coping and adaptation*. New York: Basic Books.

Cohen, F. and Lazarus, R. (1979). Coping with the stresses of illness. In G. Stine, F. Cohen, and N. Adler (Eds.), *Health psychology: A handbook*. San Francisco, CA: Jossey-Bass.

Dobzhansky, T. (1962). *Mankind evolving*. New Haven, CT: Yale University Press.

Dobzhansky, T. (1967). Changing man. *Science*, 155, 409–415.

Dubos, R. (1965). Adaptation and its dangers. In *Man adapting* (pp. 254–280). New Haven, CT: Yale University Press.

Duffy, M.E. (1987). The concept of adaptation: Examining alternatives for the study of nursing phenomenon. *Scholarly Inquiry for Nursing Practice*, 3(1), 179–192.

Fagin, C. (1987). Stress: Implications for nursing research. *Image: Journal of Nursing Scholarship*, 19(1), 38–41.

Fielo, F.M.C. (1971). *Psychosocial nursing*. New York: Macmillan.

Folkman, S. and Lazarus, R. (1980). An analysis of coping in a middle-aged community sample. *Journal of Health and Social Behavior*, 21, 219–239.

Gossen, G. and Bush, H. (1979). Adaptation: A feedback process. *Advances in Nursing Science*, 1(4), 51–65.

Gramling, L.F., Lambert, V.A., and Pursley-Crotteau, S. (1998). Coping in young women: Theoretical retroduction. *Journal of Advanced Nursing*, 28(5), 1082–1091.

Haan, N. (1969). A tripartite model of ego functioning values and clinical and research applications. *Journal of Nervous and Mental Disease*, 148, 14–30.

Hall, H.R., Neely-Barnes, S.L., Graff, J.C., Krcek, T.E., Roberts, R.J., and Hankins, J.S. (2012). Parental stress in families of children with a genetic disorder/disability and the resiliency model of family stress, adjustment, and adaptation. *Issues in Comprehensive Pediatric Nursing*, 35(1), 24–44.

Hamburg, D.A., Coelho, G.V., and Adams, J.E. (1974). Coping and adaptation: Steps toward a synthesis of biological and social perspectives. In G.V. Coelho et al. (Eds.), *Coping and adaptation*. New York: Basic Books.

Harvey, O.J. (1966). *Experience, structure and adaptability*. New York: Springer-Verlag.

Helson, H. (1959). Adaptation level theory. In S. Koch (Ed.), *Psychology: A study of a science* (Vol. 1, pp. 565–621). New York: McGraw-Hill.

Helson, H. (1964). *Adaptation level theory* (Chap. 2). New York: Harper & Row.

King, I.M. (1997). King's theory of goal attainment in practice. *Nursing Science Quarterly*, 10(4), 180–185.

Kuroki, T., Ohta, A., Sherriff-Tadano, R., Matsuura, E., Takashima, T., Iwakiri, R., and Fujimoto, K. (2011). Imbalance in the stress-adaptation system in patients with inflammatory bowel disease. *Biological Research for Nursing*, 13(4), 391–398.

Lutz, H.R., Patterson, B.J., and Klein, J. (2012). Coping with autism: A journey toward adaptation. *Journal of Pediatric Nursing*, 27(3), 206–213.

Mastal, M. and Hammond, H. (1980). Analysis and expansion of the Roy adaptation model: A contribution to holistic nursing. *Advances in Nursing Science*, 2(4), 71–81.

Minckley, B.B., Burrows, D., Ehrat, K., Harper, L., Jenkin, S.A., Minckley, W.F., Page, B., Schramm, D.E., Wood, C. (1979). Myocardial infarct stress-of-transfer inventory: Development of a research tool. *Nursing Research*, 28(1), 4–10.

Murphy, J.F. (1971). Adaptation as a unifying theory. In *Theoretical issues in professional nursing* (Chap. 4). New York: Appleton-Century-Crofts, Education Division.

Murray, R. and Zentner, J. (1975). Application of adaptation theory to nursing. In R. Murray and J. Zentner (Eds.), *Nursing concepts for health promotion*. Englewood Cliffs, NJ: Prentice-Hall.

Por, J., Barriball, L., Fitzpatrick, J., and Roberts, J. (2011). Emotional intelligence: Its relationship to stress, coping, well-being and professional performance in nursing students. *Nurse Education Today*, 31(8), 855–860.

Rabkin, J.G. and Struening, E.L. (1976). Life events, stress and illness. *Science*, 194, 1013–1020.

Redman, B.K. (1974). Why develop a conceptual framework? *Journal of Nursing Education*, 13, 2–10.

Riehl, J and Roy, C. (1974). *Conceptual models for nursing practice*. New York: Appleton-Century-Crofts.

Roy, C. (1971, April). Adaptation: A basis for nursing practice. *Nursing Outlook*, 21, 254–257.

Roy, C. (1973, March). Adaptation: Implications for curriculum change. *Nursing Outlook*, 21, 163–168.

Roy, C. (1974). The Roy adaptation model. In J. Riehl and C. Roy (Eds.), *Conceptual models for nursing practice*. New York: Appleton-Century-Crofts.

Sander, L.W. (1969). The longitudinal course of early mother-child interaction-cross-case comparison in a sample of mother-child pairs. In B.M. Foss (Ed.), *Determinants of infant behavior IV* (pp. 189–227). London, UK: Methuen.

Scott, J. (1977, February). Stress and coping: A case for intervention. *Journal of Psychiatric Nursing and Mental Health Services*, 15, 14–17.

Scott, R. and Howard, A. (1970). Models of stress. In S. Levine and N. Scotch (Eds.), *Social stress*. Chicago, IL: Aldine.

Scott, D.W., Oberst, M., and Dropkin, M. (1980). A stress-coping model. *Advances in Nursing Science*, 3(1), 9–23.

Scott, D.W., Oberst, M. and Bookbinder, M. (1984). Stress-coping response to genitourinary carcinoma in men. *Nursing Research*, 32(6), 325–329.

Selye, H. (1950). *The physiology and pathology of exposure to stress*. Montreal, Canada: ACTA Medical Publishers.

Selye, H. (1950, June 17). Stress and the general adaptation syndrome. *British Medical Journal*, 1383–1392.

Selye, H. (1964). *From dream to discovery*. New York: McGraw-Hill.

Selye, H. (1965). The stress syndrome. *American Journal of Nursing*, 65(3), 97–99.

Selye, H. (1976). The nature of adaptation. In *The stress of life* (Chap. 14). New York: McGraw-Hill.

Spielberger, C.D. (1972). Anxiety as an emotional state. In *Anxiety: Current trends in theory and research* (pp. 23–49). New York: Academic Press.

Stone, G., Cohen, F., and Adler, N. (1979). *Health psychology: A handbook*. San Francisco, CA: Jossey-Bass.

Thetford, W.N. and Schucman, H. (1971). Motivational factors and adaptive behavior. In J.A. Downey and R.C. Darling (Eds.), *Physiological basis of rehabilitation medicine* (pp. 353–371). Philadelphia, PA: W.B. Saunders.

Vailliant, G.E. (1977). *Adaptation to life*. Boston, MA: Little, Brown.

Wagner, P. (1976). Testing the adaptation model in practice. *Nursing Outlook*, 24, 682–685.

Wild, B.S. and Hanes, C. (1976). A dynamic conceptual framework of generalized adaptation to stressful stimuli. *Psychological Reports*, 37, 319–334.

Yeh, P.M., and Bull, M. (2012). Use of the resiliency model of family stress, adjustment and adaptation in the analysis of family caregiver reaction among families of older people with congestive heart failure. *International Journal of Older People Nursing*, 7(2), 117–126.

45. Role Theory

Banton, M. (1965). *Roles: An introduction to the study of social relations*. New York: Basic Books.

Bem, S. (1975). Sex roles adaptability: One consequence of psychological androgyny. *Journal of Personality and Social Psychology*, 31(4), 634–643.

Berk, B.B. and Victor, G. (1975). Selection vs. role occupancy as determinants of role-related attitudes among psychiatric aides. *Journal of Health and Social Behavior*, 16(2), 183–191.

Bertrand, A. (1972). *Social organization: A general systems of role theory perspective*. Philadelphia, PA: F.A. Davis.

Biddle, B. and Thomas, E. (Eds.). (1966). *Role theory: Concepts and research*. New York: John Wiley & Sons.

Biddle, B.J. (1979). *Role theory: Expectations, identities, and behaviors*. New York: Academic Press.

Blasi, A.J. (1971–1972). Symbolic interactionism as theory. *Sociology and Social Research*, 56, 453–465.

Blumer, H. (1969). *Symbolic interactionism: Perspective and method*. Englewood Cliffs, NJ: Prentice-Hall.

Brouse, S.H. (1985). Effect of gender role identity patterns on self concept scores from later pregnancy to early post-partum. *Advances in Nursing Science*, 7(3), 32–48.

Bunch, B. and Zahra, D. (1976). Dealing with death: The unlearned role. *American Journal of Nursing*, 76(9), 1486–1488.

Burke, P.J. and Tully, J.C. (1977). The measurement of role identity. *Social Forces*, 54, 881–897.

Burr, W.R. (1972). Role transitions: A reformulation of theory. *Journal of Marriage and the Family*, 34, 407–416.

Conway, M.E. (1978). Theoretical approaches to the study of roles. In M. Hardy and M. Conway (Eds.), *Role theory: Perspectives for the health professional*. Norwalk, CT: Appleton-Century-Crofts.

Crossan, F. and Robb, A. (1998). Role of the nurse: Introducing theories and concepts. *British Journal of Nursing*, 7(10), 608–612.

Garrosa, E., Moreno-Jiménez, B., Rodríguez-Muñoz, A., and Rodríguez-Carvajal, R. (2011). Role stress and personal resources in nursing: A cross-sectional study of burnout and engagement. *International Journal of Nursing Studies*, 48(4), 479–489.

Goffman, E. (1969). *Stigma*. Englewood Cliffs, NJ: Prentice-Hall.

Gordon, G. (1966). *Role theory and illness: A sociological perspective*. New Haven, CT: College and University Press.

Gross, N.C., Mason, W.S., and McEachern, A.W. (1958). *Explorations in role analysis: Studies of the school superintendency role*. New York: John Wiley & Sons.

Habeeb, M. and McLaughlin, F. (1977). Health care professional's role expectation and patient needs. *Nursing Research*, 26, 288–298.

Hadley, B.J. (1964). Nursing a la Weber. *Nursing Science*, 4, 95–110.

Hadley, B.J. (1967). The dynamic interactionist concept of role. *Journal of Nursing Education*, 2, 5–10.

Hall, J. (2003). Analyzing women's roles through graphic representation of narratives. *Western Journal of Nursing Research*, 25(5), 492–507.

Hanna, B. (2001). Negotiating motherhood: The struggles of teenage mothers. *Journal of Advanced Nursing*, 34(4), 456–464.

Hardy, M. and Conway, M.E. (1989). *Role theory: Perspectives for health professionals*. New York: Appleton-Century-Crofts.

Heiss, J. (1976). *Family roles and interaction: An anthology* (2nd ed.). Chicago, IL: Rand McNally.

Jones, S.L. (1976). Socialization vs. selection factors as sources of student definitions of the nurse role. *International Journal of Nursing Studies*, 13(3), 135–138.

Kassebaum, G. and Baumann, B. (1965). Dimension of the sick role in chronic illness. *Journal of Health and Human Behavior*, 6, 16–27.

Keller, N.S. (1973). The nurse's role: Is it expanding or shrinking? *Nursing Outlook*, 21, 236–240.

Levenstein, A. (1976). Role ambiguity in nursing. *Supervisor Nurse*, 7(6), 16–17.

Lewandowski, L.A. and Kramer, M. (1980). Role transformation of special care unit nurses: A comparative study. *Nursing Research*, 29(3), 170–179.

Lindersmith, A.R. and Strauss, A.L. (1968). Roles, role behavior and social structure. In A.R. Lindersmith, A.L.

Strauss, and N.K. Denzin (Eds.), *Social psychology* (3rd ed., pp. 276–298). New York: Holt, Rinehart & Winston.

Lindersmith, A.R., Strauss, A.L., and Denzin, N. (1975). *Social psychology* (4th ed.). Hinsdale, IL: Dryden Press.

Meleis, A.I. (1971). Self-concept and family planning. *Nursing Research*, 20, 299–236.

Meleis, A.I. (1975). Role insufficiency and role supplementation: A conceptual framework. *Nursing Research*, 24, 264–271.

Meleis, A.I. and Swendsen, L.A. (1978). Role supplementation: An empirical test of a nursing intervention. *Nursing Research*, 27(1), 11–18.

Mercer, R.T. (1985). The process of role attainment over the first year. *Nursing Research*, 34, 198–204.

Miyamoto, F.S. (1963). The impact of research of different conceptions of role. *Sociological Inquiry*, 33, 144–123.

Miyamoto, F.S. and Dornbush, S. (1956). A test of the symbolic interactionist hypothesis of self-conception. *American Journal of Sociology*, 61, 399–403.

Mlotshwa, L., Harris, B., Schneider, H., and Moshabela, M. (2015). Exploring the perceptions and experiences of community health workers using role identity theory. *Global health action*, 8, 28045.

Morgan, W.R.B. (1975). Role theory: An attribution theory interpretation. *Sociometry*, 38, 429–444.

Morris, C.W. (Ed.). (1962). Herbert Mead, 1863–1931. In *Mind, self and society from the standpoint of a social behaviorist*. Chicago, IL: University of Chicago Press.

Murphy, J. (1968). Psychiatric nurses and their patients: A study of role perception of performance. *Communicating Nursing Research*, 1, 139–150.

Oda, D. (1977). Specialized role development, a three phase process. *Nursing Outlook*, 25(6), 374–377.

Plutchik, R., Conte, H.R., Wells, W., and Darasu, T.B. (1976). Role of the psychiatric nurse. *Journal of Psychiatric Nursing and Mental Health Services*, 14(9), 38–43.

Porter, S.F. (1978). Interaction modeling. *Journal of Nursing Administration*, 8, 20–24.

Robischon, P. and Scott, D. (1969). Role theory and its application in family nursing. *Nursing Outlook*, 17, 52–57.

Sarbin, T.R. (1954). Role theory. In G. Lindzey (Ed.), *Handbook of social psychology, Vol. 1. Theory and method* (pp. 223–258). Cambridge, MA: Addison-Wesley.

Sarbin, T.R. and Jones, D.S. (1955, September). An experimental analysis of role behavior. *Journal of Abnormal Social Psychology*, 51, 236–241.

Swendsen, L.A., Meleis, A.I., and Jones, D. (1978). Role supplementation for new parents—A role mastery plan. *MCN, The American Journal of Maternal Child Nursing*, 3, 84–91.

Thornton, R. and Nardi, P. (1975). The dynamics of role acquisition. *American Journal of Sociology*, 80, 870–885.

Turner, R.H. (1962). Role taking: Process vs. conformity. In A. Rose (Ed.), *Human behavior and social processes*. Boston, MA: Houghton-Mifflin.

Turner, R.H. (1970). *Family interaction*. New York: John Wiley & Sons.

Turner, R.H. (1976). The real self from institution to impulse. *American Journal of Sociology*, 81(5), 989–1016.

Turner, R.H. (1978). The role and the person. *American Journal of Sociology*, 84, 1–23.

Turner, R.H. and Shosid, N. (1976). Ambiguity and interchangeability in role attribution: The effect of alter's response. *American Sociological Review*, 41, 993–1006.

Videbeck, R. and Bates, A. (1959). An experimental study of conformity to role expectations. *Sociometry*, 22(1).

Ward, C.R. (1986). The meaning of role strain. *Advances in Nursing Science*, 8(2), 39–49.

Weiss, S.J. (1983). Role differentiation between nurses and physician: Implications for nursing. *Nursing Research*, 32(3), 133–139.

46. Physiological Nursing Theory

Badgley, L.E. (1985). Therapeutic application of extra low frequency electromagnetic fields to living tissue. *Journal of Holistic Medicine*, 7(2), 135–144.

Carrieri, V.K., Lindsey, A.M., and West, C.M. (1986). *Physiological phenomena in nursing: Human responses to illness*. Philadelphia, PA: W.B. Saunders.

Feldman, H.R. (1984). Psychological differentiation and the phenomenon of pain. *Advances in Nursing Science*, 6(2), 50–57.

Janson-Bjerklie, S., Broushey, H.D., Carrieri, V.K., and Lindsey, A.I. (1986). Emotionally triggered asthma as a predictor of airway response to suggestion. *Research in Nursing and Health*, 9, 43–59.

Janson-Bjerklie, S., Carrieri, V., and Hudes, M. (1986). The sensations of dyspnea. *Nursing Research*, 35(3), 154–159.

Longworth, J. (1982). Psychophysiological effects of slow stroke back massage in normotensive females. *Advances in Nursing Science*, 4(4), 44–61.

Ng, L. and McCormick, K. (1982). Position changes and their physiological consequences. *Advances in Nursing Science*, 4(4), 13–25.

47. Critical Theory and Hermeneutics

Baker, C., Norton, S., Young, P., and Ward, S. (1998). An exploration of methodological pluralism in nursing research. *Research in Nursing and Health*, 21(6), 545–555.

Bauman, Z. (1978). *Hermeneutics and society science*. New York: Columbia University Press.

Berman, H., Ford-Gilboe, M., and Campbell, J.C. (1998). Combining stories and numbers: A methodologic approach for a critical nursing science. *Advances in Nursing Science*, 21(1), 1–15.

Boutain, D.M. (1999). Critical nursing scholarship: Exploring critical social theory with African American studies. *Advances in Nursing Science*, 21(4), 37–47.

Browne, A.J. (2000). The potential contributions of critical social theory to nursing science. *Canadian Journal of Nursing Research*, 32(2), 35–55.

Bubner, R. et al. (Eds.). (1975). Theory and practice in the light of the hermeneutic-criticist controversy. *Cultural Hermeneutics*, 2, 237–377.

Bubner, R. et al. (1976). Is transcendental hermeneutics possible? In J. Manninen and R. Tuomela (Eds.), *Essays on explanation and understanding: Studies in the foundations of humanities and social sciences* (pp. 59–77). Boston, MA: D. Reidel Publishing.

Butterfield, P.G. (1990). Thinking upstream: Nurturing a conceptual understanding of the societal context of health behavior. *Advances in Nursing Science*, 12(2), 1–8.

Dallmayr, W. (1972). Critical theory criticized: Habermas' knowledge and human interests and its aftermath. *Philosophy of Social Sciences*, 2, 211–229.

Dieckelmann, N. (2001). Narrative pedagogy: Heideggerian hermeneutical analyses of lived experiences of students, teachers and clinicians. *Advances in Nursing Science*, 23(3), 53–71.

Duffy, K. and Scott, P.A. (1998). Viewing an old issue through a new lens: A critical theory insight into the education-practice gap. *Nurse Education Today*, 18(3), 183–189.

Ekstrom, D.N. and Sigurdsson, H.O. (2002). An international collaboration in nursing education viewed through the lens of critical social theory. *Journal of Nursing Education*, 41(7), 289–294.

Eriksson, K. (1997). Understanding the world of the patient, the suffering human being: The new clinical paradigm from nursing to caring. *Advanced Practice Nursing Quarterly*, 3(1), 8–13.

Fealy, G.M. (2004). 'The good nurse': Visions and values in images of the nurse. *Journal of Advanced Nursing*, 46(6), 649–656.

Floistad, G. (1973). Understanding hermeneutics. *Inquiry*, 16, 445–465.

Fraser, N. (1987). What's critical about critical theory? In S. Benhabib and D. Cornell (Eds.), *Feminism as critique* (pp. 31–55). Cambridge, England: Polity Press.

Frye, M. (1983). On being white: Thinking toward a feminist understanding of race and race supremacy. In *The Politics of reality: Essays in feminist theory* (pp. 110–127). New York: Crossing Press.

Gadamer, H.G. (1975). Hermeneutics and social science. *Cultural Hermeneutics*, 2, 307–336.

Gadamer, H.G. (1976). *Philosophical hermeneutics*. In D.E. Linge (Ed., Trans.). Berkeley/Los Angeles/London: University of California Press.

Geanellos, R. (1998). Hermeneutic philosophy. Part I: Implications of its use as methodology in interpretive nursing research. *Nursing Inquiry*, 5(3), 154–163.

Geanellos, R. (1998). Hermeneutic philosophy. Part II: A nursing research example of the hermeneutic imperative to address forestructures/pre-understan-dings. *Nursing Inquiry*, 5(4), 238–247.

Geanellos, R. (2000). Exploring Ricoeur's hermeneutic theory of interpretation as a method of analysing research texts. *Nursing Inquiry*, 7(2), 112–119.

Georges, J.M. (2002). Suffering: Toward a contextual praxis. *Advances in Nursing Science*, 25(1), 79–86.

Georges, J.M. (2004). The politics of suffering: Implications for nursing science. *Advances in Nursing Science*, 27(4), 250–256.

Gibson, C.H. (1999). Facilitating critical reflection in mothers of chronically ill children. *Journal of Clinical Nursing*, 8(3), 305–312.

Habermas, J. (1970). On systematically distorted communication. *Inquiry*, 13, 205–218.

Habermas, J. (1970). Towards a theory of communicative competence. *Inquiry*, 13, 360–375.

Habermas, J. (1971). *Knowledge and human interests*. Boston, MA: Beacon Press.

Habermas, J. (1976). Theory and practice in a scientific society. In P. Connerton (Ed.), *Critical sociology* (pp. 331–347). New York: Penguin Books.

Habermas, J. (1977). A review of Gadamer's Truth and Method. In F.R. Dallmayr and T.H. McCarthy (Eds.), *Understanding and social inquiry* (pp. 335–363). Notre Dame, IN: University of Notre Dame Press.

Habermas, J. (1984). *The theory of communicative action* (Vol. 2). T. McCarthy (Trans.). Boston, MA: Beacon Press.

Hegel, G.W.F. (1931). *The phenomenology of mind* (2nd ed.). Translated with an introduction and notes by J.B. Baillie. London, UK/New York: Macmillan.

Heidegger, M. (1962). *Being and time*. J. MacQuarrie and E. Robinson (Trans.). London, UK: SCM Press.

Heinrich, K.T. and Witt, B. (1998). Serendipity: A focus group turned hermeneutic evaluation. *Nurse Educator*, 23(4), 40–44.

Held, D. (1980). *Introduction to critical theory*. Berkeley, CA: University of California Press.

Heslop, L. (1997). The (im)possibilities of poststructuralist and critical social nursing inquiry. *Nursing Inquiry*, 4(1), 48–56.

Holmes, C.A. and Warelow, P.J. (1997). Culture, needs and nursing: A critical theory approach. *Journal of Advanced Nursing*, 25(3), 463–470.

Holter, I.M. (1988). Critical theory: A foundation for the development of nursing theories. *Scholarly Inquiry for Nursing Practice*, 2, 223–232.

Hopton, J. (1997). Towards a critical theory of mental health nursing. *Journal of Advanced Nursing*, 25(3), 492–500.

Horkheimer, M. (1976). Traditional and critical theory. In P. Connerton (Ed.), *Critical sociology* (pp. 206–224). New York: Penguin Books.

Howard, R.J. (1982). *Three faces of hermeneutics: An introduction to current theories of understanding*. Berkeley, CA: University of California Press.

Koch, T. (1995). Interpretive approaches in nursing research: The influence of Husserl and Heidegger. *Journal of Advanced Nursing*, 21(5), 827–836.

Koch, T. and Harrington, A. (1998). Reconceptualizing rigour: The case for reflexivity. *Journal of Advanced Nursing*, 28(4), 882–890.

Manias, E. and Street, A. (2000). Possibilities for critical social theory and Foucault's work: A toolbox approach. *Nursing Inquiry*, 7(1), 50–60.

Marshall, B.L. (1988). Feminist theory and critical theory. *Canadian Review of Sociology and Anthropology*, 25(2), 208–230.

McLain, B.R. (1988). Collaborative practice: A critical theory perspective. *Research in Nursing Health*, 11, 391–398.

Mill, J.E., Allen, M.N., and Morrow, RA. (2001). Critical theory: Critical methodology to disciplinary foundations in nursing. *Canadian Journal of Nursing Research*, 33(2), 109–127.

Ruane, J. and Tood, J. (1988). The application of critical theory. *Political Studies*, 36, 533–538.

Scott, J.P. (1978). Critical social theory: An introduction and critique. *British Journal of Sociology*, 29(1), 1–20.

Thompson, J.B. and Held, D. (Eds.). (1982). *Habermas: Critical debates*. Cambridge, MA: MIT Press.

Thompson, J.L. (1987). Critical scholarship: The critique of domination in nursing. *Advances in Nursing Science*, 10(1), 27–38.

Tracy, J.P. (1997). Growing up with chronic illness: The experience of growing up with cystic fibrosis. *Holistic Nursing Practice*, 12(1), 27–35.

Ward-Griffin, C. (2001). Negotiating care of frail elders: Relationships between community nurses and family caregivers. *Canadian Journal of Nursing Research*, 33(2), 63–81.

Wilson-Thomas, L. (1995). Applying critical social theory in nursing education to bridge the gap between theory,

research and practice. *Journal of Advanced Nursing*, 21(3), 568–575.

Wilson-Thomas, L. (1995). Clinical notes. Theory and practice: Maintaining and facilitating the links after qualifying—The lecturer's view. *Journal of Clinical Nursing*, 4(1), 4.

48. Feminist Perspectives

Adams, T.L. and Bourgeault, I.L. (2003). Feminism and women's health professions in Ontario. *Women & Health*, 38(4), 73–90.

Alex, L. and Hammarstrom, A. (2004). Women's experiences in connection with induced abortion—A feminist perspective. *Scandinavian Journal of Caring Sciences*, 18(2), 160–168.

Allen, D.G., Allman, K.K.M., and Powers, P. (1991). Feminist nursing research without gender. *Advances in Nursing Science*, 13(3), 49–58.

Anderson, G.W., Monsen, R.B., and Rorty, M.V. (2000). Nursing and genetics: A feminist critique moves us towards transdisciplinary teams. *International Journal for Health Care Professionals*, 7(3), 191–204.

Anderson, J.M. (1991). Reflexivity in fieldwork: Toward a feminist epistemology. *Image: Journal of Nursing Scholarship*, 23, 115–118.

Anderson, J.M. (2000). Gender, "race," poverty, health and discourses of health reform in the context of globalization: A postcolonial feminist perspective in policy research. *Nursing Inquiry*, 7(4), 220–229.

Anderson, J.M. (2002). Toward a post-colonial feminist methodology in nursing research: Exploring the convergence of post-colonial and black feminist scholarship. *Nurse Researcher*, 9(3), 7–27.

Anderson, J.M. (2004). Lessons from a postcolonial-feminist perspective: Suffering and a path to healing. *Nursing Inquiry*, 11(4), 238–246.

Anderson, J.M. and McCann, E.K. (2002). Toward a post-colonial feminist methodology in nursing research: Exploring the convergence of post-colonial and black feminist scholarship. *Nurse Researcher*, 9(3), 7–27.

Anderson, J., Perry, J., Blue, C., Browne, A., Henderson, A., Khan, K.B., Reimer Kirkham, S., Lynam, J., Semeniuk, P., and Smye, V. (2003). "Riting" cultural safety within the postcolonial and postnational feminist project: Toward new epistemologies of healing. *Advances in Nursing Science*, 26(3), 196–214.

Andrist, L. (1997). A feminist model for women's health care. *Nursing Inquiry*, 4(4), 268–274.

Andrist, L.C. and MacPherson, K.I. (2001). Conceptual models for women's health research: Reclaiming menopause as an exemplar of nursing's contributions to feminist scholarship. *Annual Review of Nursing Research*, 19, 29–60.

Armishaw, J. and Davis, K. (2002). Women, hepatitis C, and sexuality: A critical feminist exploration. *Contemporary Nurse*, 12(2), 194–203.

Arpanantikul, M. (2003). Methodological issues. Integration of Heideggerian phenomenology and feminist methodology applied to the study of lived experience in women. *Thai Journal of Nursing Research*, 7(4), 281–293.

Arpanantikul, M. (2004). Midlife experiences of Thai women. *Journal of Advanced Nursing*, 47(1), 49–56.

Arslanian-Engoren, C. (2002). Feminist poststructuralism: A methodological paradigm for examining clinical decision-making. *Journal of Advanced Nursing*, 37(6), 512–517.

Aston, M., Price, S., Kirk, S.F. and Penney, T. (2011). More than meets the eye. Feminist poststructuralism as a lens toward understanding obesity. *Journal of Advanced Nursing*, 68(5), 1187–1194.

Banister, E. and Schreiber, R. (1999). Teaching feminist group process within a nursing curriculum. *Journal of Nursing Education*, 38(2), 72–76.

Banks-Wallace, J. (2000). Womanist ways of knowing: Theoretical considerations for research with African American women. *Advances in Nursing Science*, 22(3), 33–45.

Barbee, E.L. (1994). A black feminist approach to nursing research. *Western Journal of Nursing Research*, 16, 495–506.

Barnes, M. (1999). Research in midwifery—The relevance of a feminist theoretical framework. *Journal–Australian College of Midwives*, 12(2), 6–10.

Bartky, S.L. (1979). Toward a phenomenology of feminist consciousness. In S. Bishop and M. Weinzweig (Eds.), *Philosophy and women* (pp. 252–258). Belmont, CA: Wadsworth.

Belenky, M.F., Clinchy, B.M., Goldberger, N.R., and Tarule, J.M. (1986). *Women's ways of knowing*. New York: Basic Books.

Bender, A. and Ewashen, C. (2000). Group work is political work: A feminist perspective of interpersonal group psychotherapy. *Issues in Mental Health Nursing*, 21(3), 297–308.

Blackford, J. (2003). Cultural frameworks of nursing practice: Exposing an exclusionary healthcare culture. *Nursing Inquiry*, 10(4), 236–244.

Blackford, J. and Street, A. (2000). Nurses of NESB working in a multicultural community. *Contemporary Nurse*, 9(1), 89–98.

Blackford, J. and Street, A. (2002). Cultural conflict: The impact of western feminism(s) on nurses caring for women of non-English speaking background. *Journal of Clinical Nursing*, 11(5), 664–671.

Bleier, R. (1990). *Feminist approaches to science*. New York: Pergamon Press.

Boughton, M.A. (2002). Premature menopause: Multiple disruptions between the woman's biological body experience and her lived body. *Journal of Advanced Nursing*, 37(5), 423–430.

Bowden, P. (2000). An "ethic of care" in clinical settings: Encompassing "feminine" and 'feminist' perspectives. *Nursing Philosophy*, 1(1), 36–49.

Breines, W. (1986). The 1950s: Gender and some social science. *Sociological Inquiry*, 6(1), 69–93.

Briscoe, L. and Street, C. (2003). "Vanished twin": An exploration of women's experiences. *Birth*, 30(1), 47–53.

Byrd, M.M. and Garwick, A.W. (2004). A feminist critique of research on interracial family identity: Implications for family health. *Journal of Family Nursing*, 10(3), 302–322.

Camillo, P. (2004). Understanding the culture of primary health care: Implications for clinical practice. *Journal of the New York State Nurses' Association*, 35(1), 14–19.

Campbell, J.C. and Bunting, S. (1991). Voices and paradigms: Perspectives on critical and feminist theory in nursing. *Advances in Nursing Science*, 13(3), 1–15.

Caroselli, C. (1995). Power and feminism: A nursing science perspective. *Nursing Science Quarterly*, 8(3), 115–119.

Ceci, C. and McIntyre, M. (2001). A "quiet" crisis in health care: Developing our capacity to hear. *Nursing Philosophy*, 2(2), 122–130.

Chinn, P.L. and Wheeler, C.E. (1985). Feminism and nursing: Can nursing afford to remain aloof from the women's movement? *Nursing Outlook*, 33(2), 74–77.

Chinn, P.L. (1986). *Feminism, knowledge development, and client/environment interaction*. Doctoral Forum Proceedings, 1986. San Francisco, CA: University of California.

Chinn, P.L. (1986). Feminist nursing literature? *Cassandra: Radical Feminist Nurses News Journal*, 4, 9–11.

Chinn, P.L. (1988). From the editor: The politics of knowing [Editorial]. *Advances in Nursing Science*, 10(4), viii.

Cloyes, K.G. (2002). Agonizing care: Care ethics, agonistic feminism and a political theory of care. *Nursing Inquiry*, 9(3), 203–214.

Condon, E.H. (1992). Nursing and the caring metaphor: Gender and political influences on an ethics of care. *Nursing Outlook*, 40, 14–19.

Connell, M.T. (1983). Feminine consciousness and the nature of nursing practice: A historical perspective. *Topics in Clinical Nursing*, 5(3), 1–10.

Cook, J.A. and Fonow, M. (1986). Knowledge and women's interests: Issues of epistemology and methodology in feminist sociological research. *Sociological Inquiry*, 6(1), 2–29.

Cooper, M.C. (1982). Gilligan's different voice: A perspective for nursing. *Journal of Professional Nursing*, 5(1), 10–16.

Cowling, W.R. III and Chinn, P.L. (2001). Conversation across paradigms: Unitary-transformative and critical feminist perspectives. *Scholarly Inquiry for Nursing Practice*, 15(4), 347–365.

Crowe, M. and Alavi, C. (1999). Mad talk: Attending to the language of distress. *Nursing Inquiry*, 6(1), 26–33.

Davis, A.Y. (1989). *Women, culture and politics*. New York: Random House.

Davis, K., Taylor, B., and Furniss, D. (2001). Narrative accounts of tracking the rural domestic violence survivors' journey: A feminist approach. *Health Care for Women International*, 22(4), 333–347.

De Beauvoir, S. (1970). *The second sex*. New York: Bantam.

DeMarco, R., Campbell, J., and Wuest, J. (1993). Feminist critique: Searching for meaning in research. *Advances in Nursing Science*, 16(2), 26–38.

DeMarco, R.F., Miller, K.H., Patsdaughter, C.A., Chisholm, M., and Grindel, C.G. (1998). From silencing the self to action: Experiences of women living with HIV/AIDS. *Health Care for Women International*, 19(6), 539–552.

Diem, E. (2000). Balancing relationship and discipline: The pressing concern of mothers of early-adolescent girls. *Canadian Journal of Nursing Research*, 31(4), 87–103.

Doering, L. (1992). Power and knowledge in nursing: A feminist post-structuralist view. *Advances in Nursing Science*, 14, 24–33.

Doiron-Maillet, N. and Meagher-Stewart, D. (2003). The uncertain journey: Women's experiences following a myocardial infarction. *Canadian Journal of Cardiovascular Nursing*, 13(2), 14–23.

Donovan, J. (1985). *Feminist theory: The intellectual traditions of American feminism*. New York: Frederick Ungar.

Doran, F.M. and Cameron, C.C. (1998). Hearing nurses' voices through reflection in women's studies. *Nurse Education Today*, 18(1), 64–71.

DuBois, B. (1983). Passionate scholarship: Notes on values, knowing and method in feminist social science. In G. Bowles and R. Klein (Eds.), *Theories of women's studies*. London, UK: Routledge & Kegan Paul.

Duffy, M.E. (1985). A critique of research: A feminist perspective. *Health Care for Women International*, 6(5–6), 341–352.

Duffy, M. and Hedin, B. (1988). New directives. In N. Woods and M. Catanzano (Eds.), *Research methods for nursing science* (pp. 530–539). St. Louis, MO: C.V. Mosby.

Ehlers, V. (1999). Nursing research: Can a feminist perspective make any contribution? *Curationis*, 22(1), 22–28.

Eisenstein, Z. (1977). Developing a theory of capitalist patriarchy and socialist feminism. *The Insurgent Sociologist*, 7(3), 5–40.

Eisler, R. (1988). *The chalice and the blade: Our history, our future*. San Francisco, CA: Harper & Row.

Ellingston, L. (2003). Women's somatic styles: Rethinking breast self-examination education. *Health Care for Women International*, 24(9), 759–772.

Evans, J. (2004). Men nurses: A historical and feminist perspective. *Journal of Advanced Nursing*, 47(3), 321–328.

Evans, J.A. (2002). Cautious caregivers: Gender stereotypes and the sexualization of men nurses' touch. *Journal of Advanced Nursing*, 40(4), 441–448.

Falk-Rafael, A.R., Chinn, P.L., Anderson, M.A., Laschinger, H., and Rubotzky, A.M. (2004). The effectiveness of feminist pedagogy in empowering a community of learners. *Journal of Nursing Education*, 43(3), 107–115.

Fallon, D. (2003). Adolescents accessing emergency contraception in the A&E department—A feminist analysis of the nursing experience. *Accident & Emergency Nursing*, 11(2), 75–81.

Farganis, S. (1986). Social theory and feminist theory: The need for dialogue. *Sociological Inquiry*, 56(1), 50–68.

Farrell, G.A. (2001). From tall poppies to squashed weeds: Why don't nurses pull together more? *Journal of Advanced Nursing*, 35(1), 26–33.

Finfgeld, D.L. (2001). New directions for feminist therapy based on social constructionism. *Archives of Psychiatric Nursing*, 15(3), 148–154.

Flax, J. (1987). Postmodernism and gender relations in feminist theory. *Signs: Journal of Women in Culture and Society*, 12, 621–643.

Ford, K. and Turner, D. (2001). Stories seldom told: Paediatric nurses' experiences of caring for hospitalized children with special needs and their families. *Journal of Advanced Nursing*, 33(3), 288–295.

Francis, B. (2000). Poststructuralism and nursing: Uncomfortable bedfellows? *Nursing Inquiry*, 7(1). 20–28.

Gilligan, C. (1982). *In a different voice: Psychological theory and women's development*. Cambridge, MA: Harvard University Press.

Georges, J.M. (2002). Suffering: Toward a contextual praxis. *Advances in Nursing Science*, 25(1), 79–86.

Georges, J.M. (2003). An emerging discourse: Toward epistemic diversity in nursing. *Advances in Nursing Science*, 26(1), 44–52.

Georges, J.M. and McGuire, S. (2004). Deconstructing clinical pathways: Mapping the landscape of health care. *Advances in Nursing Science*, 27(1), 2–11.

Giarratano, G. (2003). Woman-centered maternity nursing education and practice. *Journal of Perinatal Education*, 12(1), 18–28.

Giarratano, G., Bustamante-Forest, R., and Pollock, C. (1999). New pedagogy for maternity nursing education. *Journal of Obstetric, Gynecologic, and Neonatal Nursing*, 28(2), 127–134.

Glass, N. and Davis, K. (1998). An emancipatory impulse: A feminist postmodern integrated turning point in nursing research. *Advances in Nursing Science*, 21(1), 43–52.

Glass, N. and Davis, K. (2004). Reconceptualizing vulnerability: Deconstruction and reconstruction as a postmodern feminist analytical research method. *Advances in Nursing Science*, 27(2), 82–92.

Grady, K. (1981). Sex bias in research design. *Psychology of Women Quarterly*, 5, 628–637.

Gray, D.P. (1995). A journey into feminist pedagogy. *Journal of Nursing Education*, 34, 77–81.

Green, B. (2012). Applying feminist ethics of care to nursing practice. *Journal of Nursing & Care*, 1(3), 1–4.

Guruge, S. and Khanlou, N. (2004). Intersectionalities of influence: Research the health of immigrant and refugee women. *Canadian Journal of Nursing Research*, 36(3), 32–47.

Gustafson, D.L. (2000). Best laid plans: Examining contradictions between intent and outcome in a feminist, collaborative research project. *Qualitative Health Research*, 10(6), 717–733.

Haegert, S. (2000). An African ethic for nursing? *Nursing Ethics*, 7(6), 492–502.

Hagell, E.I. (1989). Nursing knowledge: Women's knowledge. A sociological perspective. *Journal of Advanced Nursing*, 14(3), 226–233.

Hall, J.M. (2000). Women survivors of childhood abuse: The impact of traumatic stress on education and work. *Issues in Mental Health Nursing*, 21(5), 443–471.

Hall, J.M. and Stevens, P.E. (1991). Rigor in feminist research. *Advances in Nursing Science*, 13(3), 16–29.

Harding, S. (1983). Common causes: Toward a reflexive feminist theory. *Women and Politics*, 3(4), 27–42.

Harding, S. (1986). *The science question in feminism*. Ithaca, NY: Cornell University Press.

Harding, S. (Ed.) (1987). *Feminism and methodology*. Bloomington, IN: Indiana University Press.

Harding, S. (1988). Feminism confronts the sciences: Reform and transformation. In C. Bridges and N. Wells (Eds.), *Proceedings of the fifth nursing science colloquium* (pp. 73–92). Boston, MA: Boston University.

Harvin, S. (2002). While leaving abusive male partners, women engaged in a 4 stage process of reclaiming self. *Evidence Based Nursing*, 5(2), 60.

Hedin, B. (1986). Nursing, education, and emancipation: Applying the critical theoretical approach to nursing research. In P. Chinn (Ed.), *Nursing research methodology: Issues and implementation* (pp. 133–146). Rockville, MD: Aspen Systems.

Hedin, B. and Donovan, J. (1989). A feminist perspective on nursing education. *Nurse Educator*, 14(4), 8–13.

Heffern, W.A. and Austin, W. (1999). Compulsory community treatment: Ethical considerations. *Journal of Psychiatric and Mental Health Nursing*, 6(1), 37–42.

Henderson, D. (1997). Intersecting race and gender in feminist theories of women's psychological development. *Issues in Mental Health Nursing*, 18(5), 377–393.

Huntington, A.D. (2002). Working with women experiencing mid-trimester termination of pregnancy: The integration of nursing and feminist knowledge in the gynaecological setting. *Journal of Clinical Nursing*, 11(2), 273–279.

Huntington, A.D. and Gilmour, J.A. (2001). Re-thinking representations, re-writing nursing texts: Possibilities through feminist and Foucauldian thought. *Journal of Advanced Nursing*, 35(6), 902–908.

Im, E. (2001). Nursing research on physical activity: A feminist critique. *International Journal of Nursing Studies*, 38(2), 185–194.

Im, E.O. and Chee, W. (2001). A feminist critique of research on cancer pain. *Western Journal of Nursing Research*, 23(7), 726–752.

Im, E.O. and Chee, W. (2001). A feminist critique on the use of the Internet in nursing research. *Advances in Nursing Science*, 23(4), 67–82.

Im, E.O., Park, Y.S. Lee, E.O., and Yun, S.N. (2004). Korean women's attitudes toward breast cancer screening tests. *International Journal of Nursing Studies*, 41(6), 583–589.

Jackson, D., Brady, W., and Stein, I. (1999). Towards (re) conciliation: (Re)constructing relationships between indigenous health workers and nurses. *Journal of Advanced Nursing*, 29(1), 97–103.

Jackson, D., Daly, J., Davidson, P., Elliott, D., Cameron-Traub, E., Wade, V., Chin, C., and Salamonson, Y. (2000). Women recovering from first-time myocardial infarction (MI): A feminist qualitative study. *Journal of Advanced Nursing*, 32(6), 1403–1411.

Jackson, D. and Mannix, J. (2003). Mothering and women's health: I love being a mother but . . . there is always something new to worry about. *Australian Journal of Advanced Nursing*, 20(3), 30–37.

Jackson, D. and Mannix, J. (2004). Giving voice to the burden of blame: A feminist study of mothers' experiences of mother blaming. *International Journal of Nursing Practice*, 10(4), 150–158.

Jaggar, A. (1979). Political philosophies of women's liberation. In S. Bishop and M. Weinzweig (Eds.), *Philosophy and women*. Belmont, CA: Wadsworth.

Jaggar A. and Struhl, P.R. (1978). *Feminist frameworks: Alternative theoretical accounts of the relations between women and men*. New York: McGraw-Hill.

Jayaratne, T.E. (1983). The value of quantitative methodology for feminist research. In G. Bowles and R.D. Klein (Eds.), *Theories of Women's Studies* (pp. 140–161). Boston, MA: Routledge & Kegan Paul.

Joseph, G.I. and Lewis, J. (1981). *Common differences: Conflicts in black and white feminist perspectives*. Boston, MA: South End Press.

Kako, M. (2002). Students' corner. An oral history of Japanese nursing: Voices of five senior nurses who have experienced nursing since the 1950s. *Contemporary Nurse*, 12(2), 176–184.

Kane, D. and Thomas, B. (2000). Nursing and the 'F' word. *Nursing Forum*, 35(2), 17–24.

Karabenies, A., Miller, L., Nagel-Bamesberger, H., Rossiter, A., and Thompson, M. (1986). What makes a feminist social science? *Cassandra: Radical Feminist Nurses News Journal*, 4(1), 9–11.

Kathleen Croft, R. and Anne Cash, P. (2012). Deconstructing contributing factors to bullying and lateral violence in nursing using a postcolonial feminist lens. *Contemporary Nurse*, 42(2), 226–242.

Keddy, B., Sims, S.L., and Stern, P.N. (1996). Grounded theory as feminist research methodology. *Journal of Advanced Nursing*, 23(3), 448–453.

Keller, E.F. (1982). Feminism and science. In N.O. Keohane, M.Z. Rosaldo, and B.C. Gelpi (Eds.), *Feminist theory: A critique of ideology* (pp. 113–126). Chicago, IL: University of Chicago Press.

Keller, E.F. (1983). *A feeling for the organism. The life and work of Barbara McClintock*. New York: W.H. Freeman.

Keller, E.F. (1985). *Reflections on gender and science*. New Haven, CT: Yale University Press.

Kelly, P.J., Bobo, T., Avery, S., and McLachlan, K. (2004). Feminist perspectives and practice with young women. *Issues in Comprehensive Pediatric Nursing*, 27(2), 121–133.

Keohane, N.O., Rosaldo, M.Z., and Gelpi, B.C. (1981). *Feminist theory: A critique of ideology*. Chicago, IL: University of Chicago Press.

Kirkley, D.L. (2000). Is motherhood good for women? A feminist exploration. *Journal of Obstetric, Gynecologic, and Neonatal Nursing*, 29(5), 459–464.

Klein, R.D. (1983). How to do what we want to do: Thoughts about feminist methodology. In G. Bowles and R.D. Klein (Eds.), *Theories of women's studies* (pp. 88–104). Boston, MA: Routledge & Kegan Paul.

Klima, C.S. (2001). Women's health care: A new paradigm for the 21st century. *Journal of Midwifery & Women's Health*, 46(5), 285–291.

Kralik, D. (2002). The quest for ordinariness: Transition experienced by midlife women living with chronic illness. *Journal of Advanced Nursing*, 39(2), 146–154.

Kralik, D., Koch, T., and Brady, B.M. (2000). Pen pals: Correspondence as a method for data generation in qualitative research. *Journal of Advanced Nursing*, 31(4), 909–917.

Le Cornu, J. (1999). The need for counselling of women who undergo hysterectomy: A feminist perspective. *Contemporary Nurse*, 8(2), 46–52.

Lengermann, P.M. and Niegrugge-Brantley, J. (1988). Contemporary feminist theory. In G. Ritzer (Ed.), *Contemporary sociological theory* (2nd ed.). New York: Alfred A. Knopf.

Letvak, S. (2003). The experience of being an older staff nurse. *Western Journal of Nursing Research*, 25(1), 45–56.

Lewis, M.A. and Lewis, C.E. (2002). Nurse practitioners: The revolution produced by a 'gender-related destructive innovation' in health care. *Nursing and Health Policy Review*, 1(1), 63–71.

Liaschenko, J. (1999). Can justice coexist with the supremacy of personal values in nursing practice? *Western Journal of Nursing Research*, 21(1), 35–50.

Lindsay, R. and Graham, H. (2000). Relational narratives: Solving an ethical dilemma concerning an individual's insurance policy. *Nursing Ethics*, 7(2), 148–157.

Longino, H. E. (1987). Can there be a feminist science? *Hypatia: Journal of Feminist Philosophy*, 2(3), 51–64.

MacDonald, C. (2002). Nurse autonomy as relational. *Nursing Ethics*, 9(2), 194–201.

MacKinnon, C. (1982). Feminism, Marxism, method and the state: An agenda for theory. *Signs: Journal of Women in Culture and Society*, 7(3), 515–544.

MacPherson, K.I. (1983). Feminist methods: A new paradigm for nursing research. *Advances in Nursing Science*, 5(2), 17–25.

MacPherson, K.I. (1988). The missing piece: Women as partners in feminist research. *Advances in Nursing Science*, 5(2), 17–26.

Malmsten, K. (2000). Basic care, bodily knowledge and feminist ethics. *Medicine & Law*, 19(3), 613–622.

Marshall, B.L. (1988). Feminist theory and critical theory. *Canadian Review of Sociology and Anthropology*, 25(2), 208–230.

Mason, D.J., Backer, B.A., and Georges, C.A. (1991). Toward a feminist model for the political empowerment of nurses. *Image: Journal of Nursing Scholarship*, 23, 72–77.

Matthews, S. (2001). Registered male: A discussion on men in the nursing profession. *Contemporary Nurse*, 11(2–3), 231–235.

Maxwell-Young, L., Olshansky, E., and Steele, R. (1998). Conducting feminist research in nursing: Personal and political challenges. *Health Care for Women International*, 19(6), 505–513.

McCormick, J., Kirkham, S.R., and Hayes, V. (1998). Abstracting women: Essentialism in women's health research. *Health Care for Women International*, 19(6), 495–504.

McCormick, K.M. and Bunting, S.M. (2002). Application of feminist theory in nursing research: The case of women and cardiovascular disease. *Health Care for Women International*, 23(8), 820–834.

McDonald, C. (1999). Promoting the power of nursing identity. *Canadian Nurse*, 95(2), 34–37.

McDonald, C. and McIntyre, M. (2002). Women's health, women's health care: Complicating experience, language and ideologies. *Nursing Philosophy*, 3(3), 260–267.

McLoughlin, A. (1997). The "F" factor: Feminism forsaken? *Nurse Education Today*, 17(2), 111–114.

Melchior, F. (2004). Feminist approaches to nursing history. *Western Journal of Nursing Research*, 26(3), 340–355.

Mies, M. (1983). Towards a methodology for feminist research. In G. Bowles and R. Klein (Eds.), *Theories of women's studies* (pp. 117–139). London, UK: Routledge & Kegan Paul.

Moccia, P. (1988). A critique of compromise: Beyond the methods debate. *Advances in Nursing Science*, 10(4), 1–9.

Moraga, C. (1986). From a long line of vendidas: Chicanas and feminism. In T. de Lauretis (Ed.), *Feminist studies/critical studies* (Chap. 11). Bloomington, IN: Indiana University Press.

Nateetanasombat, K., Fongkaew, W., Sripichyakan, K., and Sethabouppha, H. (2004). The lived experiences of retired women. *Thai Journal of Nursing Research*, 8(2), 110–125.

Neely-Smith, S. (2003). The impact of HIV/AIDS on Bahamian women: A feminist perspective. *Health Care for Women International*, 24(8), 738–754.

Oakley, A. (1981). Interviewing women: A contradiction in terms. In H. Roberts (Eds.), *Doing feminist research* (Chap. 2). New York: Routledge & Kegan Paul.

Parker, B. and McFarlane, J. (1991). Feminist theory and nursing: An empowerment model for research. *Advances in Nursing Science*, 13(3), 59–67.

Peckover, S. (2002). Supporting and policing mothers: An analysis of the disciplinary practices of health visiting. *Journal of Advanced Nursing*, 38(4), 369–377.

Peckover, S. (2003). Health visitors' understandings of domestic violence. *Journal of Advanced Nursing*, 44(2), 200–208.

Perry, P.A. (1994). Feminist empiricism as a method for inquiry in nursing. *Western Journal of Nursing Research*, 16, 480–494.

Peter, E. (2000). The politicization of ethical knowledge: Feminist ethics as a basis for home care nursing research. *Canadian Journal of Nursing Research*, 32(2), 103–118.

Peter, E. (2002). The history of nursing in the home: Revealing the significance of place in the expression of moral agency. *Nursing Inquiry*, 9(2), 65–72.

Peter, E. and Liaschenko, J. (2013). Moral distress reexamined: A feminist interpretation of nurses' identities, relationships, and responsibilities. *Journal of Bioethical Inquiry*, 10(3), 337–345.

Peter, E. and Morgan, K.P. (2001). Explorations of a trust approach for nursing ethics. *Nursing Inquiry*, 8(1), 3–10.

Pitre, N.Y., Kushner, K.E., Raine, K.D. and Hegadoren, K.M. (2013). Critical feminist narrative inquiry: Advancing knowledge through double-hermeneutic narrative analysis. *Advances in Nursing Science*, 36(2), 118–132.

Racine, L. (2003). Implementing a postcolonial feminist perspective in nursing research related to non-western populations. *Nursing Inquiry*, 10(2), 91–102.

Racine, L., and Petrucka, P. (2011). Enhancing decolonization and knowledge transfer in nursing research with non-western populations: Examining the congruence between primary healthcare and postcolonial feminist approaches. *Nursing Inquiry*, 18(1), 12–20.

Rafael, A.R. (1999). From rhetoric to reality: The changing face of public health nursing in southern Ontario. *Public Health Nursing*, 16(1), 50–59.

Reason, P. and Rowan, J. (1981). *Human inquiry: A sourcebook of new paradigm research*. New York: John Wiley & Sons.

Reinharz, S. (1983). Experimental analysis: A contribution to feminist research. In G. Bowles and R. Klein (Eds.), *Theories of women studies*. London, UK: Routledge & Kegan Paul.

Roberts, H. (1981). *Doing feminist research*. London, UK: Routledge & Kegan Paul.

Rogers, J. and Kelly, U.A. (2011). Feminist intersectionality: Bringing social justice to health disparities research. *Nursing Ethics*, 18(3), 397–407.

Rose, H. (1983). Hand, brain, and heart: A feminist epistemology for the natural sciences. *Signs: Journal of Women in Culture and Society*, 9(1), 73–90.

Rose, H. (1986). Beyond masculinist realities: A feminist epistemology for the sciences. In R. Bleier (Ed.), *Feminist approaches to science*. New York: Pergamon Press.

Rubotzky, A.M. (2000). Nursing participation in health care reform efforts of 1993 to 1994: Advocating for the national community. *Advances in Nursing Science*, 23(2), 12–33.

Sampselle, C.M. (1990). The influence of feminist philosophy on nursing practice. *Image: Journal of Nursing Scholarship*, 22(4), 243–206.

Schuiling, K.D. and Sampselle, C.M. (1999). Comfort in labor and midwifery art. *Image: The Journal of Nursing Scholarship*, 31(1), 77–81.

Seibold, C. (2000). Qualitative research from a feminist perspective in the postmodern era: Methodological, ethical and reflexive concerns. *Nursing Inquiry*, 7(3), 147–155.

Selanders, L.C. (1998). Florence Nightingale: The evolution and social impact of feminist values in nursing. *Journal of Holistic Nursing*, 16(2), 227–243; discussion 244–246.

Sherwin, S. (1987). Concluding remarks: A feminist perspective. *Health Care for Women International*, 8(4), 293–304.

Shields, L.E. (1995). Women's experiences of the meaning of empowerment. *Qualitative Health Research*, 5(1), 15–35.

Simpson, C. (2002). Hope and feminist care ethics: What is the connection? *Canadian Journal of Nursing Research*, 34(2), 81–94.

Smith, D. (1974). Women's perspective as a radical critique of sociology. *Sociological Inquiry*, 44, 7–13.

Smith, D. (1990). *The conceptual practices of power: A feminist sociology of knowledge*. Toronto, Canada: University of Toronto Press.

Sohier, R. (1992). Feminism and nursing knowledge: The power of the weak. *Nursing Outlook*, 40, 62–66, 93.

Stacey, J. and Thorne, B. (1985). The missing feminist revolution in sociology. *Social Problems*, 32(4), 301–316.

Taylor, J.Y. (1998). Womanism: A methodologic framework for African American women. *Advances in Nursing Science*, 21(1), 53–64.

Thomas, L.W. (1995). A critical feminist perspective of the health belief model: Implications for nursing theory, research, practice, and education. *Journal of Professional Nursing*, 11(4), 246–252.

Thompson, J.L. (1985). Practical discourse in nursing: Going beyond empiricism and historicism. *Advances in Nursing Science*, 7(4), 59–71.

Thompson, J.L. (1991). Exploring gender and culture with Khmer refugee women: Reflections on participatory feminist research. *Advances in Nursing Science*, 13(3), 30–48.

Thorne, S. and Varcoe, C. (1998). The tyranny of feminist methodology in women's health research. *Health Care for Women International*, 19(6), 481–493.

Tronto, J. (1987). Beyond gender difference to a theory of care. *Signs: Journal of Women in Culture and Society*, 12(4), 644–663.

Van Herk, K.A., Smith, D., and Andrew, C. (2011). Examining our privileges and oppressions: Incorporating an intersectionality paradigm into nursing. *Nursing Inquiry*, 18(1), 29–39.

Weedon, C. (1991). *Feminist practice and post-structuralist theory*. Cambridge, MA: Basil Blackwell.

Weyenberg, D. (1998). The construction of feminist pedagogy in nursing education: A preliminary critique. *Journal of Nursing Education*, 37(8), 345–353.

Williams, S.C. and Mackey, M.C. (1999). Women's experiences of preterm labor: A feminist critique. *Health Care for Women International*, 20(1), 29–48.

Wright, N. and Owen, S. (2001). Feminist conceptualizations of women's madness: A review of the literature. *Journal of Advanced Nursing*, 36(1), 143–150.

Wuest, J. (1993). Removing the shackles: A feminist critique of noncompliance. *Nursing Outlook*, 41, 217–224.

Wuest, J. (1994). A feminist approach to concept analysis. *Western Journal of Nursing Research*, 16(5), 577–586.

Wuest, J. (1994). Professionalism and the evolution of nursing as a discipline: A feminist perspective. *Journal of Professional Nursing*, 10, 357–367.

Wuest, J. (2001). Precarious ordering: Toward a formal theory of women's caring. *Health Care for Women International*, 22(1/2), 167–193.

MIDDLE-RANGE THEORY

Acton, G.J., Irvin, B.L., Jensen, J.A., Hopkins, B.A., and Miller, E.W. (1997). Explicating middle-range theory through methodological diversity. *Advances in Nursing Science*, 19(3), 78–85.

Auvil-Novak, S.E. (1997). A middle-range theory of chronotherapeutic intervention for postsurgical pain. *Nursing Research*, 46(2), 66–71.

Bu, X. and Jezewski, M.A. (2007). Developing a mid-range theory of patient advocacy through concept analysis. *Journal of Advanced Nursing*, 57(1), 101–110.

Carr, J.M. (2014). A middle-range theory of family vigilance. *MEDSURG Nursing*, 23(4), 251–255.

Casalenuovo, G.A. (2002). Fatigue in diabetes mellitus: Testing a middle range theory of well-being derived from Neuman's theory of optimal client system stability and the Neuman systems model. *Dissertation Abstracts International*, 63, 2301B.

Chinn, P.L. (2001). Why middle-range theory? [Editorial]. *Advances in Nursing Science*, 19(3), viii.

Christie, J., Poulton, B.C., and Bunting, B.P. (2008). An integrated mid-range theory of postpartum family development: A guide for research and practice. *Journal of Advanced Nursing*, 61(1), 38–50.

Davidson, J.E. (2010). Facilitated sensemaking: A strategy and new middle-range theory to support families of intensive care unit patients. *Critical Care Nurse*, 30(6), 28–39.

Dunn, K.S. (2004). Toward a middle-range theory of adaptation to chronic pain. *Nursing Science Quarterly*, 17(1), 78–84.

Dunn, K.S. (2005). Testing a middle-range theoretical model of adaptation to chronic pain. *Nursing Science Quarterly*, 18(2), 146–156.

Dyess, S.M. and Chase, S.K. (2012). Sustaining health in faith community nursing practice: Emerging processes that support the development of a middle-range theory. *Holistic Nursing Practice*, 26(4), 221–227.

Elo, S., Kaariainen, M., Isola, A., and Kyngas, H. (2013). Developing and testing a middle-range theory of the well-being supportive physical environment of home-dwelling elderly. *The Scientific World Journal*. Article ID 945635.

Fawcett, J. (2005). Middle-range nursing theories are necessary for the advancement of the discipline. *Revista Aquichan*, 5(1), 32–43.

Fearon-Lynch, J.A. and Stover, C.M. (2015). A middle-range theory for diabetes self-management mastery. *Advances in Nursing Science*, 38(4), 330–346.

Flood, M. (2005). A mid-range nursing theory of successful aging. *Journal of Theory Construction and Testing*, 9(2), 35–39.

Forsberg, A., Lennerling, A., Fridh, I., Karlsson, V. and Nilsson, M. (2015, January-December). Understanding the perceived threat of the risk of graft rejections: A middle-range theory. *Global Qualitative Nursing Research*, 2, 1–9.

Garcia-Fernandez, F.P., Agreda, J.J., Verdu, J. and Pancorbo-Hidalgo, P.L. (2014). A new theoretical model for the development of pressure ulcers and other dependence-related lesions. *Journal of Nursing Scholarship*, 46(1), 28–38.

Gigliotti, E. (2003). The Neuman Systems Model Institute: Testing middle-range theories. *Nursing Science Quarterly*, 16(3), 201–206.

Hanson, M.D. (2004). Using data from critical care nurses to validate Swanson's phenomenological derived middle range caring theory. *Journal of Theory Construction and Testing*, 8(1), 21–25.

Hills, R.G.S. and Hanchett, E. (2001). Human change and individuation in pivotal life situations: Development and testing the theory of enlightenment. *Visions: The Journal of Rogerian Nursing Science*, 9(1), 6–19.

Kolcaba, K. (2001). Evolution of the mid-range theory of comfort for outcomes research. *Nursing Outlook*, 49(2), 86–92.

Lasiuk, G.C. and Ferguson, L.M. (2005). From practice to midrange theory and back again: Beck's theory of postpartum depression. *Advances in Nursing Science*, 28(2), 127–136.

Liehr, P. (2005). Looking at symptoms with a middle-range theory lens. *Advanced Studies in Nursing*, 3(5), 152–157.

Liehr, P. and Smith, M.J. (1999). Middle range theory: Spinning research and practice to create knowledge for the new millennium. *Advances in Nursing Science*, 21(4), 81–91.

Lenz, E.R. (1998). Beneath the surface: The role of middle-range theory for nursing research and practice: Part 2. Nursing practice. *Nursing Leadership Forum*, 3(2), 62–66.

Lenz, E.R., Pugh, L.C., Milligan, R.A., Gift, A., and Suppe, F. (1997). The middle range theory of unpleasant symptoms: An update. *Advances in Nursing Science*, 19(3), 14–27.

Marsh, J.R. (2013). A middle-range theory of postpartum depression: Analysis and application. *International Journal of Childbirth Education*, 28(4), 50–54.

McCreaddie, M. and Wiggins, S. (2009). Reconciling the good patient persona with problematic and non-problematic humour: A grounded theory. *International Journal of Nursing Studies*, 46, 1079–1091.

McEwen, M. (2002). Middle-range nursing theories. In M. McEwan and E. Wills (Eds.), *Theoretical basis for nursing* (pp. 202–205). Philadelphia, PA: Lippincott Williams & Williams.

Meleis, A.I. (2015). Transitions theory. In M.C. Smith and M.E. Parker (Eds.) *Nursing theories and nursing practice* (4th ed., pp. 361–380). Philadelphia, PA: FA Davis.

Meleis, A., Sawyer, L.M., Im, E., Messias, D.K.H., and Schumacher, K. (2000). Experiencing transitions: An emerging middle-range theory. *Advances in Nursing Science*, 23(1), 12–28.

Olsen, J. and Hanchett, E. (1997). Nurse-expressed empathy, patient outcomes, and development of middle-range theory. *Image: Journal of Nursing Scholarship*, 29(1), 71–76.

Orticio, L.P. (2007). Sensing presence and sensing space: A middle range theory of nursing. *Insight*, 32(4), 7–11.

Perry, D.J. (2015). Transcendent pluralism: A middle-range theory of nonviolent social transformation through human and ecological dignity. *Advances in Nursing Science*, 38(4), 317–329.

Peterson, S.J. and Bredow, T.S. (2004). *Middle range theories: Application to nursing theory*. Philadelphia, PA: Lippincott Williams & Wilkins.

Pickett, S., Peters, R.M. and Jarosz, P.A. (2014). Toward a middle-range theory of weight management. *Nursing Science Quarterly*, 27(3), 242–247.

Polk, L.V. (1997). Toward a middle-range theory of resilience. *Advances in Nursing Science*, 19(3), 1–13.

Riegel, B., Jaarsma, T., and Stromberg, A. (2012). A middle-range theory of self-care of chronic illness. *Advances in Nursing Science*, 35(3), 194–204.

Ryan, P. and Sawin, K.J. (2009). The individual and family self-management theory: Background and perspectives on context, process, and outcomes. *Nursing Outlook*, 57(4), 217–225.

Sanford, R.C. (2000). Caring through relation and dialogue: A nursing perspective for patient education. *Advances in Nursing Science*, 22(3), 1–15.

Sieloff, C.L., Frey, M.A., and King, I.M. (2007). *Middle range theory development using King's conceptual system*. New York: Springer Publishing Company.

Smith, M.J. and Liehr, P. (1999). Attentively Embracing Story: A middle-range theory with practice and research implications. *Scholarly Inquiry for Nursing Practice*, 13(3), 187–204.

Smith, M.J. and Liehr, P. (2003). *Middle range theory for nursing*. New York: Springer Publishing Company.

Thurmond, V.A. and Popkess-Vawter, S. (2003). Examination of a middle range theory: Applying Astin's Input-Environment-Outcome (I-E-O) model to web-based education. *Online Journal of Nursing Informatics*, 7(2).

Tsai, P.F. (2003). A middle-range theory of caregiver stress. *Nursing Science Quarterly*, 16(2), 137–145.

Whittemore, R. and Roy, Sister C. (2002). Adapting to diabetes mellitus: A theory synthesis. *Nursing Science Quarterly*, 15(4), 311–317.

Woods, S.J. and Isenberg, M.A. (2001). Adaptation as a mediator of intimate abuse and traumatic stress in battered women. *Nursing Science Quarterly*, 14(3), 215–221.

SITUATION-SPECIFIC THEORY

Chang, S.J. and Im, E.O. (2014). Development of a situation-specific theory for explaining health-related quality of life among older South Korean Adults with type 2 diabetes. *Research and Theory for Nursing Practice: An International Journal*, 28(2), 113–126.

Clingeman, E. (2007). A situation-specific theory of migration transition for migrant farmworker women. *Research and Theory for Nursing Practice*, 21(4), 220–235.

Im, E.O. (2005). Development of situation–specific theories—An integrative approach. *Advances in Nursing Science*, 28(2), 137–151.

Im, E.O. (2006). A situation-specific theory of Caucasian cancer patients' pain experience. *Advances in Nursing Science*, 29(3), 232–244.

Im, E.O. (2008). The situation-specific theory of pain experience for Asian American cancer patients. *Advances in Nursing Science*, 31(4), 319–331.

Im, E.O. (2014). The status quo of situation-specific theories. *Research and Theory for Nursing Practice*, 28(4), 278–298.

Im, E.O. (2014). Situation-specific theories from the middle-range transitions theory. *Advances in Nursing Science*, 37(1), 19–31.

Im, E.O., Chang, S.J., Nguyen, G., Stringer, L., Chee, W., and Chee, E. (2015). Korean immigrant women's physical activity experience: A situation-specific theory. *Research and Theory for Nursing Practice: An International Journal*, 29(1), 10–24.

Lee, H., Fawcett, J., Yang, J.H., and Hann, H.-W. (2012). Correlates of hepatitis B virus health-related behaviors of Korean Americans: A situation-specific nursing theory. *Journal of Nursing Scholarship*, 44(4), 315–322.

Nelson, A.M. (2006). Toward a situation-specific theory of breastfeeding. *Research and Theory for Nursing Practice*, 20(1), 9–27.

Riegel, B. and Dickson, V.V. (2008). A situation-specific theory of heart failure self-care. *Journal of Cardiovascular Nursing*, 23(3), 190–196.

Riegel, B., Dickson, V.V., and Faulkner, K.M. (2015). The situation-specific theory of heart failure self-care: Revised and updated. *The Journal of Cardiovascular Nursing.* 31(3):226–235.

Smith, J.J. and Liehr, P.R. (2014). *Middle range theory for nursing* (3rd ed.). New York: Springer Publishing Company.

Willis, D.G., DeSanto-Madeya, S., and Fawcett, J. (2015). Moving beyond dwelling in suffering a situation-specific theory of men's healing from childhood maltreatment. *Nursing Science quarterly*, 28(1), 57–63.

WEBSITES AND MEDIA ON THEORY

49. DVD Productions from the National League for Nursing

A Conversation with Virginia Henderson
Interview with Virginia Henderson about her life and work, conducted by Patricia Moccia. Available from: NLN Customer Service, National League for Nursing, 350 Hudson Street, New York, NY 10014 (800) 669–9656, ext. 138, FAX (212) 989–3710. Send Internet e-mails (queries only) to: Custserv@nln.org

Nursing in America: A History of Social Reform
Video that examines nursing's history of social reform while chronicling social, political, and economic influences that shaped American nursing. Available from: NLN Customer Service, National League for Nursing, 350 Hudson Street, New York, NY 10014 (800) 669–9656, ext. 138, FAX (212) 989–3710. Send Internet e-mails (queries only) to: Custserv@nln.org

Nursing Theory: A Circle of Knowledge
Video hosted by Patricia Moccia that examines issues related to philosophy of nursing science, particularly the relevance of nursing theory to practice. Features discussions with Patricia Benner, Virginia Henderson, Dorothea Orem, Martha Rogers, Callista Roy, and Jean Watson. Available from: NLN Customer Service, National League for Nursing, 350 Hudson Street, New York, NY 10014 (800) 669–9656, ext. 138, FAX (212) 989–3710. Send Internet e-mails (queries only) to: Custserv@nln.org

Theories at Work
Video hosted by Patricia Moccia about innovative applications of nursing theory in nurse-managed health care systems. Moccia visits centers of nursing practice around the country and talks with Dorothy Powell, Bernadine Lacey, Jean Watson, and Janet Quinn about their theory-based nursing care. Available from: NLN Customer Service, National League for Nursing, 350 Hudson Street, New York, NY 10014 (800) 669–9656, ext. 138, FAX (212) 989–3710. Send Internet e-mails (queries only) to: Custserv@nln.org

Therapeutic Touch: Healing through Human Energy Fields
A three-part video hosted by Janet F. Quinn. Part I explores the theoretical framework of therapeutic touch, defines key concepts, and highlights research studies documenting the clinical effectiveness of therapeutic touch. Part II explains the method nurses use in performing therapeutic touch, and Part III explores the clinical application of therapeutic touch in clinics, private practice, and hospitals. Available from: NLN Customer Service, National League for Nursing, 350 Hudson Street, New York, NY 10014 (800) 669–9656, ext. 138, FAX (212) 989–3710. Send Internet e-mails (queries only) to: Custscrv@nln.org

Critical Thinking in Nursing: Lessons from Tuskegee
This video examines the story of nurse Eunice Rivers and the infamous Tuskegee Syphilis Study in which 400 African American men were left untreated for the disease as part of a government study. The presentation brings forth a number of social and ethical issues that warrant critical thinking among nurses. A companion book is also available. Available from: NLN Customer Service, National League for Nursing, 350 Hudson Street, New York, NY 10014 (800) 669–9656, ext. 138, FAX (212) 989–3710. Send Internet e-mails (queries only) to: Custserv@nln.org

A Conversation on Caring with Jean Watson and Janet Quinn
A video in which Jean Watson and Janet Quinn discuss the elements of caring. Available from: NLN Customer Service, National League for Nursing, 350 Hudson Street, New York, NY 10014 (800) 669–9656, ext. 138, FAX (212) 989–3710. Send Internet e-mails (queries only) to: Custserv@nln.org

A Guide to Applying the Art and Science of Human Care
A set of two videos in which Jean Watson gives an overview of her Theory of Human Science and Human Caring and a panel, moderated by Peggy Chinn, discusses the implementation of the caring model in diverse practice and educational settings. Available from: NLN Customer Service, National League for Nursing, 350 Hudson Street, New York, NY 10014 (800) 669–9656, ext. 138, FAX (212) 989–3710. Send Internet e-mails (queries only) to: Custserv@nln.org

The Power of Nursing
A discussion of the concept of power and of nurses' relation with health policy. Available from: NLN Customer Service, National League for Nursing, 350 Hudson Street, New York, NY 10014 (800) 669–9656, ext. 138, FAX (212) 989–3710. Send Internet e-mails (queries only) to: Custserv@nln.org

Nursing in America: Through a Feminist Lens
A video in which the issues of autonomy and control are compared in relation to nurses' historic struggle for independence and feminists' battle to empower women. Available from: NLN Customer Service, National League for Nursing, 350 Hudson Street, New York, NY 10014 (800) 669–9656, ext. 138, FAX (212) 989–3710. Send Internet e-mails (queries only) to: Custserv@nln.org

50. DVD Productions from FITNE

The Nurse Theorists: Portraits of Excellence: Volume I
Series of 16 DVDs about the lives and scholarly accomplishments of notable nurse theorists. Each video contains a biographical sketch of the theorist, an interview conducted by Jacqueline Fawcett, and a summary of the nursing theory. Videotapes include: (1) Virginia Henderson, "Definition of Nursing"; (2) Dorothy Johnson, "Behavioral Systems Model"; (3) Imogene King, "Interacting System Framework"; (4) Madeline Leininger, "Transcultural Nursing Care"; (5) Myra Levine, "The Conservative Model"; (6) Betty Neuman, "Neuman Systems Model"; (7) Florence Nightingale, "Special Edition"; (8) Dorothea Orem, "Self Care Framework"; (9) Ida Orlando Pelletier, "The Deliberative Nursing Process"; (10) Hildegard Peplau, "Interpersonal Relations in Nursing"; (11) Martha Rogers, "Science of Unitary Human Beings"; (12) Callista Roy, "The Adaptations Model of Nursing"; (13) Reva Rubin, "Theory of Maternal Identity"; (14) Jean Watson, "A Theory of Caring"; (15) Margaret Newman, "Health as Expanding Consciousness"; and (16) Rosemarie Parse, "Man-Living Health." Available from: FITNE, 5 Depot Street, Athens, OH 45701, (614) 592–2511. https://www.fitne.net/nurse_theorists1.jsp

The Nurse Theorists: Portraits of Excellence: Volume II
Series of 6 DVDs about the lives and scholarly accomplishments of distinguished middle-range theorists. Each video includes interviews in which the theorist discusses her life, the evolution of her work and its impact on nursing practice and education. Videotapes include: (1) Helen Erickson, "Modeling and Role-Modeling"; (2) Merle Mishel, "Uncertainty in Illness"; (3) Nola Pender, "Health Promotion"; (4) Pamela Reed, "Self-Transcendence"; (5) Afaf Meleis, "Transitions"; and (6) Patricia Benner, "Novice to Expert." Available from: FITNE, 5 Depot Street, Athens, OH 45701, (614) 592–2511. https://www.fitne.net/nurse_theorists2.jsp

From Beginner to Expert: Clinical Knowledge in Critical Care Nursing
Dr. Patricia Benner and her research team discuss the methods and major findings of a study of clinical learning and skilled clinical judgment among critical care nurses, and the implications in terms of the process of becoming an expert nurse. Available from: FITNE, 5 Depot Street, Athens, OH 45701, (614) 592–2511.

Adaptation Model in Practice
The application of Callista Roy's adaptation model, which promotes the biological, psychological and sociological aspects of patients in relation to a constantly changing environment, is demonstrated at two different health care institutions. Available from: FITNE, 5 Depot Street, Athens, OH 45701, (614) 592–2511.

Self-Care Framework Model in Practice
This video describes Dorothea Orem's self-care deficit nursing theory and presents case studies to demonstrate the application of the theory to nursing practice. Available from: FITNE, 5 Depot Street, Athens, OH 45701, (614) 592–2511.

51. DVD Productions from the Health Sciences Consortium

Care with a Concept
This program by Mary Hale and Gates Rhodes discusses the application of Dorothea Orem's self-care conceptual model in a pediatric rehabilitation center. As Orem's model is applied, nurse-managers are enabled to evaluate the effects of the nursing care rendered. Available from: Health Sciences Consortium, 201 Silver Cedar Court, Chapel Hill, NC 27514–1517, (919) 942–8731, FAX (919) 942–3689.

52. Conference DVD's

Nurse Theorist Conference 1985
Videotaped presentations include (1) Dorothea Orem, "Presentation"; (2) Hildegard Peplau, "Nursing Science: A Historical View"; and (3) "Panel Discussion with Theorists" with Dorothea E. Orem, Callista Roy, Imogene M. King, Martha E. Rogers, Rosemarie Rizzo Parse, and Hildegard E. Peplau. Available from: Discovery International's Nurse Theorist Conferences, Veranda Communications, Inc., 4229 Taylorsville Road, Louisville, KY 40220, (502) 485–1484, FAX (502) 485–1482.

Nurse Theorist Conference 1987, Pittsburgh, PA
Videotaped presentations include (1) Hildegard Peplau, "Art and Science of Nursing: Similarities, Differences and Relations"; (2) Imogene King, "King's Theory"; (3) Rosemarie Parse, "Parse's Theory"; (4) Callista Roy, "Roy's

Model"; (5) Martha Rogers, "Rogers' Framework"; (6) Jean Watson, "Watson's Model"; (7) Rozella Schlotfeldt, "Nursing Science in the 21st Century"; and (8) "Panel Discussion with Theorists." Available from: Discovery International's Nurse Theorist Conferences, Veranda Communications, Inc., 4229 Taylorsville Road, Louisville, KY 40220, (502) 485–1484, FAX (502) 485–1482.

Nurse Theorist Conference 1989, Pittsburgh, PA
Videotaped presentations include (1) Afaf Meleis, "Being and Becoming Healthy: The Core of Nursing Knowledge"; (2) Betty Neuman, "Health as a Continuum in Neuman's Model"; (3) Rosemarie Parse, "Health as a Personal Commitment in Parse's Theory"; (4) Martha Rogers, "Evolutionary Emergence: Infinite Potential"; (5) Nola Pender, "Expressing Health Through Beliefs and Actions"; (6) Imogene King, "Health as the Goal of Nursing in King's Theory"; and (7) "Panel Discussion with Theorists." Available from: Discovery International's Nurse Theorist Conferences, Veranda Communications, Inc., 4229 Taylorsville Road, Louisville, KY 40220, (502) 485–1484, FAX (502) 485–1482.

Nurse Theorist Conference 1993, Pittsburgh, PA
Videotaped presentations include (1) Rosemarie Rizzo Parse, "Quality of Life and Becoming Human"; (2) Madeleine M. Leininger, "Quality of Life and Transcultural Nursing"; (3) Martha Rogers, "Quality of Life and the Science of Unitary Human Beings"; (4) Marlaine C. Smith, Cheryl Forchuk, Gail J. Mitchell, and Jacqueline Chapman, "Nursing Theory-based Practice and Research: A Glimpse of the Canadian Scene"; (5) Hildegard Peplau, "Quality of Life: An Interpersonal Perspective"; and (6) Imogene King, "Nursing and the Next Millennium" moderated by Marlaine C. Smith. Available from: Discovery International's Nurse Theorist Conferences, Veranda Communications, Inc., 4229 Taylorsville Road, Louisville, KY 40220, (502) 485–1484, FAX (502) 485–1482.

53. Conference Media

Nursing Theory Congress 1986, Toronto, Canada
Audiotapes of plenary sessions by Betty Neuman, Imogene King, Callista Roy, Rosemarie Parse, Martha Rogers, and Myra Levine. Other audiotapes include (1) Moyra Allen, "A Developmental Health Model: Nursing as Continuous Inquiry"; (2) Patricia James and James Dickoff, "Overview of the Concept of Theoretical Pluralism"; (3) Bonnie Holaday, "Adaptation of Johnson's Framework"; (4) Susan Taylor, "Presenting Orem's Framework"; (5) Phyllis Kritek, "Impact of Nursing Theory on the Diagnostic Process"; and (6) Marian McGee, "Criteria for Selection and Use of a Nursing Model for Clinical Practice." Available from: Audio Archives International, 100 West Beaver Creek, Unit 18, Richmond Hill, Ontario, Canada, L4B 1H4, (905) 889–6555.

Nursing Theory Congress 1988, Toronto, Canada
Audiotapes include (1) Carol Lindeman, "Nursing Theory: Elitism or Realism in 1988"; (2) Virginia Henderson, "Nursing Theory: A Historical Perspective"; (3) Jean Watson, "One Model or Many Models"; (4) Marjory Gordon, "Nursing Diagnosis: The Interface of Nursing Theory and Nursing Process"; (5) Rosemarie Parse, "Nursing Science as a Basis for Research"; (6) Phyllis Kritek and others, "Impact of Nursing Theory on the Profession"; and (7) Phyllis Kritek, "Agendas for the

Future." Available from: Audio Archives International, 100 West Beaver Creek, Unit 18, Richmond Hill, Ontario, Canada L4B 1H4, (905) 889–6555.

Nurse Theorist Conference 1985, Philadelphia, PA

Audiotapes include (1) Presentations by Dorothea Orem, Callista Roy, Imogene M. King, Martha E. Rogers, Rosemarie Rizzo Parse; (2) Hildegard Peplau, "Nursing Science: A Historical Overview"; (3) Mary Jane Smith, "Theorist: Dorothea E. Orem"; (4) S.J. Magan, "Theorist: Imogene M. King"; (5). J.R. Phillips, "Theorist: Rosemarie Rizzo Parse"; (6) A. Whall, "Theorist: Martha E. Rogers"; (7) M.H. Huch, "Theorist: Callista Roy"; (8) "Panel Discussion with Theorists"; and (9) "Small Group Discussions" led by Jean Watson, Imogene King, Rosemarie Parse, Martha Rogers, and Callista Roy. Available from: Veranda Communications, Inc., 4229 Taylorsville Road, Louisville, KY 40220, (502) 485–1484, FAX (502) 485–1482.

Nurse Theorist Conference 1989, Philadelphia, PA

Audio tapes include (1) Afaf I. Meleis, "Being and Becoming Healthy: The Core of Nursing Knowledge"; (2) Betty M. Neuman, "Health as a Continuum in Neuman's Model"; (3) Rosemarie Parse, "Evolutionary Emergence: Infinite Potential"; (4) Nola J. Pender, "Expressing Health Through Beliefs and Actions"; (5) Imogene M. King, "Health as the Goal of Nursing in King's Theory"; and (6) "Panel Discussion with Theorists." Available from: Discovery International's Nurse Theorist Conferences, Veranda Communications, Inc., 4229 Taylorsville Road, Louisville, KY 40220, (502) 485–1484, FAX (502) 485–1482.

54. Miscellaneous Media

American Academy of Nursing YouTube Channel: https://www.youtube.com/user/NursingPolicy

National League of Nursing YouTube Channel: https://www.youtube.com/channel/UCs69j-7ABCzIBfaM79KAa6A

Nursing Continuing Education (CE) Podcast: https://itunes.apple.com/podcast/nursing-continuing-education/id340841068

Nursing Theories and Models YouTube Channel: https://www.youtube.com/playlist?list=PL1E004CCBDDF0F5DC

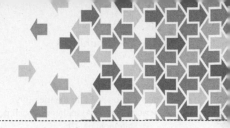

Author Index

Note: Page numbers followed by *b* and *t* indicate boxes and tables respectively

A

Abbott, C.A., on concept analysis, 345
Abdellah, F.G.
  bibliography on, 534–536
  on concept of client, 96
  on decision making process, 116
  on interaction theories, 157
  as Levine influence, 284
  need theory and, 158–159*t*
  on nursing concepts, 126
  on nursing functions, 165
  on nursing process, 100, 116
  on nursing science, abstract, 5
  on Orem influence, 206, 207
  on role nurses play, 169*t*
  on theory in education, 189
  theory of, 69, 189
Abdullah, A., on nursing theory, 34
Aber, C., on Roy, 319
Abraham, I.L., on theory testing, 192
Acorn, S., on scholarship, 16
Adam, E., as theory advocate, 74
Adams, A., on nursing concepts, 118
Adams, J., on conceptual barriers, 49
Adams, J.M., on innovative inventions, 427
Adams-Leander, S., on discipline, 86
Adams, M.
  on flexibility, 53
  on intuition, 53
Adamsen, L., on Wiedenbach, 258
Adolfsson, R., on Orem, 211
Affonso, D., on nursing, 11
Agan, R.D.
  on caring, 114
  on intuition, 138
  on knowing patterns, 138
Agreda, J.J., on middle-range theories, 376
Agronow, S.J., on role strain in faculty, 192
Agüero-Torres, H., on Orem, 218
Ahlström, G., on concept analysis, 348
Aiken, L.H., on theoretical thinking, 54
Ailinger, R.L., on Orem, 202*b*, 212
Ainsworth, M., affiliation concepts of, 273
Akhtar-Danesh, N., on concept development, 348
Akyol, A.D.
  on Orem, 208, 210
  on Roy, 322

Al-Aslamiah, Rufaida Bent Saad, as founder of Eastern
    nursing, 60
Albert, N.M., on self-care, 208
Alexander, J.W., on Johnson, 276
Algase, D. L., on nursing perspective, 86
Ali, S.
  on integrative theory, 148
  on postcolonialism, 145
Alimohammadi, N., on Roy, 322
Alizadeh, V., on situation-specific theories, 398–399
Allan, J.
  on medical model, 419
  on Orem, 211
Allan, J.D., on self-use, 103
Allcock, N., on advancing theory, 420
Allen, A., on Orem, 209
Allen, D.
  on critical theory, 144
  on health, 95, 103
  on health orientation of discipline, 91
  on knowing patterns, 135
  on nursing, 91
  on nursing concepts, 75, 141
  on nursing theory, 144
Allen, D.E., on Orlando, 237
Allen, D.G.
  on advancing theory, 421
  on knowledge development approaches, 75
  on theory development, 103
Allen, J., on medical models as theory
    source, 114
Alligood, M.R.
  on advancing theory, 419
  on behavioural system, 274
  on borrowed theory, 129
  on King, 230
  on Levine's theory, 286
  on nursing, 268
  on nursing theorists, 422
  on testing theory, 230
  on theory analysis, 183
  on theory in nursing education, 129
Allison, S.E.
  on Orem, 205, 208
    abstract, 471
Allmark, P., research to theory strategy, 366
Allvin, R., on Levine, 287

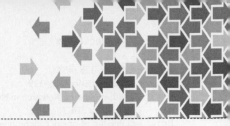

Subject Index

Note: Page numbers followed by *b*, *f* and *t* indicate boxes, figures and tables respectively